FNP Certification
Intensive Review

Maria T. Codina Leik, MSN, APRN, FNP-C, FNP-BC, AGPCNP-BC, is the president and principal lecturer at National ARNP Services, Inc. Well known for her ability to simplify complex concepts for her students, she is a popular speaker and educator. Ms. Leik previously taught in the nurse practitioner program at Florida International University Graduate School of Nursing, Miami, Florida. She is board certified by the American Nurses Credentialing Center (ANCC) and the American Academy of Nurse Practitioners Certification Board (AANPCB) in two specialties: family nurse practice and adult-gerontology primary care nurse practice. She has more than three decades of experience in clinical practice. Ms. Leik is a member of Sigma Theta Tau International Honor Society of Nursing.

FNP Certification Intensive Review

Fifth Edition

Maria T. Codina Leik, MSN, APRN, FNP-C, FNP-BC, AGPCNP-BC

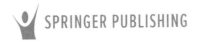
SPRINGER PUBLISHING

Springer Publishing Company, LLC
www.springerpub.com
connect.springerpub.com

VP, Assessment & Digital Solutions: Adrianne Brigido
Director, Product Development, Exam Prep: Cynthia Kitchel
Senior Director, Content Development: Taylor Ball
Senior Content Development Editor: Jennifer Ehlers
Compositor: Amnet

ISBN: 978-0-8261-7066-8
ebook ISBN: 978-0-8261-7067-5
DOI: 10.1891/9780826170675

23 24 25 26 / 5 4 3 2 1

The author and the publisher of this Work have made every effort to use sources believed to be reliable to provide information that is accurate and compatible with the standards generally accepted at the time of publication. Because medical science is continually advancing, our knowledge base continues to expand. Therefore, as new information becomes available, changes in procedures become necessary. We recommend that the reader always consult current research and specific institutional policies before performing any clinical procedure or delivering any medication. The author and publisher shall not be liable for any special, consequential, or exemplary damages resulting, in whole or in part, from the readers' use of, or reliance on, the information contained in this book. The publisher has no responsibility for the persistence or accuracy of URLs for external or third-party Internet websites referred to in this publication and does not guarantee that any content on such websites is, or will remain, accurate or appropriate.

The certifying bodies for the FNP exam are the American Academy of Nurse Practitioners Certification Board (AANPCB) and the American Nurses Credentialing Center (ANCC). AANPCB and ANCC do not sponsor or endorse this resource, nor do they have a proprietary relationship with Springer Publishing.

Library of Congress Cataloging-in-Publication Data

Names: Codina Leik, Maria T., author.
Title: FNP certification intensive review / Maria T. Codina Leik.
Other titles: Family nurse practitioner certification intensive review
Description: Fifth edition. | New York : Springer Publishing Company, LLC,
   [2025] | Preceded by Family nurse practitioner certification intensive
   review / Maria T. Codina Leik. 4th ed. 2021. | Includes bibliographical
   references and index.
Identifiers: LCCN 2023039341 (print) | LCCN 2023039342 (ebook) | ISBN
   9780826170668 (paperback) | ISBN 9780826170675 (ebook)
Subjects: MESH: Family Nurse Practitioners | Certification | Family
   Practice | Examination Questions
Classification: LCC RT82.8 (print) | LCC RT82.8 (ebook) | NLM WY 18.2 |
   DDC 610.7306/92--dc23/eng/20230921
LC record available at https://lccn.loc.gov/2023039341
LC ebook record available at https://lccn.loc.gov/2023039342

Contact sales@springerpub.com to receive discount rates on bulk purchases.

Publisher's Note: **New and used products purchased from third-party sellers are not guaranteed for quality, authenticity, or access to any included digital components.**

Printed in the United States of America.

What a great time to be a nurse practitioner.
This is our *decade, girls (and guys). I dedicate this book to you.*
What a privilege it is to be able to make a difference in someone's health.
Wow.
Of course, my grateful thanks to
Ed, Mary, Chrissy, and my parents.

CONTENTS

V. PEDIATRICS AND ADOLESCENTS REVIEW

VI. GERONTOLOGY REVIEW

VII. PROFESSIONAL ROLE REVIEW

VIII. PRACTICE TESTS

CONTRIBUTORS AND REVIEWERS

Contributors and reviewers for the fifth and previous editions:

Julie Adkins, DNP, APRN, FNP-BC, FAANP[1]
Family Nurse Practitioner, Adkins Family Practice, LLC, West Frankfort, Illinois

Donna Bowles, EdD, MSN, RN, CNE
Professor and Dean, Indiana University School of Nursing, Indiana University Southeast, New Albany, Indiana

Therese Boyd, EdD, ARNP, AGPCNP-BC
Nurse Practitioner, Clinical Assistant Professor, Florida International University, Miami, Florida

Linda Carman Copel, PhD, RN, PMHCNS, BC, CNE, NCC, FAPA, ANEF
Professor, Villanova University College of Nursing, Philadelphia, Pennsylvania

Jill C. Cash, MSN, APRN, FNP-BC
Nurse Practitioner, Vanderbilt Medical Group at Westhaven Family Practice, Franklin, Tennessee; Vanderbilt University Medical Center, Nashville, Tennessee

Tanya L. Fernandez, MS, PA-C, IBCLC
Assistant Professor, Department of Pediatrics, Child Health Associate/Physician Assistant Program, University of Colorado Anschutz Medical Campus, Aurora, Colorado

Lucille R. Ferrara, EdD, MBA, RN, FNP-BC
Professor and Director, Family Nurse Practitioner Program, Lienhard School of Nursing, Pace University, New York, New York

Susanne W. Gibbons, PhD, C-AGNP
Assistant Professor, Daniel K. Inouye Graduate School of Nursing, Uniformed Services University of the Health Sciences, Bethesda, Maryland

Frank L. Giles, PhD, CRC, CCM, NCC, LMFT
President, Giles & Associates, Inc., Madison, Mississippi

Cheryl A. Glass, MSN, WHNP, BC
Clinical Research Specialist, KEPRO, TennCare Medical Solutions Unit, Nashville, Tennessee

Elizabeth Johnston Taylor, PhD, RN
Professor, School of Nursing, Loma Linda University, Loma Linda, California

Pamela L. King, PhD, FNP, PNP
Director, Post Master's Doctor of Nursing Practice Program, Kosair Charities College of Natural and Health Sciences, Spalding University, Louisville, Kentucky

Eugene Lucas, DNP, CRNP, PMHNP-C
Associate Professor, Coordinator, Psychiatric/Mental Health Nurse Practitioner Program, Wilkes University, Wilkes-Barre, Pennsylvania

Emily Ferrara Mandernach, AGACNP, MSN, RN
Barnes-Jewish Hospital, St. Louis, Missouri

Liza Marmo, MSN, RN-BC, CCRN, ANP-C
Director, Clinical Services, Lehigh Valley Health Network, Allentown, Pennsylvania

Karen M. Myrick, DNP, APRN, ANP-BC, FNP-BC, ONP-C, FAAN
Professor of Nursing and Track Coordinator for the Orthopedics and Sports Medicine Certificate Program, University of Saint Joseph, West Hartford, Connecticut; Clinical Professor of Medicine, Frank H. Netter School of Medicine, Quinnipiac University, Hamden, Connecticut

Susanne J. Pavlovich-Danis, MSN, ARNP-C, CDE, CRRN
Director of Clinical Continuing Education, TeamHealth, Advanced Practice Registered Nurse, Plantation Medical Clinic; Nursing Professor, University of Phoenix–South Florida Campus, Miramar, Florida

[1] Deceased

JoAnne M. Pearce, MS, RNC, APRN-BC
Nursing Education Consultant, Idaho State University,
Pocatello, Idaho

Sue Polito, MSN, RN, ANPC, GNPC
Specialist Professor, Monmouth University, West Long
Branch, New Jersey

Dana R. Sherman, DNP, ARNP, ANP-BC, FNP-BC
Clinical Adjunct Faculty, Florida International University,
Advanced Practice Registered Nurse, Emergency
Department, Mount Sinai Medical Center, Miami Beach,
Florida

Elyse Watkins, DHSc, PA-C, DFAAPA, NCMP
Associate Professor, University of Lynchburg
College of Medical Science, Lynchburg, Virginia

Cirese Webster, RN, CPN, FNP-BC
Nurse Practitioner,
Metro Medical and
Midwest Physicians,
Certified Pediatric Nurse,
St. Louis Children's Hospital,
St. Louis, Missouri

PREFACE

Welcome to the fifth edition of *FNP Certification Intensive Review*. This review book is designed to help you study effectively and efficiently for the family nurse practitioner certification exams of both the American Academy of Nurse Practitioners Certification Board (AANPCB) and American Nurses Credentialing Center (ANCC).

The goal for all of my nurse practitioner (NP) certification review books is to provide you, the NP test-taker, with a tool to effectively and rapidly review and prepare for your exam. This book is also a valuable resource for current NP students and educators. Many students credit these books with helping them pass not only their certification exam but also quizzes and tests when they were students. Students report that the review book has helped them successfully pass their school's dreaded "exit" exam.

The book's format remains the same as in the popular and best-selling first four editions, with the addition of hundreds of new questions and a more navigable format. The book is styled as a "mega-review" study guide because it combines six different resources in one:

1. Certification exam information that is highly specific for both the AANPCB and ANCC exams
2. Useful test-taking techniques to help you prepare and strategize for exam day
3. Question dissection and analysis tools to help you break down questions for further study and hone critical-thinking skills
4. A thorough review of pharmacology; health promotion, screening, and disease prevention; and primary care diseases and conditions, with pertinent normal physical exam findings, danger signals, exam tips, and clinical pearls

5. *New:* Hundreds of additional end-of-chapter "knowledge check" questions designed to help you assess knowledge retention and application
6. Four full practice tests—two in print, two digital only—based on the blueprints for the AANPCB and ANCC certification exams, with answers and detailed rationales

The fifth edition has been significantly updated and features new disease topics, tables, procedures, updated clinical content, and the latest practice and treatment guidelines (note that it may take 1 to 2 years for new guidelines to appear on the certification exams). In addition, it has many full-color images of dermatologic diseases and other conditions and more than 1,200 practice questions.

Readers receive 6 months of free digital access to the interactive digital version on ExamPrepConnect (see access details on inside front cover). Features include:

- Review all the high-quality content from the book.
- Take four full-length timed practice tests.
- Build custom quizzes or study by exam topic.
- Sharpen your test-taking skills with interactive Q&A tools.
- Keep on track with your Personalized Study Plan.
- Take notes, highlight, and bookmark content.
- Use flashcards to review key terms.
- Study with your peers in the community discussion boards.
- Access everything on any device.

This book and my *AGNP Certification Intensive Review* have become the most sought-after and relied-upon review books for use in studying for both the AANPCB and ANCC certification exams. The contents and procedures in this book are designed for review purposes only. They are not intended for use in clinical practice.

Maria T. Codina Leik

ACKNOWLEDGMENTS

To my awesome editor, Adrianne Brigido, whose endless patience and support has helped me tremendously. I want to thank you and give you a big hug. I want to extend my gratitude to Springer Publishing Company and its staff.

I want to extend my deep gratitude to Ricardo G. Codina and Thelma Y. Codina. And, of course, kudos to Angelica, my assistant, who wears so many hats.

PASS GUARANTEE

If you use this resource to prepare for your exam and do not pass, you may return it for a refund of your full purchase price, excluding tax, shipping, and handling. To receive a refund, return your product along with a copy of your exam score report and original receipt showing purchase of a new product (not used). Product must be returned and received within 180 days of the original purchase date. Refunds will be issued within 8 weeks from acceptance and approval. One offer per person and address. This offer is valid for U.S. residents only. Void where prohibited. To initiate a refund, please contact Customer Service at csexamprep@springerpub.com.

I

CERTIFICATION AND EXAM INFORMATION

1 CERTIFICATION EXAM INFORMATION

AMERICAN NURSES CREDENTIALING CENTER

www.nursingworld.org/ancc
Credential: FNP-BC
Toll-Free Phone: 1-(800)-284-2378
Electronic Transcripts: aprnvalidation@ana.org

The American Nurses Credentialing Center (ANCC) is the independent credentialing body of the American Nurses Association (ANA). It is the largest nurse credentialing organization in the United States. The current edition of the ANCC Family Nurse Practitioner (FNP) exam was released on September 28, 2022.

The ANCC currently offers certification exams for the following nurse practitioner (NP) specialties: Family NP (FNP-BC), Adult-Gerontology Primary Care NP (AGPCNP-BC), Adult-Gerontology Acute Care NP (AGACNP-BC), and Psychiatric–Mental Health NP (PMHNP-BC). You must first establish an online account at the ANCC website before you can apply for any of the exams.

Prometric Computer Testing Centers

www.prometric.com/ANCC
Toll-Free Phone: (800) 350-7076
Special Conditions Department (Special Accommodations): 1-(800)-967-1139

The ANCC uses Prometric testing centers to administer its exams. Before you can schedule an appointment, you must have your candidate eligibility number; this is provided in the Authorization to Test Notice email sent to qualified candidates who meet eligibility requirements and have completed their application documentation.

You can schedule, reschedule, cancel, and/or confirm an appointment on the website or by telephone (1-800-742-8738). Prometric has 8,000 test centers in more than 180 countries, including the United States, Puerto Rico, the U.S. Virgin Islands, Canada, and the United Kingdom. There are also test centers in Africa, Asia, and Europe.

International Testing for Military Personnel
Military nurses who want to take the exam outside the United States are allowed to take their exams at one of Prometric's global testing centers.

Qualifications
One must graduate from an approved master's, postgraduate, or doctoral degree program with a specialization in family NP (plus the required minimum of 750 faculty-supervised clinical practice hours) from an institution of higher learning. The program must be accredited by the Commission on Collegiate Nursing Education (CCNE) or the Accreditation Commission for Education in Nursing (formerly known as the National League for Nursing Accrediting Commission). In addition, the candidate must possess an active RN license in any state or territory of the United States. The ANCC will, on an individual basis, accept the professional legally recognized equivalent (of NP status) from another country if the applicant meets its certification criteria. If the applicant is educated and/or licensed outside the United States, there are additional requirements.

AMERICAN ACADEMY OF NURSE PRACTITIONERS CERTIFICATION BOARD

www.aanpcert.org
Credential: FNP-C
Toll-Free Phone: 1-(855)-822-6727
Certification Administration: 1-(512)-637-0500
Email: certification@aanpcert.org
Electronic Transcripts: transcripts@aanpcert.org

The American Academy of Nurse Practitioners Certification Board (AANPCB) is an independent organization that is affiliated with the American Association of Nurse Practitioners (AANP) and the American Academy of Emergency Nurse Practitioners (AAENP).

The AANPCB currently offers three specialty exams: Family NP (FNP-C), Adult-Gerontology Primary Care NP (AGNP-C), and Emergency NP (ENP-C). The current FNP, AGNP, and ENP exams were released in January 2023. Their Adult NP exam was retired in December 2015, and their Gerontologic NP exam was retired in December 2012. A new Psychiatric-Mental Health NP (PMHNP) certification exam is slated to debut in 2024.

You must first establish an online account at their website before you can apply for the exam. Applicants enrolled in an MSN or post-master's certificate program may begin the application process 6 months before completion of the program. If you are enrolled in a DNP program, you can begin the application process as early as 1 year prior to completion of the program. But you must complete all the NP program didactic courses and supervised clinical practice hour requirements before you can sit for the exam. In addition, an official transcript showing the doctor of nursing practice (DNP) degree awarded and conferral date is required to release your exam score. The certification start date will be the date the score is released (not the date the examination was taken).

Prometric Computer Testing Centers

www.prometric.com/test-takers/search/aanpcb
Toll-Free Phone: 1-(800)-350-7076
Special Conditions Department (Special Accommodations): 1-(800)-967-1139

The AANPCB also uses Prometric testing centers to administer its exams. Before you can schedule an appointment, you must have your candidate eligibility number; this is provided in the Authorization to Test Notice email sent to qualified candidates who meet eligibility requirements and have completed their application documentation.

You can schedule, reschedule, cancel, and/or confirm an appointment on the website or by telephone (1-800-742-8738). Prometric has 8,000 test centers in more than 180 countries, including the United States, Puerto Rico, the U.S. Virgin Islands, Canada, and the United Kingdom. There are also test centers in Africa, Asia, and Europe.

Important information about applying for the ANCC and AANPCB exams is provided in Table 1.1.

EXAM BACKGROUND INFORMATION

The ANCC usually releases a new edition of their exam every 2 years. Each ANCC exam edition has several versions. The AANPCB releases a new edition of their exam annually in January; each edition has at least two versions. If you have failed the exam and retake it, you will get a different version of the exam. The version of the exam that you are taking is assigned by the testing-center computer system. For example, you may be taking a different version of the exam than your classmate even though both of you are taking the same edition of the exam on the same date and time at the same testing center.

Table 1.1 Application Timeline for Certification Exams

Timeline	Recommended Activities Before Graduation
6 months before graduation	Open an account on the ANCC and/or the AANPCB website and start the application process. Find out about the certification requirements. Download and read the General Testing Booklet, Test Content Outline, and Reference List. Visit your SBON website and read the licensure requirements for NPs in your state. Download the licensure application.
4–6 weeks before graduation	Order three to four copies of your official final transcript.
2–3 weeks before graduation	Ask the NP director of your program to sign the ANCC Education Validation form.

AANPCB, American Academy of Nurse Practitioners Certification Board; ANCC, American Nurses Credentialing Center; NP, nurse practitioner; SBON, state board of nursing.

Exam Format

The formats on the ANCC exam include "drag and drop"; multiple-select questions with five or six answer options (you are asked to select all answers that apply); "hot spot" (a picture is presented that is divided into four quadrants, and you click on the correct quadrant as the answer); color photographs of skin and eye conditions; EKG strips; and chest x-ray films. (See Chapter 2 for more information.) Most questions on the ANCC exam are still multiple choice with four answer options and only one correct answer.

Similarly, most AANPCB exam questions are the classic multiple-choice format with four answer options and only one correct answer. There may be one EKG strip, a chest x-ray film, and some multiple-select questions with five or six answer options (you are asked to select two to three answers).

The exams are computer-based tests (CBTs). Unlike the NCLEX-RN® exam, which is a computer-adaptive test, the NP exams do not shut down automatically after you have earned enough points.

Test Content Outline and Reference List

Both the ANCC and the AANPCB provide test content outlines (TCOs) and a reference list on their website. It is important that you read these documents carefully and concentrate your studies on the designated topic areas.

Total Number of Questions and Time Allowance

- ANCC FNP exam (released September 2022): There are 175 total questions. Only 150 questions are graded; 25 are pretest questions that are not scored.
  - **Total Time:** Total counted testing time is 3.5 hours.
- AANPCB: FNP exam (released January 2023): There are 150 total questions. Only 135 questions are graded; 15 questions are pretest questions that are not scored.
  - **Total Time:** Total counted testing time is 3.5 hours.

Computer Tutorial

For both exams, each testing session starts with a computer tutorial session of 10 to 15 minutes. This time is not counted as part of the testing time; it is "free" time. When the tutorial time expires, the computer will automatically start the exam, and the first question will appear on the screen. The countdown clock (upper corner of the screen) will start counting down the time. The countdown clock will not stop for "breaks," but if you need a break, inform a testing center staff member who is monitoring the testing area. Watch the time clock closely because when the allotted testing time expires, the computer will automatically shut down the exam.

Time Allotted per Question

For both the ANCC and the AANPCB certification exams, each question is allotted approximately 60 seconds. If you find yourself spending too much time on one question, pick an answer (best guess), and then "flag" it so that you can return to it later. Never leave any question unanswered. If you guess correctly, it will be counted; if you leave it blank, it will be marked as an error (0 points).

Sample Exam Questions

I highly recommend that you try the free sample exams on the ANCC's website even if you are planning to take only the AANPCB exam. The ANCC's sample exam is web-based and contains 25 questions. It can be taken as many times as desired at no charge (and it is scored every time). The AANPCB also has free questions, which are included in their candidate handbook (no answer key is provided). If you want to familiarize yourself with the format of the AANPCB exam, you can purchase their 75-item practice examination (timed at 90 minutes), which is taken online and graded. It can be taken only once. The ANCC also sells sample exam questions, but their free web-based sample exam provides a good opportunity to practice using their exam formats.

COMPARING THE ANCC AND AANPCB EXAMS

1. **What are the pass rates for the two exams?**
   ANCC FNP exam: 87%
   AANPCB FNP exam: 74%

2. **What are the major differences between the two exams?**
   There are two major differences between the exams. First, the ANCC exam contains nonclinical questions. These nonclinical questions cover many topics, such as ethical behavior, how to act in a culturally respectful manner, medical orders for life-sustaining treatment, clinical practice guidelines, third-party payers, leadership, health promotion, and many others. Second, different question formats, such as drag and drop, photographs, EKG strips, chest x-ray films, and multiple-select questions with five to six answer options, were added beginning with the 2016 ANCC exams.

   The questions on the AANPCB exam are all on clinical topics. The current version (January 2023) does not contain nonclinical topics. Most of the questions are the classic multiple-choice format with four answer options and only one correct answer, but there may be some multiple-select questions that have five to six answer options (you are asked to select two to three answers). An EKG strip and/or chest x-ray film is not always included on the exam.

3. **If I join their respective membership organizations, will I receive a discount on my fees?**
   ANCC: To be eligible, you need to be a member of the ANA. If you belong to a state nursing association, you may already be a member of the ANA. Check with your state's nursing association. To apply for membership, apply online at the ANA's website (www.nursingworld.org). A word of warning: If you are not a member, you have only 5 business days after you apply for the exam to claim the membership discount. Exam discount claims received after this time are not allowed, and "refunds will not be issued."

   AANPCB: To be eligible, you must be a member of the AANP (www.aanp.org). If you already applied for the exam as a nonmember, you have up to 30 days to apply for membership. To receive the membership discount (as a refund), inform the AANPCB by email that you are a member (certification@aanpcert.org).

4. **How do I apply for the ANCC or AANPCB certification exam?**
   For both agencies, you must initially open an online account on their website. To avoid loss of information, it is best to complete your online application within 30 days of starting it. The application forms are in editable PDF format so you can enter the information directly on your computer and then print a hard copy for your records. If you apply by mail, do not forget to photocopy the entire contents of your application package. If you plan on using the U.S. Postal Service to mail your package, it is recommended that you pay the extra fee for registered mail.

   ANCC: The ANCC accepts applications online and by email, standard mail, and fax.

   AANPCB: The AANPCB accepts applications online and by mail. Applying online does not expedite processing. The organization automatically charges a non-refundable application processing fee for all "paper" applications (PDF sent by email or printout sent by mail or fax). There is no charge for processing of supporting documents for certification and recertification (e.g., unofficial transcripts, RN license).

5. **How early can I apply for the certification exam?**
   ANCC: The ANCC allows students to apply as early as 6 months before graduation. It will not process an application until payment has cleared. A completed application must contain a copy of your RN license, an official copy of your final transcripts, and the original copy of the Validation of Education form, signed by your NP program director.

   AANPCB: Applicants enrolled in an MSN or post-master's certificate program may apply 6 months prior to graduation. DNP students may apply up to 12 months before graduation, but the AANPCB will not release the exam scores or grant certification until the MSN or DNP degrees are issued. If you apply before you graduate, you are required to submit an official copy of your current transcript (the interim transcript). The interim transcript is your most recent transcript, which contains all the coursework that you have completed up to that date. When the official final transcript is released, either you or the registrar's office of your school can mail or email it directly to the AANPCB. In addition, the AANPCB requires a hard copy of your RN license. Do not forget to download the State Board of Nursing Notification form from the board's website so that it can release your exam scores to your state board of nursing.

6. **How long does it take to process a completed application?**
   ANCC: It takes about 4 to 6 weeks to process an application. Be warned that the ANCC will not process an application until it is complete and all required documents have been received (copy of RN license, original of the signed education validation form, final transcript). If there are problems with your application, an email will be sent to you. Answer all the questions on the forms, and do not leave any blanks.

AANPCB: It generally takes between 4 and 6 weeks after you have paid the fees and submitted all the required documentation to process an application. Fill out all the questions, and do not leave any blanks or forget signatures. An error can delay your application significantly.

7. **What is the ANCC's "expedited application" process?**
This option shortens the processing time to 5 business days ($200 nonrefundable fee). Download and print the Certification Expedite Review Request form from the ANCC website and fax it to (301)-628-5233. If your school has not released your final transcript, it will delay the expedited application. The Validation of Education form can be signed by electronic signature (give your NP director's email address), and an electronic copy of your final transcript can be emailed directly by secure transmission from your school's registrar office (aprnvalidation@ana.org). Call to verify that the ANCC has received your faxed application.

Note: Mailing the ANCC "expedited" form will delay processing; it should be faxed. If you both fax and mail it, you will be charged the processing fee twice.

The AANPCB does not expedite applications.

8. **What are the final transcript and the "official" transcript?**
The final transcript is the one that is issued after you graduate from your NP program. It should indicate the type of degree you earned along with the NP specialty (e.g., family or adult-gerontology NP).

A transcript is considered official only if it remains inside the sealed envelope in which it was mailed from your college registrar's office or if it is mailed directly from their office to the certifying agency. An electronic copy of your transcript can be transmitted directly by secure transmission from the registrar's office (aprnvalidation@ana.org). Order at least three to four copies of your final transcript and keep the extras unopened to keep them official. Open one copy (yours) and check it for accuracy.

9. **What is the ANCC Validation of Education form?**
This one-page form is a requirement for ANCC applicants only. Most NP programs have this document signed in bulk by the current director of the NP program. Ideally, it should be distributed to the students before the final day of school. Only electronic-signature PDF forms will be accepted; printed, scanned, handwritten, or paper versions of this form will not be processed.

Note: It is probably a good idea for all NP students to get this document signed, even if they plan to take only the AANPCB exam. Because the ANCC requires this form, it will save you precious time in the future if you decide to apply for their exam. You will always have the option of applying quickly for the "other" certification exam if you fail the first. Do not forget that you will need another official final transcript (another good reason why you should have at least four copies).

10. **Is it possible to take the exams at any time of the year?**
You can take both certification exams at any time of the year, whenever Prometric testing centers are open.

11. **When should I schedule my exam?**
Do not wait until the last minute to schedule your exam because the testing centers in your area may no longer have the date (or the time) that you desire. Morning time slots tend to get filled very quickly. Prometric testing centers allow test takers to schedule, reschedule, or cancel an appointment on their website or by phone, but you should give them notice. A processing fee is charged if <30 days' notice is given.

Note: Avoid scheduling yourself at the time of day when you tend to get tired or sleepy. For most, this is usually after lunchtime. Simply picking the wrong time of day can cause you to fail the exam, sometimes by as little as two points.

12. **What should I do if the time slot or date that I want is no longer available?**
Look for another testing center as soon as possible. For some, it may mean a long drive to another city, but it may well be worth the extra time and effort if your Authorization to Test letter is about to expire.

13. **Can I take the exam if my name does not match my primary picture identification?**
The name that you used to register must match exactly the name on your primary picture identification with signature. If it doesn't, you will not be allowed to test. If you need to modify your name, call the ANCC as soon as possible prior to scheduling your appointment.

14. **If I have a disability, how can I obtain special testing accommodations?**
You can download the Special Accommodations form from each organization's website (ANCC and AANPCB). It requires a description of the disability and limitations related to testing. It should be dated and signed by the provider. For example, if a student has severe test-taking anxiety, a special accommodation (if approved) is an extension of the testing time. Check the agency's website for further instructions.

COMMON QUESTIONS ABOUT ANCC AND AANPCB EXAMS

1. **What are the passing scores?**
ANCC: The passing score is 350 points or higher. The maximum possible score is 500 points.

AANPCB: The passing score is 500 points or higher. AANPCB scores range from 200 to 800 points.

2. **Will I find out immediately if I pass (or fail) the exam?**
Yes, you will. After you exit the testing area, ask the proctor to print a copy of your results (pass or fail format). This is the "unofficial" score. If you pass the

exam, you will not get a number score. According to the AANPCB, a preliminary pass score at the testing center is not considered official notification. It does not indicate active certification status, and it may not be used for employment or licensure as an NP. A letter with your official score will be mailed to you at a later date, indicating the type of certification and the starting date. If you fail the exam, you will receive a scaled number score with diagnostic feedback information for each domain, such as:

- Low: Your score from this content area is below the acceptable level.
- Medium: Your score from this content area is marginally acceptable.
- High: Your score from this content area is above average.

  Concentrate your studies on the domain(s)/category(ies) in which you scored "low" or "medium."

3. **How many times a year can I retake the FNP certification exam?**

   ANCC: You can take this exam up to three times in a 12-month calendar period. You must wait at least 60 days between each exam. If you fail, you can reapply online (retest application), but wait about 5 days (after taking your exam) before you reapply online.

   AANPCB: You can take the exam up to two times per calendar year. Although there is no wait-time requirement prior to retesting, the AANPCB requires test takers to take 15 contact hours in their area(s) with the weakest score (your "areas of weakness"). Reapply for the exam online by using the Retake Application form. Note: The CE hours that you took before sitting for the certification exam are not eligible. The contact hours must be taken after you failed the exam. If you took a review course, it can be retaken again with the new dates. When you have completed the required 15 contact hours, email or fax the certificate of completion as proof. Call the AANPCB certification office first before faxing any documents.

4. **What happens if I fail the ANCC or AANPCB exam the second time?**

   You must resubmit a full application along with all the required documentation (like the first time) and pay the full test fee.

5. **What happens if my Authorization to Test letter expires, and I have not taken the exam?**

   Immediately call the certifying agency for further instructions. Both the ANCC and the AANPCB will allow you to reschedule your exam (one time only). You must pay a rescheduling fee. If you fail to test on your extended testing window, you must reapply like a new applicant and pay the full registration fee again.

6. **Is it possible to extend the testing window?**

   ANCC: You can request (one time only) a new 120-day testing window. It must occur <6 months from the last day of the initial testing window. Your request for extension to the ANCC should be received after the end of the initial 120-day testing period.

   AANPCB: You can request an extension (one time only) by sending an email to certification@aanpcert.org. If an extension is granted, it will be for 60 days only. If you do not retake the exam during that time, you must reapply to take the examination (like the first time) and pay the full fee.

7. **Is there a penalty for guessing on the exam?**

   No, there is no penalty for guessing. If you are running out of time, answer the remaining questions at random. Do not leave any questions "blank" or without an answer, because this will be marked as an error (0 points). You may earn a few extra points if you guess correctly, which can make the difference between passing and failing the exam.

8. **Is it possible to return to a question later and change its answer?**

   Yes, it is, but only if you "flag" the question. You will learn about this simple command during the computer tutorial at the beginning of the exam. Flagging a question allows the test taker to return to the question at a later time (if you want to change or review your answer). On the other hand, if you indicate to the computer that your answer is "final," then you will not be allowed to change the answer. Do not worry about forgetting to "unflag" the questions if you run out of time. As long as a question has an answer, it will be graded by the computer.

9. **Does the certifying agency inform the state board of nursing of my certification status?**

   The AANPCB and ANCC will not automatically send your scores to the state board of nursing. For both certifying agencies, you must sign their Release of Scores consent form when you apply for the exam.

10. **How can I obtain an "official" verification of my national certification for my employer?**

    Both agencies have verification request forms on their websites. If you just took the exam, the AANPCB recommends you wait at least 10 days after your testing date. A nominal fee is charged.

11. **I am getting married or divorced or otherwise changing my name. Is there a problem with changing my legal name after I applied for the exams using my birth name or married name?**

    Yes, there may be a problem. The name that you use in your application must be the same as the one listed on your primary ID (e.g., unexpired driver's license, passport, military ID). Check the agency's website or call for more details. If you get married after you applied for the exam, it is better to wait until you have taken and passed the exam before changing the name on your driver's license.

COMMON QUESTIONS ABOUT CERTIFICATION RENEWAL

1. **How long is my certification valid?**
   Certification from the ANCC as well as the AANPCB is valid for 5 years. A few months before your certification expires, both the ANCC and the AANPCB will send you a reminder letter. However, if you do not receive your reminder, you are still responsible for renewing your certification.

2. **Can I still use my professional designations after my certification expires because I forgot to renew it?**
   No, credentials cannot be used once they have expired.

3. **What should I do if I change my legal name, have a new email address, have a new telephone contact number, or move to a new address?**
   You need to update your online account at the ANCC or the AANPCB website within 30 days if there are any changes in your contact information, such as your legal name, residence address, email address, or phone number.

4. **Is there a time period that must be followed to renew certification?**
   Yes, there is. All of the contact hours and practice hours must be completed within the current 5-year certification period.

5. **When should I submit my renewal application?**
   The process can be started as early as 12 months before your certification expires. It is best to start early because if you do not have enough CE/clinical/pharmacology contact hours, you still have enough time to obtain them. Recertification applications should be submitted no later than 12 weeks prior to the expiration date of the current certification to allow time for reviewing, processing, and issuing the new certificate before the expiration of the current certification.
      Note: Save a digital or hard copy (or other proof) of all your CE hours and clinical practice hours. If you are audited, you will be asked to submit proof of your CE hours (i.e., certificates) and clinical practice hours.

6. **How many clinical hours of practice are required to renew my certification every 5 years?**
   The ANCC no longer requires clinical practice hours for recertification, although the AANPCB does require 1,000 hours of clinical practice in your area of specialty (completed in the previous 5 years before recertification), plus 100 hours CE, of which 25 hours must be pharmacology CE. If you plan to use your clinical volunteer hours as an NP, keep a notebook to record each clinical site's address, the number of hours that you practiced, and the name/signature of the supervising NP/physician. If you do not have enough clinical hours, another method you can use to recertify is to retake the examination combined with the required CE hours. For adult nurse practitioners (ANPs) and gerontological nurse practitioners (GNPs), you do not have the option to recertify by retaking the examination, because the exams for your specialty have been retired.

7. **How many CE contact hours are required for recertification?**
   ANCC: 75 contact hours of CE are required. You also need one or more of the eight ANCC renewal categories (i.e., academic credits, presentations, preceptor hours, quality improvement project, professional service, practice hours, retake exam, publication or research).
      AANPCB: 100 contact hours of CE are required.

8. **How many pharmacotherapeutic contact hours are required per renewal cycle?**
   ANCC: Of the 75 contact hours, 25 of those hours must be in pharmacotherapeutics. If you double the 75 (150 contact hours), only 25 contact hours are required.
      AANPCB: Of the 100 contact hours, 25 contact hours in advanced pharmacology are required.

9. **What happens if my certification lapsed (I forgot to renew it)?**
   There is no "grace period" or backdating. On the day when your certification expires, you are prohibited from using your designation after your name. In addition, you will have a gap in your certification dates. The ANCC recommends that you check with your state licensing board to determine whether you can continue to practice as an NP. They also recommend that you check with your employer and with the agencies that are reimbursing your services.

10. **If my specialty certification exam was retired, can I continue with my specialty designation?**
    Yes, you may. You can renew your certification only through CE and clinical hours. If you let your certification lapse, you no longer have the examination option. Unless there are other options in the future (check the websites for updates), only students who have graduated from an AGNP program are permitted to take that exam. ANPs and GNPs are not allowed to take the AGNP exam.

11. **Is there any reciprocity between the ANCC and the AANPCB?**
    No, there is not. Both the ANCC and the AANPCB discontinued their reciprocity program many years ago.

EXAM QUESTION CLASSIFICATION

American Nurses Credentialing Center
See Table 1.2 for the ANCC FNP exam domains.

American Academy of Nurse Practitioners Certification Board
See Table 1.3 for the AANPCB FNP exam domains and Table 1.4 for breakdown by patient age group.

Table 1.2 ANCC FNP Exam: Domains

Domain (Released September 2022)	% of Questions	# of Questions
Assessment	19	29
Diagnosis	17	26
Planning	19	29
Implementation	29	43
Evaluation	15	23
Total	100*	150 scored questions

ANCC, American Nurses Credentialing Center; FNP, family nurse practitioner.
*Total does not come to 100 because of rounding.
Source: Data from American Nurses Credentialing Center. (2022, September 28). (See Resources section for complete source information.)

Table 1.3 AANPCB FNP Exam: Domains

Domain (Released January 2023)	% of Questions	# of Questions
Assess	27	36
Diagnose	26	35
Plan	25	34
Evaluate	22	30
Total	100	135 scored questions

AANPCB, American Academy of Nurse Practitioners Certification Board; FNP, family nurse practitioner.
Source: Data from American Academy of Nurse Practitioners Certification Board. (n.d.). (See Resources section for complete source information.)

Table 1.4 AANPCB FNP Exam: Age Groups

Age Group	% of Questions	# of Questions
Prenatal	2	3
Pediatrics (newborn, infant, and child)	11	15
Adolescent (early and late)	14	19
Adult (young and middle)	43	58
Older adult	22	30
Elder adult	8	10
Total	100	135 scored questions

AANPCB, American Academy of Nurse Practitioners Certification Board; FNP, family nurse practitioner.
Source: Data from American Academy of Nurse Practitioners Certification Board. (n.d.). (See Resources section for complete source information.)

FAST FACTS ABOUT THE ANCC AND AANPCB EXAMS

1. The ANCC FNP exam has approximately 10% nonclinical questions, or about 15 questions (out of 150 graded questions).
2. The current AANPCB FNP exam released in January 2023 does not contain nonclinical topics.
3. The ANCC and AANPCB FNP certification exams are designed for entry-level (not expert-level) practice. Most test takers who sit for the FNP certification exams are new graduates.
4. There are 25 pilot-test questions on the ANCC exam and 15 pilot-test questions on the AANPCB exam. These questions are not graded. There is no way to identify the graded questions from the pilot-test questions.
5. New clinical information (treatment guidelines or new drugs) released within the 10 months prior to the current exam will most likely not be included.
6. Keep in mind that the questions will be on primary care disorders (e.g., primary care clinics, public health clinics). If you are guessing, avoid picking an "exotic" diagnosis as an answer.
7. The AANPCB exams will list the normal lab results when they are pertinent to a question.
8. Unlike the AANPCB, the ANCC does not list the normal lab results. If you are taking the ANCC exam, it is important to memorize some normal lab results and to write them down on scratch paper during the computer tutorial time period.
9. Expect a few questions regarding pregnancy-related topics (obstetrics). Example: Uterine involution is when the uterus contracts and shrinks in size until it returns to its prepregnancy state; the process takes about 6 weeks.
10. Learn the significance of abnormal lab results and the type of follow-up needed to further evaluate the patient.
    - Example: An elderly male patient complains of a new-onset, left-sided temporal headache accompanied by scalp tenderness and indurated temporal artery. The NP suspects temporal arteritis. The screening test is the sedimentation rate, which is expected to be much higher than normal (elevated value).
    - Example: A patient with an elevated white blood cell (WBC) count >11,000/mm³ accompanied by neutrophilia (>70%) and the presence of bands ("shift to the left") most likely has a serious bacterial infection.
11. Sometimes there will be one unexpected question relating to a dental injury. Example: A completely avulsed permanent tooth should be reimplanted as soon as possible. It can be transported to the dentist in cold milk (not frozen milk).
12. There may be a question on epidemiologic terms. Example: *Sensitivity* is defined as the ability of a test to detect a person who has the disease. *Specificity* is defined as the ability of a test to detect a person who is healthy (or to detect the person without the disease).

13. Learn the definitions of some of the research study designs. Example: A cohort study follows a group of people who share some common characteristics to observe the development of disease over time (e.g., the Framingham Nurses' Health Study).

14. Several emergent conditions that may present in the primary care area will be on the exam. Examples: Navicular (or scaphoid) fracture, acute myocardial infarction (MI), cauda equina syndrome, anaphylaxis, angioedema, meningococcal meningitis.

15. Become familiar with the names of some anatomic areas. Example: Trauma to Kiesselbach's plexus will result in an anterior nosebleed.

16. Some questions may ask about the "gold-standard test" or the diagnostic test for a condition. Example: The diagnostic or gold-standard test for sickle cell anemia, glucose-6-phosphate dehydrogenase (G6PD) anemia, and alpha or beta thalassemia is the hemoglobin electrophoresis.

17. Distinguish between first- and second-line antibiotics. Example: A 7-year-old child with acute otitis media (AOM) who is treated with amoxicillin returns in 48 hours without improvement (complains of ear pain, bulging tympanic membrane). The next step is to discontinue the amoxicillin and start the child on a second-line antibiotic such as amoxicillin–clavulanate (Augmentin) twice a day × 10 days.

18. Become knowledgeable about alternative antibiotics for penicillin-allergic patients. If the patient has a gram-positive infection, possible alternatives are macrolides, clindamycin, or quinolones with gram-positive activity such as levofloxacin or moxifloxacin.

19. If a patient has an infection that responds well to macrolides, but they think they are "allergic" to erythromycin (symptoms of nausea or gastrointestinal [GI] upset), inform them that they had an adverse reaction, not a true allergic reaction (hives, angioedema). Example: Switch the patient from erythromycin to azithromycin (usually a Z-Pak).

20. If a patient fails to respond to the initial medication, add another medication (follow the steps of the treatment guideline). Example: A patient with chronic obstructive pulmonary disease (COPD) is prescribed ipratropium bromide (Atrovent) for dyspnea. On follow-up, the patient complains that the symptoms are not relieved. The next step would be to prescribe an albuterol inhaler (Ventolin) or a combination inhaler.

21. Disease states are usually presented in their full-blown, "classic" textbook presentations. Example: In a case of acute mononucleosis, the patient will most likely be a teen presenting with the classic triad of sore throat, prolonged fatigue, and enlarged cervical nodes. If the patient is older, but has the same signs and symptoms, it is still mononucleosis (reactivated type).

22. Ethnic background may give a clue for some conditions. Example: Alpha thalassemia is more common among Southeast Asian (e.g., Filipino) people. Beta thalassemia is more common in Mediterranean people.

23. No asymptomatic or "borderline" cases of disease states are presented in the test. Example: In real life, most patients with iron-deficiency anemia are asymptomatic and do not have either pica or spoon-shaped nails. In the exam, they will probably have these clinical findings plus the other findings of anemia.

24. Become familiar with lupus or systemic lupus erythematosus (SLE). Example: A malar rash (butterfly rash) is present in most patients with lupus. These patients should be advised to avoid or minimize sunlight exposure (photosensitivity).

25. Become familiar with polymyalgia rheumatica (PMR). Example: First-line treatment for PMR includes long-term steroids. Long-term, low-dose steroids are commonly used to control symptoms (pain, severe stiffness in shoulders and hip girdle). PMR patients are also at higher risk for temporal arteritis.

26. The gold-standard exam for temporal arteritis is a biopsy of the temporal artery. Refer the patient to an ophthalmologist for management.

27. Learn the disorders for which maneuvers are used and what a positive report signifies. Example: Finkelstein's test—positive in De Quervain's tenosynovitis. Anterior drawer maneuver and Lachman maneuver—positive if anterior cruciate ligament (ACL) of the knee is damaged. The knee may also be unstable. Flexion pinch sign—positive in meniscus injuries of the knee.

28. Some conditions need to be evaluated with a radiologic test. Example: If suspected soft tissue damage in a joint, order an x-ray first (but MRI is the gold standard).

29. The abnormal eye findings in diabetes (diabetic retinopathy) and hypertension (hypertensive retinopathy) should be memorized. Learn to distinguish each one. Example: Diabetic retinopathy: Neovascularization, cotton wool spots, and microaneurysms. Hypertensive retinopathy: Atrioventricular (AV) nicking, silver and/or copper wire arterioles.

30. Become knowledgeable about physical exam "normal" and "abnormal" findings. Example: When checking deep tendon reflexes (DTRs) in a patient with severe sciatica or diabetic peripheral neuropathy, the Achilles reflex may be absent or hypoactive. Scoring: Absent (0), hypoactive (1), normal (2), hyperactive (3), and clonus (4).

31. There are only a few questions on benign or physiologic variants. Example: A benign S4 heart sound may be auscultated in some elderly patients. A geographic tongue, torus palatinus, and fishtail uvula may be seen during the oral exam in a few patients.

32. Some commonly used drugs have rare (but potentially life-threatening) adverse effects. Example: A rare but serious adverse effect of angiotensin-converting enzyme inhibitors (ACEIs) is angioedema. A common side effect of ACEIs is a dry cough (up to 10%).

33. Learn about the preferred and/or first-line drug used to treat some diseases. Example: ACEIs or angiotensin receptor blockers (ARBs) are the preferred drugs to

treat hypertension in diabetics and patients with renal disease because of their renal-protective properties.

34. When medications are used in the answer options, they will be listed either by name (generic and brand name) or by drug class alone. Example: Instead of using the generic/brand name of ipratropium (Atrovent), it may be listed as a drug class (an anticholinergic).

35. Most of the drugs mentioned in the exam are the well-recognized drugs. Examples (additional examples are listed in Chapters 2 and 3):
    * Penicillin: Amoxicillin (broad-spectrum penicillin), penicillin VK
    * Macrolide: Erythromycin, azithromycin (Z-Pak), or clarithromycin (Biaxin)
    * Cephalosporins: First-generation (Keflex), second-generation (Cefaclor, Ceftin, Cefzil), third-generation (Rocephin, Suprax, Omnicef)
    * Quinolones: Ciprofloxacin (Cipro), ofloxacin (Floxin)
    * Quinolones with gram-positive coverage: Levofloxacin (Levaquin), moxifloxacin (Avelox), gatifloxacin (Tequin)
    * Sulfa: Trimethoprim–sulfamethoxazole (Bactrim, Septra)
    * Tetracyclines: Tetracycline, doxycycline, minocycline (Minocin)
    * Nonsteroidal anti-inflammatory drugs (NSAIDs): Ibuprofen, naproxen (Aleve, Anaprox)
    * COX-2 inhibitor: Celecoxib (Celebrex)

36. Category B drugs are allowed for pregnant or lactating patients. Example: For pain relief, pick acetaminophen (Tylenol) instead of NSAIDs such as ibuprofen (Advil) or naproxen (Aleve, Anaprox). Avoid nitrofurantoin and sulfa drugs during the third trimester (these increase risk of hyperbilirubinemia).

37. The preferred treatment for cutaneous anthrax is ciprofloxacin 500 mg orally twice a day for 60 days or 8 weeks. If the patient is allergic to ciprofloxacin, use doxycycline 100 mg twice a day. Cutaneous anthrax is not contagious; it comes from touching fur or animal skins that are contaminated with anthrax spores.

38. Approximately 15% of the questions will be about infants and children. Example: The American Academy of Pediatrics (AAP) recommends that breastfed infants should be started on vitamin D during the first few days of life; then at age 4 months, iron-supplementation is recommended (formula contains vitamins/minerals so no need to supplement).

39. A common question design regarding pediatrics is to query about growth and development norms (or abnormal). Example: At the age of 6 months, infants can sit without support; roll over front to back, then from back to front; transfer objects from one hand to the other; use a raking grasp; and babble.

40. Physical exam findings in children that are abnormal with serious consequences might be included. Example: Leukocoria (white color) is noted on one eye while checking for the red reflex. Rule out retinoblastoma of the eye, which is a malignant tumor of the retina.

41. There are some questions on theories and conceptual models. Example: Stages of change or "decision" theory (Prochaska) include concepts such as precontemplation, contemplation, preparation, action, and maintenance.

42. Other health theorists who have been included on the exams in the past are (not inclusive) Alfred Bandura (self-efficacy), Erik Erikson, Sigmund Freud, Elisabeth Kübler-Ross (grieving), and others. Example: If a small child expresses a desire to marry a parent of the opposite sex, the child is in the oedipal stage (Freud). The child's age is about 5 to 6 years (preschool to kindergarten).

43. Starting at the age of about 11 years, most children can understand abstract concepts (early abstract thinking) and are better at logical thinking. Example: When performing the Mini-Mental State Exam, when the NP is asking about "proverbs," the nurse is assessing the patient's ability to understand abstract concepts.

44. Keep these good communication rules in mind: Ask open-ended questions; do not reassure patients, avoid angering them, and respect their culture. There may be two or three questions relating to abuse (e.g., child abuse, domestic abuse, elder abuse).

45. Follow national treatment guidelines for certain disorders. Note that it may take 1 to 2 years for the latest guidelines to appear on the certification exams. Following is a list of treatment guidelines used as references by the ANCC and the AANPCB.*
    * **Asthma:** Global Initiative for Asthma. (2022). *Global strategy for asthma management and prevention.* https://ginasthma.org/wp-content/uploads/2022/07/GINA-Main-Report-2022-FINAL-22-07-01-WMS.pdf
    * **COPD:** Global Initiative for Chronic Obstructive Lung Disease. (2023). *Global strategy for the diagnosis, management, and prevention of chronic obstructive pulmonary disease (2023 report).* https://goldcopd.org/2023-gold-report-2
    * **Diabetes:** Kahn, S. E. (Ed.). (2023). Standards of care in diabetes. *Diabetes Care, 46*(Suppl. 1), S1–S291. https://diabetesjournals.org/care/issue/46/Supplement_1
    * **Ethics:** Fowler, M. (2015). *Guide to the code of ethics for nurses with interpretive statements: Development, interpretation, and application* (2nd ed.). Nursesbooks.org.
    * **Healthy People:** Office of Disease Prevention and Health Promotion. (n.d.). *Healthy People 2030: Browse objectives.* https://health.gov/healthypeople/objectives-and-data/browse-objectives
    * **Health Promotion:** U.S. Preventive Services Task Force. www.uspreventiveservicestaskforce.org/uspstf
    * **Hyperlipidemia:** Grundy, S. M., Stone, N. J., Bailey, A. L., Beam, C., Birtcher, K. K., Blumenthal, R. S., Braun, L. T., de Ferranti, S., Faÿla-Tommasino, J., Forman, D. E., Goldberg, R., Heidenreich, P. A., Hlatky, M. A., Jones, D. W., Lloyd-Jones, D., Lopez-Pajares, N., Ndumele, C. E., Orringer, C. E., Peralta, C. A., ... Yeboah, J. (2019). AHA/

---

* Not an all-inclusive list.

ACC/AACVPR/AAPA/ABC/ACPM/ADA/AGS/APhA/ASPC/NLA/PCNA Guideline on the Management of Blood Cholesterol: A report of the ACC/AHA Task Force on Practice Guidelines. *Circulation*, 139(25). https://doi.org/10.1161/CIR.0000000000000625

- **Hypertension:** Whelton, P. K., Carey, R. M., Aronow, W. S., Casey, D. E., Jr., Collins, K. J., Dennison Himmelfarb, C., DePalma, S. M., Gidding, S., Jamerson, K. A., Jones, D. W., MacLaughlin, E. J., Muntner, P., Ovbiagele, B., Smith, S. C., Jr., Spencer, C. C., Stafford, R. S., Taler, S. J., Thomas, R. J., Williams, K. A., Sr., ... Wright, J. T., Jr. (2017). Guideline for the prevention, detection, evaluation, and management of high blood pressure in adults: A report of the American College of Cardiology/American Heart Association Task Force on Clinical Practice Guidelines. (2018). *Journal of the American College of Cardiology*, 71, e127–e248. https://doi.org/10.1161/HYP.0000000000000065

- **Mental Health:** American Psychiatric Association. (2022). *Diagnostic and statistical manual of mental disorders* (5th ed., text rev.). https://doi.org/10.1176/appi.books.9780890425787

- **Pediatrics:** American Academy of Pediatrics. (2017). *Bright futures: Guidelines for health supervision of infants, children, and adolescents* (E-book; 4th ed.). https://doi.org/10.1542/9781610020237

- **Sexually Transmitted Infections:** Centers for Disease Control and Prevention. (2021). *Sexually transmitted infections treatment guidelines*. https://www.cdc.gov/std/treatment-guidelines/toc.htm

46. The ANCC exam has several questions about evidence-based medicine that are designed in the drag-and-drop format. Review Chapter 2 to become familiar with this format.

47. If the question is asking for the initial or screening lab test, it will probably be a less expensive and readily available test such as the complete blood count (CBC) to screen for anemia.

MAXIMIZING YOUR SCORE

1. The first answer that "pops" into your head is usually the correct answer.

2. If you are guessing, make an educated guess. Pick what you think is the most likely answer. Try not to change it unless you are sure that you should.

3. Use the "flag" command so that you can return to a question later when you complete the exam.

4. Avoid changing too many answers. If you are not sure, then leave the answer alone. I advise my students not to change more than three answers.

5. Avoid choosing "exotic" diseases as answers if you are guessing. Remember, these are tests for primary care conditions.

6. One method of guessing is to look for a pattern. Pick the answer that does not fit the pattern. Another is to

pick the answer that you are most "attracted" to. Go with your gut feeling, and do not change the answer unless you are very sure.

7. Remind yourself to read slowly and carefully throughout the test. Avoid reading questions too rapidly. Make sure that you understand the stem of the question.

8. If you are having problems choosing or understanding the answer options, try to read them not only from the top down, but also from the bottom up (e.g., from option D to A, or from 4 to 1).

9. Eliminate the wrong answers after you have read all the answer options. If an answer option contains all-inclusive words (*all*, *none*, *every*, *never*), then it is probably wrong.

10. Be careful with certain words, such as *always*, *exactly*, *often*, *sometimes*, and *mostly*.

11. Assume that each question has enough information to answer it correctly. Questions and answers are carefully designed. Take the facts at face value.

12. The first few questions are usually harder to solve. This is a common test design. Do not let it shake your confidence. (Guess the answer if you need to, and flag it so that you can return to it later.)

13. Save yourself time (and mental strain) by reading the last sentence of long questions and case scenarios *first*. Then read the question again from the beginning. The advantage of this "backward reading" technique is that you know ahead of time what the question is asking for. When you read it again normally, it becomes easier to recognize important clues that will help you answer the question.

14. When reading a lengthy or complicated question, read it at least twice (or more) until you understand it. Do not ignore modifiers (e.g., *only*, *first*, *initial*, *preferred treatment*) because they will help you determine the correct answer. Usually, most questions can be answered without major difficulty. For some, you will have to differentiate between two possible answer options. Read the question again; you may have missed the key words that will help you to narrow it down to one answer.

15. Just because a statement or an answer is *true* does not mean that it is the correct answer. If it does not answer the stem of the question, then it is the wrong answer.

16. Design and memorize your "scratch paper" a few weeks before you take the exam. Choose what you want on it wisely. Remember to keep it brief.

17. Use the time left from the "free" computer tutorial time to write down the facts that you memorized for your scratch paper. If you run out of time, skip this step.

18. Some suggestions of facts to write down on your scratch paper are lab results (e.g., hemoglobin, hematocrit, mean corpuscular volume, platelets, WBC count, neutrophil percentage, potassium, urinalysis). Other popular choices are the murmurs, the cranial nerves, or helpful mnemonics.

19. Do not leave any of the questions blank or unanswered, because there is no penalty for guessing. Questions that are left blank are marked as errors (0 points). If you are running out of time and you are not done, quickly answer the remaining questions at random.

20. Do not change your answers unless you are very sure that you have made a mistake. Remember, the first answer that comes into your head is usually the correct answer. Do not second-guess yourself! I have had students fail the exam due to changing too many answers during their "leftover" time.

21. If you spend more than 60 seconds on a question, you are wasting time. If you are not sure, pick the most likely answer, and then flag the "difficult" question so that you can return to it later (after you finish the entire test). Look at the clock often (upper half of screen) so that you do not run out of time.

22. Most test takers who finish the exam will have several minutes left. If so, go over the exam and make sure that you have not skipped any questions. All questions should contain an answer.

23. Consider a quick break (if you have enough time) if you get too mentally fatigued. Solving 150 to 175 questions is pretty intense. If you feel "fuzzy" or tired, go to the restroom and get a drink of water, and splash cold water on your face. This can take fewer than 5 minutes. You can bring bottled water, but you have to leave it outside the testing area.

24. The countdown clock on the computer does not stop for breaks. Do not use more than 5 minutes for your quick restroom break. When the time expires, the exam will automatically be shut down by the computer.

25. If you have failed the test before, try not to memorize what you did on the previous exam you took. The answers you remember may be wrong. Pretend that you have never seen the test before so that you can start out fresh mentally.

26. Do not panic or let your anxiety take over. Learn to use a calming technique, such as deep breathing (see below), to calm yourself quickly before you take the exam.

27. Consider listening to a test-anxiety hypnosis program; use it every night for at least 2 to 3 weeks for maximum effect.

28. One of the most important pieces of advice that I can give you is to make sure that you get enough sleep the night before the exam. Aim for at least 7 to 8 hours of sleep. Better yet, make sure that you get enough sleep a few nights before, not just the night before.

29. Before the test, practice answering questions and check the rationales afterward. The ANCC has free questions per specialty that you can take online and score. Buy practice questions from the ANCC or the AANPCB (depending on which test you are taking).

30. Check out the website allnurses.com and search for examination tips from others who have taken/failed an FNP certification exam. You can also do this directly by searching online.

PREPARING FOR THE EXAM
Review Timeline

1. Start seriously reviewing for the exam at least 3 months in advance. Study time can range from 2 to 3 hours per session, or you can break it up into 1-hour segments. Be consistent. The best time to study is the time of day you are most alert.

2. Prepare a study schedule by organ system. Photocopy the table of contents of your primary care textbook. Place check marks next to the diseases that you want to concentrate on, and then schedule the date and time period for each organ system.

3. Concentrate your studies on your weaker areas. For example, if orthopedics is one of your weak areas, devote more time to it. Spend 3 days on orthopedics versus 1 day for the "easy" organ systems (since you understand them better).

4. I highly recommend that you attend at least one quality review course and buy another online review course. I teach review courses live and by webinar.

5. Buy a new notebook. If you find that you are having a problem understanding a concept, write it down in your notebook, then research it and find the answer to your question.

6. Meet with someone in your local area or by an online meeting platform who is also taking the exam. Practice quizzing each other.

7. Note the diseases and topics that I have highlighted in this book. Some organ systems have more "weight" on the exam than others. Become more familiar with these areas.

8. If you are taking the ANCC exam, I highly recommend that you devote at least 30% of your study time to learning about the nonclinical topics.

9. If you learn better in a group, organize one. Decide ahead of time what organ systems or diseases to cover together so that you do not waste time.

Testing Center Details

1. Call the testing center or confirm your appointment online 4 weeks before to verify your scheduled date and time.

2. Locate and travel to the testing center 1 to 2 weeks before taking the exam. Save the address of the testing center on your GPS or map app.

3. Arrive at least 45 to 60 minutes before your scheduled time so that you have enough time to park your car, locate the testing center, and check in for your appointment.

4. Carry acceptable forms of unexpired primary ID (photo with signature). If you do not have the proper forms of identification, you will not be allowed to take the exam.
   - Primary IDs include driver's license issued by the Department of Motor Vehicles (DMV), state ID card issued by the DMV, passport, and U.S. military ID.

- Secondary (nonphoto) IDs include cards with your name and signature (e.g., credit card, debit card, Social Security card, voter registration card, employee ID).
- Expired IDs are not acceptable.
- The name that is printed on your primary ID must match the name that you used when you applied for the exam.
- Check that both your primary and secondary IDs and the letter with your Prometric identification number match; be sure that all your IDs are inside your wallet/handbag.

5. Biometrics are used for enhanced security. The test-taking room is also monitored closely by video and microphones. Your glasses will be checked visually, and you will be asked to show your arms and ankles, as well as empty your pockets from an agreed-upon safe distance.
6. A whiteboard (8.5 × 11 inches) with a marker, or scratch paper and a pencil, will be given to you by the testing center staff (and collected after you are done). If you are given paper and tend to write a lot, ask for extra paper.
7. You can request noise-reducing headsets or earplugs; consider this option if you are sensitive to noise.
8. Cell phones, watches, cameras, pagers, jewelry (except for engagement and/or wedding ring), and food or drink are not allowed inside the testing area.
9. Testing computers are predetermined. Each test taker is assigned one small cubicle with one computer. If you are having problems seeing the computer screen, bring it to the proctor's attention as soon as possible.
10. Verify that you are given the correct examination as soon as you sit down. Check that the title and the examination code on the screen match the information sent by the testing agency for your NP specialty.
11. No food or drink is allowed inside the testing room. You can bring drinks and food (e.g., snack bars) into the building and place them outside your locker (on top of the locker) so that you do not have to open your locker. You are not permitted to unlock your locker during the testing period.
12. If you need to go to the restroom, you must first sign out with the proctor/testing staff. Remember, the time clock will continue to count down the time. It does not stop for breaks.
13. Do not forget your glasses if you need them to read text on the computer.

The Night Before the Exam

1. Avoid eating a heavy meal or consuming alcoholic drinks the night before the exam. Avoid eating 3 to 4 hours before bedtime.
2. Get enough sleep. Aim for at least 7 to 8 hours. Getting adequate sleep is probably one of the most important things you can do to help you pass the exam.
3. If you are scheduled to take your exam in the morning, set two alarms to wake you up on time. Give yourself extra time if it is a weekday (traffic congestion).

The Day of the Exam

1. Avoid eating a heavy breakfast or eating only simple carbohydrates. The best meals are a combination of a protein with a complex carbohydrate (e.g., eggs, whole-wheat bread, nuts, cheese).
2. If you get drowsy and "fuzzy" during the exam, there are several ways to "wake up" rapidly. Excuse yourself and go to the restroom to splash cold water on your face. You can perform 10 to 20 jumping jacks. Drinking cold water, a caffeinated beverage, or coffee can be very helpful. (However, don't drink too much.)
3. Avoid drinking too much fluid and do not forget to empty your bladder before the exam.
4. Wear comfortable clothing and dress in layers in case of temperature changes.
5. Jewelry is not allowed inside the testing area, except for wedding and/or engagement rings.

Test Anxiety

It is normal to feel anxious before taking an exam. A little anxiety helps us to become alert and vigilant, but too much anxiety can wear you down both emotionally and physically.

Your internal perception about how well you will do on the exam is very important. If you tend to become very anxious (or you are now more anxious because you previously failed the exam), there are calming methods that may prove helpful in controlling your anxiety. Following are some suggestions to help reduce test-taking anxiety a few weeks before the exam:

1. Make sure that you have devoted enough time for your review studies. If you feel in your gut that you have not studied "enough" or that you are not ready, it will worsen anxiety.
2. Consider taking one or two review courses.
3. Avoid negative "self-talk."
4. Improve the nutritional content of your diet, especially about 4 weeks before the exam.
5. Hypnotherapy audio files are sold online. For maximum effectiveness, it is best to listen to them daily for 2 to 4 weeks.
6. "Tapping" is another method used to counteract test anxiety (or increase self-confidence). The technique is demonstrated in videos on YouTube.

Your Panic Button

If you find yourself feeling panicky during the exam, try the following calming technique. Practice this exercise at home until you feel comfortable doing it.

1. Close your eyes. During inhalation, tell yourself gently, "I am breathing in calmness." Then hold your breath and count from 1 to 3.
2. During exhalation, tell yourself gently, "I am breathing out fear," while counting from 1 to 5.
3. Inhale deeply through your nose and exhale slowly through your mouth.
4. Complete one cycle of three inhalations and three exhalations. Repeat as needed.

2 QUESTION DISSECTION AND ANALYSIS

EVIDENCE-BASED MEDICINE

I. Discussion

Questions about evidence-based medicine (EBM) are typically designed in "drag-and-drop" format on the American Nurses Credentialing Center (ANCC) exam. They are presented as two boxes with three sections each. The example that follows illustrates this format. On the left side, three types of article summaries (or research studies) are marked A, B, and C (in the exam, they will appear as blue boxes). On the right side, you will see the rankings from 1 to 3 (in the exam, they will be yellow boxes). You "drag" one of the articles from the left-hand box and "drop" it into the correct ranking or hierarchy in the right-hand box. Your job is to rank the three research article summaries as best evidence (1), moderate evidence (2), or weakest evidence (3).

II. Example

Example of Drag-and-Drop Formatted Question

Article Summaries	Strength of Evidence (Strongest to Weakest)
A. An experimental study on 500 patients with early dementia who were given ginkgo biloba daily for 6 months versus the control group, which was given placebo pills	1
B. A specialty society opinion paper regarding the effectiveness of ginkgo biloba supplementation in dementia	2
C. A meta-analysis on MEDLINE and Cochrane databases that found 53 randomized controlled trials about ginkgo biloba use in patients with early dementia	3

III. Correct Answer

Article C is ranked 1, Article A is ranked 2, and Article B is ranked 3.

IV. Question Dissection

Best Clues

The easiest way to answer this type of question is to memorize and understand the highest level of evidence (e.g., meta-analysis, systematic review, randomized controlled

trial [RCT]) and the types of studies that have the lowest level of evidence (e.g., opinions, editorials). The "leftover" study belongs in the middle (#2 ranking). The first sentence of each article summary usually gives a clue about the study design. Notice that in option C of the example, it is a "meta-analysis"; in option A, it is an "experimental study"; and in option B, it is a "specialty society opinion paper."

I teach a three-step system to students in my review courses:

1. First, identify the research study that has the highest/best level of evidence (#1 ranking). An easy way to do this is by searching for key words in the question such as *meta-analysis, systematic review,* or *RCT* combined with *Cochrane Database of Systematic Reviews (CDSR),* MEDLINE® database, and/or Cumulative Index to Nursing and Allied Health Literature (CINAHL®).
2. Next, look for the research study that has the weakest evidence (#3 ranking). It usually contains key words such as *expert opinion, opinion, editorial,* or *specialty society.*
3. Therefore, view the study that is leftover as having the middle ranking (#2 ranking). In addition, keep in mind that if the choices do not include a meta-analysis or systemic review, then the study with the highest ranking would be an RCT or an experimental study. The ANCC exams usually have several of this type of question.

The full levels of evidence rankings are:

- Meta-analysis and/or systematic reviews (Cochrane/MEDLINE/CINAHL/PubMed)
- RCTs (used for testing medical treatment effectiveness, subjects assigned at random to either a control or treatment group)
- Experimental studies (control group, intervention group, randomization)
- Cohort/case control studies
- Retrospective chart reviews
- Expert/specialty society opinions

PHOTOGRAPHS

I. Discussion

On the ANCC exam, expect to see several color photographs of skin conditions and a few on the eyes/fundi. In the future, there may be pictures from other organ systems. The stem of the question usually will ask for the possible diagnosis, differential diagnosis, or type of treatment. If you plan to take the ANCC exam, you need to memorize how a skin condition or eye finding appears in a color photo. It is a good idea to use a search engine (e.g., Google) to look for the images. For example, you want to become familiar with the appearance of skin cancers, such as basal cell carcinoma and melanoma, and funduscopic findings in diabetes and hypertension.

II. Example

The nurse practitioner (NP) is performing a routine physical exam on a 54-year-old White male farmer who is an emigrant from Australia. The NP notices a round skin lesion on the patient's head. It has a firm texture with indurated edges and telangiectasia (Figure 2.1). The patient reports that the lesion does not itch, but it has slowly enlarged over the past few years. Which of the following conditions is most likely in this patient?

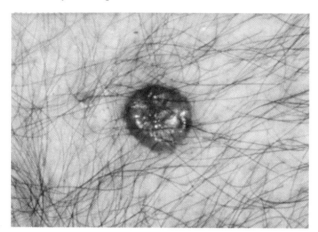

Figure 2.1 Example of an exam image.
Source: National Cancer Institute.

A. Nodular melanoma
B. Squamous cell carcinoma
C. Basal cell carcinoma
D. Actinic keratosis

III. Correct Answer: Option C

C. Basal cell carcinoma

IV. Question Dissection

Best Clues

- Notice that the skin lesion has a pearly or waxlike (shiny) appearance with telangiectasia, which is "classic" for basal cell carcinoma; some lesions may show central ulceration.
- Patient has risk factors for skin cancer, such as light-colored skin, and he is from Australia, which has high rates of skin cancer.
- The skin lesion is located on a sun-exposed area.
- It is probably not nodular melanoma, which usually has pigment such as brown or black color with irregular borders.
- Actinic keratosis is a precancer of squamous cell carcinoma and is usually located on the scalp (males), face, and back of the hands (dorsum); they appear as a crusty/scaly growth that slowly enlarges over time.
- The gold-standard test for skin cancer is the skin biopsy.

MULTIPLE-CHOICE QUESTIONS WITH MORE THAN ONE CORRECT RESPONSE

I. Discussion

Expect to see some "select all that apply" questions with five or six answer options in both the ANCC and the American Academy of Nurse Practitioners Certification Board (AANPCB) exams. The question will ask you to select all of the answers that are correct. For example, you may be asked to pick two or three differential diagnoses for a case of skin rash. The clues are given in the presentation of the signs and symptoms.

II. Example

A 75-year-old woman with mild dementia, hyperlipidemia, and emphysema is brought in by her middle-aged daughter as a walk-in patient in a community clinic with a complaint of a sudden onset of red rashes on her left lower arm and hand. During the skin exam, the NP notes that there are a few blisters. When the NP touches one of the blisters, it ruptures and drains clear serous fluid. Which of the following conditions should the NP consider in the differential diagnosis?
A. Contact dermatitis
B. Erysipelas
C. Psoriasis
D. Impetigo
E. Thermal burn

III. Correct Answer: Options A, D, and E

A. Contact dermatitis
D. Impetigo
E. Thermal burn

IV. Question Dissection

Best Clues

- Easily ruptured blisters (fragile) are a classic finding for bullous impetigo, an acute bacterial skin infection caused by *Staphylococcus* or *Streptococcus*.
- Contact dermatitis can present with just red skin or red skin with blisters. The rash can be located anywhere on the body, and it may have a pattern (like a belt) or no pattern.
- The timing of the rash is very important. Is it acute or chronic? Rule out option C (psoriasis), which is a chronic skin disease.
- Erysipelas is a type of cellulitis caused by strep. It resembles a bright-red, warm, raised rash (plaque-like) with discrete borders usually located on the face or the shins. Blistering is not present.
- A thermal burn is a burn caused by heat (e.g., fire, heat). Consider a second-degree burn in the differential diagnosis because of its acute onset. Also, the patient has mild dementia, which puts her at a higher risk for accidents.

DIAGNOSTIC IMAGING

I. Discussion

Questions about diagnostic imaging tests may appear on the exam. You may get a multiple-choice question alone or a question that is accompanied by a chest x-ray film. I recommend that you use a search engine (e.g., Google) to search for images of chest films with lobar consolidation due to community-acquired pneumonia (CAP), right middle lobe pneumonia, pulmonary tuberculosis (TB) infection, and emphysema/chronic obstructive pulmonary disease (COPD).

II. Example

A 34-year-old male smoker presents in an urgent care clinic complaining of a productive cough, chest congestion, fever, chills, and poor appetite for 1 week. Cough is productive of greenish sputum, which is sometimes tinged with a small amount of blood. Vital signs are as follows: temperature of 101.2°F, pulse of 100 beats/min, respirations of 24 breaths/min, and blood pressure (BP) of 122/88 mmHg. A radiograph of the chest is obtained (Figure 2.2). What is the most likely diagnosis in this patient?

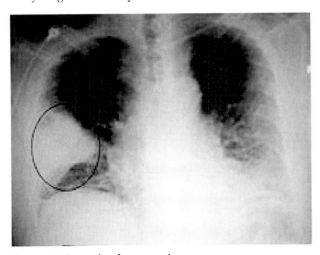

Figure 2.2 Example of an exam image.

A. Acute bronchitis
B. Right middle lobe pneumonia
C. Right lower lobe pneumonia
D. Legionella pneumonia

III. Correct Answer: Option B
B. Right middle lobe pneumonia

IV. Question Dissection

Best Clues

- The signs and symptoms of CAP include fever and cough productive of green sputum with a small amount of blood (or rust-colored sputum). Rust-colored sputum is associated with *Streptococcus pneumoniae* infection.
- Most of the middle lobe of the right lung is anatomically in the anterior chest by the right nipple area. Notice that lobar consolidation occurs in the same area.
- Patients with acute bronchitis may have chest congestion but not fever, chills, or productive cough with purulent sputum.
- Legionella pneumonia (Legionnaire's disease) is uncommon in primary care. Look for a history of exposure to "nebulized" water sources (e.g., air conditioners, fountains). Presents with pneumonia signs/symptoms that are accompanied by gastrointestinal (GI) symptoms (diarrhea, nausea/vomiting).

CULTURE

I. Discussion

There will be several questions on the ANCC exam that address culture. The questions will address knowledge of respecting diversity and inclusivity.

II. Example

The nurse practitioner (NP) is working in a primary care clinic where the patient population represents many different cultures. Which of the following should the NP consider when planning care for their patients to reflect cultural competency? (Select all that apply.)

A. Cultural diversity is limited to people of certain cultures and races.
B. Patients may be members of multiple cultural groups.
C. Cultural practices may change and evolve over time.
D. Culture may determine what behavior is acceptable for members of that group.

III. Correct Answers: Options B, C, and D

B. Patients may be members of multiple cultural groups.
C. Cultural practices may change and evolve over time.
D. Culture may determine what behavior is acceptable for members of that group.

IV. Question Dissection

Best Clues

Option A is not inclusive of all cultures and races.

Cultural competence is the ability of an individual to understand and respect values, attitudes, and beliefs that differ across cultures. Furthermore, the NP who demonstrates cultural competence also is able to consider and respond appropriately to these differences in planning, implementing, and evaluating healthcare, patient education, and health promotion.

LAB RESULTS AND DIAGNOSTIC TESTS

I. Discussion

Laboratory tests, such as hemoglobin and hematocrit, mean corpuscular volume (MCV), total white blood cell (WBC) count, percentage of neutrophils in the WBC differential, thyroid-stimulating hormone (TSH), prostate-specific antigen (PSA), and urinalysis (UA), are commonly encountered in the exams. Learn the significance of the abnormal results and the follow-up tests that are needed to evaluate them further.

The AANPCB exam does list the norms for some of the common laboratory tests. They will appear only when needed to answer a question (such as an anemia question).

In contrast, the ANCC does not list any of the normal results in its certification exams. Therefore, if you plan to take the ANCC exam, it is important that you memorize the normal results of these laboratory tests.

Be warned that lab results are also used as distractors; the labs listed may not be necessary to solve the exam question correctly. The normal results for these labs are also included in the pertinent review chapters of this book (e.g., TSH is found in Chapter 9).

II. Example

An elderly man of Mediterranean descent has a routine complete blood count (CBC) done for an annual physical. The following are his lab test results: hemoglobin is 12.0 g/dL, hematocrit is 39%, and mean corpuscular value (MCV) is 72 fL. His prostate-specific antigen (PSA) result is 3.2 ng/mL. Urinalysis (UA) shows no leukocytes and few epithelial cells. Which of the following laboratory tests are indicated for this patient?

A. Serum iron, serum ferritin, total iron-binding capacity (TIBC), and the red cell distribution width (RDW)
B. Serum vitamin B_{12} and folate level with a peripheral smear
C. CBC with white cell differential and UA
D. Urine culture and sensitivity with microscopic exam of the urine (Tables 2.1 and 2.2)

III. Correct Answer: Option A

A. Serum iron, serum ferritin, total iron-binding capacity (TIBC), and the red cell distribution width (RDW)

IV. Question Dissection

Best Clues

- Low hemoglobin and hematocrit for gender (male) and age (abnormal CBC result)
- An MCV of 72 fL, which is indicative of microcytic anemia (assessment)
- The ethnic background of the patient (demographics)
- Ignore the UA and PSA tests because they are not necessary to solve the problem

Table 2.1 List of Laboratory Norms (Adults)

CBC	Reference Ranges
Hemoglobin	
Males	13.0–17.5 g/dL
Females	12.0–16 g/dL
Hematocrit	
Males	40%–50%
Females	36%–45%
MCV	80–100 Fl
RDW	>14.5%
Platelet count	<150,000/mm³ (increased risk of bleeding, disseminated intravascular coagulation)
Reticulocytes	0.5%–1.5% of red cells (↑ acute bleeding), starting treatment for vitamin deficiencies (iron, B_{12}, folate), acute hemolytic episodes
Total WBC count	4,500–11,000/mm³ (↑ bacterial infections)
Neutrophils (or segs)	55%–70% (↑ bacterial infections)
Band forms (immature WBCs)	>5% (↑ severe bacterial infections)
	Also called "shift to the left"
Eosinophils	>3% (↑ allergies, parasitic diseases, cancer)

CBC, complete blood count; MCV, mean corpuscular volume; RDW, red cell distribution width; WBC, white blood cell.

Table 2.2 List of Blood Chemistries

Laboratory Test	Reference Ranges
TSH	>5.0 mU/L (hypothyroidism)
	<0.4 mU/L (hyperthyroidism)
PSA	<4.0 ng/mL (benign prostatic hyperplasia [BPH], prostate cancer)
Ferritin	<15 mcg/L (iron-deficiency anemia)
ESR; sed rate	Men 0–22 mm/hr Women 0–29 mm/hr Elevated (giant cell arteritis, rheumatoid arthritis [RA], lupus, inflammation)
CRP	Elevated (inflammation, autoimmune diseases, a risk factor for heart disease)
CTnT	Elevated in myocardial infarction (MI), heart damage, heart failure
	Sensitive test for myocardial cell damage (MI, unstable angina)
BNP	Elevated (elevated in heart failure)
Potassium	<3.5 or >5.5 mEq/L (critical values <2.5 or >8 mEq/L)

BNP, B-type natriuretic peptide; CRP, c-reactive protein; cTnT, cardiac troponins; ESR, erythrocyte sedimentation rate; PSA, prostate-specific antigen; TSH, thyroid-stimulating hormone.

NOTES

- You must go through three steps to answer this question correctly:

  First step: A hemoglobin of <13.5 g/dL in males (but not in females) is indicative of anemia. An MCV of 72 fL is indicative of microcytic anemia (norm 80–100 fL).

  Second step: The MCV will direct you in the differential diagnosis (microcytic, normocytic, or macrocytic).

  Third step: The differential diagnosis for microcytic anemia is iron deficiency and alpha or beta thalassemia trait or minor for the exams.
- In iron-deficiency anemia, the following results are found: Serum ferritin and serum iron levels decreased; TIBC and RDW elevated.
- In alpha or beta thalassemia trait or minor, the following results are found: Serum ferritin and serum iron levels normal; TIBC normal.
- The gold-standard test to diagnose any anemia involving abnormal hemoglobin (e.g., thalassemia, sickle cell) is the hemoglobin electrophoresis.
- The RDW is a measure of the variability in size of red blood cells (RBCs; or anisocytosis). An elevated RDW is one of the earliest indicators of iron-deficiency anemia.
- In clinical practice, rule out iron-deficiency anemia first (most common anemia in the world for all ages/races/sexes) before ordering a hemoglobin electrophoresis.

PHARMACOLOGIC CONCEPTS

I. Discussion

The current version of the exams includes more topics about pharmacology than have been included in the past. To solve a question, you need to understand key terms, their definitions, and how they are applied. There are no math problems where you must figure out the correct dose of a drug. See Chapter 3 for further discussion.

II. Examples

■ Deprescribing: The process of adjusting the dose of a medication down to the minimum effective dosage or stopping it when it is no longer needed (or if the patient's health status has changed). Deprescribing helps to decrease polypharmacy. For example, there are evidence-based deprescribing guidelines for benzodiazepines, which can be found online.

■ Pharmacogenomics/pharmacogenetics: Your genes affect how you respond (or do not respond) to a drug. It is now known that certain genes affect how the body metabolizes certain drugs. It allows us to truly "individualize" medicine.

■ Pharmacokinetics: The process by which a medication is absorbed, distributed, metabolized, and eliminated by the body.

■ Half-life: Amount of time it takes for a drug concentration to reduce to half of its original dose.

■ First-pass metabolism (first-pass effect): When an oral drug reaches the stomach, it goes to the small intestines, then to the portal circulation where it is metabolized by the liver. After the liver has metabolized the drug, it is released to the systemic circulation where it can reach the target organ(s).

WOMEN'S HEALTH

I. Discussion

Expect to see several questions addressing gynecologic conditions. The topics that are covered include recognizing and treating sexually transmitted infections (STIs), oral contraceptive issues, abnormal Pap smears, menopausal conditions, threatened abortion or early pregnancy, and many more. For example, there will be questions about vaginal disorders, such as bacterial vaginosis (BV), candida vaginitis, trichomoniasis, and atrophic vaginitis. In pregnant patients, use only medications that are U.S. Food and Drug Administration (FDA) Category A or B or those that have no adverse effect on pregnancy and lactation.

Be aware that a clinical finding can be described in detail instead of using its common name. For example, the term *clue cell* is not used in the question that follows. Instead, it is described in detail ("mature squamous epithelial cells with numerous bacteria on the cell surface and borders").

II. Example

An 18-year-old female student presents in the college health clinic complaining of a strong odor in her vagina. She reports that she had an abortion about 3 weeks ago and recently completed her prescription of antibiotics. The nurse practitioner (NP) performs a vaginal speculum exam and notes a large amount of gray to off-white discharge coating the patient's vaginal walls. It has a milk-like consistency. During microscopy, the slide reveals mature squamous epithelial cells with numerous bacteria on the cell surface and borders. The vaginal pH is 6.0. Which of the following conditions is most likely?

A. Trichomoniasis
B. Bacterial vaginosis (BV)
C. Candida vulvovaginitis
D. Hormonal changes

III. Correct Answer: Option B

B. Bacterial vaginosis (BV)

IV. Question Dissection

Best Clues

■ The vaginal pH is alkaline (pH of 6.0).
■ Rule out *Candida vulvovaginitis* because it is classified as a yeast organism (not a bacteria).
■ Rule out *Trichomoniasis* because it is a protozoan or unicellular flagellated organism.
■ The odor and discharge are not due to hormonal changes in an 18-year-old.

NOTES

■ BV has an alkaline pH (vagina normally has an acidic pH of 3.5–4.5). BV is the only vaginal condition with an alkaline pH for the exam.

■ BV is not considered an STI (it is caused by an imbalance of vaginal bacteria). The sex partner does not need to be treated. It is a vaginosis (not a vaginitis).

■ BV does not cause inflammation (the vulvovagina will not be red or irritated). The microscopy slide will have very few WBCs and a large number of clue cells.

■ The vaginal discharge in *Candida* infection is a white color with a thick and curdlike consistency. It frequently causes redness and itching in the vulvovagina because of inflammation.

■ The microscopy in candidiasis will show a large number of WBCs, pseudohyphae, and spores ("spaghetti and meatballs").

■ Candida yeast is a normal flora of the GI tract and in some women's vaginas.

■ *Trichomonas* infection (or trichomoniasis) vaginal discharge is copious, bubbly, and green in color. It causes a lot of inflammation, resulting in itching and redness of the vulvovagina. It is considered to be an STI. The sex partner also needs treatment.

■ PCR testing is now available for trichomonas and vaginal candida infections. For trichomonas, a urine specimen (males or females) is used. For vaginal candida, a vaginal swab is used.

MEDICATIONS

I. Discussion

When studying pharmacology for the exam, it is generally not important to memorize the specific drug doses. What is more important is to study a drug's "safety" issues, such as contraindications, major drug/food interactions, and well-known side effects.

You will need to be familiar with the drug's indications and the duration of treatment. Become familiar with a "first-line drug" and the alternative drug (if applicable). For example, the first-line (or preferred) drug for treating "strep" throat is still penicillin V PO × 10 days. If the patient has a penicillin allergy, macrolides and clindamycin can be used instead.

The majority of the medicines seen on the exam are the well-known drugs that have been in use for a few years to many decades (e.g., doxycycline, penicillin, amoxicillin). Memorize drug class and some representative drugs from that class. For example, in the quinolone drug class are drugs such as ofloxacin (Floxin), moxifloxacin (Avelox), and levofloxacin (Levaquin). A drug's brand name may not be used on the exam; instead, only the drug's generic name or drug class may be used. In addition, you need to become familiar with some of the FDA Category X drugs (see Chapter 3).

II. Examples

Example A

Using the drug class as the answer option:
A previously healthy 30-year-old complains of an acute onset of fever and chills accompanied by a productive cough with purulent sputum and a loss of appetite. The patient has received an antibiotic in the previous 3 months. The nurse practitioner (NP) diagnoses community-acquired pneumonia (CAP). The Infectious Diseases Society of America (IDSA) and the American Thoracic Society (ATS) treatment guidelines recommend which of the following as the preferred first-line treatment for this patient?

A. Beta lactam
B. Antitussives
C. Cephalosporins
D. Fluoroquinolones with gram-positive bacteria activity

Example B

Which of the following antibiotics is the preferred treatment for healthy adults diagnosed with uncomplicated community-acquired pneumonia (CAP)?

A. Amoxicillin 1 g PO three times a day (TID) × 5 to 7 days
B. Dextromethorphan with guaifenesin (Robitussin DM) 1 to 2 teaspoons PO four times a day (QID) as needed
C. Cephalexin (Keflex) 500 mg PO QID × 10 days
D. Levofloxacin (Levaquin) 500 mg PO daily × 7 days

Example C

The following is an example of a question about a common side effect:
Which of the following are possible side effects that may be seen in a patient who is being treated with hydrochlorothiazide for hypertension?

A. Dry cough and angioedema
B. Swollen ankles and headache
C. Hyperuricemia and hyperglycemia
D. Fatigue and depression

III. Correct Answers

Example A: Option A
A. Beta lactam

Example B: Option A
A. Amoxicillin 1 g PO three times a day (TID) × 5 to 7 days

Example C: Option C
C. Hyperuricemia and hyperglycemia

IV. Question Dissection

Best Clues

- Lack of comorbidity ("healthy adults") is an important clue in Examples A and B.
- Your knowledge of the latest IDSA and the ATS treatment guidelines helps to correctly answer Examples A and B (covered in Chapter 8).
- For Example C, you must memorize the adverse side effects of thiazide diuretics.

NOTES
- According to the IDSA and the ATS treatment guidelines, outpatient treatment of CAP in healthy patients (no comorbidities) involves amoxicillin or doxycycline.
- The side effects in Example C, option A are caused by angiotensin-converting enzyme (ACE) inhibitors. Look for a sudden or new onset of a dry cough in a patient with hypertension (without signs of the common cold). Angioedema is a rare adverse effect and can be life-threatening.
- The side effects in Example C, option B are caused by calcium channel blockers (CCBs). Look for a hypertensive patient with swollen ankles (not associated with heart failure) and headache.
- The side effects in Example C, option C are caused by thiazide diuretics (hyperuricemia and hyperglycemia).
- The side effects in Example C, option D are caused by beta-blockers. Look for a patient with a history of MI, heart failure, and/or hypertension who complains of increased fatigue and depression (avoid if possible in depressed patients, pulse <50 beats/min, second- or third-degree heart block).

U.S. CENTERS FOR DISEASE CONTROL AND PREVENTION STATISTICS

I. Discussion

It is important that you memorize the following U.S. Centers for Disease Control and Prevention (CDC) statistics. The questions will be short and to the point. Determine whether a question is asking about the most common cause of death (mortality) or whether it is asking about the most common cause of a certain disease in a population (prevalence). For example, the most common cause of cancer death overall is lung cancer (mortality), but the most common cancer overall (prevalence) is skin cancer. The most common type of skin cancer is basal cell skin cancer.

Sometimes, a question will ask about a gender-specific cause. For example, the most common cancer in females is breast cancer, and the most common cancer in males is prostate cancer (prevalence). But the cancer causing the most deaths overall for both males and females is still lung cancer (mortality).

Mortality Statistics
- Disease causing the most deaths overall: Heart disease
- Cancer with the highest mortality: Lung cancer
- Cancer with the highest mortality in males and females: Lung cancer
- Most common cause of death in adolescents: Motor vehicle crashes

Prevalence
- Most common cancer in females: Breast cancer
- Most common cancer in males: Prostate cancer
- Most common type of cancer overall (males/females): Skin cancer
- Most common type of skin cancer (males/females): Basal cell cancer
- Skin cancer with the highest mortality: Melanoma
- Gynecologic cancer (vulva, vagina, cervix, uterus, ovary): Uterine/endometrial cancer (most common gynecologic cancer); ovarian cancer (second most common gynecologic cancer)

II. Example
What is the most common type of gynecologic cancer?
A. Uterine
B. Cervical
C. Breast
D. Ovarian

III. Correct Answer: Option A
A. Uterine

IV. Question Dissection
Best Clues
- This question is based on your recall of facts that you memorized (rote memory).
- Rule out breast cancer because it is not considered a gynecologic cancer.

NOTES
- There may be a question about the gynecologic cancers. These types of cancers are located in the pelvis (labia, vagina, uterus, fallopian tubes, ovaries).
- Breast cancer is not classified as a gynecologic cancer.

BENIGN PHYSIOLOGIC VARIANTS
I. Discussion
A benign variant is a physiologic abnormality that does not interfere with bodily processes or functions. There are very few questions on benign variants. Some examples of the benign variants that have been seen on the exams include the geographic tongue, torus palatinus, and a split or fish-tail uvula (see Chapter 5). Benign variants are listed under the appropriate organ system.

II. Example
A 45-year-old female patient complains of a sore throat. Upon examination, the nurse practitioner (NP) notices a bony growth midline at the hard palate of the mouth. The patient denies any changes or pain. It is not red, tender, or swollen. She reports a history of the same growth for many years without any change. Which of the following conditions is most likely?
A. Torus palatinus
B. Geographic tongue
C. Acute glossitis
D. Leukoplakia

III. Correct Answer: Option A
A. Torus palatinus

IV. Question Dissection
Best Clues
- The description of a chronic bony growth located midline in the hard palate indicates torus palatinus.
- Rule out glossitis, geographic tongue, and hairy leukoplakia because they are all located on the tongue and not on the hard palate (roof of the mouth).

NOTES
- A torus palatinus is a benign growth of bone (an exostosis) located midline on the hard palate and covered with normal oral skin. It is painless and does not interfere with function.
- A "geographic tongue" has multiple fissures and irregular smoother areas on its surface that make it look like a topographic map. The patient may complain of soreness on the tongue after eating or drinking acidic or hot foods.
- Leukoplakia is not a benign variant. It appears as a slow-growing white plaque that has a firm to hard surface that is slightly raised on the tongue or inside the mouth. It is considered a precancerous lesion. It is due to chronic irritation of the skin or precancerous changes on the tongue and inside the cheeks. Its causes include poorly fitting dentures, chewing tobacco (snuff), and using other types of tobacco. Refer the patient for a biopsy because it can sometimes become malignant.
- Oral hairy leukoplakia (OHL) of the tongue is a painless white patch (or patches) that appears corrugated. It is usually located on the lateral aspects of the tongue (or other areas inside the mouth) and is associated with HIV and AIDS infection. It is caused by Epstein–Barr virus (EBV) infection of the tongue. It is not considered a premalignant lesion.

U.S. PREVENTIVE SERVICES TASK FORCE SCREENING GUIDELINES

I. Discussion

U.S. Preventive Services Task Force (USPSTF) screening guidelines are graded as A, B, C, D, or I (insufficient evidence or evidence is lacking or of poor quality). The highest rating is a Grade A (routine screening is advised—high certainty that the net benefit is substantial). A rating of Grade D means that the harm outweighs the benefits (or there is no benefit) to the service and the use of the service is discouraged.

Both the ANCC and the AANPCB exams use the USPSTF screening recommendations of 2018. Regarding breast cancer screening, the USPSTF (2016) currently recommends that a screening baseline mammogram (with or without clinical breast exam) start at age 50 years and then every 2 years until the age of 74 years. For women aged 40 to 49 years, mammograms should be based on individual factors (such as risk factors, preferences, risk vs. benefits of mammograms). Note that an update to the USPSTF guidelines is in progress as of October 2023. The draft recommends biennial mammogram screening for all women ages 40 to 75 years.

II. Example

What is the U.S. Preventive Services Task Force (USPSTF) screening recommendation for ovarian cancer?

A. Annual bimanual pelvic exam with pelvic ultrasound
B. Pelvic and intravaginal ultrasound
C. Intravaginal ultrasound with CA-125 tumor marker
D. The USPSTF does not recommend routine screening of women for ovarian cancer (Grade D)

III. Correct Answer: Option D

D. The USPSTF does not recommend routine screening of women for ovarian cancer (Grade D)

IV. Question Dissection

Best Clues

- Do not "overread" the question. Assume that the question is asking about routine screening of the general population.
- Transvaginal ultrasound and CA-125 are not used for routine screening.
- Although the bimanual pelvic exam is "low tech," it is being used as a distractor.

> NOTES
> - The USPSTF (2018) is against routine screening for ovarian cancer in asymptomatic women who are not known to have a high risk of hereditary cancer syndrome.
> - If there is a case scenario of an older woman who complains of vague abdominal/pelvic symptoms (stomach bloating, low-back ache, constipation) and is found to have a palpable ovary during the bimanual exam, rule out ovarian cancer.
> - Always rule out ovarian cancer in a postmenopausal woman who has a palpable ovary.

> - The next step is to order a pelvic and intravaginal ultrasound with CA-125. Refer to an oncologist.
> - The strongest risk factor for ovarian cancer (or breast cancer) is genetic predisposition, such as *BRCA1* or *BRCA2* mutations and positive family history. Absolute risk of developing ovarian cancer is 35% to 45% in women with *BRCA1* mutation. Other risk factors are age, obesity, clomiphene (Clomid) use, and early-age menarche or late-onset menopause.

FOLLOWING UP ON A PRESCRIPTION MEDICINE

I. Discussion

In these cases, a patient who is taking prescription medicine is running out of their supply or does not have refills left. The test-taker must decide what type of initial follow-up is needed. Depending on the case scenario, for a patient who is fully symptomatic due to the abrupt cessation of medicine (either due to running out of refills or due to discontinuation of health insurance), a reasonable initial action is to continue the prescription medicine.

II. Example

A 65-year-old female smoker presents with a history of Barrett's esophagus and gastroesophageal reflux disease (GERD). The patient reports that her gastroenterologist's prescription for pantoprazole (Protonix) 40 mg daily ran out a few days ago. She is complaining of severe heartburn and a sore throat. During the physical exam, the nurse practitioner (NP) notes an erythematous posterior pharynx without tonsillar discharge and mild dental enamel loss on the rear molars. What is the best initial action for the NP to follow?

A. Refer the patient to an oncologist for a biopsy to rule out esophageal cancer.
B. Give the patient a refill of her proton-pump inhibitor (PPI) prescription and advise her to schedule an appointment with her gastroenterologist.
C. Recommend that the patient take over-the-counter (OTC) famotidine (Pepcid) twice a day until she can be seen by her gastroenterologist.
D. Switch the patient's prescription to another brand of PPI because her symptoms are not improving.

III. Correct Answer: Option B

B. Give the patient a refill of her proton-pump inhibitor (PPI) prescription and advise her to schedule an appointment with her gastroenterologist.

IV. Question Dissection

Best Clues

- Rule out option A because the patient is already under the care of a gastroenterologist.
- OTC famotidine (Pepcid) is not potent enough to control the symptoms of erosive esophagitis. A PPI is the preferred treatment for erosive esophagitis.
- Do not switch the patient to another brand of PPI. Her worsening symptoms are due to rebound caused by abrupt cessation of PPI.

- The best initial action in this case is to refill the PPI prescription because the patient is fully symptomatic (erosive esophagitis) until she can see her gastroenterologist.

> **NOTES**
> - The patient's severe symptoms are caused by the sudden discontinuation of the high-dose PPI (rebound type of reaction).
> - Barrett's esophagus is the "precancerous" lesion of esophageal cancer. It is best managed by a gastroenterologist (not an oncologist).
> - Patients diagnosed with Barrett's esophagus typically have endoscopic examinations with biopsy by a gastroenterologist annually (or every 6 months for high-grade lesions).
> - Patients with Barrett's esophagus are treated with high-dose PPIs for a "lifetime."
> - The first-line treatment of mild, uncomplicated GERD is lifestyle changes (e.g., avoid eating 3–4 hours before bedtime, dietary changes, weight loss if needed).
> - If a patient is at high risk for esophageal cancer (aged 50 years or older, smoker, chronic GERD for decades), consider referral to a gastroenterologist for an upper endoscopy.

TANNER STAGES

I. Discussion

Expect to see at least one or two questions regarding Tanner stages in girls and boys. Because Tanner stage I is prepuberty and Tanner stage V is the adult pattern for both boys and girls, the only stages to memorize for the exams are Tanner stage II to Tanner stage IV.

For girls, memorize the pattern of breast development, and for boys, the genital development (testes and penis).

Girls

- Stage I: Prepubertal pattern
- Stage II: Breast bud and areola start to develop.
- Stage III: Breast continues to grow with nipples/areola (one mound/no separation).
- Stage IV: Nipples and areola become elevated from the breast (a secondary mound).
- Stage V: Adult pattern

Boys

- Stage I: Prepubertal pattern
- Stage II: Testes and scrotum start to enlarge (scrotal skin starts to get darker/more rugae).
- Stage III: Penis grows longer (length) and testes/scrotum continues to become larger.
- Stage IV: Penis become wider and continues growing in length (testes are larger with darker scrotal skin and more rugae).
- Stage V: Adult pattern

II. Example

A 14-year-old boy is brought in by his parent for a physical exam. Both are concerned about his breast enlargement. The patient denies breast tenderness. On physical exam, the nurse practitioner (NP) palpates soft breast tissue that is not tender. No dominant mass is noted. The skin is smooth, and there is no nipple discharge with massage. The patient has a body mass index (BMI) of 29. Which of the following statements is correct?

A. Advise the parent that the patient has physiologic gynecomastia and should return for a follow-up exam.
B. Order an ultrasound of both breasts to further assess the patient's breast tissue development.
C. Reassure the parent that the patient's breast development is within normal limits.
D. Educate the parent that the patient has pseudogynecomastia.

III. Correct Answer: Option D

D. Educate the parent that the patient has pseudogynecomastia.

IV. Question Dissection

Best Clues

- The boy has a BMI of 29.
- The clinical breast exam does not show palpable breast tissue. Instead, the breast palpation reveals soft fatty tissue.
- Because the breast development is not part of the Tanner stages for boys, reassurance is not appropriate in this case.

> **NOTES**
> - Physiologic gynecomastia physical exam findings will show disklike breast tissue that is mobile under each nipple/areola; the breast may be tender, and the breast can be asymmetrical (one breast larger than the other).
> - A BMI of 25 to 29.9 is considered overweight. Obesity is a BMI of 30 or higher.
> - Males with a BMI of 25 or higher are at highest risk for pseudogynecomastia.

QUESTIONS ABOUT FOOD

I. Discussion

There are basically three kinds of food-related questions on the exam. You may be asked to pick the foods that have high levels of certain minerals, such as potassium, calcium, or magnesium. Other questions will address food interactions (tetracycline and dairy), drug interactions (monoamine oxidase inhibitor [MAOI] and high-tyramine-containing foods such as fermented foods), or foods that should be avoided for a particular disease (e.g., wheat products in the case of celiac disease).

Certain foods are recommended for certain diseases (e.g., salmon/omega-3 for heart disease) because of their favorable effect. In contrast, certain foods are contraindicated for some conditions because of their adverse or dangerous effects.

II. Example

Which of the following foods are known to have high potassium content?
A. Low-fat yogurt, soft cheeses, and collard greens
B. Aged cheese, red wine, and chocolate
C. Potatoes, apricots, and brussels sprouts
D. Black beans, red meat, and citrus juice

III. Correct Answer: Option C
C. Potatoes, apricots, and brussels sprouts

IV. Question Dissection

Best Clues

- First, look at the answer options for inconsistencies in the list of foods.
- Rule out option A because it is inconsistent, and these foods do not contain high levels of potassium: low-fat yogurt and soft cheeses (calcium) with collard greens (vitamin K).
- Rule out option B because these foods have a high tyramine, not potassium, content.
- Rule out option D because it is inconsistent. Although citrus juices are high in potassium, both black beans and red meat are not (iron).
- If options A, B, and D are incorrect, then the only one left is option C (potatoes, apricots, and brussels sprouts). A large number of fruits and vegetables are rich in potassium and vitamins.

NOTES

- Foods with a high tyramine content can cause dangerous food–drug interactions with MAOI inhibitors (e.g., isocarboxazid [Marplan], phenelzine [Nardil], and tranylcypromine [Parnate]).
- Foods and supplements containing stimulants, such as caffeine, are best avoided by patients with hypertension, arrhythmias, high risk for MI, hyperthyroid disease, albuterol use, amphetamine use, and so on.
- If one of the food choices in an answer option is incorrect, rule out this option because all of the foods on the list have to be correlated.

Examples of Food Groups

1. Gluten (avoid with celiac disease/celiac sprue): Wheat (including spelt and kamut), rye, barley (breads, cereals, pasta, cookies, cakes). Gluten-free (safe) carbohydrates include corn, rice, potatoes, quinoa, tapioca, soybeans.
2. Plant sterols and stanols (reduce cholesterol, triglycerides): Sterol-fortified spreads (e.g., Benecol spread), sterol-fortified foods, wheat germ, sesame oil
3. Monounsaturated fats/fatty acids (decrease risk of heart disease): Olive oil, canola oil, some nuts (almonds,

walnuts), sunflower oil/seeds; Mediterranean diet, which is high in monounsaturated fats
4. Saturated fats or trans fats (increase risk of heart disease): Lard, beef fat (fatty steak), deep-fried fast foods
5. Omega-3 or fish oils (decrease risk of heart disease): Fatty cold-water marine fish (salmon), fish oils, flaxseed oil, and krill oil
6. Magnesium (decreases BP, dilates blood vessels): Some nuts (almonds, peanuts, cashews), some beans, whole wheat; also found in laxatives, antacids, milk of magnesia
7. Potassium (helps decrease BP): Most fruits (especially apricots, bananas, oranges, prune juice), some vegetables
8. Folate (decreases homocysteine levels and fetal neural tube defects): Breakfast cereals fortified with folate, green leafy vegetables (e.g., spinach), liver
9. Iron (treats iron-deficiency anemia): Beef, liver, black beans, black-eyed peas
10. Vitamin K (should control intake if on anticoagulants or have a clotting disorder): Green leafy vegetables (kale, collard greens, spinach), broccoli, cabbage
11. High sodium content (increases water retention, can increase BP): Cold cuts, pickles, preserved foods, canned foods, hot dogs, chips
12. Calcium (helps with osteopenia and osteoporosis, helps decrease BP): Low-fat dairy, low-fat milk, low-fat yogurt, cheeses

Common Disorders Associated With Certain Foods

1. Celiac disease: Lifetime avoidance of gluten-containing cereals such as wheat, rye, and barley is necessary. Gluten-free foods include rice, corn, potatoes, peanuts, soybeans, meat, dairy, all fruits/vegetables; most people with celiac disease can eat oats.
2. Hypertension: Maintain an adequate intake of calcium, magnesium, and potassium. Good sources of calcium include low-fat dairy, low-fat yogurt, cheeses. Sources of magnesium include wheat bread, nuts (almonds, peanuts, cashews), some beans. Sources of potassium include most fruits (apricots, bananas, oranges, cantaloupes, raisins) and green vegetables. Avoid high-sodium foods such as cold cuts, pickles, preserved foods, and canned foods.
3. Migraine headaches and MAOIs (Marplan, Nardil, and Parnate): Avoid high-tyramine foods such as aged cheeses/meats, red wine, fava beans, draft beer, fermented foods.
4. Anticoagulation therapy (i.e., warfarin sodium or Coumadin): Avoid eating large amounts of leafy green vegetables (kale/collard greens, spinach, cabbage, broccoli) and cooking with canola oil (high in vitamin K); use other oils instead. High levels of vitamin K decrease the effects of warfarin sodium.

CASE MANAGEMENT

I. Discussion

NPs lead primary care teams in the management and coordination of patients with chronic conditions. In this role, they work closely with medical case managers. Medical case managers are experienced RNs who work for hospitals, healthcare plans, and health insurance companies. Their job is essentially to coordinate the outpatient healthcare of patients with high-cost chronic conditions. The goal of case management is to decrease disease exacerbations and decrease the risk of hospitalization.

Asthma

A good outcome for children with asthma is their ability to attend school full time and to play normally every day. A poor case management outcome is if the child misses school and/or is unable to play because of poor control of asthma symptoms.

NOTES

- With asthma, a good case outcome is for the child (or adult) to return to normal function. For children, it means the child is attending school and can play daily. If the child is not able to attend school full time (frequent absences), this is a poor case management outcome.
- The risk factors for asthma fatality include a history of ED visits, frequent use of short-acting beta-agonist use (i.e., albuterol), nocturnal awakenings, increased dyspnea and wheezing, respiratory viral infection, and so on.
- Diseases that are selected for case management are usually chronic conditions, such as asthma, congestive heart failure (CHF), HIV infection, and chronic psychiatric conditions. A good outcome will show good symptom control and no exacerbations or hospitalizations.

ALL QUESTIONS HAVE ENOUGH INFORMATION

I. Discussion

Assume that all the questions on the exams contain enough information to answer them correctly. Do not read too much into a question or assume that it is missing some vital information. As far as the ANCC and AANPCB exams are concerned, all questions contain enough information to allow you to solve them correctly. There are no "trick" questions on the exam. If you think that a question is lacking some information or is incomplete, then you are "overreading" the question. Consider a patient is in good health unless a disease or other health condition is mentioned in the test question.

EMERGENT CASES

I. Discussion

The ability to recognize and initially manage emergent conditions that may present in the primary care arena is a skill that is expected of all NPs. It is important to memorize not only the presenting signs and symptoms of a given condition but also its initial management in primary care.

Learn how these conditions present so that you can recognize them in the exam. The following is a list of emergent conditions that will be on the exam. (They are discussed in detail in the "Danger Signals" sections of Chapters 5 through 23.)

Danger Signals

Cardiovascular System

- Acute MI, unstable angina
- Heart failure
- Bacterial endocarditis
- Abdominal aortic aneurysm (AAA)

Skin and Integumentary System

- Angioedema/anaphylaxis
- Stevens–Johnson syndrome
- Meningococcemia
- Rocky Mountain spotted fever (RMSF)
- Lyme disease
- Herpes zoster ophthalmicus
- Melanoma
- Basal cell carcinoma

Gastrointestinal System

- Acute abdomen (surgical abdomen)
- Acute appendicitis
- Acute pancreatitis
- Acute diverticulitis
- Acute cholecystitis
- *Clostridium difficile* infection
- Colon cancer

Men's Health

- Testicular torsion
- Priapism
- Prostate cancer

Psychosocial Mental Health

- Depression with suicidal plan
- Acute serotonin syndrome
- Malignant neuroleptic syndrome
- Homicidal plan

Nervous System

- Cerebrovascular accident (CVA)
- Temporal arteritis headache
- Subarachnoid bleeding
- Acute bacterial meningitis
- Subdural hematoma

Head, Eyes, Ears, Nose, and Throat

- Retinal detachment
- Orbital cellulitis
- Optic neuritis
- Peritonsillar abscess
- Battle sign
- Herpes keratitis
- Temporal arteritis
- Acute angle-closure glaucoma

Pulmonary System
- Anaphylaxis
- Severe asthmatic exacerbation (impending respiratory failure)
- Pulmonary emboli
- CAP
- Lung cancer

Renal System
- Acute pyelonephritis
- Acute renal failure
- Bladder cancer

Women's Health
- Dominant breast mass attached to surrounding tissue
- Ruptured tubal ectopic pregnancy
- Paget's disease of the breast
- Ovarian cancer

II. Example
An asthmatic male patient complains of a sudden onset of itching and coughing after taking two aspirin tablets for a headache in the waiting room. The patient's lips and eyelids are becoming swollen. The patient complains of feeling hot. Bright-red wheals are noted on his chest and arms and legs. Which of the following is the best initial intervention to follow?

A. Call 911.

B. Check the patient's blood pressure (BP), pulse, and temperature.

C. Give an injection of aqueous epinephrine 1:1,000 dilution (1 mg/mL) 0.5 mg IM into the vastus lateralis muscle immediately.

D. Initiate a prescription of a potent topical steroid and a Medrol Dose Pack.

III. Correct Answer: Option C
C. Give an injection of aqueous epinephrine 1:1,000 dilution (1 mg/mL) 0.5 mg IM into the vastus lateralis muscle immediately.

IV. Question Dissection
Best Clues
- The quick onset of symptoms, such as angioedema, after taking aspirin is a clue.
- The classic signs and symptoms of anaphylaxis described in this case should be noted.
- Severe anaphylactic episodes occur almost immediately or within 1 hour after exposure.

NOTES
- For treatment of anaphylaxis (in primary care), if only one clinician is present, give an injection of epinephrine 1:1,000 dilution 0.3 to 0.5 mg intramuscularly stat, and then call 911. May repeat dose within 5 minutes in case of poor response.

- ED treatment medications—administer epinephrine IM, 100% oxygen by face mask, an antihistamine (H_1 antagonist) such as diphenhydramine (Benadryl), a bronchodilator such as albuterol (short-acting beta-2 agonist), and systemic glucocorticosteroids such as prednisone.
- Patients with an atopic history (asthma, eczema, allergic rhinitis) with nasal polyps are at higher risk for aspirin and nonsteroidal anti-inflammatory drug (NSAID) allergies.
- Anaphylaxis is classified as a type I IgE-dependent reaction.
- Biphasic anaphylaxis occurs in up to 23% of cases (symptoms recur within 8–10 hours after initial episode). This is the reason why these patients are prescribed a Medrol Dose Pack and a long-acting antihistamine after being discharged from the ED.
- The most common triggers for anaphylaxis in children are foods. Medications and insect stings are the most common triggers in adults.

PRIORITIZING OTHER EMERGENT CASES
I. Discussion
During life-threatening situations, managing the airway, breathing, and circulation (the ABCs) is always the top priority. If the question does not describe conditions requiring the ABCs, then the next level of priority is the acute or sudden change in the mental status and the level of consciousness (LOC). One of the most important clues in such problems is the acute timing of onset of symptoms or the sudden change of the LOC from the patient's "baseline."

II. Example
A 16-year-old boy presents to a community clinic accompanied by his grandparent, who reports that he fell off his bike this morning. The patient now complains of a headache with mild nausea. The patient's grandparent reports that he was not wearing a helmet. The health history is uneventful. Which of the following statements is indicative of an emergent condition?

A. The patient complains of multiple painful abrasions that are bleeding on his arms and legs.

B. The patient complains of a headache that is relieved by acetaminophen (Tylenol).

C. The patient makes eye contact occasionally and answers with brief statements.

D. The patient is having difficulty with following normal conversation and answering questions.

III. Correct Answer: Option D
D. The patient is having difficulty with following normal conversation and answering questions.

IV. Question Dissection
Best Clues
- History of recent trauma that is followed by a headache with nausea.
- The patient did not wear a bicycle helmet.

NOTES
- Any recent changes in LOC, even one as subtle as difficulty with normal conversation, should cause you to pay particular attention.
- Notice the words "normal conversation." Do not overread the question and ask yourself what they mean by "normal conversation." Take it at face value.
- Changes in LOC on the test are usually subtle changes. Signs to watch for include difficulty answering questions, slurred speech, apparent confusion, inability to understand instructions/conversation, being sleepy/lethargic, and so forth.
- Even though the patient is bleeding, note that he has "abrasions," which are superficial.
- The behavior described in option C is considered "normal" for an adolescent male (or female).

GERIATRICS
I. Discussion
The ANCC does not give any information about the number of questions by age group, but the AANPCB does. Elderly patients are divided into two age categories on the AANPCB exam. Those between the ages of 65 and 84 years are the "young gerontologicals." Those age 85 years and older are the "frail elderly."

The AANPCB's Family Nurse Practitioner (FNP) exam has a total of 40 questions (30%) on gerontological topics.

II. Example
Which of the following drug classes is considered as first-line treatment for unipolar depression in the elderly?
A. Selective serotonin reuptake inhibitors (SSRIs)
B. Serotonin and norepinephrine reuptake inhibitors (SNRIs)
C. Tricyclic antidepressants (TCAs)
D. Monoamine oxidase inhibitors (MAOIs)

III. Correct Answer: Option A
A. Selective serotonin reuptake inhibitors (SSRIs)

IV. Question Dissection
Best Clues
- There are no obvious clues in this question. Answering it correctly is based on your recognizing that unipolar depression is the same disease entity as major/minor depression. Depression in bipolar patients is called *bipolar depression*.
- SSRIs are the first-line treatment for unipolar/major depression. They carry an FDA warning that they increase suicidality in children and young adults up to age 23 years.

- TCAs have many anticholinergic effects (e.g., dry mouth, sedation, arrhythmias, confusion, urinary retention).
- MAOIs have major food and drug interactions and are not first-line drugs.

CHOOSING THE BEST INITIAL INTERVENTION
I. Discussion
Numerous questions on the exam will ask test-takers about the best initial intervention to perform in a given case scenario. The question may ask you to pick out the best initial evaluation, treatment, or statement to say to a patient.

One reason why some test-takers answer these questions incorrectly is because they skip a step in the SOAPE (subjective, objective, assessment, planning, and evaluation) process. The first step of the patient evaluation is to find "subjective" information, such as asking about the patient's symptoms and other historical/demographic information. The next step is to find "objective" information. This means performing a physical examination or other tests. It is best to start out "low tech," such as performing a neurologic exam for peripheral vascular disease (PVD) or another low-tech maneuver.

For example, in a case of PVD, it makes sense to check the pulse and BP first on the lower and upper extremities before ordering an expensive test such as an ultrasound Doppler flow study. The following are examples of actions that can be done using the SOAPE mnemonic as a guide.

S: Look for Subjective Evidence
1. Interview the patient and/or family member about the history of the present illness.
2. Ask about the presentation of the illness (e.g., timing, signs and symptoms).
3. Ask whether the patient is on any medication; inquire about the past medical history, diet, and so forth.
4. Be alert for the historical findings because they provide important clues that help point to the correct diagnosis (or differential diagnosis).

O: Look for Objective Evidence
1. Perform a physical exam (general or targeted to the present complaints; examine associated systems in the differential, e.g., diabetic foot exams).
2. If applicable, perform a physical maneuver (e.g., Tinel's, Kernig's, drawer).
3. Order laboratory/other tests to "rule in" (or "rule out") the differential diagnosis.
4. If the laboratory test result is abnormal, you may be asked about the next step (such as a follow-up lab test that is more sensitive or specific).

A: Diagnosis or Assessment
1. What is the most likely diagnosis based on the history, disease presentation, and physical exam findings?
2. If applicable, figure out whether the lab or other testing results point to a more specific diagnosis (or rule out a diagnosis).
3. Decide whether the condition is emergent or not (if applicable).

P: Treatment Plan

1. Initiate or prescribe medications and symptomatic treatment (if applicable).
2. Educate the patient.
3. Recommend a follow-up visit to assess response to treatment and so on.

E: Evaluate Response to the Treatment/Intervention or Evaluate the Situation

1. Decide where there is poor or no response to treatment (or worsens).
2. Decide whether a situation is emergent.

II. Example

A 13-year-old girl with a history of mild persistent asthma and allergic rhinitis complains of a cough that has been waking her up very early in the morning. She reports that she is wheezing more than usual. She is accompanied by her mother. Her last office visit was 8 months ago. Which of the following is the best initial course of action?

A. Initiate a prescription of a short-acting beta-2 agonist QID PRN and a low-dose steroid inhaler twice a day (BID).
B. Refer the patient to an allergist for a scratch test.
C. Discuss her symptoms and other factors associated with the asthmatic exacerbation.
D. Perform a thorough physical exam and obtain blood work.

III. Correct Answer: Option C

C. Discuss her symptoms and other factors associated with the asthmatic exacerbation.

IV. Question Dissection

Best Clues

- The patient's asthma appears to be getting worse (wheezing more than usual, early-morning cough).
- There is a need to find out about precipitating factors, medication compliance, comorbid conditions, and so on.
- Always obtain a history (subjective) before performing a physical exam and labs.
- The adolescent age group starts at age 13 years (ANCC).

NOTES

The correct order of actions to follow in this case scenario is the following:

- Interview the patient/parent to find out more about the symptoms (subjective).
- Perform a thorough physical exam (objective).
- Administer a nebulizer treatment. Check peak expiratory flow (PEF) before and after treatment to assess for effectiveness.
- Initiate a prescription of a short-acting beta-2 agonist QID PRN and a low-dose steroid inhaler BID.
- Refer the patient to an allergist for a scratch test if you suspect the patient has allergic asthma (evaluation).

- Patients with asthmatic exacerbations whose PEF is <50% of predicted value after being given nebulized albuterol/saline treatments should not be discharged. Consider calling 911.
- The differential diagnosis for an early-morning cough includes postnasal drip, allergic rhinitis, sinusitis, GERD, and so forth.

SIGNS AND SYMPTOMS

I. Discussion

It is very common for a question to ask for the sign(s) and/or symptom(s) of a disease process. After a description of a disease's signs and symptoms, you may be asked about the diagnosis or about the laboratory or follow-up tests for the disease.

PICK OUT THE MOST SPECIFIC SIGN/SYMPTOM

I. Discussion

Always pick out the most specific answer to a question when it is asking about the signs and/or symptoms of a disease. Learn the unique or the most specific signs/symptoms associated with the disease. The following question is a good example of this concept.

II. Example

Which of the following is *most likely* to be found in patients with a long-standing case of iron-deficiency anemia?

A. Pica
B. Fatigue
C. Pallor
D. Irritability

III. Correct Answer: Option A

A. Pica

IV. Question Dissection

Best Clues

- The diagnosis (iron-deficiency anemia)
- Knowledge that pica is also associated with iron-deficiency anemia

---

NOTES

- If you are guessing, use common sense. Fatigue and irritability are found in many conditions.
- Pallor is also seen in many disorders such as shock, illness, and anemia.
- By the process of elimination, you are left with option A, the correct choice.
- Another specific clinical finding in iron-deficiency anemia is spoon-shaped nails (or koilonychia). Do not confuse this finding with pitted nails (psoriasis).

DERMATOLOGY

I. Discussion

Many of the questions from this area may be accompanied by a color image. One of the problems that students have with these questions is their unfamiliarity with the dermatologic terms used to describe skin conditions. A list and descriptions of primary and secondary skin lesions are found in Chapter 6.

- A *maculopapular* skin rash has both color (macular) and texture (small papules or raised skin lesions—the color ranges from red [erythematous] to bright pink)
- Maculopapular rash in a lace-like pattern (Fifth disease)
- Maculopapular rashes with papules, vesicles, and crusts (varicella zoster, herpes simplex)
- Maculopapular rashes that are oval shaped with a herald patch (pityriasis rosea)
- Vesicular rashes on an erythematous base (herpes simplex, genital herpes)

II. Example

A male nursing assistant who works in a nursing home is complaining of multiple pruritic rashes that have been disturbing his sleep at night for the past few weeks. He reports that several of the residents are starting to complain of pruritic rashes. On physical exam, the nurse practitioner (NP) notices multiple small papules, some vesicles, and maculopapular excoriated rashes on the sides and the webs of the fingers, on the waist, and on the penis. Which of the following is the most likely diagnosis?

A. Scarlatina
B. Impetigo
C. Erythema migrans
D. Scabies

III. Correct Answer: Option D

D. Scabies

IV. Question Dissection

Best Clues

- History (pruritic rashes disturb sleep at night, and individual works in a higher risk area [nursing home])
- Classic location of the rashes (finger webs, waist, penis)

NOTES

- Assume that a patient has scabies if excoriated pruritic rashes are located in the finger webs and the penis until proven otherwise. Higher risk groups are healthcare providers or people who work with large populations such as those in schools, nursing homes, group homes, or prisons.
- The usual recommendation is that all family members and close contacts be treated at the same time as the patient (spread by skin-to-skin contact). Used clothes/sheets should be washed in hot water and then dried or ironed with high heat.
- The rash of scarlatina has a sandpaper-like texture and is accompanied by a sore throat, strawberry tongue, and skin desquamation (peeling) of the palms and soles. It is not pruritic.
- The rash of impetigo initially appears as papules that develop into bullae. These rupture easily, becoming superficial, bright-red "weeping" rashes

with honey-colored exudate that becomes crusted as it dries. The rashes are very pruritic and are located on areas that are easily traumatized, such as the face, arms, or legs. Insect bites, acne lesions, and varicella lesions can also become secondarily infected, resulting in impetigo.

- Cutaneous larva migrans (creeping eruption) rashes are shaped like red raised wavy lines (serpiginous or snake-like) that are alone or a few may be grouped. They are red and very pruritic, and they become excoriated from scratching (appear maculopapular).
- The areas of the body that are commonly exposed directly to contaminated soil and sand, such as the soles of the feet, extremities, or buttocks, are the most common locations for larva migrans.
- Systemic treatment with either ivermectin once a day (for 1–2 days) or albendazole (for 3 days) is the preferred therapy for larva migrans.

CHOOSING THE CORRECT DRUG

I. Discussion

Test-takers are expected to know not only a drug's generic and/or brand name, but also its drug class. If you are familiar only with the drug's brand name or generic form, you will still be able to recognize the drug on the test because both names will be listed.

In addition, the drug's action, indication(s), common side effects, drug interactions, and contraindications are important to learn. Drugs may only be listed as a drug class.

II. Example

A 10-year-old female student complains of pain and decreased hearing in her left ear that is getting steadily worse. She has a history of allergic rhinitis and is allergic to dust mites. On physical exam, the left tympanic membrane is bulging and red with displaced landmarks. The tympanogram exam reveals a flat line. The student denies frequent ear infections, and the last antibiotic she took was 8 months ago for a urinary tract infection (UTI). She is allergic to sulfa and tells the nurse practitioner (NP) that she will not take any erythromycin because it makes her very nauseated. Which of the following is the best choice of treatment for this patient?

A. Amoxicillin 500 mg PO three times a day (TID) for 7 days
B. Pseudoephedrine (Sudafed) 20 mg PO as needed every 4 to 6 hours
C. Fluticasone (Flonase) nasal inhaler 1 to 2 sprays each nostril every 12 hours
D. Clarithromycin (Biaxin) 500 mg PO two times a day for 10 days

III. Correct Answer: Option A

A. Amoxicillin 500 mg PO three times a day (TID) for 7 days

IV. Question Dissection
Best Clues
- Red bulging tympanic membrane with cloudy fluid inside and displaced landmarks are a clue.
- Last antibiotic taken was 8 months ago and ear infections were infrequent (lack of risk factors for beta-lactamase-resistant bacteria).

> NOTES
> - This question is more complicated compared with the first example. Although the question is asking about the correct drug treatment, it also lists the signs/symptoms of the disease. In order to answer this question correctly, you must first arrive at the correct diagnosis, which is acute otitis media (AOM).
> - Amoxicillin is the preferred first-line antibiotic for both AOM and acute sinusitis in children (for patients with no risk factors for resistant organisms).
> - The ideal patient is someone who has not been on any antibiotics in the past 3 months and/or does not live in an area with high rates of beta-lactam-resistant bacteria.
> - If the patient is a treatment failure or was on an antibiotic in the previous 3 months, then a second-line antibiotic, such as amoxicillin-clavulanate (Augmentin) BID or cefdinir (Omnicef) BID, should be given.
> - If penicillin allergic, an alternative is azithromycin (Z-Pak) and clarithromycin (Biaxin) BID.
> - Pseudoephedrine (Sudafed) is for symptoms only. Do not use for infants, young children, or patients with hypertension.
> - A nasal steroid spray BID is a good adjunct treatment for this patient because of allergic rhinitis, which causes the eustachian tube to swell and become blocked.

DIAGRAMS
I. Discussion
A diagram that may be seen on the exam is of a chest with the four cardiac auscultatory areas (aortic, pulmonic, tricuspid, and mitral) marked. The diagram is used for questions on either cardiac murmurs or the heart sounds.

II. Example
Which of the following is the best location to auscultate for the S3 heart sound?
A. Aortic area
B. Pulmonic area
C. Tricuspid area
D. Mitral area

III. Correct Answer: Option D
D. Mitral area

IV. Question Dissection
Best Clues
Memorization of the S3 heart sound facts

> NOTES
> - The mitral area, sometimes called the cardiac apex, is the optimal location to hear the S3.
> - This area is located at the left fifth intercostal space, along the midclavicular line.
> - The left lateral recumbent position brings the apex closer to the wall and improves the practitioner's ability to hear the left ventricular S3.

"GOLD-STANDARD" TESTS
I. Discussion
Learn to distinguish between a screening test and a diagnostic test (the "gold standard"). Depending on the disease process, the preferred diagnostic test might be a biopsy (e.g., melanoma), a blood culture (e.g., septicemia), or an MRI scan (e.g., meniscus or labral tear, cartilage damage).

In contrast, screening tests are generally more available and cost-effective. Some examples of screening tests are the CBC (anemia), the BP (hypertension), the Mantoux test (TB), or a UA (UTI). The ideal screening test is one that can detect a disease at an early-enough stage so that it can help to decrease the morbidity and mortality. A good example of a disease with no approved screening test is ovarian cancer. Although the CA-125 and intravaginal ultrasound are widely available, these two tests are not sensitive enough to detect ovarian cancer during the early stages of the disease when it is potentially curable.

II. Example
A middle-aged male patient is having his Mantoux test result checked. A reddened area of 10.5 mm is present. It is smooth and soft and does not appear to be indurated. During the interview, the patient denies fever, cough, and weight loss. Which of the following is a true statement?
A. The Mantoux test result is negative.
B. The Mantoux test result is borderline.
C. The Mantoux test should be repeated in 2 weeks.
D. A chest x-ray and sputum culture are indicated.

III. Correct Answer: Option A
A. The Mantoux test result is negative.

IV. Question Dissection
Best Clues
- Knowledge that skin induration, not the red color, is the best indicator of a positive reaction, as redness can be irritation or local inflammation from the procedure, not indicative of infection.
- Lack of signs or symptoms of TB

> NOTES
> - When some test takers see the 10.5-mm size and the red color, they assume automatically that it is a positive result.

(continued)

NOTES *(continued)*

- The Mantoux test (TB skin test [TST]) result is negative because of the description of the soft and smooth skin (it is not indurated). Erythema alone is not an important criterion. The area must be indurated (firm texture) and of the correct size to be positive for TB.
- For pulmonary TB, a sputum culture is the gold standard. Treatment is started with at least three antitubercular drugs because of high rates of resistance. When the sputum culture and sensitivity results are available, the antitubercular antibiotic treatment can be narrowed down or changed. Another drug can be added.
- TB is a reportable disease. Noncompliant patients who refuse treatment can be quarantined to protect the public.
- A baseline LFT level and follow-up testing are recommended for patients on isoniazid (INH).

SIMILAR NAMES FOR THE SAME CONDITION

I. Discussion

Some diseases and conditions are known by two different names that are used interchangeably in both the clinical area and the literature. Sometimes the alternate name is the one being used in the exam questions. This can fool the test taker who is familiar with the disease but only recognizes it under its other name.

II. Examples

- Degenerative joint disease (DJD), or osteoarthritis
- Atopic dermatitis, or eczema
- Senile arcus, or arcus senilis
- Lupus, or systemic lupus erythematosus (SLE)
- Otitis media with effusion (OME), or middle ear effusion (MEE)
- Group A beta *Streptococcus*, or *S. pyogenes*
- Tinea corporis, or ringworm
- Enterobiasis, or pinworms
- Vitamin B_{12}, or cobalamin or cyanocobalamin
- Vitamin B_1, or thiamine
- Scarlet fever, or scarlatina
- Otitis externa, or swimmer ear
- Condyloma acuminata, or genital warts
- Tic douloureux, or trigeminal neuralgia
- Tinea cruris, or jock itch
- Thalassemia minor, or thalassemia trait (either alpha or beta)
- Giant cell arteritis, or temporal arteritis
- Psoas sign, or iliopsoas muscle sign
- Tinea capitis, or ringworm of the scalp
- Light reflex, or the Hirschberg (corneal reflex) test
- Sentinel nodes, or Virchow nodes
- Mantoux test, or TB skin test

SUICIDE RISK AND DEPRESSION

I. Discussion

All depressed patients should be screened for suicidal and/or homicidal ideation. This is true in the clinical arena as well as on the exam. Avoid picking statements that do not directly address the patient's suicidal and homicidal plans. Risk factors for suicide and depression are discussed in Chapter 15.

Incorrect answers are statements that are judgmental, reassuring to the patient, vague, or disrespectful or do not address the issue of suicide (or homicide) in a direct manner.

II. Example

A nurse practitioner (NP) working in a school health clinic is evaluating a new student who has been referred by a teacher. The student is a 16-year-old boy with a history of attention deficit disorder (ADD). He complains that his parents are always fighting, and he thinks that they are getting divorced. He reports that he is failing two classes. During the interview, he stares at the floor and avoids eye contact. He reports that he is having problems falling asleep at night and has stopped seeing friends, including his girlfriend. Which of the following statements is the best choice to ask this teen?

A. "Do you want me to call your parents after we talk?"
B. "Do you have any plans for killing or hurting yourself or other people?"
C. "Do you have any close male or female friends?"
D. "Do you want to wait to tell me about your plans until you feel better?"

III. Correct Answer: Option B

B. "Do you have any plans for killing or hurting yourself or other people?"

IV. Question Dissection

Best Clues

- Classic behavioral cues (avoidance of eye contact, insomnia, social isolation)
- Parents fighting and getting divorced

NOTES

- Option B is the most specific approach in the evaluation for suicide in this case.
- Although option C ("Do you have any close male or female friends?") is a common question asked of depressed patients, it is incorrect because it does not give specific information about specific plans of suicide or homicide.
- Always avoid picking answer choices in which an intervention is delayed. The statement "Do you want to wait to tell me about your plans until you feel better?" is a good example. This advice is applicable to all areas of the test.
- Teenagers are separating from their parents emotionally and value their privacy highly. When interviewing a teen, do it privately (without parents) and also with the parent(s) present.

OTHER PSYCHIATRIC DISORDERS

I. Discussion

Other psychiatric disorders, such as obsessive-compulsive disorder (OCD), bipolar disorder, minor depression, anxiety, panic disorder, alcohol addiction, attention deficit hyperactivity disorder (ADHD), ADD, and posttraumatic stress disorder (PTSD), may be included in the exams. Not all of these disorders are usually seen together in one exam. The most common psychiatric conditions on the exam are major depression, alcohol abuse, and suicide risk. The question may be as straightforward as querying about the correct drug treatment for the condition, as illustrated in this example.

II. Example

Which of the following drug classes is indicated as first-line treatment of both major depression and obsessive-compulsive disorder (OCD)?

A. Selective serotonin reuptake inhibitors (SSRIs)
B. Tricyclic antidepressants (TCAs)
C. Mood stabilizers
D. Benzodiazepines

III. Correct Answer: Option A

A. Selective serotonin reuptake inhibitors (SSRIs)

IV. Question Dissection

Best Clues

- Rule out benzodiazepines, which are used to treat anxiety or insomnia (process of elimination).
- Mood stabilizers, such as lithium salts, are used to treat bipolar disorder (process of elimination).
- The stem is asking for the "first-line treatment" for depression, which is the SSRIs.

NOTES

- TCAs are not first-line treatment for depression (SSRIs are first-line treatment).
- TCAs are also used as prophylactic treatment for migraine headaches, chronic pain, and neuropathic pain (i.e., tingling, burning) such as postherpetic neuralgia. Examples of TCAs are amitriptyline (Elavil), nortriptyline (Pamelor), doxepin (Sinequan), desipramine (Norpramin).
- Do not give suicidal patients a prescription for TCAs, because of the high risk of hoarding the drug and overdosing. Overdose of TCAs can be fatal (cardiac and central nervous system [CNS] toxicity).
- SSRIs are also first-line treatment for OCD, generalized anxiety disorder (GAD), panic disorder, social anxiety disorder (extreme shyness), PTSD, and premenstrual mood disorder (fluoxetine or Prozac). Examples of SSRIs are citalopram (Celexa), escitalopram (Lexapro), fluoxetine (Prozac), sertraline (Zoloft), and paroxetine (Paxil).
- Anticonvulsants, such as carbamazepine (Tegretol), are also used for chronic pain and trigeminal neuralgia.

ABUSIVE SITUATIONS

I. Discussion

Healthcare workers are required by law to report suspected and actual child abuse to the proper authorities. Abuse-related topics may include domestic violence, physical abuse, child abuse, child neglect, elderly abuse, elderly neglect, and sexual abuse.

II. Example

A 16-year-old teenager with a history of attention deficit hyperactivity disorder (ADHD) is brought in to the ED by his mother. She does not want her son to be alone in the room. The nurse practitioner (NP) doing the intake notes several burns on the teen's trunk. Some of the burns appear infected. The NP documents the burns as mostly round in shape and about 0.5 cm (centimeter) in size. Which of the following questions is most appropriate to ask the child's mother?

A. "Your son's back looks terrible. What happened to him?"
B. "Does your son have more friends outside of school?"
C. "Did you burn his back with a cigarette?"
D. "Can you tell me what happened to your son?"

III. Correct Answer: Option D

D. "Can you tell me what happened to your son?"

IV. Question Dissection

Best Clues

- Option D is the only open-ended question in the group.
- In addition, it is not a judgmental statement.

NOTES

- In general, open-ended questions are usually the correct answer in cases in which an NP is trying to elicit the history in an interview.
- "Your son's back looks terrible. What happened to him?" and "Did you burn his back with a cigarette?" are both considered judgmental questions and are always the wrong choice.
- These types of questions are more likely to make people defensive and/or hostile and cause them to end the conversation.
- "Does your son have more friends outside of school?" This question does not address the immediate issue of the burn marks on the patient's back.
- Here are some communication tips for questions on abuse. If a history is being taken, pick the open-ended question first. Interview both the patient and possible "abuser" together, and then interview the patient separately.
- Here are some communication tips for questions on depression. Pick the statement that is the most specific to find out whether the patient is suicidal or homicidal. Any answer considered judgmental or confrontational is wrong. Do not pick answers that "reassure" patients about their issues, because this discourages them from verbalizing more about it. In addition, consider the patient's cultural beliefs. Integrate them into the treatment plan if they are not harmful to the health of the patient.

THE "CAGE" MNEMONIC

I. Discussion

The CAGE is a screening tool used to screen patients for possible alcohol use disorder. A positive response to two out of four questions is highly suggestive of alcohol use disorder. In the exam, you are expected to use higher-level cognitive skills and apply the concepts of CAGE. Examples of this concept are the questions that ask you to pick the patient who is most likely (or least likely) to misuse alcohol.

CAGE Screening Tool (Two or More Positive Answers Is Suggestive of Alcoholism)
- **C:** Do you feel the need to **c**ut down?
- **A:** Are you **a**nnoyed when your friends/spouse comment about your drinking?
- **G:** Do you feel **g**uilty about your drinking?
- **E:** Do you need to drink **e**arly in the morning (eyeopener)?

II. Example
Which of the following individuals is *least likely* to have an alcohol misuse problem?
- **A.** An executive who gets annoyed if her best friend talks to her about her drinking habit
- **B.** A carpenter who drinks two cans of beer per night when playing cards with friends
- **C.** A nurse who feels shaky when she wakes up and drinks one glass of wine to feel better
- **D.** A college student who tells his friend that he drinks only on weekends but feels that he should be drinking less

III. Correct Answer: Option B
- **B.** A carpenter who drinks two cans of beer per night when playing cards with friends

IV. Question Dissection
Best Clues
- Lack of risk factor (two cans of beer at night is considered normal consumption for males); for females, the limit is one drink per day (one 12 oz beer, 5 oz wine).
- There is no description of any negative effects on the carpenter's daily functioning, social environment, or mental state.

> **NOTES**
>
> Any person who feels compelled to drink (or use drugs), no matter what the consequences are to their health, finances, career, friends, and family, is addicted to the substance.
> - "An executive who gets annoyed if her best friend talks to her about her drinking habit." This is the "A" in CAGE ("annoyed"), a good example of an alcohol misuser getting annoyed when someone close remarks about her drinking problem.
> - "A nurse who feels shaky when she wakes up and drinks one glass of wine to feel better." This is the "E" in CAGE ("eye-opener"). The patient is having withdrawal symptoms and must drink in order to feel better.
> - "A college student who tells his friend that he drinks only on weekends but feels that he should be drinking less." This fits the "C" in CAGE ("cut down"). This student is aware that he is drinking too much.

PHYSICAL ASSESSMENT FINDINGS
I. Discussion
Questions about physical exam findings are plentiful. Learn the classic presentation of disease and emergent conditions. The knowledge of normal findings, as well as some variants, is important for the exam. In addition, if the question style used is negatively worded, careful reading is essential.

II. Example
An older woman complains of a new onset of severe pain in her right ear after taking swimming classes for 2 weeks. On physical exam, the right ear canal is red and swollen. Purulent green exudate is seen inside. Which of the following is an incorrect statement?
- **A.** Pulling on the tragus is painful.
- **B.** The tympanic membrane is translucent with intact landmarks.
- **C.** The external ear canal is swollen and painful.
- **D.** Tenderness of the mastoid area may be noted during palpation.

III. Correct Answer: Option D
- **D.** Tenderness of the mastoid area may be noted during palpation.

IV. Question Dissection
Best Clues
- Positive risk factor (history of swimming)
- Classic signs (reddened and swollen ear canal with green exudate)

> **NOTES**
>
> - Acute otitis externa is a superficial infection of the skin in the ear canal. It is more common during warm and humid conditions such as swimming and summertime.
> - The most common bacterial pathogen is *Pseudomonas* (bright-green pus).
> - Otitis externa does not involve the middle ear or the tympanic membrane (translucent tympanic membrane with intact landmarks, no redness, no bulging).
> - Tenderness of the mastoid area is not a complication of otitis externa.

TWO-PART QUESTIONS
I. Discussion
There may be case scenarios that are followed by two questions. These questions are problematic because the two questions are dependent on each other.

To solve both correctly, the test-taker must answer the first portion by figuring out the diagnosis in order to solve the second question correctly.

II. Example
Part One
An adolescent male patient reports the new onset of symptoms 2 weeks after returning from a hiking trip in North Carolina. He presents with complaints of high fever, severe

headache, muscle aches, lack of appetite, and nausea. The symptoms are accompanied by a generalized red rash that is not pruritic. The rash initially appeared on both ankles and wrists and then spread toward the patient's trunk. The rash involves both the palms and the soles. Which of the following conditions is most likely?

A. Meningococcemia
B. Rocky Mountain spotted fever (RMSF)
C. Idiopathic thrombocytopenic purpura (ITP)
D. Lyme disease

Part Two
Which of the following is the best treatment plan to follow?

A. Refer the patient to the hospital ED.
B. Refer the patient to an infectious disease specialist.
C. Initiate a prescription of oral glucocorticoids.
D. Collect a blood specimen for culture and sensitivity.

III. Correct Answers
Part One: Option B
B. Rocky Mountain spotted fever (RMSF)

Part Two: Option A
A. Refer the patient to the hospital ED.

IV. Question Dissection
Best Clues
Part One
- Location and activity (south-central United States, out-door activity)
- Classic rash (red rash on both wrists and ankles that spreads centrally with involvement of the palms and the soles)
- Systemic symptoms (high fever, headache, myalgia, nausea)

Part Two
Knowledge of the emergent nature of RMSF (can cause death if not treated within the first 8 days of symptoms)

> **NOTES**
> - Early treatment is important, and empiric treatment should be started early if RMSF is suspected. Refer the patient to the closest ED as soon as possible.
> - It may be difficult to distinguish RMSF from meningococcemia before the blood culture results and the CSF culture results are available.
> - Doxycycline is the preferred agent for both children and adults.
> - RMSF is caused by dog/wood tick bite; spirochete called *Rickettsia rickettsia*. Treat with doxycycline 100 mg orally or by IV for a minimum of 7 days or longer.
> - Stage one, early Lyme disease (localized Lyme disease), is caused by ixodes (deer) tick bite; spirochete called *Borrelia burgdorferi*. Treat with doxycycline × 21 days. Majority of cases are in the mid-Atlantic and

> New England states (e.g., Connecticut, Massachusetts, New York, New Jersey, Pennsylvania).
> - ITP severity ranges from mild to severe (platelet count <30,000/mcL). Platelets are broken down by the spleen, causing thrombocytopenia. Look for easy bruising, petechiae, purpura, epistaxis, and gingival bleeding (combined with low platelet count).
> - Initial treatment for ITP is glucocorticoids (i.e., prednisone) based on platelet response.

NORMAL PHYSICAL EXAM FINDINGS
I. Discussion
A good review of normal physical exam findings and some benign variants is necessary. Pertinent physical exam findings are discussed at the beginning of each organ system review.

A good resource to use in your review is the advanced physical assessment textbook that was used in your program. Keep in mind that sometimes questions about normal physical findings are written as if they were a pathologic process. This is important to remember when you encounter these types of questions.

II. Example
A 13-year-old girl complains of an irregular menstrual cycle. She started menarche 6 months ago. Her last menstrual period was 2 months ago. She denies being sexually active. Her urine pregnancy test is negative. Which of the following would you tell the child's parents?

A. Consult with a pediatric endocrinologist to rule out problems with the hypothalamic–pituitary–adrenal (HPA) axis.
B. Advise the parents that irregular menstrual cycles are common during the first year after menarche.
C. Advise the parents that their child is starting menarche early and has precocious puberty.
D. Ask the medical assistant to get labs drawn for thyroid-stimulating hormone (TSH), follicle-stimulating hormone (FSH), and estradiol levels.

III. Correct Answer: Option B
B. Advise the parents that irregular menstrual cycles are common during the first year after menarche.

IV. Question Dissection
Best Clues
- Patient recently started menarche 6 months ago (knowledge of pubertal changes); the ovaries may not ovulate monthly (resulting in irregular periods) when starting menarche.
- The teen is not sexually active (rule out pertinent negative, such as the negative pregnancy test).

> **NOTES**
> - This question describes normal growth and development in adolescents.
> - When girls start menarche, their periods may be very irregular for several months up to 2 years.

PEDIATRICS

I. Discussion

Questions for this age group will cover common child-hood infections, growth and development milestones, and immunizations. The age group ranges from infancy and childhood into adolescence.

II. Example

A 6-year-old boy is brought to the clinic by his parents. They state that their son complains of ear pain in the right ear. He has been "fussy" and pulling on his right ear for several days. He attends school on weekdays. The nurse practitioner suspects that the child has otitis media. Which of the following is the *most objective* finding in a child with otitis media?

A. Child's fussy behavior
B. Child's verbal complaint of ear pain
C. Tympanic membrane (TM) that is erythematous
D. Impaired mobility of TM by insufflation

III. Correct Answer: Option D

D. Impaired mobility of TM by insufflation

IV. Question Dissection

The most objective finding is impaired mobility of the TM by insufflation, which is measured by a tympanogram. The other clinical signs are more subjective, such as the appearance of a bulge in the eardrum. The bulge in the TM can range from mild to a large bulge that may be accompanied by retraction of the TM. The complaint of ear pain (otalgia) and the child's fussy behavior are subjective information.

ADOLESCENCE

I. Discussion

During this period of life, numerous changes are occurring, both physically and emotionally. Adolescents are thinking in more abstract ways and are psychologically separating from their parents. The opinions of peers are more important than those of the parents. Privacy is a big issue in this age group and should be respected.

II. Example

Which of the following is the second highest cause of mortality among adolescents and young adults in this country?

A. Suicide
B. Smoking
C. Homicide
D. Illicit drug use

III. Correct Answer: Option A

A. Suicide

IV. Question Dissection

Best Clues

Rote memory (suicide is the second highest cause of mortality among adolescents)

NOTES

- According to the CDC, the number one cause of mortality in this age group is motor vehicle crashes.
- The second most common cause of mortality in adolescents in the United States is suicide, and the third is homicide.
- Screening for depression in all adolescents is recommended. Signs of a depressed teen include falling grades, acting out, avoiding socializing, moodiness, and so forth.
- Smoking is ruled out because its health effects take decades (e.g., COPD).
- Mortality from illicit drug use is more common among adults.

DIFFERENTIAL DIAGNOSIS

I. Discussion

Differential diagnoses are the conditions whose presentations share many similarities. For example, the differential diagnoses to consider for chronic cough (a cough lasting more than 8 weeks) are asthma, GERD, ACE inhibitors, chronic bronchitis, lung cancer, and lung infections such as TB (and many more). As a clinician, your ability to apply differential diagnosis is important for patient safety. In this type of question, the differential diagnoses are the distractors.

II. Example

A 67-year-old man walks into an urgent care center. The patient complains of episodes of chest pain in his upper sternum when he is climbing up stairs in his apartment building. When he stops the activity, the pain goes away. He reports that once when he was eating a steak dinner, he also experienced the chest pain. A fasting total lipid profile is ordered. The result reveals total cholesterol of 250 mg/dL, low-density lipoprotein (LDL) of 180 mg/dL, and high-density lipoprotein (HDL) of 25 mg/dL. Which of the following is most likely?

A. Acute esophagitis
B. Myocardial infarction (MI)
C. Gastroesophageal reflux disease (GERD)
D. Angina

III. Correct Answer: Option D

D. Angina

IV. Question Dissection

Best Clues

- Classic presentation (chest pain that is precipitated by exertion and is relieved by rest)
- History (several episodes of the same chest pain)
- Positive risk factors (low HDL, elevated lipid levels, age, and sex)

NOTES

All four answer options are some common conditions that can mimic angina (differential diagnoses). Rule out the pertinent negatives.

- Pain is relieved by rest (angina). If pain is not relieved by rest, consider unstable angina. Other signs include angina that occurs at rest, unpredictable episodes, increased frequency episodes, or no response to medications (e.g., nitroglycerin) that previously worked.
- Risk factors for heart disease and chest pain (angina, MI) are present.
- Physical activity aggravates the condition (angina, MI).
- There is a lack of history of aggravating factors such as intake of certain medications such as NSAIDs, aspirin, bisphosphonates, or alcohol (rule out esophagitis).
- Chest pain is not related to meals (rule out GERD).

TUBERCULOSIS
I. Discussion

Always expect a question or two regarding pulmonary TB. Expect a question that will assess your knowledge of reading the results of a tuberculin skin test (Mantoux test). Depending on the patient's history and background, a positive result may be 5, 10, or 15 mm (no risk factors for TB).

The chest radiograph of a person with active pulmonary TB or a history of pulmonary TB (lung scarring) may show cavitations that are usually located on the upper lobes. In Figure 2.3, note that the arrows are placed on the affected areas of the lungs.

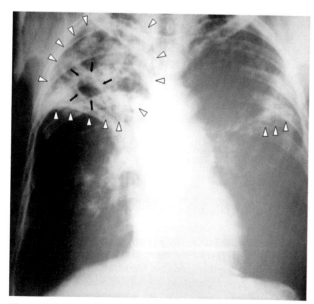

Figure 2.3 Example of an exam image.

II. Example
The chest radiograph is highly suggestive of which of the following conditions?
A. Lobar bacterial pneumonia
B. Pulmonary fibrosis
C. Pulmonary tuberculosis
D. Viral pneumonia

III. Correct Answer: Option C
C. Pulmonary tuberculosis

IV. Question Dissection
Best Clues
- Notice that there is a round, black area on the left, upper lobe. It is black because the lung tissue in the area has been destroyed by an active infection with *Mycobacterium tuberculosis*.
- Cavitations on the upper lobes of the lung are one of the classic signs of active or past TB disease.
- Pulmonary fibrosis is a lung disease where lung tissue becomes scarred (fibrosis). It is diagnosed and managed by pulmonologist. Rule out diseases that are managed by specialists.
- Lobar pneumonia does not include cavitations. It will show a white-colored patchy area on one of the lobes of the lungs.
- Bacterial pneumonia and pulmonary TB are discussed in Chapter 8.

ETHNIC BACKGROUND
I. Discussion
Ethnic background can be an important clue for certain genetic disorders. For example, Tay-Sachs, a rare and fatal genetic disorder, is most common among those of Eastern European descent.

A warning about ethnic background: It can also be used as a distractor. In most medical conditions, the patient's ethnic background does not affect the treatment plan or the patient's response to treatment. The next question is an example of this concept.

II. Example
Which of the following laboratory tests is a sensitive indicator of renal function in people of African descent?
A. Serum blood urea nitrogen (BUN)
B. Serum creatinine concentration
C. Estimated glomerular filtration rate (eGFR)
D. Serum BUN-to-creatinine ratio
The question in this example can also be phrased as, "Which of the following laboratory tests is a sensitive indicator of renal function in people of Hispanic descent? Or Asian descent?"

III. Correct Answer: Option C
C. Estimated glomerular filtration rate (eGFR)

IV. Question Dissection
Best Clues
Knowledge that the eGFR is a better test of renal function compared with the serum creatinine concentration

SENTINEL EVENTS

I. Discussion

The Joint Commission adopted a Sentinel Event Policy in 1996 to help ambulatory care centers and hospitals improve patient safety. The Commission defined a sentinel event as "a patient safety event (not primarily related to the natural course of patient's illness or underlying condition) that reaches a patient and results in any of the following: death, permanent harm, or severe temporary harm." Sentinel events require immediate investigation.

II. Example

All of the following are considered sentinel events, except:

A. Unanticipated death of a full-term infant
B. Abduction of any patient who is receiving treatment or services
C. Suicide of a patient who is receiving around-the-clock care
D. Nausea and vomiting caused by a prescription of oral erythromycin

III. Correct Answer: Option D

D. Nausea and vomiting caused by a prescription of oral erythromycin

IV. Question Dissection

Best Clues

- If you are not sure of the answer, one way to guess is to look for a pattern or for contextual clues.
- Notice that options A, B, and C all have something in common; they are all serious patient safety events.
- Option D is not considered a serious patient event. GI side effects, such as nausea/vomiting, anorexia, and abdominal pain, are not life-threatening.
- An example of a sentinel event involving medications is when a patient who is allergic to a drug (e.g., macrolides) is prescribed erythromycin, resulting in death of the patient due to anaphylaxis.

ANTIBIOTIC CASE SCENARIOS

Case 1

Penicillin-Allergic Patient With Strep Throat

An 18-year-old female patient has a positive throat culture and sensitivity (C&S) for *S. pyogenes* (group A beta streptococci). The patient reports a history of an allergic reaction to penicillin with "swollen lips" accompanied by itchy hives. Which of the following is the most appropriate treatment?

A. Clarithromycin (Biaxin) 250 mg PO twice a day × 10 days
B. Gargle with salt water three times a day
C. Cephalexin (Keflex) 250 mg PO four times a day × 10 days
D. Doxycycline 100 mg PO twice a day × 10 days

Question Dissection

Correct answer is option A: Clarithromycin (Biaxin) 250 mg PO twice a day × 10 days

Best Clues

- Positive C&S for strep
- Report of a penicillin allergy
- Rule out option B (gargling with salt water is for symptoms and will not eradicate strep); option C (penicillin-allergic patients may also be allergic to cephalosporins); and option D (doxycycline not effective for streptococcus)

Case 2

Patient With Both Mononucleosis and Strep Throat Infection

A 16-year-old high school athlete is returning for follow-up for a severe sore throat. During the physical exam, purulent exudate is noted on both tonsils. Tender lymph nodes that are 1 cm in diameter are palpable on the posterior cervical chains. The lungs are clear. The rapid strep antigen test is positive for group A beta hemolytic *Streptococcus*. The Monospot test (heterophile antibody test) is positive. What is the best *initial* clinical management of this patient?

A. Initiate a prescription of amoxicillin 500 mg PO twice a day × 10 days.

B. Initiate a prescription of penicillin V 250 mg PO three times a day × 10 days.

C. Order an Epstein–Barr virus titer to determine whether the patient has an acute or a reactivated mononucleosis infection.

D. Write a prescription for an abdominal ultrasound to determine the size of the patient's liver and spleen.

Question Dissection

Correct answer is option B: Initiate a prescription of penicillin V 250 mg PO three times a day × 10 days.

Best Clues

- Positive test results (Monospot and strep)
- Rule out option A (avoid using amoxicillin if a patient has mononucleosis, because of the risk of an amoxicillin "drug rash" that is not due to an allergy); option C (not for initial management of uncomplicated mononucleosis); and option D (not for initial management; only for cases in which the physical exam reveals an enlarged liver and/or spleen)

> **NOTES**
> - In the case of rash in mononucleosis patients who are treated with amoxicillin, it is very hard to determine whether the rash is due to a true allergy or whether the patient has a benign nonallergic drug rash. About 70% to 90% of patients with mono taking amoxicillin may break out with a "nonallergic" generalized maculopapular rash (mechanism is not well understood).
> - If a patient has both mono and strep throat, avoid using amoxicillin or ampicillin. Instead, use penicillin (if not allergic) or a macrolide to treat the patient.

CLINICAL PEARL

Of patients with true penicillin allergy, a small percentage (0.17%–8.4%) will also react to a cephalosporin.

Case 3

Patient With History of Gastrointestinal Symptoms After Taking Erythromycin

A 25-year-old healthy male patient who is a nonsmoker is diagnosed with atypical pneumonia. The patient reports a history of nausea, upset stomach, and vomiting with erythromycin. The vital signs are temperature of 99.8°F, pulse of 80/min, and respiratory rate of 16 breaths/min. What is the most appropriate treatment plan for this patient?

A. Initiate a prescription of azithromycin (Z-Pak) PO × 5 days.

B. Initiate a prescription of TMP-SMX (Bactrim) 1 tablet PO twice a day × 10 days.

C. Order a complete blood count (CBC) with differential.

D. Order a sputum for culture and sensitivity (C&S).

Question Dissection

Correct answer is option A: Initiate a prescription of azithromycin (Z-Pak) PO × 5 days.

Best Clues

- The patient has atypical pneumonia but is a healthy young adult and a nonsmoker. He is not febrile or toxic (fever is temperature of 100.4°F).
- Rule out option B (Bactrim is not effective against *Mycoplasma* or *Chlamydia* bacterial infections, but it is an excellent drug for some gram-negative infections such as UTIs); option C (ordering a CBC with differential is not necessary in this case); and option D (for community-acquired pneumonia [CAP], ordering a sputum for C&S is not recommended by the American Thoracic Society/Infectious Diseases Society of America [ATS/IDSA] treatment guidelines for CAP).

> **NOTES**
> - GI upset (nausea and vomiting, abdominal pain) is a common side effect of erythromycin—it is not an allergic reaction (such as angioedema, hives, anaphylaxis). If a patient who needs a macrolide is not allergic, azithromycin (Z-Pak) is a good choice. It usually does not cause GI side effects, has fewer drug interactions, and has a broader spectrum of activity.
> - If the patient (≥18 years) is allergic to macrolides, an alternative is doxycycline PO twice a day or new-generation quinolones (Levaquin, Avelox).

CLINICAL PEARL

Consider macrolide-resistant *S. pneumoniae* if the patient was on a macrolide in the past 3 months.

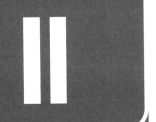

PHARMACOLOGY AND HEALTH SCREENING OVERVIEW

3

PHARMACOLOGY REVIEW

Both the current American Academy of Nurse Practitioners Certification Board (AANPCB) and American Nurses Credentialing Center (ANCC) exams now have more questions about pharmacokinetic (PK) and pharmacodynamic (PD) concepts. Pharmacotherapeutic intervention selection (picking the correct drug for a condition) includes knowledge of drug interactions, side effects, contraindications, monitoring, and patient outcomes. Learn about important primary care drug "safety issues"; for example, the drug–disease contraindication of gout (thiazide diuretics): In a case scenario about a patient with symptoms of gout and a new diagnosis or a history of hypertension, it is best not to pick a thiazide diuretic as the treatment, because they are contraindicated in gout.

For some drugs, it is required that a certain laboratory test is ordered before initiation or to monitor for adverse effects. For example, regarding angiotensin-converting enzyme inhibitors (ACEIs) (e.g., enalapril, lisinopril, captopril) and angiotensin receptor blockers (ARBs; e.g., losartan, valsartan, irbesartan), serum potassium and serum creatinine should be monitored at baseline, within the first month, and periodically, especially in the elderly, diabetics, and those with chronic kidney disease (CKD). Another example of laboratory monitoring is anticoagulation therapy and the international normalized ratio (INR) values. For patients with atrial fibrillation, the goal is to keep the INR between 2 and 3, and for patients with prosthetic heart valves, the INR goal is usually from 2.5 to 3.5.

Nonpharmacologic interventions such as alternative and herbal medicines are also included. For example, the herb feverfew is used for migraine, irregular menstrual periods, tinnitus, and other conditions.

During your review, memorize both the drug class and the representative drug(s) for that particular class. The reason is that sometimes drugs are listed by class only. Memorizing drug doses is generally not emphasized to the same extent as on the NCLEX-RN® examination.

The most common question about drugs (prescription and over the counter [OTC]) is related to disease management. These questions involve picking the correct drug to treat a condition.

The drugs that are included in the examinations are usually the "older" drugs that have been in use for several years to several decades (e.g., azithromycin, doxycycline, omeprazole, prednisone, amoxicillin). Drugs or treatment guidelines that have been recently released (past 12 months or less) will not be included on the examinations.

In the past several years, pharmacogenetic testing of patients has become more commonplace. This testing is used to determine which particular drug in various classes may be beneficial for the patient. In particular, it has been used to guide prescribing for a patient with mental health conditions such as bipolar disorder, depression, posttraumatic stress disorder (PTSD), and schizophrenia. Think of pharmacogenomics as the broader study of pharmacogenetics—pharmacogenetics refers to the individual, and pharmacogenomics may refer to a number of people with particular characteristics.

This section is not meant to be a comprehensive review of pharmacology. The goal is to help you understand pharmacologic concepts, drug names, drug classes, drug interactions, disease–drug interactions, and types of laboratory tests needed for certain medications in order to help you pass your AANPCB and ANCC certification exams.

PHARMACOLOGIC CONCEPTS

- Pharmacology: The study of the interaction between the body and drugs.
- Pharmacokinetics: The movement of drugs through the body (absorption, bioavailability, distribution, metabolism, and excretion; Figure 3.1).
- Pharmacodynamics: The study of the physiologic and biochemical effects of drugs (what a drug does to the body).
- Pharmacogenomics: The study of how a person's genes affect response to medications. Its long-term goal is to help providers select the drugs and doses best suited for each person. For example, recently the U.S. Food and Drug Administration (FDA) recommended genotyping all Asians (for HLA-B*1502) before starting carbamazepine therapy. This allele is highly associated with severe to fatal

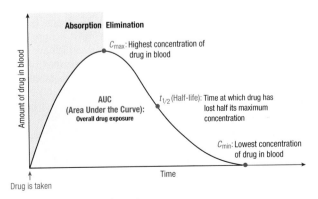

Figure 3.1 Pharmacokinetics.

carbamezapine-induced Stevens–Johnson syndrome and toxic epidermal necrolysis (mortality as high as 30%). It is most common among Chinese, but it is also present in other Asian groups (e.g., Malaysian, Thai, Filipino, Indian).

- Half-life ($t_{1/2}$): The amount of time in which drug concentration decreases by 50%.
- Area under the curve (AUC): The average amount of a drug in the blood after a dose is given. It is a measure of the bioavailability of a drug after it is administered.
- Maximum concentration (C_{max}): The peak serum concentration of a drug.
- Minimum inhibitory concentration (MIC): The lowest concentration of an antibiotic that will inhibit the growth of organisms (after overnight incubation).
- Maximum concentration: The highest concentration of a drug after a dose.
- Trough (minimum concentration): The lowest concentration of a drug after a dose.

ORAL DRUGS: FIRST-PASS HEPATIC METABOLISM (OR FIRST-PASS EFFECT)

All oral drugs (except sublingual drugs) must go through "first-pass metabolism" before they can be released and used by the body. When a drug is swallowed, it goes down the esophagus, reaches the stomach, and passes to the small intestine. When it is in the small intestine, it enters the portal circulation and reaches the liver. Inside the liver, the cytochrome P450 (CYP450) system is responsible for the biotransformation (metabolism) of the drug. When it is completed, the active drug is released to the body where it can be used. A few are also broken down in the small intestine by bacteria (e.g., oral contraceptives), in addition to being metabolized in the liver.

Some drugs that have extensive first-pass metabolism effects cannot be given by the oral route, simply because there is not enough of the active drug left. A good example is insulin, which, if given by the oral route, is completely broken down in the gastrointestinal (GI) tract (by enzymes). To bypass first-pass metabolism, insulin must be given by the parenteral route. Drug formulations that bypass first-pass metabolism are intravenous (IV) and other parenteral drugs, vaginal gels/creams, and drugs absorbed by the skin (e.g., transdermal patches, creams, ointments, gels).

DRUG METABOLISM (BIOTRANSFORMATION)

The main organ of biotransformation of drugs is the liver. The CYP450 enzyme system is the most active. CYP enzymes are found in the liver, intestines, and kidneys. The highest concentration is in the liver. Six isozymes of the P450 system are responsible for 90% of drug metabolism; these are CYP1A2, CYP2C9, CYP2C19, CYP2D6, CYP2E1, and CYP3A4. CYP3A4 and CYP2D6 are the most strongly implicated in drug metabolism issues.

The CYP450 enzyme system can either be induced (increase drug metabolism) or be inhibited (slow down drug metabolism). For example, carbamazepine (Tegretol) is a strong inducer of CYP450, resulting in numerous drug interactions. Genetic variants of the CYP450 system and receptors determine how an individual's body breaks down and reacts to a drug. The other organ systems that

are involved in drug metabolism are the kidneys, the GI tract (breakdown by gut bacteria), lungs, plasma, and skin.

DRUG EXCRETION

Renal filtration accounts for most of drug excretion. The kidney is the principle organ for drug elimination. As people age, renal drug excretion is decreased because of physiologic decline in glomerular filtration. CKD alters renal drug metabolism and increases the risk of adverse drug reactions. See Table 3.1 for drugs affected by kidney disease.

PHARMACOKINETICS: AGE-RELATED CHANGES

- Increase in fat-to-water ratio
- Decrease in albumin and plasma proteins
- Decrease in liver blood flow and size
- Decrease in some CYP450 enzyme pathways (decreased drug clearance)
- Decrease in glomerular filtration rate (GFR)

POTENT INHIBITORS: CYP450 SYSTEM

The following are some "problematic" drugs. These drugs are responsible for a large number of drug–drug interactions. Drugs that act as inhibitors slow down drug clearance (increase drug concentration). When this happens, the patient is at high risk for a drug overdose and adverse effects. When a test question is asking about a drug interaction, think of these:

- Macrolides (erythromycin, clarithromycin, telithromycin)
- Antifungals (ketoconazole, fluconazole, itraconazole)
- Cimetidine (Tagamet)
- Citalopram (Celexa)
- Protease inhibitors (saquinavir, indinavir, nelfinavir)
- Antipsychotics (clozapine, olanzapine, quetiapine)

Table 3.1 Drugs Affected by Kidney Disease

Name/Drug Class	Notes
NSAIDs	Reduction of renal blood flow will damage kidneys
ACEIs	Higher risk of hyperkalemia
Warfarin	Higher incidence of overcoagulation (INR >4). Severe CKD and ESRD at risk of hemorrhagic complications. Needs more frequent monitoring
Lithium	Increases risk of kidney injury Monitor renal function closely
Contrast dyes	Injected contrast media used with CT scans, MRIs, and angiograms can injure the kidneys
Potassium-sparing diuretics	Increased risk of hyperkalemia
Oral sodium phosphate (to cleanse bowel before colonoscopies)	FDA 2019 warning (for CKD patients): may cause sudden loss of kidney function (acute kidney injury) as well as blood mineral disturbances

ACEI, angiotensin-converting enzyme inhibitor; CKD, chronic kidney disease; ESRD, end-stage renal disease; FDA, U.S. Food and Drug Administration; INR, international normalized ratio; NSAID, nonsteroidal anti-inflammatory drug.

- Although not a drug, grapefruit juice affects the CYP450 system. Drugs that are adversely affected by grapefruit juice include statins, erythromycin, calcium channel blockers (CCBs; nifedipine, nisoldipine), antivirals (indinavir, saquinavir), amiodarone, benzodiazepines (diazepam, triazolam), cisapride, carbamazepine, and buspirone.

NARROW THERAPEUTIC INDEX DRUGS

- Warfarin sodium (Coumadin): Monitor INR.
- Digoxin (Lanoxin): Monitor digoxin level, EKG, electrolytes (potassium, magnesium, calcium).
- Theophylline: Monitor blood levels.

Table 3.2 Safety Issues Associated With Common Prescription Drugs*

Drug Class and Generic/Trade Names	Safety Issues
H$_2$ antagonists Famotidine (Pepcid) Cimetidine (Tagamet) Nizatidine (Axid)	Mental status changes with kidney disease Avoid if kidney disease with creatinine clearance of <50 mL/minute
Proton-pump inhibitors Omeprazole (Prilosec)	Increased risk of fractures (postmenopausal women), pneumonia, *Clostridium difficile* infection, hypomagnesemia, vitamin B$_{12}$ and iron malabsorption, atrophic gastritis, and kidney disease Interacts with warfarin (Coumadin), diazepam (Valium), carbamazepine (Tegretol), phenytoin (Dilantin), ketoconazole (Nizoral)
Vitamin K antagonist Warfarin (Coumadin)	Interacts with "G" herbs such as garlic, ginger, ginkgo, and ginseng; other herbs/supplements: feverfew, green tea, and fish oil; numerous drug interactions Discontinue 7 days before surgery
Thiazolidinediones Pioglitazone (Actos)	Boxed warning: Cause or exacerbate congestive heart failure in some patients; do not use if New York Health Association Class III or IV heart failure Contraindications: History of MI, stroke, bladder cancer, type I diabetes, eye or liver problems Stop if causes dyspnea, weight gain, cough (heart failure)
Atypical antipsychotics Risperidone (Risperdal) Olanzapine (Zyprexa) Quetiapine (Seroquel)	High risk of weight gain, metabolic syndrome, type 2 diabetes; monitor weight every 3 months Boxed warning: Higher mortality in elderly patients Monitor TSH, lipids, blood glucose/A1C, weight/body mass index
Bisphosphonates Alendronate (Fosamax) Risedronate (Actonel)	Erosive esophagitis (chest pain with eating, odonophagia, dysphagia, heartburn), stop immediately if symptoms of esophagitis (chest pain, difficulty swallowing, burning midback) or jaw pain (osteonecrosis); take alone upon awakening with 8-oz glass water (*not juice*) before breakfast; do not lie down for 30 minutes afterward; do not mix with other drugs Contraindications: Active GI disease (GERD, PUD), CKD, esophageal stricture/varices
Statins Atorvastatin (Lipitor) Lovastatin (Mevacor) Rosuvastatin (Crestor) Simvastatin (Zocor) Fluvastatin (Lescol) Pravastatin (Pravachol) Pitavastatin (Livalo)	Do not mix with grapefruit juice; drug-induced hepatitis or rhabdomyolysis higher if mixed with azole antifungals High-dose Zocor (80 mg) has highest risk of rhabdomyolysis (muscle pain/tenderness, muscle weakness, brown or dark red urine) Patients of Chinese descent: Higher risk myopathy or rhabdomyolysis when taking simvastatin 40 mg/d (or higher) with niacin Creatine kinase level goes up
Lincosamides Clindamycin (Cleocin)	Higher risk of CDAD
Inhaled corticosteroids	Adrenal insufficiency possible in children (long term [>6 months]; high doses, low-BMI child); suspect and test for adrenal insufficiency if symptoms (hypoglycemia, hypotension, altered mental status, weakness, Cushingoid features), growth deceleration/failure
Systemic glucocorticoids	Cataracts, osteoporosis, skin changes (telangiectasia, easy bruising), emotional lability, weight gain, high BP
Anticonvulsants Phenytoin (Dilantin)	Earliest signs of toxicity (horizontal nystagmus, unsteady gait); if severe, slurred speech, lethargy, confusion, coma; check blood level Can cause gingival hyperplasia

* List is not all-inclusive.
BMI, body mass index; CDAD, *Clostridium difficile*–associated diarrhea; CKD, chronic kidney disease; GERD, gastroesophageal reflux disease; GI, gastrointestinal; MI, myocardial infarction; PUD, peptic ulcer disease; TSH, thyroid-stimulating hormone.

- Carbamazepine (Tegretol) and phenytoin (Dilantin): Monitor blood levels.
- Levothyroxine: Monitor thyroid-stimulating hormone (TSH).
- Lithium: Monitor blood levels and TSH (risk of hypothyroidism).

BEERS CRITERIA®

Beers Criteria are used to provide guidance regarding medications that should be avoided in adults over 65 years of age. These criteria were developed in 1991 by Mark H. Beers and were adopted by the American Geriatrics Society. Starting in 2015, the guideline lists medications by organ system, therapeutic category, and drug name, and then describes rationale, quality of evidence used in decision-making, and recommendations. For instance, first-generation antihistamines (e.g., diphenhydramine, doxylamine, chlorpheniramine) that are in OTC medications for sleep are to be avoided in older adults, as they may cause dizziness and lead to falls. The most recent 2020 guideline emphasizes that the following drugs/drug classes should be avoided:

- Antipsychotics: Quetiapine, clozapine, and pimavanserin may be used with caution.
- Rivaroxaban and dabigatran: Higher bleeding risk than warfarin and other direct oral anticoagulants (DOACs).
- Tramadol: Risk of hyponatremia from syndrome of inappropriate antidiuretic hormone secretion.
- Opioids: Do not combine with benzodiazepines or gabapentinoids, as they increase the risk of severe respiratory depression.

DRUGS USED TO TREAT HEART DISEASE

CARDIAC GLYCOSIDES: DIGOXIN (LANOXIN)

- Use of digoxin has declined because of newer drugs that are more effective and safer to use. It has been replaced by ACEIs, ARBs, beta-blockers, and CCBs.
- Digoxin is now the second- to third-line drug therapy for heart failure with reduced ejection fraction (HFrEF).
- Digoxin has a narrow therapeutic range (0.5–2.0 ng/mL).
- Suspected intake of poisonous plants with cardiac glycosides (foxglove, oleander, lily of the valley): Refer to ED.
- Life-threatening effects include severe bradycardia, heart block, ventricular tachycardia, ventricular fibrillation. Approximately 30% of people with digoxin toxicity are asymptomatic.
- Signs and symptoms of digoxin overdose include initial symptoms of GI (nausea/vomiting), hyperkalemia, and bradydysrhythmias (atrioventricular [AV] blocks) or tachydysrhythmias (ventricular tachycardia/fibrillation or atrial tachycardia with 2:1 block). Others include confusion and visual changes (yellowish-green–tinged color vision).
- Laboratory tests for suspected digoxin toxicity include ordering a digoxin level, electrolytes (potassium, magnesium, calcium), creatinine, and serial EKGs.

- Treatment includes digoxin-specific antibodies, which are IgG antidigoxin antibodies that bind free digoxin in blood (Digibind, DigiFab).
- Potassium values (adult to elderly) may be critical <2.5 or >6.5 mEq/L; normal 3.5 to 5.0 mEq/L

ANTICOAGULANTS

Anticoagulation therapy is recommended for treating, preventing, and reducing the recurrence of venous thromboembolism (VTE), which results in stroke, pulmonary embolism (PE), or acute MI. The first-line agent for patients who do not have valvular disease are the DOACs, which do not require laboratory monitoring of INR and are not affected by vitamin K in the diet. For those with valvular disease or prosthetic heart valves, the only anticoagulant that can be used for chronic anticoagulation is warfarin sodium (Coumadin).

Warfarin Sodium (Coumadin)

This is a vitamin K antagonist (VKA):

- Pregnancy: Has two different pregnancy categories. Pregnant women with mechanical heart valve, it is a Category D drug. It is a Category X for all other pregnant women
- Indications: Atrial fibrillation, prosthetic heart valve, PE, deep venous thrombosis (DVT), stroke/cerebrovascular accident (CVA), heart failure (HF) and antiphospholipid syndrome
- Onset of action: Typically within 24 to 72 hours
- Atrial fibrillation, DVT, stroke/CVA: Target INR is 2.0 to 3.0 (ideal INR 2.5)
- Mechanical mitral valves (lifelong anticoagulation): Target INR is 2.5 to 3.5 (ideal INR 3.0)
- Concurrent aspirin (75–100 mg/d): For all patients on a VKA for mechanical prosthetic valves
- For initiation and stabilization of warfarin dose: Refer patient to cardiologist/anticoagulation clinic
- INR: Will increase 2 to 3 days after the first warfarin dose, but full anticoagulation effect takes longer, ranging from 5 to 7 days after initiation
- Contraindications: See Table 3.3

Consistently Stable INR
Check every 2 to 4 weeks up to every 12 weeks.

Single Out-of-Range INR
If patient has stable INR and has a single out-of-range INR ≤0.5 below or above therapeutic INR (2–3), experts suggest continuing current warfarin dose; retest INR within 1 to 2 weeks.

INR <5 With No Significant Bleeding Risk
Omit one dose and/or reduce maintenance dose slightly; recheck INR.

Signs and Symptoms: Elevated INR
Educate patient to call if prolonged bleeding from cuts, frequent nosebleeds, bloody/tarry stool, hematuria, petechiae, excessive bruising, excessive menstrual bleeding, persistent oozing/bleeding gums after brushing, sudden decrease in hemoglobin, new onset of severe headache especially after a fall (central nervous system [CNS] bleed).

Table 3.3 Drug Contraindications*

Drug Class and Generic/Trade Names	Contraindications and Notes
Vitamin K antagonist Warfarin (Coumadin)	Large esophageal varices, thrombocytopenia, recent eye/brain/trauma surgery, within 72 hours of major surgery, blood dyscrasias Careful if history of GI bleeding

ACEIs
    Enalapril (Vasotec)
    Ramipril (Altace)
    Lisinopril (Zestril)
    Captopril (Capoten)
	Avoid mixing with potassium supplements or potassium-sparing diuretics
	Avoid in pregnancy, breastfeeding, aortic stenosis, angioedema, symptomatic hypotension, severe aortic stenosis, hyperkalemia
	ACEI cough: New onset of dry cough (not accompanied by upper respiratory infection symptoms), switch to an ARB or another antihypertensive drug class

ARBs
    Candesartan (Atacand)
    Valsartan (Diovan)
    Losartan (Cozaar)
	Avoid mixing with potassium supplements
	Do not combine ACEI with ARBs
	Lower incidence of cough compared with ACEIs
	Avoid in pregnancy

Potassium-sparing diuretics
    Triamterene (Dyrenium)
    Triamterene + hydrochlorothiazide (Dyazide)
    Amiloride (Midamor)
    Spironolactone (Aldactone)
	Higher risk of hyperkalemia if combined with ACEI, potassium, or ARBs and with severe renal disease
	Diuretics may worsen urinary incontinence
	Spironolactone: Avoid combining with ACEI, ARBs, high potassium diet/supplements, salt substitutes, chronic NSAIDs (risk of hyperkalemia); gynecomastia may occur; aldosterone antagonist activity

Beta-blockers
    Propranolol (Inderal)
    Atenolol (Tenormin)
    Metoprolol (Lopressor)
    Pindolol (Visken)
	Contraindicated if patient has chronic lung diseases (asthma, COPD, emphysema, chronic bronchitis)
	Do not discontinue beta-blockers abruptly because of severe rebound (hypertensive crisis)

Phosphodiesterase 5 (PDE5) inhibitors
    Sildenafil (Viagra)
    Tadalafil (Cialis)
    Vardenafil (Levitra)
	Do not mix with nitrates (nitroglycerine, isosorbide dinitrate) and some alpha-blockers
	Erection >4 hours: Refer to ED
	Do not give within 3–6 months of a myocardial infarction, stroke

SSRIs Citalopram (Celexa)	Avoid doses >40 mg/d; can prolong QT interval For patients >60 years of age, the maximum dose is 20 mg per day

* List is not all-inclusive.

ACEI, angiotensin-converting enzyme inhibitor; ARB, angiotensin receptor blocker; COPD, chronic obstructive pulmonary disease; GI, gastrointestinal; NSAIDs, nonsteroidal anti-inflammatory drugs; SSRIs, elective serotonin reuptake inhibitors.

One Missed Dose

Take the dose as soon as possible on the same day. Do *not* double dose the next day.

Vitamin K

- Routine vitamin K₁ (phytonadione) supplementation: Not advised.
- Dietary issues: Do not forget to review patient's daily dietary intake of vitamin K foods (kale, spinach, collards/mustard/beet greens, broccoli raab); high intake of vitamin K will reduce anticoagulant effect of warfarin (will decrease INR).
- Contraindications: See Table 3.3.

Alcohol

Avoid drinking or limit to no more than one or two servings occasionally; increases risk of bleeding even if INR is in target range.

Adverse Reaction

"Purple toes syndrome" (rare); skin necrosis located in subcutaneous fat, breasts, extremities, trunk (within first few days of receiving large doses of warfarin), bleeding.

Direct Oral Anticoagulants

DOACs include direct thrombin inhibitors (dabigatran) and direct factor Xa (FXa) inhibitors (apixaban, rivaroxaban, betrixaban, edoxaban). They are preferred for their ease of use, favorable PK with fixed dosing, fewer drug interactions, and lack of monitoring requirements. DOACs exhibit comparable efficacy and significantly lower bleeding risk compared with warfarin. Clinical indications are VTE prophylaxis in various settings (atrial fibrillation, acute coronary syndromes, orthopedic surgery, others). Reversal agents (e.g., idarucizumab and andexanet alfa) reverse the anticoagulant effects of dabigatran and FXa inhibitors, respectively. Fresh frozen plasma and prothrombin complex concentrate can also be used for rapid reversal.

CLINICAL PEARLS

- It takes 10 days (platelet life span) for platelet function to return to normal after a patient stops taking clopidogrel (Plavix).
- Be aware of increased bleeding risk with certain drugs (Table 3.4).

(continued)

CLINICAL PEARLS (continued)

- Asian patients may require lower starting and maintenance doses of warfarin.
- Some genotypes require lower doses of warfarin (genetic testing is available).
- Persons older than 60 years are more likely to have larger increases in INR (after dose is increased) compared with younger patients.
- INR values <2.0 increase stroke risk sixfold.
- Mayonnaise, canola oil, and soybean oil also have high levels of vitamin K.

DRUGS USED TO TREAT HYPERTENSION

HYPERTENSION GUIDELINES

The American College of Cardiology and the American Heart Association (ACC/AHA) released new hypertension guidelines in 2021. Before diagnosing hypertension, it is important to use an average blood pressure (BP) based on two or more readings. Out-of-office readings and self-monitoring are recommended to confirm a diagnosis of hypertension (and to titrate BP-lowering medications). There is a strong emphasis on proper BP measurement technique. BP should also be checked by other methods in addition to the clinic/office readings, such as ambulatory BP monitoring (ABPM) and home BP monitoring (HBPM). Advise patient to buy a good-quality automated BP monitor for home use. Also tell patient to bring the device to the office so that it can be checked; a difference of ≤5 mmHg is acceptable.

Following are the 2021 ACC/AHA stages of hypertension:

- Normal BP: Systolic <120 mmHg and diastolic <80 mmHg
- Elevated BP: Systolic 120 to 129 mmHg and diastolic <80 mmHg
- Stage 1: Systolic 130 to 139 mmHg or diastolic 80 to 89 mmHg
- Stage 2: Systolic ≥140 mmHg or diastolic ≥90 mmHg

If there is a disparity between systolic and diastolic readings, the higher value determines the stage. For example, a patient with a BP of 130/90 mmHg has stage 2 hypertension due to diastolic of 90 mmHg. The systolic BP readings of the right and left arms should be almost the same. *White coat hypertension* is defined as BP that is consistently elevated but does not meet the definition of hypertension. Hypertension management is discussed in-depth in Chapter 7.

Preferred diets are the low-sodium DASH or Mediterranean diets. Other recommended lifestyle modifications include weight loss, exercise, relaxation, and meditation, which can be tried for 3 to 6 months in patients with elevated BP or stage 1 hypertension without underlying disorders such as diabetes.

DIURETICS

Thiazide Diuretics

- Hypertension, edema
- Hypertension accompanied by osteopenia or osteoporosis
- Recommended as first-line therapy in Black patients with hypertension
- Hydrochlorothiazide (HCTZ)
- Chlorthalidone
- Indapamide (Lozol)
- Do not combine with lithium (increased risk of lithium toxicity)
- Contraindication is sulfa allergy

Table 3.4 Drugs That Increase Bleeding Risk

Drug Class	Name
Coumarins	Warfarin sodium (Coumadin); reversal/antidote is vitamin K (phytonadione)
Direct thrombin inhibitors	Dabigatran (Pradaxa) oral; reversal/antidote is idarucizumab (Praxbind)
Factor Xa inhibitor	Rivaroxaban (Xarelto), apixaban (Eliquis); reversal antidote is andexanet alfa (Andexxa)
Heparins	Heparin, low-molecular-weight heparin (Lovenox); reversal/antidote is protamine sulfate
Antiplatelet	Clopidogrel (Plavix); no reversal agent yet, but fresh frozen plasma or cryoprecipitate seem effective
Salicylate Other medications that contain salicylate: Aspirin, magnesium salicylate (Doans Pills), salsalate (Disalcid), bismuth subsalicylate (Pepto-Bismol)	After taking aspirin, it takes 4 days for the platelet function to return to normal
NSAIDs	Discontinue for 5 to 7 days before surgery Ketorolac (Toradol); do not exceed 5 days of use Naproxen (Aleve, Naprosyn), ibuprofen (Advil, Motrin), indomethacin (Indocin), and Mefenamic acid (Ponstel) are indicated for dysmenorrhea
Ginkgo biloba, garlic, ginseng, fish oil, feverfew, Dong quai	Increase bleeding risk, especially if taken in high doses; advise patient to stop taking approximately 7 days before surgery Ginkgo biloba; stop taking at least 36 hours before surgery

NSAIDs, nonsteroidal anti-inflammatory drugs.

Adverse Effects

- Elevates plasma glucose/hyperglycemia (careful with diabetics)
- Elevates cholesterol and low-density lipoprotein (LDL) (careful if preexisting hyperlipidemia)
- Elevates uric acid (can precipitate a gout attack); HCTZ should not be used in patients with gout
- Hypokalemia (severe muscle weakness, arrhythmias)

> **NOTES**
> - Chlorthalidone is longer acting and more "effective" than HCTZ.
> - Patients with both hypertension and osteoporosis receive an extra benefit from thiazides.
> - Thiazide diuretics reduce calcium excretion by the kidneys and stimulate the osteoblasts. This helps build bone.
> - Patients with serious sulfa allergies should avoid thiazide and loop diuretics. Potassium-sparing diuretics, such as triamterene and amiloride (Midamor), are the alternative options for these patients.

Potassium-Sparing Diuretics

- Hypertension; alternative diuretic for patients with sulfa allergy
- Triamterene (Dyrenium)
- Amiloride (Midamor)
- Combination of triamterene and HCTZ (Dyazide), amiloride and HCTZ (Moduretic)
- Boxed warning for hyperkalemia, which can be fatal; higher risk with renal impairment, diabetes, elderly, severely ill
- Monitor serum potassium (baseline, during, dose changes, illness)
- See Table 3.3 for contraindications

Mineralcorticoid Receptor Antagonists

- Spironolactone (Aldactone) for hypertension, HF, hirsutism (also considered as a potassium-sparing diuretic)
- Eplerenone (Inspra)

> **NOTES**
> - Do not give potassium supplement. Avoid using salt substitutes that contain potassium.
> - Do not combine ACEIs, ARBs, or direct renin inhibitor (aliskiren); increases risk of hyperkalemia.
> - With severe renal disease/CKD, all ACEIs, ARBs, and aliskiren are contraindicated because of high risk of hyperkalemia.
> - Spironolactone adverse effects: Gynecomastia (13%) and hyperkalemia
> - Boxed warning: Increased risk of both benign and malignant tumors shown in rats

Loop Diuretics

- Edema from HF, cirrhosis, renal disease, and hypertension
- Loop diuretics are excreted via the loop of Henle of the kidneys and are more potent than HCTZ.
- More potent than thiazides but with shorter duration of action
- Furosemide (Lasix)
- Bumetanide (Bumex)
- Boxed warning for excessive amounts of furosemide may lead to profound diuresis; medical supervision required, individualized dose schedule
- Contraindications: Sulfa allergy

Adverse Effects

- Electrolytes (hypokalemia, hyponatremia, hypomagnesemia, and low levels of chlorine)
- Hypovolemia and hypotension (dizziness, lightheadedness)
- Pancreatitis, jaundice, and rash
- Ototoxicity (worsens aminoglycoside ototoxicity effect if combined)

ANGIOTENSIN-CONVERTING ENZYME INHIBITORS AND ANGIOTENSIN RECEPTOR BLOCKERS

- Hypertension, diabetes (renal protection), CKD, post-MI, HF or left ventricular HF, and HFrEF (clinical diagnosis of HF and left ventricular ejection fraction (LVEF) ≤40%)
- Improve LVEF and survival post-MI.
- Preferred agents for patients with HFrEF are the ACEIs or ARBs and mineralcorticoid receptor antagonists (spironolactone, eplerone).
- These are not to be used during pregnancy, as these drugs damage the developing fetal renin-angiotensin system and can lead to death.
- ACE inhibition blocks conversion of angiotensin I to angiotensin II (potent vasoconstrictor); ACEI suffix of *-pril*.
- ARBs block angiotensin II (less aldosterone); ARB suffix of *-sartan*
- Boxed warning; ACEIs can cause death/injury to the developing fetus.
- Contraindications include ACEI-/ARB-associated angioedema, hereditary angioedema (see Table 3.3)

Angiotensin-Converting Enzyme Inhibitors

- Ramipril (Altace)
- Lisinopril (Zestril, Prinivil)
- Benazepril (Lotensin)
- Captopril (Capoten)
- Enalapril (Vasotec)
- Fosinopril (Monopril)
- Perindopril (Aceon)
- Quinapril (Accupril)
- Trandolapril (Mavik)
- Combination of lisinopril and HCTZ (Zestoretic), enalapril and HCTZ (Vaseretic), captopril and HCTZ (Capozide), benazepril and amlodipine (Lotrel)

Angiotensin Receptor Blockers

- Losartan (Cozaar)
- Irbesartan (Avapro)
- Valsartan (Diovan)
- Candesartan (Atacand)
- Telmisartan (Micardis)

- Olmesartan (Benicar)
- Eprosartan (Teveten)
- Combination of losartan and HCTZ (Hyzaar), valsartan and HCTZ (Diovan HCT), valsartan and amlodipine (Exforge)

Adverse Effects

- Hypotension
- ACEI cough
- Hyperkalemia
- Angioedema and anaphylactoid reactions
- Acute kidney injury (AKI)

NOTES

- A fairly common (5%–20%) side effect of ACEIs is dry cough. The cough may occur a few hours after the first dose or within weeks to months. Stop the ACEI and switch to another antihypertensive drug class or switch to an ARB (diabetic, CKD, HF).
- ACEIs and ARBs are contraindicated in pregnancy, renal artery stenosis, angioedema, hyperkalemia (>5.5 mmol/L), and hypersensitivity to the drug.
- Other drugs that affect the renin-angiotensin-aldosterone system (RAAS) are the direct renin inhibitor (aliskiren) and the neprilysin inhibitor/ ARB combination (sacubitril/valsartan), which are contraindicated in patients with a history of angioedema. Do not use it within 36 hours of switching from or to an ACEI. Diabetics should avoid concomitant use of sacubitril/valsartan with aliskiren.
- ACEIs and ARBs protect the kidneys and are preferred drugs for treatment of hypertension in diabetics and patients with mild-to-moderate CKD. But if severe CKD (eGFR <60), avoid these drugs because of higher risk of hyperkalemia.
- ACEIs are first-line therapy for HF with left ventricular dysfunction (or HFrEF).
- Monitor for side effects such as hypotension, AKI (more common in elderly and diabetics), hyperkalemia, and angioedema, which can be fatal.
- Captopril is associated with agranulocytosis, neutropenia, and leukopenia (rare). Monitor complete blood count (CBC).
- Both ACEIs and ARBs are excreted in breast milk (breastfeeding mothers should avoid them).

CLINICAL PEARLS

- ACEI-induced cough and angioedema are caused by inhibition of the metabolism of bradykinin and kallikrein system, which are involved in the inflammatory process.
- Some patients are at higher risk of AKI and hyperkalemia (elderly, patients with renal artery stenosis, diabetics). Check kidney function 3 to 5 days after starting the drug.

CALCIUM CHANNEL BLOCKERS (CALCIUM ANTAGONISTS)

- Binds L-type calcium channels located on the vascular smooth muscle, cardiac myocytes, and cardiac nodal tissue (sinoatrial and AV nodes), causing vasodilation, decreased myocardial force generation (negative inotropy), decreased heart rate (negative chronotrophy), and decreased conduction velocity.
- Used to treat hypertension, angina pectoris, coronary artery spasms, supraventricular dysrhythmias, pulmonary hypertension, hypertrophic cardiomyopathy, and Raynaud's phenomenon (first line).

Dihydropyridines

- Amlodipine (Norvasc)
- Nifedipine (Procardia, Adalat CC)
- Felodipine (Plendil)
- Nicardipine (Cardene)
- Isradipine (Dynacirc)

Nondihydropyridines

- Verapamil (Calan, Verelan) should not be mixed with erythromycin and clarithromycin (drug interaction).
- Diltiazem (Cardizem)
- Contraindications are AV block (second- to third-degree block), bradycardia, HFrEF

Adverse Effects

- Headache (vasodilation)
- Peripheral edema (not due to fluid overload)
- Bradycardia (reduction in cardiac contractility)
- HF and heart block (negative iotrophic effects)
- Hypotension (profound peripheral vasodilation)
- Reflex tachycardia (only nondihydropyridines; due to reflex increase in sympathetic activity)

NOTES

- Avoid using diltiazem and verapamil (nondihydropyridine CCBs) in patients with HFrEF (can worsen it).
- Pedal edema may occur with nifedipine and amlodipine because of vasodilation. If it bothers patient, reduce dose or take it later in the day. The pedal edema is positional and improves when laying down.
- Dihydropyridine CCBs can cause peripheral edema, headaches, flushing, and lightheadedness.
- Nondihydropyridine CCBs can worsen cardiac output and cause bradycardia and constipation, which can be problematic for elderly patients.
- Hypotension and bradycardia are the main symptoms of CCB poisoning.

BETA-BLOCKERS (BETA-ANTAGONISTS)

- Hypertension, HFrEF (carvedilol), post-MI, angina, arrhythmias, and migraine prophylaxis
- Beta-blockers are preferred for treating angina pectoris and postacute MI (unless contraindicated with shock, hypotension, severe bradycardia, heart block > first-degree block, chronic pulmonary disease).

- Adjunctive treatment for hyperthyroidism/thyrotoxicosis (decreases heart rate, palpitations, tachycardia, anxiety)
- Propranolol immediate release (Inderal) or extended release (Inderal LA) and carvedilol (Coreg) are noncardioselective beta-blockers (blocks beta-1 and beta-2).
- Cardioselective beta-blockers are more potent because they block beta-1 receptors, which are found mainly in the heart; include atenolol (Tenormin) daily; metoprolol immediate release (Lopressor) or extended release (Toprol XL)
- Timolol oral (Blocadren) or timolol ophthalmic drops (glaucoma)
- See Table 3.3 for contraindications; also:
  - Asthma (causes bronchoconstriction)
  - Chronic bronchitis and chronic obstructive pulmonary disease (COPD; causes bronchoconstriction)
  - Emphysema (causes bronchoconstriction)
  - Bradycardia and AV block (second- to third-degree block)
  - Abrupt discontinuation

Adverse Effects

- Bronchospasm (blocks beta-2 receptors in the lungs)
- Bradycardia (blocks beta-1 receptors in the heart)
- Depression, fatigue (careful with elderly)
- Erectile dysfunction
- Blunts hypoglycemic response (warn diabetic patients to initially monitor blood sugars more often)
- HF
- Exacerbation of Raynaud syndrome symptoms

DIRECT RENIN INHIBITORS

- First drug in the renin inhibitor drug class; blocks action of renin
- Aliskiren (Tekturna), aliskiren/HCTZ (Tekturna HCT)
- Aliskiren does not have outcome data available to demonstrate cardiovascular disease risk reduction with its use yet.
- Contraindications include concomitant use of ACEI or ARBs, especially in diabetic patients (risk of kidney injury, hypotension, hyperkalemia), angioneurotic angioedema, pregnancy/breastfeeding, age <6 years, renal artery stenosis

NEPRILYSIN INHIBITORS AND ANGIOTENSIN II RECEPTOR BLOCKERS

- Sacubitril and valsartan (Entresto)
- Indications include adult HF (NYHA Class II-IV), pediatric HF (age >1 year)
- Boxed warning for fetal toxicity; drugs that act on the renin–angiotensin system can cause injury or death to the developing fetus; if pregnancy detected, discontinue as soon as possible
- Contraindications include concomitant use with ACEIs; concomitant use of aliskiren in diabetics, history of angioedema related to ACEI or ARB therapy, renal artery stenosis, hyperkalemia, liver disease
- Use of sacubitril/valsartan is contraindicated in patients with history of angioedema, regardless of cause.

- On Canadian labeling, additional contraindications are symptomatic hypotension prior to initiation, concomitant use of aliskiren if renal impairment (eGFR <60 mL/minute), pregnancy, or breastfeeding.

Adverse Effects

- Hypotension
- Hyperkalemia
- Angioedema
- Dizziness
- Cough

ALPHA-BLOCKERS (ALPHA-1-ADRENERGIC ANTAGONISTS)

- Relaxes smooth muscles on the bladder neck and the prostate and improves symptoms of benign prostatic hyperplasia (BPH).
- Also known as selective alpha-blockers, which end in the suffix -osin; they are all recommended as initial therapy for BPH, but only two drugs from this group can also lower BP (terazosin, doxazosin).
- Terazosin (Hytrin) can lower BP and treat BPH
- Doxazosin (Cardura) can lower BP and treat BPH
- Tamsulosin (Flomax) for BPH treatment
- Alfuzosin (Uroxatral) for BPH treatment
- Silodosin (Rapaflo) for BPH treatment
- Prazosin (Minipress) is an alpha-blocker for hypertension but not for BPH; off-label use for PTSD-related nightmares/sleep dysfunction

Adverse Effects

- Orthostatic hypotension (caution in elderly patients)
- Dizziness, syncope
- Priapism (Flomax)
- Do not give during cataract/glaucoma surgery (floppy iris syndrome).

NOTES

- Alpha-blockers are potent vasodilators. Common side effects are dizziness and hypotension. Give at bedtime at very low dose and slowly titrate up. Careful with frail elderly (risk of syncope and falls).
- Tamsulosin (Flomax) on initial dose may cause a vasovagal response, bottoming out the BP. Patients need to be warned that someone should be with them when initiating therapy.
- Alpha-blockers are not first-line choice except for males with both hypertension and BPH.

CLINICAL PEARLS

- In the United States, myocardial infarctions (MIs) are more likely to occur in the morning between 7 a.m. and 9 a.m. (70% higher). Strokes and ventricular arrhythmias also occur more frequently in the morning.
- The day of the week when most MIs occur is Monday, and the season when most MIs occur is in winter.

ANTIBIOTICS

Antibiotics are either bacteriostatic or bactericidal. Bactericidal antibiotics kill bacteria. Bacteriostatic antibiotics limit bacterial growth and replication. The result is a lower bacterial count, which helps the immune system clear the infection. Only antibiotic drug classes that are commonly used in primary care will be discussed.

TETRACYCLINES

Tetracyclines (Table 3.5) are broad-spectrum bacteriostatic antibiotics. They are effective against many aerobic gram-positive and gram-negative bacteria; they are well known for their activity against atypical bacteria/pathogens. They are absorbed mainly in the proximal small intestine and stomach. They are not used during pregnancy or lactation. Risk of neural tube defects, cleft palate, skeletal defects, and other major defects, as well as maternal hepatotoxicity.

They can cause permanent discoloration of teeth (yellow-gray-brown) if used during the last half of pregnancy (teeth develops), in infants, and in children until the age of 8 years. Short-term use of doxycycline does not cause dental staining in young children. In 2018, the Centers for Disease Control and Prevention (CDC) recommended that doxycycline be used to treat Rocky Mountain spotted fever (RMSF) in adults and children of all ages. By the age of 8 years, permanent teeth development is complete, except for "wisdom teeth" (rear molar teeth), which erupt between age 17 and 25 years.

- Doxycycline: Sexually transmitted infections (STIs), respiratory tract infections, anthrax, RMSF, ophthalmic infections, skin (acne, rosacea), adjunctive therapy in acute intestinal amebiasis, malaria prophylaxis, specific bacterial infections (e.g., plague, cholera, relapsing fever, brucellosis, typhus fever).
- Minocycline: Acne vulgaris, chlamydia (endocervix, urethra, rectum), nongonococcal urethritis, syphilis, infective endocarditis, meningococcal carrier state, community-associated methicillin-resistant *Staphylococcus aureus* (CA-MRSA; off-label use).
- Tetracycline: Adjunct in severe acne, rosacea. Avoid taking within 4 hours of an antacid, iron, zinc, calcium, magnesium, dairy, and multivitamins.

Other Tetracyclines

- Tigecycline (Tygacil): Complicated intra-abdominal infections, community-acquired pneumonia (CAP), complicated skin and skin structure infections (IV only). Boxed warning: An increase in all-cause mortality observed. Reserve for use in situations when alternative treatments are not suitable.
- Eravacycline (Xerava): Complicated intra-abdominal infections (IV only)
- Sarecycline (Seysara): Moderate-to-severe acne vulgaris (nonnodular form)
- Omadacycline (Nuzyra): CAP and skin and skin structure infections (PO, IV)

Table 3.5 Macrolides and Tetracyclines

Drug Class and Generic/Trade Names	Drug Interactions and Contraindications

Macrolides
  Erythromycin BID to QID
  Azithromycin (Z-Pak)
  Clarithromycin BID
	Many major drug interactions
	Contraindication: Myasthenia gravis (respiratory failure)
	Anticoagulants: Warfarin (Coumadin)
	Antacids: Avoid mixing; decreases effectiveness
	Benzodiazepines: Triazolam (Halcion), midazolam (Versed)
	Major: Blood levels of statins get very high (atorvastatin, simvastatin), risk of rhabdomyolysis, hepatitis
	QT prolongation: Verapamil (Calan), amlodipine (Norvasc), diltiazem (Cardizem), amiodarone, sotalol, others; QT prolongation can cause torsades de pointes and ventricular tachycardia, so diagnosis must not be missed
	Asthma: Salmeterol (Serevent), theophylline
	Others: Anticonvulsants (carbamazepine [Tegretol], phenytoin), ergotamine

Ketolide Telithromycin (Ketek) once a day	Boxed warning: Myasthenia gravis patients—do not use Do not use in children; causes liver failure; avoid if history of jaundice/hepatitis from macrolides Same drug interactions as macrolides

Tetracyclines
  Tetracycline QID
  Doxycycline BID
  Minocycline (Minocin) BID
  Tigecycline (Tygacil) IV every 12 hours
	Photosensitivity reactions (use hat, sunblock)
	If taken without water and pill gets stuck in the esophagus, it can cause esophagitis/esophageal ulceration
	Binds with iron, calcium, magnesium, zinc
	Antacids, sucralfate, and bile acid sequestrants markedly decrease absorption; oral contraceptives (may decrease effectiveness)
	Boxed warning: Increase in all-cause mortality; reserve for use in situations when alternative treatments are not suitable

BID, twice a day; QID, four times a day.

Adverse Reactions

- Photosensitivity reaction occurs with minimal sunlight exposure; avoid or minimize sunlight or UV light exposure; use sunblock, wide-brim hats, and sunglasses.
- Esophageal irritation/ulcerations can occur if the capsule becomes lodged in the esophagus; advise patient to swallow a full glass of water with each tablet/capsule.
- Pseudotumor cerebri is a rare adverse effect. It is idiopathic intracranial hypertension (intracranial pressure [ICP] elevation).
- Avoid in pregnancy, infancy, and children aged 8 years or younger. It should be avoided during breastfeeding, if possible.

> **NOTES**
> - Do not use oral tetracycline for mild acne (open/close comedones). Start with OTC topicals such as salicylic acid (Noxzema, Stridex) and benzoyl peroxide.
> - For mild acne not responding to OTC drugs, try prescription topicals (benzoyl peroxide and erythromycin [Benzamycin]), tretinoin (Retin-A), or azelaic acid cream.
> - Consider adding tetracycline after 2 to 3 months if a patient with moderate inflammatory acne is not responding to topical prescriptions (Benzamycin, Retin-A, azelaic acid).
> - Another tetracycline option is minocycline (Minocin). It can cause vertigo (more common in females) that is dose related. It usually resolves in 1 to 2 days after discontinuation of the drug.
> - Tetracycline binds to some minerals (calcium, dairy products, iron, magnesium, zinc). It is best to take it on an empty stomach. Take 1 hour before or 2 hours after a meal.
> - Tetracyclines may decrease effectiveness of oral contraceptive pills.
> - Advise patients to throw away expired tetracycline pills (they degenerate and may cause nephropathy or Fanconi syndrome).

MACROLIDES

Macrolides are mainly bacteriostatic, but can be bactericidal with high concentrations. Allergic reactions to macrolides are less common than reactions to beta-lactam antibiotics, sulfonamides, and fluoroquinolones. Anaphylaxis (type I IgE reactions) are very rare. Erythromycin has a motilin-like effect and is used as short-term treatment of gastroparesis to improve gastric emptying. Can be used during pregnancy and lactation.

They cover gram-positive cocci (except enterococci), methicillin-susceptible *Staphylococcus aureus* (*Staphylococcus aureus* MSSA), *Streptococcus pyogenes*, and atypical bacteria (e.g., mycoplasma, chlamydia). Compared with other antibiotic drug classes, macrolides (and quinolones) are associated with more drug interactions (see Table 3.5). Both erythromycin and clarithromycin (Biaxin) are potent CYP34A inhibitors, but not azithromycin (which has fewer drug interactions). Most studies do not suggest fetal risk in pregnancy with the use of most macrolides, except telithromycin. Clarithromycin is considered low risk based on human data. Telithromycin should not be used in pregnancy.

- Erythromycin (Ery-Tab, EryPed, E.E.S., Ilosone) two to four times a day
- Azithromycin (Zithromax, Z-Pak) once a day
- Clarithromycin (Biaxin) twice a day

Adverse Effects

- GI distress (diarrhea, nausea, vomiting)
- Hepatotoxicity (risk cholestatic jaundice, hepatic failure with erythromycin estolate or ethylsuccinate)
- QT prolongation (risk of torsades de pointes); at risk if preexisting prolonged QT
- May exacerbate symptoms of myasthenia gravis.

> **NOTES**
> - Erythromycin's GI side effects are common (nausea, vomiting, abdominal pain, diarrhea).
> - Azithromycin is the most well-tolerated macrolide (rare GI effects).
> - Multiple drug interactions (e.g., anticoagulants, digoxin, theophylline, astemizole, carbamazepine, cisapride, triazolam, terfenadine, atorvastatin, simvastatin).
> - Ethanol may delay absorption of erythromycin.

CLINICAL PEARLS

- Advise patients to use only one pharmacy so that all the drugs they take are in one database. This makes it easier for the pharmacy to check for drug interactions.
- May prolong INR and increase risk of bleeding if warfarin is mixed with erythromycin or clarithromycin.

CEPHALOSPORINS (CATEGORY B)

Cephalosporins and penicillins belong to the beta-lactam family (Table 3.6). They contain a beta-lactam ring in their chemical structure. Beta-lactams are bactericidal and work by interfering with the cell wall synthesis of actively growing bacteria. Some bacteria are resistant to beta-lactams because they produce beta-lactamase, an enzyme that inactivates the beta-lactam ring (beta-lactam resistance). There are five generations of cephalosporins. However, as the nurse practitioner (NP) certification exams are about primary care conditions, only the first to the third generations are covered. Oral cephalosporins are used extensively in primary care. Ceftriaxone (Rocephin) is the most commonly used parenteral cephalosporin in primary care, and it can be used in pregnancy.

First-Generation Cephalosporins

- Activity against gram-positive cocci bacteria (e.g., group A *Streptococcus*/*Streptococcus pyogenes*, *S. aureus* MSSA, *S. pneumoniae*)
- Not effective against beta-lactamase-producing strains and MRSA

Table 3.6 Cephalosporins and Penicillins*

Drug Class and Generic/Trade Names	Indications
CEPHALOSPORINS	
First-generation Cephalexin (Keflex) PO QID	Skin: Uncomplicated skin and soft tissue infections (not caused by MRSA), impetigo Pregnancy: Urinary tract infection (if sensitive)

Second-generation
  Cefuroxime axetil (Ceftin) PO BID
  Cefprozil (Cefzil) PO BID
  Cefaclor (Ceclor) PO BID
	ENT: Rhinosinusitis, otitis media
	Lungs: CAP, exacerbation of chronic bronchitis
	Avoid using cefaclor, because it does not cover common pathogens

Third-generation
  Ceftriaxone (Rocephin) IM
  Cefixime (Suprax) daily to BID
  Cefdinir (Omnicef) daily to BID
	STIs: Gonorrhea infections, pelvic inflammatory disease
	Renal: Pyelonephritis
	ENT: Acute otitis media in children, acute rhinosinusitis, otitis media
	Genitourinary: Pyelonephritis
	Lungs: CAP

PENICILLINS	
Penicillin VK PO QID Amoxicillin BID to TID Amoxicillin plus clavulanic acid (Augmentin PO BID) Benzathine penicillin G IM Dicloxacillin PO QID	Strep throat, group A streptococcal pharyngitis Otitis media (first line), rhinosinusitis Otitis media/rhinosinusitis (first to second line) Cystitis if patient is susceptible Mastitis Syphilis (first line) Penicillinase-resistant penicillin; cellulitis (not caused by MRSA), impetigo, erysipelas

*List is not all-inclusive. Oral formulations are preferred in primary care.

BID, twice a day; CAP, community-acquired pneumonia; ENT, ear, nose, and throat; IM, intramuscular; MRSA, methicillin-resistant *Staphylococcus aureus*; PO, by mouth; QID, four times a day; STIs, sexually transmitted infections; TID, three times a day; VK, V potassium.

- Poor anaerobic coverage; risk of cross-reactivity if allergic to penicillin

Second-Generation Cephalosporins

- Considered to be "broad-spectrum" antibiotics; used to treat infections caused by both gram-positive cocci (*S. pneumoniae*) and gram-negative bacilli (e.g., *Haemophilus influenzae, Moraxella catarrhalis*), such as rhinosinusitis and otitis media.
- Slightly less active against gram-positive cocci than first-generation drugs

Third-Generation Cephalosporins

- Less effective against gram-positive infections compared with first-generation cephalosporins
- Better protection against enterobacteria and gram-negative bacteria (e.g., *H. influenzae, Escherichia coli, Proteus mirabilis*) compared with first- or second-generation cephalosporins

Adverse Effects

- Hypersensitivity reactions (most common)
- Clostridioides (formerly *Clostridium difficile* infection in adults)
- Leukopenia
- Thrombocytopenia

NOTES
- Ceftriaxone (Rocephin) 500 mg IM is first-line treatment for gonorrheal infections.
- Avoid ceftriaxone in hyperbilirubinemia and preterm infants because it can cause kernicterus.

- MRSA skin infections (boils, abscesses): Do not use cephalosporins. First-line therapy is trimethoprim–sulfamethoxazole (Bactrim DS) or clindamycin. Treat for at least 5 to 10 days.
- Patients who have a true allergy to penicillin (history of anaphylaxis, angioedema) are more likely to have an allergic reaction to cephalosporins (especially first generation).
- Anaphylaxis and angioedema are type 1 IgE-mediated reactions.
- As empiric therapy, third-generation cephalosporins include indications for CNS infections, including meningitis, as they can cross the blood–brain barrier; genitourinary tract infections; bone and joint infections; CAP; and skin and soft tissue infections.

PENICILLINS

Penicillins are bactericidal and directly kill bacteria. Amoxicillin and ampicillin are broad-spectrum penicillins. They are effective against gram-positive bacteria as well as some gram-negative bacteria (*H. influenzae, E. coli, P. mirabilis*). Some bacteria produce penicillinase and inactivate penicillins. They can be used in pregnancy and lactation. In general, resistance to penicillin has been increasing in recent years.

- Penicillin VK PO three to four times a day
- Amoxicillin PO two to three times a day
- Amoxicillin plus clavulanic acid (Augmentin) PO twice a day

- Benzathine penicillin G intramuscular
- Dicloxacillin PO four times a day

Adverse Reactions
- Diarrhea
- *C. difficile*-associated diarrhea (CDAD)
- Vaginitis (usually candida)
- Stevens–Johnson syndrome

NOTES
- Avoid using amoxicillin for patients with mononucleosis (causes a generalized rash not related to allergy); use penicillin VK instead (if not allergic). If penicillin allergy, use a macrolide antibiotic.
- Dicloxacillin is for penicillinase-producing staph skin infections (mastitis and impetigo).
- Patients who have a true allergy to penicillin (history of anaphylaxis, angioedema) are more likely to have an allergic reaction to cephalosporins (especially first-generation).
- Anaphylaxis and angioedema are type 1 IgE-mediated reactions.
- Some women will experience candida vaginitis with amoxicillin. Recommend taking probiotic capsules or eating yogurt daily. If needed, suggest use of OTC miconazole.

FLUOROQUINOLONES (QUINOLONES)

Quinolones are bactericidal (Table 3.7). They are effective agents that are effective against gram-negative bacteria and atypical bacteria (*Chlamydia, Mycoplasma, Legionella*). Newer generation quinolones (levofloxacin, moxifloxacin, gatifloxacin) are also active against gram-positive bacteria and have excellent activity against streptococcal pneumonia. They have high oral bioavailability, absorbed by the higher GI tract. They have several warnings; the FDA recommends to reserve use for severe infections (except for ophthalmic solutions).

- Fluoroquinolones: Ciprofloxacin (Cipro) PO twice a day, ofloxacin (Floxin) PO twice a day
- Broad-spectrum quinolones: Levofloxacin (Levaquin) PO daily, moxifloxacin (Avelox) PO daily, gemifloxacin (Factive) PO daily
- Ophthalmic formulations: Ciprofloxacin (Ciloxan ophthalmic), ofloxacin (Ocuflox ophthalmic), moxifloxacin (Vigamox ophthalmic). Dose: One or two drops instilled into the conjunctival sacs every 2 hours while awake for 2 days, then one or two drops every 4 hours while awake the next 5 days
- Serious side effects: Increased risk of Achilles tendon rupture: Increased risk if on steroids, >60 years, or history of organ transplant. Avoid strenuous activity while on the drug. Stop drug if tendon pain/swelling develops. In 2016, the FDA warned that the serious side effects associated with fluoroquinolones generally outweigh the benefits for patients with sinusitis, bronchitis, and uncomplicated urinary tract infections (UTIs) who have other treatment options. In 2018, the FDA warned of an increased incidence of aortic dissection with the use of quinolones. They should not be used unless there is no other choice in the elderly or patients with cardiovascular disease, history of aneurysm, and hypertension.
- Contraindications: Age younger than 18 years; myasthenia gravis; pregnancy; breastfeeding; elderly; history of cardiovascular disease, aneurysm, and hypertension

Drug Interactions

Avoid concomitant use of quinolones with other QT-prolonging drugs (amiodarone, macrolides, tricyclic antidepressants [TCAs], antipsychotics, others) or with electrolyte imbalance (hypomagnesemia, hypokalemia), because these will elevate the risk of sudden death from arrhythmias (torsades de pointes).

Coadministration of minerals and antacids (aluminum/magnesium/calcium) or sucralfate drastically reduces effectiveness of quinolones because of binding (inactivation).

Table 3.7 Quinolones*

Generic/Trade Names	Indications
Ciprofloxacin (*Cipro*) BID	Anthrax infection and prophylaxis, treat pseudomonal pneumonia in cystic fibrosis Traveler's diarrhea (severe) Malignant otitis externa in patients with diabetes
Ofloxacin (Floxin) BID	Urinary tract infections, pyelonephritis, epididymitis, prostatitis
Broad-spectrum quinolones Levofloxacin (Levaquin) daily Moxifloxacin (Avelox) daily Gemifloxacin (Factive) daily	Community-acquired pneumonia, acute exacerbation of chronic bronchitis, pyelonephritis, epididymitis, prostatitis Osteomyelitis, acute bacterial rhinosinusitis (if no other treatment options), exacerbation of chronic bronchitis Intra-abdominal infections, the plague (*Yersinia pestis*)
Topical formulations Floxin Otic (gtts) Ocuflox ophthalmic (gtts)	Otitis media with perforated tympanic membrane, otitis externa Bacterial conjunctivitis

*List is not all-inclusive. Reserve fluoroquinolones for serious infections.
BID, twice a day.
Source: U.S. Food and Drug Administration. (2018). (See Resources section for complete reference information.)

Adverse Effects

- Hypoglycemia (monitor blood glucose in type 1 diabetics)
- CNS effects (headache, dizziness, insomnia, memory impairment, delirium, seizures)
- QT prolongation, torsades de pointes
- Peripheral neuropathy (can occur at any time, can last for months to years)
- Phototoxicity (advise patients to avoid excessive sunlight or UV light)
- Double vision
- Tendinopathy, tendon rupture (higher risk if on steroids, >60 years, history of organ transplantation)
- Hepatotoxicity (may cause mild elevations of aspartate aminotransferase [AST] and alanine aminotransferase [ALT])

> **NOTES**
> - Achilles tendon rupture is a serious side effect of quinolone therapy, and patients who are on steroids or >60 years are at higher risk.
> - Do not use quinolones in children (<18 years) or women who are pregnant or breastfeeding because of adverse effects on growing cartilage.
> - If a patient on quinolone reports a new onset of difficulty in walking, order an ultrasound to rule out Achilles tendon rupture or peripheral neuropathy and discontinue the medicine.
> - Bioterrorism-related inhalation of anthrax spores (postexposure prophylaxis) is treated with ciprofloxacin 500 mg every 12 hours × 60 days (treat within 48 hours). In addition, a three-dose series of anthrax vaccine is recommended.
> - Cutaneous anthrax is treated with ciprofloxacin 500 mg twice a day × 7 to 10 days.
> - Traveler's diarrhea (severe) is treated with Cipro 750 mg (single dose) or 500 mg twice a day × 3 days.
> - Ciprofloxacin has the best activity against *Pseudomonas aeruginosa* (gram negative) and is the first-line drug for treating pseudomonal pneumonia for patients with cystic fibrosis.
> - For minor infections, use antibiotics other than quinolones. Careful with use in elderly or those with hypertension and vascular disease because of risk of aortic dissection.

CLINICAL PEARL

For athletes or very physically active patients, if fluoroquinolone is needed, advise to reduce their training volume and intensity to reduce risk of Achilles tendon injury. Wait from 2 to 4 weeks after completion of fluoroquinolones before resumption of sport or activity.

SULFONAMIDES

- Sulfonamides are bacteriostatic.
- Active against gram-negative bacteria (*E. coli*, *Klebsiella*, *H. influenzae*) and some gram-positive bacteria (e.g., MRSA)
- TMP-SMX (Bactrim DS) twice a day trimethoprim is teratogenic in the first trimester, causing neural tube and cardiovascular defects, based on animal and human data.

- Erythromycin–sulfisoxazole (Pediazole)
- Other sulfa-type drugs include:
  - Diuretics (furosemide, acetazolamide, HCTZ)
  - Sulfonylureas (e.g., glyburide, glipizide)
  - COX-2 inhibitor (celecoxib [Celebrex])
  - Dapsone (for HIV, leprosy, *Pneumocystis jirovecii* infection)
  - Sulfasalazine (for rheumatoid arthritis, Crohn's disease, ulcerative colitis)
  - Silver sulfadiazine
  - Sumatriptan (Imitrex)
  - Bismuth subsalicylate
  - Nitrofurantoin (use with caution in patients with sulfa allergy)
  - Sulfites to preserve foods (wines, balsamic vinegar, beverages, deli meats)
- Contraindications include:
  - Hypersensitivity or allergy to sulfa drugs
  - Glucose-6-phosphate dehydrogenase (G6PD) anemia (a genetic hemolytic anemia) causes hemolysis.
  - Newborns and infants <2 months of age (risk of hyperbilirubinemia)
  - Pregnancy 32 weeks or later (increased risk of hyperbilirubinemia, kernicterus, hemolytic anemia in the infant)
  - Porphyria (genetic disease)

Drug Interactions

- Warfarin (increases INR)
- Astemizole (Hismanal)
- Others

Adverse Effects

- Fever and nonblistering morbilliform rash
- Stevens–Johnson syndrome

> **NOTES**
> - Patients with a UTI who are on warfarin (Coumadin) should not be given TMP-SMX (increased risk of bleeding). Monitor INR closely.
> - Pregnant patients (or suspected pregnancy) with a UTI can be treated with beta-lactams, nitrofurantoin, and fosfomycin.

CLINICAL PEARLS

- HIV patients are at high risk (25%–50%) for sulfa-related Stevens–Johnson syndrome.
- In the United States, the typical G6PD deficiency anemia patient is a person of African American descent. This patient is usually asymptomatic, but may present with hemolysis/jaundice secondary to being treated with a sulfa drug or after eating fava beans. Look for a low hemoglobin and hematocrit (H&H) and jaundice. G6PD anemia is also seen with Mediterranean ancestry.
- Sulfonamide antibiotics are the second most frequent cause of allergic drug reactions (penicillins and cephalosporins are the first).

LINCOSAMIDES

- Clindamycin is a lincosamide antibiotic that is bacteriostatic, but it is also bactericidal with some strains of bacteria.
- It is approved for treatment of streptococcal, staphylococcal, and anaerobic infections.
- It is an alternative for penicillin-allergic persons who have a gram-positive infection such as strep throat or cellulitis.
- Higher risk of clostridioides (formerly known as *C. difficile colitis*). From 0.1% to 10% of patients on clindamycin develop severe or life-threatening *C. difficile* infection.
- The most common adverse effect is diarrhea, which can occur in 2% to 20% of patients. It is usually mild and will resolve when the drug is discontinued.
- Clindamycin should be used with caution in patients who are receiving neuromuscular-blocking agents.
- Indications: Infections of the skin, skin structure, bone/joints, lower respiratory tract infections, intra-abdominal infections, sepsis, bacterial vaginosis (clindamycin in oral or vaginal cream form).

Adverse Effects

- Diarrhea
- Maculopapular rash (up to 10% of patients), including Stevens–Johnson syndrome
- Thrombophlebitis (with IV administration)

Drug and Herbal Interactions

Strong inducers of cytochrome P450 (3A) will interact, such as carbamazepine, phenytoin, rifampin/rifampicin, modafinil, St. John's wort.

OVER-THE-COUNTER DRUGS AND HERBS

TOPICAL NASAL DECONGESTANTS

Oxymetazoline Nasal Spray (Afrin) and Phenylephrine (Neo-Synephrine)

- Short-term use of topical nasal decongestants (twice a day as needed × 3 days) is considered safe treatment for nasal congestion (common cold, allergic rhinitis).
- Rhinitis medicamentosa is due to chronic use (>3 days) of nasal decongestants.

ANTIHISTAMINES (HISTAMINE ANTAGONIST OR H1 BLOCKER)

Diphenhydramine (Benadryl), Loratadine (Claritin), Cetirizine (Zyrtec), Fexofenadine (Allegra), Doxylamine (Unisom), and Chlorpheniramine (ChlorTrimeton)

- Avoid using diphenhydramine (Benadryl), cetirizine (Zyrtec), and doxylamine (Unisom) in the elderly, if possible.
- For elderly patients, use loratadine (Claritin) because it has a lower incidence of sedation.
- Cetirizine (Zyrtec) is more potent and long acting. It is very effective for acute and chronic urticaria.

Topical Antihistamines

- Nasal sprays for allergic rhinitis, seasonal allergic rhinitis, vasomotor rhinitis
- Azelastine (Astelin) nasal spray

Ophthalmic Drops

- Pruritus from allergic conjunctivitis
- Azelastine hydrochloride ophthalmic solution 0.5%

COLD, COUGH, AND/OR SINUS MEDICINES

Decongestants

- Pseudoephedrine (Sudafed) and phenylephrine
- The Combat Methamphetamine Epidemic Act passed in 2005 restricts the amount of pseudoephedrine you can buy.

Antitussives

- Dextromethorphan (Robitussin, Delsym) and benzonatate (Tessalon)
- Dextromethorphan increases risk of serotonin syndrome (major drug interaction) with monoamine oxidase inhibitors (MAOIs), selegiline (Eldepryl), SSRIs, and SNRIs
- Benzonatate can be sedating and should not be used in patients younger than 10 years
- Benzonatate is often overused due to psychoactive effects

Mucolytics

Guaifenesin and water (hydration)

CLINICAL PEARLS

- Decongestants (stimulants) are contraindicated with hypertension and coronary artery disease (CAD; angina, MI).
- Advise patients that mixing decongestants with other stimulants (caffeine, methylphenidate [Ritalin], albuterol inhaler) will cause heart palpitations, tremors, and anxiety.

NONSTEROIDAL ANTI-INFLAMMATORY DRUGS

OVER-THE-COUNTER NONSTEROIDAL ANTI-INFLAMMATORY DRUGS

- Ibuprofen (Advil, Motrin), naproxen sodium (Aleve)
- Ibuprofen available by prescription in 600-mg and 800-mg dosages

PRESCRIPTION NONSTEROIDAL ANTI-INFLAMMATORY DRUGS

- Naproxen (Naprosyn, Anaprox), diclofenac (Voltaren) oral and topical gel
- Indomethacin (Indocin), ketoprofen (Orudis), ketorolac (Toradol), etodolac (Lodine), mefenamic acid (Ponstel), diflunisal (Dolobid), nabumetone (Relafen)
- COX-2 inhibitors Celecoxib (Celebrex)
- Meloxicam (Mobic)

TOPICAL NONSTEROIDAL ANTI-INFLAMMATORY DRUGS

- Diclofenac gel 1% (Voltaren Gel), diclofenac solution 1.5% (Pennsaid), patch 1.3% (Flector)
- Skin topical for joint pain (knees, hands) from osteoarthritis/degenerative joint disease (DJD)

OPHTHALMIC NONSTEROIDAL ANTI-INFLAMMATORY DRUGS

- Seasonal allergic conjunctivitis (for itch), eye pain after cataract surgery
- Ketorolac ophthalmic (Acular), diclofenac sodium (Voltaren ophthalmic)

NONSTEROIDAL ANTI-INFLAMMATORY DRUG WARNINGS

- NSAIDs should be avoided in HF, severe heart disease, GI bleeding, and severe renal disease and during the last 3 months of pregnancy (blocks prostaglandins).
- Patients with nasal polyps and asthma can be sensitive to aspirin/NSAIDs.
- Ketorolac (Toradol) is for short-term use only (up to 5 days) per episode. First dose given intramuscular or IV, then continue orally.
- Ketorolac should not be used before surgery, with concurrent acetylsalicylic acid (ASA), in pediatric patients, in those at high risk of bleeding, or in those with active or recent GI bleed, peptic ulcer disease, suspected or confirmed cerebrovascular bleed, hemorrhagic diathesis, incomplete hemostasis, stroke, labor/delivery, and others.
- For long-term use of NSAIDs, document informed consent such as the higher risk of serious MI, stroke, emboli, GI bleeds, and acute renal failure.
- COX-2 inhibitors (celecoxib) have lower risk of GI bleeding compared with the other NSAIDs. They are not a first-line NSAID, except for patients at high risk for GI bleeding.
- Increased risk of bleeding if NSAIDs are combined with warfarin, dabigatran (Pradaxa), steroids, aspirin, alcohol, and some alternative herbs (ginkgo biloba). For long-term use, consider prescribing concurrent proton-pump inhibitors (PPIs), H_2 antagonists, or misoprostol (Cytotec). Cytotec is a synthetic prostaglandin.
- Avoid long-term use of NSAIDs if patient is on aspirin prophylaxis (interferes with aspirin's cardioprotective effect and increases risk of GI bleed).
- NSAIDs may worsen hypertension in patients who were previously well controlled.

EXAM TIP

Maximum amount of time that ketorolac (Toradol) can be used is 5 days.

SALICYLATES

- Aspirin (Bayer) 325 mg to 650 mg every 4 to 6 hours as needed
- Aspirin controlled/extended/delayed-release (enteric-coated): 650 to 1,300 mg every 8 hours (do not exceed 3.9 g/d)
  - Acute coronary syndrome: 160 to 325 mg orally; chew nonenteric-coated tablet as soon as possible (within minutes of symptoms)
  - Secondary prevention (MI, stroke): 75 to 81 mg orally daily (up to 325 mg/d)
  - Aspirin 845 mg with caffeine (BC Powder): One powder sublingually every 6 hours as needed; drink or mix powder with full glass of water
- Topical therapy of methyl salicylate and menthol (BEN-GAY gel/cream)
- Nonacetylated salicylates are salsalate (Disalcid), nabumetone (Relafen)
- For thromboembolic stroke, take immediate-release aspirin
- Do not take aspirin under the age of 12 years (Reye's syndrome)

EXAM TIPS

- Aspirin irreversibly suppresses platelet function for up to 4 days (because of irreversible acetylation). Life span of platelets is about 10 days.
- Discontinue ASA if patient complains of tinnitus (possible aspirin toxicity).

CAPSAICIN

- Capsaicin topical cream (Zostrix HP), capsaicin patch
- For temporary relief of muscle and joint pain (arthritis, sprains/strains, bruises) and neuropathic pain (postherpetic neuralgia [PHN], trigeminal neuralgia)
- May take up to 4 weeks to work; may cause temporary burning sensation; do not use on broken skin; advise patient to wash hands with soap and water immediately after using capsaicin cream and to avoid touching the eyes, nose, mouth, and genitals.

EXAM TIP

Capsaicin cream can be used to treat pain in trigeminal neuralgia and PHN.

ACETAMINOPHEN (TYLENOL)

- Adults and children ≥12 years of age; maximum dose ranges from 3,000 mg (3 g) to 3,250 mg/d or 3,900/day (almost 4 g/d)
- Considered first-line drug for pain from osteoarthritis/DJD
- For regular-strength Tylenol (325 mg), take two tablets every 4 to 6 hours as needed; do not take more than 10 tablets in 24 hours (maximum dose is 3,250 mg in 24 hours).
- For extra-strength Tylenol (500 mg each), take two caplets every 6 hours as needed; do not take more than six caplets in 24 hours (maximum dose 3,000 mg [3 g] in 24 hours).
- For extended-release Tylenol (8 hour; 650 mg each), take two caplets every 8 hours as needed; do not take more than six caplets in 24 hours (maximum dose is 3,900 mg [3.9 g] in 24 hours).

- Do not use for more than 10 days unless directed by health provider.
- Avoid if chronic hepatitis B/C/D, dehydration, liver disease, cirrhosis, heavy drinker
- Antidote for overdose is acetylcysteine (Mucomyst)
- Risk of severe liver damage if intake of three or more alcoholic drinks per day while using medication

EXAM TIP

The maximum dose for acetaminophen (Tylenol) ranges from 3 to 4 g/d.

IMMUNE SYSTEM DRUGS

GLUCOCORTICOIDS (STEROIDS)

- Oral or systemic corticosteroids are adjunct treatment for rheumatoid arthritis, lupus, other autoimmune disorders, anaphylaxis, and septic shock.
- Oral corticosteroids are first-line treatment of polymyalgia rheumatica (dramatic relief of symptoms) and temporal arteritis/giant cell arteritis, emergent conditions that require immediate treatment with high-dose corticosteroids.
- Inhaled corticosteroids are first-line treatment for asthma; short-term burst of oral steroids are used to treat exacerbations.
- If uveitis (inflammation of the middle portion of the eye) is suspected, refer to ED. Ideally it should be treated within 24 hours to reduce risk of blindness. It is a complication of autoimmune diseases such as rheumatoid arthritis, lupus, and polymyalgia rheumatica. Treated with topical steroid eye drops and/or systemic steroids.
- Topical steroids are first-line or adjunct treatment for some inflammatory skin diseases or acute cases of dermatitis such as contact dermatitis.

Systemic/Oral Steroids

- Prednisone 40 to 60 mg/day (high dose) for 3 to 4 days; can be used for short-term treatment (e.g., asthma exacerbation); there is no need to taper if patient is not on chronic steroids (oral or inhalation)
- Methylprednisolone (Medrol Dose Pack) × 7 days; does not need to be weaned
- For infants and children 2 years and younger, 20 mg/day; children 3 to 5 years: 30 mg/day; children 6 to 11 years: 40 mg/day; children 12 years and older and adolescents: oral: 1 mg/kg/day for 5 to 7 days; maximum daily dose: 50 mg/day

Topical Steroids

- Classification: Group 1 (superpotent) to Group 7 (least potent):
  - Superpotent (Group 1): Clobetasol (Temovate), halobetasol propionate (Ultravate)
  - High potency (Group 2): Halcinonide (Halog)
  - High potency (Group 3): Mometasone furoate (Elocon)
  - Medium potency (Group 4): Hydrocortisone valerate ointment (Westcort)
  - Lower-mid potency (Group 5): Desonide gel (Desonate)

- Low potency (Group 6): Alclometasone dipropionate (Aclovate)
- Least potent (Class 7): Hydrocortisone base <2% (Cortaid, Cortizone 10)
- The formulation (vehicle) helps to determine the absorption, dose, and potency; ointments are usually more potent than creams and lotions; gels are alcohol-based and can cause a burning sensation in abraded skin; solutions and foams work well in scalps.
- For thickest skin on palms and soles (superpotent to high potency)
- For medium-thickness nonfacial and nonintertriginous skin (medium to high potency)
- For thinnest skin on eyelids and genitals (low potency for limited time periods); if the lesion is in the eye area (around eye or eyelids), it can leach into the eyes and cause secondary glaucoma.
- The larger the area of skin treated, the higher the risk of systemic absorption

Side Effects of Glucocorticoids/Steroids (Chronic Use)

- Hypothalamic–pituitary–adrenal (HPA) axis suppression
- Secondary Cushing's disease (e.g., dorsal hump, rounded face)
- Osteoporosis (advise weight-bearing exercises, vitamin D, calcium 1,200 mg/d, bisphosphonates)
- Immunosuppression (increased risk of infection)
- Skin changes from long-term topical therapy (skin atrophy, striae, telangiectasia, acne, pigmentation changes)

NOTES

- Use low-potency steroids for the face, intertriginous areas, and genitals (thinner skin). Example: Use hydrocortisone cream/ointment/lotions 0.5% to 1% (OTC) to prescription strength such as hydrocortisone 2.5% (Hytone Rx).
- Avoid topical steroids around the eye area and/or eyelids. They can leach into the eye and cause secondary glaucoma (and blindness) in susceptible individuals. Refer to dermatologist.
- Use moderate- to high-potency steroids for thicker skin (scalp, soles of feet, palms of the hands) or for plaques (psoriasis). Taper potent-strength topical steroids (or will rebound).
- If higher potency steroids are necessary, refer to dermatologist, since at high risk of suppression of the HPA axis.
- Infants and young children have thinner stratum corneum than adults, so they absorb topical steroids very well, which increases risk of adverse effects.
- What is occlusion? Thick, resistant psoriatic plaques are sometimes treated by using occlusion (increases absorption 10-fold). Topical steroid is applied to the plaque and covered with dressing or plastic wrap. Ultrapotent steroids (e.g., Temovate) should not be occluded for more than 2 weeks (risk of HPA suppression).

CLINICAL PEARLS

- A severe case of poison ivy or poison oak rash may require 14 to 21 days of an oral steroid to clear.
- The most common cause of acute liver failure in the United States is acetaminophen overdose. Poison Control Center: 1-800-222-1222.

OTHER DRUGS AND SAFETY ISSUES

DRUGS THAT REQUIRE EYE EXAMINATION

Patients taking the following drugs require careful monitoring of vision because of adverse effects. Ensure that the patient has a baseline eye examination (fundi, vision). Ask about visual symptoms (more floaters, blurred vision, decreased vision, sudden visual changes). Regular eye exams by an ophthalmologist are required.

- Digoxin (yellow-to-green vision, blurred vision, halos if blood level too high)
- Ethambutol and linezolid (optic neuropathy)
- Corticosteroids (cataracts, glaucoma, optic neuritis)
- Fluoroquinolones (retinal detachment)
- Phosphodiesterase 5 (PDE5) inhibitors (cataracts, blurred vision, ischemic optic neuropathy, others)
- Isotretinoin (cataracts, decreased night vision, others)
- Topiramate (acute angle-closure glaucoma, increased ICP, mydriasis)
- Hydroxychloroquine (neuropathy; permanent loss of vision)

CISAPRIDE (PROPULSID)

- Available only by limited-access protocol in the United States
- Numerous drug contraindications (e.g., macrolides, antifungals, TCAs)
- Boxed warning for serious cardiac arrhythmias (ventricular fibrillation/tachycardia, torsades de pointes, prolongation of QT interval); check 12-lead EKG at baseline; check serum electrolytes and creatinine

THEOPHYLLINE DRUG INTERACTIONS

- Theophylline level (adults): 5 to 15 mcg/mL
- Drug interactions: Cimetidine, alprazolam, macrolides, fluvoxamine, others; avoid combining with other stimulants (theophylline, pseudoephedrine, caffeine, Ritalin)
- Disorders worsened by stimulants: Hypertension, arrhythmias, heart disease, stroke, seizures
- BPH: Causes urinary retention, worsening of symptoms (due to spasm of sphincters)
- Suspect toxicity: If persistent vomiting

AVOID ABRUPT DISCONTINUATION (TAPERING NEEDED)

Certain drugs that are used long term need to be tapered over 2 to 4 weeks or longer (Table 3.8). Abrupt discontinuation may cause seizures, headache, severe anxiety, chills, or other adverse effects.

FDA CATEGORY CLASSIFICATIONS

A new FDA Pregnancy and Lactation Labeling Rule (PLLR) went into effect on June 30, 2015. It replaced the pregnancy letter categories A, B, C, D, and X. The new labeling categories are Pregnancy, Lactation, and Females and Males of Reproductive Potential. Prescription drugs and biologics approved after June 30, 2015, used the new format immediately. Drugs/biologics approved on or after June 30, 2001, will be phased in gradually. Drugs approved prior to June 29, 2001, are not subject to the PLLR rule, but the pregnancy letter category must be removed by June 29, 2018. OTC drugs are not subject to this rule.

- Pregnancy: Includes labor and delivery; it will include information about potential risks to the developing fetus.
- Lactation: Includes drugs that should not be used during breastfeeding as well as the clinical effects on the infant. It may have information about the timing of breastfeeding to minimize infant exposure.

Table 3.8 Avoid Abrupt Discontinuation: Withdrawal Symptoms*

Drug Name or Class (Brand Name)	Withdrawal Symptoms
Venlafaxine (Effexor)	Sweating, agitation, dizziness, nausea, fatigue, tremor, restlessness
Paroxetine (Paxil)	Nausea, vomiting, diarrhea, headaches, vivid dreams, insomnia
Gabapentin (Neurontin)	Agitation, confusion, disorientation, sweating, insomnia, GI effects
Steriods (long term)	Weakness, severe fatigue, nausea, vomiting, anorexia, diarrhea
Baclofen (Lioresal)	Muscle cramps/spasms, rigidity, confusion, seizures, psychotic mania/paranoid states
Clonidine (Catapres)	Acute rebound hypertension, sudden death
Propranolol (Inderal)	Acute rebound hypertension, angina, MI, or sudden death
Benzodiazepines	Seizures, anxiety, insomnia
Opioids	Pain, anxiety, restlessness, diarrhea
SSRIs, SNRIs, atypical antipsychotics	Dizziness, nausea, headaches, irritability, anxiety, insomnia, and flu-like symptoms; should not be stopped abruptly

*List is not all-inclusive.

GI, gastrointestinal; MI, myocardial infarction; SNRI, serotonin and norepinephrine reuptake inhibitor; SSRI, selective serotonin reuptake inhibitor.

- Females and males of reproductive potential: Includes information on the drug's effect on fertility, pregnancy testing/loss (if available), and birth control.

LIST OF DRUGS TO AVOID DURING PREGNANCY

These drugs pose fetal risks that outweigh the medication's benefits:

- Finasteride (Proscar, Propecia); reproductive-aged or pregnant patients should not handle crushed/broken finasteride tablets
- Risperidone (Risperdal)
- Isotretinoin (Amnesteem)
- Warfarin sodium (Coumadin)
- Misoprostol (Cytotec)
- Androgenic hormones including combined hormonal contraceptives (pills and patches), hormone replacement therapy (HRT), testosterone
- Live virus vaccines (measles, mumps, rubella, varicella, rotavirus, FluMist)
- Folate antagonists
- Antiepileptics (except for lamotrigine and levetiracetam)
- ACEI/ARBs
- Thalidomide, diethylstilbestrol (DES), methimazole, and so on

U.S. DRUG ENFORCEMENT AGENCY

CONTROLLED SUBSTANCES ACT

- Schedule I drugs (e.g., heroin, ecstasy/MDMA, phencyclidine [PCP]) are illegal to prescribe; no currently accepted medical use; high abuse potential (Table 3.9)

- Schedule II drugs (e.g., Demerol, Dilaudid, OxyContin, cocaine, amphetamines, fentanyl)
  - Only the original prescription with the prescriber's signature (not stamped) is acceptable.
  - The total number of pills must be indicated. Write the date clearly (important); it will expire in 6 months automatically.
  - If the medication is to be taken regularly, then a new prescription is written every month because Schedule II medications cannot be refilled on the same script. For example, a patient with attention deficit hyperactivity disorder (ADHD) who is on methylphenidate (Ritalin) daily needs a new paper prescription every month. Some states now accept electronic prescribing for Schedule II drugs. Make sure the date is written clearly.
- Schedule III drugs (e.g., Tylenol with codeine, Vicodin, anabolic steroids, testosterone)
- Schedule IV drugs (e.g., benzodiazepines, Ambien, Lunesta, Soma)
- Schedule V drugs (cough medicines with <200 mg of codeine, Lomotil, Lyrica)
- Schedule III to V medications can be prescribed by verbal order over the phone, by paper prescription, or by electronic prescribing of controlled substances (EPCS).
- Rules vary by state regarding controlled substance prescriptions and the NP. Some states require that the NP must have a collaborative agreement with a physician in order to write prescriptions. The best resource is to check your state board of nursing (SBON) website.
- For all controlled substances, must have the prescriber's Drug Enforcement Agency (DEA) number with the clinic address on the pad; it cannot be predated or postdated.

Table 3.9 Common Drugs of Abuse

Drug Name	Alternate Names	Drug Effect	Notes
Cannabis	Marijuana, hash, hashish	Euphoria ("high"), more sociable, increased appetite, and slurred speech Ataxia, nystagmus, conjunctival infection (red eyes), and dilated pupils (mydriasis) Lowers sperm count; increases heart rate and BP Psychomotor effects last 12 to 24 hours	Recreational and/or medical use of marijuana is allowed in some states (e.g., Marinol).
Prescription opioids	Fentanyl, oxycodone, meperidine, hydromorphone, amphetamines	Euphoria, drowsiness, slowed breathing, pupil constriction (miosis) Overdose or combining with alcohol may cause respiratory depression, coma, death	Naltrexone can reverse effects
Dextromethorphan	Robo, robo-trip, triple C	Euphoria, slurred speech, tachycardia, possibly elevated BP and temperature, seizures, paranoia, confusion	Obtained from OTC cough and cold medications
Cocaine	Coke, crack, rock	Happy, mental alertness, paranoia, decreased appetite, insomnia, nosebleeds Pupil dilations (mydriasis), tachycardia, hypertension, angina/MI, strokes, seizures May cause midline nasal septum perforation and/or ulceration with intranasal chronic use	
Methamphetamine	Meth, crystal meth, ice, methylphenidate	Chronic use results in bruxism and severe dental caries with loss of front teeth on the upper jaw Anorexia results in drastic weight loss; pupils appear constricted	

BP, blood pressure; MI, myocardial infarction; OTC, over the counter.

PRESCRIPTION PADS

Tamper-resistant prescription pads/paper is required. If a prescription goes directly to the pharmacy (electronically, by fax, or by telephone), it does not have to be on tamper-resistant paper. It should contain the following information:

- Practitioner's name/designation/license number/ National Practitioner Identification (NPI) number
- Supervising or collaborating physician's name/designation if required
- Clinic address (if multiple sites, the sites where the NP works should be listed on the pad) and phone number(s)
- Prescription pads are ordered by the office staff; print your name, degree, designations, NPI, and/or license number on a piece of paper so that they can order you your own prescription pad

WRITING A PRESCRIPTION

- Date, patient's name, and another identifier, such as the date of birth (DOB).
- Drug name and dosage, then the route (e.g., by mouth), frequency (e.g., daily), and duration, if needed (e.g., antibiotics).
- The pharmacy automatically uses generics (if available) to fill most prescriptions. If you want a brand name to be used and do not want generic substitutions, write *no generics* on the pad.
- Write the quantity in both number and word [e.g., #30 (thirty)] and number of refills (e.g., one).
- For controlled drugs, a DEA number *must* be on the script (NPs or supervising physicians).

- For FDA Schedule II drugs, the script must be handwritten or typed on a tamper-resistant prescription paper and manually signed.
  - Schedule II drug prescriptions cannot be called in to the pharmacy. They cannot be refilled. If the patient needs the drug daily (e.g., Ritalin), then a traditional paper prescription is written every month.
  - Schedule III to V medications can be prescribed by traditional paper prescription, by verbal order over the phone, or by using the EPCS system.
- Sign prescription with your specialty initials and certification (e.g., FNP-BC) and NPI/license number (if it is not printed on your prescription pad).
- Example: How should this prescription be written (Figure 3.2)?
  - Name and DOB
  - Colace 100 mg
  - One tablet by mouth at bedtime
  - Dispense: #30 (thirty)
  - Dx: Constipation
  - Refills: None

E-PRESCRIBING

The process of sending and receiving prescriptions by electronic means. Preferred method for drug prescriptions for Medicare, Medicaid, health maintenance organizations (HMOs), and others. Clinicians write the prescription in their offices on a laptop computer or tablet using e-prescribing software. The formulary (approved medications by the health plan) is included, which makes it easier to choose the appropriate drug.

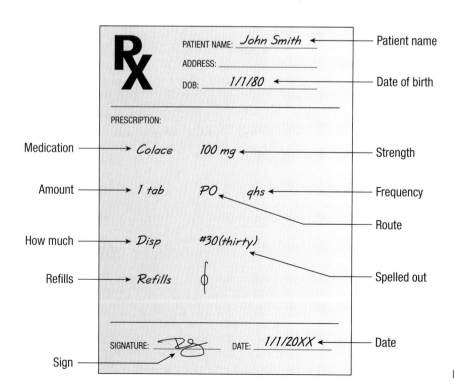

Figure 3.2 Example prescription.

THE "FIVE RIGHTS"

There are "five rights" that help to prevent or decrease the chances of a medical error:

1. Right patient
2. Right drug
3. Right dose
4. Right time
5. Right route

DRUG FORMULARIES

Medicare, Medicaid, HMOs, and other health plans have a list of preferred drugs in their formulary, which can be accessed easily through electronic prescribing. These are the drugs that will be paid in full (allowed drugs). Most generic drugs are on this list of allowed drugs. Some brand-name and newer drugs may not be paid in full, and the patient will have a higher co-pay or out-of-pocket expense. Discuss cost issues with the patient; if they cannot afford it, they will probably not take the drug. Some drug companies have special programs for high-cost or new drugs; advise the patient to check the website of the drug company.

CLINICAL PEARLS

- Maximum number of refills for Schedule III to V drugs is five refills (limit of 90 pills per refill).
- Schedule II drugs have zero refills, and maximum quantity dispensed is for 30 days only. It cannot be called in by phone. It has to be written on a traditional paper prescription pad (some states now accept electronic prescriptions). Prescription will automatically expire in 6 months.

COMPLEMENTARY AND ALTERNATIVE MEDICINE

Conventional medicine (or allopathic medicine) is also known as *modern medicine* or *Western medicine*. *Complementary and alternative medicine (CAM)* is the term for medical practices and products that are not part of standard medical care. Herbals are also called botanical medicine or phytomedicine. Examples include herbal supplements, probiotics, chiropractic, homeopathy, meditation, yoga, massage therapy, essential oils, tai chi, cupping, coining, sound/light therapy, acupuncture, acupressure. *Integrative medicine* is a total approach to medical care (mind, body, and spirit) that combines standard medicine with CAM practices that have been shown to be safe and effective.

HERBAL SUPPLEMENTS

- Echinachea (purple coneflower): Used to shorten duration of common cold or flu; avoid if history of autoimmune disease or allergic to ragweed (may cause anaphylaxis)
- Feverfew or butterbur: Migraine headache
- Cinnamon: Improves blood sugar (diabetes) and cholesterol
- Glucosamine (with/without chondroitin): Osteoarthritis
- Ginkgo biloba: Dementia, memory problems, tinnitus; affects blood-clotting; stop taking 2 weeks before surgery (including dental procedures); NSAIDs will increase risk of bleeding.
- Natural progesterone cream or sublingual capsules (from Mexican wild yam or soybeans): Premenstrual symptoms and menopausal symptoms such as hot flashes; no research on safety with long-term use
- Isoflavones (from soybeans): Estrogen-like effects
- Saw palmetto: Urinary symptoms of BPH
- Kava kava, valerian root: Anxiety and insomnia; do not mix kava kava with CNS drugs, since it will worsen the sedative effect.
- St. John's wort: Mild depression; do not use with SSRIs, sumatriptan, HIV protease inhibitors (indinavir), others.
- Turmeric: Alzheimer's disease, arthritis, cancer
- Fish or krill oil, omega-3 oil: Heart disease, high cholesterol, arthritis/joint pain (reduces inflammation)

HOMEOPATHY

The founder is the physician Samuel Hahnemann (1755–1843). This healing system is based on the "Law of Similars" or "Let likes be cured by likes."

- What is the Homeopathic Pharmacopoeia of the United States? It is a list of approved homeopathic substances used in this country.
- How are homeopathic substances made? Extremely small amounts of a substance are diluted (ultradilution). For example, the herb *Arnica montana*, which is used to treat pain and muscle aches and prevent or treat bruises, can be diluted 30 times (e.g., *A. montana* 30× dilution).

AYURVEDA

An ancient healing system from India. Food, spices, herbs, yoga, and lifestyle are believed to prevent and treat disease or injury. For example, turmeric powder is used to treat cuts and abrasions.

KNOWLEDGE CHECK: CHAPTER 3

1. Pharmacogenomics is the study of:
   A. How genes affect the ability to respond to medications
   B. How medications move through the body
   C. How medications are used in a population
   D. How medications are distributed throughout the body

2. Pharmacokinetics is the study of:
   A. How a population metabolizes a medication
   B. What type of response a person will have to a medication
   C. How a medication is metabolized in a person
   D. How a person's genes may alter a medication's response

3. Which of the following *best* describes the term *half-life*?
   A. The amount of time it takes to clear a medication from the body
   B. The time it takes for a medication to achieve its peak effect
   C. The amount of time it takes for a medication to achieve its peak concentration
   D. The time it takes for a medication to decrease its concentration by 50%

4. Which of the following *best* describes minimum inhibitory concentration?
   A. Lowest concentration of an antibiotic necessary to inhibit bacterial growth
   B. Lowest concentration of a medication needed to achieve a response
   C. Lowest concentration of a medication necessary to inhibit undesirable side effects
   D. Lowest concentration of a medication needed to inhibit first-pass metabolism

5. Which of the following *best* describes the concept of the area under the curve (AUC)? It is a measure of:
   A. How a medication is metabolized after oral ingestion
   B. How medications are cleared from the body
   C. The effect of a medication on the body
   D. The bioavailability of a medication

6. Which of the following *best* describes the concept of bioavailability?
   A. Tolerability of a medication to be given orally
   B. Way a medication is absorbed and used by the body
   C. Amount of drug necessary to achieve peak effect
   D. Way genes affect the metabolism of a medication

7. Which of the following is/are the main organ/s of biotransformation?
   A. Kidneys
   B. Small intestines
   C. Large intestines
   D. Liver

8. Which of the following *best* describes the concept of first-pass metabolism?
   A. Medications administered orally must first be metabolized in the liver.
   B. Medications given sublingually must first be metabolized in the small intestines.
   C. Medications given intramuscularly must first pass from intestine to liver before reaching general circulation.
   D. Medications given intravenously must first be metabolized in the liver.

9. Which of the following *best* describes a CYP450 inducer?
   A. An additive to a medication to increase its absorption
   B. A medication that increases the clearance of other medications
   C. A medication that decreases the clearance of other medications
   D. An additive to a medication to decrease the first-pass effect

10. Which of the following *best* describes a CYP450 inhibitor?
    A. A medication that decreases the clearance of other medications
    B. A medication that prevents the degradation of its chemical compound
    C. An additive to a medication that turns off the CYP450 system
    D. An additive to a medication that upregulates the CYP450 system

(See answers next page.)

1. A) How genes affect the ability to respond to medications

Pharmacogenomics studies how a person's genes affect the way in which a drug will affect the person.

2. C) How a medication is metabolized in a person

Pharmacokinetics includes the study of how a medication is metabolized in an individual.

3. D) The time it takes for a medication to decrease by 50%

The half-life is how much time it takes a medication to decrease its concentration in the body by 50%.

4. A) Lowest concentration of an antibiotic necessary to inhibit bacterial growth

The minimum inhibitory concentration is the lowest concentration of an antibiotic needed to inhibit bacterial growth after overnight incubation. Although the lowest concentration of a medication needed to achieve a response is a goal when prescribing medications, it is not the definition of minimum inhibitory concentration. It is also not defined by the lowest concentration needed to inhibit undesirable effects or the first-pass metabolism.

5. D) The bioavailability of a medication

The AUC is the average amount of a drug in the blood after a dose is given. It is the measure of the bioavailability of a drug after it is administered. The cytochrome P450 system is responsible for the biotransformation (metabolism) of the drug, and renal filtration accounts for most of drug excretion and clearance. The AUC is not a measure of the effect of a medication on the body.

6. B) Way a medication is absorbed and used by the body

Bioavailability refers to the amount of the drug that arrives in systemic circulation and depends on the properties of the substance and the mode of administration. It provides information as to how the body metabolizes the medication. The maximum concentration is the peak serum concentration of a drug. While genetic variants of the CYP450 system and receptors can alter how an individual's body breaks down and reacts to a drug, this concept is not referred to as bioavailability. Drug tolerability refers to the degree to which adverse effects can be tolerated by patients.

7. D) Liver

The main organ of biotransformation of drugs is the liver. The CYP450 enzyme system is the most active; the CYP enzymes are found in the liver, intestines, and kidneys, but the highest concentration is the liver. The other organ systems involved in drug metabolism are the lungs, plasma, and skin.

8. A) Medications administered orally must first be metabolized in the liver.

All oral drugs (except sublingual drugs) must go through first-pass metabolism before they can be released and used by the body. The first-pass effect is a concept used to describe when a drug is metabolized at a specific location in the body, resulting in a reduced concentration of the active drug that is able to reach its site of action (or the systemic circulation). While it's often associated with the liver, first-pass metabolism can also occur in the gastrointestinal tract, lungs, vasculature, and other tissues in the body. Drugs that are administered orally (compared to intravenously, intramuscularly, sublingually, or transdermally) undergo the first-pass effect.

9. B) A medication that increases the clearance of other medications

A CYP450 inducer is a medication that increases the clearance of other drugs, resulting in the potential for drug-drug interactions because it increases drug metabolism. A CYP450 inhibitor can slow down drug metabolism, which decreases the clearance of other medications. A CYP450 inducer is not an additive to a medication and does not decrease the first-pass effect.

10. A) A medication that decreases the clearance of other medications

A CYP450 inhibitor slows down drug metabolism, which decreases the clearance of other medications, resulting in higher drug concentrations. This can cause significant drug-drug interactions. A CYP450 inducer is a medication that increases the clearance of other drugs. A CYP450 inhibitor is not an additive to a medication and does not prevent the degradation of its chemical compound.

11. Which of the following statements *best* describes why prescribing in elderly patients must be undertaken cautiously?
    A. Drug clearance increases with age, so doses often have to be higher.
    B. Renal function decreases with age, so doses often have to be modified.
    C. A low water-to-fat ratio in elderly patients means drugs must be taken with food.
    D. A decrease in total protein with age means drugs should be taken with high-protein foods.

12. A male patient presents with a chief complaint of a cough that he has had for several weeks. He denies shortness of breath or chest pain. His previous medical history is significant for newly diagnosed hypertension. On physical exam, the lung fields are clear without any retractions. Which of the following is the most likely cause of his symptoms?
    A. Atenolol
    B. Amlodipine
    C. Diltiazem
    D. Enalapril

13. A male patient presents with intermittent heart palpitations for a few days. He reports the symptoms to be worse at night and states, "It feels like my heart is fluttering." He denies use of illicit or recreational drugs and does not drink caffeinated beverages. A review of his medication list reveals that he is taking diltiazem, chlorthalidone, tamsulosin, and trazodone. A quick review of the patient's notes indicates that he was seen a few days ago for an upper respiratory tract infection and was given clarithromycin. On physical examination, the vital signs are stable except for the pulse rate of 112 bpm. Which of the following is the *best next step* in managing this patient?
    A. Perform an EKG
    B. Perform an echocardiogram
    C. Obtain serum thyroid-stimulating hormone level
    D. Obtain a chest x-ray

14. A male patient is taking warfarin for atrial fibrillation and calls the office because he has been experiencing nosebleeds since the day before. He also reports that he cut his leg and the bleeding has not stopped. These symptoms are suggestive of which of the following?
    A. The patient likely has skipped a few doses of warfarin.
    B. The international normalized ratio (INR) is likely elevated and should be re-checked.
    C. The INR is likely subtherapeutic, and the dose should be increased.
    D. The patient likely had an increased consumption of green, leafy vegetables.

15. A 57-year-old Black male patient presents for a follow-up on his blood pressure (BP). His BP was elevated at the last two visits, and he was instructed to monitor it at home. A review of his chart and log reveals systolic BPs consistently between 140 and 145 mmHg and diastolic BPs between 95 and 100 mmHg. At the patient's visit today, an appropriately sized cuff is used, and his BP is 142/90 mmHg with a pulse of 82 bpm. His past medical history is significant for chronic obstructive pulmonary disease (COPD). Which of the following is the most appropriate *initial* intervention at this time?
    A. Lifestyle interventions (increased exercise, diet modifications) for 3 months
    B. Atenolol 50 mg once daily and continued home monitoring
    C. Spironolactone 25 mg once daily and re-evaluation in 6 months
    D. Chlorthalidone 25 mg once daily and re-evaluation in 3 months

16. Which of the following statements *best* describes first-pass metabolism?
    A. When an oral drug is swallowed, it goes through the small intestine and enters the portal circulation of the liver, where it is metabolized before it is released to the general circulation.
    B. When an oral drug is swallowed, it goes to the stomach, which breaks down the medicine so that the body can use it.
    C. When a parenteral drug is in the body, it is broken down by the liver and the kidneys before it can be used by the body.
    D. When a parenteral drug enters the body, it goes directly to the circulation, and the drug is not metabolized.

(See answers next page.)

11. B) Renal function decreases with age, so doses often have to be modified.

Age-related changes in pharmacokinetics include increase in fat-to-water ratio, decrease in albumin and plasma proteins, decrease in liver blood flow and size, decrease in some CYP450 enzyme pathways (decreased drug clearance), and decrease in glomerular filtration rate. As people age, renal drug excretion (and drug clearance) is decreased because of physiologic decline in glomerular filtration. Despite a decrease in total protein, eating high-protein foods with medications does not affect age-related drug metabolism. Drug clearance is often lower with age, so doses should be adjusted appropriately.

12. D) Enalapril

Enalapril is an angiotensin-converting enzyme (ACE) inhibitor. A fairly common side effect of ACE inhibitors is a dry cough, which may occur a few hours after the first dose or within weeks to months. If the patient had a history of asthma or chronic obstructive pulmonary disease, atenolol (a beta-blocker) might be causing bronchospasm, but the physical exam would likely reveal wheezing. Adverse effects of amlodipine, a dihydropyridine calcium channel blocker, include peripheral edema, headaches, flushing, and lightheadedness. Diltiazem, a nondihydropyridine calcium channel blocker, can worsen cardiac output and cause bradycardia and constipation.

13. A) Perform an EKG

Patients who take macrolides, particularly clarithromycin, and calcium channel blockers are at a higher risk of developing a prolonged QT interval, which can cause torsades de pointes and ventricular tachycardia. A timely EKG is essential for diagnosis. An echocardiogram may be helpful after a diagnosis is established based on the rhythm to evaluate heart function, but the EKG is the priority, along with obtaining serum electrolytes. The chest x-ray may also help to rule out other differential diagnoses (e.g., pneumonia) if the patient was presenting with worsening respiratory symptoms; however, the patient's vital signs are stable and the patient does not report a productive cough. While thyroid disease may cause atrial fibrillation, there would be other historical and physical exam findings that would prompt evaluation of thyroid-stimulating hormone.

14. B) The international normalized ratio (INR) is likely elevated and should be re-checked.

Signs and symptoms of an elevated INR include prolonged bleeding from cuts, frequent nosebleeds, bloody/tarry stool, hematuria, petechiae, excessive bruising, excessive menstrual bleeding, and persistent oozing/bleeding gums after brushing. The INR must be checked before providing any advice on changing the dose. Frequent missed doses can cause a subtherapeutic INR level. High intake of vitamin K foods (e.g., kale, spinach, collards/mustard/beet greens, broccoli rabe) can reduce the anticoagulant effect of warfarin (i.e., can decrease INR).

15. D) Chlorthalidone 25 mg once daily and re-evaluation in 3 months.

The patient is considered to have stage 2 hypertension based on his follow-up visits and BP readings; therefore, pharmacologic and nonpharmacologic therapy is warranted. The American College of Cardiology/American Heart Association guideline recommends that initial antihypertensive drug therapy in Black patients should include a thiazide-type diuretic (e.g., chlorthalidone) or a calcium channel blocker. Atenolol, a beta-blocker, should be avoided in patients with COPD due to the risk of bronchoconstriction. Spironolactone, a mineralocorticoid receptor antagonist, is preferred in primary aldosteronism and is a common add-on therapy in resistant hypertension.

16. A) When an oral drug is swallowed, it goes through the small intestine and enters the portal circulation of the liver, where it is metabolized before it is released to the general circulation.

First-pass metabolism occurs only to drugs taken orally (not including the sublingual route). It is also known as the first-pass effect. Medications given by other routes, such as parenteral, injection, via the skin, or transdermal patch, do not undergo first-pass metabolism.

17. A 68-year-old male patient of Hispanic descent has recently been discharged from the hospital with a diagnosis of stroke secondary to venous thromboemboli, deep vein thrombosis (DVT), and type 2 diabetes. His medications are listed on the discharge note as warfarin 5 mg every Monday, Wednesday, Friday, and Sunday; metformin 1 g twice a day, and aspirin 325 mg daily. Which of the following is the correct international normalized ratio (INR) value for this patient?
    A. 1.5 to 2.5
    B. 2.0 to 3.0
    C. 2.5 to 3.5
    D. 3.0 to 4.0

18. Which of the following statements is *most* true?
    A. Pharmacogenomics studies the way drugs are cleared from the body.
    B. Pharmacokinetics studies the effects of drugs on the body.
    C. Pharmacogenomics studies how variations in genes can affect drug metabolism.
    D. Pharmacodynamics studies the way drugs are delivered throughout the body.

19. An elderly patient with a history of severe mitral regurgitation has surgery for placement of a prosthetic mitral valve. Which of the following is the correct international normalized ratio (INR) value?
    A. 1.5 to 2.5
    B. 2.0 to 3.0
    C. 2.5 to 3.5
    D. 3.0 to 4.0

20. Which of the following is an adverse effect of nondihydropyridine calcium channel blockers (CCBs)?
    A. Hyperkalemia
    B. Hypertriglyceridemia
    C. Hyperuricemia
    D. Constipation

21. Which of the following *best* reflects how to monitor a medication with a narrow therapeutic index?
    A. Levothyroxine: monitor levothyroxine levels
    B. Warfarin: monitor complete blood count
    C. Levothyroxine: monitor thyroid-stimulating hormone levels
    D. Warfarin: monitor prothrombin time/partial thromboplastin time

22. An 81-year-old male patient presents with knee and shoulder pain. He has a long history of osteoarthritis and has been taking over-the-counter naproxen with minimal relief. He states that the knee pain is gradually getting worse and is limiting his ability to walk his dog. Past medical history is significant for hypertension, coronary artery disease, atrial fibrillation, and several transient ischemic attacks. Imaging is normal except for evidence of degenerative joint disease. Which of the following treatments would be the most appropriate *next step* in managing this patient?
    A. Ketorolac 20 mg orally every 4 hours #30 tablets
    B. Ibuprofen 600 mg every 8 hours #60 tablets
    C. Diclofenac gel applied to the affected areas
    D. Acetaminophen 500 mg every 4 to 6 hours as needed

23. A 77-year-old female patient presents for a follow-up on her echocardiogram, which was ordered last week. She has been having increased shortness of breath with pedal edema. The report shows that she has a left ventricular ejection fraction of 38%. Which of the following is the *most appropriate* pharmacologic intervention at this time?
    A. Valsartan and carvedilol
    B. Furosemide and atenolol
    C. Digoxin and referral to a heart failure clinic
    D. Nifedipine and hydrochlorothiazide

24. A 15-year-old female patient presents with acne. She reports using over-the-counter (OTC) products without much success. On physical examination, there are multiple open and closed comedones on her face, forehead, and chest. Which of the following would be the *best* treatment option?
    A. Oral isotretinoin
    B. Topical azelaic acid
    C. Oral tetracycline
    D. Oral spironolactone

(See answers next page.)

17. B) 2.0 to 3.0

The goal INR for a patient who has had a stroke is an INR of 2.0 to 3.0. This is the most common INR value and is also true for atrial fibrillation.

18. C) Pharmacogenomics studies how variations in genes can affect drug metabolism.

Pharmacogenomics is the study of how a person's genes impact response to medications. Pharmacokinetics is the study of the distribution of drugs in the body, and pharmacodynamics studies the effects of drugs on biochemical, molecular, and physiologic processes.

19. C) 2.5 to 3.5

The American College of Cardiology/American Heart Association guidelines for anticoagulation of patients with prosthetic valves suggest an INR of 2.5 to 3.5. These patients are at higher risk of blood clots because of the prosthetic valves.

20. D) Constipation

Constipation affects up to 25% of patients who are on nondihydropyridine CCBs (verapamil, diltiazem). It can be severe in elderly patients. It is important that the patient take soluble fiber daily (e.g., Benefiber), increase fiber intake, walk daily, and ensure adequate fluid intake. Prunes or prune juice daily is also effective. Polyethylene glycol (Miralax) can be mixed with the fiber if fiber alone is not effective. It takes 12 to 24 hours for Miralax to be effective.

21. C) Levothyroxine: monitor thyroid-stimulating hormone levels

Levothyroxine use requires regular monitoring of thyroid-stimulating hormone to ensure the patient is euthyroid. Patients on warfarin need to have their international normalized ratio monitored to ensure appropriate anticoagulation.

22. D) Acetaminophen 500 mg every 4 to 6 hours as needed

There are a few red flags with this patient, including his age and his history of transient ischemic attacks and atrial fibrillation, meaning he is likely on an anticoagulant. Nonsteroidal anti-inflammatory drugs are contraindicated in patients who are taking anticoagulants, even topical diclofenac. Concomitant use of anticoagulants and diclofenac has a risk of serious gastrointestinal bleeding higher than that for users of either drug alone, and diclofenac is indicated only for osteoarthritis of the knee.

23. A) Valsartan and carvedilol

This patient has Stage C heart failure (HF), specifically HFrEF (clinical diagnosis of HF and left ventricular ejection fraction [LVEF] ≤40%). Current American College of Cardiology/American Heart Association guidelines recommend initial pharmacologic therapy with angiotensin receptor neprilysin inhibitor (ARNIs), angiotensin-converting enzyme inhibitors (ACEIs), angiotensin receptor blockers (ARBs), beta-blockers, loop diuretics, aldosterone antagonists, hydralazine/isosorbide dinitrate (HYD/ISDN), and ivabradine. Digoxin has a narrow therapeutic index and is rarely used. Carvedilol is the preferred beta-blocker in HFrEF.

24. B) Topical azelaic acid

In patients with mild (not cystic) acne who have not responded to OTC products, topical prescription remedies are the preferred next step. Oral isotretinoin carries significant risks of teratogenicity and is indicated for severe acne. It requires participation in the iPLEDGE® REMS (Risk Evaluation and Mitigation Strategy). Oral tetracycline or minocycline could be considered after 3 to 6 months of therapy but have significant side effects. Oral spironolactone could be considered as an adjunct if other interventions fail.

25. A male patient presents with a worsening skin infection on his forearm. He has been on cephalexin for 5 days without improvement. The patient reports an allergy to aspirin and sulfa drugs. A culture is obtained that comes back as positive for methicillin-resistant *Staphylococcus aureus* (MRSA). Which of the following is the *best* treatment option?
    A. Ceftriaxone
    B. Azithromycin
    C. Ciprofloxacin
    D. Clindamycin

26. A 75-year-old female patient presents with dysuria. Her past medical history is significant for hypertension, atrial fibrillation, depression, anxiety, and osteoarthritis. Her current medications include paroxetine, warfarin, lisinopril/hydrochlorothiazide, and occasional acetaminophen. She is afebrile. Her urine dipstick shows large leukocytes, nitrates, and trace blood. A culture with sensitivity is sent to the lab. Which of the following is the *best* empiric treatment?
    A. Nitrofurantoin
    B. Levofloxacin
    C. Trimethoprim-sulfamethoxazole
    D. Amoxicillin

27. A 51-year-old female patient presents for her routine physical examination and follow-up on her blood pressure (BP). She states that she has been checking her BP at home, and it is "still in the 140s." A review of her chart indicates increasing systolic and diastolic pressures over the past year by 20 mmHg systolic and diastolic. Her history is significant for androgenic alopecia secondary to surgical menopause, depression, and a history of polycystic ovary syndrome premenopausally. She is currently taking fluoxetine for depression, spironolactone for alopecia, and transdermal estradiol from her gynecologist. At today's visit, her BP is 142/90 mmHg with an appropriately sized cuff. Which of the following would be the *most appropriate* intervention at this time?
    A. Add a low-dose angiotensin-converting enzyme inhibitor
    B. Discontinue the estrogen
    C. Add a calcium channel blocker
    D. Add triamterene

28. The Beers Criteria provide a list of potentially inappropriate medications that should be avoided in which patient population?
    A. Pediatric
    B. Adolescent
    C. Adult <65 years of age
    D. Adult ≥65 years of age

29. A patient with a past medical history of heart failure presents complaining of visual changes and noting yellow-green–tinged color vision. The patient does not remember the name of their prescribed medication. The patient's caregiver has also noted increased confusion that is different from the patient's baseline. An EKG reveals a first-degree atrioventricular (AV) block. These signs and symptoms are suggestive of an overdose of which of the following medications?
    A. Warfarin
    B. Digoxin
    C. Furosemide
    D. Lisinopril

30. A patient presents for a routine check-up. Vital signs are significant for blood pressure of 135/85 mmHg. The patient is advised to re-check their blood pressure at home and adopt appropriate dietary and lifestyle modifications. During a follow-up appointment, the patient's blood pressure is 132/79 mmHg. Based on the American College of Cardiology/American Heart Association (ACC/AHA) stages of hypertension, this patient has:
    A. Normal blood pressure
    B. Elevated blood pressure
    C. Stage 1 hypertension
    D. Stage 2 hypertension

31. A female patient who is sexually active presents with dysuria, vaginal pruritus, and a mucuopuluent cervical discharge. Nucleic acid amplification testing is positive for *Neisseria gonorrhoeae* infection. Which of the following is the *preferred* first-line agent for this patient's treatment?
    A. Ceftriaxone
    B. Cephalexin
    C. Cefuroxime
    D. Cefdinir

(See answers next page.)

25. D) Clindamycin

The first-line treatment for MRSA is trimethoprim-sulfamethoxazole, but this patient has a sulfa allergy, so it cannot be used. The alternative would be clindamycin. Ceftriaxone is indicated for gram-negative bacteria and should always be used with caution due to the risk of Achilles tendon rupture. Azithromycin covers some gram-positive and gram-negative bacteria but is not indicated for the treatment of MRSA.

26. A) Nitrofurantoin

As this patient is taking warfarin, she should not be prescribed trimethoprim-sulfamethoxazole unless it is the only option; if so, the international normalized ratio must be closely monitored. Fluoroquinolones are never indicated as first-line therapy for an uncomplicated urinary tract infection. Amoxicillin has some gram-negative coverage but resistance is high; its coverage can be augmented with the addition of clavulanic acid.

27. C) Add a calcium channel blocker

American College of Cardiology/American Heart Association guidelines recommend combination therapy for patients with stage 2 hypertension. Since the patient is already on a potassium-sparing diuretic, an angiotensin-converting enzyme inhibitor would not be appropriate. Triamterene is also potassium-sparing and thus would be inappropriate. While estrogen has been shown to increase BP, the patient should speak with her gynecologist about risks and benefits of continuing it since her new diagnosis of hypertension.

28. D) Adult ≥65 years of age

The American Geriatrics Society (AGS) provides a Beers Criteria list of potentially inappropriate medications that should be avoided in adults 65 years and older in all ambulatory, acute, and institutionalized settings of care, except hospice and palliative care settings. It is not specified to the pediatric, adolescent, or younger adult population.

29. B) Digoxin

Digoxin can be used as second- or third-line therapy for heart failure. Digoxin has a narrow therapeutic window; signs and symptoms of drug toxicity include gastrointestinal symptoms (e.g., nausea, vomiting), hyperkalemia, bradydysrhythmias (AV blocks) or tachydysrhythmias (ventricular tachycardia/fibrillation or atrial tachycardia with 2:1 block), confusion, and visual changes (yellow-green–tinged color vision). While furosemide can cause ototoxicity, it is not known to cause these side effects and changes in vision. Side effects of warfarin, an anticoagulant, include increased bleeding risk of skin necrosis, not visual changes or AV blocks. Lisinopril overdose often leads to severe hypotension; other side effects include hyperkalemia, cough, reduction in glomerular filtration rate, and angioedema and anaphylactoid reactions.

30. C) Stage 1 hypertension

The patient has stage 1 hypertension. The ACC/AHA stages of hypertension are as follows: Normal blood pressure is systolic <120 mmHg and diastolic <80 mmHg; elevated blood pressure is systolic 120 to 129 mmHg and diastolic <80 mmHg; stage 1 hypertension is systolic 130 to 139 mmHg or diastolic 80 to 89 mmHg; and stage 2 hypertension is systolic >140 mmHg or diastolic >90 mmHg.

31. A) Ceftriaxone

Ceftriaxone (a third-generation cephalosporin) is the preferred treatment regimen for gonococcal infections. Cephalexin (first generation), cefuroxime (second generation), and cefdinir (third generation) are all cephalosporins; however, ceftriaxone is the preferred first-line therapy for gonorrhea.

32. A 65-year-old patient who is currently receiving antibiotic therapy for community-acquired pneumonia presents with calf swelling and pain. The patient reports a new onset of difficulty in walking after initiation of therapy. Which antibiotic is *most likely* the cause of this advserse effect?

A. Amoxicillin
B. Doxycycline
C. Cephalexin
D. Levofloxacin

33. Which of the following is a superpotent (group 1) topical steroid?

A. Halcinonide (Halog)
B. Clobetasol (Temovate)
C. Mometasone furoate (Elocon)
D. Desonide gel (Desonate)

34. A male patient with benign prostate hyperplasia (BPH) reports increased frequency and urgency and difficulty starting urination. The patient reports taking an herbal supplement for his symptoms but cannot remember the name. Which of the following herbal supplements is commonly used in patients with BPH?

A. St. John's wort
B. Ginkgo biloba
C. Saw palmetto
D. Kava kava

35. A patient presents after a recent camping trip with complaints of a fever, headache, fatigue, and muscle pain. The patient reports a blanching erythematous rash with macules and petechiae. The rash began on the ankles and wrists and is now spreading toward the trunk. Based on this presentation, what is the preferred agent for treatment?

A. Doxycycline
B. Amoxicillin
C. Clindamycin
D. Trimethoprim-sulfamethoxazole

(See answers next page.)

32. D) Levofloxacin

Fluoroquinolones (e.g., levofloxacin) have a boxed warning due to increased risk of tendinitis and acute tendon rupture, especially in patients older than 60 years and in those who are on steroid treatment or who have received an organ transplant. Patients are advised to avoid strenuous activity while on the medication. Cephalexin (a cephalosporin), amoxicillin (a penicillin), and doxycycline (a tetracycline) are less likely to cause an acute tendon rupture compared with fluoroquinolones.

33. B) Clobetasol (Temovate)

Clobetasol (Temovate) is classified as a superpotent (group 1) topical steroid. Halcinonide is classified as high potency (group 2), mometasone furoate is high/medium potency (group 3), and desonide gel is considered medium/low potency (group 5).

34. C) Saw palmetto

Historically, extracts of the fruit from the saw palmetto (Serenoa repens), the American dwarf palm tree, have been used to treat BPH. However, with many herbal supplements, there is often both limited data to support efficacy and multiple drug interactions; thus, they are generally not recommended for treatment. St. John's wort has been used for the management of depression. Ginkgo biloba has been studied for the treatment and prevention of memory issues, cognitive impairment, and dementia. Kava kava has been used for anxiety and insomnia.

35. A) Doxycycline

The patient is presenting with the classic features of Rocky Mountain spotted fever (RMSF), a potentially lethal but curable tickborne disease. Early signs of illness are nonspecific symptoms such as fever, headache, malaise, and myalgias. A petechial or maculopapular rash develops between the third and fifth day of illness in most patients. According to the Centers for Disease Control and Prevention, doxycycline is the preferred agent for the treatment of RMSF and all other tickborne rickettsial diseases in adults and children. Of note, chloramphenicol is the only alternative agent, but it is less effective than doxycycline. Sulfa-containing drugs may worsen the clinical course and increase the risk of death in treating RMSF. Other antibiotics, such as amoxicillin and clindamycin, are not indicated or effective for the treatment of RMSF.

U.S. HEALTH STATISTICS

MORTALITY STATISTICS

Leading cause of death (all ages/sexes):
1. Heart disease
2. Cancer
3. Accidents/unintentional injuries

CANCER MORTALITY

Top three cancer deaths (all ages/sexes):
1. Lung and bronchus
2. Colon and rectum
3. Pancreas

Cancer is more common in older adults; 80% of all cancers in the United States are diagnosed in people age 55 years or older.

LEADING CAUSES OF DEATH IN ADOLESCENTS

Death rate for teen males is higher than for teen females:
- Unintentional injuries; the most common cause is motor vehicle crashes (risk is highest from 16 to 19 years of age).
- Suicide; watch for signs of depression, such as talking about suicide, saying goodbye to friends and family, social isolation, social media updates about death. Interview teen with parent, then alone (without parent). Refer to pediatric psychiatrist/therapist for further evaluation.
- Homicide; nonfatal and fatal violence are much higher among young people compared with any other age group.

LEADING CAUSES OF MORTALITY BY AGE GROUP

- Birth to 12 months: Congenital malformations
- Age 1 to 44 years: Unintentional injuries
- Age 45 to 64 years: Cancer
- Age 65 years and older: Heart disease

LIFE EXPECTANCY

According to 2023 data from the Centers for Disease Control and Prevention (CDC), in 2021, average life expectancy in the United States was 76.4 years: 73.5 years for males and 79.3 years for females.

CANCER STATISTICS

The most common cancer is skin cancer. The most common type of skin cancer is basal cell carcinoma; melanoma causes the majority of skin cancer deaths.

Most common cancer by sex (prevalence):
- Men: Prostate cancer. In men, there are more cases of prostate cancer (prevalence), but the cancer that causes the most deaths (mortality) is lung cancer. African American men and Caribbean men of African ancestry are at higher risk for prostate cancer than men of other races. Other risk factors are a first-degree relative (father or brother) with prostate cancer at an early age (younger than 65 years).
- Women: Breast cancer. In women, there are more cases of breast cancer (prevalence), but the cancer that causes the most deaths (mortality) is lung cancer.

The most common cancer among children (age 0–14 years) is leukemias; approximately three out of four cases are acute lymphocytic leukemia.

SCREENING TESTS

SENSITIVITY

- A sensitive test is very good at identifying/detecting those people who have the disease (true positive).
- An easy way to remember is to think of "sensitivity—rule in" or "SIN."

SPECIFICITY

- A specific screening test is very good at identifying/detecting those people without the disease (true negative).
- An easy way to remember is to think of "specificity—rule out" or "SPOUT."

HEALTH PROMOTION/DISEASE AND DEATH PREVENTION

PRIMARY PREVENTION (PREVENTION OF DISEASE OR INJURY/ELIMINATE OR REDUCE RISK FACTORS FOR AN ILLNESS)

- Eat a nutritious diet, exercise, and use seatbelts and helmets.
- Practice gun safety, including using safety locks for guns and keeping guns out of reach of children and teenagers.
- Federal health-promotion/disease-prevention programs include immunizations, Occupational Safety and Health Administration (OSHA) job safety laws, and Environmental Protection Agency (EPA) laws.

- Change risky behaviors (e.g., poor eating habits, tobacco use, not using condoms).
- Build a youth center in an urban high-crime area or a Habitat for Humanity house.
- Use aspirin prophylaxis for primary prevention of cardiovascular disease (CVD) in adults age 40 to 59 years who have a 10% risk or higher (who are not at increased risk of bleeding).

SECONDARY PREVENTION (EARLY DETECTION OF A DISEASE TO MINIMIZE BODILY DAMAGE)

- Screening tests (e.g., Pap smears, mammograms, complete blood count for anemia)
- Screening for depression (interviewing a patient about feelings of sadness, hopelessness)
- Screening for sexually transmitted infections (STIs), such as testing for chlamydia and gonorrhea and asking about sexual history and partners and signs/symptoms
- Screening for alcohol use disorder (interviewing a patient using the CAGE questionnaire)
- Testing for hepatitis C virus (anti-HCV) for all adults age 18 to 79 years old and for persons with risk factors such as long-term hemodialysis, received blood/blood component transfusion (before July 1992), injection drug use, HIV infection, and persistently abnormal alanine aminotransferase (ALT) levels
- Having a person with a history of myocardial infarction (MI), transient ischemic attack (TIA), or stroke take an aspirin or statin daily (to prevent a future stroke or MI)

TERTIARY PREVENTION (REDUCE IMPACT OF DISEASE OR INJURY/REHABILITATION/SUPPORT GROUPS/ EQUIPMENT)

- Support groups: Alcoholics Anonymous (AA), breast cancer support groups, HIV support groups
- Education for patients with preexisting disease (e.g., diabetes, hypertension): Avoidance of drug interactions, proper use of wheelchair or medical equipment, and so on
- Rehabilitation: Cardiac rehabilitation, physical therapy (PT), occupational therapy (OT)
- Vocational rehabilitation programs: Retrain workers for new jobs (after they have recovered as much as possible)

U.S. PREVENTIVE SERVICES TASK FORCE RECOMMENDATIONS

ASPIRIN USE TO PREVENT CARDIOVASCULAR DISEASE AND COLORECTAL CANCER (APRIL 2022)

- Age 40 to 59 years with ≥10% CVD risk: Initiate low-dose aspirin use for primary prevention of CVD in patients who are not at increased risk for bleeding with life expectancy of at least 10 years and who are willing to take low-dose aspirin daily for at least 10 years
- Age ≥60 years: Aspirin use not recommended for primary prevention.

BREAST CANCER (JANUARY 2016)

- Start baseline mammogram at age 50 years and repeat every 2 years until age 74 years. Note that an update to this recommendation was in progress as of July 2023. The draft update recommends biennial screening mammography for those ages 40 to 74 years.
- Insufficient evidence for routine mammogram in those age ≥75 years
- Does not apply to women with known genetic mutations (*BRCA1* or *BRCA2*), familial breast cancer, or a history of chest radiation at a young age or women previously diagnosed with high-risk breast lesion who may benefit from starting screening in their 40s
- Evidence is insufficient to assess the balance of benefits and harms of adjunctive screening for breast cancer using breast ultrasonography, MRI, digital breast tomosynthesis (DBT), or other methods in women identified to have dense breasts on an otherwise-negative screening mammogram.

> **NOTE**
>
> The American Cancer Society recommends that women who are at the highest risk of breast cancer (i.e., those with the *BRCA* gene) should obtain both a breast MRI and a mammogram every year, typically starting at age 30 years.
>
> *Source:* American Cancer Society. (2022, January 14). (See Resources section for complete source information.)

CERVICAL CANCER (AUGUST 2018)

Table 4.1 Cervical Cancer Screening

Patient Group	Recommendations for Pap/Liquid Cytology
Age 20 years or younger	Do not screen (even if sexually active with multiple partners); cervical cancer is rare before age 21 years
Age 21–29 years	Every 3 years with cervical cytology alone
Age 30–65 years	Every 3 years with cervical cytology alone, every 5 years with high-risk human papillomavirus (hrHPV) testing alone, or every 5 years with hrHPV testing in combination with cytology
Prior hysterectomy with removal of cervix	If hysterectomy with cervical removal was not due to cervical intraepithelial neoplasia (CIN grade 2) or cervical cancer, stop screening
Age >65 years with adequate prior screening	Do not screen if history of adequate prior screening and otherwise not at high risk for cervical cancer

Source: U.S. Preventive Services Task Force. (2018). (See Resources section for complete source information.)

COLORECTAL CANCER (MAY 2021)

- Baseline: Starting at age 45 years until age 75 years (older age is the most common risk factor)
- Age 76 to 85 years: Against routine screening, but "there may be considerations"; individualize screening as needed.
- Age ≥85 years: Do not screen.

NOTES

Several methods are acceptable for screening people with average risk of colon cancer:
- Colonoscopy every 10 years
- Flexible sigmoidoscopy or CT colonography every 5 years
- High-sensitivity fecal occult blood test (FOBT) or fecal immunochemical test (FIT) every year (if positive, needs colonoscopy)
- Stool DNA (SDNA) every 1 or 3 years (if positive, needs colonoscopy)

LIPID DISORDERS (NOVEMBER 2016)

Total lipid profile should be taken after a 9-hour (minimum) fast; universal lipid screening should be done for all adults age 40 to 75 years. Screening for asymptomatic children and adolescents younger than 20 years is not recommended (July 2023).

The U.S. Preventive Services Task Force (USPSTF) recommends the use of a low- to moderate-dose statin for adults with no history of CVD (primary prevention) when all of the following criteria are met:
- Age is 40 to 75 years.
- Patient has one or more CVD risk factors (e.g., dyslipidemia, diabetes mellitus [DM], hypertension, smoking).
- Patient has a calculated 10-year risk of a cardiovascular event of ≥10%.
- If age ≥76 years, evidence is insufficient to recommend for or against initiating a statin.
- The likelihood that a patient benefits from statin therapy depends on their absolute baseline risk of having a future CVD event.

LUNG CANCER (MARCH 2021)

- Screening for persons who smoke (20 pack-years) or who have quit in the past 15 years
- Annual screening with low-dose CT (LDCT) for patients age 50 to 80 years

- Discontinue screening once person has not smoked for 15 years or person develops a health problem that substantially limits life expectancy or the ability or willingness to have curative lung surgery

OVARIAN CANCER (FEBRUARY 2018)

- Grade D: Routine screening is not recommended.
- High-risk patients: Refer for genetic risk evaluation and counseling. Note that numerous genetic mutations and hereditary cancer syndromes may be associated with ovarian cancer, each with a different cluster of associated cancers and family history pattern. In women with a family history of ovarian or breast cancer, there may an elevated risk for a hereditary cancer syndrome, and these patients should discuss their family history with their healthcare professional.
- *BRCA1*-and/or *BRCA2*-positive mutation: Increases risk for breast cancer, male breast cancer, ovarian cancer, prostate cancer, pancreatic cancer, and melanoma.

PROSTATE CANCER (MAY 2018)

- Age 55 to 69 years: Individualize the decision to undergo periodic prostate-specific antigen (PSA) screening. Discuss the potential harms, including those associated with false-positive results, and then the potential complications of prostate biopsy (erectile dysfunction, urinary incontinence) versus the benefits. Do not screen those who do not express preference for screening.
- Age 70 years or older: Do not screen.

SKIN CANCER BEHAVIORAL COUNSELING (MARCH 2018)

- Counsel young adults, adolescents, children, and parents of young children about minimizing exposure to UV radiation for persons age 6 months to 24 years with fair skin types to reduce their risk of skin cancer.
- Education includes avoidance of sunlight from 10 a.m. to 4 p.m. and use of SPF 15 or higher sunblock, protective clothing, and wide-brim hats.

SKIN CANCER SCREENING (JUNE 2023)

The USPSTF concludes that current evidence is insufficient to assess the balance of benefits and harms of screening (visual skin examination) for skin cancer in adults.

OTHER

Routine screening is not recommended by the USPSTF for the following conditions (see Table 4.2 for a summary of USPSTF Health Screening Recommendations):
- Oral cancer
- Prostate cancer
- Testicular cancer (adolescents or adult males)

Table 4.2 U.S. Preventive Services Task Force Health Screening Recommendations

Disorder	Baseline	Recommendations
Abdominal aortic aneurysm (December 2019)	Men age 65–75 years who have smoked	One-time screening with ultrasonography in men age 65–75 years who have smoked; individualize for men who never smoked
Breast cancer (January 2016)	Start at age 50 years Note: 2023 draft update recommends start at age 40 years. Age 75 years or older*	Mammogram every 2 years (biennial) until age 74 years Stop routine screening; individualize*
Blood pressure in adults (April 2021)	Start at age 18 years or older	Obtain measurements outside of clinical setting for diagnostic confirmation before starting treatment
Colon/colorectal cancer (May 2021)	Start at age 45 years; continue until age 75 years Age 76–85 years Age older than 85 years	High-sensitivity FOBT or FIT every year, or flexible sigmoidoscopy or CT colonography every 5 years, or SDNA every 1–3 years (if positive, needs colonoscopy), or colonoscopy every 10 years Individualize* Stop routine screening
Depression in adolescents (May 2016)	Adolescents (12–18 years)	Start screening for major depressive disorder at age 12–18 years
Depression in adults (January 2023)	General adult population	Include pregnant and postpartum patients
Diabetes mellitus type 2 (August 2021)	Screen for prediabetes and type 2 diabetes in adults age 35 to 70 years who have overweight or obesity	Applies to adults in primary care settings who are not "high risk"; patients with risk factors (e.g., PCOS, GDM) can undergo screening at younger age
Hepatitis C virus infection (March 2020)	Age 18–79 years	Screen adults age 18–79 years
HIV infection (June 2019)	Age 15–65 years Pregnant people	Screen; younger adolescents and older adults who are at increased risk should also be screened Screen; including those in labor or delivery whose HIV status is unknown
Latent tuberculosis (May 2023)	Asymptomatic adults at increased risk of infection	Screen
Lung cancer (March 2021)	Age 50–80 years with history of smoking	LDCT if currently smokes with 20-pack-year history *or* quit in the past 15 years
Obesity in adults (September 2018); obesity in children and adolescents (June 2017) Note: Update in progress	Start at age 6–18 years	Offer or refer for intensive behavioral interventions
Sexually transmitted infections (August 2020)	Start at the onset of sexual activity	High-intensity behavioral counseling for sexually active adolescents and adults who are at high risk for STIs
Skin cancer (April 2023)	Insufficient evidence	Routine screening not recommended; individualize*
Osteoporosis (June 2018)	Start at age 65 years or older	May start earlier if a younger woman has a fracture risk equal to or greater than that of a 65-year-old White woman (e.g., from chronic use of steroids)
Ovarian cancer (February 2018)	Against routine screening	Do not screen for ovarian cancer except high risk
Pancreatic cancer (August 2019)	Asymptomatic adults	Do not screen
Syphilis infection (September 2022)	Asymptomatic adults and adolescents Pregnant people	Screen persons who are at increased risk of infection Early screening for syphilis infection in all pregnant people; congenital syphilis can occur at any time during pregnancy or birth

*Decision to screen is based on risk factors, life expectancy (>10 years), and risk versus benefits.
FIT, fecal immunochemical test; FOBT, fecal occult blood test; GDM, gestational diabetes mellitus; LDCT, low-dose computed tomography; PCOS, polycystic ovary syndrome; SDNA, stool DNA; STI, sexually transmitted infection.
Source: Data from U.S. Preventive Services Task Force. (n.d.). (See Resources section for complete source information.)

RISK FACTORS

BREAST CANCER
- Age 50 years or older (most common risk factor)
- Previous history of breast cancer
- *BRCA1* or *BRCA2* gene mutation
- History of high-dose radiation therapy to the chest at a young age (such as treatment for Hodgkin lymphoma)
- Two or more first-degree relatives with breast cancer
- Early menarche, late menopause, nulliparity (longer exposure to estrogen)
- Obesity (adipose tissue can synthesize small amounts of estrogen)

CERVICAL CANCER
- Multiple sex partners (defined as more than four lifetime partners)
- Younger age of onset of sex (immature cervix easier to infect)
- Immunosuppression and smoking

COLORECTAL CANCER
- History of familial polyposis (multiple polyps on colon)
- First-degree relative (parent, sibling, or child) diagnosed with colon cancer at younger than 60 years
- History of chronic inflammatory bowel disease (ulcerative colitis, Crohn's disease)

PROSTATE CANCER
- Age 50 years or older
- Genetic predisposition
- First-degree relative with prostate cancer

SEXUALLY TRANSMITTED INFECTIONS
- Having anal, vaginal, or oral sex without a condom
- Having sex while under the influence of alcohol or drugs
- Having anonymous partners or multiple sexual partners
- Earlier age of onset of sex
- New partners (defined as <3 months)
- History of STI
- Homelessness

VACCINES AND IMMUNIZATIONS

HEPATITIS B VACCINE
- Total of three doses (0, 1, 6 months); first vaccine given at birth (monovalent hepatitis B vaccine)
- Requires a minimum interval of 4 weeks between doses one and two
- If series is not completed, catch up until three-dose series is completed; the Centers for Disease Control and Prevention (CDC) does not recommend a restart of the hepatitis B series.
- See Table 4.3 for a summary of CDC immunization recommendations for hepatitis B and other conditions in adults age 19 years or older.

> **VACCINE FACT**
>
> *If a patient had only one dose of hepatitis B vaccine, and is off the recommended dosing schedule, what is recommended?*
>
> Do not restart the hepatitis B series again. If only one dose, give the second dose. Catch up until the three-dose series is completed.

SEASONAL INFLUENZA VACCINE
- Start giving the influenza injection at the end of October of each year (fall to winter season).
- According to 2023 CDC guidance, as long as influenza viruses circulate, vaccination should continue to be offered, even into January or later. Most seasons, influenza activity peaks in January or later.
- All healthcare personnel should get vaccinated annually.
- If a person with an egg allergy *only* experiences hives, an influenza vaccine can be administered.

Formulations

Inactivated and Recombinant Influenza Vaccines (Injectable)
- Trivalent influenza vaccine or quadrivalent vaccines given by intramuscular injection in the arm are preferred. There are intradermal and nasal forms of these vaccines.
- High-dose trivalent influenza vaccine for people age 65 years or older (Fluzone High-Dose).
- Recombinant trivalent influenza vaccine that is egg-free approved for persons age 18 years and older (Flublok).
- Quadrivalent influenza vaccine protects against four types of flu virus (broader protection). Different vaccines are approved for different age groups, ranging from 6 months old to children, adults, and elderly.

Live Attenuated Influenza Vaccine
- Live attenuated influenza vaccine (LAIV) is approved for use in nonpregnant healthy persons age 2 to 49 years.
- Some antivirals (amantadine, rimantadine, zanamivir, or oseltamivir) should be avoided 48 hours before vaccination because they interfere with antibody production. Do not give aspirin to children within the 4 weeks following vaccination.

LAIV Contraindications
- Pregnancy, chronic disease (e.g., asthma, chronic obstructive pulmonary disease [COPD], renal failure, diabetes, immunosuppression)
- Children on aspirin therapy (age 2–17 years)
- Children age 2 to 4 years who have asthma or a history of wheezing in the past 12 months

Contraindications (All Types of Influenza Vaccine)
- Infants age 6 months or younger
- People with severe, life-threatening allergies to components of the influenza vaccine (e.g., gelatin, gentamicin,

Table 4.3 CDC Immunization Recommendations for Adults and Teens Age 19 Years or Older (2023)*

Vaccine	Schedule/Population	Notes
COVID-19	Two or three primary series and booster	Primary series two doses given at 0 and 308 weeks (depending on manufacturer). Booster dose, see www.cdc.gov/vaccines/covid-19/clinical-considerations/interim-considerations-us.html for up-to-date information
Hepatitis B	Two, three, or four doses depending on vaccine or condition	If incomplete series, do not restart; if had one dose, give the second dose during the visit; if had two doses, give the third dose.
Tetanus/diphtheria (Td) Tetanus/diphtheria/acellular pertussis (Tdap)	Every 10 years for lifetime	Substitute one-time dose of Tdap for Td booster (once in a lifetime). "Dirty" wounds, give tetanus booster if last dose more than 5 years ago. Contaminated/"dirty" wounds that either are unvaccinated or did not complete primary series should be given TIG (tetanus immune globulin) for prophylaxis.
Flu (influenza) Inactivated IIV4 or influenza recombinant (RIV4) OR Live attenuated influenza vaccine (LAIV) intranasal** Quadrivalent flu vaccine	Once a year For healthy persons (not pregnant) age 2–49 years Age 65 years and older	Give in fall/winter season. Do not give if pregnant or immunocompromised or if caregiver of severely immunocompromised persons (or avoid contact with these persons for 7 days after getting live flu vaccine). Any one of quadrivalent high-dose inactivated influenza vaccine (HD-IIV4), quadrivalent recombinant influenza vaccine (RIV4), or quadrivalent adjuvanted inactivated influenza vaccine (aIIV4) is preferred. If none of these three vaccines is available, then any other age-appropriate influenza vaccine should be used.
Varicella**	Two doses if born 1980 or later	First dose at age 12–15 months. Second dose at age 4–6 years.
Zoster recombinant	Two doses	First dose (RZV, Shingrix) for healthy adults age 50 years or older; separate second dose by 2–6 months.
Meningococcal A, C, W, Y (MenACWY)	One or two doses depending on indication. Booster may be recommended.	Age 19–23 years. Immunocompromise, travel to high-risk areas, first-year college students in residential housing, military recruits, not previously immunized (Menactra, Menveo, or MenQuadfi)
Meningococcal B (MenB)	Two to three doses depending on vaccine and indications	Adolescents and young adults age 16–23 not at increased risk for meningococcal disease (Bexsero, Trumenba).
Pneumococcal polysaccharide vaccine (PCV15, PCV20, PPSV23)	1 dose PCV15 followed by PPSV23 or 1 dose PCV20	Age 65 years and older who have not previously received a dose of PCV 13, PCV 15, or PCV20, or whose vaccination history is not known. Refer to updated CDC mobile app for most up-to-date information: www.cdc.gov/vaccines/vpd/pneumo/hcp/pneumoapp.html

*List is not all-inclusive.
**Live virus vaccine contraindications apply.
Source: Centers for Disease Control and Prevention. (2023). (See Resources section for complete source information.)

preservative), which are not related to an egg allergy, should not be given influenza vaccine (egg allergy-related reactions are discussed below).

Safety Issues

- If severe reaction (hypotension, wheezing, nausea/vomiting, reaction requiring epinephrine or emergency medical attention) occurs after eating eggs or food containing eggs, vaccine should be administered in an inpatient or outpatient medical setting (clinics, hospitals, health departments, physician offices)

under the supervision of a healthcare provider who is able to recognize and manage severe allergic conditions.
- According to the CDC in 2020, if patient experienced *only* hives previously, they can receive the influenza vaccine. People with egg allergies no longer need to be observed for an allergic reaction for 30 minutes after receiving the flu vaccine.
- Age-appropriate recombinant (RIV) or cell-cultured flu vaccines are an option for patients who refuse egg-based influenza vaccine.

- Use caution or avoid influenza vaccine if there is a history of Guillain–Barré syndrome within 6 weeks of previous vaccination.

> **VACCINE FACTS**
>
> **1. How long does it take for the flu vaccine to become effective?**
> It takes about 2 weeks after being vaccinated to develop antibodies.
>
> **2. How long does immunity from influenza vaccine last?**
> Protection is thought to persist for at least 6 months. Early vaccination (in July or August) will likely result in suboptimal immunity before the end of the influenza season, especially in older adults.

PNEUMOCOCCAL VACCINE

- Pneumococcal polysaccharide vaccine (PPSV23 or Pneumovax): All adults age 65 years or older or those at high risk for pneumococcal disease (age 2–64 years). If received dose before age 65, should receive one final dose of the vaccine at age 65 years or older. Administer this last dose at least 5 years after prior dose. PPSV23 is 50% to 85% effective.
- Pneumococcal conjugate vaccine (PCV13 or Prevnar): All children younger than 2 years receive a series of four doses (2, 4, 6, and 12–15 months) or those who are at high risk of pneumococcal disease. PCV13 (Prevnar) is also recommended for adults age 19 years or older with immunocompromising conditions, cerebrospinal fluid (CSF) leaks, or cochlear implants. For adults age 65 years or older who want to receive PCV13, give dose at least 1 year after PPSV23.
- Highest risk (of fatal pneumococcal infection): Chronic diseases (alcoholism, diabetes, CSF leaks, asthma, chronic hepatitis); anatomical or functional asplenia (including sickle cell disease); immunocompromised or on medications causing immunocompromised state; generalized malignancy or cancers of the blood (leukemia, lymphoma, multiple myeloma); renal diseases (e.g., chronic renal failure, nephrotic syndrome); history of organ or bone marrow transplant

> **VACCINE FACTS**
>
> **1. What vaccine is recommended for persons who are 65 years of age?**
> Give Pneumovax (PPSV23) at 65 years of age. If patient presents in the fall/winter season, also offer influenza vaccine. If immunocompromising condition, CSF leak, or cochlear implant, do not give PPSV23.
>
> **2. If a person is vaccinated with Pneumovax before age 65 years, what is recommended?**
> Give a booster dose of Pneumovax 5 years after the initial dose.

SHINGLES VACCINE

Shingrix (Recombinant Zoster Vaccine)

- Shingrix is the shingles vaccine for adults age 50 years or older.

- Shingrix requires two injections from 2 to 6 months apart.
- The Advisory Committee on Immunization Practices (ACIP) recommends that people who previously received Zostavax (now-discontinued shingles vaccine) should receive Shingrix.
- You can get Shingrix even if you have had shingles, received Zostavax, or are not sure that you had chickenpox.
- Shingrix causes a strong response from the immune system, and side effects, such as a sore arm, headache, fever, stomach pain, or nausea, may occur.
- If the second dose of Shingrix is delayed by more than 6 months after the first dose, do not restart the series. Give the second dose.
- Risk factors (shingles) include older age (≥60 years); immunocompromise (HIV, steroids, chemotherapy); leukemia or lymphoma
- Contraindications include currently having shingles; pregnancy or breastfeeding; negative varicella zoster titer (CDC recommends person should get chickenpox vaccine instead)

> **VACCINE FACTS**
>
> **1. What is the vaccine for shingles prophylaxis?**
> Shingrix is the vaccine for shingles prophylaxis. Shingrix is 90% effective against shingles. At age 50 years or older (even if history of shingles), a person needs a total of two doses of Shingrix.
>
> **2. Can a person who has never had chickenpox develop shingles?**
> No, they cannot. If the person becomes infected with the varicella zoster virus, it will manifest initially as chickenpox.
>
> **3. How long are persons with shingles contagious?**
> Shingles is infectious until all the skin lesions are dry and crusted. Follow contact precautions. About half of cases of shingles occur in persons age 60 years or older.

TETANUS VACCINES (TDAP AND TD)

- Give every 10 years for lifetime.
- For "dirty"/contaminated wounds, give a booster if the last dose was more than 5 years prior.
- Use DTaP form in infants and children younger than 7 years.
- For those age 7 years and older, use only tetanus and diphtheria (Td) or the tetanus, diphtheria, acellular pertussis (Tdap) forms of the vaccine; give one Tdap dose (lifetime) to replace one Td dose.
- Give DTaP by IM route to infants and children younger than 7 years.
- Give Td by IM route; start using at age 7 years.
- Give Tdap by IM route.

Safety Issue

History of Guillain–Barré syndrome within 6 weeks of previous dose. Be careful with pertussis component if progressive or unstable neurologic disorder or uncontrolled seizures.

VARICELLA VACCINE

- Varicella live attenuated virus (Varivax) is given by SC route and requires two doses. First dose given in infancy at 12 to 15 months (do not give to infants younger than 12 months). The second dose is given at age 4 through 6 years.
- Adolescents (age 13 years or older) and adults need two doses given 4 to 8 weeks apart.
- Advise patients not to get pregnant for 1 month after getting vaccine.
- A new combination vaccine called the MMRV (measles, mumps, rubella, varicella; ProQuad) contains both chickenpox and the MMR vaccines (only for age 12 years or younger).
- For postexposure prophylaxis, vaccine should ideally be given within 72 hours post exposure but may be given up to 5 days (120 hours) after incident (in healthy, previously unvaccinated person).
- Reactions include mild rash or several small chickenpox rashes that can occur after vaccination (contagious, avoid immunocompromised people).
- Acceptable proof of varicella immunity includes documentation of two doses of varicella vaccine, written diagnosis of chickenpox or shingles based on healthcare provider diagnosis, positive laboratory varicella titer (IgG ELISA), and birth in the United States before 1980.
- Routine testing for varicella immunity after two doses is not recommended.

Safety Issues
Avoid giving to pregnant patients, patients with immunosuppression or who are on drugs that affect the immune system (steroids, biologics such as Humira or Enbrel), or patients having radiation treatment or with any type of cancer.

HEALTHCARE PERSONNEL VACCINATION RECOMMENDATIONS
These recommendations also apply to students who are in training to become healthcare providers.

Td or Tdap
Give one-time dose of Tdap to all healthcare workers who have not received it previously (regardless of when previous dose of Td was received). Pregnant healthcare workers need to get a dose of Tdap during each pregnancy.

MMR
Proof of immunity is necessary (born before 1957, laboratory confirmation such as positive titers). If not vaccinated for MMR, two doses are needed (at least 28 days apart).

Varicella
Proof of immunity is necessary (positive varicella titer; documentation of two doses of varicella vaccine or diagnosis of varicella by physician/healthcare provider).

Hepatitis B
If incomplete hepatitis B series (fewer than three doses), complete the series (do not restart). Obtain hepatitis B virus surface antibody (anti-HBV) serologic test 1 to 2 months after the final dose.

Influenza
All healthcare personnel should have an annual influenza shot during the fall/winter.

Bacillus Calmette–Guérin
Bacillus Calmette–Guérin (BCG) is a vaccine against tuberculosis (TB) infection. BCG is made from live attenuated (or weakened) *Mycobacterium tuberculosis*. Healthcare workers should consider this vaccine if a high percentage of TB patients are infected with TB strains resistant to both isoniazid and rifampin. Vaccination with BCG can produce a false positive with the TB skin test (Mantoux).

THE NATIONAL VACCINE INJURY COMPENSATION PROGRAM

The Vaccine Injury Compensation Program (VICP) is a federal program created to compensate people who have been injured by certain vaccines. Call 1-800-338-2382 or visit the VICP website at https://www.hrsa.gov/vaccine-compensation

CLINICAL PEARLS

- Without treatment, about 1 in 10 people with latent TB infection will develop TB disease.
- Antibodies against influenza take about 2 weeks to develop after vaccination. The flu vaccine can be offered even into January or later because the flu season can last until May.
- For patients age 65 years or older, the higher-dosed vaccines (Fluad, Fluzone High-Dose) are more effective.
- Baloxavir marboxil (Xofluza) is a new single-dose antiviral drug approved by the U.S. Food and Drug Administration (FDA) for treatment of acute uncomplicated influenza within 2 days of illness onset in people age ≥12 years who are otherwise healthy or are at high risk of developing complications from an influenza infection.
- Remind patients to get the influenza vaccine by the end of October. Vaccinating too early (e.g., July, August) may lead to reduced protection against influenza later in the season, particularly among older adults.

KNOWLEDGE CHECK: CHAPTER 4

1. According to the U.S. Preventive Services Task Force (USPSTF) guidelines, which of the following is the screening test for lung cancer for a 70-year-old male patient with a 35 pack-year history of cigarette smoking?
   A. Chest radiograph
   B. MRI of the lungs
   C. Helical low-dosed CT scan
   D. Lung biopsy

2. After receiving the inactivated influenza injection, how many weeks does it take for antibodies to develop in the body?
   A. 1
   B. 2
   C. 3
   D. 4

3. A 40-year-old female patient who is sexually active is being seen by the nurse practitioner (NP) for her annual gynecologic exam. The patient reports that she has been sexually active with two male partners for several months. The NP uses liquid cytology for her Pap exam with cotesting. What is the best explanation for cotesting?
   A. The lab will test for the human papillomavirus (HPV) on the same sample used for the Pap test.
   B. Chlamydia and gonorrhea testing is done after the Pap test on the same visit.
   C. HIV testing is performed after the gynecologic pelvic exam.
   D. Liquid cytology testing is performed during the gynecologic exam.

4. Which of the following is considered a risk factor for colorectal cancer?
   A. Inflammatory bowel disease
   B. Irritable bowel syndrome
   C. Body mass index >24
   D. Late menarche

5. Which of the following is *true* regarding a screening test with high sensitivity?
   A. It can correctly identify an individual who has the disease.
   B. It can correctly identify an individual who does not have the disease.
   C. Subjects with a positive screening test truly have the disease.
   D. Subjects with a negative screening test truly do not have the disease.

6. Which intervention is an appropriate example of secondary prevention of disease?
   A. Daily exercise
   B. Screening for sexually transmitted infections
   C. Cardiac rehabilitation
   D. Gun safety measures

7. A 72-year-old female patient is seen by the nurse practitioner (NP) for a routine physical exam. When discussing preventive screenings, which recommendation will the NP make regarding breast cancer screening?
   A. Breast cancer screenings are no longer indicated due to patient age.
   B. An MRI of the breast should be done every 2 years.
   C. A mammogram should be completed yearly.
   D. A mammogram should be completed every other year.

8. While providing education on skin cancer, which behavioral modification will the nurse practitioner recommend?
   A. Using sun protection factor (SPF) 10 sunscreen daily
   B. Avoiding morning sunlight between 8 a.m. and 10 a.m.
   C. Wearing a wide-brimmed hat while in direct sunlight
   D. Applying oil-based moisturizer before going outdoors

(See answers next page.)

1. C) Helical low-dosed CT scan

Helical low-dosed CT scan is the preferred test to screen for lung cancer. The USPSTF recommends annual screening for lung cancer with low-dose computed tomography (LDCT) in adults age 50 to 80 years who have a 20 pack-year smoking history and currently smoke or have quit within the past 15 years.

2. B) 2

It takes up to 2 weeks to build immunity after the flu vaccine.

3. A) The lab will test for the human papillomavirus (HPV) on the same sample used for the Pap test.

Cotesting is when a HPV test and a Pap test are done at the same time using the same specimen to check for cervical cancer. The Pap test will look for abnormal cervical cells, and the HPV test will test for high-risk HPV types (#16, #18). Women age 30 to 65 years may have an HPV/Pap co-test every 5 years. If cotesting is not done, then the Pap test can be repeated every 3 years until age 65 years.

4. A) Inflammatory bowel disease

Inflammatory bowel diseases such as ulcerative colitis and Crohn disease are considered risk factors for colon cancer. Irritable bowel syndrome, a functional disorder in which the colon tissue is normal, is not a risk factor for colon cancer. Body mass index >24 does not place a patient at increased risk of colon cancer. Late menarche is a risk factor for breast cancer but not for colon cancer.

5. A) It can correctly identify an individual who has the disease.

A test with high sensitivity is very good at identifying individuals who have the disease; therefore, fewer cases of the disease are missed. High specificity is the ability of a test to correctly identify an individual who does not have the disease. Positive predictive value is the probability that subjects with a positive screening test truly have the disease. Negative predictive value is the probability that subjects who have a negative screening test truly do not have the disease.

6. B) Screening for sexually transmitted infections

Secondary prevention involves screenings for early detection of a disease in order to minimize the effects on the body. Screening for sexually transmitted infections would be a secondary prevention technique to help detect infection and allow earlier treatment. Daily exercise and gun safety measures are primary prevention strategies to avoid injury or disease before it occurs. Cardiac rehabilitation is a tertiary prevention strategy to reduce the impact of a disease that has already occurred.

7. D) A mammogram should be completed every other year.

Current recommendations suggest that patients between the ages of 50 and 74 years should obtain a mammogram to screen for breast cancer every other year. Yearly mammograms are no longer recommended. The age at which screening may cease in the absence of other risk factors is age 75 years. The evidence is currently insufficient to recommend the use of adjunctive screening methods such as ultrasound or MRI as a routine screening.

8. C) Wearing a wide brimmed hat while in direct sunlight

Behavioral counseling should be provided to reduce the risk of skin cancer. Behavioral interventions to recommend include using a sunscreen with SPF 15 or higher, avoiding sunlight between 10 a.m. and 4 p.m. when the sun's rays are most direct, and using protective clothing such as long sleeves and pants and wide-brimmed hats. Sunscreen with SPF of less than 15 offers minimal protection. Application of oil-based products can increase the risk for sunburns and skin damage.

9. A 66-year-old female patient is seen by her primary care provider for routine preventive care. She has a 10 pack-year history of smoking and denies any specific symptoms or health complaints. Which screening will the nurse practitioner order for this patient?
   A. DEXA scan
   B. Pelvic ultrasound to evaluate the ovaries
   C. Pap exam with cotesting
   D. Chest radiograph

10. A parent brings their 1-year-old child in for a well-child exam. Upon review of vaccinations, the nurse practitioner (NP) notes that the patient received a dose of hepatitis B immunization at birth and then was not brought back to the clinic for follow-up and further immunizations. How will the NP proceed with immunizations?
    A. Restart the series, with the first dose given in the office today
    B. Obtain hepatitis B titers and restart the series if negative
    C. Give a second dose of the vaccine today and a third dose in 8 weeks
    D. Provide a single booster dose

11. The nurse practitioner (NP) is discussing prostate cancer screening with a patient during the yearly physical exam. Which history provided by the patient would the NP recognize as a risk factor for prostate cancer?
    A. Age of 45 years
    B. Brother with prostate cancer
    C. History of sexually transmitted infections (STIs)
    D. Body mass index (BMI) of 31

12. A patient presents to the clinic in August, requesting the influenza vaccine. They received their previous vaccine in October of last year. After evaluating and discussing the vaccine with the patient, the nurse practitioner recommends that the patient wait until October to receive the vaccine. What is the rationale for this timing?
    A. A new vaccine formulation becomes available in October.
    B. Vaccination must occur at least 1 full year after the prior vaccine was received.
    C. Patients have an increased likelihood of vaccine reactions in warmer temperatures.
    D. Later vaccination ensures that protection coincides with influenza season.

13. Which patient will the nurse practitioner advise to receive the Shingrix vaccine series?
    A. 55 years old with active herpes zoster infection
    B. 38 years old and pregnant
    C. 60 years old and previously received Zostavax
    D. 45 years old with diabetes mellitus

14. A nurse practitioner (NP) received the Bacillus Calmette-Guérin (BCG) vaccine 10 years ago while working in an area with endemic tuberculosis (TB). Which test should the NP undergo for routine TB screening?
    A. Chest x-ray
    B. Mantoux test
    C. Acid-fast bacilli culture
    D. Interferon-gamma release assay

15. A 35-year-old pregnant patient presents to the clinic to obtain the influenza vaccination. Which vaccine formulation should be administered?
    A. Quadrivalent injectable influenza vaccine
    B. High-dose trivalent injectable vaccine
    C. Live attenuated influenza vaccine
    D. Monovalent injectable influenza vaccine

16. For which patient will the nurse practitioner prescribe a low-dose statin for primary prevention of cardiovascular disease (CVD)?
    A. 50 years old with diabetes and a 15% risk of CVD over 10 years
    B. 65 years old with a prior myocardial infarction (MI)
    C. 60 years old with hypertension and a 5% risk of CVD over 10 years
    D. 35 years old with family history of CVD

17. Which of the following is considered to increase risk for development of cervical cancer?
    A. Two or more lifetime partners
    B. Initial onset of intercourse at age 25 years
    C. Body mass index (BMI) >30
    D. HIV infection

(See answers next page.)

9. A) DEXA scan

Screening for osteoporosis should begin at age 66 years or older for those at average risk, making a DEXA scan an appropriate test for this patient. Routine screening for ovarian cancer with ultrasound is not recommended in any group. Pap exam is recommended only until the age of 65 years and would no longer be indicated for this patient. Chest radiograph is no longer recommended as a screening for lung cancer because helical low-dose CT is now preferred; however, this patient has less than a 20 pack-year history and would not meet screening criteria.

10. C) Give a second dose of the vaccine today and a third dose in 8 weeks

Currently the Centers for Disease Control and Prevention do not recommend restarting the hepatitis B vaccine series for individuals that did not receive all three doses. Instead, the patient should receive the next dose in the office today and then be scheduled for a third dose to complete the series. Titers are unnecessary as completing the three-dose series is still currently recommended despite any current titer levels. A single booster would not be sufficient for this patient as only one dose of the three-dose series has been received.

11. B) Brother with prostate cancer

Risk factors for prostate cancer include age older than 50 years, first-degree relative with a history of prostate cancer, and genetic predisposition to prostate cancer. An age of 45 years is not a risk factor for prostate cancer. Additionally, there is no known connection between STIs or BMI and prostate cancer at this time.

12. D) Later vaccination ensures that protection coincides with influenza season.

Protection from the influenza vaccine is thought to last for approximately 6 months. Although the new vaccine formulation for the year generally becomes available in July or August, vaccination at this time may lead to suboptimal immunity before the end of influenza season, which peaks from December until February, but may not end until May. Vaccination does not have to be timed based on the prior vaccination. Vaccine reactions can occur at any time of the year; however, these occur in only a small percentage of patients.

13. C) 60 years old and previously received Zostavax

Patients age 50 years or older should receive the Shingrix vaccine. This should be provided even to patients who previously received Zostavax. A patient should not receive the vaccine while they have an active shingles outbreak (herpes zoster infection) or while pregnant or breastfeeding. There is no current indication for Shingrix to be administered to individuals younger than 50 years.

14. D) Interferon-gamma release assay

Individuals who have received a prior BCG vaccine may have a false-positive TB skin test (Mantoux) and should be screened using an alternate method. The interferon-gamma release assay (TB blood test) is preferred for screening as it does not result in false positives with prior vaccination. Chest x-rays can be completed to follow up on a positive interferon-gamma release assay but are not generally recommended as the preferred screening for latent TB. Acid-fast bacilli cultures are completed from sputum samples of patients with suspected or known TB, but these would not detect latent TB in a screening capacity.

15. A) Quadrivalent injectable influenza vaccine

A trivalent or quadrivalent injectable virus vaccine is recommended for all individuals receiving vaccination who are younger than 65 years. A high-dose trivalent injectable vaccine would be preferred for individuals age 65 years and older, but not for pregnant patients. The live attenuated influenza vaccine is used in individuals age 2 to 49 years, but it is contraindicated in pregnancy. The monovalent injectable influenza virus vaccine provides protection against influenza A only and is no longer used.

16. A) 50 years old with diabetes and a 15% risk of CVD over 10 years

A low-to-moderate–intensity statin is recommended for adults age 40 to 75 years with one or more CVD risk factors (including hypertension, hyperlipidemia, and diabetes) and a 10-year risk of CVD of 10% or greater. Statins are not generally recommended in those with a risk of less than 10%, but lifestyle interventions would be discussed. Patients younger than 40 years should be evaluated based on personal risk factors and lipid levels, but statins are not generally recommended as primary prevention. For individuals with a prior cardiovascular event (e.g., MI, cerebral vascular accident), high-intensity statins are recommended.

17. D) HIV infection

Immunosuppressive conditions, such as HIV, increase the risk for development of cervical cancer. Additionally, having four or more lifetime partners increases the risk, as does early or young onset of sexual intercourse. BMI is not a factor in development of cervical cancer.

18. A 65-year-old female patient is seen in the clinic for a routine examination. During review of her immunizations, it is determined that she received the pneumococcal polysaccharide vaccine (PPSV23) at age 63 years due to a new diagnosis of chronic obstructive pulmonary disease (COPD). What will the nurse practitioner recommend in regard to further pneumonia vaccination?
    A. A booster should be given every 10 years.
    B. No further pneumonococcal vaccine is indicated.
    C. An additional dose should be given 5 years after the first.
    D. A booster should be given now at age 65 years.

19. Which of the following is an indication for the meningococcal vaccine?
    A. Entrance into a public school system
    B. Travel to Canada
    C. Moving to residential college housing
    D. Frequent hiking and camping

20. A 20-year-old pregnant female patient is seen in the clinic for her initial prenatal exam. She reports a history of two prior sexual partners and denies any current symptoms or illness. Which screening will the nurse practitioner recommend?
    A. Cervical cytology
    B. HIV screening
    C. Cervical cytology with high-risk human papillomavirus (HPV) testing
    D. Tuberculosis (TB) screening

(See answers next page.)

18. C) An additional dose should be given 5 years after the first.

PPSV23 is given to adults age 65 years and older and to those with certain high-risk conditions. All adults who have received a previous dose of the vaccine should receive a final dose of PSSV23 after the age of 65 years; however, this should be given at least 5 years after the previous dose. An additional booster would not be warranted now as it has only been 2 years since the last dose. Boosters are not given every 10 years for pneumonia vaccines; instead, Tdap boosters are provided every 10 years.

19. C) Moving to residential college housing

The meningococcal vaccine is indicated for first-year college students entering residential college housing, as well as for individuals entering the military and living in military barracks, individuals with immunocompromise, and individuals traveling to high-risk areas such as sub-Saharan Africa. Children beginning public school require other common childhood vaccines but are not at increased risk for meningitis and are not typically vaccinated for this disease. Canada is not a country with increased risk for meningitis requiring vaccination. Hiking, camping, and outdoor activities do not increase risk for meningitis.

20. B) HIV screening

HIV screening is recommended for all pregnant individuals and therefore would be indicated for this patient. Pap testing with cervical cytology and Pap testing with HPV cotesting are not recommended for women younger than 21 years, even when they are sexually active. TB screening is not routinely completed in pregnant patients and would not be indicated unless the patient expressed concern about symptoms or exposure.

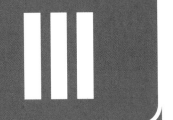

SYSTEMS REVIEW

DANGER SIGNALS

ACUTE ANGLE-CLOSURE GLAUCOMA

Older adult patient with acute onset of severe eye pain accompanied by headache, nausea/vomiting, halos around lights, lacrimation, and decreased vision. Examination reveals mid-dilated, oval-shaped pupil(s). The cornea appears cloudy. Fundoscopic examination reveals cupping of the optic nerve. If the rise in intraocular pressure (IOP) is slower, patient may be asymptomatic. An ophthalmologic emergency. Refer to ED.

AURICULAR HEMATOMA

Direct blunt trauma to the ear that can cause bleeding in the auricular cartilage. The hematoma should be drained as soon as possible. If the hematoma is not drained, it can result in cauliflower ear. It is more common in wrestlers, boxers, and mixed martial arts fighters.

AVULSED TOOTH

Considered a dental emergency for permanent teeth. The sooner the avulsed tooth is reimplanted, the better the outcome. If primary tooth (baby tooth) in a young child, do not reimplant. If permanent tooth, avoid touching root and handle only the crown. Rinse tooth in normal saline; irrigate socket with normal saline, and reimplant tooth. Afterward, have patient hold tooth or bite down on gauze, and refer to dentist as soon as possible. Store tooth in cool milk or saline, or store inside cheek (buccal sulcus) if unable to reimplant.

BASILAR SKULL FRACTURE

Temporal bone is most commonly fractured. Linear fracture most common, followed by depressed and basilar skull fractures. Causes in adults include falls, assaults, car collisions, and penetrating missiles. Periorbital ecchymosis ("raccoon eyes") and mastoid ecchymosis (Battle sign) appear about 1 to 3 days after trauma. Physical exam after trauma does not show these two signs immediately. Assess for clear rhinorrhea or otorrhea, discharge from the ear or nose suggesting a cerebrospinal fluid (CSF) leak. Another common finding in basilar skull fractures is hemotympanum (blue to purple color of the tympanic membrane [TM]), which is caused by blood inside the middle ear. These findings are highly suggestive of a serious head injury. Additional clinical findings are determined by brain hemorrhage, brain injury, and/or cranial nerve (CN) injury. Refer to ED.

CHOLESTEATOMA

Patient may be asymptomatic or may complain of hearing loss and intermittent ear discharge (otorrhea) from one ear that is purulent and foul smelling. On examination, there is perforation of the TM on the superior quadrant and a cauliflower-like or pearly-white mass (Figure 5.1). Another presentation is an intact TM with missing landmarks with the white mass visible behind the TM. Tympanogram will be abnormal (straight line). History of chronic or recurrent otitis media infection. The mass is not cancerous, but it can erode into the bones of the face and damage the facial nerve (CN VII). Treated with antibiotics and surgical excision and repair. Refer to otolaryngologist.

DIPHTHERIA

Infectious disease caused by gram-positive bacillus *Corynebacterium diphtheriae*. Sore throat, malaise, low-grade fever, cervical lymphadenopathy, and possible swelling of the submandibular region and anterior neck ("bull neck"). In one third of cases, the posterior pharynx, tonsils, uvula, and soft palate are coated with a gray to yellow pseudomembrane that is hard to displace. Very contagious. Contact prophylaxis required. Refer to ED.

HERPES SIMPLEX KERATITIS

Acute onset of severe eye pain, photophobia, tearing, and blurred vision in one eye. Often diagnosed based on physical examination. Classified by infectious epithelial keratitis (most common), stromal keratitis, endotheliitis, and neurotrophic keratopathy. Necrotizing stromal keratitis may progress to corneal perforation. Treatment depends on if episode is caused by active viral replication or immune response to past infection. Often, antiviral medications are indicated.

HERPES ZOSTER OPHTHALMICUS

Herpes zoster involvement of the ophthalmic division of the trigeminal nerve (CN V). Herpes zoster ophthalmicus begins with headache, malaise, and fever with unilateral eye involvement or hypesthesia in the affected eye or forehead. Accompanied by vesicular lesions, which signify involvement of the nasocilliary branch of the trigeminal nerve (one side of forehead, eyelids, and tip of nose). Potentially sight-threatening condition. Refer to ED.

INFECTIOUS KERATITIS

Soft contact lens user presents with severe eye pain, eyelid swelling, reduced visual acuity, and photophobia. Assess

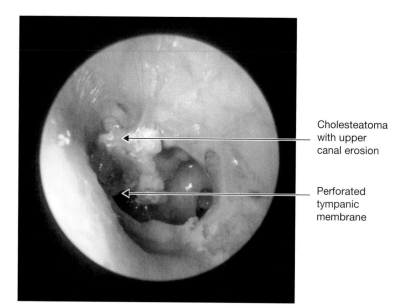

Cholesteatoma with upper canal erosion

Perforated tympanic membrane

Figure 5.1 Cholesteatoma with upper canal erosion.
Source: Image courtesy of Michael Hawke, MD.

visual acuity, pupil size and reactivity, and any lesions or foreign bodies on cornea. Slit lamp evaluation to assess for a corneal perforation. Bacterial keratitis (95% of all contact lens infections) predominantly due to *Pseudomonas*, followed by *Staphylococcus*, or *Streptococcus*. Can permanently impair vision because of scarring or perforation. Most serious complication of contact lens use; considered an ophthalmologic emergency. Refer to ED.

OPTIC NEURITIS

Two thirds of cases occur in female patients in their 20s, 30s, or 40s. Highly associated with multiple sclerosis (MS). Patient often reports loss of visual acuity over hours to days. Color vision is affected, and a central scotoma (blind spot central vision) is common. May be accompanied by other neurologic symptoms (e.g., afferent pupillary defect). Complains of daily fatigue on awakening that worsens as the day goes on. Higher-than-normal temperature will worsen symptoms (Uhthoff phenomenon). Has recurrent episodes. Refer to neurologist.

ORBITAL CELLULITIS

Acute onset of erythematous swollen eyelid with proptosis (bulging of the eyeball) and pain in affected eye. Unable to perform full range of motion (ROM) of the eyes (abnormal extraocular movement [EOM] exam) with pain on eye movement. Look for history of recent rhinosinusitis or upper respiratory infection (URI). Caused by acute bacterial infection of the orbital contents (fat and ocular muscles). More common in young children than adults. Serious complication. Refer to ED.

PERITONSILLAR ABSCESS

Collection of pus between the palatine tonsil and the pharyngeal muscles. Severe sore throat and difficulty swallowing, odynophagia (pain on swallowing), trismus (jaw muscle spasm making it difficult to open mouth), drooling, and a muffled ("hot potato") voice. Unilateral swelling of the peritonsillar area and soft palate. Affected area is markedly swollen and appears as a bulging red mass with the uvula displaced away from the mass. Accompanied by malaise, fever, and chills. Refer to ED.

RETINAL DETACHMENT

Sudden onset of floaters (or black dots in the vision) associated with sudden flashes of light (photopsia). Painless; often presents as a missing portion of the monocular visual field (shadow or "like a curtain being pulled down"). Central vision may be intact or lost if macula is detached. Refer to ED.

VESTIBULAR SCHWANNOMA (ACOUSTIC NEUROMA)

Patient in 50s to 60s presents with unilateral hearing loss (sensorineural) and tinnitus, which has been present for about 3 to 4 years. Complains of unsteadiness while walking and episodes of veering or tilting that vary in severity. Caused by Schwann cell–derived tumor of the acoustic nerve (CN VIII). If facial nerve (CN VII) involved, may have facial paresis and paresthesias. Refer to neurologist.

VIRCHOW'S NODE

Enlarged and hard left-sided supraclavicular node(s) associated with malignancy, especially in adults age 40 years or older. Highly suggestive of cancers of the stomach, colon, pancreas, gallbladder, kidneys, ovaries, testicles, prostate, or lymphoid tissue. The left supraclavicular lymph node drains via the thoracic duct, abdomen, and thorax. Workup includes a thorough history, physical exam, laboratory testing, and imaging. Refer to oncology/surgery for a biopsy.

NORMAL FINDINGS

EYES

The *fundus* is the interior surface visible by fundoscopic exam (ophthalmoscopy). Fundus exam provides ability to view the following anatomic structures:

- Peripheral retina: Fundal background should be a deep red color, without exudate or hemorrhages.
- Optic nerve: Round sphere with sharp margins, an orange/pink neuroretinal rim, and a central white depression (physiologic cup). Cup should not be more than half the size of the disc diameter (if larger, consider glaucoma).
- Macula: Dark, flat spot located in the exact center of the posterior portion of the retina. Responsible for central vision, sharpest vision (20/20 vision), and color vision. Center of the macula is called the fovea centralis. It contains only cones and is area of highest visual acuity. Diseases of the macula cause loss of central vision.
- Vasculature: Blood vessels arise from the nasal side of the optic disc. Arteries are brighter red and narrower than veins; A:V ratio = 2:3 or 4:5. Should not be tortuous or have hemorrhages.

Normal anatomy of the eye also includes:

- Palpebral conjunctiva: Mucosal lining inside eyelids
- Bulbar conjunctiva: Mucosal lining covering the outer surface of the eyes
- Cones: For color perception, sharpest vision (20/20 vision)
- Rods: For low-light vision (night vision), peripheral vision

EARS

- Bones (ossicles) of the ear: Malleus, incus, and stapes. The stapes is the smallest bone in the body.
- TM: Appears as translucent off-white to gray color with the "cone of light" intact. The lateral process of the malleus is located at the upper quadrant of the TM and lies in front of the pars flaccida (Figure 5.2). The pars tensa is located on the lower aspect and appears to bulge slightly. It is the area of the TM where the cone of light is visible.

- Pinna: Has a large amount of cartilage. Blunt trauma can result in a hematoma, which should be drained as soon as possible to avoid damage to the cartilage of the ear. If untreated, it can result in cauliflower ear.
- Tragus: A small cartilage flap of tissue on the front of the ear.
- Cartilage: Found on the nose and ears. Does not regenerate. Refer injuries to plastic surgeon.
- Cerumen: Ear wax; the color can range from yellow to dark brown.

NOSE

- Kiesselbach's plexus: Vasculature of the nasal septum. Located on the anterior inferior aspect of the nose (lower one third). Responsible for up to 90% of nosebleeds.
- Turbinates: Erectile structures in the lateral wall composed of mucosa and spongy bone, covered by mucous membrane. Only the inferior nasal turbinates are usually visible. The medial and superior turbinates are not visible without special instruments. Bluish, pale, and/or boggy nasal turbinates are seen in allergic rhinitis.
- Cartilage: Lower third of the nose is cartilage. Cartilage tissue does not regenerate.
- Septum: Perforation of the nasal septum can result from inhalation of cocaine, which is a potent vasoconstrictor. Refer to plastic surgeon for repair.

SINUSES

Sinuses are air-filled cavities in the skull. There are four types: ethmoid and maxillary (both present at birth), frontal (age 5 years), and sphenoid (age 12 years) (Figure 5.3). By age 12 years, a child's sinuses are nearly at adult proportions.

MOUTH

Mucous membranes are pink to dark pink and moist. Look for ulcers, fissures, leukoplakia, and inflammation. If the gums are red and swollen, the patient may have gingivitis (gums may bleed when brushing teeth) or be taking

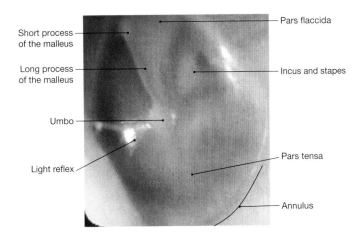

Short process of the malleus

Long process of the malleus

Umbo

Light reflex

Pars flaccida

Incus and stapes

Pars tensa

Annulus

Figure 5.2 Left tympanic membrane.

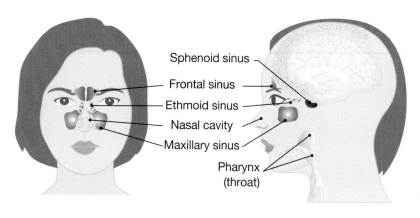

Figure 5.3 Paranasal sinuses.
Source: From Gawlik, K. S., Melnyk, B. M., & Teall, A. M. (Eds.). (2021). (See Resources section for complete source information.)

phenytoin (Dilantin) for seizures (gingival hyperplasia). The tongue should not be red or swollen (glossitis). A normal adult has 32 teeth.

- Vermilion border: Vermilion border is at the edges of the lips. The corners of the lips are called the *oral commissures* (cheilosis, perleche).
- Buccal mucosa: Mucosal lining inside the mouth
- Soft palate: Area where uvula, tonsils, and anterior of throat are located
- Hard palate: "Roof" of the mouth

SALIVARY GLANDS

There are three salivary glands: parotid, submandibular, and sublingual. The glands may become infected (sialadenitis, sialadenosis, mumps) or can become blocked with calculi ("stone"; sialolithiasis).

TONSILS

Also known as the *palatine tonsils*; tonsils are made up of lymphoid tissue. Oval-shaped glands with small pore-like openings that may secrete thick white exudate (mononucleosis) or purulent exudate that is a yellow-to-green color (strep throat).

POSTERIOR PHARYNX

Retropharyngeal lymph nodes that are mildly enlarged and distributed evenly on the back of the throat (allergies, allergic rhinitis). The *uvula* should be in midline position; is displaced if infected and abscessed (peritonsillar abscess).

LYMPH NODES

- Anterior cervical nodes (superficial chain) drain the lymph from the skin and superficial surfaces of the anterior neck.
- The anterior cervical lymph nodes can become enlarged with viral or bacterial infections (strep throat).
- Posterior cervical nodes (superficial chain) drain the scalp, neck, and skin of the upper thoracic area.
- Mononucleosis can cause posterior cervical lymphadenopathy.
- See Figure 5.4 for the lymph nodes of the head and neck.

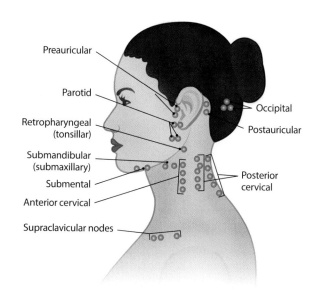

Figure 5.4 Lymph nodes of the head and neck.
Source: From Gawlik, K. S., Melnyk, B. M., & Teall, A. M. (Eds.). (2021). (See Resources section for complete source information.)

ABNORMAL FINDINGS

EYE TERMINOLOGY

- Hyperopia: "Farsightedness"; distance vision is intact, but near vision is blurry.
- Myopia: "Nearsightedness"; near vision is intact, but distance vision is blurry.
- Amblyopia: Also called "lazy eye." Usually starts in infancy. The affected eye has reduced vision. Refer to ophthalmologist.
- Miosis: Excessive constriction of the pupil of the eye.
- Ptosis: Drooping of the upper eyelid.

CATARACTS

- Opacity of the lens of the eye, which can be central (nuclear cataract) or on the sides (cortical cataract) or the back (posterior subcapsular cataract).

- Occur more frequently with increasing age (most occur after age 60 years); however, cataracts can appear at any age from infants (congenital cataracts) through adults to the elderly secondary to poor nutrition, metabolic insults, excessive sunlight or radiation exposure, trauma, and certain medications.
- Painless, progressive process; symptoms include difficulty with glare (with headlights when driving at night or in sunlight), halos around lights, difficulty with distance vision, and blurred vision.

DIABETIC RETINOPATHY

Microaneurysms and "hard exudates" (leakage of lipid and protein material) are the initial detectable signs of diabetic retinopathy. *Neovascularization* (development of new blood vessels) results in:

- Small flame-shaped and blot hemorrhages and intraretinal infarcts ("cotton wool" or "soft exudates"; Figure 5.5) distal to the occlusion
- Irregular changes in venous caliber; tortuosity of blood vessels and proliferation of networks of fragile new vessels
- Capillary leakage can contribute to retinal thickening and can progress to macular edema.

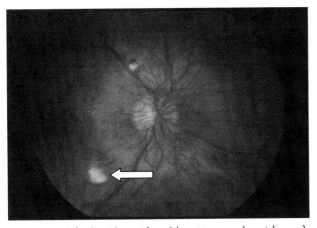

Figure 5.5 Diabetic retinopathy with cotton-wool spot (arrow).
Source: National Institutes of Health and National Eye Institute.
(See Resources section for complete source information.)

DISC CUPPING

Optic nerve cupping is associated with glaucoma. It is caused by increased IOP, and it is measured by using the "cup-to-disc" ratio. The "cup" of the optic disc is the center, and the surrounding area is the "disc." As glaucoma progresses, the cup-to-disc ratio becomes abnormal.

ECTROPION

Eyelid is turned outward or sags away from the eye (Figure 5.6A). It causes irritation and eye dryness. More common in the elderly.

ENTROPION

Eyelid (usually the lower eyelid) is turned inward (Figure 5.6B). The eyelashes continuously rub against the cornea, causing irritation, watery eyes, redness, pain, and/or foreign body sensation. More common in the elderly.

HYPERTENSIVE RETINOPATHY

- Mild: Generalized retinal arteriolar narrowing, arteriolar wall thickening, arteriovenous nicking ("nipping"), and opacification of the arteriolar wall ("copper wiring"; Figure 5.7)
- Moderate: Hemorrhages, either flame- or dot-shaped, cotton-wool spots, hard exudates, and microaneurysms
- Severe: The above symptoms plus optic disc edema (papilledema). Requires rapid lowering of blood pressure.

PAPILLEDEMA

Optic disc swollen with blurred edges due to increased intracranial pressure (ICP) secondary to bleeding, brain tumor, abscess, pseudotumor cerebri

PHYSIOLOGIC GAZE-EVOKED NYSTAGMUS

- On prolonged, extreme lateral gaze, a few beats of nystagmus that resolve when the eye moves back toward midline in healthy patients is often normal.
- Can also be caused by brain lesions

HEARING LOSS

Conductive Hearing Loss (Outer Ear and Middle Ear)

Any type of obstruction (or conduction) of sound waves will cause conductive hearing loss. Other causes include blockage of the outer ear (ceruminosis, otitis externa) or fluid inside the middle ear (otitis media, serous otitis media).

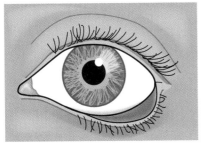
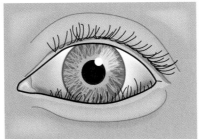

(A)   (B)   **Figure 5.6** (A) Ectropion. (B) Entropion.

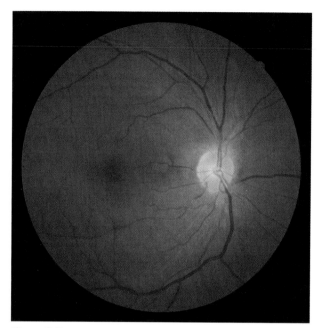

Figure 5.7 Hypertensive retinopathy.
Source: Image courtesy of Frank Wood.

Sensorineural Hearing Loss (Inner Ear)

Damage or aging of the cochlea/vestibule (presbycusis, Ménière's disease) and/or of the nerve pathways causes sensorineural hearing loss. Other causes are ototoxic drugs (e.g., oral aminoglycosides, erythromycin, tetracyclines) and stroke. Usually results in permanent hearing loss.

FISHTAIL OR SPLIT UVULA

- Uvula is split into two sections and resembles a fishtail.
- May be a sign of an occult cleft palate (rare).

GEOGRAPHIC TONGUE

- Tongue surface has a maplike appearance; patches may move from day to day.
- Patient may complain of soreness with acidic or spicy foods.

TORUS PALATINUS

- Painless bony protuberance midline on the hard palate (roof of the mouth); may be asymmetric; skin should be normal.
- Does not interfere with normal function.

ORAL HAIRY LEUKOPLAKIA

- Unusual disease of the lingual squamous epithelium; not considered a premalignant lesion.
- Lesions are corrugated painless plaques on the lateral aspects of the tongue that cannot be scraped off (Figure 5.8).
- Often seen in immunocompromised patients (e.g., HIV infection)
- Associated with Epstein–Barr virus (EBV) infection

KOPLIK'S SPOTS

- Clusters of small whitish, grayish, or bluish elevations with an erythematous base, typically seen on the buccal mucosa opposite the molar teeth (Figure 5.9).
- Pathognomonic for measles

ORAL LEUKOPLAKIA

- Although regarded as benign and not dangerous, certain instances of leukoplakia indicate initial signs of oral cancer forming next to the growths.
- Bright-white to light-gray plaques on the tongue, floor of mouth, or inner cheeks (buccal mucosa) caused by chronic irritation, such as from tobacco use (smoked and smokeless) and alcohol drinking.
- Chewing or smoking tobacco, alcohol use disorder, and human papillomavirus (HPV) are risk factors for oral cancer. Refer to oral surgeon for biopsy.

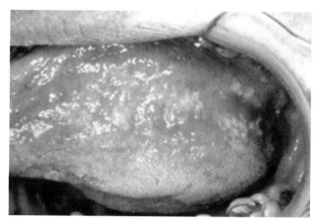

Figure 5.8 Oral hairy leukoplakia.
Source: National Cancer Institute. (See Resources section for complete source information.)

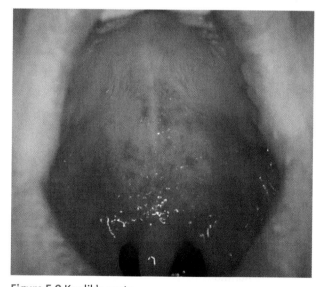

Figure 5.9 Koplik's spots.
Source: Heinz F. Eichenwald, MD/Centers for Disease Control and Prevention.

APHTHOUS STOMATITIS (CANKER SORES)

Painful shallow ulcers on soft tissue of the mouth that usually heal within 7 to 10 days (Figure 5.10). Cause is unknown; however, minor trauma such as biting the inside of the cheek, acidic foods, and stress are thought to be causative. Treat symptoms with "magic mouthwash" (combination of liquid diphenhydramine, viscous lidocaine, and glucocorticosteroid). Swish, hold, and spit every 4 hours as needed. Other options include Orabase cream/ointment (OTC).

NASAL POLYPS

- Painless, soft, mucus-filled lobular lesions found inside the nose and paranasal sinuses.
- "Grape-like" appearance with boggy, pale, enlarged turbinate; causes nasal symptoms and allergy symptoms (e.g., itchy, watery eyes); patient may have chronic sinus infections.
- Common in patients with cystic fibrosis and allergic fungal sinusitis.
- Intranasal or oral glucocorticoids may be used as treatment. If poor response or recurrent sinus infection, refer to an ear, nose, and throat (ENT) specialist for surgical treatment.

EXAM TIP

Koplik's spots are seen in rubeola (measles). Think of the letter *o* as a spot (as in Koplik's spot).

EVALUATION AND TESTING

VISION TESTING

Distance Vision

The Snellen chart measures central distance vision.
- If the person cannot read, can use the Tumbling E chart. Patient must stand 20 feet away from the chart.

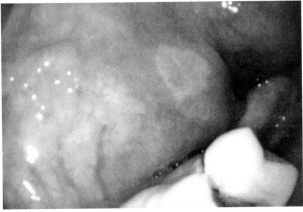

Figure 5.10 Aphthous stomatitis (canker sore).
Source: From Gawlik, K. S., Melnyk, B. M., & Teall, A. M. (Eds.). (2021). (See Resources section for complete source information.)

- If the patient wears glasses, test the vision with the glasses in both eyes (OU), the right eye (OD), and the left eye (OS).
- Abnormal result is two-line difference between each eye; fewer than four letters out of six correct.

Visual Test Results

- Definition of a Snellen test result 20/60: The top number (or numerator) is the distance in feet that the patient stands from the Snellen or picture eye chart (always 20 feet and never changes). The bottom number (or denominator) is the number of feet at which the patient can see compared with a person with normal vision of 20/20 or less. The number changes, dependent on patient's vision. In this example, the patient can see at 20 feet what a person with normal vision can see at 60 feet.
- Definition of legal blindness: A best corrected vision of 20/200 or less or a visual field of less than 20 degrees (tunnel vision).

Near Vision

Near visual acuity can be measured with the Rosenbaum pocket vision screening card or by having the patient read a newspaper or magazine held 14 inches (at arm's length) from the eyes.

Peripheral Vision

- Use the "visual fields of confrontation" exam.
- Look for blind spots (scotoma) and peripheral visual field defects.

Color Blindness

Use the Ishihara chart for color vision testing.

Testing of Children

By age 6 years, visual acuity (retina or CN II) is 20/20 in both eyes. Use the Snellen chart with the child standing 20 feet away from the chart. If the child's vision is not at least 20/30 in either eye by age 6 years, refer to ophthalmologist.

HEARING TESTS

Table 5.1 Types of Hearing Loss: Results of Weber and Rinne Tests

Results	Weber Test	Rinne Test
Normal	No lateralization (hears sound equally in both ears)	AC > BC
Sensorineural loss (e.g., Presbycusis, Ménière's disease)	Lateralization to "good" ear (sound is heard louder in the ear that is normal)	AC > BC
Conductive loss (e.g., otitis media, cerumen, perforation of tympanic membrane)	Lateralization to "bad" ear (sound is heard louder in the affected ear)	BC > AC

AC, air conduction; BC, bone conduction.

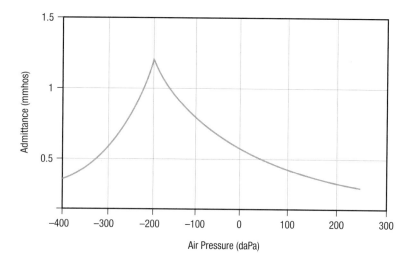

Figure 5.11 Tympanogram result (normal peak).

Weber Test

- Place the tuning fork midline on the forehead. Ask the patient if the sound is louder in one ear or the other.
- Normal finding is no lateralization; sound heard equally in both ears. Lateralization (hearing the sound in only one ear, or sound louder in one ear) is an abnormal finding.

Rinne Test

- Place tuning fork first on mastoid process (bone conduction [BC]), then at front of the ear (air conduction [AC]). Time each area.
- Normal finding is AC lasting longer than BC (i.e., can hear longer in front of ear than on mastoid bone).

Tympanogram

Objective measure to test for presence of fluid inside middle ear (results in a straight line vs. a peaked shape). Acute otitis media (AOM) and serous otitis media will show a straight line on testing (Figure 5.11).

DISEASE REVIEW

EYES

Age-Related Macular Degeneration

Usually asymptomatic during the early stages. Caused by gradual damage to the pigment of the macula (area of central vision) that results in severe visual loss or blindness. Leading cause of blindness in the elderly. More common in smokers.

Age-related macular degeneration (AMD) can be either atrophic (dry form) or exudative (wet form). The dry form of AMD is more common and is less severe compared with the wet form. The wet form of AMD is responsible for 80% of vision loss (choroidal neovascularization).

Classic Case

Elderly smoker complains of gradual or sudden and painless loss of central vision in one or both eyes. Reports that straight lines (doors, windows) appear distorted or curved. Peripheral vision is usually preserved.

Treatment Plan

- Diagnosis and testing via dilated eye exam, fluorescein angiography, optical coherence tomography, and/or Amsler grid (focus eye on center dot and view grid 12 inches from eyes). A patient with wet AMD will see center of grid as distorted with bent, wavy lines.
- Both wet and dry AMD can be treated with the Age-Related Eye Disease Studies (ARES) formula, a combination of ocular vitamins and minerals. Patients should consult their ophthalmologist before taking ocular vitamins.
- Wet AMD can be treated with vascular endothelial growth factor (VEGF) inhibitors (prevent new blood vessels from forming) and/or photodynamic therapy.
- Refer to ophthalmologist.

Angle-Closure Glaucoma

Caused by narrowing or closure of the anterior chamber angle, leading to inadequate drainage, elevated IOP, and damage to the optic nerve. Medical emergency that must be treated to prevent permanent blindness.

Classic Case

Older patient complains of acute onset of decreased/blurred vision with severe eye pain and frontal headache that is accompanied by nausea and vomiting. Patient may also complain of halos around lights.

Objective Findings

Eyes are fixed and mid-dilated, cloudy pupil (4–6 mm) that looks more oval than round. Pupil reacts slowly to light. Conjunctival injection with increased lacrimation. Corneal edema or cloudiness. A shallow anterior chamber.

Treatment Plan

Refer to ED.

Anterior Uveitis (Iritis)

Insidious onset of eye pain with conjunctival injection (redness; note that *injection of the eye* means the superficial blood vessels of the conjunctiva are prominent [red eyes]) located mainly on the limbus (junction between cornea and sclera). Frequently occurs in association with other infections and inflammatory diseases such as rheumatoid arthritis (RA), lupus, ankylosing spondylitis, sarcoidosis, or syphilis. Symptoms can be nonspecific and depend on the portion of the uveal tract involved.

Treatment Plan

Refer to ophthalmologist for management as soon as possible within 24 hours. Anterior uveitis can result in blindness.

Blepharitis

Chronic condition caused by inflammation of the eyelids (hair follicles, meibomian glands). Associated with seborrheic dermatitis and rosacea. Lid may be colonized by staphylococcal bacteria. Intermittent exacerbations. Patient complains of itching or irritation in the eyelids (upper/lower or both), gritty sensation, eye redness, and crusting.

Treatment Plan

- Gently scrub eyelid margins with diluted baby shampoo and warm water until resolves. Consider topical antibiotic solution (erythromycin eye drops) to eyelids two or three times/day (lid hygiene). Commercial eyelid scrub products are available.
- Apply warm compress to eyelids two to four times/day during exacerbations to soften debris and relieve itching.
- Limit trigging factors such as allergens, cigarette smoking, and contact lenses.
- Refer to ophthalmologist for more severe symptoms; treatment may require topical antibiotic ointment (e.g., bacitracin) or oral antibiotic therapy (e.g., doxycycline).

Chalazion

A chronic inflammation of the meibomian gland (specialized sweat gland) of the eyelids. It may resolve spontaneously in 2 to 8 weeks.

Classic Case

Patient complains of a gradual onset of a small, superficial nodule on the upper eyelid that feels like a bead and is discrete and movable (Figure 5.12). Painless. Can slowly enlarge over time. If chalazion is large, it can press on the cornea and cause blurred vision.

Treatment Plan

- May take several weeks to resolve if untreated. Place warm compresses on eyelid at least twice a day to facilitate drainage. Antibiotics often not indicated.

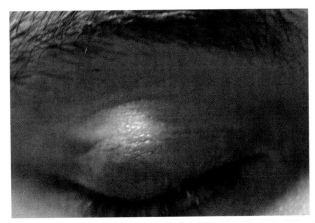

Figure 5.12 Chalazion.

- If it does not resolve over 1 to 2 months, refer to ophthalmologist for possible incision and curettage or glucocorticoid injection.

Corneal Abrasion

Trauma to the eye resulting in interruption of epithelial surface. Patient complains of acute onset of severe eye pain with tearing and redness. Reports feeling of a foreign-body sensation on the surface of the eye. Always ask any patient with eye complaints whether they wear contact lenses.

Objective Findings

Normal visual acuity. A round reactive pupil associated with mild conjunctival injection, tears, and/or corneal defect. Staining defect on fluorescein examination. Contact lens–associated abrasions are usually in the center and are round.

Treatment Plan

- Use topical ophthalmic antibiotic with pseudomonal coverage (especially if contact lens user), such as ciprofloxacin (Ciloxan), ofloxacin (Ocuflox), or trimethoprim–polymyxin B (Polytrim), applied to affected eye for 3 to 5 days.
- Do not patch eye. Follow up in 24 hours. If not improved, refer to ED or ophthalmologist.

Herpes Simplex Keratitis

Patient complains of acute onset of severe eye pain, photophobia, and blurred vision in affected eye. Presentation often unilateral. Diagnosis often based on clinical history and examination findings without lab testing. Infection permanently damages corneal epithelium, which may result in corneal blindness.

Objective Findings

Conjunctivitis, decreased corneal sensation, and characteristic dendritic lesions of the cornea. Fluorescein staining appears as fernlike with branching pattern.

Treatment Plan

Treatment depends on whether the episode is caused by active viral replication or immune response to past infection. Epithelial herpes simplex keratitis, use antiviral therapy. Stromal keratitis, combination therapy with a topical glucocorticoid and antiviral treatment. Do not use topical glucocorticoids when active herpes simplex virus (HSV) epithelial disease is present.

Hordeolum (Stye)

An external hordeolum is an abscess of a hair follicle and sebaceous gland in the upper or lower eyelid. An internal hordeolum involves inflammation of the meibomian gland. May have history of blepharitis.

Classic Case

Patient complains of acute onset of a swollen, red, and warm abscess on the upper or lower eyelid involving one hair follicle that gradually enlarges. May spontaneously rupture and drain purulent exudate. Infection may spread to adjoining tissue (preseptal cellulitis).

Treatment Plan

- Most resolve spontaneously and do not require specific intervention.
- Hot compresses for 5 to 10 minutes two to three times a day until it drains.
- If infection spreads (preseptal cellulitis), start empiric antibiotic therapy. Refer to ophthalmologist for incision and drainage (I&D).

Infectious Keratitis

Patient complains of acute onset of red eye, blurred vision, watery eyes, photophobia, and sometimes a foreign-body sensation in affected eye. History of using contacts past prescribed time schedule, sleeping with contact lenses, bathing/showering or swimming with contacts, extended lens use, and/or poor disinfection practices.

Objective Findings

Red, painful eye in any contact lens wearer.

Treatment Plan

- Always check visual acuity and check pupils with penlight. Rule out penetrating trauma, retained foreign body, and contact lens–associated eye infections. If suspect bacterial infection, obtain C&S of eye discharge.
- Flush eye with sterile normal saline to remove any foreign body. Evert eyelid to look for foreign body. If unable to remove, refer.
- Stop contact lens use. Do not patch eye. Urgent ophthalmologic referral. Initiation of topical empiric antibiotic therapy. Avoid glucocorticoids.
- Consider pain prescription (hydrocodone with acetaminophen; prescribe enough for 48 hours of use).
- Consider topical pain medication (ketorolac tromethamine [Acular] 1 gtt four times a day (QID); contraindicated if allergy to nonsteroidal anti-inflammatory drugs [NSAIDs]).

Open-Angle Glaucoma

Open-angle glaucoma is characterized by progressive peripheral visual field loss followed by central field loss (late manifestation). Patients rarely experience symptoms as long as central vision is preserved. While not always, can be associated with increased IOP secondary to increased aqueous production and/or decreased outflow.

Classic Case

Mostly seen in elderly patients, especially those who are have diabetes. Usually asymptomatic during early stages. Gradual changes in peripheral vision (lost first) and then central vision. May complain of missing portions of words when reading. Ophthalmoscopic examination reveals "cupping," the optic nerve taking on a hollowed appearance. If fundoscopic exam shows cupping, IOP is too high. Refer to ophthalmologist.

Treatment Plan

- Check IOP (use tonometer). Normal range is 8 to 21 mmHg.
- IOP ≥30 mmHg is considered very high. Urgent referral within 24 hours to ophthalmologist or referral to ED.

Medications

- Xalatan (Latanoprost): Topical prostaglandin eye drops (increase aqueous outflow)
- Timolol 0.5% (Betimol): Beta-blocker eye drops (decrease aqueous production).
- Ocular side effects: Hyperemia or a burning sensation in the eyes.
- Contraindications: Asthma, emphysema, chronic obstructive pulmonary disease (COPD), second- or third-degree heart block, heart failure; side effects in these patients are similar to those associated with systemic therapy (worsening of heart failure, bradycardia, heart block, increased airway resistance).

Complications

- Second leading cause of blindness in the world (after cataracts).
- Leading cause of irreversible blindness and leading cause of blindness among African Americans

Pinguecula

A raised, yellow-to-white, small, round lesion arising at the limbal conjunctiva next to the cornea. Arises from the limbus and remains confined to the conjunctiva without corneal involvement. Located on the nasal and temporal side of the eye. Caused by chronic sun exposure.

Pterygium

A yellow, triangular (wedge-shaped) thickening of the conjunctiva that extends across the cornea on the nasal side (Figure 5.13). Results from chronic sun exposure. Sometimes called *surfer's eye*. Can be red or inflamed at times. Patient may complain of foreign body sensation in the eye.

Treatment Plan (for Both Pinguecula and Pterygium)

- Manage symptoms with topical ophthalmologic lubricants (artificial tears) as needed for irritation.
- Recommend use of good-quality sunglasses (100% protection against ultraviolet A [UVA] and ultraviolet B [UVB] radiation).
- Remove surgically if the growth encroaches on cornea and affects vision.

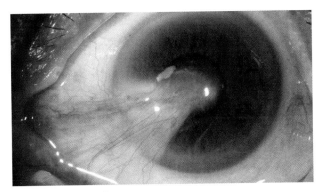

Figure 5.13 Pterygium.
Source: Image courtesy of J. M. Vargas.

Sjögren's Syndrome
Chronic autoimmune disorder characterized by decreased function of the lacrimal and salivary glands. It can occur alone or with another autoimmune disorder (e.g., RA).

Classic Case
Persistent daily symptoms of dry eyes and dry mouth (xerostomia) for >3 months. Patient complains of chronic dry eyes and a sandy or gritty sensation (keratoconjunctivitis sicca). Has used over-the-counter (OTC) artificial tears more than three times per day. Marked increase in dental caries; oral examination shows swollen and inflamed salivary glands.

Treatment Plan
Use OTC tear-substitute eye drops three times daily (TID). Refer to multidisciplinary team for evaluation and management, such as an ophthalmologist (keratoconjunctivitis sicca), dentist (dental caries), rheumatologist, and oral medicine specialist.

Subconjunctival Hemorrhage
Blood that is trapped underneath the conjunctiva and sclera secondary to broken arterioles. Can be caused by coughing, sneezing, heavy lifting, vomiting, or local trauma or can occur spontaneously. Resolves within 1 to 3 weeks (blood reabsorbed) like a bruise, with color changes from red, to green, to yellow. Increased risk if patient is on aspirin or anticoagulants or has hypertension.

Classic Case
Patient complains of sudden onset of bright-red blood in one eye after an incident of severe coughing, sneezing, or straining. May also be due to trauma such as a fall. Denies visual loss and pain.

Treatment Plan
- Spontaneous, nontraumatic subconjunctival hemorrhage: Watchful waiting and reassurance of patient. Most are not associated with intraocular injury. Follow up until resolution.
- Traumatic subconjunctival hemorrhage: Rule out underlying retinal trauma and open globe injury.

EARS AND SINUSES
Acute Bacterial Rhinosinusitis
Inflammation of the nasal cavity and paranasal sinuses; generally lasts less than 4 weeks. The maxillary and frontal sinuses are most affected. History of a "bad cold" or flare-up of allergic rhinitis. Fluid is trapped inside the sinuses, causing secondary bacterial (e.g., *S. pneumoniae, H. influenzae*) or viral infection. Antibiotics rarely needed; viral infections are causative in most cases.

Classic Case
Patient complains of unilateral facial pain or upper molar pain (maxillary sinus) with nasal congestion for 10 days or longer with purulent nasal and/or postnasal drip. If frontal sinusitis, pain is located over the frontal sinus. May report hyposmia (reduced ability to smell). Postnasal drip cough worsens when supine and may interfere with sleep. Self-treatment with OTC cold and sinus remedies provides no relief of symptoms.

Objective Findings
- Posterior pharynx: Purulent dark-yellow to green postnasal drip
- Sinuses: Tender to palpation on the front cheek (maxillary) or on frontal sinus area above the inner canthus of the eye. Erythema or edema over the involved cheekbone or periorbital area.
- If seen with allergy flare-up: Possible swollen (boggy) nasal turbinates
- Fever: Seen more often in children than adults
- Transillumination (frontal and maxillary sinuses): Positive ("glow" of light on infected sinus is duller compared with normal sinus); in transillumination, turn off the light (darkened room). Place a bright light source directly on the surface of the cheek (on maxillary sinus). Instruct patient to open mouth and look at the roof of the mouth (hard palate) for a round glow of light. Compare both sides. The affected sinus has no glow or duller glow compared with the normal sinus. For frontal sinusitis, place the light under the supraorbital ridge in the medial aspect and compare glow of light.

Treatment Plan
- Symptomatic treatment without antibiotics if mild, uncomplicated acute bacterial rhinosinusitis (ABRS) in healthy patient. Generally, self-limiting disease. Treatment is symptom management with oral fluids and, if needed, saline nasal irrigations. Follow up in 10 days

(if better, no antibiotics needed). If symptoms are worse (or have not resolved) on follow-up visit, initiate antibiotic treatment if a bacterial infection is suspected.

- Treat with antibiotics if there are severe symptoms (toxic, high fever, pain, purulent nasal or postnasal drip for ≥2 to 3 days, maxillary toothache, unilateral facial pain, sense of bad odor in nose [cacosmia], initial symptom improved, then worsening of symptoms), patient is immunocompromised, or symptoms present for >10 days (or have worsened).

Antibiotic Treatment
First-Line (Adults)
- Choice of antibiotic is based on the most common bacteria associated with ABRS
- Amoxicillin–clavulanate (Augmentin) (500 mg/125 mg PO three times daily or 875 mg/125 mg PO twice daily [BID]). Treatment of children is covered in Section V of this book.

Penicillin Allergy or Alternative Antibiotics
- Doxycycline BID 100 mg PO twice daily
- For those who can tolerate cephalosporins, a third-generation oral cephalosporin (cefixime 400 mg daily or cefpodoxime 200 mg twice daily) with or without clindamycin (300 mg every 6 hours) is an alternative

Symptomatic or Adjunct Treatment
Recommended for rhinosinusitis or otitis media (discussed below).
For pain or fever:
- Naproxen sodium (Anaprox DS) PO BID or ibuprofen (Advil) PO QID as needed (PRN)
- Acetaminophen (Tylenol) every 4 to 6 hours PRN
For drainage:
- Increased oral fluids will thin mucus
- Oral decongestants such as pseudoephedrine (Sudafed) or pseudoephedrine combined with guaifenesin (Mucinex D)
- Topical decongestants (i.e., Afrin), to be used for 3 days maximum or will cause rebound
- Saline nasal spray (Ocean spray) one or two times every 2 to 3 hours PRN
- Steroid nasal spray (Flonase, Vancenase) if allergic rhinitis
- Mucolytic (guaifenesin) and increase fluid to thin mucus
For cough:
- Dextromethorphan (Robitussin) QID
- Benzonatate (Tessalon Perles) prescription; swallow pills with water; do not crush, suck, or chew; toxic for children younger than 10 years (seizures, cardiac arrest, death)
- Increase intake of fluids, avoid exposure to cigarette smoke and alcohol
- The use of systemic steroids is not recommended

Treatment Failure
If symptoms persist despite treatment (purulent nasal discharge, sinus pain, nasal congestion, fever), re-examine patient and possibly switch to another antibiotic. If recurrent sinusitis, refer to otolaryngologist. Nasal irrigation may help: Use only sterile water (not tap water) with saline packet.

Serious Complications of Rhinosinusitis and Otitis Media
- Mastoiditis: Red and swollen mastoid that is tender to palpation.
- Preorbital or orbital cellulitis (more common in children): Swelling and redness at periorbital area, double vision or impaired vision, and fever. Abnormal extraorbital muscles (EOM) movement of affected orbit (check CNs, EOM). Altered level of consciousness (LOC) or mental status changes.
- Meningitis: Acute onset of high fever, stiff neck, severe headache, photophobia, toxicity. Positive Brudzinski or Kernig sign.
- Cavernous sinus thrombosis: Patient complains of acute onset of severe headache that interferes with sleep, abnormal neurologic exam, confusion, febrility. Life-threatening emergency with high mortality.

Acute Otitis Media
Most cases occur in childhood. An acute, suppurative infection of the middle ear cavity with bacterial pathogens due to mucus that becomes trapped in the middle ear; secondary to temporary eustachian tube dysfunction. The infection is usually unilateral but may at times involve both ears. Most have middle ear effusion (MEE). See above for serious complications.

Organisms
- *Streptococcus pneumoniae* and *Hemophilus influenzae* are the common bacterial pathogens in both adults and children.
- Group A *Streptococcus, Staphylococcus aureus*, and *Moraxella catarrhalis* are less frequent causes.

Classic Case
Patient complains of ear pain (otalgia), popping noises, muffled hearing. Recent history of a cold or flare-up of allergic rhinitis. Adult infections usually develop much more slowly than in children. Afebrile, or a low-grade fever. May be accompanied by rupture of the TM (reports blood and pus seen on pillowcase on awakening with relief of ear pain). In adults, an upper respiratory tract infection or exacerbation of seasonal allergic rhinitis often precedes the onset of AOM.

Objective Findings
- With otoscopy, shows bulging TM; reduced mobility of the TM when pneumatic pressure is applied; may also see erythematous TM and/or partial or complete opacification of the TM
- Decreased mobility with flat-line tracing on tympanogram
- If TM is ruptured, purulent discharge from affected ear (and relief of ear pain)
- A conductive hearing loss may be demonstrated: Weber exam shows lateralization to the "bad"/affected ear; Rinne test result is BC > AC.

Treatment Plan

Antibacterial therapy: Amoxicillin-clavulanate is first-line treatment for any age group (if no antibiotics in the prior month). Give amoxicillin-clavulanate 875 mg/125 mg PO twice daily.

- With penicillin allergy, acceptable alternatives include a second- or third-generation cephalosporin (e.g., cefdinir).
- Most patients will respond in 48 to 72 hours. If no response to treatment, re-examine and use high-dose amoxicillin-clavulanate (if not used initially), a second- or third-generation cephalosporin, or another agent.
- In addition to antibiotic, treat symptoms of ear pain (otalgia) and eustachian tube dysfunction (becomes swollen due to inflammation and cannot drain). Patient will complain of a "plugged-up" ear (MEE) and decreased hearing in affected ear (temporary). When fluid in the middle ear drains, hearing will become normal.
- See previous discussion for symptomatic or adjunct treatment.

Bullous Myringitis

May mimic AOM, but the pathology is limited to the TM and does not affect the contents of the middle ear. Infectious condition characterized by the presence of blisters (bullae) on a reddened and bulging TM. Conductive hearing loss. Caused by different types of pathogens (mycoplasma, virus, bacteria).

Otitis Externa (Swimmer's Ear)

Also known as external otitis. Infection and inflammation of the skin of the external ear canal (rarely fungal). More common during warm and humid weather. Other risk factors include trauma (e.g., from cotton swabs), occlusive devices (e.g., hearing aids), allergic contact dermatitis (e.g., from shampoos), and dermatologic conditions (e.g., psoriasis).

Organisms

Several bacteria can cause external otitis, but it is most often caused by:

- *Pseudomonas aeruginosa* (gram-negative)
- *Staphylococcus epidermidis* (gram-positive)
- *S. aureus* (gram-positive)

Classic Case

Patient complains of external ear pain, swelling, discharge, pruritus, and hearing loss (if ear canal is blocked with pus). History of recent activities that involve swimming or getting ears wet.

Objective Findings

Ear pain and tenderness with manipulation of the external ear or tragus. Purulent green discharge. Erythematous and swollen ear canal that is very tender to the touch.

Treatment Plan

- Cleanout of the external ear canal is the first essential step in treatment.
- Mild disease with an intact TM is characterized by minor discomfort and pruritis and minimal canal edema. Treat with a non-antibiotic acidifying agent and glucocorticoid (e.g., acetic acid-hydrocortisone).
- Moderate disease with an intact TM is characterized by intermediate degree of pain and pruritis; canal may be partially occluded. Treat with a topical antibiotic and a glucocorticoid (e.g., ciprofloxacin-hydrocortisone) for 1 week.
- Severe disease with an intact TM is characterized by intense pain, and canal is completely occluded from edema. Treat with a topical antibiotic and a glucocorticoid (e.g., ciprofloxacin-hydrocortisone) for 1 week with wick placement.
- Treat immunocompromised patients with combined topical and systemic antibiotics rather than topical therapy alone.
- For non-intact TM, treatment with a topical fluoroquinolone (e.g., ciprofloxacin) or oral antibiotics (e.g., levofloxacin 500 mg PO once daily).
- Keep water out of ear during treatment. Hearing aids and other devices should not be worn until pain and discharge subsides.

Otitis Media With Effusion

Middle ear fluid without active infection. May follow AOM. Can also be caused by chronic allergic rhinitis, recent viral infection, or barotrauma. Patient complains of ear pressure, popping noises, and muffled hearing in affected ear. Often, characterized by a temporary conductive hearing loss and aural fullness typically without pain.

Objective Findings

- TM may appear normal or slightly erythematous.
- TM is intact and may or may not be retracted (depending on chronicity).
- Fluid behind the TM is often yellow or clear. An air-fluid level and/or bubble may be seen.

Treatment Plan

- Majority will resolve over the course of 12 weeks; can be managed with observation
- Symptom management with oral decongestants (pseudoephedrine or phenylalanine), antihistamines, and/or nasal corticosteroids.
- Steroid nasal spray BID to TID × few weeks or saline nasal spray PRN
- Myringotomy with tympanostomy tubes may be considered for persistent symptomatic effusions lasting longer than 12 weeks

CLINICAL PEARLS

- MEEs can persist for 8 weeks or longer after treatment of AOM.
- Allergy pillow covers, allergy mattresses, and high-efficiency particulate air (HEPA) allergy filters for air conditioners are recommended for patients with allergic rhinitis. Many are allergic to dust mites, an indoor allergen.

- Treatment for moderate otitis externa is ciprofloxacin-hydrocortisone (topical antibiotic combined with a steroid).
- Common bacterial pathogens in otitis externa are *P. aeruginosa*, *S. epidermidis*, and *S. aureus*.

Vertigo

- Vertigo is a symptom, not a diagnosis, of illusory movement. Result of asymmetry in the vestibular system due to damage to or dysfunction of the labyrinth, vestibular nerve, or central vestibular structures in the brainstem.
- There are two types of vertigo. Peripheral vertigo (most common) is caused by disorders of the vestibular apparatus of the inner ear or by the inflammation of vestibular nerve (CN VIII). The most common are benign paroxysmal positional vertigo (BPPV), vestibular neuritis, and Ménière's disease. Central vertigo is associated with serious to life-threatening conditions such as stroke (cerebellar or brainstem bleeding), MS, infections, or tumor.

- A person with vertigo will describe the sensation of the room spinning or of rotational movement. May be associated with nystagmus; presence helps confirm vertigo, but absence does not rule out. May also be associated with nausea and vomiting and postural and gait instability.
- It is important to assess if the person has vertigo or other types of dizziness such as near syncope, hypoglycemia, orthostatic hypotension, cerebrovascular disease, and arrhythmias. Table 5.2 lists the differential diagnoses of vertigo.

- Cholesteatoma presents in affected ear either with retracted TM (primary acquired) or result of TM perforation (secondary acquired). Patient presents with hearing loss, vertigo, and/or otorrhea.
- Cerumen removal is indicated for patients with symptoms (e.g., hearing loss, earache, ear fullness, itchiness). Cerumenolytics are safe to use (e.g., mineral oil, hydrogen peroxide, carbamide peroxide).

Table 5.2 Differential Diagnoses of Vertigo

Condition	Characteristics	Assessment and Treatment
Ménière's disease	Peripheral vestibular disorder attributed to excess endolymphatic fluid pressure causing episodic inner ear dysfunction Triad of recurrent vertigo, tinnitus, and progressive hearing loss; may have nausea/vomiting with episodes. No associated neurologic symptoms.	Initial treatment involves lifestyle changes. Salt restriction (2–3 g/day); avoid triggers (e.g., MSG and nicotine); minimize intake of caffeine, alcohol (one serving/day). Vestibular suppressant PRN; antiemetic medication PRN. Persistent attacks, refer to ENT specialist; consider vestibular rehabilitation or pharmacotherapy for refractory symptoms.
BPPV	Peripheral vertigo due to calcium carbonate crystals (otoconia) trapped in the semicircular canals. Abrupt onset with brief episodes of vertigo that last <1 minute induced by sudden head movements and positions. Risk factors are head trauma, high-intensity aerobics, bike riding in rough trails. Common cause of vertigo; more common in those older than 60 years.	Dix–Hallpike maneuver is gold-standard test to identify posterior canal BPPV (most common subtype). Treatment with a particle repositioning maneuver: Epley maneuver or Semont maneuver. Antiemetics: Meclizine PO q4–8h (vertigo); prochlorperazine IM, rectal suppository, or PO (nausea/vomiting). Advise to avoid sleeping on the side of the affected ear for several days.
Vestibular schwannoma (acoustic neuroma)	CN VIII (vestibular portion) tumors. Schwann cell–derived tumors. Account for 80–90% of CPA tumors in adults. Symptoms are slow and insidious. Two major symptoms with cochlear nerve involvement (95% of patients) are chronic hearing loss (average duration 4 years) and chronic tinnitus. If trigeminal nerve is compressed (17%), symptoms are facial numbness and pain. With vestibular nerve involvement (61%), causes unsteadiness while walking. Facial nerve involvement (6%) causes facial paresis and taste disturbances.	Diagnosis suggested by presence of asymmetric sensorineural hearing loss or other CN deficits. Weber and Rinne tests, hearing testing (audiometry best initial screening test), CN testing. MRI or CT to detect CPA tumor. Refer to ENT specialist; surgical removal, radiation therapy, hearing rehabilitation.

(continued)

Table 5.2 Differential Diagnoses of Vertigo (*continued*)

Condition	Characteristics	Assessment and Treatment
Vestibular neuritis (labyrinthitis)	Due to inflammation of the vestibular portion of the eight CNs caused by viral or bacterial infection. Sudden onset of severe vertigo with nausea, vomiting, and gait impairment. Labyrinthitis with unilateral hearing loss. Episodes can last from hours to days.	HINTS and, if indicated, MRI to rule out vascular event. Steroid taper; vestibular suppressants and antiemetics PRN for symptom management in the first 24 to 48 hours. If suspect bacterial infection, treat with broad-spectrum antibiotic, and refer to ENT specialist.
Cerebellar infarction or hemorrhage (cerebellar stroke)	Sudden onset of severe headache, vertigo, nausea/vomiting, motor deficits, impaired gait, imbalance, impaired control arm/leg movements, slurred speech (dysarthria). High mortality.	Call 911. MRI is gold standard for diagnosing infarction on the brain.

BPPV, benign paroxysmal positional vertigo; CN, cranial nerve; CPA, cerebellopontine angle; ENT, ear, nose, and throat; h, hour; HINTS, Head Impulse test, Nystagmus, Test of Skew; IM, intramuscular; MSG, monosodium glutamate; PO, orally; PRN, as needed; q, every.

Maneuvers

- Dix–Hallpike maneuver: Gold-standard clinical test for BPPV disease. A positive finding is rotary nystagmus with latency of limited duration. Assuming affected ear is on the right, with the patient sitting on the examination table (facing forward, with eyes open), turn the patient's head 45 degrees to the right. While standing behind the patient and supporting the patient's head with one hand, rapidly move the head from an upright to "head hanging" position, where the patient's head is at least 10 degrees below horizontal. To achieve complete dependency of the patient's head during the maneuver, the patient should be positioned in such a way that their shoulders meet the head of the table when they are reclined (Figure 5.14). There are many YouTube videos and websites that depict how to do this maneuver.
- Epley maneuver: This maneuver can be done in the clinic or at home by the patient. See Figure 5.15 for instructions on how to perform the maneuver.

CLINICAL PEARLS

- Special caution with geriatric patients, since antivertigo medications (e.g., meclizine) are antihistamines and may cause dizziness and sedation (increased risk of falls).
- It is important to distinguish if a patient with vertigo has peripheral vertigo (vestibular apparatus disorder) versus central vertigo, which can be serious to life-threatening (cerebellar stroke, brainstem bleeding).

NOSE

Allergic Rhinitis

Also known as allergic rhinosinusitis. Inflammatory changes of nasal mucosa due to allergy. Increases risk of sinusitis. May have intermittent, seasonal, or daily symptoms. Atopic family history (asthma, eczema). May be allergic to dust mites (daily symptoms), mold and grasses (summer), ragweed pollen (fall), cockroach dander (older buildings in urban areas), and others. May affect sleep and quality of life. Affects 10% to 30% of adults and children in the United States. Classified by temporal pattern (intermittent or persistent) and by severity (mild or moderate-severe).

Classic Case

Patient complains of chronic or seasonal nasal congestion with clear mucus rhinorrhea or postnasal drip. Coughing due to postnasal drip worsens when supine. Accompanied by itching of the eyes, nose, and palate and frequent sneezing. Some people produce a clicking sound to clear mucus inside their throat (palatal click).

Objective Findings

Nose has blue-tinged or pale and boggy nasal turbinates. Mucus clear. Posterior pharynx reveals thick mucus, with colors including clear, white, yellow, or green (rule out sinusitis). Undereye "circles" due to subcutaneous venodilation. Dennie-Morgan lines (accentuated lines or folds below the lower lids) suggest associated allergy. Transverse nasal crease from frequent rubbing (allergic salute). Posterior pharynx may show "cobblestoning" (hyperplastic lymphoid tissue). More common in children, "allergic facies" may appear as highly arched palate, open mouth due to mouth breathing, and dental occlusion.

Treatment Plan

Clinical diagnosis suggested by history, symptoms, and physical examination. First-line treatment is topical nasal sprays:

- Glucocorticoid nasal sprays (OTC) are the most effective single-agent maintenance therapy. Fluticasone (Flonase) twice a day, triamcinolone (Nasacort Allergy 24HR), one or two sprays once a day.
- If only partial relief, another option is topical antihistamine nasal spray with azelastine (Astelin) daily or twice a day.
- If no relief, consider combination product (azelastine and fluticasone nasal spray).
- Use cromolyn sodium nasal spray three times a day (less effective than steroids).

Use decongestants (e.g., pseudoephedrine [Sudafed]) as needed. Do not give to infants/young children. Consider oral antihistamines as needed. Second-generation

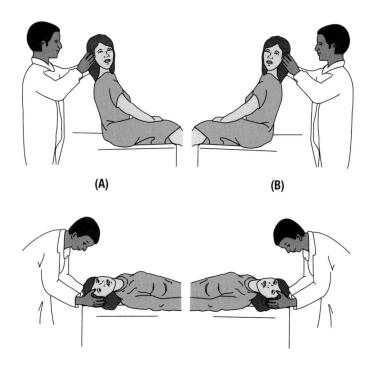

Figure 5.14 (A) Dix–Hallpike positioning maneuver to the right. (B) Dix–Hallpike maneuver to the left.
Source: Adapted from Armitage, A. (2015). (See Resources section for complete source information.)

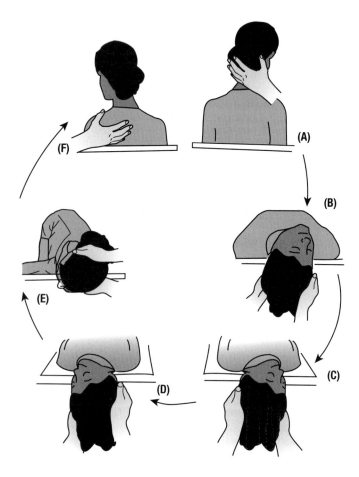

Figure 5.15 Epley maneuver. (A) With the patient sitting on the examination table (facing forward, eyes open), turn the patient's head 45 degrees toward the affected ear. (B) While standing behind the patient and supporting the patient's head with one hand, rapidly move the head from an upright to "head hanging" position, where the patient's head is at least 10 degrees below horizontal. (C) Maintain for 30 seconds or until any nystagmus and vertiginous symptoms subside. (D) Reposition hands on either side of the patient's head and turn the patient's head 90° away from the affected ear, placing it at 45 degrees toward the opposite shoulder. (E) Ask the patient to roll onto their shoulder on the unaffected (left) side, with the help of an assistant. While the patient rolls onto their shoulder, maintain the patient's head at its 45-degrees orientation to the shoulder. As the patient rolls, their face will be directed to the floor. Patient should keep this position until the nystagmus and vertigo subside, or 30 seconds have passed, and then sit up (F).
Source: Adapted from Armitage, A. (2015). (See Resources section for complete source information.)

antihistamines (OTC) are less sedating. Cetirizine (Zyrtec), loratadine (Claritin) orally once daily or as needed. Be careful with diphenhydramine (Benadryl), a first-generation sedating antihistamine. Ideally, eliminate environmental allergens. With dust mite allergies, avoid using ceiling fans; no stuffed animals or pets in bed; use a HEPA filter for air conditioners, use room filters, and so on. Refer to allergist.

Complications
- Recurrent sinusitis
- AOM

Epistaxis (Nosebleeds)
Anterior nasal bleeds are milder and more common than posterior nasal bleeds. Most episodes are self-limiting. Anterior nasal bleeds are the result of bleeding from Kiesselbach's plexus (vascular area), which is located anteriorly on the lower one third of the nose. Posterior nasal bleeds can lead to severe hemorrhage. Aspirin or NSAID use, cocaine use, severe hypertension, and use of anticoagulants (e.g., warfarin sodium [Coumadin]) place patients at higher risk. (Intranasal cocaine use can cause nosebleeds and nasal septum perforation.)

Classic Case
Patient complains of acute onset of nasal bleeding secondary to trauma (e.g., nose picking). Bright-red blood may drip externally through the nasal passages and/or the posterior pharynx. Profuse bleeding can result in vomiting of blood.

Treatment Plan
- Evaluate the airway, hemodynamic stability, and need for further urgent evaluation.
- Apply direct pressure on the front of the nose for several minutes.
- For anterior bleeding, examine nose with nasal speculum. Consider cauterization with silver nitrate or electrocautery. If unsuccessful, nasal packing (e.g., nasal tampons, gauze packing, nasal balloon catheters) to tamponade the local bleeding. Use of nasal decongestants (i.e., Afrin) may help hasten hemostasis.
- Consider posterior bleeding in patients who continue to bleed after anterior packing. Referral and/or hospitalization for observation and posterior packing with nasal balloon catheter or a Foley catheter.

Complications
Synechiae (intranasal adhesions), aspiration, angina, myocardial infarction, and hypovolemia.

Rhinitis Medicamentosa
- Prolonged use of topical nasal decongestant sprays (>3 days) causes rebound effects that result in severe and chronic nasal congestion.
- Patients present with daily severe nasal congestion and nasal discharge (clear, watery mucus). Physical examination with swollen, red nasal mucous membranes.

Treatment Plan
- Stop use of nasal decongestants. Prevent future occurrences by limiting use to a maximum of about 5 days and not exceeding the recommended frequency; use as few doses as possible.
- Encourage use of nasal saline spray to control symptoms.

Septal Perforation
A hole on the nasal septum (cartilage) that can range in size from small to large. Shining a light on one nostril will transilluminate both sides. One of the most common causes is snorting or inhalation of cocaine, a potent vasoconstrictor, which can cause ischemia. Other causes are trauma, prior septal surgery, untreated septal hematomas, and self-induced lesions.

EXAM TIPS
- Inhalation of an illicit substance such as cocaine can cause septal perforation(s).
- For allergic rhinitis, topical steroid nasal spray (e.g., Flonase) is first-line treatment.

THROAT AND MOUTH
Cheilitis
Acute or chronic inflammation of the lips often involving the lip vermilion and the vermilion border, the surrounding skin, and/or the oral mucosa. Often a result of contact irritants or allergens, chronic sun exposure, infection, or atopic disease. Many different forms.

Angular Cheilitis
Painful skin fissures and maceration at the corners of the mouth due to excessive moisture and secondary infection with *Candida albicans* (yeast) or bacteria (*Staphylococcus aureus*).
- More common in the elderly with dentures.
- Less common causes include nutritional deficiencies (vitamins B_2 [riboflavin], B_3 [niacin], B_6 [pyridoxine], or B_9 [folic acid]), lupus, autoimmune disease (Sjögren's syndrome), irritant dermatitis, and squamous cell carcinoma, as well as pacifier use, lip licking, and thumb sucking in children.

Treatment Plan
- Check vitamin B_{12} level; consider checking other B vitamins (B_3, B_6, B_9).
- Remove underlying cause. Check if dentures fit correctly; if loose, refer to dentist.
- If yeast infection is suspected, microscopy with potassium hydroxide (KOH). If positive (pseudohyphae and spores), treat with topical azole ointment (e.g., clotrimazole, miconazole) twice a day.
- If suspect staphylococcal infection, order C&S. If positive, treat with topical mupirocin ointment twice a day.
- When infection has cleared, apply barrier cream with zinc or petroleum jelly at night. High rate of recurrence.

Infectious Mononucleosis

- Infection by EBV (herpesvirus family). Peak ages of acute infection in the United States are between 15 and 24 years. After acute infection, EBV lies latent in oropharyngeal tissue. Can become reactivated and cause symptoms. Virus is shed mainly through saliva.
- Classic triad is fever, pharyngitis, lymphadenopathy (>50% cases). Other findings include splenomegaly, palatal petechiae, and occasionally a generalized maculopapular, urticarial, or petechial rash.

Classic Case

Teenage patient presents with history of sore throat, enlarged posterior cervical nodes, symmetric lymphadenopathy, and fatigue (several weeks). Tonsillar exudate, with color of exudate ranging from white to gray-green. Fatigue may last weeks to months. May have abdominal pain due to hepatomegaly and/or splenomegaly. History of intimate kissing.

Objective Findings

- Complete blood count (CBC): Atypical lymphocytes and lymphocytosis (a differential count >50%); repeat CBC until resolves
- Liver function tests (LFTs): Elevated aminotransferases are seen in majority of patients but self-limited
- Heterophile test (e.g., the Monospot) or EBV-specific antibody testing: Often, positive but the Monospot test can be repeated since it can be negative during the first week of illness
- Nodes: Large cervical nodes that may be tender to palpation
- Pharynx: Erythematous
- Tonsils: Inflamed, sometimes with cryptic exudate (off-white color)
- Hepatomegaly and splenomegaly: Avoid vigorous palpation of abdomen until resolves
- Skin: Occasionally a generalized red maculopapular rash is present.

Treatment Plan

- In acute stages, limit physical activity (e.g., exercise, weightlifting) and refrain from sport activities during early illness. Splenic rupture is most likely within 2 to 21 days. Gradually, resume noncontact sports 3 weeks from symptom onset. For strenuous contact sports, recommendations include waiting a minimum of 4 weeks after illness onset. Routine imaging is not needed in most patients, but an abdominal ultrasound may be considered to document resolution of splenomegaly.
- Treat symptoms. Rarely do EBV infections require more than supportive therapy.
- Avoid close contact such as kissing; sharing toothbrush, fork, spoon, or knife; or using the same glass.

Complications

- Most acute symptoms resolve in 1 to 2 weeks. Fatigue and poor functional status can persist for months.
- Splenomegaly/splenic rupture is a rare but serious complication of mononucleosis.

- If airway obstruction, patient may need to be hospitalized for observation. Consider corticosteroids and consult to otolaryngologist.
- Neurologic complications include Guillain–Barré syndrome, aseptic meningitis, optic neuritis.
- If blood dyscrasias (atypical lymphocytes), repeat CBC until lymphocytes are normalized.

Mumps (Parotitis)

Often, a school-aged child or college-aged young adult with acute onset of fever, headache, fatigue, myalgia, and anorexia. Usually 16 to 18 days (range 12 to 25) from exposure to onset of symptoms. Mumps is the classic virus to cause parotitis. Within 48 hours, the salivary/parotid gland(s) become(s) swollen and tender. It can be unilateral or bilateral. The cheek appears puffy, and the angle of the jaw on the involved side appears swollen. The swelling and tenderness usually subside in about 1 week. Highly infectious; transmitted by respiratory droplets, direct contact, or fomites. Usually self-limiting with recovery within a few weeks. Complications are rare and include orchitis or oophoritis, neurologic conditions (e.g., meningitis, encephalitis, deafness), and others. Mumps is a nationally notifiable disease; report all cases to local or state health department.

Streptococcal Pharyngitis/Tonsillopharyngitis (Strep Throat)

An acute infection of the pharynx and/or palatine tonsils caused by group A streptococcal bacteria (*Streptococcus pyogenes*). Acute pharyngitis is one of the most common conditions encountered in outpatient practice. Keep in mind that the most common pathogen of acute pharyngitis is often viral (e.g., rhinovirus, adenovirus, COVID-19, respiratory syncytial virus [RSV]) and group A streptococcus (GAS). Suspect viral etiology (or coinfection) if cough and symptoms such as stuffy nose, rhinitis with clear mucus (coryza), and watery eyes.

Classic Case

All ages are affected, but most common in children. Abrupt onset of fever (temperature >100.4°F/38°C), sore throat, pain on swallowing, and mildly enlarged submandibular nodes. Purulent, patchy tonsillar or pharyngeal exudate. Anterior cervical nodes mildly enlarged and tender (anterior cervical adenitis). Adult patient may report that their child attends preschool.

> **NOTE**
>
> Centor criteria are a clinical decision tool used to help diagnose GAS in adults. Criteria for strep throat include tonsillar exudate, tender anterior cervical adenopathy, fever, and absence of cough. One point is given for each criterion; the likelihood of GAS increases with each point. Patients with <3 Centor criteria are unlikely to have GAS pharyngitis.

Objective Findings

- Pharynx is dark pink to bright red. Adults usually afebrile (or mild fever).

- May have tonsillar exudate that is yellow-to-green color. May have petechiae on the hard palate (roof of the mouth). Anterior cervical lymph nodes mildly enlarged.

Treatment Plan

- Rule out: Other viral pathogens (e.g., COVID-19). Rapid antigen detection testing (RADT) and/or throat culture
- First-line adults: Oral penicillin V 500 mg two to three times a day × 10 days
- First-line children: Oral penicillin V or amoxicillin (often preferred for taste)
- Penicillin or beta-lactam allergy: Clindamycin and macrolides are alternatives; selection based on drug allergy and local antibiotic resistance rates
- Throat pain and fever: Ibuprofen (Advil) or acetaminophen (Tylenol)
- Symptomatic treatment: Saltwater gargles, throat lozenges; drink more fluids
- Repeat culture or RADT after antibiotic treatment (test of cure): History of rheumatic fever; patients who acquired infection during an outbreak of acute rheumatic fever or poststreptococcal glomerulonephritis; patients who acquired infection during a group outbreak in close-contact setting
- Prevention: Hand hygiene, covering mouth when coughing or sneezing

Complications

- Suppurative complications include otitis media, peritonsillar cellulitis or abscess, sinusitis, meningitis, bacteremia, and necrotizing fasciitis. *Peritonsillar abscess* is a displaced uvula, red bulging mass on one side of anterior pharyngeal space, dysphagia, and fever. Refer to ED *stat*.
- Nonsuppurative complications include acute rheumatic fever, poststreptococcal glomerulonephritis, and reactive arthritis. *Acute rheumatic fever* is an inflammatory reaction to strep infection that may affect the heart and the valves, joints, and brain. *Poststreptococcal glomerulonephritis* is abrupt onset of proteinuria, hematuria, dark-colored urine, and red blood cell (RBC) casts in urine, accompanied by hypertension and edema.

EXAM TIPS

- Acute or reactivated mononucleosis can present with generalized maculopapular rash, enlarged tonsils with cryptic exudate (white or darker color), sore throat, or enlarged cervical nodes that are tender to the touch.
- Avoid contact sports for about 4 weeks to avoid splenic rupture after infectious mononucleosis.

KNOWLEDGE CHECK: CHAPTER 5

1. A patient presents for their annual routine eye exam. Which of the following findings on fundoscopy examination warrants rapid lowering of the blood pressure?
   A. Arteriovenous nicking
   B. Cotton-wool spots
   C. Papilledema
   D. Microaneurysms

2. Inhalation of cocaine can cause which of the following conditions?
   A. Nasal polyps
   B. Allergic rhinitis
   C. Rhinitis medicamentosa
   D. Nasal septal perforation

3. A patient presents with fever, generalized fatigue, and anorexia. Upon physical assessment, white-gray lesions are noted with an erythematous base on the buccal mucosa of about 2 mm in size. This clinical finding suggests:
   A. Epstein-Barr virus
   B. Herpes zoster
   C. Mumps
   D. Measles

4. The nurse practitioner (NP) uses the Snellen chart to evaluate the patient's visual acuity, which is 20/50. How does the NP explain this finding to the patient?
   A. The denominator is the distance in feet at which the patient stands from the Snellen chart.
   B. The patient can read letters while standing 20 feet from the chart that the average person could read at 50 feet.
   C. The numerator is dependent on the patient's vision.
   D. The patient can read letters while standing 50 feet from the chart that the average person could read at 20 feet.

5. Which of the following bedside tests can be used to identify cerebrospinal fluid (CSF) in patients who present with otorrhea or rhinorrhea?
   A. Beta-2 transferrin examination
   B. Halo test
   C. Head impulse test
   D. Test of skew

6. A middle-aged adult presents with anxiety and dizziness. They complain that upon getting out of bed that morning, they had severe dizziness and almost fell because "the room was spinning so much." The patient's gait is unstable with some swaying noted. They report becoming very dizzy and having problems with balance when moving their head quickly. The patient denies trauma, hypertension, tinnitus, hearing loss, and fever. The Romberg test is positive. Which of the following conditions is *most* likely?
   A. Benign paroxysmal positional vertigo (BPPV)
   B. Ménière's disease
   C. Acoustic neuroma
   D. Cerebrovascular accident (CVA)

7. Regarding the previous case, which of the following tests will help diagnose this patient?
   A. Lachman
   B. Dix-Hallpike
   C. Obturator
   D. Finkelstein

8. Where is Kiesselbach's plexus located?
   A. Posterior area of the pharynx
   B. Superior lateral area of the maxillary sinus
   C. Anterior inferior area of the nasal septum
   D. Submandibular area of the mouth

(See answers next page.)

1. C) Papilledema

All patients with newly diagnosed hypertension should receive a fundoscopy because the retina is the only part of the vasculature that can be visualized noninvasively. Ocular diseases directly related to hypertension are progressive and can be classified by their degree of severity. Arteriovenous nicking alone indicates mild hypertensive retinopathy, whereas cotton-wool spots, hemorrhages, and microaneurysms are indicative of moderate hypertensive retinopathy. Severe hypertensive retinopathy is indicated by swelling of the optic disc (papilledema), alongside retinal hemorrhages, hard exudates, cotton-wool patches, microaneurysms, and arteriovenous nicking. The presence of papilledema warrants rapid lowering of the blood pressure. It occurs when increased intracranial pressure spreads to the optic nerve sheath. Urgent diagnosis, evaluation, and treatment are needed to prevent serious complications.

2. D) Nasal septal perforation

Snorting or inhalation of cocaine is a common cause of nasal septal perforation. Chronic cocaine use can also lead to a plethora of other complications, including neurologic, psychiatric, cardiovascular, pulmonary, gastrointestinal, and reproductive system effects.

3. D) Measles

Measles, a highly contagious viral illness, is characterized by the clinical stages of incubation (6 to 21 days), prodrome, exanthem (red maculopapular rash), and recovery. The prodrome phase is characterized by fever, malaise, anorexia, conjunctivitis, coryza, and cough. Patients may develop Koplik's spots, which are 1- to 3-mm whitish, grayish, or bluish lesions with an erythematous base. These are often found on the buccal mucosa opposite the molar teeth. They generally last 12 to 72 hours and are pathognomonic for measles.

4. B) The patient can read letters while standing 20 feet from the chart that the average person could read at 50 feet.

The Snellen chart is used to evaluate visual acuity. The top number (or numerator) is the distance in feet at which the patient stands from the Snellen or picture eye chart (always 20 feet). The bottom number (or denominator) changes and is dependent on the patient's vision. This patient can see at 20 feet what a person with normal vision can see at 50 feet.

5. B) Halo test

In patients with suspected craniofacial trauma, the clinician should inspect the nose and ears for drainage. If present, rhinorrhea and otorrhea should be tested for the presence of CSF. The halo test (also called the ring or target sign) is a quick bedside tool that may be used to determine the presence of CSF. A drop of fluid is placed on a tissue; a rapidly expanding ring of clear fluid around red blood suggests a positive test. While this is considered a nonspecific finding, it may be helpful to identify patients who may need a higher level of care and neuroimaging to confirm a CSF leak. A CSF leak may be diagnosed when CSF proteins, such as beta-2 transferrin, are found by laboratory analysis of a collected sample. While this is highly specific and sensitive for a CSF leak, it involves analysis by immunohistochemcial assays and cannot be performed at the bedside. The HINTS examination (which includes the head impulse test, evaluation for direction-changing nystagmus, and a test of skew) can be used to suggest central rather than peripheral vertigo in patients.

6. A) Benign paroxysmal positional vertigo (BPPV)

BPPV is the most common cause of vertigo in the United States. It is caused by calcium carbonate crystals in the semicircular canals. An initial treatment is the Epley maneuver, in which the head is turned sequentially, which helps to move the crystals in the semicircular canals by gravity. Several repositioning maneuvers may be needed at the same visit; recurrences can occur. There is no tinnitus or hearing loss, so Ménière's disease and acoustic neuroma can be ruled out. There is no limb weakness or slurred speech, so a stroke (CVA) can also be ruled out.

7. B) Dix-Hallpike

The Dix–Hallpike test or maneuver is the gold-standard test for benign paroxysmal positional vertigo (BPPV). It is positive if classic rotary nystagmus is seen with latency (limited duration). The Lachman maneuver is a test for the anterior cruciate ligament (ACL) of the knee. The obturator test is used for acute appendicitis. The Finkelstein test is used to assess for De Quervain's tenosynovitis.

8. C) The anterior inferior area of the nasal septum

Kiesselbach's plexus is a vascular network of four arteries that supply the nasal septum. It is located on the anterior inferior area of the nasal septum (lower one third of the nose). When there is trauma to this area (e.g., from picking the nose), it can cause rupture of tiny blood vessels, which causes an anterior epistaxis or a nosebleed.

9. What is the first-line treatment for allergic rhinitis?
   A. Saline nasal spray
   B. Oral antihistamine
   C. Topical nasal decongestant spray
   D. Topical nasal steroid spray

10. Which of the following conditions is classified as sensorineural hearing loss?
    A. Presbycusis
    B. Otitis media
    C. Ceruminosis
    D. Otitis externa

11. A 40-year-old male patient presents with a 2-day history of foreign body sensation and excessive tearing of the right eye. What type of exam is recommended initially?
    A. Cardiac
    B. Visual
    C. Neurologic
    D. Cerebellar

12. An 80-year-old female patient with a history of hypertension, atrial fibrillation, and type 2 diabetes presents to the clinic with a complaint of painless bright-red blood on the right eye, which she noticed upon awakening. She denies falling, visual changes, visual loss, eye pain, headache, coryza, and fever. The visual exam is normal, and both pupils are equal and reactive to light and accommodation. The funduscopic exam does not show bleeding. Which of the following conditions is most likely?
    A. Hyphema
    B. Subconjunctival hemorrhage
    C. Ectropion
    D. Blepharitis

13. A 16-year-old athlete has recently been diagnosed with infectious mononucleosis. During the abdominal exam, the nurse practitioner (NP) identifies an enlarged spleen. Abdominal ultrasound confirms this finding. The patient wants to know when they can go back to playing football. Which of the following responses by the NP is the *most* appropriate?
    A. "You may return to playing contact sports when your sore throat is gone."
    B. "You should avoid all sports and exercise for the next 2 weeks."
    C. "You may not play contact sports for 4 to 6 months."
    D. "You may return to exercise and sports in 4 to 6 weeks after your splenomegaly is resolved."

14. A patient presents with severe eye pain. The patient is reluctant to open the eye due to photophobia. They report working on their house earlier in the day and feeling something fall into their eye. The nurse practitioner performs a visual acuity and fundus examination. Which of the following diagnostic studies is indicated next?
    A. Ultrasonography
    B. Fluorescein examination
    C. CT scan
    D. MRI

15. A patient presents with a headache, severe eye pain, visual disturbances, and halos around lights. Physical assessment reveals conjunctival redness and cloudiness of the cornea. Emergent ophthalmologic examination is necessary. Which of the following diagnostic tests is indicated?
    A. Dilated fundus examination
    B. Pachymetry
    C. Fluorescein examination
    D. Measurement of intraocular pressure

(See answers next page.)

9. D) Topical nasal steroid spray

The first-line treatment for allergic rhinitis is a topical nasal steroid spray, which is used once or twice per day. Allergic rhinitis can be seasonal (e.g., due to ragweed, mold, or pollens), or it can be due to an indoor allergen, such as dust mites. If it is severe or accompanied by asthma, referral to an allergist for allergy testing is helpful. Topical nasal decongestant spray (e.g., Afrin) is for short-term use only because it can result in a rebound effect with worsening of symptoms (rhinitis medicamentosa).

10. A) Presbycusis

Presbycusis is a type of sensorineural hearing loss that is caused by normal aging of the auditory system. It initially affects the ability to hear higher-pitched sounds (i.e., high frequency). It has a gradual onset, and over time it affects lower frequencies as well. Speaking is an example of a higher-frequency sound. Common symptoms of presbycusis include setting the volume of TVs or radio high and having difficulty hearing in noisy environments. A hearing aid can help. Otitis media, ceruminosis, and otitis externa are some of the causes of conductive hearing loss.

11. B) Visual

Any patient who is complaining of new onset of eye symptoms should have a visual exam first. Distance vision can be checked by using the Snellen chart. Near vision is tested by asking a patient to read a paragraph of a book or newspaper. The eye exam also includes an inspection of the surface of the eye, pupillary reflex, and red reflex. A fluorescein exam is performed to look for a corneal abrasion, which appears as pooling of the dye that is visualized using a blue light in a darkened room.

12. B) Subconjunctival hemorrhage

A subconjunctival hemorrhage is caused by blood that is trapped between the sclera and the conjunctiva. The patient's history of atrial fibrillation is highly suggestive of anticoagulation therapy, which increases her risk of bleeding. Hypertension and diabetes are also risk factors. A hyphema is blood that is trapped in the anterior chamber of the eye (the space between the cornea and the iris); it is usually painful. Ectropion is the eversion of the lower eyelids, which can cause irritation but no bleeding. Blepharitis presents on the edge of an eyelid as a painful abscess.

13. D) "You may return to exercise and sports in 4 to 6 weeks after your splenomegaly is resolved."

Most reported cases of splenic rupture occurred in athletes who returned to play within 3 weeks of the illness. Many sports medicine clinicians will restrict all exercise for the first 3 weeks of reported symptoms. After 3 weeks, when the fever is gone and the athlete feels better, they can gradually return to exercise and athletics. Therefore, the instruction to avoid exercise or sports for 4 to 6 weeks after illness onset is probably based on this timeline. The patient should return for a follow-up visit at 4 to 6 weeks to confirm that the splenomegaly has resolved. The best test to confirm that the spleen and/or liver size is back to normal is the abdominal ultrasound.

14. B) Fluorescein examination

This patient is presenting with signs and symptoms consistent with a corneal abrasion (severe eye pain, reluctance to open the eye due to photophobia, foreign body sensation). Fluorescein examination is used to confirm the diagnosis of corneal abrasion after completion of visual acuity, penlight, and fundus assessment. Fluorescein staining and examination with Wood's light or a slit-lamp can identify surface eye injuries, such as corneal abrasions. More detailed imaging such as a CT scan of the orbits is preferred for patients with serious traumatic eye injuries (e.g., open globe, intraocular or intraorbital foreign body, traumatic optic neuropathy, orbital fracture, orbital compartment syndrome). While a bedside ultrasonography of the globe and orbit may detect serious eye injuries, a working diagnosis of corneal abrasion can be made based on this patient's history, physical findings, and lack of signs of a more serious disorder. An MRI is not the preferred initial imaging modality and may be contraindicated in patients who have a metal foreign body.

15. D) Measurement of intraocular pressure

This patient is presenting with signs and symptoms of acute primary-angle closure glaucoma. The clinical presentation often includes decreased vision, halos around lights, headache, severe eye pain, nausea, and vomiting. Clinical signs that suggest a rapid increase in intraocular pressure include conjunctival redness, corneal edema or cloudiness, a shallow anterior chamber, and a mid-dilated pupil (4 to 6 mm) that reacts poorly to light. Diagnosis begins with emergent examination of both eyes by an ophthalmologist, including the following tests: visual acuity, evaluation of the pupils, measurement of intraocular pressure, slit-lamp examination of the anterior segments, visual field testing, gonioscopy, and undilated fundus examination. Pupillary dilation can exacerbate angle-closure glaucoma and should be deferred when diagnosis is suspected. Fluorescein examination is used to confirm the diagnosis of a corneal abrasion after completion of visual acuity, penlight, and fundus assessment. Pachymetry is the measurement of corneal thickness, which is indicated in patients with open-angle glaucoma to further evaluate their risk of development and progression.

16. A patient presents with hearing loss and tinnitus. The patient denies a spinning sensation but notes unsteadiness while walking. During the physical assessment, the patient is found to have asymmetric sensorineural hearing loss. This finding suggests which diagnosis?
    A. Ménière's disease
    B. Vestibular schwannoma
    C. Benign paroxysmal positional vertigo
    D. Labyrinthitis

17. Which of the following is the *best* initial screening test for vestibular schwannoma?
    A. Audiometry
    B. Weber test
    C. Rinne test
    D. Vestibular testing

18. A patient presents with unilateral ear pain, a sensation of ear fullness, and muffled hearing. The physical assessment is notable for a bulging, erythematous tympanic membrane with reduced mobility on otoscopy. These findings suggest which diagnosis?
    A. Otitis media with effusion
    B. Otitis externa
    C. Acute otitis media
    D. Bullous myringitis

19. A patient presents with chronic eye irradiation and dryness. Physical assessment reveals outward turning of the eyelid. This finding describes which condition?
    A. Xanthelasma
    B. Entropion
    C. Hordeolum
    D. Ectropion

20. A patient presents with conductive hearing loss secondary to otitis media. What findings are expected with the Rinne and Weber tests?
    A. Weber lateralizes to good ear
    B. Bone conduction > air conduction
    C. No lateralization noted on the Weber test
    D. Air conduction > bone conduction

21. Which of the following structures of the eye is responsible for color perception?
    A. Cones
    B. Rods
    C. Optic nerve
    D. Macula

22. A patient presents with a severe sore throat, fever, and a "hot potato," or muffled, voice. The patient is drooling due to difficulty opening the mouth. Unilateral swelling and a bulging red mass are noted on physical examination. These findings are suggestive of which diagnosis?
    A. Epiglottis
    B. Acute pharyngitis
    C. Infectious mononucleosis
    D. Peritonsillar abscess

23. Which of the following is a common bacterial pathogen found in otitis externa?
    A. *Streptococcus pneumoniae*
    B. *Haemophilus influenzae*
    C. *Pseudomonas aeruginosa*
    D. *Moraxella catarrhalis*

24. A patient presents with reduced hearing, tinnitus, and fullness in the affected ear. The patient reports frequent spontaneous episodes of vertigo, each lasting at least 30 to 45 minutes. Audiometry confirms sensorineural hearing loss in the affected ear. Which of the following is the first-line treatment for this diagnosis based on the clinical findings?
    A. Vestibular rehabilitation therapy
    B. Lifestyle modification including salt restriction
    C. Pharmacotherapy with diuretics
    D. Glucocorticoid therapy for symptom management

(See answers next page.)

16. B) Vestibular schwannoma

Asymmetric sensorineural hearing loss often indicates vestibular schwannoma. Patients with symptomatic cochlear nerve involvement often present with hearing loss and tinnitus. Those with vestibular nerve involvement may complain of unsteadiness while walking. Most patients do not experience true spinning vertigo. Patients with Ménière's disease experience vertigo as a rotatory spinning or rocking with nausea and vomiting, hearing loss, and tinnitus. Patients with benign paroxysmal positional vertigo present with recurrent episodes of vertigo provoked by certain head movements. Labyrinthitis presents as rapid onset of severe vertigo with nausea, vomiting, and gait instability.

17. A) Audiometry

Audiometry is the best initial screening test for the diagnosis of vestibular schwannoma because only 5% of patients with vestibular schwannoma have a normal test. Results often reveal an asymmetric sensorineural hearing loss. The Weber and Rinne tests can be useful to suggest a hearing impairment. Vestibular testing has limited utility as a screening test in comparison with audiometry.

18. C) Acute otitis media

Typically, in adults, the clinical manifestations of acute otitis media are unilateral and include otalgia (ear pain) and decreased or muffled hearing. Diagnosis is by otoscopy, which reveals a bulging tympanic membrane with reduced mobility. Often, the tympanic membrane is erythematous. Otitis media with effusion presents with yellow, clear fluid behind the tympanic membrane with or without viscous bubbles and/or retraction of the tympanic membrane. Otitis externa often presents with ear pain, pruritis, discharge, and hearing loss. Otoscopy reveals an edematous and erythematous external ear canal. Bullous myringitis does not affect the contents of the middle ear; the tympanic membrane will present as thickened and erythematous.

19. D) Ectropion

Chronic eye inflammation is often seen on the physical examination of a patient with blepharitis, which can lead to structural changes such as entropion (inward turning of eyelid) or ectropion (outward turning of eyelid). Xanthelasma are soft, yellow plaques often appearing symmetrically on the medial aspects of the eyelids and may be associated with hypercholesterolemia. A hordeolum (stye) is an acute inflammation of the eyelid that presents as a localized painful and erythematous swelling or nodule.

20. B) Bone conduction > air conduction

An abnormal Rinne test (bone conduction > air conduction) is seen in patients with conductive hearing loss. The Weber test suggests sensorineural hearing loss if the sound lateralizes to the good side; conductive hearing loss is suggested if the sound lateralizes to the bad side.

21. A) Cones

Rods and cones are the photoreceptor cells within the eye. Cones function in bright light and are more numerous in the central region of the retina. The stimulation of different combinations of blue, green, and red cones provides color vision. Rods function in dim light and occur more frequently in the periphery of the retina. The optic nerve (cranial nerve II) is the sensory nerve that transmits the neural-visual impulses from the retina to the brain. The macula is in the center of the posterior portion of the retina. Within the macula, the fovea centralis contains only cones and is the area of highest visual acuity.

22. D) Peritonsillar abscess

These findings are suggestive of a peritonsillar abscess, a collection of pus between the palatine tonsil and the pharyngeal muscles. Common symptoms include a severe sore throat; a fever; a "hot potato," or muffled, voice; drooling; and trismus. Physical assessment reveals an enlarged tonsil with deviation of the uvula. Epiglottis also presents with fever and drooling; however, airway stridor and respiratory distress are more common, along with "sniffing" posture. Acute pharyngitis causes nonspecific symptoms such as a sore throat and cervical lymphadenopathy. Infectious mononucleosis presents with fever, pharyngitis, adenopathy, fatigue, and atypical lymphocytosis.

23. C) Pseudomonas aeruginosa

The most common pathogens responsible for external otitis are *Pseudomonas aeruginosa, Staphylococcus epidermidis*, and *S. aureus*. The most causative organisms in acute otitis media are *S. pneumoniae, H. influenzae, and M. catarrhalis.*

24. B) Lifestyle modification including salt restriction

This patient is presenting with findings supporting the clinical diagnosis of Ménière's disease. Patients experience progressive hearing loss with vestibular symptoms, including spontaneous episodes of vertigo that last 20 minutes to 12 hours and occur two or more times, and fluctuating aural symptoms (reduced hearing, tinnitus, or fullness). Audiometry confirms sensorineural hearing loss. Initial therapy includes lifestyle modifications such as salt restriction and limiting of caffeine and alcohol consumption. Vestibular rehabilitation and pharmacotherapy may be considered with patients with persistent disequilibrium and refractory symptoms.

25. A patient presents with fever, pharyngitis, adenopathy, fatigue, and atypical lymphocytosis. Physical assessment is notable for splenomegaly and a generalized maculopapular rash. Based on these findings, treatment includes which of the following?
    A. Acetaminophen and nonsteroidal anti-inflammatory drugs (NSAIDs) for symptom management
    B. Initiation of antiviral therapy (e.g., acyclovir [Zovirax])
    C. Administration of corticosteroids
    D. Hospitalization for monitoring of possible splenic rupture

26. When palpating lymph nodes, a red flag that requires further investigation is lymph nodes that are:
    A. Bilateral
    B. Less than 1 cm in size
    C. Hard and fixed
    D. Located in the axillary region

27. A patient presents with unilateral ear pain and decreased hearing. The patient reports a recent upper respiratory tract infection. Otoscopic examination reveals a bulging tympanic membrane (TM) with reduced mobility. There is partial opacification of the TM. The patient does not report a penicillin allergy. Based on these symptoms, which medication is indicated for first-line therapy?
    A. Cefdinir (Omnicef)
    B. Amoxicillin-clavulanate (Augmentin)
    C. Doxycycline (Adoxa)
    D. Clarithromycin (Biaxin)

28. Which of the following can be used to test color vision?
    A. Ishihara test
    B. Rosenbaum card
    C. Snellen chart
    D. Confrontation testing

29. A patient with a history of ankylosing spondylitis presents with eye pain and redness. Slit examination reveals the presence of leukocytes in the anterior chamber. This finding suggest which disease?
    A. Optic neuritis
    B. Subconjunctival hemorrhage
    C. Anterior uveitis
    D. Orbital cellulitis

30. A patient presents with a chief complaint of redness and crusting near the corners of their mouth. Physical assessment is significant for scaling, erythema, and fissuring at the corners of the mouth. Culture is positive for staphylococcal infection. Treatment includes which of the following therapies?
    A. Mupirocin ointment
    B. Lip moisturizer
    C. Topical corticosteroids
    D. Miconazole ointment

31. Optic neuritis is highly associated with which condition?
    A. Mumps
    B. Diphtheria
    C. Measles
    D. Multiple sclerosis

32. The clinician notices clear fluid draining from the patient's nose and periorbital ecchymosis after a blow to the head that occurred 2 days ago. What type of injury does the clinician expect?
    A. Epidural hematoma
    B. Subdural hematoma
    C. Basilar skull fracture
    D. Cerebral contusion

(See answers next page.)

25. A) Acetaminophen and nonsteroidal anti-inflammatory drugs (NSAIDs) for symptom management

The patient is presenting with the classic clinical manifestations of infectious mononucleosis. Initial treatment involves supportive therapy and symptomatic treatment with fluids and proper nutrition, along with acetaminophen or NSAIDs to manage fever, throat discomfort, and malaise. If there are signs of impending airway obstruction (noted by dyspnea or increased work of breathing), corticosteroids and emergent consultation may be indicated. Antiviral treatment has no effect on latent infection or ability to cure the infection. Unless there are other symptoms to suggest impending rupture (e.g., intense abdominal pain; pale, clammy skin), hospitalization is not required.

26. C) Hard and fixed

When palpating lymph nodes, the characteristics of lymph nodes that are considered red flags and warrant further investigation include hard, fixed, and matted; greater than 1 cm in size; located in the supraclavicular, infraclavicular, iliac, popliteal, or epitrochlear regions; generalized or unilateral; and/or associated with systemic symptoms (e.g., weight loss, fever, night sweats).

27. B) Amoxicillin-clavulanate (Augmentin)

This patient is presenting with the signs and symptoms consistent with acute otitis media (unilateral otalgia and decreased hearing). Otoscopic examination is required for diagnosis, often revealing a bulging, opacified, erythematous tympanic membrane. Antibiotics are recommended for treatment; amoxicillin-clavulanate (Augmentin) is preferred for first-line therapy in patients with no penicillin allergy. Alternative agents for patients with a mild penicillin allergy include second- or third-generation cephalosporins (e.g., cefdinir [Omnicef]) or doxycycline (Adoxa) or clarithromycin (Biaxin) for those with a known allergy to cephalosporins.

28. A) Ishihara test

Color vision testing can be achieved with pseudo-isochromatic plates, such as those available with the Ishihara and the Hardy-Rand Rittler tests. The Snellen chart evaluates visual acuity. A Rosenbaum card can be used to measure near vision. Confrontation testing of the visual fields is used to screen for visual field defects.

29. C) Anterior uveitis

Anterior uveitis is characterized by pain and redness (primarily at the junction between the cornea and the sclera) and the presence of leukocytes in the anterior chamber of the eye on slit lamp examination. Visual loss may vary.

Uveitis is often a manifestation of many systemic inflammatory conditions, including spondyloarthritis (such as ankylosing spondylitis and reactive arthritis), sarcoidosis, and other systemic and rheumatic diseases. Optic neuritis presents as painful, monocular visual loss over several hours to a few days. Orbital cellulitis is characterized by eyelid swelling, pain with eye movements, proptosis, and chemosis. Subconjunctival hemorrhage is often caused by a trauma or contact lens use and presents as a focal, flat, red region on the ocular surface due to blood collection between the sclera and the conjunctiva.

30. A) Mupirocin ointment

This patient is presenting with symptoms of angular cheilitis, which is inflammation of the skin and labial mucosa located at the lateral commissures of the mouth. Clinical features include erythema, maceration, scaling, and fissures at the corners of the mouth. Treatment includes maintaining oral hygiene and treatment of bacterial or fungal infection. Mupirocin ointment can be used to treat staphylococcal infection. If potassium hydroxide (KOH) preparation is positive, an antifungal (e.g., miconazole) ointment can be used. Once the infection has cleared, a barrier cream or petrolatum can help protect and moisturize the skin. Topical corticosteroids can help treat eczematous cheilitis, plasma cell cheilitis, cheilitis glandularis, and cheilitis granulomatosa.

31. D) Multiple sclerosis

Multiple sclerosis is highly associated with optic neuritis. Mumps is the classic virus that can cause parotitis. Diphtheria can be associated with a sore throat, fever, cervical lymphadenopathy, and markedly swollen neck ("bull neck") along with a gray pseudomembrane that adheres tightly to the tissue. Measles are associated with Koplik's spots.

32. C) Basilar skull fracture

Basilar skull fractures involve at least one of the five bones that compose the base of the skull: the cribriform plate of the ethmoid bone, the orbital plate of the frontal bone, the petrous and squamous portion of the temporal bone, and the sphenoid and occipital bones. Clinical signs may include retroauricular or mastoid ecchymosis (Battle's sign), periorbital ecchymosis (raccoon eyes), cerebral spinal fluid (CSF) leakage from nose (rhinorrhea) and ears (otorrhea), and hemotympanum (blood behind the tympanic membrane). While similar neurologic deteriorations may occur with epidural or subdural hematoma or cerebral contusion, CSF leaks (manifested as otorrhea or rhinorrhea) are a specific characteristic of a basilar skull fracture.

33. A patient presents with difficulty reading signs that are far away. The patient reports that "things look blurry" until they are able to get close enough to read clearly. This presentation suggests the patient is likely experiencing:
    A. Hyperopia
    B. Amblyopia
    C. Presbyopia
    D. Myopia

34. A patient presents with a painful red eye, decreased vision, halos around lights, and a headache. Fundoscopic examination reveals cupping of the optic disc. Which of the following diagnostic tests is considered the gold-standard method for diagnosis of this condition?
    A. Fluorescein staining
    B. Gonioscopy
    C. CT of the orbits
    D. Slit lamp examination

35. Which of the following is considered a cause of peripheral vertigo?
    A. Cerebellar infarction
    B. Ménière's disease
    C. Benign paroxysmal positional vertigo
    D. Vestibular neuritis

36. A patient presents with eye redness and irritation. Visual assessment is significant for a triangular (wedge-shaped) thickening of conjunctival tissue that extends onto the corneal surface. This finding is commonly associated with which of the following?
    A. Eye trauma
    B. Aging-related change
    C. Chronic sun exposure
    D. Smoking

37. A patient presents with episodes of sneezing, rhinorrhoea, nasal obstruction, and postnasal drip. The patient appears fatigued with undereye circles noted. Physical assessment is significant for pale and boggy nasal turbinates with cobblestoning along the posterior pharynx. These findings suggest which of the following disease processes?
    A. Blepharitis
    B. Rhinitis medicamentosa
    C. Sjögren's syndrome
    D. Allergic rhinitis

38. The clinician receives a call from a patient who reports experiencing an avulsed tooth after being hit by a baseball. Attempt at manual reimplantation was unsuccessful. The clinician urges the patient to seek care and prioritizes which of the following?
    A. Sterilizing and scrubbing the tooth to keep it clean
    B. Transporting the tooth in tap water
    C. Handling the tooth by the periodontal ligament and avoiding touching the crown
    D. Placing the avulsed tooth in cold milk during transport

(See answers next page.)

33. D) Myopia

Myopia ("nearsightedness") is a refractive disorder resulting in blurred distance vision. Hyperopia ("farsightedness") is a refractive disorder resulting in difficulty with near vision. Presbyopia ("aging sight") occurs when the lens loses its normal accommodating power and can no longer focus on objects at arm's length or closer. This affects visual acuity and is often secondary to the natural aging process. Amblyopia ("lazy eye") is caused by abnormal early visual development leading to reduced visual acuity in the affected eye.

34. B) Gonioscopy

This patient is presenting with signs and symptoms concerning for angle-closure glaucoma with characteristic atrophy of the optic nerve head ("cupping"). Untreated, it can lead to increased intraocular pressure and damage to the optic nerve, resulting in vision loss and blindness. Gonioscopy is the gold-standard method to diagnose angle-closure glaucoma. Fluorescein staining can help assess for a corneal abrasion. A CT is preferred for patients with serious traumatic eye injuries. A slit lamp examination is the gold standard when assessing the anterior segment of the eye or to facilitate foreign body removal. It can diagnose conditions such as corneal epithelial defect, keratoconjunctivitis, hyphema, hypopyon, lens dislocation, herpetic infections, and iritis.

35. D) Vestibular neuritis

Peripheral vertigo is caused by disorders of the vestibular apparatus of the inner ear or by the inflammation of the vestibular nerve (CN VIII). The most common are benign paroxysmal positional vertigo, vestibular neuritis, and Ménière's disease. Central vertigo (20% of cases) is associated with serious to life-threatening conditions as a result of lesions affecting the brainstem and cerebellum; the most common are vestibular migraine and vascular etiologies (e.g., transient ischemic attack, stroke, multiple sclerosis, infections, tumor).

36. C) Chronic sun exposure

This patient is presenting with symptoms suggestive of a pterygium, which is characterized by a triangular wedge of conjunctival tissue that extends onto the corneal surface, causing eye redness and irritation. Pterygium is commonly associated with chronic sun exposure, specifically ultraviolet light. Other inciting factors include abnormal expression of tumor suppressor genes, presence of angiogenesis-related factors, human papillomavirus infection, hereditary factors, and abnormal human leukocyte antigen expression.

37. D) Allergic rhinitis

Allergic rhinitis is characterized by nasal congestion with clear mucous rhinorrhea and/or a postnasal drip, frequent sneezing, and nasal itching. Physical exam findings often reveal blue-tinged or pale and boggy nasal turbinates, undereye darkening due to subcutaneous venodilation, and hyperplastic lymphoid tissue lining the posterior pharynx, resulting in a cobblestone appearance. Rhinitis medicamentosa can present with nasal congestion and discharge as a result of prolonged (>3 days) use of topical nasal decongestant sprays, which causes a rebound effect resulting in severe and chronic nasal congestion. Blepharitis is a chronic condition caused by inflammation of the eyelids (hair follicles, meibomian glands) causing itching and/or irritation. Sjögren's syndrome is a chronic autoimmune disorder characterized by decreased function of the lacrimal and salivary glands.

38. D) Placing the avulsed tooth in cold milk during transport

Avulsed permanent teeth should be replanted immediately if possible. If the tooth cannot be replaced in the socket, it should be handled carefully by the crown to prevent damage to the periodontal ligament. The tooth should not be sterilized or scrubbed; instead, debris should be gently removed by rinsing with saline or tap water. The tooth should be kept in place by having the patient hold it or bite down on gauze. Appropriate storage solutions include culture media; however, it is not widely available. Cold milk is an appropriate alternative, as is saliva. Tap water should not be used due to its low osmolality.

39. A patient presents with a sensation of aural fullness and decreased hearing. The patient denies significant pain but reports a recent viral infection. Otoscopic examination reveals an intact tympanic membrane (TM) with clear yellow fluid behind the TM. Treatment for this condition includes which of the following interventions?

A. Observation and supportive therapy with oral decongestants

B. Treatment with amoxicillin-clavulanate (Augmentin)

C. Topical antibiotic ear drops

D. Immediate referral for ear, nose, and throat evaluation

40. Which of the following components of the ocular system is the area of highest visual acuity?

A. Fovea centralis

B. Fundus

C. Peripheral retina

D. Optic nerve

(See answers next page.)

39. A) Observation and supportive therapy with oral decongestants

This patient is presenting with otitis media with effusion, which is characterized by hearing loss and a sense of aural fullness. Otoscopy examination indicates the presence of middle ear fluid and an intact (or retracted) tympanic membrane (TM) without evidence of active infection. Management often involves supportive care because most effusions resolve over 12 weeks. Treatment for symptoms includes antihistamines, oral decongestants, and/or nasal corticosteroids. Myringotomy with tympanostomy tubes may be considered in some patients. Acute otitis media requires antibiotic therapy with amoxicillin-clavulanate (Augmentin) or second- or third-generation cephalosporins for those with mild penicillin allergies. Topical antibiotics may be indicated in addition to oral therapy for those with a ruptured TM in acute otitis media. Referral is indicated in patients with recurrent acute otitis media, persistent hearing loss, or chronic TM perforation.

40. A) Fovea centralis

The macula can be visualized on the fundal exam; it is a dark, flat spot in the exact center of the posterior portion of the retina. In the center of the macula is the fovea centralis, which contains only cones and is the area of highest visual acuity or resolution. The fundus of the eye is the interior surface visible by the ophthalmoscopic exam. The retina is the innermost layer of the eyeball, a neurosensory layer attached to the posterior pole of the eye. The peripheral retina can be seen during the fundal exam; it should be a deep red color, without exudate or hemorrhages. The optic nerve is seen as a round sphere with sharp margins on the fundal exam. It is a sensory nerve (cranial nerve II) that transmits the neural-visual impulses from the retina to the brain.

DANGER SIGNALS

ACRAL LENTIGINOUS MELANOMA

Subtype of melanoma that is most common in darker-pigmented individuals. These dark brown-to-black lesions are located on the nail beds (subungual), palmar and plantar (sole of foot) surfaces, and rarely the mucous membranes. Subungual melanomas look like longitudinal brown-to-black bands on the nail bed (Figure 6.1).

ACTINIC KERATOSIS

Older-to-elderly fair-skinned adults complain of numerous dry, round, and red-colored lesions with a rough texture that do not heal. Lesions are slow growing. Most common locations are sun-exposed areas, such as the cheeks, nose, face, neck, arms, and back. The risk is highest for those with light-colored skin, hair, and/or eyes. In some cases, a precancerous lesion of squamous cell carcinoma is a possibility. Patients with early-childhood history of severe sunburns are at higher risk for skin cancer (squamous cell carcinoma, basal cell carcinoma [BCC], melanoma).

ANAPHYLAXIS (ANGIOEDEMA, HIVES)

A severe, life-threatening hypersensitivity reaction, anaphylaxis is caused by immunoglobulin E (IgE)– and immunoglobulin G (IgG)–mediated reactions, as well as immune complex/complement-mediated mechanisms. In the outpatient setting, anaphylaxis is mostly caused by food allergies but can also be caused by insect stings and certain drugs. It is characterized by acute onset (minutes to several hours) with symptoms such as flushing, hives, angioedema, dyspnea, wheezing, tachycardia or bradycardia, hypotension, hypoxia, or cardiac arrest. Immediate treatment with epinephrine (1 mg/mL) 0.3 to 0.5 mg intramuscularly (IM) can be given on the mid-outer thigh. The condition can repeat every 5 to 15 minutes if the response is poor to treatment. In the setting of anaphylaxis, there are *no* absolute contraindications to epinephrine. Call 911.

BASAL CELL CARCINOMA

Common skin cancer arising from basal layer of epidermis. Clinical presentation classified as nodular, superficial, and morpheaform. Nodular form of BCC typically presents on face as a pink or flesh-colored papule with a pearly or translucent quality and a telangiectatic vessel. Superficial form of BCC mostly occurs on the trunk as slightly scale, non-firm macules, patches, or thin plaques light red to pink in color with an atrophic or ulcerated center that does not heal (Figure 6.2). Morpheaform are smooth, flesh-colored, or very light pink papules or plaques that are usually atrophic, firm, or indurated with ill-defined borders. Most common risk factor for BCC is exposure to ultraviolent radiation in sunlight.

BROWN RECLUSE SPIDER BITES

Brown recluse spiders (*Loxosceles reclusa*) are found mostly in the midwestern and southeastern United States.

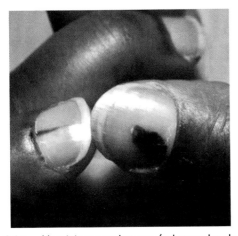

Figure 6.1 Acral lentiginous melanoma (subungual melanoma).
Source: Centers for Disease Control and Prevention/Carl Washington, MD, Emory University School of Medicine; Mona Saraiya, MD, MPH.

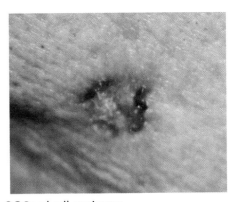

Figure 6.2 Basal cell carcinoma.
Source: Gawlik, K. S., Melnyk, B. M., & Teall, A. M. (2021). (See Resources section for complete source information.)

Systemic symptoms include fever, chills, nausea, and vomiting. Deaths are rare but have occurred in young children (younger than age 7 years). Any child with systemic signs should be hospitalized (the condition may cause hemolysis).

Most spider bites are located on the arms, upper legs, or trunk (underneath clothing). Bite may feel like a pinprick (or be painless). The bitten area becomes swollen, red, and tender, and blisters appear within 24 to 48 hours. Central area of bite becomes necrotic (purple-black eschar). When the eschar sloughs off, it leaves an ulcer, which takes several weeks to heal.

ERYTHEMA MIGRANS (EARLY LYME DISEASE)

The classic lesion is an expanding red rash with central clearing that resembles a target. The "bull's-eye" or target rash usually appears within 7 to 14 days after a deer tick bite (range: 3–30 days). The rash feels hot to the touch and has a rough texture. Common locations are the belt line, axillary area, behind the knees, and groin area. It is accompanied by flu-like symptoms. The lesion spontaneously resolves within a few weeks. It is most common in the northeastern regions of the United States. Use of DEET-containing repellent on skin and permethrin on clothing and gear can repel deer ticks.

MELANOMA

Dark-colored moles with uneven texture, variegated colors, and irregular borders with a diameter of 6 mm or larger are observed (Figure 6.3). They may be pruritic. If melanoma is in the nail beds (subungual melanoma), it may be very aggressive. Lesions can be located anywhere on the body, including the retina. Risk factors include family history of melanoma (10% of cases), extensive/intense sunlight exposure, blistering sunburn in childhood, tanning beds, high nevus count/atypical nevus, and light skin/eyes.

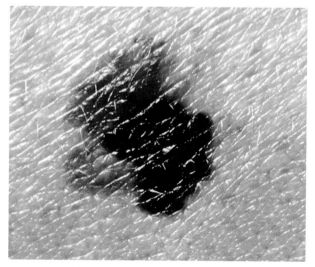

Figure 6.3 Melanoma.
Source: National Cancer Institute.

MENINGOCOCCEMIA (MENINGITIS)

Acute systemic meningococcal disease can manifest as meningitis with or without meningococcemia or meningococcemia without clinical evidence of meningitis. Meningitis is an inflammatory disease of the leptomeninges (the tissues surrounding the brain and spinal cord). Meningococcemia is a systemic bloodstream infection caused by *Neisseria meningitidis* (gram-negative bacterium) that can progress very rapidly without treatment. Symptoms include sudden onset of sore throat, cough, fever, headache, stiff neck, photophobia, and changes in level of consciousness (LOC; drowsiness, lethargy to coma). In some cases, there is abrupt onset of petechial (small red spots) to hemorrhagic rashes (pink to purple colored) in the axillae, flanks, wrist, and ankles. Hypotension and shock are common. In up to 25% of cases, cutaneous hemorrhage and disseminated intravascular coagulopathy (DIC) are seen. Procalcitonin is usually elevated in bacterial meningitis. Fulminant cases can result in death within hours of symptom onset. Mortality rate of bacterial meningitis is about 13%. The risk is higher for those who live in close quarters, such as first-year college students residing in dormitories, nursery or day care, and military barracks; individuals with asplenia, defective spleen (sickle cell anemia), HIV infection, or complement immune-system deficiencies; and infants (3 months to 1 year). The Centers for Disease Control and Prevention (CDC) recommends vaccination for these higher risk groups and for adolescents (age 11–18 years). Follow aerosol droplet precautions. Prophylaxis should be given as soon as possible after exposure (e.g., rifampin). Ceftriaxone is recommended initial therapy.

ROCKY MOUNTAIN SPOTTED FEVER

Rocky Mountain spotted fever (RMSF) presents with abrupt onset of high fever, chills, severe headache, nausea/vomiting, photophobia, myalgia, and arthralgia followed by a rash that erupts 2 to 5 days after onset of fever. The rash consists of small red spots (petechiae) that start to erupt on the wrist, forearms, and ankles (sometimes the palms and soles). It rapidly progresses toward the trunk until it becomes generalized (approximately 10% of RMSF patients do not develop a rash). See Figure 6.4 and Table 6.1. Most cases of RMSF occur from spring to early summer when outdoor activity is highest. Most common rickettsial infection in the United States; most prevalent in the southeastern and south-central states in rural and suburban populations. Incidence increases with age. Mortality rate has decreased since availability of tetracycline antibiotics. First-line treatment is doxycycline (both children and adults). Use of DEET-containing repellent on skin and permethrin on clothing and gear can repel dog and deer ticks.

SHINGLES INFECTION OF THE TRIGEMINAL NERVE (HERPES ZOSTER OPHTHALMICUS)

This is a sight-threatening condition caused by reactivation of the herpes zoster virus with involvement of the ophthalmic branch of the trigeminal nerve (cranial nerve

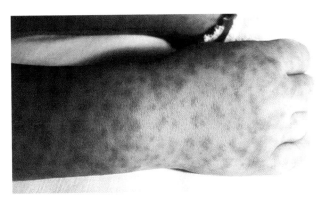

Figure 6.4 Rocky Mountain spotted fever (later-stage rash).
Source: Centers for Disease Control and Prevention.

[CN] V; Figure 6.5). Patients report sudden eruption of multiple vesicular lesions (which rupture into shallow ulcers with crusts) that are located on one side on the scalp and forehead and the sides and tip of the nose. If herpetic rash is seen on the tip of the nose, suspect shingles until proved otherwise. The eyelid on the same side is swollen and red. Patients complain of photophobia, eye pain, and blurred vision. This is more common in elderly patients. Refer to an ophthalmologist or the ED as soon as possible.

STEVENS–JOHNSON SYNDROME AND TOXIC EPIDERMAL NECROLYSIS

Stevens–Johnson syndrome (SJS) and toxic epidermal necrolysis (TEN) lesions appear like a target (or a "bull's-eye"). Multiple lesions erupt abruptly and can include

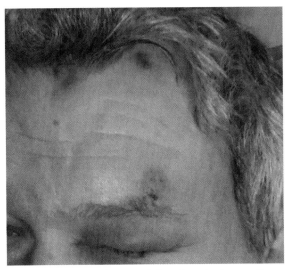

Figure 6.5 Shingles infection of the trigeminal nerve (herpes zoster ophthalmicus).

ill-defined skin lesions with erythematous macules with purpuric centers, hives, blisters (bullae), petechiae, purpura, and necrosis and sloughing of the epidermis. Extensive mucosal surface involvement (eyes, nose, mouth, esophagus, and bronchial tree) are often observed. There could be a prodrome of fever with flu-like symptoms 1 to 3 days before rashes appear. SJS is less severe (involves <10% body skin) compared with TEN (involves >30% body

Table 6.1 Comparison of Common Skin Rashes

Disease	Description
Impetigo	"Honey-colored" crusts, fragile bullae, pruritic
Measles	Koplik's spots are small, white, round spots on a red base on the buccal mucosa by the rear molars and appear 2 to 3 days before onset of symptoms
Scabies	Very pruritic, especially at night; serpiginous rash on interdigital webs, waist, axilla, penis
Scarlet fever	"Sandpaper" rash with sore throat (strep throat)
Tinea versicolor	Hypopigmented round-to-oval macular rashes, most lesions on upper shoulders/back, not pruritic
Pityriasis rosea	Starts with a "herald" patch, a single round or oval, sharply delimited, pink-colored lesion (2–5 cm); progresses to "collarette" of scale with lesion clearing centrally; develops into a "Christmas tree" pattern rash (rash on cleavage lines)
Molluscum contagiosum	Smooth papules 2–5 mm in size that are dome shaped with central umbilication with a white "plug"
Erythema migrans	Red target-like lesions that grow in size, some central clearing, early stage of Lyme disease
Meningococcemia*	Purple to dark-red painful skin lesions all over body, acute-onset high fever, headache, LOC changes, rifampin prophylaxis for close contacts
Rocky Mountain spotted fever* (*Rickettsia rickettsii* from tick bite)	Red spot–like rashes that first break out on the hand/palm/wrist and foot/sole/ankle, acute-onset high fever, severe headache, myalgias
Brown recluse spider bite	Bite area becomes swollen, tender, and red; blister appears within 24 hours; center of lesion may form a purple-to-black eschar, about 10%–20% become necrotic.

*These are life-threatening and Centers for Disease Control and Prevention-reportable diseases.
LOC, level of consciousness.

skin). The most common triggers are medications such as allopurinol, anticonvulsants (lamotrigine, carbamazepine, phenobarbital), sulfonamides, and oxicam nonsteroidal anti-inflammatory drugs (NSAIDs). Mortality rate ranges from 10% (SJS) to 50% (TEN). Risk factors include HIV infection (100-fold higher risk), genetics, systemic lupus erythematosus, and malignancies.

SUBUNGUAL HEMATOMA

Direct trauma to the nail bed results in pain and bleeding that is trapped between the nail bed and the fingernail/toenail. If the hematoma involves >25% of the area of the nail, there is a high risk of permanent ischemic damage to the nail matrix if the blood is not drained. May be simple or accompanied by significant injury (e.g., fingertip avulsion, mallet finger). One method of draining (trephination) a subungual hematoma is to straighten one end of a steel paperclip or use an 18-gauge needle and heat it with a flame until it is very hot. The hot end is pushed down gently (90-degree angle) until a 3- to 4-mm hole is burned on the nail. The nail is pressed down gently until most or all of the blood is drained or suctioned with a smaller needle. Blood may continue draining for 24 to 36 hours. Draining (trephination) of a subungual hematoma involves placing one or more holes in the nail to allow for blood to drain. Complete a neurovascular exam and tendon assessment for evidence of disruption at the join. Large subungual hematomas should receive radiographs. May require prophylactic antibiotics and hand surgery consultation; assess tetanus immunization status.

EXAM TIPS

- Treatment for adult with recluse spider bite is antibiotic on wound, cold packs, and NSAIDs.
- Subungual hematoma can be drained by trephination.

NORMAL FINDINGS

ANATOMY OF THE SKIN

The skin has three layers—epidermis, dermis, and subcutaneous.

- Epidermis: No blood vessels; gets nourishment from the dermis. Consists of two layers: Top layer consists of keratinized cells (dead squamous epithelial cells). Bottom layer is where melanocytes reside and vitamin D synthesis occurs.
- Dermis: Consists of blood vessels, sebaceous glands, and hair follicles.
- Subcutaneous layer: Is composed of fat, sweat glands, and hair follicles.
- Apocrine glands: Type of sweat gland located mainly in the axilla and groin.
- Eccrine glands: Major sweat glands of the body, widely distributed but greatest in the hands, soles of the feet, and forehead; helps with heat dissipation and thermoregulation.

SKIN EXAMINATION: DARKER COLORED SKIN

Urticaria and wheals can appear paler than surrounding skin (palpate for induration and warmth). Very dry dark skin can appear ashy to gray in color (check arms and legs). Skin conditions that are more common in people of African background are keloids, hyperpigmentation, and traction alopecia (due to chronic tight hair braiding). Jaundice may be harder to assess in darker skinned patients; assess oral mucosa and sclera.

Pseudofolliculitis barbae (barber's itch), often referred to as "razor bumps" or "ingrown hairs," is a common cutaneous condition that develops with the removal of facial hair (most frequently due to shaving). It is caused by inflammation from the curly hair growing back into the skin. Most prevalent in males post-puberty with a predisposition for those with curly hair. The treatment is to let the beard hair grow for 3 to 4 weeks. Advise patient to avoid shaving beard hair too short and too close to the skin.

People with darker skin require longer periods of sun exposure to produce vitamin D. A deficiency during pregnancy results in infantile rickets (brittle bones, skeletal abnormalities).

SKIN LESIONS

DERMATOLOGIC TERMS

- Acral: Distal portions of the limbs (i.e., the hand or feet [acral melanoma])
- Annular: Ring-shaped (e.g., ringworm, or tinea corporis)
- Exanthem: Cutaneous rash
- Extensor: The skin area that is outside of the joint (e.g., front of knee, back of elbow)
- Flexor: The area of the skin on top of the joint with skin folds (e.g., back of knees, antecubital space)
- Flexural: Skin flexures are body folds (eczema affects flexural folds)
- Intertriginous: An area where two skin areas touch or rub each other (e.g., axilla, breast skin folds, anogenital area, between the fingers/digits)
- Maculopapular rash: Rash with color (usually pink to red) with small bumps that are raised above the skin (viral rashes)
- Morbilliform: Rash that resembles measles (pink rash with texture)
- Nummular: Coin-shaped, round (nummular eczema)
- Purpura: Bleeding into the skin; small bleeds are petechial (RMSF), and larger areas of bleeding are ecchymoses or purpura (meningococcemia)
- Serpiginous: Shaped like a snake (e.g., larva migrans)
- Verrucous: Wartlike
- Xerosis: Dry skin

SCREENING FOR MELANOMA

The "A, B, C, D, E" of melanoma:

- **A** (asymmetry)
- **B** (border irregular)

- **C** (color varies in the same region)
- **D** (diameter >6 mm)
- **E** (enlargement or change in size)

Other symptoms to watch for include intermittent bleeding with mild trauma and new onset of itching.

SKIN CANCER STATISTICS

Skin cancer is the most common cancer in the United States. Basal and squamous cell carcinoma are the most common types of skin cancer. Melanoma is the third most common type of skin cancer but most fatal because of its tendency to metastasize.

SKIN LESION REVIEW

Primary Skin Lesions

- Macule: Flat nonpalpable lesion <1 cm in diameter. Example: Freckles (ephelis), lentigo or lentigines (plural)
- Papule: Palpable solid lesion ≤1 cm in diameter. Example: Nevi (moles), acne, small cherry angiomas
- Plaque: Flattened, elevated lesion with variable shape >1 cm in diameter. Example: Psoriatic lesions
- Vesicle: Elevated superficial skin lesion <1 cm in diameter, filled with serous or hemorrhagic fluid. Example: Herpetic lesions
- Bulla: Elevated superficial blister filled with serous fluid and >1 cm in size (large vesicles). Example: Impetigo, second-degree burn with blisters, SJS lesions
- Pustule: Small, circumscribed skin papules containing purulent fluid. Example: Acne pustules

Secondary Skin Lesions

- Primary lesion that changes: Complication of a primary lesion or injury
- Lichenification: Thickening of the epidermis with exaggeration of normal skin lines due to chronic itching (eczema)
- Scale: Flaking skin (psoriasis)
- Crust: Dried exudate, may be serous exudate (impetigo)
- Ulceration: Full-thickness loss of skin (decubiti or pressure injury)
- Scar: Permanent fibrotic changes following damage to the dermis (surgical scars)
- Keloids/hypertrophic scar: Overgrowth of scar tissue; more common in Blacks, Asians

SKIN: CLINICAL FINDINGS

Urticaria (Hives)

Erythematous and raised skin lesions with discrete borders that are irregular, oval, or round (Figure 6.6). Lesions

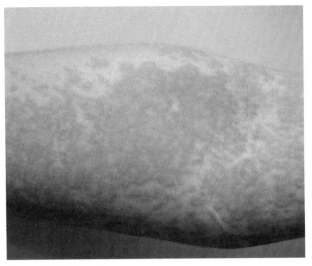

Figure 6.6 Urticaria.
Source: Courtesy of James Heilman, MD.

become more numerous and enlarge over minutes to hours, and then they disappear. They may occur as one episode or recurrent (usually daily) episodes that resolve in 24 hours and then recur. Skin that is compressed (e.g., with tight bra straps) may have lesions that assume a shape (such as linear-shaped lesions under bra strap). Urticaria is considered chronic if it lasts longer than 6 weeks. Most cases are self-limited. Urticaria has multiple etiologies (e.g., medications, viral/bacterial infections, insect bites, latex allergies); if the cause is eliminated, the urticaria will often resolve. If associated with angioedema or progresses to anaphylaxis, it can be life-threatening.

Seborrheic Keratoses

Soft, wartlike, fleshy growths in the trunk that are located mostly on the back. Skin lesions look like they are "pasted" on the skin. Lesions on the same person can range in color from light tan to black. They start to appear during middle age (or later) and become more numerous as patient gets older. They are generally painless.

Xanthelasma

Raised, soft, yellow-colored plaques that are usually painless and located symmetrically under the brow or upper and/or lower lids of the eyes on the medial sides (Figure 6.7). If the patient is younger than 40 years of age, rule out hyperlipidemia. Approximately 50% of patients with xanthelasma have hyperlipidemia. If the xanthomas are located on the fingers, it is pathognomonic for familial hypercholesterolemia. Order a fasting (8–12 hours) lipid profile. The condition is also known as *plane xanthomas*.

Melasma (Mask of Pregnancy)

Bilateral brown- to tan-colored macules and patches located on sun-exposed skin (e.g., upper cheeks, malar area, forehead, and chin). Common in female patients of reproductive age but can also be seen in male patients. Risk factors include genetics, exposure to sunlight, skin

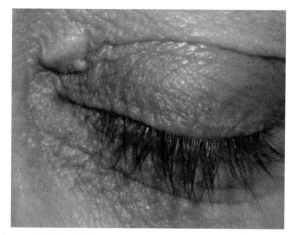

Figure 6.7 Xanthelasma.
Source: Courtesy of Klaus D. Peter.

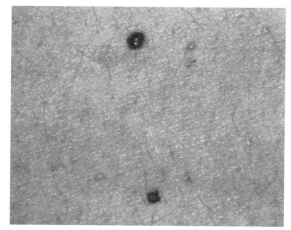

Figure 6.8 Cherry angiomas.
Source: Centers for Disease Control and Prevention/F. Gilbert, MD.

phototype, and hormonal factors (e.g., pregnancy, use of oral contraceptives). Stains can be permanent but can lighten over time.

Vitiligo

Loss of epidermal melanocytes. White patches of skin (hypopigmentation) with irregular shapes that gradually develop, coalesce, and spread over time. It is chronic and progressive and can be located anywhere on the body. Lesions may remain stable or can be associated with flare-ups. Risk factors are presence of autoimmune disease (e.g., Graves' disease, Hashimoto's thyroiditis, rheumatoid arthritis [RA], psoriasis, pernicious anemia). Condition is more obvious and disfiguring in patients with darker skin. Refer to dermatologist for treatment options (e.g., topical steroids, light therapy). Advise patients to use sunscreen and avoid prolonged sun exposure (makes white patches more obvious). It can have a major impact on patients' self-image and self-esteem.

Cherry Angioma

Benign small and smooth round papules that are a bright cherry-red color (Figure 6.8). Sizes range from 1 to 4 mm. Lesions are due to a nest of malformed arterioles in the skin. They blanch with pressure and are more common in middle-aged to older patients. No treatment is necessary, since the condition is benign.

Lipoma

Soft, fatty cystic tumors that are usually painless and are located in the subcutaneous layer of the skin. Most are located on the neck, trunk, and arms. Lipoma is the most common type of benign soft tissue tumor. Tumors are round or oval shape and measure 1 to 10 cm or more, and they feel smooth with a discrete edge. They are asymptomatic unless they become too large or are irritated or ruptured. Surgical excision is an option.

Nevi (Moles)

Round macules to papules (junctional nevi) in colors ranging from light tan to dark brown. Their borders may be distinct or slightly irregular. They are often concentrated on the trunk and lower extremities. Junctional nevi are macular or minimally raised with colors ranging from brown to black. Compound nevi appear as pigmented papules and vary in color from tan to medium brown.

Xerosis

Inherited skin disorder that results in extremely dry skin and may involve mucosal surfaces such as the mouth (xerostomia) or the conjunctiva of the eye (xerophthalmia).

Acanthosis Nigricans

Diffuse velvety thickening of the skin that is usually located behind the neck and on the axilla (Figure 6.9). It is associated with diabetes, metabolic syndrome, obesity, and cancer of the gastrointestinal (GI) tract.

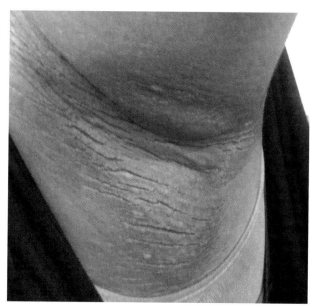

Figure 6.9 Acanthosis nigricans.
Source: Courtesy of Masryyy.

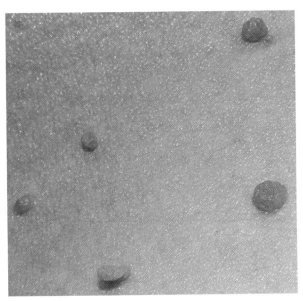

Figure 6.10 Acrochordon (skin tags).
Source: Courtesy of Jmarchn.

Acrochordon (Skin Tags)

Painless and pedunculated outgrowths of skin that are the same color as the patient's skin (Figure 6.10). Common locations are the neck and axillary area. When twisted or traumatized (e.g., gets caught on a necklace), the outgrowth can become necrotic and drop off the skin. Incidence increases with age. More common in diabetics and patients who are obese.

TOPICAL STEROIDS

- Topical corticosteroids are essential in inflammatory and autoimmune skin disease (e.g., atopic dermatitis, allergic contact dermatitis, psoriasis, vitiligo, lichen planus, discoid lupus erythematosus).
- Avoid combination antifungal/topical steroids in cases of suspected fungal etiology because they can risk incomplete resolution of the fungal infection.
- Steroids range in potency from class 1 (super potent) to class 7 (least potent); see Table 6.2 for list of topical steroids.
- Steroids are most effective when applied within 3 minutes after bathing.
- Sensitive skin—face, genitals, intertriginous areas (under breasts, intergluteal folds, inner thighs)—can absorb more of the topical steroid.
- For children and areas with sensitive skin, do not use fluorinated topical steroids. Use class 7 (least potent) topical steroids, such as 0.5% to 1% hydrocortisone. Class 6 (mild-potency) steroids, such as fluocinolone acetonide (Synalar cream/solution), are prescription drugs. Proceed to next step if over-the-counter (OTC) hydrocortisone is not working. Avoid potent or super-potent topical corticosteroids in children younger than 12 years, except in specific cases.
- Hypothalamic–pituitary–adrenal (HPA) axis suppression may occur with excessive or prolonged use (>2 weeks), especially in infants and children, or with use of potent

Table 6.2 Common Topical Steroids

Name	Potency	Frequency
Halobetasol propionate 0.5% (Ultravate)	Class I (super-high)	Daily–BID (max 2 weeks)
Halcinonide 0.1% (Halog)	Class II (high)	BID–TID
Triamcinolone acetonide 0.5% (Kenalog)	Class III (medium-high)	BID–TID
Mometasone furoate 0.1% (Elocon)	Class IV (medium)	BID–QID
Desonide 0.05% (Desonate)	Class V (low-medium)	BID–QID
Fluocinolone acetonide 0.01% (Synalar)	Class VI (low)	BID–QID
Hydrocortisone 1% (OTC; no Rx needed)	Class VII (least potent)	BID–QID

BID, twice daily; OTC, over the counter; QID, four times daily; Rx, prescription; TID, three times daily.

to ultrapotent topical steroids. These agents can cause striae, skin atrophy, telangiectasia, acne, and hypopigmentation.

General Recommendations

- Super-high potency: Use for severe dermatoses (psoriasis, severe eczema) on non-facial and non-intertriginous areas for up to 2 weeks. Works well on palms, scalp, and soles, which have thicker skin.
- Medium-high potency: Use on mild-to-moderate non-facial and non-intertriginous areas
- Low-medium potency: Use on larger areas that need treatment.
- Low-potency: Can use on eyelid and genital areas for limited duration. Ophthalmic form of topical steroid is used on eyelids.

DISEASE REVIEW

ACNE VULGARIS (COMMON ACNE)

Acne is inflammation and infection of the pilosebaceous units. Has multifactorial causes, such as high androgen levels, bacterial infection with cutibacterium (formerly known as *Propionibacterium acnes*), follicular hyperproliferation, and genetic influences. Lesions are located mainly on the face, shoulders, chest, and back. Highest incidence during puberty and adolescence.

Mild Acne (Topicals Only)

Scattered open comedones (blackheads) and closed comedones (noninflammatory acne), with or without small papules (<5 mm), are considered mild acne. First-line treatment includes topical retinoids, benzoyl peroxide, and topical antibiotics.

- Mild comedonal acne: Tretinoin topical (Retin-A)
- Mild papulopustular and mixed acne: Topical retinoid and topical antimicrobials (e.g., benzoyl peroxide

gel with or without topical clindamycin [Cleocin]) *or* benzoyl peroxide and topical antibiotic (for those who cannot tolerate a retinoid)

- Start at lowest dose: Tretinoin topical (Retin-A) 0.25% cream every other day at bedtime × 2 to 3 weeks, then daily application at bedtime; alternative is azelaic acid or salicylic acid (OTC)

Retinoids also help decrease facial wrinkles and hyper- or hypopigmentation. Advise patients that acne may worsen (first few weeks of use) with topical retinoids. In about 4 to 6 weeks, acne improves and clears up. The facial skin can become red and irritated (dryness, itch, peeling) in the first few weeks of use. Photosensitivity reaction is possible (use sunscreen). If no improvement in acne within 8 to 12 weeks, consider using alternative topical therapies: topical dapsone, minocycline, or clascoterone.

Moderate Acne (Topicals Plus Antibiotic)
Presence of papules and pustules (inflammatory lesions) with comedones is considered moderate acne.

Treatment
- Systemic therapy: Commonly used for moderate to severe acne; options include oral isotretinoin, oral antibiotics, and oral hormonal therapies (oral contraceptives and spironolactone).
- Combination with systemic therapy and topical therapy: Often recommended (with the exception of oral isotretinoin). Topical agents include retinoids, benzoyl peroxide, and other agents (topical antibiotics, topical dapsone or clascoterone, salicylic acid, and azelaic acid).
- Patients with severe, extensive, nodular acne vulgaris: Oral isotretinoin (retinoid) is recommended for initial therapy because it is the only medication that can permanently alter the course of acne vulgaris. Patients may require combination with systemic glucocorticoid.
- Isotretinoin is teratogenic and contraindicated in pregnancy: Participation in a Risk Evaluation and Mitigation Strategy (REMS) program is required for therapy in the United States with the goal of eliminated fetal exposure to isotretinoin (iPLEDGE):
  - Patients must use two forms of reliable contraception. Prescribe 1-month supply only. Monthly pregnancy testing with results shown to pharmacist is necessary before refills. Pregnancy test is needed 1 month after treatment is discontinued.
  - Discontinue if the following are present: Severe depression, visual disturbance, hearing loss, tinnitus, GI pain, rectal bleeding, uncontrolled hypertriglyceridemia, pancreatitis, hepatitis.
- If no improvement: Consider addition of oral antibiotics (e.g., tetracycline antibiotics such as minocycline, doxycycline) at a duration of about 3 to 4 months. Tetracyclines (Category D) can cause permanent discoloration of growing tooth enamel. Not given during pregnancy or to children up to the age of 8 years.
- Others: Certain oral contraceptives (Desogen, Yaz) are indicated for acne.
- Role of diet: Limited evidence that some types of dairy (e.g., skim milk) may affect acne.

ACTINIC KERATOSES
Precancerous precursor that can progress to squamous cell carcinoma. The risk of progression is low, but about 60% of cutaneous squamous cell carcinomas arise from pre-existing actinic keratoses. Most likely to develop in older adults with fair skin and a history of chronic sun exposure (UV light) and sunburn.

Classic Case
Older-to-elderly adult complains of numerous dry, round, and pink-to-red lesions with a rough and scaly texture that do not heal. Lesions are slow growing and become more numerous with age; most common locations are sun-exposed areas, such as the cheeks, nose, face, neck, arms, and back.

Treatment Plan
Refer to dermatologist for biopsy (gold-standard diagnosis). Treatment ranges from surgery and cryotherapy to topical medications (e.g., fluorouracil cream 5% [5-FU], imiquimod). If there are only a small number of lesions, they can be treated with cryotherapy. With larger numbers, 5-FU cream is used over several weeks. It selectively destroys sun-damaged cells in the skin. Treatment with 5-FU cream (Efudex) causes inflammation that appears as erythema (redness), oozing, crusting, scabs, and soreness, which disappears in a few weeks.

BIOTERRORISM
Anthrax
Infection caused by *Bacillus anthracis* (gram-positive rods). Reportable disease. There are three types of anthrax: cutaneous, GI, and pulmonary. Cutaneous anthrax (most common) lesion(s) begins as a papule that enlarges in 24 to 48 hours and develops eschar (necrosis) and ulceration. Usually lesions are located on the arms, neck, or face. Check for history of exposure or handling animals or hides, hair, or wool. Pulmonary anthrax (inhalational anthrax) is caused by inhaling aerosolized spores through (a) working with animals, wool, or animal hides/hair or (b) bioterrorism. Fulminant inhalational anthrax causes death within days. Symptoms are flu-like and associated with cough, chest pain with cough, hemoptysis, dyspnea, hypoxia, and shock.

- Cutaneous anthrax (without systemic involvement): Doxycycline twice a day, ciprofloxacin twice a day (preferred for pregnant, lactating, and postpartum patients), levofloxacin once a day. Alternatives include: clindamycin.
- Postexposure prophylaxis (bioterrorism suspected): Doxycycline 100 mg orally twice a day or ciprofloxacin; duration ranges from 42 to 60 days.

- Case-fatality rate of cutaneous anthrax: <2% with antibiotic therapy; mortality increases from 16% to 39% without treatment. The mortality rate for pulmonary anthrax is higher as most patients present late in the course of their illness. Prior to 2001, mortality rates were as high as 90%. Between 2001 to 2021, about 53% of patients survived.
- Pathogens that have high mortality rates, are easily spread, and are airborne (i.e., aerosolized route): Can be used for bioterrorism.
- Highest risk pathogens: Anthrax bacilli (*Bacillus anthracis*), smallpox virus, botulism (*Clostridium botulinum*), plague (*Yersinia pestis*), viral hemorrhagic fevers (Ebola, Marburg).

Smallpox (Variola Virus)
Infection targets respiratory and oropharyngeal mucosal surfaces. "Eliminated" in 1977. Incubation period of 2 weeks. Flu-like signs and symptoms. Numerous large nodules appear mostly in the center of the face and on the arms and legs. The antiviral tecovirimat (Tpoxx) is the first antiviral indicated for the treatment of smallpox. Mortality rate is 20% to 50%.

Smallpox Vaccine
If vaccine is given within 2 to 3 days postexposure, it can lessen severity of illness. Vaccinia immune globulin (e.g., for pregnant, immunosuppressed) is available from special clinics.

CLINICAL PEARLS

- The U.S. Food and Drug Administration (FDA) recommends that health providers avoid prescribing oral ketoconazole (Nizoral PO) for fungal skin and nail infections because the harm (e.g., serious liver damage, adrenal insufficiency, and drug interactions) outweighs the benefit. Topical ketoconazole shampoo is safe.
- Use ophthalmic-grade sterile cream and ointments for rashes near the eyes.
- Patients with scarlet fever are at higher risk for developing postglomerular nephritis.
- Recurrences of tinea pedis and tinea cruris infection are common; they are also frequently seen concurrently.
- Patients on anti-tumor necrosis factor (TNF) biologics are at higher risk for melanoma and squamous cell skin cancer.
- Most cases of rabies in the United States are from wild animals such as bats, raccoons, skunks, and foxes.

BITES: HUMAN AND ANIMAL
Human Bites
The bite that involves the most pathogens. Watch for closed-fist injuries of the hands (may involve joint capsule and tendon damage). *Eikenella corrodens* and numerous bacteria may be involved.

Dog and Cat Bites
Pasteurella multocida (gram negative) most common pathogen in cat and dog bites. Dog bites also carry *capnocytophaga canimorsus* (gram negative). Cat bites have a higher risk of infection than dog bites. Signs of infection are redness, swelling, and pain, and systemic symptoms may develop within 12 to 24 hours.

Treatment Plan (Both Human and Animal Bites)
- Amoxicillin–clavulanate (Augmentin) 875 mg/125 mg orally twice a day × 10 days.
- If penicillin allergy, doxycycline twice a day, Bactrim DS twice a day *plus* coverage for anaerobes combine with metronidazole (Flagyl) twice a day or clindamycin three times a day.
- Irrigate copiously with sterile saline. All bites and infected wounds should be sent for culture and sensitivity (C&S).
- Do not suture wounds at high risk for infection, such as puncture wounds, wounds >12 hours old (24 hours on face), infected bite wounds, cat bites.
- Tetanus vaccine required if last dose was >5 years ago. Use Tdap vaccine (tetanus, diphtheria, and acellular pertussis, if never had Tdap) in patients older than 7 years.
- Follow up with patient within 24 to 48 hours after treatment.

Rabies
- Consider bites from bats, raccoons, skunks, foxes, and coyotes (domestic animals can also have rabies). If dog bite, check if dog has received rabies vaccine recently (within 1 year).
- Rabies rarely seen in rodents such as mice, rats, hamsters, guinea pigs, or rabbits.
- Rabies immune globulin *plus* rabies vaccine may be required. Call local health department for current guidelines. Consider if wild animal acts abnormally tame, produces copious saliva, attacks without provocation, or looks ill.

EXAM TIPS

- Preferred antibiotic for human, dog, and cat bites is amoxicillin–clavulanate (Augmentin).
- Know anthrax prophylaxis.

BURNS
The traditional classification of burns as first, second, third, or fourth degree has been replaced according to depth of tissue injury, which reflects the healing potential and need for surgical grafting. Current designation of burn depth includes superficial, partial-thickness (characterized as superficial or deep), and full-thickness burns. The term *fourth degree* is still used to describe the most severe burns extending into underlying tissue with involvement of muscle and/or bone. Minor burn criteria are outlined in Table 6.3.

Table 6.3 Minor Burn Criteria (American Burn Association)*

Burn Type	Description
Partial-thickness burns	<10% of TBSA in patients 10–50 years of age <5% of TBSA in patients younger than 10 or older than 50 years of age
Full-thickness burns	<2% of TBSA in any patient without other injury
All of the above criteria *plus*	May not involve face, hands, perineum, or feet May not cross major joints May not be circumferential No suspicion of inhalation injury No suspicion of high-voltage injury

*If patient meets these criteria, refer to ED or burn center.
TBSA, total body surface area.

Superficial-Thickness Burns
- Involve only epidermal layer; may be caused by UV exposure (e.g., sunburn).
- Erythema only (no blisters); painful (e.g., sunburns, mild scalds), dry, blanches with pressure.
- Cleanse with mild soap and water (or saline); cold packs for 24 to 48 hours.
- Intact skin does not require topical antibiotics; apply a topical OTC anesthetic such as benzocaine if desired or aloe vera gel. Dressings are often not required; healing time 3 to 6 days.

Partial-Thickness Burns
- Involve the epidermis and portions of the dermis: May be caused by scald (spill or splash), flame, oil, or grease.
- Superficial partial thickness: Form blisters within 24 hours between epidermis and dermis, moist, red, weeping, blanches with pressure, painful to temperature, air, and touch; healing time 7 to 20 days.
- Deep partial thickness: Extend into deeper dermis, damaging hair follicles and glandular tissue; almost always blister, wet or waxy dry, variable color (patchy to white or red), blanching with pressure may be sluggish; painful to pressure only; healing time >21 days.
- Do not rupture blisters: Use water with mild soap or normal saline to clean broken skin (not hydrogen peroxide or full-strength Betadine)
- Topical antibiotic: Should be applied to any non-superficial burn to prevent infection (such as Polysporin [bacitracin zinc and polymyxin B]). Apply antimicrobial cream once to twice a day until the burn is healed. After skin is healed, consider using topical zinc oxide daily for 1 to 2 weeks to protect area from sunlight. Do not expose recently healed burned skin to sunlight (causes hyperpigmentation).
- Apply: Nonadherent dressings (e.g., Adaptic, Xeroform), a second layer of fluffed dry gauze, and an outer layer of elastic gauze roll (e.g., Kerlix).

Full-Thickness Burns
- Extend through and destroy all layers of the dermis.
- Common causes are scald, flame, steam, oil, grease, chemical, electrical.
- Appearance is waxy white to leathery gray to charred and black, dry and inelastic, no blanching with pressure.
- Treatment is referral to burn center.

Deeper Injury (Fourth Degree)
- Initial assessment is to rule out airway and breathing compromise. Smoke inhalation injury is a medical emergency. Entire skin layer, subcutaneous area, and soft tissue fascia may be destroyed. Potentially life-threatening.
- Requires referral to a burn center.

Methods of Estimation: Total Percentage of Body Surface Area

Child
Because children have larger heads and smaller lower extremities, the total percentage of body surface area (TBSA) is more accurately estimated using the Lund-Browder chart (Figure 6.11B).

Rule of Nines: Adult
- Arms/head: 9% each (Figure 6.11A)
- Legs/trunk: 18% each leg, anterior trunk, and posterior trunk

Example
A 40-year-old chef suffers hot oil burns while cooking. He reports that he immediately went to the kitchen sink to cool off his burns. The nurse practitioner notes that the patient has bright-red skin on the right arm and right thigh. The skin on the patient's chest and abdomen has several blisters that are red, weeping, and blanch with pressure. What is this patient's diagnosis?

Answer
Superficial-thickness burns on the right arm (9%) and right thigh (9% instead of 18% because it is only on the thigh) with partial-thickness burns (likely superficial partial thickness) on the chest and abdomen (anterior trunk 18%). The TBSA is 36%.

Criteria for Burn Center Referral
- Partial-thickness burns greater than 10% of TBSA
- Burns involving the face, hands, feet, genitalia, perineum, or major joints
- Full-thickness burns
- Electrical and chemical burns
- Inhalation injury
- Burn injury in patients with pre-existing comorbidities
- Any patient with burns and concomitant trauma
- Children in hospitals without qualified personnel or equipment
- Burn injury in patients who require special social or rehabilitative interventions

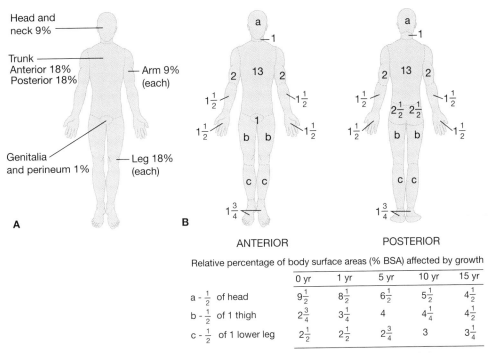

Figure 6.11 Estimating percentage of total body surface area affected by burns. (A) Rule of nines; (B) Lund-Browder chart.
Source: Furstein, J. S. (2022). (See Resources section for complete source information.)

CARBUNCLES (MULTIPLE ABSCESSES)

Carbuncles are several boils that coalesce to form a large boil or abscess. Sometimes they may form several "heads." They are usually treated with systemic antibiotics.

CELLULITIS

Acute skin infection of the deep dermis and underlying tissue, usually caused by gram-positive bacteria. There are two forms of cellulitis (purulent and nonpurulent). Points of entry are skin breaks, insect bites, abrasions, or preexisting skin infections (tinea pedis, impetigo). Community-acquired methicillin-resistant *Staphylococcus aureus* (MRSA) strain (USA300 MRSA) is a virulent strain that causes aggressive skin infections.

- Orbital cellulitis and peritonsillar cellulitis: Refer to ED for parenteral antibiotics. Discussed in Chapter 5.
- Purulent form of cellulitis: *S. aureus* (gram positive). Community-acquired MRSA now common. Most cases are located on the lower leg.
- Non-purulent form of cellulitis: Usually due to streptococci (but may also be staphylococcal).
- Cat bites: *P. multocida* (gram negative).
- Dog bites: *P. multocida, P. canis, Capnocytophaga.*
- Puncture wounds (foot): Contaminated with soft foam liner material or puncture wounds through sneakers. May be at risk for infection with *Pseudomonas aeruginosa*.
- *Vibrio vulnificus*: Exposure of wound to brackish water or saltwater (or eating raw oysters/clams) from the Gulf Coast or Chesapeake Bay can cause infection with this bacterium. Leading cause of shellfish-associated death in the United States.

> **NOTE**
>
> People with liver disease, immunocompromised status, or those who are pregnant should avoid eating raw or undercooked oysters or clams due to the possibility of *V. vulnificus* infection. High mortality rate from *V. vulnificus* septicemia.

Classic Case

Acute onset of diffused pink- to red-colored skin that is poorly demarcated with advancing margins. The lesion feels warm to the touch, and it may become abscessed, or it may be fluctuant (pointing) or draining pus. Abscess (boils) usually due to *Staphylococcus* or MRSA. Infection may spread to lymph node chains (lymphangitis); this appears like red streaks radiating from the infected area. May involve lymphadenopathy. Patient may have systemic symptoms. Lower limb is a common location.

Labs

- C&S advancing edge of lesion (if fluid or pus, vesicles, drainage)
- Complete blood count (CBC) if fever or signs of systemic illness (refer to ED)

Treatment Plan

- If toxic, rapid progression, immunocompromised, diabetic, or concern for joint involvement or osteomyelitis, refer to ED for parenteral antibiotics.
- For immunocompetent patients with non-purulent cellulitis without systematic toxicity and no risk factors for MRSA, oral options include dicloxacillin, flucloxacillin, cephalexin, and cefadroxil.

- For immunocompetent patients with purulent cellulitis without severe sepsis but with a risk factor for MRSA, oral options include trimethoprim-sulfamethoxazole, amoxicillin combined with doxycycline, or linezolid.
- Elevate affected limb, manage predisposing conditions, local wound care.

Risk Factors and Indications for MRSA Infection

- Systemic signs of toxicity: Fever, hypotension
- Cellulitis: With purulent drainage or exudate
- Immunocompromising condition: Neutropenia, immunosuppressive drugs
- Recent hospitalization, residence in long-term care facility
- Specific risk factors: Known MRSA history, HIV infection, IV drug use, homelessness, recent antibiotic use
- Environmental exposures: Military service, incarceration, living in crowded conditions or close contact with a person recently colonized for MRSA, childcare centers, contact sports or sharing equipment

Follow-Up

Follow up with the patient within 48 hours. Patients treated with oral antibiotics usually start to show improvement in 48 to 72 hours. Refer cellulitis cases if:

- Systemic symptoms develop (e.g., fever, toxic) or worsen.
- The cellulitis is unresponsive to treatment within 48 hours.
- Cellulitis is spreading quickly or is a small lesion with black center (gangrene) associated with severe pain (concern for necrotizing fasciitis).
- Patient has diabetes, is immunocompromised, or is taking anti-TNF agents (RA).

Complications

Bacteremia, endocarditis, septic arthritis or osteomyelitis, metastatic infection, sepsis, and toxic shock syndrome.

EXAM TIPS

- For immunocompetent patients with purulent cellulitis without severe sepsis but with a risk factor for MRSA, administer trimethoprim-sulfamethoxazole.
- Differentiate erysipelas versus cellulitis.

DERMATITIS: ATOPIC (ECZEMA)

Chronic inherited skin disorder marked by extremely pruritic rashes that are located on the hands, flexural folds, and neck (older child to adult). The rashes are exacerbated by stress and environmental factors (e.g., winter). The condition is associated with atopic disorders such as asthma, allergic rhinitis, and multiple allergies (check for family history of atopy).

Classic Case

Infants up to 2 years of age have a larger area of rash distribution compared with teens and adults. The rashes are typically found on the cheeks, entire trunk, knees, and elbows. Older children and adults have rashes on the hands, neck, and antecubital and popliteal space (flexural folds). The classic rash starts as multiple small vesicles that rupture, leaving painful, bright-red, weepy lesions. The lesions become lichenified from chronic itching and can persist for months. Fissures form that can be secondarily infected with bacteria.

Treatment

General approach to therapy:

- Oral antihistamines for pruritus are diphenhydramine (Benadryl) and hydroxyzine (Vistaril).
- Avoid drying skin/xerosis because it will exacerbate eczema (e.g., no hot baths, harsh soaps, chemicals, wool clothing). Avoid trigger factors, manage stress and anxiety.
- Hydrating baths (avoid hot water/soaps) followed immediately by application of skin lubricants (Eucerin, Keri Lotion, Crisco, mineral oil). Do not wait until skin is dry before applying.

Mild to moderate disease: Topical steroids and emollients are first-line treatment:

- Mild disease: Low potency, classes V and VI (e.g., hydrocortisone 2.5%)
- Moderate disease: Medium- to high-potency, classes III and IV (e.g., triamcinolone acetonide 0.1%)
- Face and skin folds: Recommend topical calcineurin inhibitors, which are at higher risk for skin atrophy.
- Ear canal: Corticosteroid-based ophthalmic solutions

DERMATITIS: CONTACT

Inflammatory skin reaction caused by direct contact with an irritating external substance; can be a single lesion or generalized rash (e.g., sea bather's itch). There are two types: irritant and allergic. Common offenders are poison ivy (Rhus dermatitis), nickel, latex rubber, chemicals, and the like. Onset can occur within minutes to several hours after skin contact.

Classic Case

Acute onset of one to multiple bright-red and pruritic lesions that evolve into bullous or vesicular lesions; they easily rupture, leaving bright-red moist areas that are painful. Patient may complain of burning or stinging. When rash dries, it becomes crusted, very pruritic, and lichenified from chronic itching. The shape may follow a pattern (e.g., a ring around a finger) or have asymmetric distribution.

Treatment

- Stop exposure to substance. Topical steroids applied once to twice a day × 1 to 2 weeks. If skin is lichenified or does not involve face or flexural areas, use high-potency steroid (triamcinolone, halcinonide), calamine lotion, or oatmeal baths (Aveeno) as needed.
- Consider referral to an allergist for patch testing.

EXAM TIPS

- Practice identifying skin diseases by photograph. Review images of the skin cancers, psoriasis, tinea versicolor, tinea corporis, and candida rash (satellite lesions).
- Differentiate between contact dermatitis and atopic dermatitis. The best clue is the unilateral location and the shape of the lesions in contact dermatitis.

DERMATOPHYTE (TINEA) INFECTIONS

Infection of superficial keratinized tissue (skin, hair, nails) by tinea organisms (Figure 6.12). Tinea trichophyton, microsporum, and epidermophyton are classified as dermatophytes. Tinea infection is classified by location.

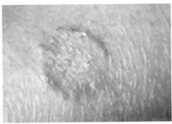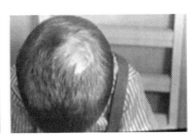

Figure 6.12 Tinea infections (ringworm).
Source: Courtesy of Corina G; Centers for Disease Control and Prevention; Lucille K. George, MD/CDC.

Most cases of tinea can be treated with topical antifungal medication except for tinea capitis and moderate-to-severe onychomycosis or tinea unguium (toenails).

Labs
- Fungal culture of scales/hair/nails or skin lesions
- Potassium hydroxide (KOH) slide microscopy (low–medium power) reveals pseudohyphae and spores

Treatment Plan
- Treatment of limited infection: Most dermatophyte infections can be managed with topical antifungal treatments (e.g., azoles, allylamines, ciclopirox, butenafine, and tolnaftate).
- Treatment of extensive infection or those refractory to initial treatment: Recommend oral antifungal therapy (e.g., terbinafine, fluconazole, and griseofulvin). Oral therapy is recommended for infections extending into follicles, the dermis (e.g., tinea capitis, tinea barbae), or the nails.
- Treatment of dermatophyte infections: Nystatin is not effective. Generally, topical corticosteroids are not recommended.

Tinea Capitis
Black dot tinea capitis (BDTC) is the most common type in the United States. African American children are at higher risk. Spread by close contact and fomites (shared hats, combs). Systemic treatment only (topicals are not effective).

Classic Case
School-aged child with an asymptomatic scaly patch that gradually enlarges. The hairs inside the patch break off easily by the roots (looks like black dots), causing patchy alopecia. Black dot sign: Broken hair shafts leave a dot-like pattern on scalp.

Treatment Plan
- Determine baseline liver function tests (LFTs) and repeat 2 weeks after initiating systemic antifungal treatment.
- Gold standard is oral antifungal therapy with griseofulvin (first-line therapy for *Microsporum* species), terbinafine (recommended for *Trichophyton*), fluconazole, and itraconazole.
- Avoid hepatotoxic substances (alcohol, statins, acetaminophen).
- Avoid sharing combs, headgear, towels, pillows, and clothes with others.

Complications
Kerion: Inflammatory and indurated lesions that permanently damage hair follicles, causing patchy alopecia (permanent).

Tinea Pedis (Athlete's Foot)
Two types are scaly and dry form or moist type (strong odor). Dry type has scales. The scales can include the entire sole, edges of the foot, or the toes only. Moist lesions occur between toe webs and have a strong unpleasant odor. Recurrences are common. Tinea pedis can spread to the fingernails of the dominant hand from scratching feet (two feet–one hand syndrome). Ensure feet are dry after showering or bathing (can use blow-dryer to dry feet). Treatment is topical antifungal therapy.

Tinea Corporis
Refers to epidermal dermatophyte infections in sites other than the feet, groin, face, or hand. Clinical features include ringlike pruritic rashes with a ring of fine scales that slowly enlarge with some central clearing (see Figure 6.12). Most cases respond to topical azole antifungals (topical terbinafine 1%, butenafine 1%) for 2 to 3 weeks. Oral treatment is an alternative for extensive or refractory disease.

Tinea Cruris ("Jock Itch")
Perineal and groin area has pruritic red rashes with fine scales; may be mistaken for candidal infection (bright-red rashes with satellite lesions) or intertrigo (bright-red diffused rash due to bacterial infection). Initial therapy includes topical antifungal agents.

Tinea Manuum (Hands)
Pruritic round rashes with fine scales found on the hands. Usually infected from chronic scratching of foot that is also infected with tinea (athlete's foot). Treatment is similar to tinea pedis (initial therapy is topical antifungals).

Tinea Barbae (Beard Area)
Beard area is affected. Scaling occurs with pruritic red rashes. Oral antifungal therapy is necessary.

Onychomycosis (Nails)
The nail becomes opaque, yellow or brown discoloration, and thickened with scaling under the nail (hyperkeratosis).

Also known as *tinea unguium*. It is usually caused by dermatophytes, but it can become infected with yeast and molds. The most common type is called distal subungual onychomycosis. Nail may separate from nail bed (onycholysis). Great toe is the most common location.

Labs
Fungal cultures of affected nails for confirmation of infection; KOH slide for microscopy.

Medications
- Not all patients with onychomycosis require treatment: Indications include a history of repeated lower extremity cellulitis, diabetes, immunosuppression, and nail pain or discomfort.
- Mild to moderate cases: Oral terbinafine, however, may cause drug interactions and systemic effects. Recommended to start topical antifungals such as efinaconazole (Jublia) and ciclopirox (Penlac). Apply Penlac nail lacquer × several weeks. Works best in mild cases on fingernails.
- Moderate to severe cases: Administer oral terbinafine (Lamisil) × 6 weeks (fingernail) or 12 weeks (toenail) or itraconazole for 1 week per month for 2 months (fingernail) or 1 week per month for 3 months (toenail).

EARLY LYME DISEASE
Erythema migrans is a rash at the site of the bite of an *Ixodes* tick infected with *Borrelia burgdorferi*. The rash begins usually 7 to 14 days after the bite in 80% of patients. If untreated, infection can spread systemically and affect multiple organ systems. May have only rash or rash may be accompanied by flu-like symptoms.

Classic Case
Described in "Danger Signals" section.

Labs
Two-step (two-tier) testing recommended (designed to be done together):
- First step is enzyme immunoassay (EIA); if negative, no further testing is recommended.
- If first test is positive (or equivocal/indeterminate), the second step test is the indirect immunofluorescence assay (IFA, or immunoblot test or "western blot" test).
- If both EIA and IFA tests are positive, patient likely has Lyme disease. Serologic testing alone cannot establish nor exclude the diagnosis of Lyme disease. It is important to take into account the stage of disease when interpreting the results.
- Antibody tests may be false negative the first 4 to 6 weeks (infection present but no antibodies yet).

Treatment Plan
- Early Lyme disease only: Doxycycline twice a day × 10 days (first-line drug for both adults and children)
- Alternative: Amoxicillin 500 mg three times a day or cefuroxime axetil (Ceftin) 500 mg twice a day × 14 days

Complications
- Neuropathy (e.g., facial palsy), impaired memory
- Lyme arthritis, chronic fatigue

ERYSIPELAS
A subtype of cellulitis involving the upper dermis and superficial lymphatics that is usually caused by group A *Streptococcus*. For facial erysipelas, assume it is infected with MRSA and choose an antibiotic that is effective against MRSA.

Classic Case
Sudden onset of one large hot and indurated red skin lesion that has clear demarcated margins. It is usually located on the lower legs (the shins) but may involve the cheeks or ear (may see butterfly involvement of the face or Milian's ear sign; Figure 6.13). It is accompanied by fever, chills, severe malaise, and headache. May cause enlargement of regional lymph nodes. Hospitalization is recommended, since patient may be bacteremic.

FOLLICULITIS
Infection of hair follicle(s) with purulent material in the epidermis. May involve several follicles. Small (1-mm) round lesions filled with pus with erythema. Usually,

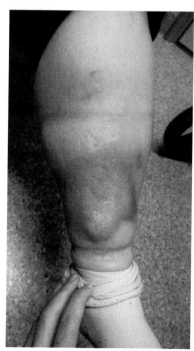

Figure 6.13 Erysipelas.
Source: Courtesy of Mikael Häggström, MD.

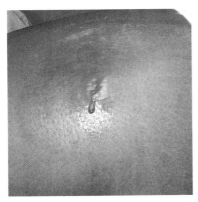

Figure 6.14 Furuncle or boil (caused by methicillin-resistant *Staphylococcus aureus*).
Source: Centers for Disease Control and Prevention.

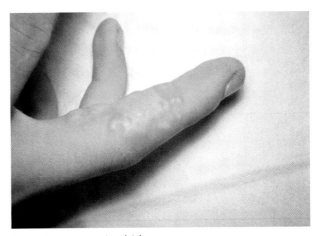

Figure 6.15 Herpetic whitlow.
Source: Courtesy of James Heilman, MD.

self-limiting. Avoid shaving or scrubbing area. Consider mupirocin (Bactroban) ointment or cream.

FURUNCLES (BOILS)

An infected hair follicle that fills with pus (abscess). May have started out as folliculitis that worsened. It looks like a round red bump and is hot and tender to the touch (Figure 6.14). When it is fluctuant, it can rupture and drain purulent green-colored discharge. Apply antibiotic ointment twice a day and cover with dressing until healed.

- For small boils, use warm compress twice a day. If abscess is >2 cm, incising and draining of abscess and/ or empiric antibiotic treatment may be adequate.
- If located over a joint, refer to ED for plain radiograph (x-ray) of joint to rule out osteomyelitis. Best imaging method is MRI to detect bone infection.

HERPETIC WHITLOW

Herpetic whitlow is a viral skin infection of the finger(s) caused by herpes simplex (type 1 or type 2) virus infection and results from direct contact with either a cold sore or genital herpes lesion.

Classic Case

Patient complains of an acute onset of extremely painful red bumps and small blisters on the sides of the finger, the cuticle area, or on the terminal phalanx of one or more fingers (Figure 6.15); may have recurrent outbreaks. Ask patient about coexisting symptoms of oral herpes or genital herpes.

Treatment Plan

These infections gradually heal over 2 to 3 weeks but can recur.

- Self-limited infection: Analgesics or NSAIDs for pain as needed
- Severe infections or immunocompetent patients: Treat with acyclovir (Zovirax)

Patient Education

- Avoid sharing personal items, gloves, and towels.
- Cover skin lesions completely with large adhesive bandage until they heal.

HIDRADENITIS SUPPURATIVA

Chronic and recurrent inflammatory disorder of the apocrine glands that results in painful nodules, abscesses, and pustules in locations such as the axilla (most common location), mammary area, perianal area, and groin (Figure 6.16). More common in women. Associated risk factors include genetics, smoking, and obesity. No cure. Classified by stages: Stage I disease (nodule, abscess formation without sinus tracts or scarring), Stage II (recurrent abscesses with skin tunnels and scarring), and Stage III (multiple interconnected tracts, abscesses, scarring, diffuse involvement).

Classic Case

Patient complains of recurrent episodes of painful, large, inflamed, dark-red nodules, abscesses, and pustules. Ruptured lesions drain purulent, malodorous discharge. Pain resolves when the abscess drains and heals. Lesions take from 10 to 30 days to heal. History of recurrent episodes on the same areas in the axilla results in sinus tracts, keloids, and multiple scars. Patient may be anxious and/or depressed. Persistent disease characterized by inflammatory plaques, epithelialized skin, end-stage "tombstone" comedones, and "rope-like" scarring.

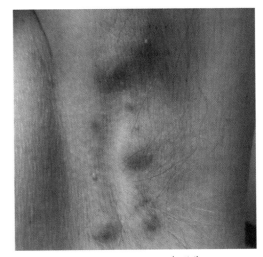

Figure 6.16 Hidradenitis suppurativa (mild).

Treatment Plan
- Warm compresses, topical and/or oral pain medication for pain
- Daily wound and skin care.
- Smoking cessation, weight loss if obesity.

Stage I disease:
- Initial therapy: Topical clindamycin
- Failure of initial therapy: Oral tetracycline 500 mg twice a day or minocycline twice a day for 7 to 10 days

Stage II to III disease:
- Initial therapy: Oral tetracycline for moderate inflammatory burden; combination therapy with clindamycin and rifampin for extensive disease
- Failure of initial therapy: Oral retinoids, dapsone, adalimumab, and infliximab
- For skin tunnels, recurrent nodules, and severe refractory disease: May require surgical excision as well as other medical therapies (e.g., biologic agents)

IMPETIGO

Acute contagious superficial bacterial infection often caused by gram-positive bacteria (beta *Streptococcus* or *Staphylococcus aureus*). Most common bacterial skin infection in young children ages 2 to 5 years. More common in hot and humid environments (summer, subtropics, tropics). It can appear on normal skin or skin breaks (scratches, insect bites, acne, varicella lesions). If infection is due to beta *Streptococcus* (*S. pyogenes*), postglomerular nephritis is a potential complication. Variants include: bullous, nonbullous (most common), and ecthyma.

Classic Case
Acute onset of itchy pink-to-red lesions, which evolve into vesiculopustules that rupture. Bullous impetigo appears as large blisters that rupture easily. After rupture, red, weeping, shallow ulcers appear. When serous fluid dries up, it looks like lesions covered with honey-colored crusts (see Table 6.1). Can present with a few (two to three) to multiple lesions.

Labs
C&S of crusts/wound.

Treatment Plan
- For limited lesions, topical mupirocin (three times daily) and topical retapamulin (twice daily).
- For numerous lesions, cephalexin (Keflex) four times a day, dicloxacillin four times a day × 10 days. If penicillin allergic, erythromycin 250 mg four times per day or clindamycin.
- Clean lesions with antibacterial soap, Betadine, or chlorhexidine (Hibiclens), then apply topical antibacterial to lesions.
- For infection prevention, shower/bathe daily with antibacterial soap until healed. Do not share towels. Handwashing to reduce spread.
- For children in day care, do not return to school until 48 to 72 hours after initiation of treatment.

MENINGOCOCCEMIA

A serious life-threatening bloodstream infection caused by *N. meningitidis* (gram-negative diplococci) that are spread by respiratory droplets. Bacterial meningitis is a medical emergency. Mortality rate of 10% to 15%. Use droplet precautions. Do not delay treatment if high index of suspicion—refer to ED *stat*.

Classic Case
Described in "Danger Signals" section.

Prophylaxis
- Indicated for close contacts as early as possible (ideally less than 24 hours and no greater than 14 days after exposure)
- Regimens for antimicrobial prophylaxis include rifampin 5 mg/kg/dose every 12 hours, ciprofloxacin, and ceftriaxone
- Close contacts are defined as being in close proximity to patient (<3 feet) who has had prolonged contact (>8 hours) or directly exposed to patient's oral secretions, going back to 7 days before onset of patient's symptoms until 24 hours after initiation of antibiotic
- Meningococcal vaccination as follows:
  - The CDC recommends that all 11- and 12-year-old adolescents receive a meningococcal conjugate vaccine (MenACWY) with a booster dose at 16 years.
  - A serogroup B meningococcal vaccine (MenB) is recommended for adolescents and young adults (16 through 23 years old) who have a complement component deficiency, functional or anatomic asplenia, or complement inhibitor. MenB vaccines are not approved for use in people under 10 years old.
  - Younger children (down to 2 months old) and adults should receive MenACWY vaccines (or MenB vaccine if older than 10 years old) if they are at increased risk for meningococcal disease. such as freshman college students living in dormitories, military recruits, persons with asplenia or a nonfunctioning spleen (e.g., sickle cell), patients on eculizumab (Soliris), or others.

Labs
- Lumbar punctures—culture cerebrospinal fluid (CSF)
- Blood cultures, throat cultures, and the like (do not delay treatment to wait for lab results)
- CT scan or MRI of the brain

Treatment Plan
- Ceftriaxone (Rocephin) 2 g IV every 12 hours
- Hospital admission, isolation precautions, supportive treatment

Complications
- Tissue infarction and necrosis (e.g., gangrene of the toes, foot, fingers) causing amputation
- Death

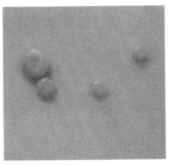 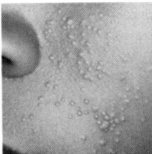 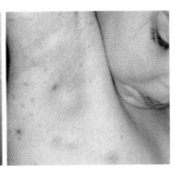

Figure 6.17 Molluscum contagiosum.
Source: Centers for Disease Control and Prevention.

MOLLUSCUM CONTAGIOSUM

Dome-shaped papules (2- to 5-mm diameter) with central umbilication (white plug; Figure 6.17). Caused by skin infection with the poxvirus. Spread by skin-to-skin direct contact. More common in children. In immunocompetent host, it usually clears up in 6 to 12 months. Considered a sexually transmitted infection (STI) if lesions are located on the genitals in sexually active adolescents and adults.

NECROTIZING FASCIITIS ("FLESH-EATING" BACTERIA)

Reddish to purple-colored lesion that increases rapidly in size. May have bullae. Infected area appears indurated ("woody" induration) with complaints of severe pain on affected site. Refer to ED.

PARONYCHIA

Acute local bacterial skin infection of the proximal or lateral nail folds (cuticle) that resolves after the abscess drains. Often, causative bacteria are *S. aureus*, *S. pyogenes*, or *P. aeruginosa* (gram negative). Chronic cases are associated with coexisting onychomycosis (fungal infection of nails; Figure 6.18).

Classic Case

Patient complains of acute onset of a painful and red swollen area around the nail on a finger; a superficial abscess is often present. The most common locations are index finger and thumb. Reports a history of picking a hangnail, biting off hangnail, or trimming of the cuticle during a manicure.

Treatment Plan

- Without abscess, soak affected finger or toe in warm water for 20 minutes three times a day.
- Apply topical antibiotic, such as triple antibiotic or mupirocin, to the affected finger after soaking.
- With abscess, incision and drainage (use no. 11 surgical blade), or use the beveled edge of a large-gauge needle to gently separate the cuticle margin from the nail bed to drain the abscess.

PITYRIASIS ROSEA

Self-limiting illness (6–8 weeks). This skin condition may be caused by a viral infection.

Classic Case

Patient complains of oval lesions with fine scales that follow skin lines (cleavage lines) of the trunk or a "Christmas tree" pattern (see Table 6.1). Salmon-pink color in White people. May be pruritic. A "herald patch" is the first lesion to appear and is largest in size; appears 2 weeks before full breakout. It is a single round-to-oval shape and about 2 to 5 cm in diameter (Figure 6.19).

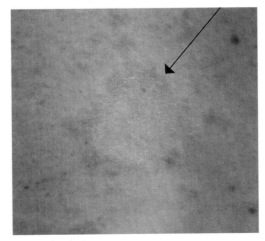

Figure 6.19 Pityriasis rosea.
Source: Courtesy of James Heilman, MD.

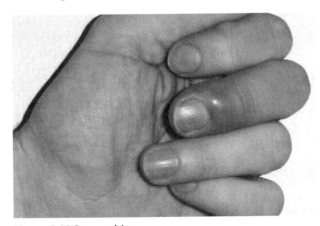

Figure 6.18 Paronychia.

Treatment Plan

- Most patients do not require treatment. Advise patient that lesions will take about 4 weeks to resolve. Mild itching can be treated with medium-potency topical corticosteroids.
- If high risk of STI, check rapid plasma reagent (RPR) to rule out secondary syphilis.

PSORIASIS

Inherited skin disorder in which squamous epithelial cells undergo rapid mitotic division and abnormal maturation. The rapid turnover of skin produces the classic psoriatic plaque (Figure 6.20). There are several phenotypes, such as plaque, guttate, erythrodermic, and pustular psoriasis. Patients with psoriasis are at risk for psoriatic arthritis, an inflammatory musculoskeletal disease.

Special Findings

- Koebner phenomenon: New psoriatic plaques form over areas of skin trauma
- Auspitz sign: Pinpoint areas of bleeding in the skin when scales from a psoriatic plaque are removed

Classic Case

Patient complains of pruritic erythematous plaques covered with fine silvery-white scales along with pitted fingernails and toenails. The plaques are distributed in the scalp, elbows, knees, sacrum, and intergluteal folds. Partially resolving plaques are pink-colored with minimal scaling. Patient with psoriatic arthritis will complain of painful red, warm, and swollen joints (migratory arthritis) in addition to the skin plaques.

Treatment

- Limited disease: Topical steroids and emollients; alternatives include topical retinoids (tazarotene), tar preparations (psoralen drug class), topical vitamin D, and anthralin; localized phototherapy
- Severe disease: Phototherapy, systemic agents such as methotrexate, cyclosporine, and biologics agents such as TNF-alpha inhibitors (etanercept, adalimumab)

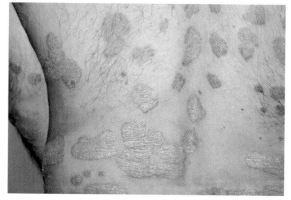

Figure 6.20 Psoriasis.
Source: Gawlik, K. S., Melnyk, B. M., & Teall, A. M. (2021). (See Resources section for complete source information.)

Boxed Warnings

- Topical tacrolimus: Rare cases of malignancy (including skin and lymphoma), use sunblock, avoid if patient is immunocompromised
- Biologics/antitumor necrosis factor agents: Humira, Enbrel, and Remicade are associated with higher risk of serious/fatal infections, malignancy, tuberculosis (TB), fungal infections, and sepsis (baseline purified protein derivative [PPD], CBC with differential)

Complications

- Guttate psoriasis (drop-shaped lesions): Form of psoriasis often resulting from a beta-hemolytic *Streptococcus* group A infection (usually due to "strep" throat)
- Pustular psoriasis: Can be associated with life-threatening complications (e.g., renal, hepatic, or respiratory abnormalities and sepsis)

EXAM TIPS

- An example of an antimetabolite or disease-modifying antirheumatic drug (DMARD) is methotrexate.
- Know diagnosis and treatment of hidradenitis suppurativa.

ROCKY MOUNTAIN SPOTTED FEVER

Caused by the bite of a dog tick (wood tick) that is infected with the parasite *Rickettsia rickettsii*. If high index of suspicion, do not delay treatment (do not wait for lab results). Treatment most effective if started within first 5 days of symptoms. Doxycycline is the first-line treatment for all age groups. Check if resident of the southeastern or south-central states (North Carolina, Tennessee, Oklahoma, Arkansas, and Missouri) or visitor to or vacationer in these states. Early diagnosis and treatment with doxycycline are critical to survival. RMSF is a reportable disease.

Classic Case

Described in "Danger Signals" section. RMSF can be difficult to diagnose due to nonspecific signs and symptoms in early stages of the infection, and, initially, diagnosis is based on signs and symptoms. Always take a thorough history and include important areas such as travel history (especially from areas where RMSF is endemic) and exposure factors (brushy or woody areas with high grasses and leaf litter). Ask about exposure to dogs.

Labs

- Early diagnosis is based on clinical suspicion and requires prompt empiric therapy as soon as the diagnosis is suspected.
- Definitive diagnosis is based on antibody titers to *R. rickettsii* (by indirect fluorescent IgG antibodies or IFA assay).
- IgG IFA assays on paired acute and convalescent serum samples collected 2 to 4 weeks apart to demonstrate evidence of a four-fold seroconversion. RMSF cannot be confirmed using a single acute antibody result. Antibodies to *R. ricketsii* might remain elevated for many months after disease has resolved.

Red spot–like rashes that start on the hands/palms and feet/soles accompanied by fever, headache, and myalgia suggest RMSF.

Treatment Plan
- Presumptive treatment with doxycycline is recommended in patients of all ages, including children <8 years of age. Children ≤45 kg are dosed by weight.
- The decision of initiating antibiotic therapy for RMSF should be based on signs and symptoms along with a careful patient history (exposure in brushy, woody areas with high grasses and leaf litter, endemic areas). Laboratory testing can be done later.
- First-line treatment (adults and children) is doxycycline 100 mg orally or 200 mg IV every 12 hours × 72 hours. The American Academy of Pediatrics (AAP) states that doxycycline can be given for RMSF for short durations (<21 days) regardless of age.

Complications
- Death
- Neurologic sequelae (e.g., hearing loss, paraparesis, neuropathy)

NOTES
How to remove a tick:
1. Use fine-tipped tweezers to grasp the part of the tick closest to the skin.
2. Pull it upward with steady, even pressure. Do not twist or jerk (Figure 6.21).
3. After removing the tick, clean bite area with rubbing alcohol, iodine scrub, or soap and water. Dispose of the tick by flushing it into toilet. Do not crush the tick with bare fingers.

   Not effective: Painting the tick with nail polish or petroleum jelly or using heat to make the tick detach. The goal is to detach the tick as quickly as possible after it is found.

- Doxycycline is the drug of choice for RMSF and all other tickborne rickettsial diseases for both children and adults.
- *Never* delay or withhold treatment based on the laboratory test results, even if initially negative result. Antibody titers are frequently negative in the early phase of the infection.
- Tick bites are often painless; do not rule out RMSF even if patient does not remember a tick bite, especially if history of being in areas that are woody or brushy with leaf litter and high grasses.

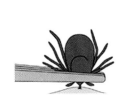
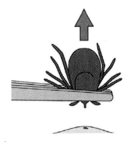

Figure 6.21 Proper tick removal.
Source: Centers for Disease Control and Prevention.

ROSACEA (ACNE ROSACEA)
Chronic and relapsing inflammatory skin disorder that is more common in people with light-colored skin. There are four subtypes of rosacea: erythematotelangiectatic, papulopustular, phymatous, and ocular. First-line management is aimed at symptom control and avoidance of triggers that cause exacerbations (e.g., spicy foods, alcohol, sunlight). Patients with rosacea have sensitive skin; advise to avoid irritating skin products (toners, alpha hydroxyl acids, strong soaps) and apply skin moisturizer frequently.

Classic Case
Light-skinned adult to older patient with Celtic background (i.e., Irish, Scottish, English) complains of chronic and small acne-like papules and pustules around the nose, mouth, and chin. Telangiectasias may be present on the nasal area and cheeks. Patient blushes easily. Patient usually is blond or red-haired and has light-colored eyes. Some have ocular symptoms such as red eyes, "dry eyes," or chronic blepharitis (ocular rosacea).

Treatment Plan
Sensitive skin, avoid scrubbing, strong soaps, cosmetic products that irritate the skin.

Medications
- Mild to moderate disease: Topical metronidazole (Metrogel), azelaic acid (Azelex), or ivermectin.
- Moderate to severe disease: Oral tetracycline or minocycline for 4 to 12 weeks. Alternative antibiotics are clarithromycin with doxycycline for inflammatory lesions.

Complications
- Rhinophyma: Hyperplasia of tissue at the tip of the nose from chronic severe disease
- Ocular rosacea: Blepharitis, conjunctival injection, lid margin telangiectasia

SCABIES
Infestation of the skin by the *Sarcoptes scabiei* mite. The female mite burrows under the skin to lay her eggs; transmitted by close contact. May be asymptomatic the first 4 to 8 weeks after infestation. Even after treatment, the pruritus may persist for 2 to 4 weeks (sensitivity reaction to mites and their feces). Higher incidence in crowded conditions (e.g., nursing homes) and in the homeless.

- Classic scabies: Most common; associated with relatively low mite burden.
- Crusted scabies (also known as Norwegian scabies): A severe form of scabies that affects the elderly and immunocompromised; associated with much higher mite burden. Lesions are covered with fine scales (looks like white plaques) and crusts; involves the nails (dystrophic nails), scalp, body; absent-to-mild pruritus; very contagious. Itching may be absent.

Classic Case

Patient complains of pruritic rashes located in the interdigital webs of the hands, axillae, breasts, buttock folds, waist, scrotum, and penis. Severe itching that is worse at nighttime and interferes with sleep (see Table 6.1). Other family members may also have the same symptoms.

Objective Findings

The rash appears as serpiginous (snakelike) or linear burrows. Lesions can be papular, vesicular, or crusted (Figure 6.22).

Labs

Scrape burrow or scales with glass slide; use coverslip (wet mount). Look for mites or eggs.

Treatment Plan

- Permethrin 5% (Elimite): Apply cream from the neck to the sole of the feet after bathing or showering. Wash off after 8 to 14 hours. Repeat treatment in 7 days. Permethrin can be applied to the scalp and face (sparing the eyes and mouth) in infants and young children.
- Crusted scabies: Combination treatment with permethrin and ivermectin.
- Persons in the same household: Treat everyone at the same time. Any clothes/bedding used 3 days before and during treatment should be washed and dried using the hot settings. Another option is to place the items in a plastic bag that is sealed for at least 72 hours.
- Pruritus: Usually improves in 48 hours but can last up to 2 to 4 weeks (even if mites are dead). Can treat itching with Benadryl and topical steroids.

Figure 6.22 Scabies.
Source: Centers for Disease Control and Prevention/Joe Miller.

- Long-term care facility: Treat all patients, staff, family members, and frequent visitors for scabies.

SUPERFICIAL CANDIDIASIS

Superficial skin infection from the yeast *Candida albicans*. Environmental factors that promote overgrowth include increased warmth and humidity, friction, obesity, diabetes, and decreased immunity. It can infect skin and mucous membranes (thrush, vaginitis) or can be a systemic infection. Intertrigo/intertriginous areas of the body (or apposed areas of skin that rub together) can be infected by fungal (candidal intertrigo) and/or bacterial organisms.

Classic Case
External (Skin)

Adult with obesity complains of bright-red and shiny lesions that itch or burn, located on the intertriginous areas (under the breast in females, axillae, abdomen, groin, the web spaces between the toes). The rash may have satellite lesions (small red rashes around the main rash).

Oropharyngeal Candidiasis (Thrush)

Patient complains of a severe sore throat with white adherent plaques with a red base that are hard to dislodge on the pharynx. Thrush in "healthy adults" who are not on antibiotics may signal an immunodeficient condition.

Treatment Plan

- For skin infections, nystatin powder and/or cream in skin folds (intertriginous areas) twice a day. OTC topical antifungals include miconazole and clotrimazole. Prescription required for terconazole and ciclopirox.
- Keep skin dry and aerated.
- For mild thrush, administer clotrimazole troches (one troche dissolved in mouth slowly five times/day) or miconazole mucoadhesive buccal tablets.
- Another option is nystatin (Mycostatin) oral suspension for oral thrush (swish and swallow) four times a day.
- For moderate-to-severe thrush (or recurrent disease), oral fluconazole is the preferred systemic antifungal agent.

TINEA VERSICOLOR

Superficial skin infection caused by yeasts *Pityrosporum orbiculare* or *P. ovale*.

Classic Case

Patient complains of multiple hypopigmented round macules on the chest, shoulders, and/or back that "appear" after skin becomes tan from sun exposure. The condition is asymptomatic (Figure 6.23).

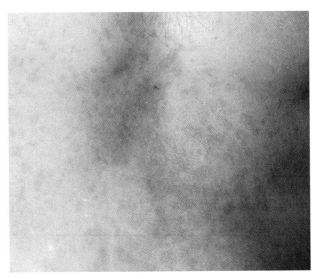

Figure 6.23 Tinea versicolor.
Source: Centers for Disease Control and Prevention/Lucille K. George, MD.

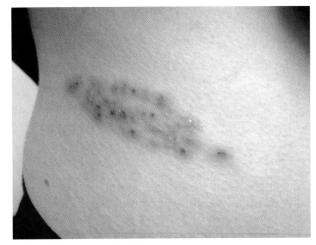

Figure 6.24 Shingles.

Labs
KOH slide: Hyphae and spores.

Medications
Topical selenium sulfide and topical azole antifungals such as ketoconazole (Nizoral) and terbinafine (Lamisil) cream twice a day × 2 weeks. Advise patients that hypopigmented spots will not spontaneously disappear after treatment (may take several months for pigment to fill in).

VARICELLA-ZOSTER VIRUS INFECTIONS
Chickenpox (varicella) and herpes zoster (shingles) are both caused by the varicella-zoster virus (VZV). The primary infection is called *chickenpox* (varicella), and the reactivation of the infection is known as *shingles* (herpes zoster). After primary infection (chickenpox), the virus becomes latent within a dermatome (sensory ganglia) and is kept under control by an intact immune system.
- Chickenpox: Contagious 1 to 2 days before the onset of the rash until all of the lesions have crusted over (chickenpox and shingles). Duration of illness is 2 weeks.
- Shingles: Contagious with the onset of the rashes until all the lesions have crusted over.

Classic Cases
Chickenpox/Varicella
Prodrome of fever, pharyngitis, and malaise that is followed within 24 hours by the eruption of pruritic vesicular lesions in different stages of development over a period of 4 days. The rash starts on the head and face and quickly spreads to the trunk and extremities. It takes 1 to 2 weeks for the crusts to fall off and the skin to heal.

Shingles
Elderly or older adults report acute onset of groups of papules and vesicles on a red base that rupture and become crusted. Crusted lesions follow a dermatomal pattern on one side of the body. Patients complain of pain, which can be quite severe. Some with prodrome may have severe pain/burning sensation at the site before the breakout. Shingles can last 2 to 4 weeks, but when the lesions crust by 7 to 10 days, they are no longer considered infectious. Immunocompromised and elderly patients are at higher risk for postherpetic neuralgia (PHN). Early treatment reduces risk. Treat within 48 to 72 hours after onset of breakout if patient is older than age 50 or immunocompromised. Completely cover lesions until dry and crusted (Figure 6.24).

Labs
Signs and symptoms of herpes zoster infection are usually distinctive enough to make an accurate clinical diagnosis once the rash has appeared. In atypical cases or if suspect disseminated herpes zoster (lesions that are seen outside the primary dermatomes), lab testing is helpful. The most sensitive test for VZV is polymerase chain reaction (PCR).

Medications
- Varicella: Antiviral therapy (e.g., valacyclovir) is recommended for immunocompetent individuals and pregnant patients due to the increased risk of complications.
- Uncomplicated herpes zoster: Acyclovir (Zovirax) 800 mg five times per day or valacyclovir (Valtrex) 1000 mg three times a day × 7 days. Most effective when started 48 to 72 hours after the appearance of the rash.

Complications
- PHN: More common in elderly and immunocompromised patients. Treat PHN with tricyclic antidepressants (TCAs; e.g., low-dose amitriptyline), anticonvulsants (e.g., Depakote), or gabapentin three times a day. Apply lidocaine 5% patch (Lidoderm) to intact skin.
- Herpes zoster ophthalmicus (CN V): Can result in corneal blindness. Refer immediately to ophthalmologist or ED (described in "Danger Signals" section).

- Others: If Ramsay Hunt syndrome (herpes zoster oticus) triad of ipsilateral facial paralysis, ear pain, and vesicles in the ear canal and auricle, refer to neurologist.

Vaccines

- Varicella vaccine: The CDC recommends two doses of varicella vaccine for children, adolescents, and adults. Children should receive the first dose at 12 through 15 months and the second dose at age 4 through 6 years old. Adolescents and adults should receive two doses 4 to 8 weeks apart. Contraindications include hstory of bone marrow malignancy, primary or acquired immunodeficiency, receiving high-dose immunosuppressive therapy, moderate or severe concurrent illness, or may be pregnant. Check the CDC guidelines for a full list of contraindications.
- Shingrix vaccine (recombinant zoster vaccine): Two doses are recommended for immunocompetent adults aged 50 years or older whether or not they have a history of herpes zoster or received a prior dose of Zostavax (no longer available in the United States). Contraindications include history of allergic reaction to any component of the vaccine and person with an acute episode. Recommend delay vaccine during pregnancy.

WOUNDS

A wound is a disruption or damage to the skin. There are four phases involved in wound healing (Table 6.4). Some of the factors that impair the wound-healing process are older/mature age, poor nutrition, impaired immune system, impaired mobility, stress (affects immune system), diabetes, certain medicines (drugs that impair clot formation, steroids), pressure loading, cigarette smoking, and secondary bacterial infection.

Types of Wound Closure

- Primary closure: Wounds caused by clean, sharp objects may undergo primary closure up to 12 to 18 hours from time of injury. Wound can be closed by suturing

Table 6.4 Phases of Wound Healing

Phase	Healing Event
Hemostasis	Constriction of local blood vessels, platelet aggregation, fibrin (clot) formation
Inflammation	Macrophages and lymphocytes proliferate, presence of inflammatory mediators such as cytokines and leukotrienes
Proliferation	Proliferation of basal and epithelial cells (angiogenesis)
Remodeling	Remodeling of collagen, scar formation (cicatrix)

or applying tissue glue or butterfly strips (so that edges of wounds are well approximated). Causes the least amount of scarring.

- Secondary intention: Wound is left open with formation of granulation tissue and scarring. Wound heals from the bottom of the wound up. Wound edges are not well approximated. Causes more scarring than primary closure.
- Tertiary intention (delayed primary closure): Wounds with heavy contamination or poor vascularity (crush injuries) are best left open to heal by secondary intention (granulation) and wound contraction. Then the wound edges are approximated in 3 to 4 days. Produces the most scar tissue.

High-Risk Wounds That May Warrant Referral

- Infected wounds (pus is present, wound that is not healing, devitalized tissue, wound becomes hot and swollen)
- Closed-fist injuries; refer to ED or urgent care clinic, especially if joint is involved (septic joint)
- Facial wounds with risk of cosmetic damage (e.g., large wound, bites, cartilage injury)
- Suspected foreign body or embedded object in wound that cannot be removed
- Injury to a joint capsule; if joint capsule penetrated, joint can become infected
- Electrical injuries
- Paint-gun or high-pressure wounds
- Chemical wounds (especially alkali-related damage) of the eyes or skin
- Suspected physical or child abuse
- Wounds with cosmetic concerns (cartilage wounds in the ears, nose); cartilage does not heal; refer to plastic surgeon or ED

Infected Wounds

- Do not suture infected wounds (open >24 hours).
- Absolute contraindication to wound closure is presence of cellulitis or abscess (e.g., redness, warmth, swelling, and pain with or without pus drainage).

Clenched-Fist Injuries

Clenched-fist injuries have a high risk of infection to joints (e.g., knuckles), fascia, nerves, and bones (osteomyelitis; especially if punched in the mouth or bitten by a human).

Test distal pulses, skin color, range of motion (ROM), tendon damage, nerve damage, and fracture. Obtain x-ray of the hand to rule out foreign body (i.e., teeth) and fracture. Sometimes, ultrasound is used to view foreign bodies that do not show up on x-rays.

Retained Foreign Bodies
- There is higher risk of infection. If unable to remove or located in a high-risk area, refer to ED.
- Plain x-ray is first-line imaging test. Ultrasound or soft-tissue x-rays are routine if suspected object or object does not show on x-rays (radiolucent).
- Small glass splinters or particles, wood splinters, thorns, fish bones, and plastics may not be visible on x-rays.

Minor Burn (Superficial and Partial Thickness)
1. Wash area with water and mild soap.
2. Using sterile tongue blade, apply thin layer of 1% silver sulfadiazine (Silvadene) topical antibiotic to burned area.
3. Cover burned area with nonstick gauze (e.g., Telfa). Secure with stretch-conforming gauze (e.g., Kerlix).
4. Apply Silvadene antimicrobial cream once to twice a day until the burn is healed. After skin is healed, consider using topical zinc oxide daily for 1 to 2 weeks to protect area from sunlight. Do not expose recently healed burned skin to sunlight (causes hyperpigmentation).
5. See Burns section for additional details.

Wound Care
1. During history, ask about mechanism of injury and other details about the incident.
2. Check for allergy to iodine, rubber, latex, or lidocaine. If patient has rubber or latex allergy, do not use latex gloves. Use silicone-based disposable gloves.
3. Do not forget tetanus prophylaxis. If last dose was >5 years ago, give Tdap booster.
4. Irrigate wound with normal saline and/or wash area with mild soap and water. Remove dirt.
5. Assess wound for neurovascular and tendon damage. Check distal pulses. Check ROM. Check sensation (sharp and dull). Depending on injury, rule out foreign body.
6. Specific treatment depends on the type of wound and patient characteristics.

Referral of Wounds
- Closed-fist injuries or crush injuries: Refer to hand surgeon.
- Cartilage damage or wounds with cosmetic effects: Refer to plastic surgeon.
- Compromised hosts: Consider diabetes, absent/dysfunctional spleen, and immunocompromise.

PRIMARY CARE PRACTICE: COMMON PROCEDURES

Informed consent should be obtained (verbal or written) prior to performing any procedure. Discuss the benefits and risks of the procedure, including bleeding risk, infection, scarring, depigmentation, damage to underlying structures (e.g., blood vessels, nerves), recurrence, or incomplete treatment of the lesion.

LOCAL ANESTHESIA
- Common types of anesthetics: Lidocaine 1% (plain or mixed with epinephrine), bupivacaine, mepivacaine, and procaine. Lidocaine is the most commonly used anesthetic for local infiltration.
- Drug: Lidocaine 1% (plain) onset of action is 2 to 5 minutes. Duration of action is 30 minutes to 2 hours. Advise patient that they will feel a burning sensation at the start of the injection; this will disappear.
- Contraindications: Do not administer if the amount of anesthetic needed to provide adequate analgesia exceeds the maximal safe total dose and/or the patient has had generalized urticaria or anaphylaxis with previous administration of local anesthesia.
- Adverse complications: Complications may arise if patient has an allergic reaction or infection, solution is injected directly into blood vessel, or there is injury to nerves and tendons in the area.
- Examples of anesthesia use: Use anesthesia for wounds that need suturing, incisions (e.g., embedded splinter or paronychia), abscess drainage, foreign body removal form the skin, and biopsy.

Direct Infiltration
1. Clean the lead with povidone-iodine or chlorhexidine solution and allow it to dry.
2. For open wounds, put a few drops of anesthetic into the wound and then place the needle into the subcutaneous layer by inserting through the wound margin.
3. Slowly infiltrate the edges of the wound, then withdraw slightly to move it to another area. The amount of lidocaine that is used varies based on the size of the wound and the location.
4. For intact skin, place the needle through the skin into the subcutaneous layer.
5. Slowly inject small volumes. Aspiration is not necessary prior to each infiltration unless the area is close to major blood vessels.
6. After a few minutes, lightly test the skin to ensure adequate anesthesia.

Digital Nerve Block: Finger Web Space Block
1. Clean web space on each side of the involved finger with alcohol, povidone iodine, or chlorhexidine solution and allow to dry.
2. Draw up about 3 mL of plain lidocaine 1% from vial using a 5- to 10-mL syringe with an 18-gauge needle. Then change needle to smaller gauge (25- to 30-gauge, 1½ inches).
3. Place needle in perpendicular position above web space and insert into subcutaneous tissue space.
4. Slowly retract the plunger to avoid injecting into one of the digital blood vessels. Inject slowly and use small amounts to infiltrate the tissues surrounding the dorsal nerve.

5. Slowly, advance the needle straight through the web space toward the palmar surface. Inject while advancing the needle, a total of about 1 to 1.5 mL of anesthetic.

6. Instruct patient that it may take 5 to 10 minutes for the anesthesia to become effective. Ask patient if area is numb (test by using tip of needle to test sensation) before suturing.

SUTURING

General Rules

- Do not suture puncture wounds or human or animal bites.
- Do not suture heavily contaminated wounds.
- Lacerations >12 hours old are at higher risk for infection. Do not suture infected wounds.
- Do not suture wounds that have been open >24 hours (high bacterial load).

Types of Sutures and Needles

For example, skin laceration:

- Use nonabsorbable synthetic suture (i.e., nylon, Prolene).
- Preferred needle type to suture skin is a curved cutting needle.
- Suture size; the United States Pharmacopeia (USP) classifies suture by diameter size with decreasing diameters correlated to decreasing USP sizes. Suture sizes smaller than 0 are denoted with increasing numbers of zeros. The more zeros (e.g., 5–0 is equal to 00000), the smaller the diameter. Suture sizes range from 1.0 to 12–0; the smallest diameter suture used in human surgery is 11–0 (about the size of human hair) and is used to repair small blood vessels. The preferred suture size for a skin laceration repair is 3–0 to 5–0.

Suture Placement

1. Evert the edges of the wound by inserting needle at 90-degree angle (ensures that wound edges are well approximated).
2. Use needle holder to hold needle. Use forceps to grab wound edges.
3. Usually, simple sutures are used on skin lacerations. Each suture is individually tied, then cut (simple interrupted sutures).
4. When cutting suture thread, do not cut too short. Leave a short tail (easier to remove).
5. Nonabsorbable synthetic sutures are preferred for lacerations/wounds of the skin.
6. Use staples on scalp lacerations.

Suture Removal

Suture removal depends on the anatomic site; see guidelines that follow. Sutures that are left beyond 10 days may develop scars that resemble a "railroad track." Clean and prep the area. Use forceps and lift suture from the skin. Cut suture with scissors. Use forceps to grasp the knot and pull the suture gently out of the wound.

- Face, neck: 5 days
- Scalp: 7 to 10 days
- Trunk and upper extremities: 7 days
- Lower extremities: 8 to 10 days
- Digits, palm, and sole: 10 to 14 days

> **NOTE**
>
> Do not suture deep puncture wounds, animal bites (except if cosmetic area like the face), or actively bleeding wounds (will form a subcutaneous hematoma). Control bleeding first, especially arterial bleeds.

SKIN BIOPSY

Punch Biopsy

- Check for history of bleeding disorder and use of drugs that affect bleeding time (aspirin, warfarin). Patients with international normalized ratio (INR) >2.5 should not be biopsied. Check scar history (e.g., history of keloids or hypertrophic scarring).
- Refer to dermatologist for facial biopsies, biopsy of areas with cartilage, suspected melanoma, history of keloid/hypertrophic scarring.
- Ask whether patient is allergic to lidocaine or rubber/latex (use silicone gloves).

Procedure

1. "Prep" skin site with alcohol, chlorhexidine, or another cleaning agent and allow to dry.
2. Using a syringe, draw lidocaine 1% and epinephrine 1:100).
3. Inject slowly under the epidermis until a small bleb is formed. The color of the skin over the bleb area becomes paler due to the vasoconstricting effect of epinephrine.
4. Check site for numbness by using the point of the syringe and testing sensation on the bleb area. The skin will become numb within 5 to 10 minutes (lasts about 30–120 minutes).
5. Using a 3-mm skin punch, position instrument at 90 degrees (perpendicular to the skin).
6. Twist the punch instrument gently using a "drilling" motion until it has pierced the epidermis (there should be about ½ inch of the blade visible on top of the skin).
7. Remove from skin and lift plug gently with forceps (do not crush). Use a scalpel to cut the plug at the base. Immediately place it on the biopsy specimen container. Do not forget to label the specimen cup with the patient's name, location of the biopsy site, and the type of tissue obtained.
8. Cover area with sterile 2 × 2 gauze held with tape (if bleeding) or with adhesive bandage if minimal bleeding. Instruct patient to change bandage once a day.
9. Instruct patients to keep the site dry. Instruct to avoid submerging site in water (avoid tub baths, swimming, hot tubs) until it is healed. Site will scab within a few days.

CRYOTHERAPY (CRYOSURGERY)

- Cryotherapy causes ice crystals to form inside the cells and destroys them. It rarely requires anesthesia. There are several methods that can be used such as open spray, dipstick, contact, and the tweezer technique.
- The expected outcome is blistering of the treated area with the first 12 to 24 hours and crusting. The blistered skin will be shed, and a shallow ulcer will be left, which will heal within a few days.

Contraindications

- Area has impaired circulation and/or neuropathy, open wounds, cold hypersensitivity (Raynaud phenomenon, cold urticaria, cryobulinemia, and paroxysmal cold hemoglobinuria), angina, or severe cardiac disease.
- Certain locations should be avoided, such as the eye area, vermilion border of the lip, the nail matrix, and areas with cartilage. An adverse effect is hypopigmentation, although darker skinned individuals can develop hyperpigmentation. Other effects are scarring, alopecia, and tissue distortion.

EXAM TIPS

- Be familiar with psoriasis and Koebner phenomenon, RMSF, meningococcemia, erythema migrans (Lyme disease), contact dermatitis, and rosacea.
- The American Academy of Nurse Practitioners Certification Board (AANPCB) exam is all multiple-choice with one answer for each question. The American Nurses Credentialing Center (ANCC) exam has more variety in the questions, with some having one correct answer, some having a "select all that apply" approach, and others featuring images (think of an EKG strip or pictures of a region of the body).

NOTE

The procedure descriptions provided in this chapter are designed for review purposes only. They are not intended for use in clinical practice.

KNOWLEDGE CHECK: CHAPTER 6

1. In which of the following patients is the Shingrix vaccine indicated?
   A. A 60-year-old patient experiencing an acute episode of herpes zoster
   B. A 35-year-old immunocompetent patient who is pregnant
   C. A 55-year-old patient with a history of liver transplant 8 months ago who is on maintenance immunosuppressant medications
   D. A 45-year-old patient with no past medical history who is also receiving a COVID-19 vaccine

2. A patient with hidradenitis suppurativa presents with inflammatory lesions and multiple abscess formations without skin tunnels or scarring. This would be classified as which stage of the disease?
   A. II
   B. III
   C. I
   D. More information necessary to determine stage

3. Based on the stage identified in the previous question, initial therapy for this patient includes which of the following?
   A. Doxycycline
   B. Topical clindamycin
   C. Metformin
   D. Spironolactone

4. Which of the following phases of wound healing is characterized by fibroblasts that accumulate and build upon fibrin matrix to produce wound contraction and scar formation and produce essential elements such as collagen?
   A. Hemostasis
   B. Inflammation
   C. Proliferation
   D. Remodeling

5. A patient presents with a severe sunburn to their chest. The skin is intact, and the site is dry and red and blanches with pressure. In general, first-line treatment for this type of burn includes which of the following?
   A. Application of topical zinc oxide after the skin heals
   B. Cleansing of the wound with povidone-iodine and then covering it with a dressing
   C. Cleansing of the wound with mild soap and room-temperature water
   D. Application of a topical antimicrobial agent

6. In the "ABCDE" screening for melanoma, E stands for:
   A. Edema
   B. Enlargement
   C. Effusion
   D. Erythema

7. Which of the following is a reportable disease?
   A. Molluscum contagiosum
   B. Rocky Mountain spotted fever
   C. Scarlet fever
   D. Scabies

8. A high school student who is on the wrestling team complains of multiple bumps on the lower left arm. The patient denies pruritus, pain, or discomfort from the lesions. During the skin exam, the nurse practitioner notices multiple smooth-domed papules that are 2 to 5 mm in diameter with central umbilication. Which diagnosis is *most* likely?
   A. Molluscum contagiosum
   B. Acne vulgaris
   C. Verruca vulgaris
   D. Basal cell carcinoma

(See answe

1. C) A 55-year-old patient with a history of liver transplant 8 months ago who is on maintenance immunosuppressant medications

According to the Centers for Disease Control and Prevention (CDC), the Shingrix vaccine (recombinant zoster vaccine) is recommended for immunocompetent adults age 50 years or older whether or not they have a history of herpes zoster or have received a prior dose of Zostavax (no longer available in the United States). For solid organ transplant recipients, administer the vaccine at least 6 to 12 months after transplantation when there is evidence of stable graft function and the patient is on maintenance immunosuppression. The vaccine is contraindicated in patients with a history of severe allergic reaction to any component of the vaccine and those who are experiencing an acute episode of herpes zoster. Providers should delay vaccination until after pregnancy. Shingrix can be administered concomitantly with other adult vaccines (at different anatomic sites) but is not recommended for patients younger than 50 years.

2. C) I

A clinical staging system is used to classify patients with hidradenitis suppurativa. Stage I disease involves abscess formation without sinus tracts or scarring; Stage II is defined by recurrent abscesses with skin tunnels and scarring; and Stage III is characterized by multiple interconnected tracts, abscesses, and scarring, with diffuse involvement across an entire area.

3. B) Topical clindamycin

Patients with Stage I disease (inflammatory lesions without skin tunnels or scarring) should be started on topical clindamycin as the initial medical treatment. If initial therapy fails, oral tetracycline (e.g., doxycycline) can be prescribed. Alternative treatment options include anti-androgenic drugs (e.g., oral contraceptives and spironolactone) and metformin, which may be used alone or in combination with antibiotic therapy.

4. D) Remodeling

During remodeling, fibroblasts accumulate and build upon fibrin matrix to produce wound contraction and scar formation and produce essential elements such as collagen. Hemostasis involves constriction of local blood vessels, platelet aggregation, and fibrin (clot) formation. During inflammation, macrophages and lymphocytes proliferate, and inflammatory mediators such as cytokines and leukotrienes are present. The proliferation phase involves proliferation of basal and epithelial cells (angiogenesis).

5. C) Cleansing of the wound with mild soap and room-temperature water

This patient is presenting with a superficial burn due to exposure to ultraviolet light (recent sunburn). Treatment of minor burns includes cooling with room-temperature water or ice packs to provide some pain relief. Direct application of ice should be avoided as this can increase pain and burn depth. Burn wounds should be cleaned with mild soap and tap water. Daily application of zinc oxide may be desirable following partial-thickness burns; applying it to the healed skin for 1 to 2 weeks offers additional protection. Some skin disinfectants (e.g., povidone-iodine) can inhibit the healing process and are often not recommended. Treatment for superficial burns often does not require dressings. Additionally, superficial burns rarely develop invasive infections and do not require a topical antimicrobial agent (only required for partial- or full-thickness burns).

6. B) Enlargement

The ABCDE screening of melanoma includes asymmetry, border irregularity, color variety, diameter >6 mm, and enlargement or evolving change in size.

7. B) Rocky Mountain spotted fever

Spotted fever rickettsioses, including Rocky mountain spotted fever, is a nationally notifiable condition. Molluscum contagiosum, scarlet fever, and scabies are not reportable.

8. A) Molluscum contagiosum

Molluscum contagiosum is caused by the poxvirus. It is highly contagious and spreads by autoinoculation, skin-to-skin contact (as in wrestling), sexual contact, and sharing towels. It is a self-limited infection in immunocompetent patients. It resolves in 6 to 12 months. Acne does not typically appear on the lower arm. Verruca vulgaris is the common wart; in this case, the appearance is not wartlike. It also does not resemble basal cell cancer (pearly edges, telangiectasia, papule, or central ulceration).

9. An adult patient presents with blood under the nail of the great toe that involves approximately 50% of the nail area. The patient reports dropping a hammer accidentally on the toe about 5 hours ago. Which of the following is the recommended next step?
   A. Biopsy to rule out melanoma
   B. None; no action needed
   C. Trephination
   D. Nail removal

10. Which of the following would the nurse practitioner omit from a potential care plan for a patient diagnosed with plaque psoriasis?
    A. Topical corticosteroids
    B. Vitamin D analogs
    C. Ultraviolet light therapy
    D. Oral antibiotics

11. Which of the following is considered a precursor lesion for squamous cell skin cancer?
    A. Atopic dermatitis
    B. Actinic keratosis
    C. Seborrheic keratosis
    D. Nevi

12. Molluscum contagiosum is caused by:
    A. Herpesvirus
    B. Poxvirus
    C. *Staphylococcus aureus*
    D. *Haemophilus influenzae*

13. An older adult patient with a past medical history of a venous leg ulcer presents with skin erythema, edema, and warmth on their left lower extremity. Purulent drainage is noted. The patient reports recent antibiotic use for community-acquired pneumonia. The patient's vital signs are stable, and there is no concern for systemic illness. Which of the following antibiotic regimens is appropriate for this patient?
    A. Trimethoprim-sulfamethoxazole
    B. Dicloxacillin
    C. Doxycycline
    D. Cephalexin

14. Which of the following is a super-high potency (group 1) topical steroid?
    A. Halcinonide cream
    B. Mometasone furoate
    C. Fluocinolone acetonide
    D. Halobetasol propionate

15. An older patient who has diabetes mellitus presents with a concern for an outgrowth of skin on their neck. The patient complains that it commonly gets caught on jewelry. This patient is likely presenting with which of the following?
    A. Cherry angioma
    B. Nevi
    C. Acrochordon
    D. Lipoma

16. A middle-aged adult presents with soft yellow plaques that are symmetrically located on the medial aspects of the eyelids. This finding prompts which of the following interventions?
    A. Skin biopsy
    B. Check of lipid panel
    C. Allergy testing
    D. Ophthalmology consult

17. A patient with a history of severe sunburn presents with asymmetric depigmented macules and patches that are various shades of white. The lesions lack clinical signs of inflammation and are generalized around the face and hands. This presentation suggests which of the following?
    A. Vitiligo
    B. Psoriasis
    C. Seborrheic keratoses
    D. Urticaria

(See answers next page.)

9. C) Trephination

Trephination is a procedure in which a small hole is drilled on top of the nail so that the blood can drain. An 18-gauge needle is used to drain the blood to prevent permanent ischemic damage to the nail bed, which can lead to permanent loss of the toenail. Nail removal may be necessary but is not indicated initially. There are no signs and symptoms concerning for melanoma.

10. D) Oral antibiotics

Oral antibiotics are not used to treat plaque psoriasis (the most common type of psoriasis), because the condition is not caused by bacterial infection. Topical corticosteroids, vitamin D analogs (calcipotriene ointment), and ultraviolet light therapy (with UVB light) are methods used to treat psoriasis.

11. B) Actinic keratosis

Actinic keratosis (AK) is the precursor lesion of squamous cell carcinoma of the skin. It is caused by chronic sunlight exposure or chronic indoor tanning (UV rays). Several to many lesions are common. It is located in sun-exposed areas, such as the face, the dorsum of the arms and hands, and the chest. It appears as a small dry, scaly-to-rough patch of skin that does not go away, and it may bleed with trauma. Only about 5% to 10% of AK will turn into skin cancer, but it can become invasive. Atopic dermatitis and eczema are pruritic and appear on hands, knees, and other areas. Seborrheic keratosis looks like soft warts "pasted" on the skin; most are located on the back and can range in color from tan to black. It does not itch or hurt and is benign.

12. B) Poxvirus

Molluscum contagiosum is caused by a poxvirus infection of the skin. Herpesvirus can cause herpetic whitlow, a viral infection of the hand. *Staphylococcus aureus* (gram positive) and *Haemophilus influenzae* (gram negative) are types of bacteria but do not cause molluscum contagiosum. They can cause cellulitis.

13. A) Trimethoprim-sulfamethoxazole

The patient is presenting with signs and symptoms of cellulitis. Predisposing factors associated with risk for cellulitis include a skin barrier disruption due to trauma (e.g., venous leg ulcer). Cellulitis presents as areas of skin erythema, edema, and warmth that are nearly always unilateral. The lower extremities are the most common areas of involvement. Cellulitis can be purulent or non-purulent. Patients without signs or symptoms of sepsis can be managed outpatient with antibiotics. This patient has an indication for methicillin-resistant *Staphylococcus aureus* (MRSA) coverage due to their recent antibiotic use. Patients without severe sepsis with an indication for MRSA coverage should be treated with trimethoprim-sulfamethoxazole or amoxicillin plus doxycycline. Patients without severe sepsis without an indication for MRSA coverage can be treated with dicloxacillin, cephalexin, or cefadroxil.

14. D) Halobetasol propionate

Halobetasol propionate is a super-high potency (class 1) topical steroid. Halcinonide is high potency (class 2), mometasone furoate is medium potency (class 4), and fluocinolone acetonide is low potency (class 6).

15. C) Acrochordon

The patient is presenting with acrochordon, commonly known as a skin tag. This outgrowth of normal skin appears as a pedunculated lesion on a narrow stalk. They are common in adults, especially those with diabetes mellitus; they commonly occur in areas of friction such as the neck and the axilla, inframammary, and inguinal regions. A cherry angioma is a benign, small, smooth, round papule that is a bright cherry-red color. A lipoma presents as soft, painless subcutaneous nodules ranging in size from 1 to more than 10 cm. They are the most common benign soft-tissue neoplasms. Nevi (moles) are round macules to papules in colors ranging from light tan to dark brown due to benign proliferations of the nevus cell, a type of melanocyte.

16. B) Check of lipid panel

The patient is presenting with xanthelasma, which are soft yellow plaques that usually appear symmetrically on the medial aspects of the eyelid. They are most common in middle-aged to older adults and tend to be painless. It is recommended to obtain a lipid profile because dyslipidemia is present in about 50% of adults with xanthelasma. A skin biopsy is not necessary; however, surgical excision can be performed for cosmetic reasons. Allergy testing is not indicated because this condition is not due to an allergic reaction. The patient should continue with their regular eye exams, but an ophthalmology consult is not necessary unless the patient is experiencing vision changes.

17. A) Vitiligo

This patient is presenting with clinical features consistent with vitiligo. These asymptomatic, depigmented macules and patches lack signs of inflammation; lesions can appear anywhere but usually localize near the face, hands, and genitals. Vitiligo may show more than one shade of white based on the patient's skin color. Psoriasis presents with sharply defined, erythematous plaques with overlying, coarse scales. Seborrheic keratoses present as well-demarcated, round or oval lesions with a dull, verrucous surface and a typical "stuck-on" appearance. Urticaria presents as erythematous and raised skin lesions with discrete borders.

18. Which of the following is a palpable lesion measuring <1 cm in diameter?
    A. Macule
    B. Plaque
    C. Papule
    D. Vesicle

19. A patient presents with numerous lesions that started as papules and have progressed to vesicles surrounded by erythema. There are pustules that have broken and formed thick, adherent crusts with a golden appearance. The lesions are numerous and generalized on the face. Treatment for these lesions includes which of the following?
    A. Topical mupirocin
    B. Cephalexin
    C. Topical retapamulin
    D. Levofloxacin

20. A female patient presents with a history of a "herald" patch: a single, oval, sharply delimited, pink-colored lesion on the back that is about 3 cm in diameter. The patient reports that as the lesion progressed, central clearing was noted. After a few days, oval-shaped lesions with fine scales developed following skin lines and assembled a morphologic pattern similar to a "Christmas tree." This suggests which of the following conditions?
    A. Scabies
    B. Chickenpox
    C. Cellulitis
    D. Pityriasis rosea

21. Herpetic whitlow is a viral infection of the hand caused by which of the following?
    A. Herpes simplex virus
    B. *Neisseria meningitidis*
    C. Variola virus
    D. Varicella zoster virus

22. A patient presents with a rash after camping in the woods. The patient reports that they found a tick on their leg and that the rash started about a week after the bite. The rash is near the popliteal fossa and is warm to the touch and pruritic. Central clearing is noted, suggesting a target or bull's eye appearance. Treatment includes which of the following?
    A. Cephalexin
    B. Vancomycin
    C. Doxycycline
    D. Levofloxacin

23. Which of the following is a secondary lesion?
    A. Plaque
    B. Vesicle
    C. Pustule
    D. Lichenification

24. A patient presents with sharply defined, erythematous plaques with overlying coarse scales near the extensor elbows and knees. The patient denies joint pain but reports pruritis near the plaques. After removal of the scale, visualization of pinpoint bleeding is noted. This finding suggests which of the following?
    A. Auspitz sign
    B. Koebner phenomenon
    C. Development of psoriatic arthritis
    D. Progression of disease

25. In which of the following situations should the patient be referred to a burn center?
    A. Partial-thickness burns less than 10% of total body surface area (TBSA)
    B. Inhalation injury
    C. Partial-thickness burns less than 2% of TBSA without another injury
    D. Child with burn injury in a hospital with qualified personnel and equipment

26. Which of the following terms applies to dry skin?
    A. Purpura
    B. Annular
    C. Morbilliform
    D. Xerosis

(See answers next page.)

18. C) Papule
Papules are palpable, discrete lesions measuring <1 cm in diameter. Macules are nonpalpable lesions measuring <1 cm that vary in pigmentation from the surrounding skin. Plaques are elevated lesions that are >1 cm in diameter. Vesicles are small (<1 cm in diameter), circumscribed skin papules that are filled with clear serous or hemorrhagic fluid.

19. B) Cephalexin
This patient is presenting with the clinical features suggestive of impetigo. Topical therapies (e.g., mupirocin, retapamulin) are first-line treatments for impetigo if there are a *limited number* of lesions. Oral therapy is indicated for patients with *numerous* impetigo lesions. Cephalexin and dicloxacillin are recommended as first-line therapy options. Fluoroquinolones (e.g., levofloxacin) should not be used to treat impetigo; methicillin-resistant *Staphylococcus aureus* (MRSA) resistance is widespread to this class, and resistance can develop while on therapy.

20. D) Pityriasis rosea
A "herald" or "mother" patch is present in 50% to 90% of cases of pityriasis rosea. The eruption begins as a single round or oval, sharply delimited, pink-colored lesion on the chest, neck, or back about 2 to 5 cm in diameter. Central clearing is noted as the lesion becomes scaly. A few days later, oval lesions appear in crops on the trunk and proximal areas of the extremities with the long axes oriented along lines of cleavage of the skin, resembling a "Christmas tree" distribution. Scabies causes pruritic rashes and serpiginous or linear burrows with papular, vesicular, or crusted lesions. Chickenpox presents with a vesicular rash, which is usually pruritic; the lesions begin as macules and progress to papules followed by vesicles with a pustular component. Cellulitis presents as areas of skin erythema, edema, and warmth that are nearly always unilateral, and the lower extremities are the most common areas of involvement.

21. A) Herpes simplex virus
Herpetic whitlow is a viral infection of the hand caused by herpes simplex virus (HSV-1 and HSV-2). Meningococcemia is an infection caused by *Neisseria meningitidis*. Variola virus is the causative agent of smallpox. Primary infection with the varicella zoster virus causes chickenpox.

22. C) Doxycycline
This patient is presenting with erythema migrans, a rash that appears at the site of the tick bite (usually about 7 to 14 days after the bite). Central clearing is classic for erythema migrans. All patients with erythema migrans should be treated for Lyme disease. The preferred regimen includes doxycycline, amoxicillin, or cefuroxime. Antibiotics such as first-generation cephalosporins (e.g., cephalexin), quinolones (e.g., levofloxacin), and vancomycin should not be used because they are not effective against Lyme disease.

23. D) Lichenification
Primary lesions represent the initial pathologic change and include macules, papules, plaques, nodules, telangiectasia, purpura, pustules, vesicles, wheals, scale, atrophy, and hyperpigmentation. Secondary lesions represent changes from the skin disorder due to secondary external forces and include excoriation, lichenification, edema, scale, crust, fissue, and erosion.

24. A) Auspitz sign
This clinical presentation suggests chronic plaque psoriasis, the most common form of psoriasis with symmetrically distributed, cutaneous plaques. Koebner phenomenon and Auspitz sign are common findings in chronic plaque psoriasis and do not indicate progression of disease. Koebner phenomenon describes the development of skin disease in areas of skin trauma (also seen with lichen planus and vitiligo). Auspitz sign refers to the visualization of pinpoint bleeding after removal of a scale overlying a psoriatic plaque. Psoriatic arthritis is common in patients with psoriasis; however, the patient does not present with joint pain or stiffness.

25. B) Inhalation injury
Criteria for burn center referral include partial-thickness burns greater than 10% of TBSA; burns involving the face, hands, feet, genitalia, perineum, or major joints; full-thickness burns; electrical and chemical burns; inhalation injury; burn injury in patients with pre-existing comorbidities; burns and concomitant trauma; children in hospitals without qualified personnel or equipment; and burn injury in patients who require special social or rehabilitative interventions.

26. D) Xerosis
Xerosis (dry skin) is common in older adults and in people living in northern climates. Purpura are red-purple lesions that do not blanch under pressure. Annular lesions are figurate lesions with a ring-like morphology. Morbilliform describes a rash that resembles measles, with numerous erythematous macules and papules.

27. An adult patient presents after a cooking accident with hot oil. The patient presents with burns to their bilateral anterior arms and upper anterior chest. Using the rule of nines, what is the percentage of burned body surface area?
    A. 18%
    B. 9%
    C. 27%
    D. 21%

28. A burn that extends deeper into the dermis and damages hair follicles and glandular tissue is classified as:
    A. Superficial
    B. Superficial partial thickness
    C. Deep partial thickness
    D. Full thickness

29. A patient presents to the clinic after a hand laceration. The patient was chopping wood and accidentally pierced through the palmar surface of their hand. After the nurse practitioner cleans and sutures the wound, they advise the patient to return for suture removal in how many days?
    A. 5
    B. 10 to 14
    C. 3
    D. 21 to 28

30. A child presents with multiple scaly patches with hair loss. Multiple black dots are present at follicular orifices within areas of alopecia. First-line treatment for this condition includes which of the following?
    A. Fluconazole
    B. Ketoconazole
    C. Nystatin
    D. Griseofulvin

31. Tinea manuum is a dermatophyte infection that often occurs in association with:
    A. Tinea pedis
    B. Tinea barbae
    C. Tinea capitis
    D. Tinea cruris

32. A male patient presents with visually prominent acne with many comedones and large inflamed papules (>5 mm in diameter) with associated acne scarring. The severe, extensive, nodular acne has caused significant psychologic distress. Which of the following would be an appropriate treatment option for this patient?
    A. Isotretinoin plus topical retinoids
    B. Spironolactone
    C. Isotretinoin
    D. Topical benzoyl peroxide

33. An older patient presents with a rash characterized by erythematous papules near the thoracic dermatome. The patient reports that the rash has progressed to grouped vesicles or bullae that have started to become pustular. The patient reports a deep burning and a stabbing pain sensation. These symptoms most likely suggest which of the following?
    A. Chickenpox
    B. Herpes zoster
    C. Erythema migrans
    D. Contact dermatitis

34. A patient with diabetes and a prior history of cellulitis presents with yellow to brown discoloration of more than 50% of the nail of the great toe. The nail is opaque and thickened with separation of the nail plate from the nail bed. First-line treatment for this condition includes which of the following?
    A. Topical efinaconazole
    B. Oral ketoconazole
    C. Topical ciclopirox
    D. Oral terbinafine

35. The combination of several inflamed follicles into a single inflammatory mass with purulent drainage is:
    A. Carbuncle
    B. Folliculitis
    C. Furuncle
    D. Skin abscess

(See answers next page.)

27. A) 18%

Using the rule of nines, each anterior arm is 4.5%, and the upper anterior chest is 9% (4.5 + 4.5 + 9 = 18%).

28. C) Deep partial thickness

Deep partial-thickness burns extend into the deeper dermis and damage hair follicles and glandular tissue. Superficial burns involve only the epidermal layer of skin. Superficial partial-thickness burns form blisters between the epidermis and dermis. Full-thickness burns extend through and destroy all layers of the dermis and often extend into the underlying subcutaneous tissue.

29. B) 10 to 14

The timing of suture removal varies according to anatomic site. Suture removal for the digits, palms, and soles should occur in about 10 to 14 days. The face and neck require suture removal in 5 days, scalp 7 to 10 days, trunk and upper extremities 7 days, and lower extremities 8 to 10 days.

30. D) Griseofulvin

This patient is presenting with tinea capitis. The most common manifestation is scaly patches with alopecia and patches of alopecia with black dots at follicular orifices that represent broken hairs. The most commonly used therapies in children are oral griseofulvin and oral terbinafine; griseofulvin is considered first-line therapy based on its efficacy. Oral fluconazole can be used as an alternative therapy but is less frequently used and is not considered first line. Oral ketoconazole is no longer recommended due to its risk of severe liver injury and drug interactions. Nystatin is not effective for dermatophyte infections (it is indicated for cutaneous *Candida* infections).

31. A) Tinea pedis

Tinea manuum is a dermatophyte infection of the hand and often occurs in association with tinea pedis in a presentation referred to as "two feet—one hand syndrome." Tinea barbae is a dermatophyte infection of beard hair, tinea capitis is a dermatophyte infection of scalp hair, and tinea cruris is a dermatophyte infection of the crural fold.

32. C) Isotretinoin

This patient is presenting with clinical features consistent with moderate to severe acne vulgaris. The visually prominent acne consistent of many comedones, inflamed papules or nodules (lesions >5 mm), or pustules and associated scarring support moderate to severe involvement. Moderate to severe acne is often treated systemically. Oral isotretinoin is indicated for severe, recalcitrant, nodular acne, as well as less severe acne that is resistant to other treatments or associated with scarring. It is the only medication that can permanently alter the course of acne and cause long-term remissions. Isotretinoin is typically given as a monotherapy; combination with topical therapy is not recommended. Other systemic options for moderate to severe acne include oral antibiotics, oral contraceptives, and spironolactone. Oral contraceptives and spironolactone are indicated for postmenarchal female patients. Topical benzoyl peroxide is an effective option for mild acne.

33. B) Herpes zoster

Herpes zoster is characterized by a rash that starts as erythematous papules in single or several contiguous dermatomes (most often in the thoracic and lumbar areas). The predominant feature is grouped vesicles or bullae that then become pustular. Chickenpox usually includes a prodrome of fever, malaise, or pharyngitis followed by a generalized vesicular rash, which is usually pruritic. Central clearing is considered classic for erythema migrans, a rash that appears at the site of the tick bite. While contact dermatitis is also associated with a sensation of burning and pain, it often manifests as erythema, edema, vesicles, and oozing generally limited to the area that has been in contact with an irritant.

34. D) Oral terbinafine

The patient is presenting with clinical features suggestive of onychomycosis. Treatment is not necessary for all patients but is recommended for patients with diabetes or a history of cellulitis, patients with pain or discomfort with infected nails, immunosuppressed patients, and patients who desire treatment for cosmetic purposes. This patient meets the criteria for moderate to severe dermatophyte onychomycosis because the dermatophyte onychomycosis involves more than 50% of the nail. First-line treatment is oral terbinafine. Topical therapies (e.g., efinaconazole, ciclopirox) are treatment options for mild to moderate onychomycosis. Oral ketoconazole is not recommended due to the risk of life-threatening hepatotoxicity, adrenal insufficiency, and multiple drug interactions.

35. A) Carbuncle

A carbuncle is a combination of several inflamed follicles into a single inflammatory mass with purulent drainage. Folliculitis is a superficial bacterial infection of the hair follicles with purulent fluid in the epidermis. A furuncle is a well-circumscribed, painful, suppurative inflammatory nodule that involves hair follicles and usually occurs from preexisting folliculitis. A skin abscess is a collection of pus within the dermis and underlying skin tissues.

36. Which of the following patients is at increased risk for meningococcal disease?
   A. Traveler vacationing in Ireland
   B. Female high school student who is transgender
   C. Patient in the U.S. living with HIV infection with a low CD4 count
   D. College student living in a private apartment

37. Which of the following is an absolute contraindication to wound closure?
   A. Deep stab wounds
   B. Wounds caused by clean, sharp objects
   C. Wounds older than 24 hours that were insufficiently cleansed
   D. Wounds with presence of cellulitis or abscess

38. A patient presents with a bite wound to the right hand after being bitten by an unfamiliar dog. There is no erythema, swelling, or purulent drainage noted. Which of the following is the agent of choice for antibiotic prophylaxis?
   A. Amoxicillin-clavulanate
   B. Doxycycline plus metronidazole
   C. Moxifloxacin
   D. None; antibiotic prophylaxis not indicated

39. Where are the apocrine sweat glands primarily located?
   A. Palms of the hands
   B. Soles of the feet
   C. Forehead
   D. Axillary and anogenital areas

40. A patient presents after a recent camping trip with complaints of a fever, headache, malaise, and myalgias. The patient reports a blanching erythematous rash with macules (1 to 4 mm in size) and petechiae. The rash began on the ankles and wrists and is spreading toward the trunk. Based on this presentation, the preferred agent for treatment is which of the following?
   A. Chloramphenicol
   B. Doxycycline
   C. Amoxicillin
   D. Clindamycin

41. A patient with cutaneous plaques complains of pruritis. The plaques are limited to the bilateral elbows with a characteristic thick, silvery scale. Which of the following options should be recommended *first*?
   A. Topical corticosteroids
   B. Methotrexate
   C. Phototherapy
   D. Adalimumab

42. Which form of psoriasis is often preceded by streptococcal infection?
   A. Pustular
   B. Chronic plaque
   C. Guttate
   D. Erythrodermic

43. An immunocompetent patient who recently finished a course of antibiotics presents with a cottony feeling in the mouth, loss of taste, and pain during swallowing. Upon physical exam, white plaques are noted on the buccal mucosa and the oropharynx. This presentation suggests which of the following?
   A. Meningococcemia
   B. Oropharyngeal candidiasis
   C. Acute pharyngitis
   D. Impetigo

(See answers next page.)

36. C) Patient in the U.S. living with HIV infection with a low CD4 count

Risk factors for meningococcal disease include previous viral infection, household crowding, and smoking. Certain groups are at an increased risk, such as those with persistent complement component deficiencies, those who use complement inhibitors, those with asplenia (including sickle cell disease), those living with HIV infection, biologists exposed to *Neisseria meningitidis*, travelers to countries where the disease is hyperendemic or epidemic (specifically sub-Saharan Africa), college students living in residence halls and military recruits (likely due to the overcrowded living conditions), and men who have sex with men.

37. D) Wounds with presence of cellulitis or abscess

An absolute contraindication to wound closure is the presence of cellulitis or abscess (erythema, warmth, swelling, and pain with or without pus drainage). Primary closure is often seen for wounds caused by clean, sharp objects that close up to 12 to 18 hours from the time of injury. Secondary closure is indicated for deep stab or puncture wounds, contaminated wounds, abscess cavities, wound presentation after a significant delay, and non-cosmetic animal bites. Delayed primary closure would be considered for uncomplicated wounds that present after the safe period for primary closure (e.g., wounds older than 24 hours that were insufficiently cleansed).

38. A) Amoxicillin-clavulanate

Antibiotic prophylaxis is indicated for patients with lacerations undergoing primary closure or wounds undergoing surgical repair; wounds on the hands, face, or genital area; wounds in close proximity to a bone or joint or with underlying venous compromise (vascular grafts); immunocompromise (including diabetes); deep puncture wounds or laceration; and wounds associated with crush injury. The preferred antibiotic agent is amoxicillin-clavulanate for the prevention of infection due to animal-bite wounds. An alternative regimen is doxycycline plus metronidazole. Monotherapy with moxifloxacin is not recommended due to its insufficient evidence of effectiveness.

39. D) Axillary and anogenital areas

The apocrine sweat glands are located mainly in the axilla and groin. Dormant until puberty, they release water, salt, fatty acids, and proteins into hair follicles. Eccrine glands are the major sweat glands of the body, widely distributed but greatest in the hands, soles of the feet, and forehead. They help with heat dissipation and thermoregulation.

40. B) Doxycycline

The patient is presenting with the classic features of Rocky Mountain spotted fever, a potentially lethal but curable tick-borne disease. Early signs of illness are nonspecific, such as fever, headache, malaise, and myalgias. A petechial or maculopapular rash develops between the third and fifth day of illness in most patients. Doxycycline is the preferred agent for the treatment of Rocky Mountain spotted fever. Chloramphenicol is the only known alternative agent but is less effective than doxycycline. Amoxicillin and clindamycin are not indicated for the treatment of Rocky Mountain spotted fever.

41. A) Topical corticosteroids

The patient is presenting with chronic plaque psoriasis characterized by the thick, silvery scale and symmetrically distributed cutaneous plaques. The patient is presenting with mild (or limited) disease, which can often be managed with topical agents. Moderate to severe disease is involvement of more than 5% to 10% of body surface area; involvement of the face, palm or sole; or disease that is otherwise disabling. Topical corticosteroids and emollients are recommended for limited plaque psoriasis. For patients with moderate to severe disease, phototherapy or systemic therapies such as retinoids, methotrexate, cyclosporine, and biologic immune-modifying agents (e.g., adalimumab) are recommended.

42. C) Guttate

Guttate psoriasis is often preceded by a streptococcal infection; evidence has supported an association between new-onset guttate psoriasis and acute streptococcal pharyngitis in 56% to 97% of patients. The other forms of psoriasis are not preceded by a streptococcal infection.

43. B) Oropharyngeal candidiasis

Immunocompetent patients are at risk for oropharyngeal candidiasis especially in those treated with antibiotics or inhaled corticosteroids. Patients often complain of a cottony feeling in the mouth, loss of taste, and pain during swallowing. The physical exam reveals white plaques on the buccal mucosa, palate, tongue, and/or oropharynx (pseudomembranous form). Patients with meningococcemia may also present with a sore throat as well as a petechial rash on the trunk and lower portions of the body, fever, nausea, headache, and myalgias. Acute pharyngitis often presents with a fever, tonsillar exudates, tender cervical lymphadenopathy, and a rash. Impetigo often manifests as pustules that have broken and formed thick, adherent crusts with a golden appearance.

44. A patient with a history of frequent nail biting presents with a rapid onset of painful erythema and swelling of the proximal and lateral nail folds. The patient denies any past medical history. Physical examination reveals a superficial abscess. Initial treatment includes which of the following?

A. Topical antibiotics

B. Warm water or antiseptic soaks

C. Oral antibiotic therapy with Methicillin-resistant *Staphylococcus aureus* (MRSA) coverage

D. Incision and drainage

45. A patient presents with an intensely pruritic eruption with small, excoriated papules near the fingers, wrists, and axillae. The patient reports that the itching is worse at night and that other members of the household have similar symptoms. The patient reports living in a highly populated apartment building. The patient's presentation suggests which of the following conditions?

A. Tinea corporis

B. Molluscum contagiosum

C. Classic scabies

D. Stevens-Johnson syndrome

(See answers next page.)

44. D) Incision and drainage

This patient is presenting with paronychia, an acute local bacterial skin infection of the proximal or lateral nail folds. Risk factors include manicuring, nail biting, and picking at a hangnail. Paronychia with an abscess is treated with incision and drainage. For paronychia without abscess, treatment includes topical antibiotics and warm water or antiseptic soaks (e.g., chlorhexidine, povidone-iodine) multiple times per day. Empiric oral antibiotic therapy may be indicated in patients with or without an abscess with persistent inflammation after initial treatment. However, this patient does not have a risk factor that indicates the need for MRSA coverage (e.g., recent hospitalization, HIV infection, IV drug use, military service, crowded living conditions).

45. C) Classic scabies

Classic scabies manifests as an intensely pruritic rash with small, excoriated papules. Common sites include the fingers, wrists, axillae, areolae, waist, genitalia, and buttocks. Patients often report itching that worsens at night and other household members with similar symptoms. Risk factors include crowded conditions. Tinea corporis refers to epidermal dermatophyte infections in sites other than the feet, groin, face, or hand. It manifests as pruritic, circular, erythematous scaling patches that spread with central clearing. Molluscum contagiosum causes a chronic, localized infection characterized by firm, dome-shaped papules on the skin. Stevens-Johnson syndrome lesions are severe mucocutaneous reactions, often triggered by medications, characterized by extensive necrosis and detachment of the epidermis.

DANGER SIGNALS

ABDOMINAL AORTIC ANEURYSM

Majority of patients with abdominal aortic aneurysm (AAA) are asymptomatic. If not ruptured but has symptoms, patient will complain of abdominal, back, or flank pain. A ruptured AAA is suspected in patients with classic triad of acute abdominal pain, abdominal distention, and hemodynamic instability. The person at highest risk is an older white male who is a current or former smoker with hypertension (HTN). Incidental finding on chest x-ray may show widened mediastinum, tracheal deviation, and obliteration of aortic knob (thoracic aortic dissection). Initial imaging test is abdominal ultrasound.

ACUTE CORONARY SYNDROME

Acute coronary syndrome (ACS) refers to clinical presentations ranging from ST-elevation myocardial infarction (STEMI) to non–ST-elevation myocardial infarction (NSTEMI) and unstable angina. The classic presentation is a middle-aged to older man who complains of onset of constant chest or substernal discomfort lasting more than 15 minutes that is described as squeezing, tightness, crushing, a knot in the center of the chest, heavy pressure ("an elephant sitting on my chest"), or band-like. Some report that pain radiates to the inner aspect of one or both arms, shoulders, neck, and/or jaw. The pain can radiate to the back (interscapular region). It is provoked by physical exertion, emotional upset, or eating a heavy meal. The patient may be diaphoretic and complain of palpitations, shortness of breath, nausea, and/or vomiting. Some women, older adults and those with diabetes may have atypical presentations such as epigastric discomfort, indigestion, nausea and/or vomiting, new-onset fatigue, and dizziness. At other times, the pain is unpredictable or gets worse with rest (unstable angina). The best initial diagnostic test is the 12-lead EKG. Some patients with myocardial infarction (MI) may have a normal to nonspecific EKG. Assess airway, breathing, and circulation. All patients with suspected ACS should be given an aspirin dose of 162 to 325 mg to chew and swallow, unless contraindicated. Call 911.

BACTERIAL ENDOCARDITIS

Bacterial endocarditis is also known as *infective endocarditis*. Risk factors include cardiac factors (e.g., valvular abnormalities), underlying conditions (e.g., IV drug use, indwelling cardiac device, immunosuppression), or a recent dental or surgical procedure. Most commonly caused by *Staphylococcus aureus* as well as streptococci and enterococci. Patient presents with fever and chills that are associated with a new-onset murmur, anorexia, and weight loss. Associated skin findings are found mostly on the fingers/hands and toes/feet. There are subungual hemorrhages (splinter hemorrhages on the nail bed), petechiae on the palate, painful violet-colored nodes on the fingers and toes (Osler nodes), and nontender red spots on the palms/soles (Janeway lesions). Funduscopic exam may show Roth spots (retinal hemorrhages). First test done for suspected bacterial endocarditis is the transthoracic echocardiogram.

HEART FAILURE

Older adult patient reports being short of breath and lightheaded with minimal exertion, which can progress to dyspnea at rest. Easily fatigued even with light exertion. Symptoms often due to excess fluid accumulation; complains of feeling short of breath when lying down (orthopnea) and/or episodes of sudden awakening from sleep (recumbent position) due to severe shortness of breath, which is relieved with upright/sitting position (paroxysmal nocturnal dyspnea). Peripheral edema caused by fluid retention. Can be accompanied by poor appetite and abdominal discomfort. Multiple causes, including left ventricular (LV) dysfunction, right ventricular (RV) dysfunction, valvular heart disease, pericardial disease, obstructive lesion in heart or great vessel, or high-output heart failure. Decompensation can be caused by increased sodium intake and noncompliance with medications. Physical exam findings include lung crackles, wheezing, tachypnea, tachycardia, S3 gallop, paradoxical splitting of S2, jugular vein distention (JVD), peripheral edema, ascites, hepatomegaly, splenomegaly (due to right-sided failure), and hypoxia. Heart failure caused by LV dysfunction is categorized by LV ejection fraction (EF): heart failure with reduced ejection fraction (HFrEF), defined as an EF of 40% or less (also known as systolic heart failure); heart failure with EF of 41% to 49%, defined as heart failure with mid-range EF; heart failure with preserved ejection fraction (HFpEF), defined as an EF of 50% or higher (also known as diastolic heart failure).

STABLE VERSUS UNSTABLE ANGINA

Stable angina refers to chest discomfort that occurs predictable and reproducibly; it is usually of brief duration (2–5 minutes) and is relieved by rest and/or nitroglycerin. It may be precipitated by exercise, emotional upset, heavy meals, or lifting heavy objects. Unstable angina occurs after minimal activity, or it can occur at rest. The episodes become more frequent, severe, or prolonged, and it does not respond to rest or nitroglycerin. Unstable angina and acute NSTEMI differ in whether the ischemia is severe enough to cause sufficient myocardial damage resulting in the presence (or absence) of elevated serum biomarkers. Unstable angina is present in patients with ischemic symptoms suggestive of ACS with no elevation in troponins and with or without EKG changes indicative of ischemia.

EXAM TIPS

- Rule out AAA in an older male who has a pulsatile abdominal mass that is more than 3 cm in width.
  The next step is to order an abdominal ultrasound and CT.
- Learn the signs/symptoms of bacterial endocarditis.

NORMAL FINDINGS

ANATOMY
Position of the Heart
The right ventricle is the chamber of the heart that lies closest to the sternum. The lower border of the left ventricle is where the apical impulse is generated. The heart is roughly the size of a large adult fist. The apex beat is caused by the left ventricle. The point of maximal impulse (PMI) is located at the apex, at the fifth intercostal space (ICS) by the midclavicular line on the left side of the chest.

Displacement of the Point of Maximal Impulse
- Severe left ventricular hypertrophy (LVH) and cardiomyopathy: The PMI is displaced laterally on the chest and is larger (>3 cm) in size and more prominent.
- Pregnancy, third trimester: As the uterus grows larger, it pushes up against the diaphragm and causes the heart to shift to the left of the chest anteriorly. The result is a displaced PMI that is located slightly upward on the left side of the chest. May hear S3 heart sound during pregnancy.

Deoxygenated Blood
- Enters the heart through the superior vena cava and inferior vena cava
- Right atrium → tricuspid valve → right ventricle → pulmonic valve → pulmonary artery → the lungs → alveoli (red blood cells [RBCs] pick up oxygen and release carbon dioxide)

Oxygenated Blood
- Exits the lungs through the pulmonary veins and enters the heart
- Left atrium → mitral valve → left ventricle → aortic valve → aorta → general circulation

Systole and Diastole
The mnemonic to use is "motivated apples." These two words give you several clues. They will remind you of the names of the valves (which produce the sound) and the type of valve (atrioventricular [AV] or semilunar valve).

Motivated (S1 Heart Sound)	Apples (S2 Heart Sound)
M (mitral valve)	A (aortic valve)
T (tricuspid valve)	P (pulmonic valve)
AV (atrioventricular valves)	S (semilunar valves)

HEART SOUNDS

S1 (Systole)
- "Motivated" (M = Mitral and T = Tricuspid and AV = AV valves)
- The "lub" sound (of "lub-dub")
- Closure of the mitral and tricuspid valves
- Aortic/pulmonic (semilunar) valves open

S2 (Diastole)
- "Apples" (A = Aortic and P = Pulmonic and S = Semilunar valves)
- The "dub" sound (of "lub-dub")
- Closure of the aortic and pulmonic (semilunar) valves
- Mitral/tricuspid (AV) valves open

S3 Heart Sound
- Usually indicative of heart failure or congestive heart failure (CHF)
- Occurs during early diastole (also called a "ventricular gallop" or an "S3 gallop")
- Sounds like "Kentucky"
- Always considered abnormal if it occurs after age 40 years
- Can be a normal finding in children, pregnant patients, and some athletes (>35 years of age)

S4 Heart Sound
- Generally, abnormal in young adults and children
- Increased resistance due to a stiff left ventricle; usually indicates LVH
- Considered a normal finding in some older adults (slight stiffness of left ventricle)
- Occurs during late diastole (also called an "atrial gallop" or "atrial kick")
- Sounds like "Tennessee"
- Best heard at the apex (or apical area; mitral area) using the bell of the stethoscope

Stethoscope Skills
Bell of the Stethoscope
- Low tones such as extra heart sounds (S3 or S4)
- Mitral stenosis

Diaphragm of the Stethoscope
- Mid- to high-pitched tones such as lung sounds
- Mitral regurgitation (MR)
- Aortic stenosis (AS)

Benign Variants
Physiologic S2 Split
Best heard over the left upper sternal border; caused by splitting of the aortic and pulmonic components. A normal finding if it appears during inspiration and disappears at expiration.

S4 in Older Adults

Some healthy older adult patients have an S4 (late diastole) heart sound, also known as the "atrial kick" (the atria have to squeeze harder to overcome resistance of a stiff left ventricle). If there are no signs or symptoms of heart/valvular disease, it is considered a normal variant. Pathologic S4 is associated with LVH due to increased resistance from the left ventricle. S4 is always abnormal when it is palpable, regardless of patient age.

EXAM TIPS

- S3 is a sign of CHF; S4 is a sign of LVH.
- A physiologic split S2 is best heard at the pulmonic area (upper left sternum).

ABNORMAL FINDINGS

PATHOLOGIC MURMURS

- Murmurs have been closely linked to a multitude of diseases.
- An echocardiography is indicated in patients with cardiac symptoms and any cardiac murmur, as well as asymptomatic patients with a diastolic murmur, a grade 3 or greater systolic murmur, or a systolic murmur in combination with other abnormal physical exam findings (e.g., systolic click, reduced carotid upstroke).

SOLVING QUESTIONS: HEART MURMURS

To solve a murmur question correctly, only two pieces of information are needed.

- Look for the timing of the murmur (systole or diastole).
- Look for the location of the murmur (aortic, Erb's point, or mitral area).
- All the murmurs seen on the exams will fit into the two mnemonics below.

Timing

Systolic Murmurs

Use the "MR. PASS" (mitral regurgitation/physiologic [systolic flow murmur]/aortic stenosis = systolic) mnemonic (see below).

Diastolic Murmurs

Use the "MS. ARD" (mitral stenosis/aortic regurgitation = diastolic) mnemonic (see below).

Location

Auscultatory Areas

It is necessary to memorize the locations of the auscultatory areas in order to correctly identify a heart murmur.

EXAM TIPS

- All murmurs with "mitral" in their names are only described as located: On the apex (or apical area) of the heart *or* on the fifth ICS on the left side of the sternum medial to the midclavicular line.
- On the exam, only the systolic murmurs radiate (to the axilla in MR and to the neck with AS).

Mitral Area

- The mitral area is also known as the *apex* (or *apical area*) of the heart.
- Fifth left ICS is approximately 8 to 9 cm from the midsternal line and slightly medial to the midclavicular line.
- PMI or the apical pulse is located in this area.

Aortic Area

- The aortic area is the second ICS to the right side of the upper border of the sternum.
- The location of the aortic area can also be described as *the second ICS by the right side of the sternum at the base of the heart*. It can also be described as a murmur that is located on the right side of the upper sternum.

Erb's Point

Erb's point is located at the third to fourth ICS on the left sternal border.

Heart Murmurs: Mnemonics

MR. PASS (Systolic Murmurs)

- Systolic murmurs are also described as occurring during S1, or as holosystolic, pansystolic, early systolic, late systolic, or mid-systolic murmurs.
- Compared with diastolic murmurs, these murmurs are louder and can radiate to the neck or axillae.

MR. (Mitral Regurgitation)

- May be early systolic, mid-systolic, or pansystolic (or holosystolic) murmur
- Best heard at the apex (or apical area) of the heart
- May radiate to the base or axilla
- Often, soft, low-pitched, and decrescendo murmur (use the diaphragm of the stethoscope)

P (Physiologic Murmur)

- Systolic flow murmur
- Often heard in children and those with thin chest wall
- Also known as functional murmur, as it is heard in the absence of any cardiac abnormality

AS (Aortic Stenosis)

- A mid-systolic ejection murmur
- Best heard at the second ICS at the right side of the sternum
- May radiate to the neck
- A harsh and noisy murmur (use diaphragm of stethoscope). Patients with AS should avoid physical overexertion, because there is increased risk of sudden death. Refer to cardiologist.
- AS is monitored by serial cardiac sonograms with Doppler flow studies. Surgical valve replacement needed if it worsens.

MS. ARD (Diastolic Murmurs)

- Diastole is also known as the *S2 heart sound, early diastole, late diastole,* or *mid-diastole.*
- Diastolic murmurs are always indicative of heart disease (unlike systolic murmurs).

MS (Mitral Stenosis)

- A low-pitched diastolic rumbling murmur
- Best heard at the apex (or apical area) of the heart
- Also called an *opening snap* (use bell of the stethoscope)

- There are usually two questions regarding heart murmurs on the exam.
- Learn to use the mnemonics "MR. PASS" and "MS. ARD." If an apical/apex murmur occurs during S1, it is MR (MR. PASS). If an apical/apex murmur occurs during S2, it is MS (MS. ARD).

AR (Aortic Regurgitation)

- A high-pitched diastolic murmur (use diaphragm of the stethoscope)
- Often heard over the left sternal border or over the right second interspace, while the patient sits and leans forward with the breath held in full expiration
- If AR is due to a diseased aortic valve, the murmur is located at the third ICS by the left sternal border (Erb's point).
- If AR is due to an abnormal aortic root, the murmur is best heard at the right upper sternal border (aortic area).

Heart Murmurs: Grading System

- Grade I: A very soft murmur heard only under optimal conditions.
- Grade II: A mild to moderately loud murmur.
- Grade III: Loud murmur that is easily heard once the stethoscope is placed on the chest.
- Grade IV: Louder murmur. First time that a thrill is present. A thrill is like a "palpable murmur."
- Grade V: Very loud murmur heard with edge of stethoscope off the chest. Thrill is more obvious.
- Grade VI: Murmur is so loud that it can be heard even with the stethoscope off the chest. The thrill is easily palpated.

- Memorize the mnemonic "motivated apples" to help you remember the names of the valves that are responsible for producing S1 and S2.
- When grading murmurs, be aware that the first time a thrill is palpated is at grade IV.

DISEASE REVIEW

BACTERIAL ENDOCARDITIS

Bacterial endocarditis, also known as infective endocarditis, may be acquired in the community or by healthcare exposure. Risk factors include older age (>60 years), male sex, infection drug use, poor dentition or dental infection as well as comorbid conditions (e.g., structural heart disease, previous history of bacterial endocarditis, chronic hemodialysis, HIV infection). Three most common bacterial pathogens are staphylococci, streptococci, and enterococci. Often, categorized as native valve infective endocarditis or prosthetic valve infective endocarditis.

Classic Case

An adult male presents with fever, chills, anorexia with weight loss, and malaise that are associated with subungual hemorrhages (splinter hemorrhages on nail bed) and tender violet-colored nodules on the fingers and/or on toes (Osler's nodes). Palms and soles may have tender red spots on the skin (Janeway lesions). Some patients may have a heart murmur. May not present with all of the preceding symptoms. Another clue is to look for cardiac risk factors such as a prosthetic valve, history of valvular or congenital heart disease, cardiac device, IV drug use, IV lines, recent dental or surgical procedure. Maintain high index suspicion due to high mortality. Patient may present with rapidly progressive symptoms or subacute chronic disease with low-grade fever and nonspecific symptoms.

Treatment Plan

- Refer to cardiologist and infectious disease or ED for hospitalization and IV antibiotics.
- Diagnostic tools include microbiologic data with blood cultures and echocardiography.
- Complete blood count (CBC) (elevated white blood cells [WBCs]) and erythrocyte sedimentation rate >20 mm per hour (elevated).
- Management includes timely administration of effective antimicrobial therapy, monitoring valve function, assessing potential sources of infection, identifying candidates for surgery, and preventing recurrent bacterial endocarditis.
- Parenteral antibacterial treatment for native valve endocarditis can range from 4 to 6 weeks.

Complications

Cardiologic and neurologic complications, valvular destruction, myocardial abscess, septic emboli, metastatic infection, system immune reactions, and death

Endocarditis Prophylaxis

Box 7.1 Considerations for Endocarditis Prophylaxis

High-Risk Conditions

- Prosthetic heart valves or prosthetic valve repair material
- Previous history or recurrent bacterial endocarditis
- Implanted durable mechanical circulatory support device (e.g., ventricular assist device)
- Cardiac transplant patients who develop cardiac valvopathy
- Certain types of congenital heart disease

Invasive Procedures

- Invasive dental or invasive oral procedure: procedures involving manipulation of gingival tissue, the periapical region of the teeth, or perforation of the oral mucosa, tooth extraction, dental abscess drainage, and routine dental cleaning

- Preferred oral regimen: Give 1 hour before procedure: Amoxicillin 2 g PO × 1 dose (adults)
- IV option: Ampicillin 2 g IM or IV or cefazolin or ceftriaxone 1 g IM or IV

Penicillin Allergy
- Oral: Cephalexin 2 g or clarithromycin (Biaxin) 500 mg or cephalexin (Keflex) 2 g
- IV: Cefazolin or ceftriaxone 1 g IM or IV

CARDIAC ARRHYTHMIAS

EKG Interpretation

You may see EKG strip images on your exam. You will be asked to interpret the strip at a basic, or entry, level as a nurse practitioner. Occasionally, an arrhythmia will be described without a strip, such as an "irregularly irregular rhythm with no visible P waves (AF)." Because family and adult-gerontology nurse practitioners (NPs) function in the primary care area, most common arrhythmias are included. You are not expected to interpret an EKG strip with AV block or other complex arrhythmias. Just like in dermatology where you remember a rash by appearance, you can memorize the appearance of a rhythm by its EKG strip. The important ones to memorize (EKG appearance) are atrial fibrillation (AF) (irregularly irregular rhythm with no P waves; Figure 7.1), anterior wall MI (ST segment elevation in leads V2 to V4), ventricular tachycardia (jagged irregular QRS), and the norms such as sinus rhythm and sinus arrhythmia.

Acute ST-Elevation Myocardial Infarction

STEMI is characterized by hyperacute T waves, which are tall, peaked, and symmetric; elevation of the ST segment in contiguous leads (depending on the location of the MI); and often the development of Q waves and T wave inversions. EKG changes include ST segment elevation and Q waves (Figure 7.2). Wide QRS complex on leads V2 to V4 resembles a "tombstone."

Acute Non-ST-Elevation Myocardial Infarction

EKG characterized by T wave flattening or inversion, which precedes ST-segment depression. Q waves are often absent; and the ST and T wave duration varies.

Atrial Fibrillation and Atrial Flutter

AF is the most common cardiac arrhythmia in the United States. It is a major cause of stroke. AF is an abnormal electrical conduction in the atria that causes quivering of the upper chambers and results in ineffective pumping of the heart. AF with rapid ventricular response (RVR) is a potential sequela of AF and can lead to hemodynamic instability during critical illness. Atrial flutter is when the atria beat regularly, but faster than usual, such as four atrial beats per one ventricular beat. Both have similar treatments. The hallmark sign of this arrhythmia is a "sawtooth-like" EKG tracing. Paroxysmal AF (intermittent or self-terminating) describes episodes that terminate within 7 days or less (usually <24 hours); it is usually asymptomatic.

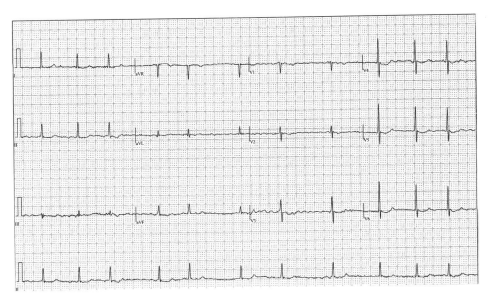

Figure 7.1 Atrial fibrillation. Atrial fibrillation has absence of P waves and an irregularly irregular ventricular rate.

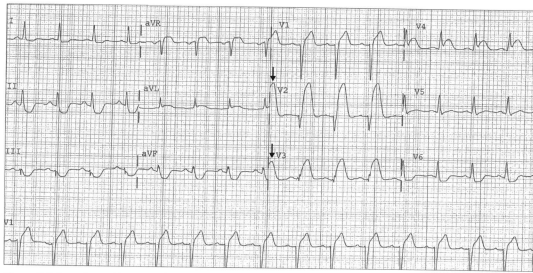

Figure 7.2 Anterior wall myocardial infarction.

Risk Factors

- AF: HTN, coronary artery disease (CAD), valvular heart disease, ACS, hyperthyroidism, heart failure, hypertrophic cardiomyopathy, congenital heart disease, venous thromboembolic disease, diabetes, chronic kidney disease, obstructive sleep apnea, obesity, metabolic syndrome, and others (e.g., family history, genetic factors, alcohol intake, night shift work, caffeine)
- Atrial flutter: Can occur after antiarrhythmic drug initiation, after an acute MI, post-cardiac surgery, after AF ablation.

Classic Case

Patient reports a sudden onset of heart palpitations described as feeling like "a fish is flopping in my chest" or "drums are pounding in my chest" that is accompanied by feelings of weakness, dizziness, and tachycardia. There is often fatigue and a reduction of exercise capacity. May complain of dyspnea, chest pain, and feeling like passing out (presyncope or rarely syncope). Rapid and irregular pulse may be more than 110 beats/min with hypotension. AF can be paroxysmal and stop spontaneously (within 7 days), or it can be long standing and persistent (12 months or longer). If patient is hemodynamically unstable (chest pain/angina, hypotension, heart failure, cold clammy skin, acute kidney failure) with a new onset of AF with severe symptoms, call 911.

Treatment Plan

- Search for underlying cause. Every patient with AF needs to be evaluated for anticoagulation therapy. The CHA$_2$DS$_2$-VASc score is a tool that will help determine whether a patient needs anticoagulation therapy.
  - CHA$_2$DS$_2$-VASc: C (CHF), H (HTN), A (age >75 years), D (diabetes), S$_2$ (stroke/transient ischemic attack [TIA]), V (vascular disease), A (age 65–74 years), S (sex: females at higher risk).
  - CHA$_2$DS$_2$-VASc scoring system: Score of 0 is low risk. Score of 2 or more requires anticoagulation. Some physicians will treat patients with a score of 1.

- Diagnostic test is the 12-lead EKG (does not show discrete P waves, irregularly irregular rhythm).
- Diagnostic evaluation is EKG, thyroid-stimulating hormone (TSH), serum electrolytes (calcium, potassium, magnesium, sodium), renal function, B-type natriuretic peptide (rule out heart failure), troponin (rule out MI). Obtain digoxin level (if on digoxin).
- Consider 24-hour (or longer) Holter monitor.
- Order echocardiogram (rule out valvular pathology, which increases risk of stroke).
- Lifestyle modifications include avoiding stimulants (caffeine, nicotine, decongestants) and alcohol.

Medications

- Patients are referred to cardiologist for medical management. An option for new-onset AF with stable patients is cardioversion (first 48 hours) or rate control.
- Management varies on the basis of AF severity and symptoms.
- For rate control, use beta-blockers (e.g., metoprolol), calcium channel blockers (CCBs; e.g., diltiazem), digoxin.
- For rhythm control, use amiodarone (Pacerone) to maintain normal sinus rhythm. Note that amiodarone has a U.S. Food and Drug Administration (FDA) black box warning for pulmonary toxicity, hepatic injury, hyper- or hypothyroidism, visual impairment, peripheral neuropathy, and worsened arrhythmia.

For anticoagulation:

- Warfarin (Coumadin; vitamin K antagonist) is the agent of choice in patients with severe rheumatic MS, any type of mechanical heart valves, with bioprosthetic valve recently implanted, and patients with drug interactions with other agents. Target international normalized ratio (INR) 2.0 to 3.0, annual time in therapeutic range (TTR) >70%.
- Initial daily dose equal to or less than 5 mg, but frail, sensitive, or patients older than 70 years should take lower dose (2.5 mg).

Table 7.1 Warfarin Therapy: Drug Interactions That Can Increase International Normalized Ratio (INR)*

Drug Class	Examples
Glucocorticoids	Methylprednisolone, prednisone
SSRIs and SNRIs	Fluoxetine, sertraline, duloxetine, fluvoxamine, venlafaxine
Fluoroquinolones	Ciprofloxacin, levofloxacin, moxifloxacin, norfloxacin
Macrolides	Azithromycin, clarithromycin, erythromycin
Penicillins	Amoxicillin, amoxicillin-clavulanate
Azole antifungals	Fluconazole, miconazole
Statins	Fluvastatin, lovastatin, rosuvastatin, simvastatin
Other medications	Tramadol, fenofibrate, trimethoprim-sulfamethoxazole

*Not an all-inclusive list
SNRI, serotonin–norepinephrine reuptake inhibitor; SSRI, selective serotonin reuptake inhibitor.

- Full anticoagulation effect can take 3 days. Check INR every 2 to 3 days until therapeutic for 2 consecutive checks, then recheck weekly, and so on until INR is stable at 2 to 3. Check every 4 weeks when stable.
- You may wish to check the institutional protocols or refer to anticoagulation clinic. If you do not have experience with anticoagulation, best to refer to cardiologist.
- If you suspect a bleeding episode, check the INR with the prothrombin time (PT), partial thromboplastin time (PTT), and CBC (check platelets).
- Drug interactions for warfarin are provided in Table 7.1.
- Direct-acting anticoagulants (DOACs) are first-line agents for nonvalvular AF.
- DOACs include dabigatran (Pradaxa), rivaroxaban (Xarelto), edoxaban (Savaysa), and apixaban (Eliquis). Advise patients to take medications on schedule and not skip doses. Do not require INR monitoring, have no major dietary restrictions, and have fewer drug interactions.
- Platelet inhibitors such as clopidogrel (Plavix), either alone or in combination with aspirin and other anticoagulants, may be better tolerated but are less effective than DOACs and warfarin.
- Alcohol abstinence lowers the risk of recurrent AF even among regular drinkers.

Complications
- Death caused by thromboembolic event (e.g., stroke, pulmonary embolism [PE]), CHF, angina, and others. Risk of stroke/death is higher in older adult patients.
- Warfarin-associated intracerebral hemorrhage has very high mortality; for this reason DOACs are preferred in older adults because of the reduced risk in comparison to warfarin. It is a medical emergency. Call 911.
- If warfarin-associated life-threatening bleeding episode, stop warfarin and all anticoagulants such as acetylsalicylic acid (ASA) and nonsteroidal anti-inflammatory

drugs (NSAIDs). Treat with vitamin K, 4-factor prothrombin complex concentrate (PCC, inactivated), and/or fresh frozen plasma. Check INR, PT, and PTT. Patient will need emergent care in the acute care setting.
- For DOAC-associated life-threatening bleeding episode, life-threatening bleeding caused by rivaroxaban (Xarelto) and apixaban (Eliquis) can be treated with andexanet alfa (Andexxa). Bleeding caused by dabigatran (Pradaxa) is treated with idarucizumab (Praxbind).

Anticoagulation Guidelines

Table 7.2 Elevated International Normalized Ratio (INR)

INR	Presence of Bleeding	Action
<4.5	None	Skip next dose and/or reduce slightly the maintenance dose. Check INR once or twice a week when adjusting dose. Do not give vitamin K. If INR elevation is minimal, often maintenance dose does not need to be reduced.
4.5–10	None or not clinically significant bleeding	Hold one or two doses, with or without administration of low-dose oral vitamin K (1–2.5 mg). Monitor INR every 2–3 days until it is stable. Decrease the warfarin maintenance dose.

Source: Adapted from Hull, R. D., & Garcia, D. A. (2020). (See Resources section for complete source information.)

Atrial Fibrillation
INR: 2.0 to 3.0

Synthetic/Prosthetic Valves
INR: 2.5 to 3.5

Patient Education: Dietary Sources of Vitamin K (Warfarin Only, Does Not Apply to Direct-Acting Anticoagulants)
- Advise patients to be consistent with their day-to-day consumption of vitamin K–rich foods.
- Give patient a list of foods with high levels of vitamin K. This includes greens such as kale, collard, mustard, spinach, and iceberg or romaine lettuce; brussels sprouts; potatoes.
- Only one serving per day is recommended for very high vitamin K–rich foods.

Paroxysmal Supraventricular Tachycardia
EKG shows tachycardia with peaked QRS complex with P waves present. When having an episode, has regular but rapid heartbeat, which starts and stops abruptly (intermittent episodes). Can be misdiagnosed as a panic or anxiety attack. Paroxysmal supraventricular tachycardia (PSVT)

is a subset of the narrow QRS complex tachycardias with regular ventricular response. There are several types, such as Wolff–Parkinson–White (WPW) syndrome and atrial tachycardia. The EKG of a patient with WPW has a short PR interval and a widened QRS complex and paroxysmal tachycardia. WPW increases risk of death; refer to cardiologist for catheter ablation. Episodes can be precipitated by digitalis toxicity, alcohol, hyperthyroidism, caffeine intake, and illegal drug use.

EXAM TIPS

- The PR interval (atrial depolarization) duration is 0.12 to 0.20 seconds (3–5 small boxes).
- In AF, the goal is INR of 2 to 3. If INR is between 4.01 and 4.99, hold one dose. Do not give vitamin K.

Classic Case

Patient complains of an abrupt onset of palpitations ("feels like fluttering in my chest"), rapid pulse, lightheadedness, shortness of breath, and anxiety. May feel weak and fatigue or faint. Rapid heart rate can range from 150 to 250 beats/min. Reports previous episodes that resolved spontaneously. Can start in childhood or older; it may resolve spontaneously or reoccur at a later time.

Treatment Plan

Check EKG. If it shows WPW syndrome or is symptomatic, refer to cardiologist. If hemodynamically unstable, may require electrical cardioversion. Call 911.

The 2015 American College of Cardiology (ACC)/Heart Rhythm Society guidelines recommend vagal maneuvers for acute treatment of supraventricular tachycardia. There are several methods.

- Vagal maneuvers: Carotid sinus massage (patient supine, monitor vital signs). If a carotid massage is done in a clinical setting, continuous 12-lead EKG during the procedure. Responses are changes in heart rate or rhythm and/or blood pressure (BP) after sinus massage. Contradictions to sinus massage are TIA or stroke within previous 3 months, presence of carotid bruits, and so forth.
- Valsalva's maneuver: Hold one's breath and strain hard, maintain strain for 10 to 15 seconds, then release it and breath normally.

Sinus Rhythm and Sinus Arrhythmia

Sinus arrhythmia is a common variation of normal sinus rhythm. It is more common in healthy children and young adults. The P waves show uniform morphology (Figure 7.3).

CLINICAL PEARLS

- Major bleeding episodes can occur even with a normal INR. Order an INR with the PT and PTT if you suspect bleeding.
- It may take up to 3 days after changing the warfarin dose to see a change in the INR.
- Warfarin (Coumadin) is an FDA category X drug. It is teratogenic.

DEEP VEIN THROMBOSIS

Venous thromboembolism (VTE) can present as deep vein thrombosis (DVT) of the lower extremity and PE. A proximal DVT is a thrombus located in the popliteal, femoral, or iliac veins; a distal DVT refers to a thrombus in the calf veins (peroneal, posterior, anterior tibial, and muscular veins).

Virchow triad proposes that VTE occurs as a result of:

1. Alterations in blood flow: For example, stasis that occurs during prolonged travel, immobility/bedrest, CHF
2. Alterations in blood components: Often, secondary to an inherited or acquired hypercoagulable state (e.g., Factor V Leiden deficiency, prothrombin gene mutations)
3. Vascular endothelial injury: For example, cell injury from the severe acute respiratory syndrome coronavirus 2 (SARS-CoV-2) virus

Acquired risk factors include prior thromboembolism; immobilization; oral contraceptive use; pregnancy; bone fractures, especially of the long bones; trauma; recent surgery; and malignancy.

Classic Case

A patient with risk factors for DVT complains of gradual onset of swelling on a lower extremity after a history of travel (more than 3 hours) or prolonged immobility. The patient complains of a painful and swollen lower extremity that is red and warm. If patient has PE, it is accompanied by abrupt onset of chest pain, dyspnea, dizziness, or syncope. Many patients are asymptomatic.

- Unprovoked DVT: No identifiable risk factors
- Provoked DVT: Caused by known event (e.g., surgery, major surgery, hospitalization)

Diagnostic and Treatment Plan

- CBC, platelets, clotting time (PT/PTT, INR), D-dimer level, chest x-ray, EKG, Wells score.
- Compression ultrasonography with Doppler is the diagnostic test of choice.

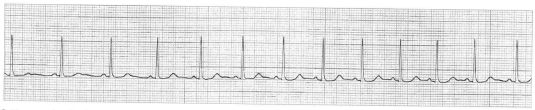

Figure 7.3 Sinus arrhythmia.

- May require hospital admission but can be managed outpatient if hemodynamically stable with a low risk of bleeding and no severe renal insufficiency. Patient should have good caregiver support for the administration and maintenance of anticoagulant therapy.
- Treatment options include anticoagulation with either low-molecular-weight heparin (enoxaparin; Lovenox) subcutaneous; heparin subcutaneous or by IV infusion (if hospitalized), then warfarin PO (Coumadin); or DOACs.
- Selection for anticoagulation depends on location of DVT, risk of bleeding and embolization, and comorbid conditions.
- For recurrent DVT or in older adults, anticoagulation may be indefinite.

Complications
- Acute pulmonary embolism, recurrent DVT, post-thrombotic syndrome, death
- Stroke and other embolic episodes

EXAM TIP

Learn DVT risk factors.

HEART FAILURE

Numerous causes and precipitating factors such as an acute MI, CAD, HTN, fluid retention, valvular abnormalities, cigarette smoking, diabetes, and arrhythmias. Heart failure caused by LV dysfunction is categorized by LV EF: HFrEF, defined as an EF of 40% or less (also known as systolic heart failure), heart failure with EF of 41% to 49% defined as heart failure with mid-range EF; HFpEF, defined as an EF of 50% or higher (also known as diastolic heart failure).

Left Heart Failure
- Pulmonary crackles with or without an S3 gallop, bibasilar rales (rales on lower lobes of the lungs), cough, dyspnea, decreased breath sounds, dullness to percussion
- Paroxysmal nocturnal dyspnea, orthopnea, nocturnal nonproductive cough, wheezing (cardiac asthma), HTN, and fatigue are symptoms of both left and right heart failure

Right Heart Failure
- Dyspnea, fatigue, chest discomfort, abdominal distention with a positive fluid wave
- RV heave, a loud P2, often tricuspid regurgitation (holosystolic murmur over left lower sternal border)
- Normal JVD is 4 cm or less
- Enlarged spleen and enlarged liver, right upper quadrant discomfort due to acute hepatic congestion
- Peripheral edema with cool skin

Diagnostic Evaluation
- Chest x-ray may show increased heart size, interstitial and alveolar edema, Kerley B lines, and other signs of pulmonary edema.
- 12-lead EKG, cardiopulmonary exercise testing
- Cardiac troponin T or I

- B-type natriuretic peptide (BNP) and N-terminal pro-BNP (NT-proBNP) often elevated with HF, but there are limitations (e.g., often increased in patients with renal failure)
- Blood urea nitrogen (BUN), serum creatinine and electrolytes, CBC, liver function tests, fasting blood glucose
- Echocardiogram (often with Doppler flow study)
- Cardiac catheterization is definitive diagnostic test for right heart failure

EXAM TIP

The S3 heart sound is a sign of HF, although it can also be heard in pregnant people and children/young adults.

Treatment Plan
- Goals of management: Reduce symptoms, increase functional status, and reduce the risk of hospital admission.
- HFpEF: Diuretic (often loop diuretic) to relieve symptoms of volume overload (dyspnea, peripheral edema). For symptomatic patients with elevated BNP, treatment with both a sodium-glucose co-transporter 2 (SGLT2) inhibitor and a mineralocorticoid receptor antagonist (MRA) is recommended; add sacubitril-valsartan with poorly controlled HTN.
- HFrEF: Combination treatment with diuretic, angiotensin-converting enzyme inhibitor (ACEI) or angiotensin receptor blocker (ARB), or angiotensin receptor-neprilysin inhibitor (ARNI; sacubitril-valsartan/Entresto), and a beta-blocker.
- Acute decompensated heart failure: Refer to ED (treatment may include IV diuretics, supplemental oxygen and assisted ventilation, vasodilators, inotropes, or vasopressor therapy).
- Patients with HF: Often managed by cardiologists or at a heart clinic. If patient presents in acute distress, refer to ED.
- New York Heart Association (NYHA) system: Use to classify patient's degree of cardiac disability (Table 7.3).

EXAM TIPS
- Memorize presentation of a patient with NYHA class II heart disease.
- First-line medication for stable HF is an ACEI or ARB.

Table 7.3 New York Heart Association Functional Capacity Ratings

Classification	Degree of Disability
Class I	No limitations on physical activity
Class II	Ordinary physical activity results in fatigue, exertional dyspnea
Class III	Marked limitation in physical activity
Class IV	Symptoms are present at rest, with or without physical activity

Source: Data from American Heart Association (2011).

Lifestyle Modifications

- Medication adherence and daily symptom monitoring.
- Restrict or abstain from alcohol. Smoking cessation if smoker; weight loss.
- Restrict sodium to less than 2 to 3 g/d.
- Fluid restriction (1.5–2 L/d) may help some patients.
- Weight should be checked daily to detect fluid accumulation.
- Cardiac rehabilitation and routine exercise therapy.

> **NOTES**
>
> Here is an easy way to remember whether a sign or symptom is from the left or right side of the heart:
>
> Both *left* and *lung* start with the letter *L*. Symptoms are lung related, such as dyspnea, orthopnea, and paroxysmal nocturnal dyspnea.
>
> Right-sided heart failure symptoms are GI related (anorexia, nausea, and right upper quadrant abdominal pain).

HYPERLIPIDEMIA

Most patients are asymptomatic until they develop atherosclerotic cardiovascular disease (ASCVD). The treatment guidelines have been updated to the *2018 Guideline on the Management of Blood Cholesterol: Executive Summary* (a report of the ACC/American Heart Association (AHA) Task Force on Clinical Practice Guidelines). The ACC's new ASCVD Risk Estimator Plus tool is available online at http://tools.acc.org/ASCVD-Risk-Estimator-Plus/#!/calculate/estimate. Note that this tool may underestimate 10-year and lifetime risk for persons from some race/ethnic groups such as American Indian, some Asian (e.g., South Asian), and some Hispanic (e.g., Puerto Rican) persons.

EXAM TIPS

- First-line treatment for hyperlipidemia is lifestyle, but presence of ASCVD or equivalents requires drug therapy as well.
- If patient has markedly high triglycerides (500 mg/dL or higher), priority is to lower triglycerides due to the increased risk of acute pancreatitis.

Screening Guidelines

- For adults at higher cardiovascular risk, it is suggested to perform follow-up lipid screening in males between the ages of 25 to 30 and females between the ages of 30 to 35.
- For adults at lower cardiovascular risk, it is suggested to perform follow-up lipid screening in males at age 35 and in females at age 45.
- The U.S. Preventive Services Task Force (USPSTF) recommends initiation of a statin in adults aged 40 to 75 years who have one or more CVD risk factor (e.g., dyslipidemia, diabetes, HTN) and an estimated 10-year CVD risk of 10% or greater.
- For adults age 76 years and older with no history of CVD, do not screen (insufficient evidence).

Total Cholesterol

- Normal: <200 mg/dL
- Borderline high: 201 to 239 mg/dL
- High: >240 mg/dL

High-Density Lipoprotein Cholesterol

- >40 mg/dL normal in men
- >50 mg/dL normal in women
- >60 mg/dL associated with lower risk of heart disease
- <40 mg/dL associated with increased risk of CAD even if normal low-density lipoprotein (LDL) or cholesterol. Genetic causes are probably the most common reason for low high-density lipoprotein cholesterol (HDL-C).
- Do not focus treatment on HDL-C alone (aim for lowering the LDL); little evidence between raising HDL-C and decreased rates of heart disease or stroke.
- Medications that increase high-density lipoprotein (HDL) include fibrates (gemfibrozil), niacin, and some high-dose statins. Although niacin can increase HDL (and decrease triglycerides), there is no data demonstrating that this effect confers a cardiovascular benefit. Low doses of niacin (vitamin B_3) in over-the-counter (OTC) multivitamins or B-complex vitamins have not been implicated.
- Lifestyle modifications include engaging in regular moderate cardiovascular/aerobic exercises most days of the week, losing weight, eating healthy fats (salmon, tuna, nuts), eliminating trans fats, and stopping smoking.

Low-Density Lipoprotein Cholesterol

- Optimal: <100 mg/dL
- LDL: <130 mg/dL for low-risk patients with fewer than two risk factors
- Heart disease or diabetes: <70 mg/dL

Triglycerides

- Normal level is <150 mg/dL.
- Hypertriglyceridemia is defined as a serum/plasma level of >150 mg/dL.
- Very high levels can be due to genetic (primary) and acquired (secondary) disorders; both often coexist.
- Possible causes are metabolic syndrome, DM, familial hypertriglyceridemia, alcohol use disorder, hyperthyroidism, kidney disease, medications.
- Medications that increase triglycerides include anabolic steroids, oral estrogens, diuretics, second-generation antipsychotics, glucocorticoids, antiretrovirals, tamoxifen, isotretinoin, nonselective beta-blockers (e.g., propranolol).
- High risk of acute pancreatitis if level ≥1,000 mg/dL.
- Lifestyle modifications include decreasing sugar and simple carbohydrates, avoiding alcoholic drinks, following low-fat diet, eating fish with omega-3 (salmon, sardines) twice a week, losing weight, and increasing aerobic-type physical activity.

Triglycerides >500 mg/dL

- Avoid alcohol if very high triglycerides because it can precipitate acute pancreatitis.
- Identify causation, such as certain medications (see the preceding list) and past medical history.
- In general, patients with hypertriglyceridemia also require lowering of low-density lipoprotein cholesterol (LDL-C) to reduce ASCVD risk. Most LDL-C–lowering drugs also reduce fasting triglyceride levels.

- Nonpharmacologic measures include managing HTN, smoking cessation, exercise, weight loss, diet modification, alcohol use cessation.
- For moderate hypertriglyceridemia (fasting triglyceride 150 to 499 mg/dL), add marine omega-3 fatty acid therapy for patients with high ASCVD risk
- For moderate to severe hypertriglyceridemia (fasting triglyceride 500 to 900 mg/dL), marine omega-3 fatty acid therapy for patients with high ASCVD risk and fibrate therapy (e.g., fenofibrate [Tricor], gemfibrozil [Lopid])
- For severe hypertriglyceridemia (fasting triglyceride ≥1,000 mg/dL), extreme dietary fat restriction, alcohol abstinence, and LDL-lowering therapy
- Niacin is not routinely used to treat patients with hypertriglyceridemia given limited benefit and risk of adverse effects.
- Statins are primarily used to reduce ASCVD risk but can have some triglyceride-lowering effects. High intensity satin therapy can lower triglyceride levels by 25% to 30% in patients with triglyceride levels <400 mg/dL.

CLINICAL PEARL

Diets that improve serum lipids are the Mediterranean diet, Dietary Approaches to Stop Hypertension (DASH) diet, vegetarian diet, low-carbohydrate diet, and low–trans-fatty acid diet.

Treatment Plan

- First-line treatment is lifestyle changes (exercise most days of the week, diet low in saturated fat, weight loss, smoking cessation), but in the presence of ASCVD and other factors, initiate statin therapy with lifestyle changes.
- Reduce dietary salt intake and learn about the DASH diet (low salt, low saturated fat <30%).
- Encourage use of soluble fiber in diet (e.g., inulin, guar gum, fruit, vegetables) to enhance lowering of LDL (lowers LDL by blocking absorption in GI tract up to 10%).
- For patients with hypertriglyceridemia, treatment includes assessment of ASCVD risk and management of LDL-C.
- Lipid abnormalities associated with increased risk of coronary heart disease (CHD): elevated total cholesterol and LDL cholesterol, low HDL cholesterol, and hypertriglyceridemia.
- Lifestyle modifications include decreasing sugar and simple carbohydrates, avoiding alcoholic drinks, following a low-fat diet, eating fish with omega-3 (salmon, sardines) twice a week, losing weight, and increasing aerobic-type physical activity.

American College of Cardiology and American Heart Association Updated Guidelines

The notes reflect the *2018 Guideline on the Management of Blood Cholesterol: Executive Summary* (a report of the ACC/AHA Task Force on Clinical Practice Guidelines). The current guideline does include content from the previous guideline (2014). See Table 7.4 for the summarized guideline and Table 7.5 for statin intensity dosages.

Table 7.4 ACC/AHA Updated Guideline on the Treatment of Blood Cholesterol (2018)

Characteristics	Statin Intensity
Clinical ASCVD	High intensity
Very high risk ASCVD*	High intensity
Severe primary hypercholesteremia with LDL >190 mg/dL	High intensity
Patient with diabetes age 50–75 years with LDL >70 mg/dL	High intensity
Patient with diabetes age 40–75 years with LDL >70 mg/dL	Moderate intensity
Patient age 40–75 years with 10-year ASCVD risk >7.5% with risk-enhancing factors	Moderate intensity
Patient age 40–75 years with 10-year ASCVD risk 7.5%–19.9% with risk-enhancing factors	Moderate intensity

*Defined as a history of multiple major ASCVD events or one major ASCVD event with multiple high-risk conditions.
ACC, American College of Cardiology; AHA, American Heart Association; ASCVD, atherosclerotic cardiovascular disease; HDL, high-density lipoprotein; LDL, low-density lipoprotein.

Table 7.5 Statin Intensity Dosages

High-Intensity Statins	Moderate-Intensity Statins	Low-Intensity Statins
Lower LDL ≥50% Atorvastatin (Lipitor) 40–80 mg/d* Rosuvastatin (Crestor) 20–40 mg/d	*Lower LDL 30%–50%* Atorvastatin 10–20 mg/d Rosuvastatin (Crestor) 5–10 mg/d Simvastatin (Zocor) 20–40 mg/d Pravastatin (Pravachol) 40–80 mg/d Lovastatin (Mevacor) 40 mg/d Fluvastatin 40 mg BID	*Lower LDL <30%* Simvastatin 10 mg/d Pravastatin 10–20 mg/d Lovastatin 20 mg/d Fluvastatin 20–40 mg/d

*Initiation at 80 mg/d is not recommended by the U.S. Food and Drug Administration; increases risk of myopathy/rhabdomyolysis. Start at lower dose and titrate up to 80-mg dose (if tolerated).
LDL, low-density lipoprotein.

Very High Risk for Future Atherosclerotic Cardiovascular Disease Events

- Recent ACS (within the past 12 months)
- History of MI
- History of ischemic stroke
- Symptomatic peripheral arterial disease (PAD; history of claudication with ankle-brachial index [ABI] <0.85 or previous revascularization or lower extremity amputation)
- High-risk conditions: age ≥65 years, heterozygous familial hypercholesterolemia, history of prior coronary artery bypass surgery or percutaneous coronary intervention, diabetes mellitus (DM), HTN, chronic kidney disease (CKD), current smoking, persistently elevated LDL-C despite maximal therapy, history of CHF

High-Risk Conditions

- Age ≥65 years
- History of prior coronary artery bypass surgery or percutaneous coronary intervention (PCI), CHF, HTN
- DM
- Current smoking
- CKD (estimated glomerular filtration rate [eGFR] 15–59 mL/min)
- Persistently elevated LDL of ≥100 mg/dL despite statin therapy and ezetimibe

Secondary Prevention (Presence of ASCVD)

Patients with any form of clinical ASCVD (history of MI, CAD, angina, stroke/TIA, PAD, coronary revascularization):

- Encourage high-intensity statin (or maximally tolerated statin therapy) and healthy lifestyle
- Decrease LDL level by 50%

Very high risk ASCVD (defined as a history of multiple major ASCVD events or one major ASCVD event with multiple high-risk conditions):

- High-intensity statin
- LDL goal of 70 mg/dL
- If already on high-intensity dose of statin and not at goal (LDL >70 mg/dL), add a non-statin such as ezetimibe/Zetia.
- If on statin and ezetimibe and LDL remains >70 mg/dL, adding a proprotein convertase subtilisin/kexin type 9 (PCSK9) inhibitor is reasonable (although long-term safety >3 years is unknown).

Diabetic patients with LDL of ≥70 mg/dL:

- Age 40 to 75 years, moderate-intensity statin therapy (without calculating 10-year ASCVD risk)
- Age 50 to 75 years, can use high-intensity statin to reduce LDL by 50% or more.
- Severe primary hypercholesterolemia (LDL of 190 mg/dL or higher):
- Age 20 to 75 years, high-intensity statin (without calculating 10-year ASCVD risk)
- If on high-intensity statin and LDL ≥100 mg/dL, add ezetimibe (Zetia).
- If multiple risk factors for ASCVD, consider adding a PCSK9 inhibitor to statin.

- Assess adherence and percentage response to LDL-lowering medications and lifestyle changes:
  - Repeat lipid measurement in 4 to 12 weeks after statin initiation or dose adjustment.
  - Repeat every 3 to 12 months as needed.

EXAM TIPS

- An adult (21–75 years) with any type of ASCVD (e.g., CAD, PAD, stroke, TIA) is given high-intensity statins such as atorvastatin 40 to 80 mg or rosuvastatin 20 to 40 mg.
- An adult with LDL >190 mg/dL (without ASCVD or DM) is a candidate for high-intensity statin dosing.

Primary Prevention (No ASCVD)

- If 10-year ASCVD risk of 7.5% or 19.9% (intermediate risk), age 40 to 75 years with LDL 70 mg/dL to 189 mg/dL (without DM): Assess risk-enhancing factors for ASCVD (Box 7.2). If decision to start statins uncertain, check the coronary artery calcium (CAC) score. If the CAC score is 1 to 99, favor starting statin therapy. Initiate moderate-intensity statin therapy to reduce LDL-C by 30%–49%.
- If 10-year ASCVD risk of 20% or higher (high risk), age 40 to 75 years with LDL 70 mg/dL to 189 mg/dL (without DM): Initiate statin therapy to reduce LDL-C by 50%.

When to Refer

Rule out familial hypercholesterolemia (FH) if presence of extensor tendon xanthomas (Achilles, subpatellar, or hand extensor tendons).

Box 7.2 Risk-Enhancing Factors for Atherosclerotic Cardiovascular Disease

- Family history of premature ASCVD
- Persistently elevated LDL-C levels of ≥160 mg/dL
- Metabolic syndrome
- Chronic kidney disease (CKD)
- History of preeclampsia or premature menopause (age <40 years)
- High-risk ethnic groups such as South Asian (from India, Pakistan, Sri Lanka, Nepal, Bangladesh)
- Chronic inflammatory disorders (e.g., psoriasis, RA, chronic HIV)
- Persistent triglyceride elevations
- Elevated C-reactive protein of ≥2.0 mg/L
- Ankle-brachial index (ABI) ≤0.9

ASCVD, atherosclerotic cardiovascular disease; LDL-C, low-density lipoprotein cholesterol; RA, rheumatoid arthritis.

Lipid-Lowering Medications
HMG-CoA Reductase Inhibitors (Statins)
- HMG-CoA reductase is the enzyme in the liver that is responsible for cholesterol synthesis. Statins inhibit this enzyme, which results in decreased lipoprotein production. HMG-CoA reductase inhibitors (statins) are best at lowering LDL, and some can increase HDL and decrease triglycerides at higher doses.
- Start at lower doses (if able) and titrate up slowly to the recommended dose to minimize adverse effects. Check baseline liver function testing before starting patient on statins. Some patients may not tolerate high-intensity statins (e.g., muscle pains, weakness) but can tolerate moderate-intensity statins.
- If patient is at very high risk for ASCVD or has severe primary hypercholesteremia (LDL >190 mg/dL) and is not at LDL goal, switch to high-dose statin. A PCSK9 inhibitor (Repatha, Praluent) can be used in the highest risk primary prevention patients who are not able to tolerate statin therapy.
- Examples include Pravastatin (Pravachol), lovastatin (Mevacor), simvastatin (Zocor), atorvastatin (Lipitor), rosuvastatin.
- With simvastatin and lovastatin drug interactions (high risk of rhabdomyolysis), avoid grapefruit juice; fibrates; antifungals (itraconazole, ketoconazole); macrolides (erythromycin, clarithromycin, telithromycin); amiodarone (Cordarone), some CCBs (diltiazem, amlodipine, verapamil)
- Combination regimens of a statin with ezetimibe (Zetia) or a PCSK9 inhibitor may be indicated if further reductions in LDL-C is needed.

Nicotinic Acid
- Nicotinic acid (niacin) is not routinely used for patients with elevated LDL-C. Niacin lowers lipoprotein(a) levels by about 25% and can be used in patients with lipoprotein(a) excess and hypercholesterolemia who have elevated LDL-C levels.
- Flushing occurs in 80% of patients and pruritis, paresthesia, and nausea occur in about 20%. Pre-administering aspirin or ibuprofen prior to dosing can minimize effects.
- Niacin can increase the risk of myopathy in patients receiving statins, as well as increase risk of hepatotoxicity.

Fibrates
- Gemfibrozil (Lopid), fenofibrate (Tricor), bezafibrate (Bezalip). Do not use with severe renal disease.
- Reduces production of triglycerides by the liver and increases production of HDL.
- Very good agents for lowering triglycerides by as much as 50% and elevating HDL level by 5% to 20%; however, not routinely recommended to lower LDL-C or to raise HDL-C in the absence of hypertriglyceridemia.
- Side effects include occasional increases in creatinine phosphokinases, myopathy, rhabdomyolysis (rare), drug-induced liver injury (monitor liver function panel).

Bile Acid Sequestrants
- Cholestyramine (Questran Light), colestipol (Colestid), colesevelam (Welchol)
- Work locally in the small intestine; interfere with fat absorption, including fat-soluble vitamins (vitamins A, D, E, and K)
- Alternative drug for patients who cannot tolerate statins, fibrates, and niacin
- If used alone, it is not as effective as statins in lowering LDL; no hepatotoxicity.
- Side effects include bloating, flatulence, abdominal pain; start at low doses and titrate up slowly. Side effects mainly from the GI tract; advise patient to take multivitamin tablets daily.

Cholesterol-Absorption Inhibitors
- Ezetimibe (Zetia); most commonly prescribed LDL-C lower agent after statins
- Absorbs cholesterol from the small intestines; combination of a statin with ezetimibe recommended for some patients
- Contraindications include active liver disease, unexplained persistent elevation of alanine aminotransferase (ALT) and aspartate aminotransferase (AST)
- Can be taken alone or combined with a statin or fibrate (e.g., simvastatin [Vytorin])
- Side effects include diarrhea, joint pains, tiredness

Proprotein Convertase Subtilisin/Kexin Type 9 Inhibitors
Human monoclonal antibodies that can decrease LDL by as much as 60%. Reduction of risk of MI, stroke, and unstable angina. Can be used alone or with other lipid-lowering therapies (statins, ezetimibe). Subcutaneous injection every 2 to 4 weeks. Current guidelines recommend adding PCSK9 to statins for patients at very high risk of ASCVD, recent ACS (within 12 months), multiple MIs, or strokes. Examples include evolocumab (Repatha), alirocumab (Praluent).

EXAM TIP

Educate patients to avoid alcohol and acetaminophen (hepatotoxic) use.

Complications of Lipid-Lowering Medications
Rhabdomyolysis
Acute breakdown and necrosis of skeletal muscle and the release of intracellular muscle components into the circulation. Often, causes acute kidney injury due to the nonprotein heme pigment that is released from either myoglobin or hemoglobin that is toxic to the kidney. Triad of muscle pain (myalgia), weakness, and red-to-brown urine. The muscles involved are usually the thighs, calves, shoulders, and lower back. Most common causes in adult include:

trauma, infections, drugs (illicit and prescribed), alcohol, and surgery. Most commonly prescribed medications associated with rhabdomyolysis are: lipid-lowering agents, psychiatric medications, certain antibiotics, antihistamines, and others (e.g., colchicine, glucocorticoids)

- Labs: Order creatine kinase if markedly elevated (at least five times the upper limit of normal from 1,500 to >100,000 IU/L).
- Urinalysis: Reddish-brown color (myoglobinuria) and proteinuria in up to 45%.
- Other labs: Include serum electrolytes, BUN, creatinine, LFTs (often elevated), and EKG.

Acute Drug-Induced Hepatitis

- Anorexia, nausea, dark-colored urine, jaundice, fatigue, flu-like symptoms
- Labs are elevated ALT and AST
- Discontinue statin and other hepatotoxic substances. Stop alcohol intake.
- Avoid prescribing statins to patients with alcoholism.
- Advise patient to report symptoms of hepatitis or rhabdomyolysis. If present, tell patient to stop the drug and call or go to ED.

CLINICAL PEARLS

- Statins may cause side effects, which are often reversible upon discontinuation of statin therapy. These include: hepatic and renal dysfunction, muscle injury, as well as behavioral and cognitive effects.
- Patients on simvastatin and lovastatin should avoid grapefruit juice. Also, they should not mix these two statins with macrolides.
- Muscle pain (mild to severe) from rhabdomyolysis is usually located on the calves, thighs, lower back, and/or shoulders. Urine will be darker than normal (reddish-brown color). Rule out rhabdomyolysis if patient on a statin complains of muscular pain with dark-colored urine.

HYPERTENSION

HTN is defined as a BP above 130/80 mmHg. The majority have primary (or essential) HTN. About 5% to 10% have secondary HTN. Nonpharmacologic treatment is now recommended for the majority of adults who are newly classified as having HTN. In the presence of risk factors (e.g., diabetes, CAD, HTN), pharmacologic therapy is recommended along with lifestyle changes.

The American Nurses Credentialing Center (ANCC) uses the treatment described in the 2017 ACC/AHA Guideline for Prevention, Detection, Evaluation, and Management of High Blood Pressure in Adults. In contrast, the American Academy of Nurse Practitioners Certification Board (AANPCB) uses both the 2017 ACA/AHA HTN treatment guideline and the older Joint National Committee (JNC) 8 guideline (available on my website: www.npreview.com). See Table 7.6.

Correct Blood Pressure Measurement

- Instruct patient to avoid smoking or caffeine intake 30 minutes before measurement and to not cross their legs (increases systolic blood pressure [SBP]).
- Begin BP measurement after at least 5 minutes of rest (mercury sphygmomanometer preferred over digital machines).
- Two or more readings separated by 2 minutes should be averaged per visit.
- Higher number determines BP stage (BP 140/100 is stage 2 instead of stage 1; Table 7.7).

Hypertension Screening

- Starting at age 18 years, screen BP every year. If normal BP, recheck in 1 year.
- If presence of risk factors for HTN, screen at least semi-annually (twice a year).

Blood Pressure, Peripheral Vascular Resistance, and Cardiac Output

Any change in the peripheral vascular resistance (PVR) or cardiac output (CO) results in a change in BP (increase/decrease). Examples include:

- Na+ (sodium): Water retention increases vascular volume, resulting in increased CO (BP increases).
- Angiotensin I to angiotensin II: Angiotensin II increases vasoconstriction and will increase PVR (BP increases).
- Sympathetic system stimulation: Epinephrine and cortisol secretion cause tachycardia and vasoconstriction (BP increases).
- Alpha-blockers, beta-blockers, CCBs: Drugs decrease PVR from vasodilation (BP decreases).

In pregnancy:

- Systemic vascular resistance is lowered because of hormones (BP declines during the first trimester and then slowly rises).
- HTN during pregnancy and preeclampsia are risk factors for future HTN and CVD. Preeclampsia is a potentially dangerous condition for the pregnant patient and fetus. As such, the USPSTF recommends screening all pregnant patients for preeclampsia by measuring BP at every prenatal visit.
- The S3 heart sound is common in the third trimester of pregnancy.
- Drugs used to control BP in pregnancy are methyldopa, nifedipine, and/or labetalol. ACE inhibitors, ARBs, or direct renin inhibitors should be avoided.

Labs

- Kidneys: Creatinine, eGFR, urinalysis, urinary albumin to creatinine ratio
- Endocrine: Thyroid-stimulating hormone (TSH), serum free T4, fasting blood glucose
- Serum electrolyte: Potassium (K^+), sodium (Na^+), calcium (Ca^{2+})

Table 7.6 Comparison of Treatment Guidelines for Hypertension

Recommendations	JNC 8 (2014)	ACC/AHA (2017/2018)
Initiation of pharmacologic therapy	Adults ≥60 years Initiate if SBP ≥150 or DBP ≥90 mmHg Goal: SBP <150, DBP <90	Recommended in patients with clinical CVD and in adults with estimated ASCVD risk of 10% or higher with an average SBP ≥130 mmHg and an average DBP ≥80 mmHg
	Adults <60 years Initiate if SBP ≥140 mmHg or DBP ≥90 mmHg Goal: SBP <140, DBP <90	Recommended in adults with no history of CVD and with an estimated 10-year ASVCD risk <10% and SBP ≥140 mmHg or DBP ≥90 mmHg
Patients with CKD	Adults ≥18 years Initiate if SBP ≥140 mmHg or DBP ≥90 mmHg Initial therapy: ACEI or ARB Goal: SBP <140, DBP <90	Initial therapy: ACEI (or ARB if not tolerated) Goal: 130/80
Patients with diabetes mellitus	Adults ≥18 years Initiate if SBP ≥140 mmHg or DBP ≥90 mmHg Goal: SBP <140, DBP <90	Initiate if BP ≥130/80 mmHg Goal: SBP <130, DBP <80 First line: Diuretic, ACEI, ARB, or CCB
Non-African American population	First line: Thiazide diuretic, CCB, ACEI, or ARB	First line: Thiazide diuretic, CCB, ACEI, or ARB
African American population	Initial therapy: Thiazide diuretic or CCB	Initial therapy: Thiazide diuretic or CCB

ACC, American College of Cardiology; ACEI, angiotensin-converting enzyme inhibitor; AHA, American Heart Association; ARB, angiotensin receptor blockers; ASCVD, atherosclerotic cardiovascular disease; CCB, calcium channel blocker; CKD, chronic kidney disease; CVD, cardiovascular disease; DBP, diastolic blood pressure; JNC, Joint National Committee; SBP, systolic blood pressure
Source: Data from Whelton et al. (2018); James (2014). (See Resources section for complete source information.)

Table 7.7 Blood Pressure Stages Based on 2017 ACA/AHA HTN Treatment Guideline

BP Category	SBP		DBP
Normal	<120 mmHg	*and*	<80 mmHg
Elevated	120–129 mmHg	*and*	<80 mmHg
Stage 1	130–139 mmHg	*or*	80–89 mmHg
Stage 2	140 mmHg or higher	*or*	90 mmHg or higher

ACC, American College of Cardiology; AHA, American Heart Association; BP, blood pressure; DBP, diastolic blood pressure; HTN, hypertension; SBP, systolic blood pressure.

- Heart: Cholesterol, HDL, LDL, triglycerides (complete lipid panel)
- Anemia: CBC
- To rule out cardiomegaly: Baseline EKG and chest x-ray
- Calculate: 10-year atherosclerotic CVD risk
- Echocardiography

How to Diagnose Hypertension

Diagnosis requires integration of multiple BP readings, the use of appropriate technique, and the use of measurements made outside of the usual office setting. While uncommon, HTN can be diagnosed in a patient who presents with hypertensive urgency or emergency (i.e., in patients with SBP ≥180 mmHg or diastolic blood pressure (DBP) ≥120 mmHg; or a patient who presents with an initial SBP ≥160 mmHg or DBP ≥100 mmHg with target end-organ damage. Diagnosis should be confirmed in all other patients using out-of-office BP measurements (suspected white coat syndrome). Ambulatory BP monitoring is considered the gold standard out-of-office BP measurement. Diagnosis is confirmed if mean home SBP is ≥130 mmHg or DBP ≥80 mmHg and validated in the office. Diagnosis can also be confirmed by at least three office-based BP measurements spaced over a period of time with a mean of SBP is ≥130 mmHg or DBP ≥80 mmHg.

Self-Measured Blood Pressure

Self-measured blood pressure (SMBP) is a useful adjunct to supplement office readings. Advise patient to buy an automatic BP machine. Advise patients to buy an appropriately sized BP cuff (patient should measure diameter of upper arm). If cuff is too small for arm, it will falsely elevate the BP. BP kiosk readings are acceptable. Advise patient to check BP at different times of the day and during work. Instruct patient to bring their BP diary during visits if titrating medications.

Evaluation of Hypertension: Rule Out Target Organ Damage

Look for the following clinical findings and complications of HTN.

Microvascular Damage

Eyes (hypertensive retinopathy; Figure 7.4):

- Mild: Generalized retinal arteriolar narrowing, arteriolar wall thickening, arteriovenous nicking ("nipping"), and opacification of the arteriolar wall ("copper wiring")
- Moderate: Hemorrhages, either flame or dot-shaped, cotton-wool spots, hard exudates, and microaneurysms
- Severe: The above symptoms plus optic disc edema (papilledema). Requires rapid lowering of BP.

Kidneys:

- Microalbuminuria and proteinuria
- Elevated serum creatinine, BUN, and abnormal eGFR
- Peripheral or generalized edema due to sodium and fluid retention

Macrovascular Damage

Heart:

- S3 (CHF)
- S4 (LVH)
- Heart failure (both reduced and preserved ejection fraction)
- Carotid bruits (narrowing due to plaque, increased risk of CAD)
- CAD and acute MI
- Decreased or absent peripheral pulses (PAD)
- Ischemic heart disease, including MI

Brain:

- Ischemic stroke, TIAs
- Intracerebral hemorrhage

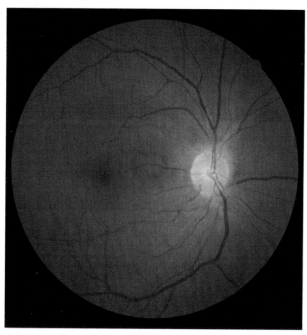

Figure 7.4 Hypertensive retinopathy with arteriovenous nicking.

Source: Image courtesy of Frank Wood.

Secondary Hypertension

In about 5% to 10% of patients with HTN, there is a secondary, specific, and remediable cause. If the condition is correctable and/or treatable, then the HTN will resolve. The causes of secondary HTN can be classified into three major groups:

1. Renal (renal artery stenosis, polycystic kidneys, primary kidney disease)
2. Endocrine (hyperthyroidism, primary aldosteronism, pheochromocytoma, Cushing's syndrome)
3. Other causes (obstructive sleep apnea, coarctation of the aorta, oral contraceptives, chemotherapeutic agents)

Renal artery stenosis is more common in younger adults. Middle-aged adults are more likely to have endocrine-related disorders. CKD is more common in older adult patients.

Rule out secondary cause and maintain a high index of suspicion if the following:

- Age younger than 30 years in patients without obesity with a negative family history and no risk factors for HTN
- Severe HTN or acute rise in BP (previously stable patient)
- Resistant HTN despite treatment with at least three antihypertensive agents
- Malignant HTN (severe HTN with end-organ damage such as retinal hemorrhages, papilledema, acute renal failure, and severe headache)

Other secondary causes include coarctation of the aorta and sleep apnea:

- Coarctation of the aorta is one of the major causes of secondary HTN in young children but is often detected in adulthood.
- Systolic BP is higher on the legs (normal finding) because it takes more force to circulate the blood back to the heart. But with coarctation of the aorta, the opposite is found. If there is a narrowed aorta in the abdomen (abdominal aorta), the part of the body above the narrowed aorta (the arms) will have higher BP and bounding pulses. The part of the body below the narrowed aorta (the legs) will have lesser blood flow, so the SBP on the legs will be lower, and the pulses will be weaker. Look for delayed or diminished femoral pulses (check both radial and femoral pulse at the same time and compare).
- With sleep apnea, sleep partner will report severe snoring with apneic episodes during sleep. Marked hypoxic episodes during sleep increase BP.

Clinical Findings of Secondary Hypertension

Kidneys

- Patients with CKD tend to be edematous due to sodium retention (high BP from fluid overload); edema typically resolves after fluid removal with diuretics. ACE inhibitor or ARB is first-line therapy for CKD patients with proteinuria (protein excretion above 500–1,000 mg/day).
- Bruit epigastric, abdomen, or flank area (renal artery stenosis)
- Enlarged kidneys with cystic renal masses (polycystic kidney)
- Increased creatinine and decreased eGFR (renal insufficiency to acute kidney failure), abnormal urinalysis

Endocrine

Primary hyperaldosteronism is also known as Conn syndrome. Aldosterone helps control BP by sodium retention and loss of potassium. The most common cause is an aldosterone-producing adenoma (usually benign) and, less commonly, adrenal cancer. Treatment is surgical removal of tumor.

- HTN with hypokalemia (low K+) usually the only sign of this condition (due to urinary potassium wasting).
- Normal to elevated sodium levels (high/normal Na+)

In hyperthyroidism, weight loss, tachycardia, fine tremor, moist skin, and anxiety are common symptoms. Check EKG for new onset of AF. Check TSH.

Pheochromocytoma is characterized by excessive secretion of catecholamines (severe HTN, arrhythmias); labile increase in BP accompanied by palpitations; and sudden onset of anxiety, sweating, and severe headache. Order plasma-free metanephrine (high-risk patient) or urine metanephrines fractionated (low risk).

Hypertensive Urgency

A hypertensive urgency is defined as an SBP >180 mmHg and/or DBP >120 mmHg without target organ damage (Table 7.8). A common reason is noncompliance with antihypertensive therapy. If there is no clinical (or laboratory) evidence of new or worsening target organ damage, restart or intensify antihypertensive drug therapy with close follow-up.

Hypertensive Emergency

A hypertensive emergency is defined as a SBP >180 mmHg and/or DBP >120 mmHg (see Table 7.8) with clinical findings of target organ damage, such as nausea and vomiting, increased intracranial pressure (ICP), cerebrovascular accident (CVA)/TIA, MI, acute PE, acute renal failure, retinopathy (flame-shaped hemorrhages), papilledema, or acute severe low-back pain (dissecting aorta). Call 911.

Masked Hypertension

Defined as office SBP 120 to 129 mmHg with normal DBP <80 mmHg after 3-month lifestyle modification trial, while daytime home measurement BP is 130/80 mmHg or higher.

Isolated Systolic Hypertension in the Older Adult

- Prevalence is as high as 70% to more than 80% in adults older than 60 to 65 years. Defined as SBP ≥160 mmHg with a DBP <90 mmHg.
- Caused by loss of recoil in the arteries (atherosclerosis), which increases PVR.

Table 7.8 Hypertensive Crises

Hypertensive Crises	SBP		DBP
Hypertensive urgency	>180 mmHg	and/or	>120 mmHg *without* target organ damage
Hypertensive emergency	>180 mmHg *plus* target organ damage	and/or	>120 mmHg *plus* target organ damage

DBP, diastolic blood pressure; SBP, systolic blood pressure.

- Pulse pressure (SBP–DBP) increases in this disorder due to diminished arterial compliance.
- Emphasize nonpharmacologic treatment, especially dietary salt restriction and weight loss as needed. Initiate drug therapy if lifestyle changes are not sufficient. Treat BP in older or frailer patients carefully; start at lower doses and titrate up slowly so that it takes about 3 to 6 months.
- Initial monotherapy with a low-dose thiazide diuretic, a CCB (long-acting dihydropyridine), or an ACEI or ARB.

Orthostatic Hypotension

Orthostatic and post-prandial hypotension are a result of autonomic dysfunction due to conditions that affect the central and peripheral nervous system, volume depletion, or the use of anti-hypertensives and other medications. Older adult patients are at higher risk for orthostatic hypotension due to a less active autonomic nervous system and slower metabolism of drugs by the liver (prolongs half-life of drugs). To evaluate for orthostatic hypotension:

- Check BP in supine, sitting, and standing positions.
- Diagnosis of a reduction of 20 mmHg or more in systolic pressure and/or a reduction of 10 mmHg or more in diastolic pressure within 2 to 5 minutes of standing (after a 5-minute period of supine rest).
- Ask patient if dizzy or lightheaded with changes in position.
- Check for polypharmacy, carefully review the medication history, and search for meds that lower BP.

EXAM TIPS

- Learn to distinguish the findings in hypertensive retinopathy (copper and silver wire arterioles, arteriovenous nicking) from those in diabetic retinopathy (neovascularization, cotton-wool spots, microaneurysms). Arteriovenous nicking occurs when a retinal vein is compressed by an arteriole that causes the venule to collapse.
- To assess orthostatic hypotension, measure after changing positions from supine, sitting, to standing.

Guidelines for the Prevention, Detection, Evaluation, and Management of High Blood Pressure in Adults*

Management

1. First, assess 10-year risk for heart disease using the ASCVD. Risk Estimator Plus calculator at http://tools.acc.org/ASCVD-Risk-Estimator-Plus/#!/calculate/estimate.
2. Reassess in 1 month for effectiveness of BP-lowering medication therapy.
3. If goal is met at 1 month, reassess in 3 to 6 months.

*Based on the 2017 ACC/AHA/AAPA/ABC/ACPM/ACS/APHA/ASH/ASPC/NMA/PCNA guidelines.

4. If goal is not met after 1 month, consider different medication or titration.

5. Continue with monthly follow-up until BP control is achieved.

Normal
- SBP <120 mmHg and DBP <80 mmHg
- Encourage heart-healthy lifestyle. Evaluate yearly.

Elevated
- SBP 120 to 129 mmHg and DBP <80 mmHg
- Recommend heart-healthy lifestyle and weight loss if needed. Reassess in 3 to 6 months.
- No more "prehypertension" stage; instead, it is known as *elevated BP*.

Hypertension: Stage 1
- SBP 130 to 139 mmHg or DBP 80 to 89 mmHg
- Goal BP <130/80 mmHg
- Clinical ASCVD or estimated 10-year CVD risk *less than 10%*, start with healthy lifestyle recommendations and reassess in 3 to 6 months.
- Risk greater than 10% or known clinical cardiovascular disease (or diabetes, CKD), lifestyle recommendations and BP-lowering medication. Re-assess in 1 month. If BP goal is met, assess and optimize adherence to therapy.

Hypertension: Stage 2
- SBP 140 mmHg or higher or DBP 90 mmHg or higher
- Goal BP <130/80 mmHg
- Lifestyle changes and BP-lowering medications (two medications of different classes). Reassess BP in 1 month.
- If goal is met after 1 month, reassess in 3 to 6 months.
- If goal is not met after 1 month, consider different medications or titration.
- Continue monthly follow-up until BP control is achieved.

EXAM TIPS

- In isolated systolic HTN in older adults, preferred medications are low-dose thiazide diuretic or CCB (long-acting dihydropyridine).
- Memorize the side effects of diuretics.

Lifestyle Modifications
First-line therapy for HTN, hyperlipidemia, and type 2 DM:
- Lose weight if body mass index [BMI] over 25 kg/m².
- Stop smoking. Reduce stress level.
- Reduce dietary sodium to <1.5 g per day (1,500 mg/d).
- Maintain adequate dietary intake of potassium (>3,500 mg/day) in patients with normal kidney function.
- Limit alcohol intake to 1 ounce (30 mL), up to two drinks or less per day for men; 0.5 ounce, up to one drink or less per day for women.
- Eat fruits and vegetables, as well as low-fat dairy products, selected fish and meats, nuts, and soy products.

DASH Diet (Dietary Approaches to Stop Hypertension)
Recommended for elevated BP and HTN. Goal is to eat foods rich in potassium, magnesium, and calcium. Reduce red meat and processed foods. Eat more whole grains and legumes. Eat more fish and poultry. This diet is high in fruits and vegetables, has moderate low-fat dairy, and is low in animal protein.
- Grains: Seven to eight daily servings
- Fruits and vegetables: Four to five daily servings
- Nuts, seeds, and dry beans: Four to five servings per week
- Fats, oils, or fat-free dairy products: Two to three daily servings
- Meat, poultry, and fish: Two or fewer daily servings
- Sweets: Try to limit to fewer than five servings per week
- Avoid high-sodium foods: Cold cuts, ready-made foods, any pickled foods (cucumbers, eggs, pork parts)

Dietary Sources of Minerals
- Calcium (low-fat dairy)
- Potassium (most fruits and vegetables)
- Magnesium (dried beans, whole grains, nuts)
- Omega-3 oils (anchovy, krill, salmon, flaxseed)

Exercise
Advise that aerobic physical activity will reduce LDL cholesterol and BP.
- Frequency: Three or four sessions per week
- Intensity: Moderate to vigorous (50%–80% of exercise capacity)
- Duration: 40 minutes average
- Modalities: Walking, treadmill, cycling, rowing, stair climbing; include resistance exercises for 2 to 3 days (e.g., elastic bands, weight machines, dumbbells)

Antihypertensive Medications
Diuretics
- Diuretics reduce sodium reabsorption at various sites in the nephron, which increases urinary sodium and water losses. Provides a decrease in blood volume, venous pressure, and preload (cardiac filling).
- Four major classes based on the site in which they act: thiazide-type, loop, potassium-sparing, and diuretics that act in the proximal tubule (e.g., acetazolamide, mannitol). Monitor electrolytes, especially sodium (Na+) and potassium (K+).

Thiazide Diuretics
- Control BP by inhibiting reabsorption of sodium and chloride ions in the distal tubules of the kidneys.
- Have a favorable effect with osteopenia/osteoporosis (slows down demineralization) by slowing down calcium excretion by the kidneys.
- Can cause photosensitivity reaction (avoid sunlight).
- All thiazides contain sulfa compounds. Avoid if patient has a sulfa allergy.

Side Effects

"Hyper":

- Hyperglycemia (use caution in patients with diabetes)
- Hyperuricemia (can precipitate a gout attack; contraindicated in gout)
- Hypertriglyceridemia and hypercholesteremia (check lipid profile)

"Hypo":

- Hypokalemia (potentiates digoxin toxicity, increases risk of arrhythmias)
- Hyponatremia (hold diuretic, restrict water intake, replace K+ loss)
- Hypomagnesemia

Contraindications

- Gout
- Hypotension
- Hypokalemia
- Renal failure
- Lithium treatment
- Sensitivity to sulfa drugs and thiazides

Examples

- Hydrochlorothiazide 12.5 to 25 mg PO daily
- Chlorthalidone (Hygroton) 12.5 to 25 mg PO daily
- Indapamide (Lozol) PO daily
- Chlorothiazide (Diuril) daily or divided dose

Loop Diuretics

Inhibit the sodium–potassium–chloride pump of the kidney in the loop of Henle.

Side Effects

- Hypokalemia (potentiates digoxin toxicity, increases risk of arrhythmias)
- Hyponatremia (hold diuretic, restrict water intake, replace K+ loss)
- Hypomagnesemia
- Possibly altered excretion of lithium and salicylates

Contraindications

- Anuria (kidney failure)
- Sensitivity to loop diuretics

Examples

- Furosemide (Lasix) PO twice a day (BID)
- Bumetanide (Bumex) PO BID

Sulfa Allergy and Diuretics

If patients are allergic to sulfa, they may have cross-sensitivity to loop diuretics and other diuretics (including thiazides and carbonic anhydrase inhibitors, such as acetazolamide). Other drugs with sulfa are sulfonylureas, sulfa antibiotics, sulfasalazine, and some protease inhibitors (darunavir, fosamprenavir). May also be sensitive to topical sulfas (ophthalmic drops) or topical silver sulfadiazine (Silvadene).

Aldosterone Receptor Antagonist Diuretics

- Action: Spironolactone antagonizes the action of aldosterone. Increases elimination of water in the kidneys and conserves potassium. Drug class also known as *mineralocorticoid receptor antagonists* or *antimineralcorticoids*.
- Indications: Resistant HTN, heart failure, hirsutism, acne, precocious puberty, primary aldosteronism
- Risk of hyperkalemia: Increased in combination with ACEIs, ARBs, potassium supplements, or NSAIDs. Monitor carefully for hyperkalemia and avoid combination therapy if possible.

Side Effects

- Gynecomastia, galactorrhea
- Hyperkalemia
- Gastrointestinal (GI; vomiting, diarrhea, stomach cramps), postmenopausal bleeding, erectile dysfunction

Contraindications

- Hyperkalemia (serum potassium >5.5 mEq/L)
- Renal insufficiency (serum creatinine >2.0 mg/dL in men or >1.8 mg/dL for women)
- Type 2 DM with microalbuminuria

Examples

- Spironolactone (Aldactone) daily
- Eplerenone (Inspra) daily

EXAM TIPS

- A side effect of spironolactone is gynecomastia; usually reversible after discontinuation of therapy.
- Women with HTN and osteopenia/osteoporosis should receive thiazides. Thiazides help bone loss by slowing down calcium loss (from the bone) and stimulating osteoclasts.

Beta-Blockers

- Action: Binds with beta-receptors on the heart and peripheral blood vessels. Decreases vasomotor activity, decreases CO, and inhibits renin (kidneys) and norepinephrine release.
- Two types of beta-receptors in the body: B1 (cardiac effects) and B2 (e.g., lungs, vascular smooth muscle).
- Avoid abrupt discontinuation after chronic use: Acute withdrawal can lead to increased sympathetic activity. Wean slowly. May precipitate angina and MI.

Contraindications

- Asthma, COPD, chronic bronchitis, emphysema (chronic lung disease)
- Second- and third-degree heart block (okay to use with first-degree block)
- Sinus bradycardia

Other Uses

- Acute MI: Reduces mortality during acute MI and post-MI
- Migraine headache: For prophylaxis only (not for acute attacks)
- Glaucoma: Reduces intraocular pressure (Betimol ophthalmic drops for open-angle glaucoma)
- Tachycardia: Target heart rate <100 beats/min
- Angina pectoris: Treats symptoms
- Post-MI: Decreases mortality
- Hyperthyroidism/thyroid storm and pheochromocytoma: Controls symptoms until primary disease is treated
- Essential tremor: Treat symptoms with nonselective beta-blocker propranolol

Examples

- Beta-blockers: Ends with -olol
- Cardioselective beta-blockers (B1 receptors): Atenolol (Tenormin), metoprolol (Lopressor), bisoprolol (Zebata)
- Nonselective beta-blockers (inhibits both B1 and B2 receptors): Propranolol (Inderal), timolol, pindolol
- Some beta-blockers have both alpha- and beta-blocking action: Labetalol (Normodyne) and carvedilol (Coreg)

Calcium Channel Blockers

- CCBs are used to treat HTN, angina, and arrhythmias.
- Block voltage-gated calcium channels in cardiac smooth muscle and the blood vessels. Results in systemic vasodilation.
- The non-dihydropyridines (e.g., verapamil, diltiazem) are less potent vasodilators but have greater depressive effect on cardiac conduction and contractility (negative inotropic effect).
- The dihydropyridines (e.g., nifedipine, nicardipine) are potent vasodilators with little to no negative impact on contractility or conduction.

Side Effects

- Headaches (due to vasodilation)
- Ankle edema (caused by vasodilation and considered benign)
- Heart block or bradycardia (depresses cardiac muscle and AV node)
- Reflex tachycardia (seen with dihydropyridines such as nifedipine)
- Constipation (seen with non-dihydropyridines)

Contraindications

- Sick sinus syndrome
- Second- and third-degree heart block (okay to use with first-degree block)
- Bradycardia
- HFrEF

Examples

- Dihydropyridine CCBs (-pine ending): Nifedipine (Procardia XL) daily; amlodipine (Norvasc) daily; felodipine (Plendil) daily
- Non-dihydropyridine CCBs: Verapamil (Calan SR) daily or BID; diltiazem (Cardizem CD) daily

Angiotensin-Converting Enzyme Inhibitors and Angiotensin Receptor Blockers

- ACEIs: Inhibit activity of angiotensin-converting enzyme, which decreases conversion of angiotensin I to II (more potent vasoconstrictor)
- ARBs: Block the effect of angiotensin II
- Preferred drugs (monotherapy or combined with other drug classes) for: Diabetes, CKD, congestive HFrEF, and after MI, especially those with heart failure or reduced systolic function

EXAM TIPS

- Use ACEIs or ARBs for DM, CKD, and heart failure. May cause a dry cough.
- Become familiar with dietary sources of magnesium, potassium, and calcium.

Pregnancy Category C (First Trimester) and Category D (Second and Third Trimesters)

Fetal kidney malformations, fetal hypotension, fetal death

Side Effects

- Dry hacking cough (occurs in 5%–20% of patients with ACEIs; about one third as many patients treated with ARBs)
- Hyperkalemia, angioedema (rare but may be life-threatening)

Contraindications

- Both ACEI and ARBs are contraindicated in pregnancy
- Patients who are on both ACEI and ARB are at a higher risk for adverse effects; thus, combined therapy should not be considered in the treatment of HTN.
- Renal artery stenosis precipitates acute renal failure if given ACEI or ARB
- Hyperkalemia is also a side effect of ACEIs and ARBs; combined will have additive effect

Examples

- ACEIs: Ramipril (Altace) once a day in one or two divided doses; benazepril (Lotensin) once a day initially; enalapril (Vasotec) once a day in one or two divided doses; fosinopril (Monopril) once a day
- ARBs: Losartan (Cozaar) once a day in one or two divided doses; candesartan (Atacand) once a day in one or two divided doses; olmesartan (Benicar) once a day in one or two divided doses; ibesartan (Avapro) once a day
- Combination antihypertensive drugs: ACEIs or ARBs are combined with other drug classes such as CCBs or thiazide diuretics

EXAM TIPS

- In bilateral renal artery stenosis, ACEIs or ARBs will precipitate acute renal failure.
- Avoid combining ACEIs with potassium-sparing diuretics (e.g., triamterene, spironolactone) because of increased risk of hyperkalemia.

Alpha-1 Blockers/Antagonists
- Also known as *alpha-adrenergic blockers*; suffix of *-zosin*.
- Potent vasodilators
- Not a first-line choice for HTN; consider in male patients with both HTN and benign prostatic hyperplasia (BPH). Alpha-blockers relax smooth muscle found on the bladder neck and prostate gland and relieve obstructive voiding symptoms such as weak urinary stream, urgency, and nocturia.
- Give at bedtime. Start at very low doses and titrate up slowly until good BP control. Advise patient to get out of bed slowly to prevent postural hypotension.

Side Effects
- "First-dose orthostatic hypotension" is common (warn patient).
- Side effects are dizziness and postural hypotension (common side effect).
- May cause severe hypotension and reflex tachycardia.

Examples
- Terazosin (Hytrin): Used for both HTN and BPH (starting dose 1 mg PO at bedtime)
- Doxazosin (Cardura): Used for both HTN and BPH
- Tamsulosin (Flomax): Used for BPH only

EXAM TIP

Alpha-blockers are not first-line drugs for HTN, except if patient has preexisting BPH.

Direct Renin Inhibitors
- Inhibit the renin-angiotensin system (RAS) by blocking renin. Reduces renin activity by about 75%.
- Do not combine aliskiren (Tekturna) with ACEI or ARB (higher risk hyperkalemia). May be used as third-line agent in patients who do not tolerate ACEI or ARBs.
- Avoid in pregnancy.

Examples
- Aliskiren (Tekturna) once a day
- Aliskiren and hydrochlorothiazide once a day

Angiotensin Receptor-Neprilysin Inhibitors (ARNIs)
- New drug class for the treatment of HFrEF
- Combination of neprilysin inhibitor (sacubitril) with ARB (valsartan)

Example
- Sacubitril/valsartan (Entresto)
- See Table 7.9 for a summary of antihypertensive drugs and their side effects.

Goals of Pharmacology Therapy
Goal of medication therapy is to prescribe the least number of medications possible at the lowest dosage to attain and maintain goal BP. First-line agents include thiazide diuretics, CCBs, ACEI, or ARBs (according to 2017 ACC/AHA Guidelines).

- Can initiate with one or two antihypertensive medications (combined or two separate agents). Treatment goal for initial treatment is 1 month; then increase dose, followed by adding a second drug. Continue to assess month until goal BP is reached.
- Referral to cardiology may be indicated for patients unable to attain goal BP, as well as for patients with multiple comorbidities.

Special Considerations According to 2017 ACC/AHA Guidelines
- Adults with HFrEF and HTN should be prescribed GDMT (Guideline-directed Medical Therapy; diuretics, beta-blockers, ACEI, or ARBs) titrated to attain a BP less than 130/80 mmHg. Non-dihydropyridine CCBs are not recommended.
- With DM, all first-line classes (e.g., diuretics, ACEIs, ARBs, CCBs) are useful and effective for a BP goal 130/80 or less.
- In CKD, ACEI (or ARB if not tolerated) for BP goal less than 130/80 mmHg.
- For African Americans (including patients with DM), thiazides or CCBs may be more effective.
- See Table 7.10 for more information.

CLINICAL PEARLS

- For BP control, most patients may require at least two medications in addition to lifestyle modifications.
- About 5% to 20% of patients on ACEIs will develop a dry cough.
- ACEI cough is more common in women.

MITRAL VALVE PROLAPSE
The classic finding is mid-systolic or non-ejection click accompanied by a late systolic or holosystolic murmur (murmur of MR). Patients with mitral valve prolapse (MVP) are at higher risk for severe MR, bacterial endocarditis, and arrhythmias. Best diagnostic test is transthoracic 3D echocardiography (3D-TTE). Patients with symptoms and auscultatory features of MVP have MVP syndrome.

Classic Case
Tall, thin adult female patient complains of fatigue, palpitations, and lightheadedness (orthostatic hypotension) that is aggravated by heavy exertion. The patient may have dyspnea, dizziness, exercise intolerance, panic, and anxiety disorders. May have atypical or nonanginal chest pain. Dyspnea is the most common symptom. Often, patients are asymptomatic. Rule out Marfan's syndrome if patient with pectus excavatum, hypermobility of the joints, and arm span greater than height.

Treatment Plan
- Asymptomatic MVP often does not require treatment. MVP is usually benign.
- Lifestyle changes include avoiding caffeine and stimulants, alcohol, and cigarettes; aerobic exercise training; reducing stress.

Table 7.9 Antihypertensive Drugs and Side Effects*

Drug Class	Examples	Side Effects/Notes
Alpha-adrenergic antagonists (alpha-blockers)	Doxazosin Prazosin Terazosin	Orthostatic hypotension
Angiotensin-converting enzyme inhibitors	Benazepril Enalapril Lisinopril Ramipril	Dry cough, angioedema, hyperkalemia Careful with CKD, renovascular disease Do not use during pregnancy
Angiotensin-receptor blockers	Candesartan Irbesartan Losartan Valsartan	Hyperkalemia Do not use during pregnancy
Angiotensin receptor–nephrilysin inhibitors	Sacubitril with valsartan (Entresto)	Hypotension, hyperkalemia, cough, angioedema
Beta-adrenergic antagonists (beta-blockers)	Alpha-beta blockade: Carvedilol, labetalol Beta selective: Atenolol, metoprolol Non–beta selective: Propranolol, nadolol	Bradycardia, fatigue, insomnia, erectile dysfunction, bronchospasm (asthma, COPD)
Dihydropyridine CCBs	Amlodipine Felodipine Nicardipine Long-acting nifedipine Nisoldipine	Headache, flushing, tachycardia, dose-dependent pedal edema Short-acting agents can cause reflex tachycardia
Loop diuretics	Bumetanide Furosemide Torsemide	Hypokalemia, hyponatremia, hyperuricemia, dehydration
Nondihydropyridine CCBs	Diltiazem Verapamil	Worsening cardiac output, bradycardia, constipation
Potassium-sparing diuretics	Aldosterone antagonists: spironolactone, eplerenone Amiloride Triamterene	Hyperkalemia, hyponatremia, dehydration
Thiazide diuretics	Chlorthalidone Hydrochlorothiazide Indapamide	Hypokalemia, hyponatremia, hyperuricemia, hypercalcemia, dehydration

*Not an all-inclusive list.
CCB, calcium channel blocker; CKD, chronic kidney disease; COPD, chronic obstructive pulmonary disease.

Table 7.10 Compelling Indications and Recommended Drug Classes

Condition	Recommended Drug Class
Diabetes mellitus	ACEI,*† ARB, thiazide diuretic,*† dihydropyridine CCB*
Chronic kidney disease (eGFR <60 mL/min)	ACEI,*† ARB
Heart failure with reduced ejection fraction	Diuretics, ARNI, ACEI,*† ARB, BB
After acute myocardial infarction	BB, ACEI,*† aldosterone

*High coronary artery disease (CAD) risk.
†High risk for recurrent stroke.
ACEI, angiotensin-converting enzyme inhibitor; ARB, angiotensin receptor blocker; ARNI, angiotensin receptor-nephrilysin inhibitor; BB, beta-blocker; CCB, calcium channel blocker; eGFR, estimated glomerular filtration rate.

- MVP with palpitations can be treated with beta-blockers.
- Echocardiography recommended for patients with clinical exam suggestive of MVP or those with family history of MVP.

OBESITY

All patients should have their BMI and, if indicated, abdominal obesity calculated (Table 7.11). Evaluate for metabolic syndrome and type 2 DM. In the United States, more than one third (39.8%) of adults have obesity (18.5% youth). As of 2015 and 2016 (latest data), the prevalence of obesity in men age 40 to 59 is 40.8% and in women aged 40 to 59 is 44.7%. Hispanic (47%) and non-Hispanic Black (46.8%) people have a higher prevalence of obesity compared with non-Hispanic White people (37.9%). The prevalence of obesity in Canada is rising. By 2016, more

Table 7.11 Body Mass Index

Classification	BMI
Underweight	<18.5
Normal weight	18.5–24.9
Overweight	25–29.9
Obese	≥30

BMI, body mass index.
Source: Data from Centers for Disease Control and Prevention.

than 22% of men and 20% of women had obesity. Nauru (Oceania) has the highest obesity rate in the world at 61% (2016).

Obesity may increase risk of mortality and other health risks, including type 2 DM, HTN, dyslipidemia, CHD, sleep apnea, and decreased mobility.

Abdominal Obesity
The "apple-shaped" body type is considered more dangerous for health compared to the "pear-shaped" body type.

Waist Circumference
- Males: ≥40 inches (102 cm)
- Females: ≥35 inches (88 cm)

Treatment Plan
- Dietary therapy and lifestyle and behavioral modifications for weight management.
- There are many "dietary" methods (e.g., Weight Watchers, keto, Nutrisystem, Atkins) and apps (e.g., Noom, Weight Watchers) that help promote weight loss. It depends on patient preferences.
- Meal delivery services (e.g., Blue Apron, Hello Fresh, Green Chef) can deliver fresh meals to homes. They make cooking easier because the ingredients are provided, although the cost may be prohibitive.
- Forty minutes of moderate to vigorous physical activity at least three to four times per week. Walking 10,000 steps per day is a popular method of exercise. Use of smart watches that track steps and exercise is helpful.
- There are many online social support group sites for weight loss on the internet.
- Therapies *not recommended* by experts are liposuction (it does not improve insulin sensitivity or risk factors for heart disease), herbal dietary supplements, and very-low-calorie diets (<1,000 kcal/day).

PERIPHERAL ARTERIAL DISEASE
Gradual (decades) narrowing and/or occlusion of medium-to-large arteries in the lower extremities. Blood flow to the extremities gradually decreases over time; patient may present with no symptoms or signs suggestive of ischemic damage secondary to arterial insufficiency (gangrene of the toes/foot). Higher risk with HTN, smoking, diabetes, male sex, hyperlipidemia, and family history of atherosclerosis.

Classic Case
Older patient who has a history of smoking and hyperlipidemia complains of worsening pain on ambulation (intermittent claudication) that is instantly relieved by rest. Over time, symptoms worsen until the patient's walking distance is greatly limited. Atrophic skin changes. Some have skin discoloration/gangrene on one or more toes or a nonhealing wound/ulcer. May complain of ischemic rest pain that involves the digits and forefoot and typically occurs at night. Often, report physical inactivity and alterations in pain perception.

Objective Findings
- Skin: Atrophic changes (shiny and hyperpigmented ankles that are hairless and cool to the touch); extremity ulcerations, dry or wet gangrene of the toe(s) or part of foot
- Cardiovascular: Decreased-to-absent dorsal pedal pulse (may include popliteal and posterior tibial pulse), increased capillary refill time (>3 seconds), and bruits over partially blocked arteries

Ankle-Brachial Index
ABI is used to evaluate severity of PAD and is predictive of CHD and cerebrovascular disease. For most patients, a score of ≤0.9 is diagnostic for PAD. In general, ABI score of 0.91 to 1.3 excludes significant occlusive arterial disease.

To measure ABI in each lower extremity:
- The patient should rest for 15 to 30 minutes prior to measuring the ankle pressure.
- Measure the dorsalis pedis and posterior tibial artery pressures at the ankle using the continuous wave Doppler. Repeat the process for both lower extremities.
- Measure the systolic brachial artery pressure bilaterally around the upper arm and using the continuous wave Doppler.
- Divide the higher ankle pressure (dorsalis pedis or posterior tibial artery) in each lower extremity by the higher of the two brachial artery systolic pressures.

Treatment Plan
- Goal to lower risk of cardiovascular disease progression and complications.
- Encourage smoking cessation (smoking causes vasoconstriction) and daily ambulation with exercise therapy.
- Pharmacologic therapy to improve walking includes cilostazol (Pletal), a phosphodiesterase inhibitor (direct vasodilator); can be taken with aspirin or clopidogrel. Grapefruit juice, diltiazem, and omeprazole can increase serum concentration if taken together. Pentoxifylline (Trental) is another option but effect is marginal (compared with cilostazol).
- Options for revascularization (if indicated for severe cases) include percutaneous angioplasty or surgical bypass.

Complications
- Gangrene of foot and/or lower limb with amputation
- Increased risk of CAD and cardiac disease progression
- Increased risk of carotid plaquing (check for carotid bruits)

PULSUS PARADOXUS

Defined as a fall in SBP of more than 10 mmHg during the inspiratory phase. Also known as a *paradoxical pulse*. It is an important physical sign of cardiac tamponade. Certain pulmonary and cardiac conditions that impair diastolic filling can cause an exaggerated decrease of the intrathoracic pressure during inspiration.

Pulmonary Cause

Asthma, emphysema (increased positive pressure)

Cardiac Cause

Cardiac tamponade, pericarditis, cardiac effusion (decreases movement of left ventricle)

RAYNAUD'S PHENOMENON

Reversible vasospasm of the peripheral arterioles on the fingers and toes due to an exaggerated response to cold temperature or emotional stress. Cause is unknown. Associated with an increased risk of autoimmune disorders (e.g., thyroid disorder, pernicious anemia, rheumatoid arthritis). Most patients are females, younger age groups, and have family members with Raynaud's. Patients with no underlying disease have "primary" Raynaud's phenomenon. Secondary Raynaud's phenomenon occurs in patients with concurrent autoimmune disease such as lupus erythematosus and scleroderma. Spontaneous remission of Raynaud's phenomenon may occur. During evaluation, check distal pulses, sensory perception, and ischemic signs (ischemic ulcers at the fingers/toes).

Classic Case

A middle-aged woman complains of chronic and recurrent episodes of color changes on her fingertips in a symmetric pattern (both hands and both feet). The colors range from white (pallor) and blue (cyanosis) to red (reperfusion). Complains of numbness and tingling. Attacks last for several hours. Hands and feet become numb with very cold temperatures. Some have livedo reticularis, which is violaceous mottling or reticular pattern of the skin of the arms and legs. Ischemic changes may be present after a severe episode such as shallow ulcers (that eventually heal) on some of the fingertips.

Treatment Plan

- Avoid touching cold objects and being in cold weather; avoid stimulants (e.g., caffeine). Maintain whole body warmth. Use thermal underwear, layered clothing, hat, gloves/mittens, and hand warmers.
- Smoking cessation is important and management of emotional stress.

- Initial pharmacologic therapy includes CCBs (e.g., nifedipine [Adalat], amlodipine [Norvasc]). Alternative options include phosphodiesterase type 5 inhibitors, topical nitrates, losartan, or fluoxetine.
- Avoid vasoconstricting drugs (e.g., sumatriptan, ergots, pseudoephedrine/decongestants, amphetamines; agent used to treat attention-deficit hyperactivity disorder).

Complications

Small ulcers in the fingertips and toes

EXAM TIPS

- Think of the colors of the American flag as a reminder for Raynaud's phenomenon. Medications include CCBs (nifedipine, amlodipine).
- Learn the definition of pulsus paradoxus.

SUPERFICIAL THROMBOPHLEBITIS

Inflammation of a superficial vein and confirmed thrombosis. Higher risk with varicose veins, vein excision/ablation, pregnancy and estrogen therapy, prior vein thrombosis, and malignancy and hypercoagulable states. Some patients may have coexistent DVT.

Classic Case

Adult patient complains of an acute onset of an indurated vein (localized redness, swelling, and tenderness). Usually located on the extremities. The patient is afebrile with normal vital signs.

Objective Findings

- Indurated cord-like vein that is warm and tender to the touch with a surrounding area of erythema.
- Often, a palpable nodular cord due to thrombus within affected vein.
- Degree of inflammation varies depending on the length of the vein affected.

Treatment Plan

- Supportive measures for uncomplicated phlebitis: Administer NSAIDs, such as ibuprofen or naproxen sodium (Anaprox DS)
- Warm compresses. Elevate limb.
- Ultrasound if suspected thrombus to rule out presence of coexistent DVT.
- Consider anticoagulation based on patient's risk for VTE.

KNOWLEDGE CHECK: CHAPTER 7

1. What is the *most* common cause of death for people with diabetes mellitus?
   A. Unintentional injuries or accidents
   B. Pancreatic cancer
   C. Cardiovascular disease
   D. Hypoglycemia

2. According to the Virchow triad, which of the following contributes to development of a venous thromboembolism?
   A. Presence of telangiectasias
   B. Venous stasis
   C. Hypocoagulability
   D. Vasodilation

3. A patient presents for a routine check-up complaining of mild symptoms such as fatigue and dyspnea while walking or climbing stairs rapidly. The patient reports a slight limitation of physical activity but feels comfortable at rest. These symptoms suggest which of the following New York Heart Association (NYHA) Functional Classifications of heart failure?
   A. I
   B. II
   C. III
   D. IV

4. The echocardiogram of a patient with heart failure with left ventricular (LV) dysfunction reveals an ejection fraction (EF) of 55%. This constitutes which of the following?
   A. Heart failure with preserved ejection fraction (HFpEF)
   B. Heart failure with mid-range ejection fraction (HFmrEF)
   C. Right-sided heart failure
   D. Heart failure with reduced ejection fraction (HFrEF)

5. An older adult male patient with past medical history significant for tobacco use presents for a routine physical examination. A pulsatile abdominal mass is palpated on routine physical examination. The patient denies any symptoms. Which of the following is the recommended initial diagnostic modality based on this patient presentation?
   A. CT of the abdomen
   B. MRI
   C. Focused Assessment with Sonography in Trauma (FAST) exam
   D. Abdominal ultrasound

6. Which of the following is the *most* common microbial cause of infective endocarditis in the United States and most developed countries?
   A. *Pseudomonas aeruginosa*
   B. *Staphylococcus aureus*
   C. *Escherichia coli*
   D. *Klebsiella pneumoniae*

7. In which of the following scenarios is antibiotic prophylaxis indicated for the prevention of infective endocarditis?
   A. A patient with a prosthetic heart valve receiving placement of orthodontic brackets
   B. A cardiac transplant recipient with no cardiac valvopathy who plans to have a tooth extracted
   C. A patient with previous infective endocarditis who plans to have a dental abscess drained
   D. A patient with a ventricular assist device who presents with bleeding from trauma to the oral mucosa

8. A patient presents with feelings of palpitations, fatigue, dizziness, and mild dyspnea. A 12-lead EKG is obtained, revealing an irregularly irregular ventricular rhythm with absent P waves. This finding suggests which cardiac arrhythmia?
   A. Atrial fibrillation
   B. Paroxysmal supraventricular tachycardia
   C. Sinus arrhythmia
   D. First-degree heart block

(See answers next page.)

1. C) Cardiovascular disease

Diabetes mellitus is a significant risk factor for cardiovascular disease, which is the most common cause of death among adults with diabetes mellitus.

2. B) Venous stasis

The Virchow triad proposes that venous thromboembolism is a result of alterations in blood flow (e.g., stasis), vascular endothelial injury, and alterations in the components of the blood (e.g., inherited or acquired hypercoagulable state). Telangiectasias are superficial "spider veins" that do not cause deep vein or superficial thrombosis. Hypocoagulability would contribute to bleeding rather than embolism. Vasodilation—the widening of blood vessels—increases blood flow, which is typically not a condition contributing to thrombus formation and is not a part of Virchow's triad.

3. B) II

The NYHA Functional Classification is used to describe the functional status of patients with heart failure, with severity ranging from Class I to Class IV. Class I is characterized by no symptoms and no limitation in physical activity; Class II involves mild symptoms and slight limitation during ordinary activity; Class III involves marked limitation in activity due to symptoms (even when walking short distances) but comfort at rest; Class IV is characterized by severe limitations and experiencing symptoms at rest.

4. A) Heart failure with preserved ejection fraction (HFpEF)

Heart failure caused by LV dysfunction is categorized by LV EF: HFrEF is defined as an EF of 40% or less (also known as systolic heart failure); heart failure with EF of 41% to 49% is defined as HFmrEF; and HFpEF is defined as an EF of 50% or higher (also known as diastolic heart failure). Left-sided heart failure is primarily caused by left heart pathologies (e.g., LV, mitral valve, or aortic valve dysfunction). Right-sided heart failure is caused by right heart conditions (e.g., pulmonary hypertension; right ventricle, pulmonic valve, or tricuspid dysfunction).

5. D) Abdominal ultrasound

This patient is presenting with clinical features suggestive of an abdominal aortic aneurysm (AAA). Male sex, older age, and smoking history increase the risk. Many patients with AAA have no symptoms. Often, a palpated pulsatile abdominal mass is noted on routine physical examination (30% of asymptomatic AAAs). The abdominal ultrasound is recommended as the first diagnostic modality for most asymptomatic patients; it is noninvasive and cost-effective for diagnosis in asymptomatic patients. For symptomatic patients who are hemodynamically stable, a CT of the abdomen (preferably with contrast) is recommended as the initial diagnostic modality. For symptomatic patients who are hemodynamically unstable, the FAST exam is recommended. FAST is an ultrasound technique used to evaluate both abdominal and thoracic cavities. It is used to detect the presence of blood or fluid (effusion) in the pericardial space. An MRI is not usually indicated as first line due to its cost, availability, and time restraints.

6. B) *Staphylococcus aureus*

Worldwide, the three most common causes of infective endocarditis are staphylococci, streptococci, and enterococci. *S. aureus* is the most common cause of infective endocarditis in the United States and most developed countries. Streptococci is a common cause in community-acquired infective endocarditis, and staphylococci is a common cause of healthcare-associated infective endocarditis.

7. C) A patient with previous infective endocarditis who plans to have a dental abscess drained

Patients with a high-risk condition or implanted device are recommended to receive antibiotic prophylaxis prior to invasive dental or oral procedures. Placement of orthodontic brackets is not an invasive procedure. Cardiac transplant recipients who plan to have a tooth extracted require antibiotic prophylaxis only if they have developed cardiac valvopathy.

8. A) Atrial fibrillation

Atrial fibrillation is diagnosed by interpretation of the 12-lead EKG; it is characterized by an irregularly irregular ventricular rhythm with a lack of discrete P waves. QRS complexes are narrow, and the baseline between successive QRS complexes shows irregular coarse fibrillatory waves. Paroxysmal supraventricular tachycardia presents with narrow QRS complexes that are intermittent, start and stop abruptly, and have a regular ventricular response. Sinus arrhythmia is characterized by an irregularity in the rate of normal sinus rhythm. First-degree heart block is a result of delayed or slowed AV conduction presenting as a prolonged PR interval (>200 ms at resting heart rates).

9. A patient presents complaining of leg pain that occurs while walking but is relieved by rest after a few minutes. Upon physical examination, the patient's skin appears pale, dry, shiny, and hairless. The patient has an ulceration on the tip of the big toe. Based on this presentation, which of the following initial diagnostic tests is indicated?
   A. Lower extremity duplex ultrasound
   B. CT scan of the lower extremity
   C. Exercise testing
   D. Ankle-brachial index

10. Upon cardiac auscultation, a loud murmur is heard with an associated palpable precordial thrill. This intensity can be classified as which grade of heart murmur?
    A. II
    B. IV
    C. V
    D. III

11. A patient presents for a routine physical examination. Cardiac auscultation reveals a systolic, harsh, blowing murmur at the second right intercostal space that radiates to the neck. This suggests which heart murmur?
    A. Mitral stenosis
    B. Aortic regurgitation
    C. Aortic stenosis
    D. Mitral regurgitation

12. According to the 2017 American College of Cardiology (ACC)/American Heart Association (AHA) Guidelines, a patient has stage 1 hypertension in which of the following scenarios?
    A. Blood pressure 135/85 mmHg
    B. Blood pressure 118/75 mmHg
    C. Blood pressure 145/95 mmHg
    D. Blood pressure 129/79 mmHg

13. A patient presents complaining of the sudden onset of cold fingers and toes. The patient reports pain and a sharply demarcated color change of the skin (first white, followed by blue) when exposed to cold surfaces or temperatures. The patient has tried nonpharmacologic management with no improvement. Based on this patient's presentation, which of the following would be indicated for treatment?
    A. Captopril
    B. Prazosin
    C. Methyldopa
    D. Amlodipine

14. A patient presents with a blood pressure (BP) of 185/125 mmHg and complains of chest discomfort, shortness of breath, and nausea with vomiting. Which of the following is the next step in treatment?
    A. This is considered a hypertensive urgency, and the blood pressure should be slowly lowered.
    B. This is considered a hypertensive emergency, and the patient should be referred to the ED *stat*.
    C. This is considered a hypertensive emergency, and the blood pressure should be quickly lowered.
    D. This is considered a hypertensive urgency, and the patient should be referred to the ED *stat*.

15. An African American patient with diabetes mellitus has recently been diagnosed with hypertension. Initial pharmacologic therapy includes which of the following?
    A. Metoprolol
    B. Ramipril
    C. Hydrochlorothiazide
    D. Losartan

16. Upon routine laboratory evaluation, a 60-year-old patient is found to have a fasting triglyceride level of 550 mg/dL. The patient has diabetes mellitus and hypertension. Which of the following is the appropriate treatment for this patient?
    A. Niacin
    B. No treatment and re-assess in 3 months
    C. Fibrate therapy
    D. Omega-3 fatty acids

(See answers next page.)

9. D) Ankle-brachial index

The patient is presenting with clinical features suggesting lower extremity peripheral artery disease. Intermittent claudication is classically defined as muscle pain that is induced by exercise and relieved with rest. Physical exam findings are often significant for a nonhealing wound or ulcer; skin discoloration or gangrene; and dry, shiny, hairless skin due to diminished blood flow. Diagnosis of arterial stenosis or occlusion (as a result of peripheral artery disease) is confirmed with the ankle-brachial index (a result ≤0.9 has a high degree of sensitivity and specificity for diagnosis). Exercise testing can be obtained if patients with a classic history of claudication have a normal resting ankle-brachial index. Additional vascular imaging (such as a duplex ultrasound or CT) is generally not necessary for establishing a diagnosis of peripheral artery disease but can be useful to identify treatment therapies for intervention.

10. B) IV

A grade IV murmur is characterized as a loud murmur with a palpable precordial thrill. A grade II murmur is a soft murmur that is readily detectable. A grade V murmur is a very loud murmur that is audible with the stethoscope placed lightly on the chest and occurs with a palpable precordial thrill. A grade III murmur is a loud murmur but without a palpable precordial thrill.

11. C) Aortic stenosis

The murmur of aortic stenosis often presents as a systolic ejection murmur, typically heard best at the base of the heart in the aortic area (right intercostal space), where it has a harsh quality. The murmur may also radiate. Think "MR. ASS," for systolic murmurs; remember to think of aortic murmurs when they occur at the second or third intercostal space (or the base of the heart).

12. A) Blood pressure 135/85 mmHg

According to the 2017 ACC/AHA Guidelines, normal systolic blood pressure is <120 mmHg, and normal diastolic blood pressure is <80 mmHg. Elevated blood pressure is systolic blood pressure of 120 to 129 mmHg and diastolic blood pressure of <80 mmHg. Stage 1 is systolic blood pressure of 130 to 139 mmHg or diastolic blood pressure of 80 to 89 mmHg. Stage 2 is defined as systolic blood pressure of ≥140 mmHg or diastolic blood pressure of ≥90 mmHg.

13. D) Amlodipine

This patient is presenting with symptoms consistent with Raynaud's phenomenon. Often, nonpharmacologic therapy is the initial approach (e.g., avoiding cold exposure and vasoconstricting drugs, smoking cessation). Pharmacologic therapy can be used in combination for patients to provide control of symptoms. Initial pharmacologic therapy includes dihydropyridine calcium channel blockers (e.g., amlodipine, nifedipine). Alternative options include phosphodiesterase type 5 inhibitors, topical nitrates, losartan, or fluoxetine. Therapies lacking efficacy, such as behavioral therapy, complementary and alternative medicine, angiotensin-converting enzyme (ACE) inhibitors, prazosin, and methyldopa, are not recommended due to lack of sufficient evidence supporting benefit.

14. B) This is considered a hypertensive emergency, and the patient should be referred to the ED *stat*.

A hypertensive emergency is severe hypertension (BP ≥180/120 mmHg) with evidence of acute end-organ damage. Common findings that suggest acute target organ damage include acute head injury or trauma; generalized or focal neurologic symptoms; fresh flame hemorrhages, exudates, or papilledema; nausea and vomiting; chest discomfort/pain; acute, severe back pain; dyspnea; pregnancy; or use of drugs that can produce a hyperadrenergic state. Management of the choice of agent and BP goal varies according to the cause, but treatment often includes ICU admission for continuous monitoring of blood pressure and parenteral administration of an antihypertensive agent. The BP should not be lowered too quickly because ischemic damage can occur (the vascular beds have reset their autoregulatory threshold to the higher level of blood pressure). A hypertensive urgency is severe hypertension but with no acute end-organ damage.

15. C) Hydrochlorothiazide

In African American adults with hypertension without heart failure or chronic kidney disease, including those with diabetes mellitus, initial treatment should include a thiazide-type diuretic or calcium channel blocker.

16. D) Omega-3 fatty acids

For patients with moderate to severe hypertriglyceridemia (fasting triglyceride 500 to 900 mg/dL) with high atherosclerotic cardiovascular disease (ASCVD) risk, the appropriate treatment is icosapent ethyl (omega-3 fatty acid). If, after treatment, the level remains greater than 500 mg/dL or the patient is not at high ASCVD risk, fibrate therapy should be added. High ASCVD risk is defined as established ASCVD or diabetes mellitus plus two additional ASCVD risk factors (e.g., age ≥50 years, cigarette smoking, hypertension). Niacin is not routinely recommended given its limited benefit and risk of adverse effects.

17. A patient with Marfan syndrome presents for a routine physical examination. Physical assessment is significant for a non-ejection click and a systolic murmur of mitral regurgitation. Diagnosis for this suspected condition is confirmed by which of the following modalities?
    A. 12-lead EKG
    B. Echocardiography
    C. Chest x-ray
    D. Ultrasound

18. A patient with a prosthetic heart valve is about to undergo routine dental cleaning. The patient has no allergies. Which of the following is *most preferred* for the prevention of infective endocarditis?
    A. Nothing; routine dental cleaning is not an indication for antibiotic prophylaxis
    B. Clindamycin
    C. Amoxicillin
    D. Cephalexin

19. Which of the following antihypertensive agents is contraindicated in pregnancy?
    A. Enalapril
    B. Methyldopa
    C. Nifedipine
    D. Labetalol

20. A patient with hypertension presents with a headache. Blood pressure is 185/115 mmHg. Which finding on fundoscopic exam mandates rapid lowering of blood pressure?
    A. Retinal arteriolar narrowing
    B. Microaneurysms
    C. Arteriovenous nicking ("nipping")
    D. Papilledema

21. A patient presents with palpitations and reports feeling light-headed. The patient's blood pressure is 115/75 mmHg. A 12-lead EKG reveals a heart rate of 125 beats per minute along with narrow QRS complexes that are less than 120 milliseconds in duration. Initial treatment includes which of the following?
    A. Synchronized cardioversion
    B. Vagal maneuver
    C. Adenosine
    D. Diltiazem

22. A patient who recently had a hip surgery presents with right lower extremity swelling, pain, and warmth. The patient has a positive D-dimer level. Based on this presentation, which of the following is the diagnostic test of choice?
    A. Repeating D-dimer in 1 week
    B. CT venography
    C. Compression ultrasonography with Doppler
    D. Magnetic resonance venography (MRV)

23. A patient with hypertension presents complaining of an episode of severe heavy chest pain that lasted for 30 minutes while watching television. The patient denies any current chest pain. A 12-lead EKG reveals normal sinus rhythm with a rate of 72 beats/min. A troponin I is negative. Which of the following describes this patient's diagnosis?
    A. ST-elevation myocardial infarction (STEMI)
    B. Unstable angina
    C. Non–ST-elevation myocardial infarction (NSTEMI)
    D. Stable angina

24. Which of the following is a diastolic murmur?
    A. Mitral regurgitation
    B. Aortic stenosis
    C. Mitral stenosis
    D. Mitral valve prolapse

(See answers next page.)

17. B) Echocardiography

Mitral valve prolapse is prevalent in patients with connective tissue disorders, such as Marfan syndrome, and should be suspected in patients with a nonejection click (single or multiple) with or without a systolic murmur of mitral regurgitation. Diagnosis is confirmed via transthoracic echocardiogram (as well as transesophageal echocardiogram) and allows for evaluation of the subvalvular structures, assessment of mitral regurgitation, and identification of hemodynamic status.

18. C) Amoxicillin

Patients with a prosthetic heart valve undergoing invasive dental or oral procedures (including routine dental cleaning) should be prescribed an oral antibiotic regimen for the prevention of endocarditis prior to the procedure. The preferred agent is amoxicillin; cephalexin is an alternative option if the patient is allergic to penicillin. Clindamycin is no longer recommended for antibiotic prophylaxis prior to dental procedures.

19. A) Enalapril

According to the American College of Cardiology (ACC)/American Heart Association (AHA) Guidelines, patients with hypertension who become pregnant (or plan to be pregnant) should be transitioned to methyldopa, nifedipine, and/or labetalol. Angiotensin-converting enzyme (ACE) inhibitors, angiotensin receptor blockers (ARBs), or direct renin inhibitors should not be used in those with hypertension who become pregnant.

20. D) Papilledema

The history and physical examination in patients presenting with severely elevated blood pressure should include a thorough fundoscopic exam to evaluate for signs of target organ damage. The ocular effects from hypertension can be classified as mild, moderate, or severe. "Mild" is characterized by generalized retinal arteriolar narrowing, arteriolar wall thickening, arteriovenous nicking ("nipping"), and opacification of the arteriolar wall ("copper wiring"). "Moderate" is classified by hemorrhages; either flame- or dot-shaped, cotton-wool spots; hard exudates; and microaneurysms. "Severe" involves some or all of the previous symptoms plus optic disc edema (papilledema). This finding requires rapid lowering of blood pressure.

21. B) Vagal maneuver

Supraventricular tachycardia is dysrhythmia defined by a narrow complex (QRS <120 milliseconds) at a rate greater than 100 beats per minute. For hemodynamically stable patients with supraventricular tachycardia, vagal maneuvers have been found to be a safe and easily performed diagnostic test as well as an effective first-line treatment intervention according to the 2015 American College of Cardiology (ACC)/American Heart Association (AHA)/Heart Rhythm Society Guidelines. If the patient is unstable, consider immediate synchronized cardioversion. If vagal maneuvers are ineffective, consider treatment with adenosine or diltiazem (as a second-line option).

22. C) Compression ultrasonography with Doppler

Deep vein thrombosis (DVT) of the lower extremity should be suspected in patients who have clinical manifestations (e.g., pain, warmth, edema) and risk factors (e.g., recent surgery) for thrombus. A positive D-dimer level (≥500 ng/mL) is suggestive of a DVT. The diagnostic test of choice in patients with suspected DVT is the compression ultrasonography with Doppler. Alternative imaging with CT or MRI can be used if there is uncertainty after ultrasonography.

23. B) Unstable angina

The patient is likely experiencing unstable angina, specifically rest angina, which generally lasts longer than 20 minutes. Stable angina refers to chest discomfort that occurs predictably at a certain level of exertion but is relieved by rest or nitroglycerin. A STEMI is unlikely as the 12-lead EKG does not reveal ST elevation at the J point in two contiguous leads. Findings consistent with NSTEMI would reveal new down-sloping ST depression in two contiguous leads and/or T wave inversion in two contiguous leads with prominent R wave or R/S ratio >1. Additionally, NSTEMI is distinguished from unstable angina by the presence of elevated serum biomarkers.

24. C) Mitral stenosis

Mitral stenosis and aortic regurgitation are diastolic murmurs. Mitral regurgitation and aortic stenosis are systolic murmurs. Patients with mitral valve prolapse often have a nonejection click (single or multiple) with or without a systolic murmur of mitral regurgitation.

25. A 45-year-old patient with diabetes mellitus with a 10-year atherosclerotic cardiovascular disease (ASCVD) risk of 8% presents for routine laboratory work. The lipid panel is significant for low-density lipoprotein (LDL) cholesterol 100 mg/dL. Which type of therapy is indicated for this patient?
A. Moderate-intensity statin
B. High-intensity statin
C. Fibrate
D. Cholesterol-absorption inhibitor

26. Which of the following is considered a high-intensity statin?
A. Atorvastatin 10 mg
B. Pravastatin 20 mg
C. Simvastatin 30 mg
D. Rosuvastatin 20 mg

27. A patient who recently received intravenous antibiotic therapy presents with tenderness, pain, and erythema along the course of a superficial vein in an upper extremity. Initial treatment includes which of the following?
A. Therapeutic anticoagulation
B. Extremity elevation, warm compresses
C. Antimicrobial therapy
D. Surgical drainage and vein excision

28. A patient presents with dyspnea and chest discomfort. Physical assessment is significant for jugular venous distention, peripheral edema, ascites, and hepatosplenomegaly. Based on this presentation, a definitive diagnosis can be made by which of the following modalities?
A. Cardiac catheterization
B. Cardiovascular MRI
C. Cardiac CT scan
D. Echocardiography

29. The point of maximal impulse is located at the:
A. Third intercostal space on the left sternal border
B. Second intercostal space to the right side of the upper border of the sternum
C. Second intercostal space in the left midclavicular line
D. Fifth intercostal space in the left midclavicular line

30. A patient with severe primary hypercholesterolemia presents for a routine checkup. The patient has been compliant with the prescribed high-intensity statin regimen; however, the low-density lipoprotein cholesterol (LDL-C) is 120 mg/dL. Which of the following therapies will be added next?
A. Fibrate agent
B. Ezetimibe
C. PCSK9 inhibitor
D. Niacin

31. Combination therapy of an angiotensin-converting enzyme (ACE) inhibitor with an angiotensin receptor blocker (ARB) or a direct renin inhibitor should be avoided due to increased risk for:
A. Hypokalemia
B. Hypernatremia
C. Hyperkalemia
D. Hypocalcemia

32. A patient presents complaining of palpitations, fatigue, and mild shortness of breath. A 12-lead EKG reveals rapid, regular atrial activity in a sawtooth pattern at about 300 beats/min and a regular ventricular rate of about 155 beats/min. Which of the following agents can be used for rate control for this arrhythmia?
A. Diltiazem
B. Digoxin
C. Amlodipine
D. Amiodarone

33. A patient with chronic kidney disease (CKD) stage 3 has been recently diagnosed with hypertension. First-line pharmacologic treatment includes which of the following agents?
A. Metoprolol
B. Lisinopril
C. Nifedipine
D. Terazosin

(See answers next page.)

25. A) Moderate-intensity statin

For adults age 40 to 75 years with diabetes mellitus and LDL cholesterol ≥70 mg/dL at a 10-year ASCVD risk of ≥7.5%, start moderate-intensity statin therapy. Fibrate therapy is indicated for high triglycerides. Cholesterol-absorption inhibitors (e.g., ezetimibe) may be reasonable in patients who are on maximally tolerated statin therapy and whose LDL cholesterol levels remain ≥70 mg/dL.

26. D) Rosuvastatin 20 mg

High-intensity statins are atorvastatin 40 to 80 mg and rosuvastatin 20 to 40 mg. Atorvastatin 10 to 20 mg is a moderate-intensity statin. Pravastatin 10 to 20 mg is a low-intensity statin. Simvastatin 20 to 40 mg is a moderate-intensity statin.

27. B) Extremity elevation, warm compresses

This patient is presenting with signs of phlebitis, an inflammation of a superficial vein. Treatment includes symptomatic care (e.g., extremity elevation, warm or cool compresses, compression stockings, pain management). For patients with suspected thrombosis, an ultrasound is recommended to rule out coexistent deep vein thrombosis (DVT), in which case anticoagulation may be needed based on the patient's risk factors. In patients with more complicated disease, additional antimicrobial treatments or surgery may be indicated.

28. A) Cardiac catheterization

This patient is presenting with signs and symptoms of right heart failure (e.g., dyspnea, fatigue, chest discomfort, abdominal distention with a positive fluid wave, jugular venous distention, peripheral edema, ascites, hepatosplenomegaly, tricuspid murmur, S3 gallop). The definitive test for diagnosis of right heart failure is a cardiac catheterization. Echocardiography is essential for evaluation and workup but does not establish or exclude the diagnosis of heart failure. A cardiovascular MRI can be helpful to assess right ventricular structure and function, as well as a CT scan if MRI is unavailable.

29. D) Fifth intercostal space in the left midclavicular line

The point of maximal impulse is located at the apex, at the fifth intercostal space in the left midclavicular line.

30. B) Ezetimibe

High-intensity statin therapy is indicated for patients with severe primary hypercholesterolemia (LDL-C level ≥190). If the LDL-C level remains ≥100 mg/dL, adding ezetimibe is a reasonable next step. A PCSK9 inhibitor can be considered if the LDL-C level on statin *plus* ezetimibe remains ≥100 mg/dL and the patient has multiple factors that increase risk of atherosclerotic cardiovascular disease (ASCVD) events. Niacin and fibrates are triglyceride-lowering drugs and have mild LDL-lowering action; however, they are not routinely recommended in combination with statin therapy.

31. C) Hyperkalemia

Do not use ACE inhibitors in combination with ARBs or direct renin inhibitors due to increased risk of hyperkalemia, especially in patients with chronic kidney disease or those on potassium supplements or potassium-sparing drugs. There is also a risk for acute renal failure in patients with severe bilateral artery stenosis.

32. A) Diltiazem

The patient is experiencing atrial flutter, an abnormal cardiac rhythm characterized by rapid, regular atrial depolarizations (about 300 beats/min) and a regular ventricular rate (about 150 beats/min). Typical P waves are absent, and the atrial activity presents as a sawtooth pattern in leads II, III, and aVF. Rate control in atrial flutter involves administration of a non-dihydropyridine calcium channel blocker (e.g., verapamil, diltiazem) or a beta-blocker. Digoxin is used less frequently due to its side effects and toxicity (it is indicated with concurrent heart failure). Amiodarone, an antiarrhythmic agent, is rarely used as a rate control agent. Reversion to normal sinus rhythm is often accomplished by catheter ablation for definitive treatment (cardioversion is also reasonable). Ibutilide is the drug of choice for pharmacologic reversion as an alternative option.

33. B) Lisinopril

First-line pharmacologic therapy for adults with hypertension and CKD (stage 3 or higher or stage 1 with albuminuria or elevated albumin-to-creatinine ratio) is an angiotensin-converting enzyme (ACE) inhibitor (e.g., lisinopril) or an angiotensin receptor blocker (ARB) if an ACE inhibitor is not tolerated. Metoprolol is a beta-blocker, nifedipine a calcium channel blocker, and terazosin is an alpha-1 blocker.

34. Which micronutrient should an individual with primary hypertension increase in their diet?
    A. Calcium
    B. Chloride
    C. Potassium
    D. Sodium

35. After antihypertensive therapy is initiated, a patient's blood pressure should be rechecked after how many months?
    A. 1
    B. 2
    C. 3
    D. 4

36. An older adult male patient who is a smoker is newly diagnosed with primary hypertension. He has a history of emphysema and second-degree AV block. His blood pressure from the previous visit is 145/80 mmHg. During the current visit, his blood pressure is 155/80 mmHg. What is the next step?
    A. Start patient on atenolol (Tenormin) 50 mg once a day and reassess in 3 months
    B. Start patient on felodipine (Cabren) 2.5 mg once a day and reassess in 2 months
    C. Start patient on chlorthalidone (Thalitone) 12.5 mg daily and reassess in 1 month
    D. Nothing; no action or treatment needed at this time

37. Which of the following is a risk-enhancing factor for atherosclerotic cardiovascular disease (ASCVD)?
    A. Acute kidney injury
    B. Low-density lipoprotein cholesterol (LDL-C) greater than 140 mg/dL
    C. Menopause
    D. C-reactive protein (CRP) of 2.0 mg/L or greater

38. The nurse practitioner is assessing a patient's risk for developing atherosclerotic cardiovascular disease (ASCVD) by using the American College of Cardiology's ASCVD Risk Estimator Plus tool. The estimate provided by the tool is likely to be *most* accurate if the patient is of which racial/ethnic background?
    A. American Indian
    B. South Asian
    C. Puerto Rican
    D. White

39. A patient with a history of atrial fibrillation is prescribed warfarin. Routine labs reveal an international normalized ratio (INR) of 8. The patient denies any signs or symptoms of bleeding. Which of the following is the *most* appropriate action?
    A. Hold warfarin indefinitely, and check INR weekly.
    B. Administer fresh frozen plasma to correct supratherapeutic INR.
    C. Skip the next dose and slightly increase the maintenance dose.
    D. Hold warfarin for two doses, and administer low-dose oral vitamin K.

40. A patient with substernal chest pain presents complaining that it feels like "an elephant is sitting on my chest." A 12-lead EKG reveals ST-elevation in leads V2 to V4. This presentation is suggestive of which of the following?
    A. Atrial fibrillation
    B. Wolff-Parkinson-White syndrome
    C. Anterior wall myocardial infarction
    D. Atrial flutter

(See answers next page.)

34. C) Potassium

Individuals with primary hypertension should increase potassium in their diet, aiming for 3,500 to 5,000 mg/d preferably from dietary sources. Foods high in potassium include avocados, sweet potatoes (yams), coconut water, bananas, oranges, watermelon, cantaloupe, honeydew, apricots, grapefruit, dark leafy vegetables (spinach/broccoli), and edamame (boiled soybeans). A higher level has been found to diminish the effect of sodium on blood pressure. Excessive absorption of sodium accounts for the increase in blood pressure noted with age and is associated with an increased risk of stroke, cardiovascular disease, and adverse outcomes.

35. A) 1

The 2017 American College of Cardiology/American Heart Association guidelines recommend follow-up in 1 month after initiating (or titrating) an antihypertensive. When blood pressure is under control, a follow-up visit can occur in 3 months.

36. C) Start patient on chlorthalidone (Thalitone) 12.5 mg daily and reassess in 1 month

First-line agents for treatment of hypertension include thiazide diuretics, calcium channel blockers (CCBs), and angiotensin-converting enzyme inhibitors and angiotensin II receptor blockers. The patient has emphysema, so beta-blockers such as atenolol (Tenormin) cannot be used. He also has a second-degree AV block, which is a contraindication to CCBs such as felodipine (Cabren).

37. D) C-reactive protein (CRP) of 2.0 mg/L or greater

Risk-enhancing factors for ASCVD include elevated CRP of ≥2.0 mg/L, chronic kidney disease (not acute injury), persistently elevated LDL-C levels of 160 mg/dL or greater, history of preeclampsia or *premature* menopause, metabolic syndrome, family history of early ASCVD, ankle-brachial index less than or equal to 0.9, and high-risk ethnicity.

38. D) White

The ASCVD Risk Estimator Plus is an online tool that can estimate the 10-year and lifetime risk for developing ASCVD. It can underestimate risk for members of some groups, including American Indians, Puerto Ricans, and individuals of South Asian descent.

39. D) Hold warfarin for two doses, and administer low-dose oral vitamin K.

If the INR is 4.5 to 10, warfarin should be held for one or two doses and low-dose oral vitamin K (1–2.5 mg) may be administered. Monitor INR every 2 to 3 days until it is stable, and decrease the warfarin maintenance dose. If the INR is <4.5, skip the next dose and/or reduce slightly the maintenance dose (however, if INR is mildly elevated, the maintenance dose often does not need to be reduced). Check INR once or twice a week when adjusting the dose. Do not give vitamin K. If the INR is >10, warfarin should be held; oral vitamin K (2.5–5 mg) can be administered, depending on bleeding risk. Monitor INR daily and resume warfarin at a lower dose once the INR is therapeutic. Non-bleeding patients should not be given fresh frozen plasma or four-factor prothrombin complex concentration (PCC). Indications include bleeding risk or when reversal is needed (e.g., for surgery).

40. C) Anterior wall myocardial infarction

An EKG characterized by ST-segment elevation or Q waves in one or more precordial leads (V1 to V6) and leads I to aVL suggests anterior wall ischemia. The EKG of a patient with Wolff-Parkinson-White syndrome has a short PR interval and a widened QRS complex and paroxysmal tachycardia. Atrial fibrillation is associated with an irregularly irregular ventricular rhythm with the absence of distinct P waves. Atrial flutter is characterized by rapid, regular atrial depolarizations with a characteristic "saw-tooth-like" EKG tracing.

8

RESPIRATORY SYSTEM REVIEW

ACUTE ASTHMA EXACERBATION

An asthmatic patient presents with tachypnea (>20 breaths/min), tachycardia or bradycardia, cyanosis, and anxiety. The patient appears exhausted, fatigued, and diaphoretic and uses accessory muscles to help with breathing. Physical exam reveals "quiet" lungs with no wheezing or breath sounds audible and potential cyanosis as a late sign. When speaking, the patient may speak only one or two words (cannot form complete sentence because needs to breathe).

ACUTE CARBON MONOXIDE POISONING

Mild-to-moderate cases of carbon monoxide poisoning can present with headache, the most common symptom. It can be accompanied by nausea, malaise, and dizziness. In some cases, it may resemble a viral upper respiratory infection (URI). Symptoms are variable and can range from mild confusion to coma. There may be a cherry-red appearance of the skin and lips, but it is considered an "insensitive sign." Severe toxicity can present with seizures, syncope, or coma. Diagnosis is based on history and physical examination in conjunction with elevated carboxyhemoglobin level measured by co-oximetry of an arterial blood gas sample. A venous sample can be used, but it is less accurate.

COVID-19

Infection is caused by the SARS-CoV-2 virus. Symptoms appear 2 to 14 days after exposure and may include fever, chills, headache, myalgia, cough, and shortness of breath, and are accompanied by fatigue, diarrhea, nausea, and/or vomiting. For some, the presenting symptom is the sudden loss of taste and/or smell. Some have cold-like symptoms such as sore throat, nasal congestion, and rhinitis. Persons with underlying medical conditions such as heart or lung disease or diabetes are at higher risk of developing more serious complications. Most people have mild illness and can recover at home. Advise patient to call their primary care provider for testing instructions and treatment. Close contacts need to self-quarantine for up to a 14-day duration. Patients with serious symptoms (e.g., trouble breathing, confusion) may need hospitalization.

LUNG CANCER

Majority of patients have advanced disease on presentation. Cough (50%–75%) in a smoker or former smoker that persists should raise suspicion. Hemoptysis and dyspnea may accompany cough. Some have chest pain, which is described as a dull, achy, persistent pain; some have shoulder and/or bone pain. Recurrent pneumonia on the same lobe might be a sign of local tumor obstruction. Can present with weight loss, anorexia, fatigue, and fever. Horner syndrome (pupil constriction with ptosis) may present in some patients and prompts an urgent MRI. Symptoms depend on location(s) and tumor metastases. Non–small-cell lung cancer is the most common type (85%). Screen for lung cancer with annual low-dose computed tomography (LDCT) in adults age 50 to 80 years who have a 20 pack-year smoking history and currently smoke or have quit in the past 15 years.

PULMONARY EMBOLISM

A form of venous thromboembolism; refers to the obstruction of the pulmonary artery (or one of its branches) by either thrombus, tumor, air, or fat material. A patient complains of sudden onset of dyspnea and coughing. Cough may be productive of pink-tinged frothy sputum. Other symptoms are tachycardia, pallor, and feelings of impending doom. Any condition that increases risk of blood clots can increase the risk of pulmonary embolism (PE). These patients often have a history of atrial fibrillation, estrogen therapy, smoking, surgery, cancer, pregnancy, long bone fractures, and prolonged inactivity.

BREATH SOUNDS

- Vesicular breath sounds: Soft and low-pitched; heard bilaterally over most of the peripheral fields.
- Bronchial breath sounds: Louder and higher in pitch; heard over the lower aspect of the trachea and over the manubrium.
- Bronchovesicular: Intermediate intensity and pitch; heard over major bronchi in the midchest area or between the scapula.
- Tracheal: Highest and loudest pitch; heard over the upper aspect of the trachea and anterior aspect of the neck.

RESPIRATORY RATE

- Normal number of breaths per minute in adults is 12 to 20 breaths/min.
- Women tend to have slightly higher rates than men.
- A very small increase in partial pressure of carbon dioxide ($PaCO_2$) will affect the respiratory rate. But high

levels of carbon dioxide (>70–80 mmHg) can depress respiration and cause headaches, restlessness, unconsciousness, and death.

TACHYPNEA

- Increased respiratory rate has many causes, including increased oxygen demand, hypoxia, and increased $PaCO_2$.
- Many conditions can cause tachypnea, such as pain, fear, fever, physical exertion, asthma, pneumonia, PE, and hyperthyroidism.

EGOPHONY

- Normal: Ask the patient to say the sound "eee" while listening with the stethoscope. Will hear "eee" clearly instead of "bah." The "eee" sound is louder over the large bronchi because larger airways are better at transmitting sounds; lower lobes have a softer sounding "eee."
- Abnormal: Will hear "bah" sound when egophony is present. This finding suggests the presence of consolidation or fluid in the lungs.

TACTILE FREMITUS

Instruct patient to say "99" or "one, two, three"; use finger pads to palpate lungs and feel for vibrations.
- Normal: Stronger vibrations are palpable on the upper lobes and softer vibrations on lower lobes.
- Abnormal: The findings are reversed; may palpate stronger vibrations on one lower lobe (i.e., consolidation); asymmetric findings are always abnormal.

WHISPERED PECTORILOQUY

Instruct patient to whisper "99" or "one, two, three." Auscultate both lungs.
- Normal: The whispered voice will be distant and muffled.
- Abnormal: If there is lung consolidation, the whispered words are clearly heard on the lower lobes of the lungs.

PERCUSSION

Use middle or index finger as the pleximeter finger on one hand. The finger on the other hand is the hammer.
- Normal: Resonance is heard over normal lung tissue.
- Hyperresonance: Very loud sound, low in pitch and longer in duration. Occurs with chronic obstructive pulmonary disease (COPD), emphysema (overinflating).
- Tympanic: Loud and high-pitched drum-like sound. Normal when percussed across the abdomen. Abnormal when found in the chest wall (suggests pneumothorax).
- Dull tone: Bacterial pneumonia with lobar consolidation, pleural effusion (fluid or tumor). A solid organ, such as the liver, sounds dull.

PULMONARY FUNCTION TESTING

Pulmonary function testing (pre- and post-bronchodilator) is the gold-standard test for asthma and COPD. Measures obstructive versus restrictive dysfunction.
- Forced expiratory volume in 1 second (FEV1): Amount of air that a person can forcefully exhale in 1 second.
- Forced vital capacity (FVC): Total amount of air that can be exhaled during the FEV1 test.
- FEV1/FVC ratio: Proportion of a person's vital capacity that the person is able to expire in 1 second. Most important for detecting airflow obstruction in diseases like asthma and COPD.
- Obstructive dysfunction (reduction in airflow rates): As in asthma, COPD (chronic bronchitis and emphysema), bronchiectasis
- Restrictive dysfunction (reduction of lung volume due to decreased lung compliance): As in pulmonary fibrosis, pleural disease, diaphragm obstruction

DISEASE REVIEW

ASTHMA

A disease characterized by chronic airway inflammation. Defined by the history of respiratory symptoms that vary over time (wheezing, shortness of breath, chest tightness, cough) accompanied by variable expiratory airflow limitation. Reversible airway obstruction and increased responsiveness to stimuli (internal or external). Genetic predisposition with positive family history of allergies, eczema, and allergic rhinitis (atopy or atopic history). Exacerbations can be life-threatening. Rule out allergic asthma (refer for allergy testing), gastroesophageal reflux disease (GERD), rhinitis, sinusitis, and stress.

Classic Case

A young-adult patient with asthma complains of worsening symptoms exacerbated by a trigger (exercise, cold air, exposure to inhaled allergens). The patient with uncontrolled asthma may report using an albuterol inhaler more than normal (three or more times/day) to treat the symptoms. Complains of shortness of breath, wheezing, and chest tightness that is sometimes accompanied by a dry cough at night and early morning (e.g., 3 a.m.) that interrupts sleep.

Objective Findings

- Lungs: Wheezing with prolonged expiratory phase (high-pitched, musical whistling sound). As asthma worsens, the wheezing occurs during both inspiration and expiration. With severe bronchoconstriction, breath sounds are faint or inaudible.
- Cardiovascular: Tachycardia, rapid pulse.

Trigger Factors for Asthma

- Viral URIs, airborne allergens
- Airborne allergens such as dust mites, mold, cockroaches, furry animals, pollens
- Food allergies such as to sulfites, red and yellow dye, seafood

- Irritants such as cold air, cold weather, and fumes from chemicals or smoke, smoking, illicit drug use, wood-burning stove
- Emotional stress, exercise (exercise-induced asthma)
- GERD (reflux of acidic gastric contents irritates airways)
- Medications such as aspirin or other nonsteroidal anti-inflammatory drugs (NSAIDs), beta-blockers and angiotensin-converting enzyme (ACE) inhibitors, certain eye drops
- Genetics, atopy
- Risk factors for severe asthma include previous hospitalization requiring intubation or ICU admission, multiple ED visits in the past year, recent history of poorly controlled asthma

Treatment Goals (All Patients With Asthma)
- Optimize asthma symptoms to perform usual activities with no limitations (e.g., attend school full time, play normally, work full-time, no job absence due to asthmatic symptoms)
- Prevent exacerbation
- Minimize use of rescue medicine (<2 days a week albuterol use)
- Avoid ED visits/hospitalization
- Maintain near-normal pulmonary function (reduce permanent lung damage); prevent loss of lung function (or, for children, prevent reduced lung growth)
- Minimize medication adverse effects

Treatment Plan
At initial visit, assess asthma control to determine if therapy should be adjusted. At each visit, assess symptoms, proper medication technique, patient adherence, and patient concerns.

EXAM TIPS

- Expect questions about asthma (diagnosis, treatment). Memorize an asthma stage because you may get "numbers" and have to figure out the asthma severity of a patient. Suggest memorizing Step 3 (e.g., FEV1 of 60%–80%).
- First-line drugs for asthma are inhaled corticosteroids (ICSs); they treat lung inflammation.

Asthma Medications
"Rescue" or "Reliever" Medicine for Acute Exacerbations
Administration of a rapid onset beta2-agonist, either short-acting beta2-agonists (SABA) (e.g., albuterol, levalbuterol) or long-acting beta2-agonists (LABA) (e.g., formoterol), for acute exacerbations. Under the Global Initiative for Asthma (GINA) of 2020, the preferred reliever is LABA in combination with ICS (e.g., budesonide-formoterol).
- SABAs in metered dose inhaler (MDI), MDI with spacer, or by nebulizer:
  - Albuterol (Ventolin HFA) or pirbuterol (Maxair), two inhalations every 4 to 6 hours as needed

- Levalbuterol (Xopenex HFA), two inhalations every 4 to 6 hours as needed; less likely to cause cardiac stimulation (fewer palpitations, less tachycardia)
  - Quick onset (15–30 minutes) and lasts about 4 to 6 hours
  - Used for quick relief (of wheezing) but does not treat underlying inflammation
  - With nebulizer, give up to three treatments every 20 minutes as needed; short course of oral corticosteroids may be needed for exacerbations (Medrol Dose Pack)
  - Used for treatment of exercise-induced asthma
- Inhaled glucocorticoid-formoterol: Usual dose of budesonide-formoterol is one to two inhalations, which can be repeated every 20 minutes for 1 hour.

Long-Term Control Medications for Asthma
LABAs (used alone) increase the risk of death from asthma. Combination of LABA and ICS is safer. Examples include fluticasone with salmeterol (Advair), budesonide with formoterol (Symbicort; see Table 8.1).

Sustained-Release Theophylline (Theo-24)
- Drug class is methylxanthine. Used as an adjunct drug. Acts as a bronchodilator.
- Monitor levels to reduce risk of toxicity. The drug has multiple drug interactions, including:
  - Adenosine, alcohol, allopurinol, clarithromycin
  - Cimetidine, erythromycin, estrogen, verapamil, rifampin, propranolol
  - Anticonvulsants such as phenytoin, diazepam, carbamazepine, ketamine, lithium
  - Check blood levels; peak serum concentration is 10 to 20 mg/dL

EXAM TIPS

- Chronic use of high-dose inhaled steroids can cause osteoporosis, growth failure in children, glaucoma, cataracts, immune suppression, hypothalamic–pituitary–adrenal suppression, and other effects.
- Do not use LABAs (salmeterol, formoterol) for rescue treatment.

Spacers or Chambers
Use of a "spacer" or "chamber" (AeroChamber) is encouraged. It will increase delivery of the aerosolized drug to the lungs and minimize oral thrush (for inhaled steroids).

Asthma Classification, Stepwise Approach, and Treatment Guidelines (Age ≥12 Years)
The National Asthma Education and Prevention Program's (NAEPP) "Expert Panel Report III: Guidelines for the Diagnosis and Management of Asthma" is the original guideline that was released in August 2007 and was updated in 2020. GINA also provided an updated asthma management and prevention guideline in 2020. Both GINA and NAEPP base initial therapy on assessment of

Table 8.1 Asthma: Long-Term Control Medications

Drug Class	Generic Name (Brand Name) Dosing	Side Effects/Adverse Effects
Inhaled corticosteroids	Triamcinolone (Azmacort) BID Budesonide (Pulmicort) BID Fluticasone (Flovent) BID	Oral thrush (gargle or drink water after use); use with spacer; HPA axis suppression, glaucoma, others.
Long-acting beta2-agonists	Salmeterol (Serevent) BID Formoterol (Foradil) BID	Warn patients of increased risk of asthma deaths; not to be used as monotherapy; use as LABA + ICS combinations (see next entry).
Combination of ICS with LABA	Salmeterol–fluticasone (Advair HFA, Advair Diskus) BID Budesonide–formoterol (Symbicort) Mometasone–formoterol (Dulera)	Preferred GINA 2020 medication is ICS–formoterol for reliever (rescue drug) or daily as treatment (Steps 1, 2, 3).
Leukotriene receptor antagonists/inhibitors	Montelukast (Singulair) daily Zafirlukast (Accolate) BID Zileuton (Zyflo) daily	Neuropsychologic effects (agitation, aggression, depression, others). Monitor liver function tests (zileuton).
Mast cell stabilizers (cromoglycates)	Cromolyn sodium (Intal) QID Nedocromil sodium (Tilade) QID	Cromolyn (Intal) and nedocromil (Tilade) inhalers have been discontinued in the United States; cromolyn (generic) for nebulization still available. Mild local throat irritation and cough may occur.
Methylxanthines	Theophylline (not used often) daily; starting dose 300 mg/day BID	Sympathomimetic. Avoid with seizures, hypertension, stroke. Several drug interactions; monitor drug levels.
Anti-immunoglobulin E antibodies	Dupilumab (Dupixent) Omalizumab (Xolair)	Risk of anaphylaxis, urticaria, and injection site reactions. May increase risk of cardiovascular events (e.g., TIA, CVA, MI, pulmonary emboli).
Systemic oral corticosteroids	Prednisone Prednisolone Methylprednisolone	Short course for 5–7 days. May require a taper before discontinuation. Can be used for exacerbations.

BID, twice a day; CVA, cerebrovascular accident; GINA, Global Initiative for Asthma; HPA, hypothalamic–pituitary–adrenal; ICS, inhaled corticosteroid; LABA, long-acting beta2-agonist; MI, myocardial infarction; QID, four times a day; TIA, transient ischemic attack.

asthma symptoms, respiratory impairment, and risk of poor asthma outcomes, but the specific categories vary. NAEPP determines asthma severity using spirometry or peak flow values whereas GINA defines severity based on the level of treatment required to control symptoms and exacerbations (Table 8.2).

Summary: Asthma Treatment

NAEPP 2020: Intermittent asthma should be treated with SABA (e.g., albuterol) as needed (PRN). Starting in Step 2, add low-dose ICS. In Step 3, add LABA to low-dose ICS (use combination medications Advair, Symbicort). Continue using SABA as PRN drug.

GINA 2020: Preferred reliever/rescue medication is ICS–formoterol (or ICS–LABA):

- Albuterol or SABA monotherapy is discouraged, but it can be used as an alternative rescue drug. GINA does not advise against their use as an add-on reliever/rescue drug.
- An ICS–LABA can be used as both maintenance (daily) treatment and a rescue inhaler. Extra inhalations can be used for breakthrough asthma symptoms. For severe persistent asthma, refer to asthma specialist.

- GINA recommends budesonide or beclomethasone as the ICS and formoterol as the LABA (Symbicort in the United States).

EXAM TIPS

- According to NAEPP, in intermittent asthma, night awakenings occur two or more times per month.
- Memorize factors needed to figure out peak expiratory flow (PEF; height, age, sex; use HAS mnemonic).

Patient Education

- Review and observe inhaler technique (use spacer if patient has problems).
- Teach about rescue medications and long-term controller medications.
- Develop a written asthma action plan; partner with patient and family.
- Control and limit exposure to allergens if allergic asthma; consider immunotherapy with allergist.
- Teach how to use spirometer; recognize worsening.

Table 8.2 Asthma Classifications

National Asthma Education and Prevention Program: Expert Panel Working Group (NAEPP, 2020)		Global Initiative for Asthma (GINA)	
Asthma Symptoms/Lung Function	**Therapy**	**Asthma Symptoms**	**Therapy**
Intermittent Asthma/Step 1		**Step 1**	
■ Symptoms: 2× or less/week ■ Nocturnal awakenings: 2× or less/month ■ Normal FEV1 ■ Exacerbations: 1× or less/year	SABA PRN	Infrequent asthma symptoms (less than 2×/week)	■ Low-dose ICS with rapid onset LABA (preferred) *or* ■ Low-dose ICS with SABA
Mild Persistent Asthma/Step 2		**Step 2**	
■ Symptoms: More than 2 days/week but not daily ■ Nocturnal awakenings: 3 to 4×/month ■ Minor interference with activities ■ Normal FEV1 ■ Exacerbations: 2× or more/year	■ Low-dose ICS daily and SABA PRN *or* ■ Low-dose ICS-SABA *or* ICS *plus* SABA (given together) PRN	Asthma symptoms or need for reliever inhaler more than 2×/week	■ Low-dose ICS PRN (preferred) *or* ■ Low-dose ICS daily and SABA PRN Note: Alternative options available
Moderate Persistent Asthma/Step 3		**Step 3**	
■ Symptoms: Daily ■ Nocturnal awakenings: >1/week ■ Daily need for SABA ■ Some activity limitation ■ FEV1 60% to 80% predicted ■ Exacerbations: 2× or more/year	■ Combination low-dose ICS daily and 1 to 2 inhalations PRN up to 12 inhalations/day (preferred) Note: Alternative options available	Troublesome asthma symptoms most days, nocturnal awakening due to asthma ≥1 times/month, risk factors for exacerbations	■ Low-dose ICS as maintenance and reliever therapy (preferred) *or* ■ Low-dose ICS-LABA combination daily and SABA PRN *or* ■ Low-dose ICS plus LTRA daily and SABA PRN Note: Alternative options available
Severe Persistent Asthma/Steps 4 to 6		**Steps 4 and 5**	
■ Symptoms: All day ■ Nocturnal awakenings: Nightly ■ Need for SABA several times/day ■ Extreme limitation in activity ■ FEV1 <60% predicted ■ Exacerbations: 2× or more/year	*Step 4* ■ Combination medium dose ICS daily and 1 to 2 inhalations as needed to 12 inhalations/day (preferred) Note: Alternative options available *Step 5* ■ Medium- to high-dose ICS-LABA plus LAMA daily and SABA PRN (preferred) Note: Alternative options available *Step 6* ■ High-dose ICS-LABA daily; consider LAMA as substitute or as additional therapy ■ Oral glucocorticoids ■ Possible addition of asthma biologics	Severely uncontrolled asthma with three or more of the following: Daytime asthma symptoms more than 2×/week; nocturnal awakening due to asthma; reliever needed for symptoms more than 2×/week; or activity limitation due to asthma *or* An acute exacerbation	*Step 4* ■ Medium-dose ICS as maintenance and reliever therapy (preferred) *or* ■ Medium dose ICS-LABA daily and SABA PRN Note: Alternative options available *Step 5* ■ Medium-dose ICS as maintenance and reliever therapy plus LAMA daily (preferred) *or* ■ Medium-dose ICS-LABA plus LAMA daily and SABA PRN ■ Assess asthma phenotype and evaluate for possible addition of asthma biologics Note: Alternative options available

FEV1, forced expiratory volume in 1 second; ICS, inhaled corticosteroid (glucocorticoid); LABA, long-acting beta2-agonist; LAMA, long-acting muscarinic antagonist; LTRA, leukotriene receptor antagonist; MDI, metered dose inhaler; PRN, as needed; SABA, short-acting beta2-agonist.
Source: Adapted from Fanta, C. H., & Barrett, N. A. (2023). (See Resources section for complete source information.)

- Effective management requires preventive approach with regularly scheduled visits, monitoring pulmonary function, control of comorbid conditions, and ongoing education.

Exercise-Induced Bronchoconstriction (Exercise-Induced Asthma)

Acute bronchoconstriction occurring during or immediately after exercise. Up to 90% of asthmatics may have exercise-induced bronchoconstriction (EIB). Leukotrienes, histamine, and interleukin levels are increased. Premedicate 5 to 20 minutes before exercise with two puffs of a SABA (albuterol [Ventolin], levalbuterol [Xopenex], pirbuterol [Maxair]). Effect will last up to 4 hours.

Asthmatic Exacerbation: Emergency Management

- Respiratory distress: Tachypnea, using accessory muscles (intercostals, abdominal) to breathe, talks in brief/fragmented sentences, severe diaphoresis, fatigue, agitation.
- Lungs: Minimal to no breath sounds audible during lung auscultation. PEF <40%. Lips/skin are blue tinged (cyanosis). Check O_2 saturation. Use supplemental oxygen.
- Give nebulizer treatment: Albuterol 0.5% solution by nebulizer every 20 to 30 minutes up to three doses. Albuterol can be given by MDI with spacer, four to eight puffs every 20 minutes for three doses.
- After nebulizer treatment(s): Listen for breath sounds. If inspiratory and expiratory wheezing is present, this is a good sign (signals opening up of airways). If there is a lack of breath sounds or wheezing after a nebulizer treatment, this is a bad sign (patient is not responding). Call 911.
- For moderate-to-severe exacerbations: Oral glucocorticoids are recommended (e.g., prednisone 40–60 mg for 5 to 7 days). If patients are also taking inhaled glucocorticoids, there is no need to taper the dose for glucocorticoid courses lasting 3 weeks or less.
- Consider: Adding inhaled ipratropium to inhaled SABA and one-time infusion of magnesium sulfate.
- Refer to ED: If poor to no response to nebulizer treatment (PEF <40% of expected), call 911. If no response to nebulizer treatment, impending respiratory arrest, give Epi-Pen (if concern for anaphylaxis). Call 911.

Peak Expiratory Flow Rate

- Maximal rate that a patient can exhale during a short maximal expiratory effort after a full inspiration.
- Measures effectiveness of treatment, worsening symptoms, and exacerbations. During expiration, patient is instructed to blow hard using the spirometer. Patients are asked to monitor and record their PEF two to four times daily for 2 weeks (ideally when asthma is controlled). The results are reviewed to determine the patient's personal best PEF value (generally the highest value).
- PEF is based on height (H), age (A), and sex (S), or HAS.

Asthma Self-Management

Asthma action plan forms are available online for free.
- Green zone: 80% to 100% of personal best PEF. No wheeze or cough. Sleeps through the night. Can work and play. Continue daily controller medications.
- Yellow zone: 50% to 80% of personal best PEF. Mild wheeze, tight chest, coughing at night. Exposure to known trigger or first signs of a cold, implement the treatment plan discussed with clinician to regain control.
- Red zone: <50% of personal best PEF, signifies "warning or medical alert." Breathing hard and fast, nasal flaring, trouble speaking. In children, ribs show from using accessory muscles. Administer supplemental oxygen. First-line bronchodilator treatment (e.g., albuterol by MDI with spacer or nebulizer). Onset of action <5 minutes. If not effective, call 911.

EXAM TIPS

- Rescue short-acting bronchodilators should be prescribed to all patients for immediate symptom relief.
- Ipratropium (Atrovent) is a short-acting antimuscarinic or SAMA.

CLINICAL PEARLS

- Pulse oximetry oxygen saturation of ≤90% suggests severe hypoxemia during an asthma exacerbation. Call 911.
- A near-normal pulse oximetry may be present in a patient with impending respiratory failure due to hypercapnia (bedside capnometry may be better method to monitor).

CHRONIC OBSTRUCTIVE PULMONARY DISEASE

COPD is a chronic lung disease characterized by the permanent loss of elastic recoil of the lungs, alveolar damage, airflow limitation, chronic inflammation, and changes in the pulmonary vasculature. Chronic and progressive dyspnea is the most characteristic symptom of COPD. The most common cause is chronic cigarette smoking. Women are more susceptible to developing COPD and emphysema.

Most patients have a mixture of emphysema and chronic bronchitis; one or the other may dominate. Many have an asthmatic component that overlaps their COPD; this is known as asthma–COPD overlap syndrome (ACOS). Pulmonary hypertension (cor pulmonale) may develop in the later stages of the disease. COPD was the sixth leading cause of death in the United States in 2020.

Chronic Bronchitis

Defined as coughing with excessive mucus production for 3 or more months for a minimum of 2 or more consecutive years. There is airway hypersecretion and inflammation.

Chronic Obstructive Asthma

Airway inflammation resulting in hyperreactivity. The contribution of each disease (chronic bronchitis, emphysema, asthma) varies in each individual.

Emphysema

Irreversible enlargement and alveolar damage with loss of elastic recoil result in chronic hyperinflation of the lungs. Expiratory respiratory phase is markedly prolonged.

Risk Factors

- Chronic cigarette smoking (up to 80% of patients with COPD have a history of smoking)
- Asthma and increased airway responsiveness to allergens, antioxidant deficiency, tuberculosis (TB)
- Environmental or occupational exposure (e.g., coal dust, grain dust) (up to 20% of patients)
- Alpha-1 anti-trypsin deficiency (AATD); patients have severe lung damage at earlier ages; alpha-1 trypsin protects lungs from oxidative and environmental damage. The World Health Organization (WHO) recommends all patients with a diagnosis of COPD should be screened at least once.

Classic Case

A middle-aged to older adult with a history of many years of cigarette smoking presents with history of a viral URI, which has exacerbated their COPD symptoms. Complains of worsening dyspnea, which is accompanied by a chronic cough that is productive of large amounts of tenacious sputum. Walking up stairs or physical exertion worsens the dyspnea. May have wheezing and chest tightness.

A "blue bloater" is a patient with chronic bronchitis with a bluish tinge to their skin (due to chronic hypoxia and hypercapnia). A "pink puffer" is a patient with emphysema with pink skin color (adequate oxygen saturation) who is thin and tachypneic and uses accessory muscles to breath and pursed-lip breathing. Many have barrel chest.

Objective Findings

- Emphysema component: Increased anterior–posterior diameter, decreased breath and heart sounds, use of accessory muscles to breathe, pursed-lip breathing, prolonged expiratory phase, and weight loss
- Chronic bronchitis component: Chronic cough productive of large amounts of sputum; lung auscultation will reveal expiratory wheezing, rhonchi, and coarse crackles
- Percussion: Hyperresonance
- Tactile fremitus and egophony: Decreased
- Spirometry: Post-bronchodilator FEV1/FVC <0.7 (lung function <70%) is the cutoff score for diagnosing COPD.
- Chest x-ray (CXR): Flattened diaphragms with hyperinflation; bullae sometimes present
- Note: Clubbing of the digits is not typical in COPD and suggests other comorbidities

Treatment Plan

The 2023 Global Initiative for Chronic Obstructive Lung Disease (GOLD) treatment guidelines are listed in Table 8.3. Each patient should be classified in one of three groups (A, B, or E).

Table 8.3 Initial Pharmacologic Treatment of COPD: GOLD Guidelines (2023)

Patient Group (Category)	Recommendations
Group A Less symptomatic patients at low risk of exacerbation (mMRC grade <2 or CAT score <10)	Either a short- or a long-acting bronchodilator (preferred)
Group B More symptomatic patients at low risk of exacerbation (mMRC grade ≥2 or CAT score ≥10)	LAMA and LABA combination
Group E High risk of exacerbation (≥2 exacerbations per year or one or more leading to hospitalization)	LAMA and LABA combination Consider LAMA, LABA, and ICS if eosinophils ≥300 cells/mcL

CAT, COPD Assessment Test; COPD, chronic obstructive pulmonary disease; GOLD, Global Initiative for Chronic Obstructive Lung Disease; LABA, long-acting beta2-agonist; LAMA, long-acting muscarinic antagonist; mMRC, modified Medical Research Council dyspnea scale.
Source: Global Initiative for Chronic Obstructive Lung Disease. (2023). (See Resources section for complete source information.)

EXAM TIPS

- The preferred choice of therapy for mild COPD (Group A) is a long-acting bronchodilator.
- COPD/smoker with pneumonia is at higher risk for *Haemophilus influenzae* bacteria.

Pharmacologic Treatment

Treatment Tips

SABAs are recommended for all patients with COPD for relief of dyspnea and early treatment of exacerbations. Bronchodilators (beta2-agonists and muscarinic antagonists) include the following:

- SABAs: Albuterol, levalbuterol (Xopenex), pirbuterol (Maxair)
- LABAs: Salmeterol, formoterol, vilanterol
- Short-acting anticholinergics (SAMAs): Ipratropium (Atrovent)
- Long-acting muscarinic antagonists (LAMAs) or long-acting anticholinergics: Tiotropium bromide (Spiriva), umeclidinium powder (Ellipta), glycopyrrolate (Seebri Neohaler). Available as combination LAMA plus LABA formulations.

Long-term monotherapy with oral corticosteroids is not recommended. Selective phosphodiesterase-4 inhibitor, roflumilast (Daliresp), can be used to reduce risk of COPD exacerbations in patients with severe COPD. It is not a bronchodilator.

Long-term oxygen therapy is recommended for chronic hypoxemia (pulse oxygen saturation [PaO_2] ≤55 mmHg) or if PaO_2 is ≤88%. Titrate oxygen so that PaO_2 is 88% to 92%. Improved survival with continuous oxygen use compared with nocturnal oxygen use.

Safety Issues

- SABAs (albuterol, levalbuterol, or metaproterenol): May cause adverse cardiac side effects (palpitations, tachycardia). Use with caution if patient has hypertension, angina, and/or hyperthyroidism. Avoid combining with caffeinated drinks.
- Anticholinergics (ipratropium [Atrovent], tiotropium [Spiriva]): Avoid if patient has narrow-angle glaucoma, benign prostatic hyperplasia (BPH), or bladder neck obstruction.
- Phosphodiesterase-4 inhibitor: Contraindicated in moderate-to-severe liver impairment. Associated with increase in psychiatric adverse reactions such as insomnia, depression, suicidal ideation, and weight loss.

General Treatment of Chronic Obstructive Pulmonary Disease

- Smoking cessation is *very important*; options include nicotine patches or gum, bupropion (Zyban) or varenicline (Chantix), patient education, and behavioral counseling.
- Vaccinations, including annual influenza, pneumococcal, and COVID-19 vaccination.
- Pulmonary hygiene (e.g., postural drainage) or pulmonary rehabilitation.
- Regular review of correct inhaler technique.
- Treat lung infections aggressively.
- Physical activity.
- Supplementation with antioxidants such as vitamins C and E, zinc, and selenium can improve muscle strength among patients with COPD.

Management of Stable Chronic Obstructive Pulmonary Disease

Once COPD has been diagnosed, effective management should be based on an individualized assessment of current symptoms and future risks. Reduce and relieve symptoms:

- Improve exercise tolerance.
- Improve health status *and* prevent disease progression, prevent and treat exacerbations, and reduce mortality.

Management of Exacerbations

- First, assess pulse oxygen saturation. An exacerbation of COPD is defined as an acute event characterized by dyspnea and/or cough and sputum that worsen over <14 days.
- Patients with characteristics of a moderate-to-severe exacerbation (increased dyspnea, increased sputum/viscosity, increased sputum purulence) should be hospitalized, as they are at higher risk of death.
- Inhaled short-acting bronchodilator therapy (e.g., SABA, albuterol), with or without SAMAs, are recommended

for initial treatment. Maintenance therapy with long-acting bronchodilators should be started. ICS can be considered to the double bronchodilator regimen in patients with frequent exacerbations.

- If at home, use inhalers with spacer device. If needed, add oral glucocorticoids, such as prednisone 40 mg daily × 5 days.
- The most common cause of exacerbations appears to be respiratory tract infections (viral or bacterial). Suspect secondary bacterial infection if acute onset of fever, purulent sputum, increased wheezing, and dyspnea. Initiate appropriate antibiotic and/or antiviral treatment as indicated.
- CXRs are useful in excluding alternative diagnoses (e.g., pneumonia, PE, pneumothorax).
- An EKG and cardiac troponins may aid in the diagnosis of coexisting cardiac problems.
- Spirometry tests are not recommended during an exacerbation because they can be difficult to perform, and measurements are not accurate enough.
- Noninvasive mechanical ventilation should be the initial mode of ventilation used in patients with COPD.
- Healthcare providers should strongly enforce stringent measures against active cigarette smoking. Patients hospitalized because of exacerbations of COPD are at increased risk for deep vein thrombosis (DVT) and PE; thromboprophylactic measures should be enhanced.

Referral

- Moderate-to-severe COPD
- Severe exacerbations or rapid progression
- Unable to take adequate oral intake

CLINICAL PEARLS

- Low body mass index (BMI) is associated with worse outcomes in patients with COPD. Consider nutritional supplementation (e.g., Ensure) in underweight patients.
- When you are treating a COPD patient, pick an antibiotic that has coverage against both *H. influenzae* (gram negative) and *Streptococcus pneumoniae* (gram positive).

LUNG INFECTIONS

Acute Bronchitis

Acute lower respiratory infection of the large airways (bronchi) with no evidence of pneumonia (Table 8.4). Usually self-limited. Highest incidence in late fall and winter. Causes include adenovirus, influenza, coronavirus, respiratory syncytial virus (RSV), parainfluenza, and human metapneumovirus.

Classic Case

A young adult male complains of a cough that is keeping him awake at night. Cough is mainly dry but can be productive of either purulent or non-purulent sputum. The patient may have frequent paroxysms of coughing; may have low-grade fever and/or chest pain with cough. May

Table 8.4 Lung Infections

Disease	Signs and Symptoms
Community-acquired pneumonia No. 1: *Streptococcus pneumoniae* (gram positive)	Acute onset. High fever and chills. Productive cough and large amount of green-to rust-colored sputum. Pleuritic chest pain with cough. Crackles; decreased breath sounds, dull. CBC: leukocytosis; elevated neutrophils. Band forms may be seen. CXR reveals lobar infiltrates.
Atypical pneumonia No. 1: *Mycoplasma pneumoniae*	Gradual onset. Low-grade fever. Headache, sore throat, cough, wheezing, rash (sometimes). CXR: interstitial to patchy infiltrates.
Viral pneumonia influenza, RSV	Fever, cough, pleurisy, shortness of breath. Scant sputum production. Myalgias. Diminished breath sounds, rales.
Acute bronchitis	Paroxysms of dry and severe cough that interrupts sleep. Cough: dry to productive. Light-colored sputum. Can last up to 4–6 weeks. No antibiotics. Treat symptoms.
Tuberculosis (TB disease)	Cough lasting 3 weeks or longer. Pleuritic chest pain. Hemoptysis with fatigue, weight loss, anorexia, fever/chills, night sweats.
Pertussis (whooping cough)	Intermittent cough that becomes more severe with inspiratory whoop; may be followed by post-tussive vomiting. Cough worse at night; persists for 2–6 weeks or longer. Infants may have mild cough followed by vomiting; complications include apnea and respiratory distress.
COVID-19	Cough, myalgias, and headache; may also have diarrhea, sore throat, and smell/taste abnormalities. Some with only mild upper respiratory symptoms. Others with more serious pneumonia have fever, cough, dyspnea, and infiltrates on chest imaging.

CBC, complete blood count; CXR, chest x-ray; RSV, respiratory syncytial virus.

have nasal congestion, sore throat, headache, wheezing, and rhonchi (clears with coughing). Average duration of cough is 18 days (range of 1 to 3 weeks). May report history of a common cold before onset of bronchitis symptoms.

Symptomatic treatment for acute bronchitis. Do not use antibiotics to treat acute bronchitis.

Objective Findings
- Lungs: Ranges from clear to severe wheezing (prolonged expiratory phase), rhonchi
- Percussion: Resonant
- CXR (to rule out pneumonia): Normal
- Fever: Afebrile to low-grade
- In 40% of patients: Bronchospasm and bronchial hyperreactivity

Treatment Plan
- Treatment is symptomatic. Increase fluids and rest; stop smoking (if smoker).
- Administer dextromethorphan BID to QID, benzonatate (Tessalon Perles) PRN (antitussives).
- Administer guaifenesin PRN (expectorant/mucolytic).
- For wheezing, use albuterol inhaler (Ventolin) QID or nebulized treatment PRN.
- For severe wheezing, consider short-term oral steroid.
- Throat lozenges as needed.

Complications
- Exacerbation of asthma (increased risk of status asthmaticus)
- Pneumonia from secondary bacterial infection (pneumococcus, mycoplasma, others)

Atypical Pneumonia
An infection of the lungs by atypical bacteria. More common in children and young adults. Seasonal outbreaks (summer/fall). Highly contagious. Also known as *walking pneumonia*.

- Recognize presentation of bacterial pneumonia versus atypical pneumonia.
- The top two bacteria in atypical pneumonia are *M. pneumoniae* and *Chlamydia pneumoniae*.

Organisms
- *M. pneumoniae:* Non-pulmonary complications may occur (e.g., hemolytic anemia, meningitis, encephalitis, urticaria). Transmitted via respiratory droplets. Gold standard for diagnosis is polymerase chain reaction (PCR) of sputum or oropharyngeal swab.
- *Chlamydophila pneumoniae:* Common in school-age children, rates range from <1% to 20% in adults; causes fever, shortness of breath, cough, and tachypnea.
- *Legionella pneumoniae:* Found in areas with moisture such as those that are air conditioned (hospitalize, more

severe with higher mortality); causes a severe type of pneumonia called *Legionnaires disease*. Fatality rate 5% to 10%. *Legionella* infection can also cause Pontiac fever. Risk factors include age ≥50 years; smoking; chronic lung disease such as COPD; immune system disorders; underlying illness such as diabetes, renal failure, or hepatic failure.

Classic Case
A young adult complains of several weeks of fatigue, accompanied by coughing that is mostly nonproductive. May be accompanied by headache and low-grade fever. Gradual onset of symptoms. Reports history of a cold before onset of bronchitis (sore throat, clear rhinitis, and low-grade fever). Older patients may have more severe disease.

Objective Findings
- Auscultation: Wheezing and diffused crackles/rales
- Nose: Clear mucus (may have rhinitis of clear mucus)
- Throat: Erythematous without pus or exudate
- CXR: Reticulonodular and/or unilateral or bilateral patchy opacities
- CBC: May have normal results
- Consider testing for *Legionella:* If patient fails outpatient therapy for community acquired pneumonia (CAP), has severe symptoms, or frequently travels. If suspected, order a urinary antigen test for *Legionella pneumophilia.*

Treatment Plan
- Azithromycin (Z-Pak) × 5 days or clarithromycin (Biaxin) 500 mg PO BID × 7 to 10 days
- Doxycycline 100 mg PO BID × 7 to 10 days
- Levofloxacin (Levaquin) 750 mg PO × 5 to 7 days
- Antitussives (dextromethorphan, benzonatate, honey) PRN
- Increased fluids and rest

Common Cold (Viral Upper Respiratory Infection)
Self-limiting infection (range of 4 to 10 days). More common in crowded areas and in small children. Transmission is by respiratory droplets and fomites. Highly contagious. Most contagious from days 2 to 3. Most cases occur in the winter months.

Classic Case
Patient has acute onset of fever, sore throat, frequent sneezing in early phase accompanied by nasal congestion, runny eyes, and rhinorrhea of clear mucus (coryza). The patient may complain of headache. Spontaneous resolution expected within 4 to 10 days.

Objective Findings
- Nasal turbinates: Swollen with clear mucus (may also have blocked tympanic membrane)
- Anterior pharynx: Reddened

- Cervical nodes: Smooth, mobile, and small nodes (≤0.5 cm) in the submandibular and anterior cervical chain
- Lungs: Clear

Treatment Plan
- Treat symptoms, increase fluids and rest, wash hands frequently
- Analgesics (acetaminophen) or NSAIDs (ibuprofen) for fever and aches PRN
- Oral decongestants (e.g., pseudoephedrine [Sudafed]) PRN
- Topical nasal decongestants (e.g., Afrin) can be used BID up to 3 days PRN only; do not use for >3 days due to risk of rebound nasal congestion (rhinitis medicamentosa)
- Antitussives (e.g., dextromethorphan [Robitussin]) PRN
- Antihistamines (e.g., diphenhydramine [Benadryl]) for nasal congestion PRN

Complications
- Acute sinusitis
- Acute otitis media

Community-Acquired Pneumonia in Adults
CAP is an acute lung infection that results in inflammatory changes and damage to the lungs. Risk factors include older age, chronic comorbidities, viral respiratory infection, impaired airway protection (e.g., dysphagia), smoking, and other lifestyle factors. It is the most common cause of focal infiltrate on a CXR (lobar pneumonia).

Organisms
- Most common bacterial cause is *Streptococcus pneumoniae* (gram positive). Other causes include *H. influenzae* (gram negative), atypical bacteria (e.g., *Mycoplasma pneumoniae*), and respiratory viruses (e.g., influenza, parainfluenza, RSV)
- *Pseudomonas aeruginosa* (gram negative) is an uncommon cause of CAP but may appear in patients with cystic fibrosis

Classic Case
An older adult presents with sudden onset of a high fever (>100.4°F) with chills, anorexia, and fatigue that is accompanied by a productive cough with purulent sputum (rust-colored sputum seen with streptococcal pneumonia). The patient complains of sharp stabbing chest pain (pleuritic chest pain) with coughing and dyspnea. Elderly patients may have atypical symptoms (e.g., afebrile or low-grade fever, no cough or mild cough, weakness, confusion).

EXAM TIPS
- The top two bacteria in CAP are *S. pneumoniae* and *H. influenzae.*
- Rust-colored or blood-tinged sputum means *S. pneumoniae* more likely.

Objective Findings

- Inspection: Increased work of breathing, tachypnea, tachycardia
- Auscultation: Rhonchi, crackles, and wheezing
- Percussion: Dullness over affected lobe
- Tactile fremitus and egophony: Increased
- Whispered pectoriloquy: Abnormal (whispered words louder)

Labs

- CXR is the gold standard (definitive) test for diagnosing CAP, not sputum culture; repeat within 6 weeks to document clearing.
- CXR result shows lobar consolidation in classic bacterial pneumonia (Figure 8.1).
- Order a posttreatment CXR to ensure clearing of infection.
- Sputum for culture and sensitivity (C&S) and Gram stain is not recommended for CAP.
- Order CBC for leukocytosis (>10.5×10^9/L) with a possible shift to the left (increased band forms).

Defining Severity and Site of Care

The Pneumonia Severity Index and CURB-65 can be used to assess severity scores and guide clinical decision-making. CURB-65 is based on a total of 5 points with each category as 1 point; 0 to 1 point indicates low severity; 2 points suggests moderate severity; and 3 to 5 points is considered high severity (risk of death 15 to 40%).

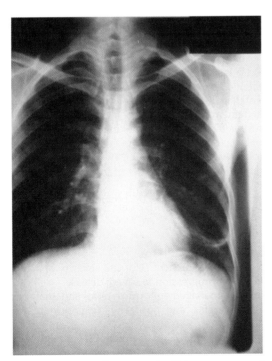

Figure 8.1 Early signs of pneumonia. This anteroposterior chest x-ray reveals signs of early left lower lobe pneumonia, with lobar consolidation.
Source: Image courtesy of Thomas Hooten, MD/Centers for Disease Control and Prevention.

C (*confusion*)
U (blood *urea* nitrogen >19.6 mg/dL)
R (*respiration* >30 breaths/min)
B (*blood* pressure <90/60 mmHg)
Age 65 years or older

Patients with a poor prognosis should be referred for hospitalization:

- Age 60 years or older, acute mental status changes, multiple comorbidities
- Multiple lobar involvement
- Acute mental status change
- Alcohol use disorder (aspiration pneumonia)

Treatment Plan

If no comorbidities (patients age <65 years who are otherwise healthy with no risk factors for drug-resistant *S. pneumoniae* infection, methicillin-resistant *Staphylococcus aureus* (MRSA), or *Pseudomonas*; no recent hospitalization or parenteral antibiotics within past 90 days), American Thoracic Society (ATS)/Infectious Diseases Society of America (IDSA) recommends:

- First-line monotherapy of amoxicillin 1 g PO TID × 5 to 7 days *OR*
- Doxycycline 100 mg PO BID × 5 to 7 days; *OR*
- Macrolide (if local resistance rates are <25%); azithromycin 500 mg PO on first day, then 250 mg PO daily; *OR* clarithromycin 500 mg PO BID or extended-release 1,000 mg PO daily
- Note that amoxicillin plus a macrolide (or doxycycline) can be prescribed to target atypical pathogens.

If there are comorbidities (e.g., alcohol use disorder; congestive heart failure [CHF]; chronic heart, lung, liver, or kidney disease; antibiotics in previous 3 months; diabetes; splenectomy/asplenia) or high rates (>25%) of local pneumococcal resistance, recommendations are for:

- Combination therapy (beta-lactam plus macrolide or doxycycline): Amoxicillin–clavulanate 875/125 mg PO BID *OR* extended-release 2,000/125 mg PO BID; *PLUS* either a macrolide (preferred) *OR* doxycycline: azithromycin 500 mg PO on first day, then 250 mg PO daily; *OR* clarithromycin 500 mg PO BID or extended-release 1,000 mg PO daily; *OR* doxycycline 100 mg PO BID
- Alternatives: Include cephalosporin *PLUS* a macrolide or doxycycline
- Monotherapy (respiratory fluoroquinolone) for patients who cannot use any beta-lactam: Levofloxacin 750 mg PO daily; *OR* moxifloxacin 400 mg PO daily; *OR* gemifloxacin 320 mg PO daily

EXAM TIP

Outpatient CAP diagnosis is based on presentation, signs and symptoms, and CXR. Do not order sputum for C&S; instead, order CXR. CBC is not required for diagnosis.

Prevention

- Influenza vaccine for all persons >50 years or if in contact with persons who are at higher risk of death from pneumonia or who are healthcare workers.

- In the United States, two kinds of vaccines prevent pneumococcal disease—pneumococcal conjugate vaccines (PCV13, PCV15, and PCV20) and pneumococcal polysaccharide vaccine (PPSV23).
- Pneumococcal vaccination is recommended for all adults age 19 through 64 years with certain medical conditions and all adults older than 65 years (see the text that follows).

Pneumococcal Conjugate Vaccines

- PCV13 or PCV15 is recommended for all children <2 years or those 5 through 18 with certain medical conditions.
- For those who have never received any pneumococcal conjugate vaccine, PCV15 or PCV20 is recommended for adults age ≥65 years and those 19 through 64 years with certain medical conditions.
- Adults who have already received PCV13 (at any age) and PPSV23 (at or after the age of 65 years) have the option to get PCV20.

Pneumococcal Polysaccharide Vaccine

- More than 80% of healthy adults who receive PPSV23 develop antibodies after vaccination; overall, the vaccine has been found to have 60% to 70% effectiveness; reduced efficacy can be seen in patients with chronic illnesses or immunodeficiency.
- PPSV23 is recommended for children age 2 through 18 years with certain medical conditions and for adults age 19 years or older who receive PCV15.
- PPSV23 should be given at least 1 year after the PCV15 dose. If PCV20 is used, a dose of PPSV23 is not indicated.
- Shared clinical decision-making for future doses for patients who have already completed the series with PCV13 and PPSV23.

Adults Age 19 to 64 Years With Chronic Medical Conditions

Pneumococcal vaccination is recommended in adults age 19 to 64 years with certain medical conditions (for all-inclusive list, visit the CDC website):

- Impaired immunity: Splenectomy, asplenia, or diseased spleen; alcoholism; HIV infection; cigarette smoking; diabetes mellitus
- Chronic heart, lung, liver, and renal disease: Asthma, congenital heart disease, emphysema, COPD, CHF, cirrhosis
- Blood disorders: Sickle cell anemia; malignancy (Hodgkin's lymphoma, multiple myeloma)

COVID-19

COVID-19 is caused by a severe acute respiratory syndrome coronavirus 2 (SARS-CoV-2). Globally, over 500 million confirmed COVID-19 cases have been reported. Primarily spread via direct person-to-person respiratory transmission. Several variants have emerged, increasing the potential for transmissibility. Information about COVID-19 is constantly evolving; latest evidence and guidelines can be found on WHO and CDC websites.

Classic Case

Patient presents with cough, fever, myalgias, and headache. Associated symptoms include diarrhea, sore throat, and smell or taste abnormalities (an unusual symptom compared with other common-cold syndromes). Report of a general health decline. The Delta and Omicron variants seem to cause more respiratory symptoms, such as nasal congestion and sneezing. A serious manifestation of the disease is pneumonia with fever, cough, dyspnea, and infiltrates on CXR.

Objective Findings

- Fever: Not universal finding; conjunctivitis
- Dermatologic findings: Reports of maculopapular/morbilliform, urticarial, and vesicular eruptions and transient livedo reticularis; reddish-purple nodules on the digits ("COVID toes")
- CBC: Often, lymphopenia, leukocytosis, leukopenia, thrombocytopenia
- LFTs: May show elevated aminotransaminase and lactate dehydrogenase levels
- Inflammatory markers: Elevated ferritin, C-reactive protein, and erythrocyte sedimentation rate
- Abnormalities: In coagulation panel; elevated D-dimer
- CXR: May be normal or abnormal with consolidation and non-solid nodules
- Chest CT: May have non-solid nodules with mixed consolidation, pleural thickening

Risk Factors for Acute Illness

- Age ≥65 years
- Comorbidities such as asthma, cancer, cystic fibrosis, cerebrovascular disease, chronic lung/liver/kidney disease, diabetes mellitus, disabilities, HIV, heart conditions, pregnancy, sickle cell disease, transplant patients, TB
- Mental health disorders such as depression, schizophrenia, dementia
- Lifestyle factors such as smoking, physical inactivity
- Males have higher number of critical cases and deaths
- African American, Hispanic, and Southern Asian individuals have a high number of infections and deaths in the United States
- Use of corticosteroids or other immunosuppressive medications
- Genetic factors

Treatment Plan

- Coordinated approach: To assess severity of symptoms and risk of progression to severe disease
- Symptom management: Antipyretics and analgesics for fever, myalgias, and headaches (e.g., acetaminophen, NSAIDs)
- Supportive care: Increase fluids, OTC cough suppressants (e.g., dextromethorphan), rest; recovery may vary depending on health status of patient, infection control, and self-isolation
- Symptomatic adults who are at increased risk for severe disease: Early treatment with nirmatrelvir-ritonavir within 5 days of symptom onset (alternative: remdesivir)

- Dexamethasone, prednisone, or other corticosteroids: Not recommended for non-hospitalized patients not receiving supplemental oxygen for COVID-19
- Counsel patients on warning symptoms that prompt further care: New-onset dyspnea, dizziness, mental status changes

Primary Prevention
- CDC recommends COVID-19 vaccinations for children and teenagers age 6 months to 17 years and adults age 18 years and older.
- Four vaccines are approved in the United States—Pfizer-BioNTech, Moderna, Novavax, and Johnson & Johnson's Janssen (recommended only in certain situations). Pfizer and Moderna have developed updated bivalent COVID-19 boosters.
- COVID-19 vaccine recommendations vary based on age, first vaccine received, and length of time since the last dose. Review the latest guidelines online for your practice area.
- In general, for adults age 18 years and older, first dose is followed by a second dose 3 to 8 weeks later; a third dose, a bivalent booster, is recommended at least 2 months after the second primary series dose or last booster.

Complications
- Respiratory failure: Acute respiratory distress syndrome
- Thromboembolic events: DVT and PE
- Cardiac complications: Arrhythmias, myocardial injury, heart failure, shock
- Neurologic complications: Encephalopathy
- Inflammatory complications: Persistent fevers, elevated inflammatory markers and proinflammatory cytokines, secondary infections

CLINICAL PEARLS

- If you suspect CAP based on clinical signs and symptoms but patient has a negative CXR/radiograph, treat them with antibiotics as appropriate.
- Macrolides given to infants <1 month of age at risk for developing infantile hyperpyloric stenosis (IHPS).
- Suspect pertussis in a "healthy" adult with no fever who has been coughing for >2 to 3 weeks, especially if previously treated with an antibiotic (that was not a macrolide) and is getting worse (rule out pneumonia first).
- Emphasize importance of adequate fluid intake (best mucolytic, thins out mucus).
- Lung cancer can present as recurrent pneumonia (due to mass blocking bronchioles).
- If *S. pneumoniae* macrolide resistance >25%, do not use macrolide monotherapy. See CAP treatment guidelines notes.

Differential Diagnoses for Cough

Table 8.5 Differential Diagnoses: Cough

Condition	Signs and Symptoms
Bacterial pneumonia	Fever, tachypnea, or tachycardia, productive cough. CXR shows lobar consolidation. May have pleuritic chest pain with cough.
Postnasal drip	Ticklish sensation in back of the throat, clearing throat often, cough worsens when supine. May have rhinosinusitis with purulent (or non-purulent) PND.
Asthma	Shortness of breath or dyspnea, wheezing, dry cough; acute symptoms respond to SABA.
Gastroesophageal reflux	Heartburn after large or fatty meals or with empty stomach; worsens when supine. Cough may be present.
Heart failure	Shortness of breath/dyspnea that worsens with exertion or physical activity, pitting edema, and dry cough. Physical exam may show S3, elevated JVD.
Pulmonary embolism	New onset of dyspnea, hemoptysis, pleuritic chest pain. Vital signs with tachycardia, tachypnea. May have signs of DVT.
Lung cancer	Cough in a person with risk factors such as long-term cigarette smoking (≥30-pack-year history). Weight loss.
ACE inhibitor use	Nonproductive cough in a person with hypertension, diabetes, or CKD. Can start within 1 week of starting medication.

ACE, angiotensin-converting enzyme; CKD, chronic kidney disease; CXR, chest x-ray; DVT, deep vein thrombosis; JVD, jugular vein distention; PND, postnasal drip; SABA, short-acting beta2-agonist.

Pertussis
Also known as *whooping cough*. Caused by *Bordetella pertussis* bacteria (gram negative). A highly contagious coughing illness of at least 14 days duration with one of the following findings: paroxysmal coughing, inspiratory whooping, or post-tussive vomiting without apparent cause. Illness can last from a few weeks to months. Unvaccinated children and adults with expired vaccinations are at the highest risk for pertussis. Neonates and infants are at highest risk of death. Pertussis has three stages (catarrhal, paroxysmal, and convalescent).
- First stage: Catarrhal stage (lasts 1–2 weeks). If treated at this stage, can shorten disease course (if treated within 3 weeks of onset).
- Second stage: Paroxysmal coughing (lasts 2–4 weeks). Treatment has little influence on disease but is useful to prevent disease spread.
- Third stage: Convalescent stage (lasts 1–2 weeks). Treatment goal is to eradicate carriage state/disease spread. Antibiotic will not shorten illness at this stage.

Classic Case

Previously healthy patient presents with a severe hacking cough of >2 weeks' duration. Initial symptoms are low-grade fever and rhinorrhea with a mild cough (catarrhal stage). Cough becomes severe with inspiratory "whooping" sound. Patient may vomit afterward. Cough is worse at night. Infants have atypical presentation of no whooping with minimal to no cough. Apnea is more common in infants.

Labs

- Less than 2 weeks of cough: Nasopharyngeal swab for culture (gold standard laboratory test) and PCR for *B. pertussis*; sensitivity for culture is highest during the first 2 weeks of illness.
- 2 to 4 weeks of cough: Perform both culture and PCR; sensitivity for culture declines but PCR is effective for up to 4 weeks.
- More than 4 weeks of cough: Only serology is useful.
- CBC: Elevated white blood cells (WBCs) and marked lymphocytosis (up to 80% lymphocytes in WBC differential).
- CXR: Should be negative; if positive, likely a secondary bacterial infection.

Treatment Plan

For adolescents or adults with *cough duration of 3 weeks or less*, pregnant patients near term, immunocompromised adolescents or adults, and those older than 65 years presenting *up to 6 weeks following symptom onset.*

First-line treatment is macrolides.

- Azithromycin (Z-Pak) 500 mg on day 1, then 250 mg daily from days 2 to 5 (drug of choice of very young infants)
- Clarithromycin (Biaxin) BID × 7 days
- When macrolides are given to infants <1 month of age, monitor for IHPS and other adverse events. For persons ≥2 months of age, an alternative to macrolides is trimethoprim–sulfamethoxazole.
- Alternative is trimethoprim–sulfamethoxazole (Bactrim DS) PO BID × 14 days (infants >1 month of age given × 7-day duration and dosed by weight)

Additional therapy includes postexposure prophylaxis for close contacts and respiratory droplet precautions. Antitussives, mucolytics, rest, and hydration; frequent small meals.

EXAM TIP

Know presentation and treatment of pertussis (whooping cough).

Prevention

- Infants and children: CDC recommends five doses of DTaP (diphtheria, tetanus, and whooping cough)
- Adolescents: Single dose of Tdap (tetanus, diphtheria, and whooping cough), preferably at age 11 to 12 years
- Pregnant patients: Single dose of Tdap during every pregnancy, preferably during the early part of gestational weeks 27 through 36.
- Adults: To those who have never received Tdap, administer a single dose of Tdap followed by a Td or Tdap booster every 10 years.

Complications

Sinusitis, otitis media, pneumonia, fainting, rib fractures.

Tuberculosis

An infection caused by *Mycobacterium tuberculosis* bacteria. Most common site of infection is the lungs. Other sites include the pleurae, kidneys, brain, lymph nodes, adrenals, and bone. Most contagious forms are pulmonary TB, pleural TB, and laryngeal TB (coughing spreads aerosol droplets). CXR (reactivated TB) will show cavitations and adenopathy and granulomas on the hila of the lungs.

- High-risk populations: Persons from high-prevalence countries; migrant farm workers; users of illicit drugs; persons who are homeless; residents of penitentiaries, nursing homes, and adult living facilities; persons who are HIV positive or immunocompromised.
- Tuberculosis infection: Previously known as latent tuberculosis infection. An intact immune system causes macrophages to sequester the bacteria in the lymph nodes (mediastinum) in the form of granulomas. Asymptomatic and noninfectious.
- Tuberculosis disease: Previously known as active tuberculosis. Refers to the presence of signs or symptoms reflecting illness due to *M. tuberculosis*. Contagious; TB bacteria are actively replicating and damaging the body.
- Miliary TB: Also known as *disseminated TB disease*. Progressive, widely disseminated hematogenous TB; infects multiple organ systems. More common in younger children (<5 years) and older persons. CXR will show classic small, firm white nodules resembling millet seeds.
- Multidrug-resistant TB (MDR TB): Bacteria resistant to at least two of the best anti-TB drugs—isoniazid (INH) and rifampin (considered first-line drugs)—and possibly additional antituberculous agents.
- Extensively drug-resistant TB: Resistance to isoniazid, rifampin, a fluoroquinolone, and at least one second-line injectable agent or resistance to either bedaquiline or linezolid.
- Prior Bacillus Calmette-Guérin (BCG) vaccine: Attenuated vaccine to prevent tuberculosis. After vaccination, most individuals have a tuberculin reaction of 3 to 19 mm for up to 3 months. This reaction decreases over time. Interferon-gamma release assay (IGRAs) testing is the preferred method of testing for people who received the BCG vaccine to identify distinction of a positive reaction.

Classic Case

An adult patient from a high-risk population complains of fever, anorexia, fatigue, and night sweats along with a mild nonproductive cough (early phase). Aggressive infections (later sign) have productive cough with blood-stained sputum (hemoptysis) along with weight loss (late sign).

EXAM TIPS

- A purified protein derivative (PPD) result may be listed as 9.5 mm. If the patient falls under the 10-mm group, then it is negative (by definition) unless the patient has the signs/symptoms and/or CXR findings suggestive of TB.
- Memorize the criteria for the 5-mm and 10-mm results.

Treatment Plan

- TB is a reportable disease. Report TB to local health department for contact tracing as soon as possible.
- Assess for signs and symptoms of TB (cough, night sweats, weight loss). If symptoms present, the patient likely has active TB disease. Patients with latent TB infection (LTBI) do not have symptoms and cannot spread the infection to others.
- Patients with both LTBI and TB disease should be treated. Treatment reduces the risk that LTBI will progress to TB disease, which can be fatal without appropriate treatment. A high priority for LTBI should be given to those with a positive TB blood test, certain groups with a positive tuberculin skin test (TST) of 5 mm or more (e.g., HIV-positive persons, organ transplant recipients, immunocompromised patients), and certain groups with a TST reaction of 10 mm or more (e.g., intravenous drug users, residents of high-risk settings, persons from high-risk countries).
- Order CXR (assess for upper lobe cavitations and mediastinal adenopathy).
- Check baseline liver function tests and monitor. Provide education on alcohol cessation, if indicated.
- All patients with TB should be tested for HIV infection. A patient with untreated LTBI and HIV is more likely to develop TB disease.
- Four CDC-recommended treatment regimens for LTBI use isoniazid, rifapentine, and/or rifampin. The preferred duration is the short-course, rifamycin-based, 3- or 4-month regimen in comparison to the 6- or 9-month isoniazid monotherapy.
- Duration of treatment for active TB disease can be 4, 6, or 9 months. Treatment depends on drug susceptibility results, coexisting medical conditions, and potential for drug interactions. The 6- to 9-month treatment regimen includes four drugs: isoniazid, rifampin, ethambutol, and pyrazinamide.
- Several treatment regimens are available. Optimal therapy involves referral to infectious disease expert. Consult the CDC's TB website (www.cdc.gov/TB).

Directly Observed Treatment

- Mandatory for noncompliant patients. Success is dependent on medication compliance.

- Patient is observed by a nurse when they take the medications. Mouth, cheek, and area under the tongue are checked to make sure the pill was swallowed adequately.

Drug Adverse Effects

- Isoniazid (INH): Give with pyridoxine (vitamin B_6) to decrease risk of peripheral neuritis, neuropathy, hepatitis, seizures.
- Ethambutol (ETH): Optic neuritis, rash. Avoid if patient has eye problems. Eye exam at baseline.
- Pyrazinamide (PZA): Hepatitis, hyperuricemia, arthralgias, rash
- Rifampin (RIF): Hepatitis; thrombocytopenia; orange-colored tears, saliva, and urine; drug interactions

Labs

Tuberculosis Skin Test (Mantoux Test)

Assess the intradermal delayed-type hypersensitivity response. Inject 0.1 mL of 5TU-PPD subdermally. Measure the reaction by the width of the induration, not the erythema. See Table 8.6.

Table 8.6 Tuberculosis Skin Test Results (Mantoux or the Purified Protein Derivative)

Size	Scenario With Positive Reaction
<5	HIV infection plus close contact of active contagious case
≥5 mm	HIV (+)
	Recent contact with infectious TB cases
	CXR with fibrotic changes consistent with previous TB disease
	Immunocompromised (e.g., organ transplant, bone marrow transplant, renal failure, patients on biologic drugs)
≥10 mm	Recent immigrants (within past 5 years) from high-prevalence countries (Latin America, Asia [except Japan], Africa, India, Pacific islands)
	Child <4 years of age or children/adolescents exposed to high-risk adult: Injection drug user, healthcare worker, homeless person
	Employees or residents from high-risk congregate settings (e.g., jails, nursing homes)
	Persons with conditions that increase risk of reaction (e.g., chronic renal failure, diabetes mellitus, some malignancies, IV drug users, underweight, silicosis)
≥15 mm	Healthy individuals age >4 with no risk factors for TB

CXR, chest x-ray; TB, tuberculosis.

Blood Tests for Tuberculosis

- QuantiFERON-TB Gold in-tube test or the T-SPOT TB test (also known as IGRAs): Blood tests that measure gamma-interferon (from lymphocytes).
- IGRA test results: Available within 24 hours (only one visit required). If history of previous BCG vaccination, IGRA blood tests preferred.

Sputum Tests for Tuberculosis

- Deep cough specimen from the lower respiratory tract of at least 5 to 10 mL: Collect three specimens in an 8- to 24-hour interval (at least one obtained in the early morning).
- Sputum nucleic acid amplification test (NAAT): Rapid test (1–3 days).
- Sputum for C&S: Gold standard for diagnosing pulmonary TB infection; can take up to 8 weeks to grow.
- Acid-fast bacilli (AFB) smear: Positive AFB is not diagnostic, but it is suggestive of TB infection. It is a rapid test, and results can be obtained 1 to 2 days. It helps to strengthen diagnosis of TB before sputum C&S results are available (takes up to 8 weeks for result).
- Order sputum for NAAT, C&S, and AFB smear: If active TB infection suspected.

Booster Phenomenon

A person with LTBI can have a false-negative reaction to the TST or the PPD if they have not been tested for many years. Two-step TST is recommended by the CDC:

- When the TST/PPD is done the first time, if there is no reaction, it may be a false negative.
- Repeat the PPD (1–4 weeks later) on the opposite forearm. Positive reaction suggests the booster phenomenon.
- Follow up with CXR and inquire about signs/symptoms of TB infection. If no symptoms of active TB disease and negative CXR, offer LTBI prophylaxis.
- If the second PPD is negative, the person likely has a true negative test result (does not have a TB infection).

CLINICAL PEARLS

- The QuantiFERON-TB Gold in-tube and the T-SPOT TB tests are available at public health clinics.
- Never treat TB with fewer than three drugs.
- According to the CDC, on average, about 10 contacts are listed for each index person with infectious TB.
- Persons with HIV infection with CD4 <500 or patients who are taking tumor necrosis factor antagonists (or biologics) are at very high risk for active TB disease after initial exposure (primary TB).
- The TST is considered both valid and safe to use throughout pregnancy.
- Younger children are more likely than older children to develop life-threatening forms of TB disease.

CHEST X-RAY INTERPRETATION

You may see images of plain CXR films on the exam. Here are some basics. X-rays are radiation (gamma rays) that pass through the human body and hit a metal target (the film cassette). Depending on the type of tissue density, they are absorbed differently. The darker the color, the lower the tissue density (e.g., air in lungs). X-rays can be plain or contrasted. In the PA view, the x-ray goes through the back to the front (with the patient standing up); see Figure 8.2 for an example. The spinal column is more visible with this view. For the anterior–posterior (AP) view, the x-ray goes through the front of the chest toward the back. Lateral view is the view from the side of the chest. A systematic approach of reading chest films should be followed every time. Compare the present film with the old films (if available).

EXAM TIP

You may be asked to identify an image of a CXR of a patient with pulmonary TB or bacterial pneumonia. See Figure 8.3 for an example of a TB x-ray.

APPEARANCE

- Air: Appears as black color (low density so less absorption) over lung field
- Bones: Appear as white to gray
- Metals: Bright white (high absorption)
- Tissue: Different grayish shades (medium absorption)
- Fluid: Grayish to whitish
- Tissues visible: Trachea, bronchus, aorta, heart, lungs, pulmonary arteries, diaphragm, gastric bubble, ribs

ABNORMAL CONDITIONS

- Emphysema: Black color in the hilum (above the clavicles), a lot of black color in hyperinflated lungs, blunted costovertebral angle (CVA; diaphragm flat instead of dome shaped).
- Lobar pneumonia/bacterial pneumonia: Grayish to white areas on a lobe or lobes of lung (consolidation) from purulent fluid.
- TB: Upper lobe with cavitation (black round holes), fibrosis (scarring), and pulmonary infiltrates (fluid) in active TB disease (Figure 8.3).
- Left ventricular hypertrophy (LVH)/cardiomyopathy: Heart occupies more than 50% of the chest diameter; it is enlarged.
- Silhouette sign: Displacement of the normal silhouette in the chest film. For example, displacement of the para-aortic line can be caused by an aortic aneurysm or dissection/rupture.

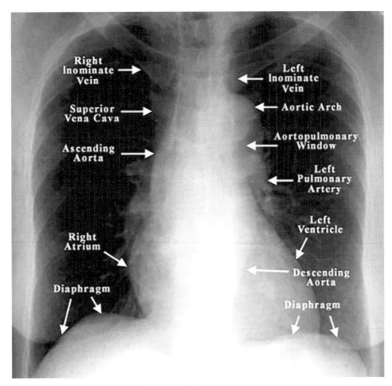

Figure 8.2 Sample posterior–anterior chest x-ray with labeled anatomy.

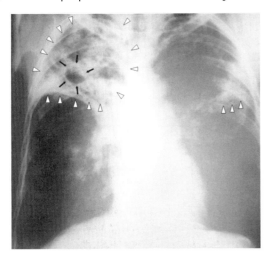

Figure 8.3 Chest x-ray: tuberculosis.
Source: Centers for Disease Control and Prevention.

EXAM TIPS

- Memorize the appearance of a posterior–anterior (PA) CXR of a person with healed pulmonary TB. The classic findings are pulmonary nodules and/or cavitations (round black holes) on the upper lobes with or without fibrotic changes (scars).
- With right middle-lobe pneumonia, look for consolidation (white-colored area) on the right middle lobe, which is located at about the same level as the right breast on the front of the chest.

CLINICAL PEARLS

- During a severe asthmatic exacerbation, it is hard to hear breath sounds, and you may not hear any wheezing. Administer albuterol nebulizer treatment and listen for wheezing, which means patient's airways are opening.
- Ask asthmatic patient how many times they use their albuterol (SABA) inhaler. If using more than twice per week, patient likely has poorly controlled asthma or is having an exacerbation.
- If you suspect allergic asthma, check serum immunoglobulin G allergy panels (e.g., mold allergy, grass allergy panels). Refer to allergist for scratch testing (more sensitive than blood allergy panels) and treatment.
- Consider supplementing with calcium with vitamin D 1,200 mg tabs daily for menopausal women and other high-risk patients (for osteoporosis) such as males who are on medium- to high-dose inhaled steroids long term.
- Consider bone-density testing in males or females who are on chronic steroids to rule out osteopenia or osteoporosis.
- Annual eye exams if on long-term steroids due to higher risk of cataracts and glaucoma.

KNOWLEDGE CHECK: CHAPTER 8

1. Which of the following influences peak expiratory flow rate?
   A. Age
   B. Body mass index
   C. Weight
   D. Temperature

2. Which of the following is *true* regarding tuberculosis (TB)?
   A. Duration of treatment is 10 to 12 months.
   B. It is a reportable disease.
   C. Treatment is required for active disease and monitoring for latent TB.
   D. Treatment consists of monotherapy with isoniazid.

3. Which of the following is a restrictive lung disease?
   A. Asthma
   B. Chronic obstructive pulmonary disease (COPD)
   C. Bronchiectasis
   D. Pulmonary fibrosis

4. Which of the following physical exam findings can confirm the diagnosis of community-acquired pneumonia?
   A. Crackles on chest auscultation
   B. Egophony
   C. Tachypnea
   D. None of the above

5. A 35-year-old patient with no past medical history presents with fever and productive cough. Vital signs are significant for temperature 38.8°C, heart rate 115, respiratory rate 20 breaths/min, blood pressure 115/75 mmHg, and pulse oximetry 98% on room air. Physical examination is significant for crackles (rales) present in the right lung field. Chest x-ray shows a right middle lobe infiltrate. Which of the following is the appropriate initial pharmacologic management?
   A. Ceftriaxone plus azithromycin
   B. Amoxicillin
   C. Levofloxacin
   D. Amoxicillin-clavulanate plus doxycycline

6. A younger child with an unknown vaccination history presents with symptoms similar to an upper respiratory infection. The child's parent reports sudden episodes of coughing and posttussive vomiting. An inspiratory whoop is heard on physical examination. These clinical features are suggestive of which respiratory condition?
   A. Acute bronchitis
   B. Atypical pneumonia
   C. Pertussis
   D. Tuberculosis

7. In which situation would a tuberculin skin test reaction be considered positive?
   A. ≥5 mm in a patient who received a liver transplant
   B. ≥10 mm in a healthy patient older than 5 years
   C. ≥5 mm in a patient with diabetes mellitus
   D. ≥5 mm in a patient who is incarcerated

8. Which of the following sounds is typically heard over normal lung tissue?
   A. Dullness
   B. Tympany
   C. Flatness
   D. Resonance

9. A young adult patient who is otherwise healthy with no comorbidities presents with a cough that has lasted for 2 weeks with posttussive emesis. Culture and polymerase chain reaction (PCR) are pending. Which of the following is the *most* appropriate medical management for this patient?
   A. It has been 2 weeks, so antibiotic therapy is not necessary.
   B. Azithromycin should be given orally for 5 days.
   C. Antibiotic therapy should be delayed until culture results have confirmed diagnosis.
   D. Oral erythromycin four times daily should be started.

(See answers next page.)

1. A) Age
Normal values for peak expiratory flow rate depend on height, age, and sex (HAS). Weight, body mass index, and temperature have no influence.

2. B) It is a reportable disease.
TB is a reportable disease; the nurse practitioner should contact the local health department for contact tracing after diagnosis. Treatment regimens can be 4, 6, or 9 months, and each consists of multidrug therapy. Both active and latent forms of the disease require treatment.

3. D) Pulmonary fibrosis
Restrictive lung diseases (reduction of lung volume due to decreased lung compliance) include pulmonary fibrosis, pleural disease, and diaphragm obstruction. Obstructive lung diseases (reduction in airflow rates) include asthma, COPD (chronic bronchitis and emphysema), and bronchiectasis.

4. D) None of the above
A posteroanterior and lateral chest x-ray is used for diagnosis in a patient suspected of having community-acquired pneumonia. Diagnosis is established by the presence of opacity on chest imaging in a patient with associated symptoms (e.g., fever, dyspnea, cough, sputum production). Rarely is the diagnosis of community-acquired pneumonia based on clinical features alone (e.g., tachycardia, tachypnea, crackles, tactile fremitus, egophony) due to their limited (and relatively nonspecific) diagnostic accuracy.

5. B) Amoxicillin
The patient is presenting with symptoms and a chest x-ray consistent with a diagnosis of community-acquired pneumonia. According to American Thoracic Society/Infectious Diseases Society of America guidelines for otherwise healthy adults <65 years with no recent antibiotic use, monotherapy with amoxicillin is indicated as first-line treatment, and monotherapy with either doxycycline or a macrolide (if local resistant rates are <25%) as second-line alternatives. For patients with comorbidities age 65 years or older or recent antibiotic use, amoxicillin-clavulanate is recommended. While fluroquinolones (e.g., levofloxacin) are routinely used to treat community-acquired pneumonia, their use is not recommended in ambulatory patients due to concern for the development of fluroquinolone resistance among respiratory pathogens. Combination therapy with ceftriaxone plus a macrolide (e.g., azithromycin) is indicated for patients with community-acquired pneumonia admitted to a general medical unit without suspicion for *Pseudomonas* or other drug-resistant pathogens.

6. C) Pertussis
The classic presentation of pertussis generally occurs in unvaccinated children and includes paroxysms of coughing, an inspiratory whoop, and posttussive vomiting. There is nothing to suggest high risk factors for tuberculosis in this patient; tuberculosis often presents with fever, anorexia, fatigue, night sweats, and nonproductive cough. While patients with acute bronchitis and atypical pneumonia often present with a cough, the total presentation of paroxysms of coughing, inspiratory whoop, and posttussive vomiting are more specific to pertussis.

7. A) ≥5 mm in a patient who received a liver transplant
A tuberculin skin test reaction size of ≥5 mm in an immunosuppressed patient, such as one who has received an organ transplant, is considered a positive reaction. A size of ≥10 would be considered a positive reaction in a patient who is incarcerated, a patient who has diabetes mellitus, and a healthy patient younger than 4 years.

8. D) Resonance
Resonance is the hollow sound heard over normal lung tissue filled with air. Flatness is normally heard over solid areas such as bones. Tympany is a loud and high-pitched drumlike sound that is normally heard when percussing across the abdomen. It is abnormal when found in the chest wall (suggests pneumothorax). Dullness is heard over a dense area or solid organ (e.g., heart, liver) as a medium-intensity pitch. It is considered abnormal over lung tissue because it is often due to fluid or consolidation (e.g., pneumonia, masses or tumors, pleural effusions, hemothorax, empyema).

9. B) Azithromycin should be given orally for 5 days.
This patient is presenting with a concern for pertussis—a cough illness lasting at least 2 weeks with paroxysms of coughing, inspiratory whoop, and posttussive emesis. Pertussis is highly contagious, so empiric antibiotic therapy is recommended once there is clinical suspicion of pertussis without awaiting diagnostic testing results. Antibiotic therapy (e.g., azithromycin, clarithromycin) is recommended for all patients who present within 3 weeks of cough onset. Trimethoprim-sulfamethoxazole is an alternative. Antibiotics are recommended after 3-week cough onset for pregnant patients and immunocompromised adults.

10. A patient with chronic obstructive pulmonary disease (COPD) has a history of three moderate exacerbations and one hospitalization over the past 6 months. Which initial pharmacologic regimen is appropriate for this patient?
    A. A bronchodilator
    B. Long-acting beta2-agonist (LABA) and inhaled corticosteroids (ICS)
    C. LABA and long-acting muscarinic antagonist (LAMA)
    D. LAMA

11. Which of the following is recommended for lung cancer screening according to the U.S. Preventive Services Task Force (USPSTF)?
    A. Low-dose CT scan
    B. Chest x-ray
    C. PET scan
    D. MRI of the chest

12. The nurse practitioner performs a physical assessment of a patient. While auscultating over the peripheral lung fields, they hear breath sounds that are of soft intensity and low pitched, with a rustling quality during inspiration and softer sound during expiration. These findings suggest which breath sound?
    A. Tracheal
    B. Bronchial
    C. Bronchovesicular
    D. Vesicular

13. A patient presents complaining of troublesome asthma symptoms on most days. They also report that their asthma symptoms wake them up at night several times each month. Based on the Global Initiative for Asthma (GINA) guidelines, this patient meets the criteria for which step?
    A. 1
    B. 2
    C. 3
    D. 4

14. A patient presents with symptoms of a headache, malaise, low-grade fever, and cough. The patient also reports nonpulmonary symptoms such as mild erythematous rashes and myalgia. Lab abnormalities suggest hemolysis. Which of the following tests is preferred for diagnosis?
    A. Polymerase chain reaction (PCR) from a nasopharyngeal swab
    B. Direct Coombs test
    C. Chest x-ray
    D. Serology markers

15. A young adult patient with no past medical history presents with a cough that awakens them throughout the night. The cough is mainly dry and has persisted for 1 week; the patient also reports a headache, nasal congestion, and a mild sore throat. The patient does not have a fever, and no tachypnea or signs of parenchymal consolidation are noted on physical exam. These findings suggest which medical management?
    A. Antibiotic therapy
    B. Throat lozenges and guaifenesin
    C. Oral corticosteroids
    D. Albuterol

16. How does tuberculosis (TB) infection differ from TB disease?
    A. A patient with TB disease has no symptoms.
    B. Only patients with TB infection need treatment.
    C. A patient with TB infection does not have symptoms.
    D. Patients with TB infection are highly contagious.

17. A patient presents with concern for an asthma exacerbation. The patient is tachypneic, heart rate is 125 beats/min, and the patient is using accessory muscles to assist breathing. Which of the following diagnostic tools should be used to assess the severity of the asthma attack?
    A. Peak flow meter (or spirometer)
    B. Pulse oxygen saturation
    C. Arterial blood gas
    D. Chest x-ray

(See answers next page.)

10. C) LABA and long-acting muscarinic antagonist (LAMA)

This patient can be categorized as group E due to their history of exacerbations and recent hospitalization. For group E patients, LABA and LAMA together is the preferred choice for initial therapy rather than using either agent alone. The use of LABA and ICS in COPD patients is not recommended. Group A patients should be offered a bronchodilator treatment.

11. A) Low-dose CT scan

According to the USPSTF, screening for lung cancer with an annual low-dose CT scan is recommended for adults age 50 to 80 years who have a 20 pack-year smoking history and currently smoke or have quit in the past 15 years. While the other imaging techniques can be used for further evaluation and work-up, the low-dose CT scan is recommended as an initial screening tool.

12. D) Vesicular

Vesicular breath sounds are soft and low pitched; they are heard bilaterally over most of the peripheral fields. Bronchial breath sounds are louder and higher in pitch and heard over the lower aspect of the trachea and over the manubrium. Bronchovesicular breath sounds are of intermediate intensity and pitch and are heard over major bronchi in the midchest area or between the scapula. Tracheal breath sounds are of the highest and loudest pitch and are heard over the upper aspect of the trachea and anterior aspect of the neck.

13. C) 3

The patient meets criteria for Step 3 according to the GINA guidelines due to occurrence of troublesome symptoms most days and nocturnal awakening more than once per month. Step 1 involves infrequent asthma symptoms (less than 2×/week); Step 2 involves asthma symptoms or need for reliever inhaler more than 2×/week; and Step 4 involves severely uncontrolled asthma with three or more of the following: daytime asthma symptoms more than 2×/week, nocturnal awakening due to asthma, reliever needed for symptoms more than 2×/week, or activity limitation due to asthma.

14. A) Polymerase chain reaction (PCR) from a nasopharyngeal swab

The patient is presenting with signs and symptoms suggestive of *Mycoplasma pneumoniae* infection. In addition to upper respiratory tract symptoms, patients often present with extrapulmonary manifestations such as dermatologic and musculoskeletal features and hemolysis on lab work. Nucleic acid amplification tests are the diagnostic tests of choice; these include direct DNA amplification tests (PCR from nasopharyngeal swab or sputum) and multiplex assays. A direct Coombs test can be used to support diagnosis in the setting of hemolysis; however, it is not routinely recommended as hemolysis is often self-limited and mild. Findings on a chest x-ray are not specific enough to definitely distinguish *M. pneumoniae* from other types of pneumonia. Serology can be used as an alternative or adjunct to molecular testing.

15. B) Throat lozenges and guaifenesin

This patient is presenting with signs and symptoms suggestive of acute bronchitis. A clinical diagnosis can be suspected in a patient presenting with a persistent cough who does not have symptoms of pneumonia (e.g., fever, tachypnea, signs of consolidation) or chronic obstructive pulmonary disease. Treatment includes supportive care (symptom management), as symptoms are often self-limiting. Treatment includes throat lozenges, hot tea, and smoking cessation; dextromethorphan or guaifenesin can be used for cough relief. Acute bronchitis is caused by viruses, so antibiotic therapy is not indicated and can contribute to antibiotic resistance. Oral corticosteroids are not recommended due to limited evidence and adverse effects. Inhaled beta2-agonists, such as albuterol, should be reserved for patients with wheezing and underlying pulmonary disease.

16. C) A patient with TB infection does not have symptoms.

A patient with TB infection has no symptoms, cannot spread TB to others, usually has a positive TB skin test reaction or positive TB blood test, and may develop TB disease if they do not receive treatment. Patients with TB disease have active TB bacteria, so they are contagious and symptomatic, and they usually have a positive TB skin test reaction, positive TB blood test, abnormal chest x-ray, or positive sputum or culture. They require treatment.

17. A) Peak flow meter (or spirometer)

The best method to objectively assess the severity of an asthma attack is measurement of maximal expiratory airflow with a peak flow meter (or spirometer). Pulse oxygen saturation testing provides a noninvasive screening test for hypoxemia. Arterial blood gas to assess for hypercapnia is not necessary in most patients. It may be more appropriate in patients who are more critically ill with worsening respiratory status or show signs of hypercapnia (e.g., depressed consciousness). A chest x-ray is not routinely recommended during acute asthma attacks because the findings are often nonspecific.

18. In regard to the scenario in question 17, which of the following is the first-line treatment?
    A. Montelukast
    B. Albuterol
    C. Theophylline
    D. Magnesium sulfat

19. Which of the following can cause a false-positive tuberculin skin reaction test?
    A. Pneumococcal conjugate vaccine (PCV13)
    B. Moderna COVID-19 vaccine
    C. Pneumococcal polysaccharide vaccine (PPSV23)
    D. Bacillus Calmette-Guérin (BCG) vaccination

20. A 67-year-old adult with no immunocompromised conditions asks about their pneumococcal vaccine schedule. The patient reports a history of receiving the PPSV23 vaccine and wants to know if they need any additional pneumococcal vaccines. Based on Centers for Disease Control and Prevention (CDC) guidelines, this patient should receive:
    A. A second dose of PPSV23
    B. PCV20 within 6 months of receiving the PPSV23 vaccine
    C. PCV20 at least 1 year after the most recent PPSV23 vaccine
    D. PCV15 at least 2 years after the most recent PPSV23 vaccine

21. A 50-year-old patient with chronic obstructive pulmonary disease (COPD) presents for their annual physical exam. The patient has no history of previous pneumococcal vaccines. Which of the following is recommended based on Centers for Disease Control and Prevention (CDC) guidelines?
    A. PCV20
    B. Nothing; pneumococcal vaccination not required for patient <65 years
    C. PPSV23 followed by PCV15 8 weeks later
    D. PCV20 followed by PPSV23 1 year later

22. Which of the following is the *most* sensitive diagnostic test to detect tuberculosis (TB)?
    A. Sputum acid-fast bacilli smear
    B. Tuberculin skin test
    C. Chest x-ray
    D. Sputum for culture and sensitivity

23. A patient with chronic obstructive pulmonary disease (COPD) denies frequent symptoms and reports no exacerbations this year. The patient's COPD Assessment Test (CAT) score is 6. Based on these findings, the preferred initial pharmacologic management for this patient includes:
    A. Long-acting bronchodilator therapy
    B. Short-acting bronchodilator therapy
    C. Dual bronchodilator therapy (long-acting muscarinic antagonist-long-acting beta2-agonist [LAMA-LABA])
    D. Combination therapy (LAMA-LABA-inhaled corticosteroid [ICS])

24. A patient with asthma presents with symptoms requiring the use of a short-acting beta2-agonist (SABA) three times per week, about four nocturnal awakenings per month due to asthma, minor interference of normal activities, and forced expiratory volume in the first second (FEV1) measurements within normal range. This presentation is consistent with which category of asthma severity based on National Asthma Education and Prevention Program (NAEPP) guidelines?
    A. Intermittent
    B. Mild persistent
    C. Moderate persistent
    D. Severe persistent

25. On chest radiographic interpretation, air appears as which color?
    A. Black
    B. Diminished white
    C. Gray
    D. Bright white

26. A patient presents with an acute onset of fever, sore throat, nasal congestion, and rhinorrhea. The patient denies nausea and vomiting and is able to tolerate oral intake. Upon physical examination, the nasal turbinates are swollen with clear mucus. The cervical lymph nodes are small, tender, and mobile in the submandibular area. Which of the following is the appropriate treatment plan for the patient based on this presentation?
    A. Azithromycin
    B. Referral to ED for intravenous (IV) fluids
    C. Symptom management with acetaminophen and nasal decongestants
    D. Amoxicillin

(See answers next page.)

18. B) Albuterol

During an acute exacerbation, all patients with hypoxemia should be treated with supplemental oxygen. Prompt administration of an inhaled short-acting beta2-agonist (SABA; albuterol) is recommended either by nebulization or metered dose inhaler with a spacer. Systemic glucocorticoids are recommended for patients who are refractory to intensive bronchodilator therapy as well as adding inhaled muscarinic antagonist (e.g., ipratropium) to inhaled SABA for patients with a severe exacerbation. Magnesium sulfate is recommended for patients with a life-threatening exacerbation or severe exacerbation not responding to initial therapy. Leukotriene receptor antagonists (e.g., montelukast) are recommended for chronic asthma, but initiation is not indicated during an acute exacerbation. Methylxanthines (e.g., theophylline) are not recommended for acute asthma exacerbation due to limited efficacy.

19. D) Bacillus Calmette-Guérin (BCG) vaccination

BCG vaccination can be used as an attenuated vaccine to prevent tuberculosis (TB) and other mycobacterial infections. It is the most widely administered vaccine around the world and is most effective in mycobacteria-naïve newborns and infants. Patients who have received the BCG vaccination may have a false-positive tuberculin reaction of 3 to 19 mm for up to 3 months. This reaction decreases over time. The pneumonia and COVID-19 vaccines have not been shown to cause a false-positive TB test. Other causes of false-positive tests include non-tuberculous mycobacteria infection.

20. C) PCV20 at least 1 year after the most recent PPSV23 vaccine

Per CDC guidelines, for adults 65 years or older who have only received PPSV23, one dose of PCV15 or PCV20 should be administered at least 1 year after the most recent PPSV23 vaccination. An additional dose is not recommended.

21. A) PCV20

Per CDC guidelines, pneumococcal vaccination is recommended for adults age 19 through 64 years with certain medical conditions (such as chronic lung disease, including COPD, asthma, and emphysema), immunocompromised conditions, or certain risk factors. For those who have not received any pneumococcal vaccine, the CDC recommends one dose of PCV15 or PCV20. If PCV15 is used, a dose of PPSV23 should be given at least 1 year later (or 8 weeks later if patient has an immunocompromising condition). A dose of PPSV23 is not indicated if PCV20 is used.

22. D) Sputum for culture and sensitivity

Culture-based testing is the most sensitive tool to detect TB and the gold standard for diagnosis of drug-resistant TB. A tuberculin skin test and interferon-gamma release assay are used for diagnosis of TB infection; a positive result supports a diagnosis of active TB disease, but a negative result does not rule out active TB disease. A sputum acid-fast bacilli smear is the most rapid and inexpensive TB diagnostic method. A chest x-ray is a useful tool and part of the initial approach when evaluating a patient with suspected TB; however, active pulmonary TB cannot be distinguished from inactive disease on chest x-ray alone.

23. A) Long-acting bronchodilator therapy

This patient is in the group A category based on their minimal symptoms (CAT score <10) and low risk of exacerbation (0 to 1 per year). Long-acting bronchodilator therapy (e.g., LAMA) is preferred over short-acting bronchodilators alone. A LABA is an appropriate alternative depending on the patient's symptoms and risk for adverse effects. Patients in group B benefit from dual bronchodilator therapy (LAMA-LABA); patients in group E who are hospitalized with elevated eosinophils may benefit from combination therapy (LAMA-LABA-ICS).

24. B) Mild persistent

Mild persistent asthma is characterized by symptoms more than twice weekly, about three to four nocturnal awakenings per month, use of SABAs more than 2 days of the week, minor interference with activities, and FEV1 measurements within normal range.

25. A) Black

Air is low density so less is absorbed, and it will appear as a dark, black color; bones appear as white to gray; metals are bright white (high absorption); and tissue and fluid appear as different shades of gray.

26. C) Symptom management with acetaminophen and nasal decongestants

The patient is presenting with signs and symptoms consistent with an upper respiratory infection (common cold). Treatment involves symptom management with fluids, rest, analgesics, oral decongestants, topical nasal decongestants, antitussives, and antihistamines. Because this patient is tolerating oral intake, IV fluids are not necessary. Antibiotics are not indicated for a viral infection.

27. During the physical exam, the nurse practitioner (NP) asks the patient to whisper a short phrase while auscultating the peripheral lung fields. The nurse practitioner notes that the whispered voice sounds clear and loud. This finding is suggestive of which of the following?
    A. Considered a normal finding
    B. Area of consolidation in the lung suggestive of pneumonia
    C. Possible air in the lungs suggestive of pneumothorax
    D. Tumor causing bronchial obstruction

28. A patient with chronic obstructive pulmonary disease (COPD) and a history of smoking presents with a sudden onset of dyspnea and pleuritic chest pain. Physical exam findings include decreased chest excursion on the left side, diminished breath sounds, decreased tactile fremitus, and tympanic sounds during lung auscultation. The patient's vital signs are stable on room air. Which of the following is an appropriate diagnostic modality for this patient presentation?
    A. Chest x-ray
    B. Chest CT scan
    C. Pleural ultrasonography
    D. Pulmonary function tests

29. A patient presents with infrequent asthma symptoms (e.g., <2 times/week). According to the Global Initiative for Asthma (GINA), therapy for step 1 patients with asthma includes which of the following?
    A. Low-dose inhaled corticosteroids (ICS) with long-acting beta2-agonists (LABA)
    B. Low-dose ICS and short-acting beta2-agonists (SABA) as needed
    C. Medium-dose ICS
    D. SABA as needed

Questions 30 and 31 apply to this case. A middle-aged adult male smoker with chronic obstructive pulmonary disease (COPD) presents to the clinic complaining of several days of fever, loss of appetite, coughing, and chest pain. The cough is productive of purulent sputum. Physical examination reveals a temperature of 102.0°F (39.0°C), pulse of 88, and respiratory rate of 24. The lung exam reveals crackles on the lower right lobe and wheezing in the upper airways.

30. Which of the following bacteria is *most* likely to be the infectious agent?
    A. *Streptococcus pneumoniae* and *Mycoplasma pneumoniae*
    B. *Staphylococcus aureus* and *Mycoplasma pneumoniae*
    C. *Haemophilus influenzae* and *Streptococcus pneumoniae*
    D. *Legionella pneumophilia* and *Haemophilus influenzae*

31. What is the preferred treatment for the patient's condition?
    A. Amoxicillin
    B. Doxycyline
    C. Amoxicillin-clavulanate (Augmentin) plus a macrolide
    D. Azithromycin (Z-Pak) plus a fluoroquinolone

32. Isoniazid therapy is associated with possible adverse events. Which of the following events can be minimized or prevented with simultaneous intake of pyridoxine?
    A. Hepatic toxicity
    B. Peripheral neuropathy
    C. Urticaria
    D. Nausea and vomiting

33. Which of the following is a major risk factor for fatal asthma?
    A. Exercising in cold weather
    B. Smoking or vaping
    C. Multiple hospital admissions in past year
    D. Allergy to pet dander and dust mites

(See answers next page.)

27. B) Area of consolidation in the lung suggestive of pneumonia

Whispered pectoriloquy is used as an auscultation technique during the respiratory component of the physical exam. The patient whispers a few numbers or a short phrase while auscultating. A normal finding is to hear distant and muffled whispered voices. However, if there is consolidation in an area of lung, the whispered voice will sound clear and loud because sound transmits better through dense consolidation than through air. Tachypnea, crackles (rales), decreased bronchial breath sounds, bronchophony, whispered pectoriloquy, increased tactile fremitus, and/or dullness to percussion are suggestive of pneumonia. Decreased tactile fremitus is seen with pneumothorax and a tumor causing bronchial obstruction.

28. A) Chest x-ray

The patient is presenting with signs and symptoms concerning for a pneumothorax (gas in the pleural space). It should be suspected in patients with acute dyspnea and pleuritic chest pain, especially in patients with risk factors (e.g., COPD, smoking history). Diagnostic imaging for most stable patients includes a chest radiography. Bedside pleural ultrasonography is indicated in patients who are hemodynamically unstable or in severe respiratory distress. While a chest CT scan is the most accurate diagnostic method, it is recommended when the diagnosis is unclear following chest radiography. Pulmonary function tests are not routinely recommended or performed during diagnosis or treatment.

29. A) Low-dose inhaled corticosteroids (ICS) with long-acting beta2-agonists (LABA)

According to GINA, step 1 asthma is treated with low-dose ICS with rapid-onset LABA (e.g., budesonide-formoterol combination). According to National Asthma Education and Prevention Program (NAEPP) guidelines, step 1 is treated with only a SABA as needed, and step 2 is treated with a low-dose ICS and SABA as needed. According to GINA, step 4 treatment involves medium-dose ICS as maintenance and reliever therapy.

30. C) *Haemophilus influenzae* and *Streptococcus pneumoniae*

People with COPD or emphysema and those who smoke are more likely to have *H. influenzae* as the predominant organism along with *S. pneumoniae*.

31. C) Amoxicillin-clavulanate (Augmentin) plus a macrolide

The patient has community-acquired pneumonia (CAP) with comorbidities (smoker, COPD), which are risk factors for *Haemophilus influenzae* (gram-negative). Also assume the presence of *Streptococcus pneumoniae* (gram-positive) because it is the most common bacteria seen in CAP. The preferred treatment for patients with comorbidities who are older than 65 years is combination therapy with beta-lactams (i.e., amoxicillin–clavulanate, cefpodoxime, or cefuroxime) plus a macrolide or doxycycline or monotherapy with a respiratory fluoroquinolone (i.e., levofloxacin, moxifloxacin, or gemifloxacin).

32. B) Peripheral neuropathy

Isoniazid competes with pyridoxine (vitamin B_6) as a cofactor for synthesis of synaptic neurotransmitters, resulting in neurologic adverse effects such as peripheral neuropathy, paresthesias, and ataxia.

33. C) Multiple hospital admissions in past year

Multiple hospital admissions in the past year with ICU admission and/or intubation is a major risk factor for fatal asthma. Other major risk factors are ED visits in the past year or recent history of poorly controlled asthma.

34. What is the preferred reliever medication for asthma according to the Global Initiative for Asthma (GINA) 2020 treatment guideline?
    A. Low-dose inhaled corticosteroids (ICS) with formoterol
    B. Short-acting beta2-agonists (SABA)
    C. Long-acting beta2-agonists (LABA)
    D. Leukotriene receptor antagonist

35. A patient presents with dyspnea on exertion and pleuritic chest pain. The patient recently had surgery for a femur fracture and reports limited mobility since discharge from the hospital. These symptoms are suggestive of which of the following?
    A. Lung cancer
    B. Pulmonary embolism
    C. Heart failure
    D. Asthma

(See answers next page.)

34. A) Low-dose inhaled corticosteroids (ICS) with formoterol

According to GINA asthma treatment guidelines (2020), the preferred reliever (or rescue) medicine is a low-dose ICS with formoterol or an ICS-LABA combination. The combination of rapid-onset LABA (formoterol) and low-dose ICS (e.g., budesonide) is effective as both a controller and a reliever to improve asthma symptom control and reduce exacerbations that require hospitalization. SABA is the alternative, but it should be used with an ICS. ICS-LABA combination inhalers are used as relievers and also as preventive (maintenance) treatment.

35. B) Pulmonary embolism

This patient is presenting with a clinical suspicion for a pulmonary embolism due to their recent history of surgery and immobility. Classic symptoms include dyspnea at rest or with exertion, pleuritic pain, cough, orthopnea, calf or thigh pain with swelling, wheezing, and hemoptysis. Patients with asthma often present with shortness of breath or dyspnea, wheezing, and dry cough. Patients with heart failure often present with dyspnea that worsens with exertion, pitting edema, and dry cough. New-onset weight loss and cough in a patient with risk factors such as long-term cigarette smoking (≥30-pack-year history) are suggestive of lung cancer.

DANGER SIGNALS

ADRENAL CRISIS

Mineralocorticoid and glucocorticoid deficiency can lead to the development of adrenal crisis. Most commonly presents with symptoms of shock secondary to cardiovascular collapse, abdominal tenderness, fever, and weight loss; patient may be hyperpigmented due to chronic corticotropin hypersecretion and have serum electrolyte abnormalities. Life-threatening emergency that requires immediate treatment.

DIABETIC KETOACIDOSIS AND HYPEROSMOLAR HYPERGLYCEMIC STATE

Serious acute complications of diabetes characterized by uncontrolled hyperglycemia. Patients with diabetic ketoacidosis (DKA) present with classic triad of anion gap metabolic acidosis, ketonemia, and hyperglycemia. Serum glucose concentration usually less than 800 mg/dL, often between 350 to 500 mg/dL. Signs of volume depletion in both DKA and hyperosmolar hyperglycemic state (HHS) include decreased skin turgor, dry axillae and oral mucosa, low jugular venous pressure, tachycardia, and, if severe, hypotension. Patients with DKA may present with abdominal pain, fruity breath odor, and Kussmaul respirations. Neurologic symptoms are more common in HHS. Refer to ED.

HYPERPROLACTINEMIA

Can be a sign of a pituitary adenoma. Slow onset. Women may present with amenorrhea. Galactorrhea in both males and females. Physiologic causes include pregnancy, breastfeeding, and stress. Serum prolactin is elevated. When the tumor is large enough to cause a mass effect, the patient may complain of headaches and vision changes.

HYPOGLYCEMIA

Hypoglycemia refers to blood glucose that is <70 mg/dL. Patient complains of weakness, hand tremors, and anxiety and feels like having a syncopal episode. Difficulty concentrating. More common in people with type 1 diabetes mellitus (DM; only 5% to 10% of DM is type 1, average of two episodes per week). If severe hypoglycemia is uncorrected, it will progress to coma.

For diabetic individuals, the American Diabetes Association (ADA) defines level 1 hypoglycemia (glucose alert) as fasting blood sugar (FBS) of <70 mg/dL but >54 mg/dL. Level 2 hypoglycemia is blood glucose of <54 mg/dL. A blood glucose of this level is sufficiently low to indicate serious, clinically important hypoglycemia. Level 3 is a severe event characterized by altered mental and/or physical status requiring assistance for treatment of hypoglycemia. Nondiabetic hypoglycemia is rare and is either reactive (diet related) or fasting (disease related).

MYXEDEMA COMA

Medical emergency with high mortality rate. Severe hypothyroidism with progression to decreased mental status, hypothermia, and other symptoms secondary to slowing of function in multiple organs (e.g., bradycardia, hypoglycemia, hypotension, hypoventilation). Early recognition and treatment is essential. If suspected, check serum thyroxine (T4) (usually low); thyroid-stimulating hormone (TSH) (may be high); and cortisol.

PHEOCHROMOCYTOMA

A pheochromocytoma is a rare hormone-releasing adrenal tumor. It generally occurs in persons age 20 to 50 years but can appear at any age. Random episodes of headache (can be mild to severe), diaphoresis, and tachycardia accompanied by hypertension (HTN). Episodes resolve spontaneously. In between attacks, patient's vital signs are normal. Triggers include physical exertion, anxiety, stress, surgery, anesthesia, changes in body position, or labor and delivery. Foods high in tyramine (some cheeses, beers, wines, chocolates, dried or smoked meats) as well as monoamine oxidase inhibitors (MAOIs) and stimulant drugs are other triggers.

THYROID CANCER

A single thyroid nodule, usually located on the upper half of one lobe in a patient, may be accompanied by enlarged cervical lymph node lump, swelling, or pain. May complain of hoarseness and problems with swallowing (dysphagia, dyspnea, or cough). Radiation therapy during childhood for certain cancers (Wilms's tumor, lymphoma, neuroblastoma) and/or a low-iodine diet increases risk. Higher prevalence in women (2.5:1). Highest incidence from age 20 to 55 years. Positive family history of thyroid cancer. Metastasis is by lymph route.

TYPE 1 DIABETES MELLITUS

Common chronic disease in childhood but can occur in all age groups. Often presents with recent onset of persistent thirst (polydipsia) with frequent urination (polyuria) and weight loss. Feeling of hunger even though eating an increased amount of food. May be accompanied by blurred vision (osmotic effect on the lens). Breath may have a fruity odor. Large number of ketones in urine. Patients present with DKA and neurologic symptoms, such as drowsiness and lethargy, which can progress to coma. May report a recent viral-like illness before the onset of symptoms. Diagnosis in children and adolescents peaks from ages 4 to 6 years and again from ages 10 to 14 years.

NORMAL FINDINGS

- The endocrine system works as a negative feedback system. If a low level of active hormones occurs, it stimulates production. Inversely, if the level of hormones is high, it stops production.
- The hypothalamus stimulates the anterior pituitary gland into producing the stimulating hormones (such as follicle-stimulating hormone [FSH], luteinizing hormone [LH], or TSH [or thyrotropin]).
- These stimulating hormones tell the target organs (e.g., ovaries, thyroid) to produce active hormones (e.g., estrogen, thyroid hormone) (Box 9.1).
- High levels of these active hormones work in reverse. The hypothalamus directs the anterior pituitary into stopping production of the stimulating hormones (e.g., TSH, LH, FSH).

Box 9.1 Endocrine System: Target Organs

Thyroid (TSH): T3 and T4
Ovaries/Testes (FSH/LH): Estrogen, progesterone, androgens, testosterone
Adrenal cortex (ACTH): Glucocorticoids, mineralocorticoids
Body (GH): Somatic growth
Uterus (oxytocin): Uterine contractions, bonding
Kidneys (vasopressin): Blood volume
Pineal (melatonin): Circadian rhythm
Breast (prolactin): Milk production

ACTH, adrenocorticotropic hormone; FSH, follicle-stimulating hormone; GH, growth hormone; LH, luteinizing hormone; TSH, thyroid-stimulating hormone.

ENDOCRINE GLANDS

These glands interact to form the hypothalamic–pituitary–adrenal (HPA) axis.

Hypothalamus
Coordinates the nervous and endocrine system by sending signals via the pituitary gland. The gland interacts to form the HPA axis. Produces neurohormones that stimulate or stop production of pituitary hormones.

Pituitary Gland
Located at the sella turcica (base of the brain). Stimulated by the hypothalamus into producing the stimulating hormones such as FSH, LH, TSH, adrenocorticotropic

hormone (ACTH), and growth hormone (GH). It has two lobes (anterior and posterior).

Anterior Pituitary Gland (Adenohypophysis)
The anterior pituitary gland produces hormones that directly regulate the target organs (e.g., ovaries, testes, thyroid, adrenals).
- FSH: Stimulates the ovaries to enable growth of follicles (or eggs); production of estrogen
- LH: Stimulates steroid release from the ovaries, ovulation, and the release of progesterone after ovulation by the corpus luteum; stimulates the testicles (Leydig cells) to produce testosterone
- TSH: Stimulates thyroid gland; production of triiodothyronine (T3) and thyroxine (T4)
- GH: Stimulates somatic growth of the body
- ACTH: Stimulates the adrenal glands (two portions of gland: medulla and cortex); production of glucocorticoids (cortisol) and mineralocorticoids (aldosterone)
- Prolactin: Affects lactation and milk production
- Melanocyte-stimulating hormone: Production of melatonin in response to UV light; highest levels at night between 11 p.m. and 3 a.m.

Posterior Pituitary Gland
Secretes antidiuretic hormone (vasopressin) and oxytocin, which are made by the hypothalamus but stored and secreted by the posterior pituitary.

Thyroid Gland
A butterfly-shaped organ (two lobes) located below the prominence of the thyroid cartilage (Adam's apple). It is 2 inches long, and the lobes are connected by the isthmus. Uses iodine to produce T3 and T4.

Parathyroid Glands
Located behind the thyroid glands (two glands behind each lobe). Produces parathyroid hormone (PTH), which is responsible for the calcium balance of the body by regulating the calcium loss or gain from the bones, kidneys, and gastrointestinal (GI) tract (calcium absorption).

Pineal Gland
Pea-sized gland located inside the brain that produces melatonin. Melatonin regulates the sleep–wake cycle. Darkness stimulates melatonin production, and light suppresses it.

DISEASE REVIEW

ADDISON'S DISEASE
Addison's disease, or primary adrenal insufficiency, is a rare disease in which the adrenal glands do not produce enough essential hormones, resulting in mineralocorticoid and glucocorticoid deficiency. Often the cause of autoimmune destruction of the adrenal gland. If left untreated, patients can develop an adrenal crisis as a result of physical stress, such as injury, infection, or illness. This is an endocrinologic emergency due to an acute deficiency of the adrenal hormone cortisol, requiring immediate recognition and treatment.

Classic Case

Patient presents with nonspecific symptoms of fatigue, weight loss (usually secondary to anorexia), GI side effects (nausea, vomiting, abdominal pain, diarrhea and/or constipation), amenorrhea, myalgia, and psychiatric changes (e.g., depression, psychosis). Other common findings include postural hypotension, salt craving, and hyperpigmentation (characteristic finding). Patients presenting in adrenal crisis will present in vasodilatory shock (dehydration, hypotension, acute abdomen, unexplained fever, tachycardia).

Labs

- Electrolyte abnormalities: Hyponatremia, hyperkalemia, hypercalcemia (rare)
- Blood glucose: Hypoglycemia may occur after prolonged fasting
- Complete blood count (CBC): Normocytic anemia, eosinophilia
- Establishing the diagnosis: Serum ACTH, renin, cortisol, and aldosterone concentrations. The standard high-dose (250 mcg) ACTH stimulation test excludes primary adrenal insufficiency and most patients with secondary adrenal insufficiency.
- Primary adrenal insufficiency: Inappropriately low serum cortisol and a very high simultaneous plasma ACTH concentration.
- Secondary (i.e., pituitary disease) and tertiary (hypothalamic disease) adrenal insufficiency: When both the serum cortisol and plasma ACTH concentrations are inappropriately low.
- Corticotropin-releasing hormone (CRH): Can be used to differentiate between secondary and tertiary adrenal insufficiency.
- Secondary or pituitary-related adrenal insufficiency: Little or no ACTH response.
- Tertiary: Exaggerated and prolonged ACTH response (due to lack of CRH from the hypothalamus).

Treatment Plan

- Chronic primary adrenal insufficiency: Replacement of glucocorticoids (e.g., hydrocortisone, dexamethasone, or prednisone) and mineralocorticoids (often fludrocortisone). Dehydroepiandrosterone (DHEA) therapy may be considered for some women with impaired mood or sense of well-being.
- Monitoring of therapy: Use the lowest dose that relieves symptoms; monitor plasma ACTH concentrations.
- Adrenal crisis: Patients require immediate administration of IV fluids (normal saline or dextrose-containing fluid if hypoglycemic) and administration of glucocorticoid (often IV hydrocortisone).
- Until crisis resolves: Patients require intensive supportive care. Intubation and mechanical ventilation may be indicated due to decreased level of consciousness (LOC), and use of vasopressors may be necessary to maintain perfusion.

Special Considerations

- Minor illness: Two or three times the maintenance glucocorticoid dose for 3 days (3x3 rule).

- Surgical procedures or severe illness: May need additional coverage depending on the severity of the operation (e.g., graded doses of hydrocortisone).
- Emergency preparedness: All patients should wear a medical alert bracelet; keep supplies for emergency glucocorticoid injections.

CUSHING'S SYNDROME

Cushing's syndrome is either ACTH dependent (more common) or independent. Most common cause is iatrogenic Cushing's due to excess exogenous administration of glucocorticoids. Second most common form is Cushing's disease, a subset of Cushing's syndrome, which is pituitary hypersecretion of ACTH. Patients often develop a characteristic appearance due to increased adipose tissue in certain locations: face (moon face), neck (buffalo hump), and above the clavicles. Dermatologic symptoms include easy bruising, striae, skin atrophy, cutaneous fungal infections, acne, and hyperpigmentation. Patient may complain of weight gain and edema, menstrual changes, hirsutism, lethargy, abnormal glucose tolerance, and HTN. Increased risk for osteoporosis, fracture, venous thromboembolism, and EKG abnormalities. Presence and severity of symptoms vary based on the cause, degree, duration of hypercortisolism, presence or absence of androgen excess, and presence of adrenal carcinoma.

Labs

- Electrolyte abnormalities: Hypokalemia, hypernatremia
- Blood glucose: Glucose intolerance; overt hyperglycemia (10%–15%)
- CBC: May see a leukocytosis, an elevated white blood count
- Check: Serum ACTH, cortisol, and aldosterone concentrations
- Initial first-line tests: Late-night salivary cortisol (two measurements), 24-hour urinary free cortisol excretion (two measurements), or the overnight 1 mg dexamethasone suppression test
- Low index of suspicion: Initial testing with one of the first-line tests
- High index of suspicion: Initial testing with two or three of the first-line tests

Treatment Plan

- Goal of therapy: Reverse signs, symptoms, and comorbidities of Cushing's syndrome by reducing cortisol secretion to normal; eradicate any tumor; avoid permanent dependence on medication or hormone deficiency.
- Acute management: Manage electrolyte balance and supportive care of symptoms.
- Exogenous Cushing's syndrome: Tapered discontinuation of glucocorticoids is indicated for patients with Cushing's syndrome secondary to long-term corticosteroid treatment.
- Cushing's disease: May require surgical intervention to excise pituitary tumor or pituitary irradiation. Medical management often is the primary treatment option if patient is not a surgical candidate or if symptoms do not resolve after excision.

- Adrenalectomy: Definitive treatment for ACTH-secreting pituitary or ectopic tumors
- Associated symptoms: Gradually resolve over a period of 2 to 12 months after effective cure of Cushing's syndrome. HTN, osteoporosis, and glucose intolerance improve but may require additional therapy.

EXAM TIPS

- Symptoms of Cushing's syndrome include moon face with buffalo hump, acne, poor wound healing, purple striae, hirsutism, HTN, weakness, amenorrhea, impotence, headache, polyuria and thirst, labile mood, frequent infections
- Symptoms of Addison's disease include hyperpigmentation in buccal mucosa and skin creases, diffuse tanning and freckles, orthostasis and hypotension, scant axillary and pubic hair

DIABETES MELLITUS

A chronic metabolic disorder affecting the body's metabolism of carbohydrates. Untreated, can progress to microvascular and macrovascular damage and immune system effects.

- Microvascular damage: Retinopathy, nephropathy, and neuropathy
- Macrovascular damage: Atherosclerosis, heart disease (coronary artery disease, myocardial infarction [MI])

Type 1 Diabetes Mellitus

The massive destruction of B-cells in the islets of Langerhans results in an abrupt cessation of insulin production. Often, patients present with new onset of polydipsia, polyuria, and weight loss with hyperglycemia and ketonemia. Can also present with DKA, a metabolic result of insulin deficiency, glucagon excess, and counterregulatory hormonal responses to stressful triggers. Ketoacidosis results from lipolysis, resulting in fruity breath. Most common chronic disease in childhood, but one fourth of cases are diagnosed as adults. Type 1 diabetes in adults accounts for about 5% to 10% of cases.

Type 2 Diabetes Mellitus

Progressive decreased secretion of insulin (with peripheral insulin resistance) resulting in a chronic state of hyperglycemia and hyperinsulinemia. Most patients are asymptomatic with hyperglycemia noted on routine lab testing. Rarely, patients can present with HHS, marked by hyperglycemia, severe dehydration, and obtundation, but without ketoacidosis. Has strong genetic component. Most common type of diabetes; represents >90% of U.S. cases.

Metabolic Syndrome

- Other names are insulin-resistance syndrome and syndrome X.
- Affected people have higher risk of type 2 DM and cardiovascular disease (CVD).
- Includes presence of any three of the following five traits:
  - Male waist circumference: >40 inches (102 cm); female waist circumference: >35 inches (88 cm)
  - HTN: Blood pressure [BP] ≥130/85 mmHg or drug treatment for elevated BP

- Triglycerides: Level ≥150 mg/dL or drug treatment for elevated triglycerides
- Serum high-density lipoprotein (HDL) cholesterol: <40 mg/dL in males and <50 mg/dL in females or drug treatment for low HDL cholesterol
- Hyperglycemia: Fasting plasma glucose (FPG) ≥100 mg/dL or drug treatment for elevated blood glucose

Risk Factors for Type 2 Diabetes Mellitus (Screen These Patients)

Consider testing in adults with body mass index (BMI) ≥25 kg/m² (or ≥23 kg/m² in Asian American individuals) who have one or more of the following risk factors:

- Family history: Especially those with a first-degree relative with diabetes
- Fat distribution: Central abdominal obesity
- Lifestyle factors: Sedentary lifestyle, smoking, sleep duration, dietary patterns (higher consumption of red meat, processed meat, and sugar-sweetened beverages)
- High-risk medical conditions: CVD, hyperuricemia, polycystic ovary syndrome, HTN, hyperlipidemia, HIV
- High-risk race/ethnicity: Hispanic, African American, Latino, Native American, Asian American, Pacific Islander
- History: Gestational diabetes or infant weighing >9 lbs. at birth
- Impaired fasting blood sugar/glucose (IFG) or impaired glucose tolerance (IGT): Considered at higher risk for type 2 DM (prediabetes)

Increased Risk of Diabetes Mellitus (Criteria for Prediabetes)

- Glycosylated hemoglobin (A1C) between 5.7% and 6.4%; defined as the average blood glucose levels over previous 3 months; no fasting required; test measures excess glucose that attaches to the hemoglobin of the red blood cells
  OR
- Fasting glucose of 100 to 125 mg/dL (impaired FPG)
  OR
- Two-hour oral glucose tolerance test (OGTT; 75 g load) of 140 to 199 mg/dL

Diagnostic Criteria for Diabetes Mellitus

- A1C ≥6.5%
  OR
- FPG ≥126 mg/dL (fasting is no caloric intake for at least 8 hours)
  OR
- Classic symptoms of hyperglycemia (polyuria, polydipsia, polyphagia) plus random blood glucose ≥200 mg/dL
  OR
- Two-hour plasma glucose ≥200 mg/dL during an OGTT with a 75-g glucose load

Labs

- Glycated hemoglobin (hemoglobin A1C) is the most widely used to estimate mean blood glucose, diagnose diabetes, and monitor the efficacy of treatment.
- Point-of-care blood glucose testing

- Lipid profile at time of diagnosis, at an initial medical evaluation, and every 5 years if under the age of 40 years or more often if indicated
- Monitor for increased urinary albumin excretion yearly. Urine albumin-to-creatinine ratio is the preferred screening test for evaluating for protein excretion and detect for progression of kidney disease
- Check electrolytes (e.g., potassium, magnesium, sodium), serum creatinine, liver function panel, and TSH

Treatment Plan

- Lifestyle changes are first-line treatment (see "Preventive Care Recommendations").
- At every visit, check vital signs, weight and BMI, blood glucose; perform physical assessment
- Assess pedal pulses, ankle reflexes, and skin for acanthosis nigricans, insulin injection or insertion sites, lipodystrophy
- BP control is important to prevent CVD and to minimize progression of diabetic nephropathy and retinopathy. Use of antihypertensives, such as angiotensin-converting enzyme inhibitors (ACEIs), angiotensin receptor blockers (ARBs), or angiotensin receptor-neprilysin inhibitor (ARNI), with tighter control of blood glucose decreases progression and lowers mortality from kidney disease.
- Pharmacotherapy as needed for glycemic control (see "Medications for Diabetes").
- Reasonable goal of therapy is an A1C value of ≤7%. Obtain an A1C at least twice yearly in patients who are meeting treatment goals and have stable glycemic management. Less stringent goals are acceptable for some (frail older adults, history of severe hypoglycemia, extensive comorbidity, limited life expectancy). A1C goal of up to 8% is acceptable. A more stringent goal of A1C <6% is recommended in pregnancy.
- A fasting blood glucose (FBG) of 80 to 130 mg/dL and a postprandial glucose (90 to 120 minutes after a meal less than 180 mg/dL are generally given as targets (Table 9.1)

Medications for Diabetes

Biguanides

- First line for DM type 2 is metformin (Glucophage). It decreases gluconeogenesis and intestinal absorption of glucose and improves insulin sensitivity.
- Metformin is preferred initial therapy because of glycemic efficacy, promotion of modest weight loss, low incidence of hypoglycemia, general tolerability, and favorable cost.
- Metformin may cause GI side effects, such as diarrhea and nausea.
- Long-term use is associated with reversible vitamin B_{12} deficiency; periodically assess lab values with chronic use.
- Use caution in patients after bariatric surgery, those with existing CVD (e.g., heart failure), hepatic or renal impairment, and stress-related states (e.g., fever, trauma, infection, surgery).

Table 9.1 Recommendations for Nonpregnant Adult Patients With Diabetes

Test	Goal
Blood pressure	<130/80 mmHg
LDL cholesterol	<70 mg/dL
A1C	<7% (although exceptions exist for certain populations)
Fasting blood glucose	80–130 mg/dL
Postprandial glucose (~2 hours after meal)	<180 mg/dL

Note: Insufficient evidence to clearly identify a threshold for LDL-cholesterol. The American Diabetes Association recommends that for patients with diabetes, aged 40–75 at higher cardiovascular risk, target LDL cholesterol goal of <70 mg/dL.
A1C, glycosylated hemoglobin; LDL, low-density lipoprotein.
Sources: Data from ElSayed et al. (2023), S97-S110; ElSayed et al. (2023), S158-S190. (See Resources section for complete source information.)

- Monitor renal function (serum creatinine, glomerular filtration rate [GFR], urinalysis [UA]) and liver function tests [LFTs].
- Increased risk of lactic acidosis (pH <7.25), which occurs during hypoxia, hypoperfusion, renal insufficiency.
- For intravenous (IV) contrast dye testing, hold metformin on day of procedure and 48 hours after. Check baseline creatinine and recheck after procedure. If serum creatinine remains elevated after the procedure, do not restart metformin. Serum creatinine must be normalized before drug can be resumed.

EXAM TIPS

- If patient is on metformin 500 mg daily and A1C is high (>7%), increase dose to metformin 500 mg BID. If A1C is still high (>7%) after dose adjustment, increase dose to metformin 1,000 mg BID.
- If taking maximum dose of metformin (1 g BID) and glycemic control is inadequate, can use combination therapy with additional oral agents such as a sulfonylurea, glipizide (Glucotrol XL) 5 mg PO daily (do not exceed maximum dose of glipizide 20 mg/day).

Sulfonylureas

- Stimulate the beta cells of the pancreas to secrete more insulin; reduces glucose output from the liver; insulin sensitivity is increased.
- Used as initial therapy when there are contraindications to metformin, severe hypoglycemia, and maturity onset of the young (MODY).
- Generally used in combination with other oral hypoglycemic drugs in patients who fail initial therapy with lifestyle intervention and metformin

- First generation is chlorpropamide (Diabinese) daily or BID. Long half-life (12 hours). Not commonly used because of high risk of severe hypoglycemia.
- Second-generation is glipizide (Glucotrol, Glucotrol XL), maximum dose of 40 mg/day; glyburide (DiaBeta), maximum dose of 20 mg/day; glimepiride (Amaryl), maximum dose of 8 mg/day.
- Adverse effects:
  - Hypoglycemia (diaphoresis, pallor, sweating, tremor); especially after exercise or a missed meal, when the dose is too high, with the use of longer-acting drugs, undernourished patients, alcohol use, kidney or cardiac impairment, concurrent therapy with other medications (e.g., salicylates, sulfonamides, warfarin), and hospitalization
  - Skin reactions; increased risk of photosensitivity (use sunscreen), rash, erythema, pruritis
  - Avoid if impaired hepatic or renal function (monitor LFTs, serum creatinine)
  - Causes weight gain (monitor weight and BMI)

Thiazolidinediones

- Enhances insulin sensitivity by acting on adipose and muscle tissue and the liver to reduce glucose utilization and decrease glucagon production (gluconeogenesis). Take daily with meal at breakfast.
- Pioglitazone (Actos) and rosiglitazone (Avandia) are available.
- Not prescribed as initial therapy. Often, combined as second-line or third-line therapy when other oral agents are not adequately controlling blood glucose.
- U.S. Food and Drug Administration (FDA) boxed warning; do not use with New York Heart Association (NYHA) class III and class IV heart disease, symptomatic heart failure. Not recommended for patients with symptomatic heart failure.
- Precautions:
  - Causes fluid retention and edema (increase the risk of heart failure and adverse atherosclerotic cardiovascular events).
  - Use caution if bladder cancer or history of bladder cancer (UA, urine cytology), active liver disease, type 1 DM, pregnancy.
  - Causes weight gain (monitor weight and BMI).
  - Increase fracture risk.
- Check LFTs.

EXAM TIPS

- First-line oral medication for type 2 DM is metformin (Glucophage).
- Actos can cause fluid retention, which may precipitate congestive heart failure (CHF). Contraindicated if history of heart failure or NYHA class III or IV (moderate to severe heart failure).

Meglitinide (Glinides)

- Stimulates pancreatic cells to increase secretion of insulin
- Repaglinide (Prandin) and nateglinide (Starlix) are glucose-lowering drugs indicated for patients with type 2 diabetes

- Precautions:
  - Rapid-acting with a very short half-life (<1 hour)
  - Recommended before meals
  - Side effects are bloating, abdominal cramps, diarrhea, flatulence, weight gain
  - May cause hypoglycemia (less risk than sulfonylureas)
  - Use caution in patients with chronic liver (metabolized by the liver) or advanced kidney disease

Bile-Acid Sequestrants

- Colesevelam (Welchol) is a bile acid sequestrant that lowers low-density lipoprotein (LDL) cholesterol also plays a beneficial role to improve glycemia
- Not routinely recommended given modest glucose-lowering effectiveness and cost
- Take with meals; side effects are GI related, such as nausea, bloating, constipation, increased triglycerides
- Side effects are a common reason for noncompliance; start patient on a low dose and titrate up slowly
- Kidney and liver effects (check serum creatinine, GFR, LFTs)

Alpha-Glucosidase Inhibitor

- Slows intestinal carbohydrate digestion and absorption and reduces postprandial blood glucose concentrations
- Does not cause hypoglycemia; modest effect on A1C level
- GI side effects are flatulence, diarrhea

Glucagon-Like Peptide-1 Receptor Agonists (GLP-1 RAs)

- Stimulate GLP-1, causing an increase in insulin production and inhibiting postprandial glucagon release (decreases postprandial hyperglycemia); slow gastric emptying (increases satiety and reduces food intake)
- Exenatide (Byetta) twice a day or liraglutide (Victoza) once-a-day injections (subcutaneous [SC])
- Reduce CVD events/death; slow progression and death from kidney disease
- Cause weight loss, suppress appetite; low risk of hypoglycemia
- Adverse effects are mostly GI (e.g., nausea, vomiting, diarrhea)
- May cause pancreatitis (monitor amylase, lipase); associated with benign and malignant thyroid C cell tumors in animals
- Avoid if personal or family history of medullary thyroid carcinoma, multiple endocrine neoplasia 2A or 2B

Sodium-Glucose Cotransporter-2 Inhibitors (SGLT2 Inhibitors)

- Expressed in the proximal tubules and mediates about 90% glucose reabsorption; promotes the renal excretion of glucose; increases glucosuria
- Canagliflozin (Invokana), dapagliflozin (Farxiga), empagliflozin (Jardiance)
- Effective in all stages of type 2 DM; generally, do not cause hypoglycemia
- Reduce CVD events/death; help to slow progression of chronic kidney disease (CKD)

- Causes polyuria, weight loss, hypotension (volume depletion), vulvovaginal candidal infections
- Avoid in patients with frequent bacterial urinary tract infections or yeast infections, low bone density and high risk for fractures and falls, foot ulceration (e.g., neuropathy, foot deformity, vascular disease), and factors predisposing to DKA (increases the risk)
- Monitor serum creatinine after 3 months and then annually or as clinically indicated

Dipeptidyl Peptidase-4 Inhibitors (DPP-4 Inhibitors)
- Inhibits the enzyme, dipeptidyl peptidase-4 (DPP-4); enhancement of glucose-dependent insulin secretion, slowed gastric emptying, and reduction of postprandial glucagon
- Sitagliptin (Januvia), saxagliptin (Onglyza), linagliptin (Tradjenta), and alogliptin (Nesina)
- Not considered initial therapy
- Some evidence suggest an increased risk of adverse atherosclerotic CVD outcomes
- FDA warning; may cause joint pain that can be severe and disabling (may occur early or months after initiation of therapy); may cause angioedema, urticaria, acute pancreatitis, increase risk of inflammatory bowel disease
- Appears to be effective in patients with CKD

NOTE

Combination therapy with GLP-1 receptor agonists and dipeptidyl peptidase 4 (DPP-4) should be avoided; there is no additive glucose-lowering effects.

Amylin Analog
- Decreases glucagon secretion, regulates postprandial glucagon, slows gastric emptying, leads to feeling satiety early, causes weight loss
- Pramlintide (SymlinPen 120; SymlinPen 60) is an amylin analog that is administered by mealtime subcutaneous injection; reproduces the actions of the naturally occurring peptide hormone, amylin, and controls glucose without causing weight gain
- Approved for use in patients also taking prandial insulin who have type 1 or type 2 diabetes
- FDA boxed warning; use with insulin increases the risk of severe hypoglycemia
- Requires patient training, careful patient instruction, and insulin dose adjustments

Insulin Therapy
For specific information about types of insulin, see Table 9.2. This is not an all-inclusive list.

Rapidly-Acting Insulin
Humalog (insulin lispro).

Short-Acting Insulin
- Regular insulin
- Injected subcutaneously 30 minutes before the meal to best cover postprandial glycemia

Table 9.2 Pharmacokinetics of Commonly Used Insulin

Insulin Type	Onset (Starts at)	Effective Peak	Duration (Mean)*
Prandial Insulin			
Rapid-acting analogs Insulin lispro/ aspart/glulisine	15 to 30 min	1–3 hr	4–6 hr
Short-acting regular human insulin	30 min	1.5–3.5 hr	8 hr
Insulin Type	**Half-Life**	**Effective Peak**	**Duration (Mean)**
Basal Insulin			
Intermediate NPH Human NPH	4.4 hr	4–6 hr	12 hr
Basal insulin analogs Insulin glargine (Lantus) U-100	12 hours	None	20 to >24 hours
U-300	19 hours	None	20 to >24 hours
Insulin detemir (Levemir)	5 to 7 hours	3 to 9 hours	6 to 24 hours

*Times are based on broad estimates and are designed for use in the nurse practitioner certification exams. Caution in clinical practice. All insulins can cause hypoglycemia and weight gain.
NPH, neutral protamine hagedorn.

- Can be used intravenously in inpatient settings for the treatment of DKA or HHS

Intermediate-Acting Insulin
- Neutral protamine hagedorn (NPH) delays the release of the insulin into the bloodstream.
- Intermediate-acting insulin (NPH) needs to be administered at least twice a day.
- If mixing NPH and regular insulin, use the mixture immediately. Regular (clear) insulin should be drawn up before the NPH (cloudy) insulin.
- Rapid-acting insulin can be mixed with NPH, but it should be used 15 minutes before a meal.

Premixed Insulin
- Humulin 70/30 (70% NPH insulin, 30% regular insulin)
- Often not prescribed for the treatment of type 1 diabetes; may be appropriate with those who are noncompliant with an intensive regimen

Basal Insulin
- Results in the slower absorption and longer duration of action
- Lantus (insulin glargine), Levemir (insulin detemir)
- Give once a day at the same time

Insulin Pumps
Insulin pumps require intensive training and can be expensive. However, new technologies have made it easier to

use insulin pumps to improve glycemic control. Can be used for both type 1 and type 2 diabetics. Patients should remove pump when swimming or showering.

Injection Sites
- Insulin can be injected in the abdomen, leg, arm, or buttock; absorption is fastest into the abdominal wall
- A clean site without evidence of infection, inflammation, skin breakdown, fibrosis, or lipohypertrophy should be used
- Injection sites should be rotated

CLINICAL PEARLS

- All patients with type 1 DM require insulin treatment.
- Patients with type 2 DM require initial treatment with insulin if they present with symptomatic (e.g., weight loss, polydipsia, polyuria) or severe hyperglycemia (FBG >250 mg/dL, random blood glucose consistently >300 mg/dL, A1C>9%) with ketonuria. If presenting without ketonuria or spontaneous weight loss, insulin (or a GLP-1) is an option, along with metformin.
- If there is difficulty distinguishing the type of diabetes or the patient has diabetes secondary to pancreatic insufficiency (e.g., cystic fibrosis, chronic pancreatitis), insulin is often indicated.
- Many patients with type 2 DM have difficulty maintaining glycemic control on oral agents alone because they become less effective as beta cell function declines. Patients with persistent hyperglycemia with lifestyle interventions and metformin can add a second oral or injectable agent, such as insulin. It is always effective and preferred in insulin-deficient, catabolic diabetes (e.g., polyuria, polydipsia, weight loss).
- Initiating insulin should not represent a personal failure and patients should be educated that many type 2 DM patients will eventually require exogenous insulin due to a decline in insulin production.

EXAM TIPS

- If presence of CVD and/or CKD, or heart failure with reduced ejection fraction (HFrEF), consider an SGLT2 inhibitor and/or GLP-1 receptor agonist.
- If persistent hyperglycemia and patient is on multiple oral agents (e.g., metformin and sulfonylurea), consider starting patient on insulin.

General Management of Diabetes
Preventive Care Recommendations
- Lifestyle interventions: Encourage weight loss (7% of body weight), regular physical activity (150 min/week), smoking cessation.
- CDC recommendations: Influenza, pneumococcal, Tdap, hepatitis B, zoster, and COVID-19 vaccinations.

- Pneumococcal polysaccharide vaccine (PPSV23): One dose, ages 19 to 64 years; once the patient is ≥65 (and ≥1 year after PCV13 and >5 years after previous dose of PPSV23), give second dose. Revaccinate every 10 years.
- Pneumococcal conjugate vaccine (PCV13): One dose, ages 19 to 64 years; once the patient is ≥65 (and ≥1 year after PPSV23), give PCV13.
- Aspirin 81 mg: If high risk for MI, stroke (if <30 years, not recommended).
- Ophthalmologist: Yearly dilated eye exam needed. If type 2, eye exam at diagnosis; if type 1 DM, first eye exam needed 5 years after diagnosis.
- Podiatrist: Refer to once or twice a year, especially with older diabetics.
- BP: Goal is 130/80 mmHg.
- Dental/tooth care: Important (poor oral health associated with heart disease).
- Pharmacotherapy: To improve and/or maintain the lipid profile

Dietary and Nutrition Recommendations
- Advise females not to exceed one alcoholic drink per day and males two drinks per day.
- Monitor carbohydrate intake (i.e., carbohydrate counting). Include carbohydrates from fruits, vegetables, whole grains, legumes, and low-fat milk.
- Protein-intake goals should be individualized (about 0.8 g/kg body weight per day).
- Reduce intake of trans fats (will lower LDL and increase HDL), such as most fried foods and junk foods. Mono- and polyunsaturated fats (e.g., those found in fish, olive oil, nuts) are relatively protective.
- Various diets are acceptable (Mediterranean, low fat, low carbohydrate, vegetarian).
- Fiber intake should be at least 14 g per 1,000 calories daily; higher fiber intake may improve glycemic control.
- Avoid sugar-sweetened beverages.
- Refer patient to a registered dietitian or diabetes educator to learn about carbohydrate counting and advice to help with adherence to diet.
- Routine vitamin supplementation of antioxidants is not yet advised.

Illness and Surgery
- Requires frequent self-monitoring of blood glucose.
- Do not stop taking antidiabetic medicine. Keep taking insulin or oral medications as scheduled unless FBG is lower than normal.
- Eat small amounts of food every 3 to 4 hours to keep FBG as normal as possible.
- Contact healthcare provider if dehydrated, vomiting, or diarrhea for several hours; blood glucose is >300 mg/dL; changes in LOC (feel sleepier than normal/cannot think clearly); fruity breath, urine with 1+ or higher ketones).

Exercise
- Increases glucose utilization by the muscles. Patients may need to check uptake and blood glucose more frequently and eat simple carbohydrates (e.g., candy, juice) before

the activity and complex carbohydrates (e.g., granola bars) afterward to prevent postexercise hypoglycemia.

■ If patient does not compensate (e.g., reducing the dose of insulin, increasing caloric intake, snacking before and after), there is an increased risk of hypoglycemia within a few hours. Example: If patient exercises in the afternoon, high risk of hypoglycemia at night/bedtime if they do supplement blood glucose with snacks, eating more food at dinner, or lowering insulin dose.

Complications of Diabetes

Dawn Phenomenon

Proposed to result from diurnal secretion patterns of hormones, particularly increased GH at midnight to 2 a.m. This tends to antagonize the actions of insulin in the early morning hours. The result is high FBG concentrations. To determine if insulin dosing needs to be adjusted, examine glucose patterns at least 3 to 4 hours after the last meal or snack and insulin bolus, as well as at 3 a.m. Ask the patient about evening snacking and bedtime insulin bolusing for food. Inadequate correction can cause hyperglycemia.

Diabetic Retinopathy

Neovascularization (new growth of arterioles in retina), microaneurysms (dot and blot hemorrhages due to neovascularization), cotton-wool spots or soft exudates (nerve fiber layer infarcts), and hard exudates.

■ Patients with type 1 DM: Screen after age 10 years.
■ Patients with type 2 DM: Refer to ophthalmologist shortly after diagnosis; then eye exam needed every 6 to 12 months.

Diabetic Foot Care

■ Patients with peripheral neuropathy should wear appropriate and protective shoes to minimize the risk of foot injury.
■ Referral to a podiatrist at least once a year.
■ Wear shoes that fit properly. Never go barefoot.
■ Check feet daily, especially the soles of the feet (use mirror).
■ Trim nails squarely (not rounded) to prevent ingrown toenails.
■ Report redness, skin breakdown, or trauma to healthcare provider immediately (main cause of lower leg amputations in the United States).
■ Check feet:
  • Vibration sense (128-Hz tuning fork): Place on bony prominence of the big toe (metatarsophalangeal [MTP] joint); if unable to sense vibration or asymmetry, patient has peripheral neuropathy
  • Light and deep touch, numbness: Place at right angle on plantar surface, push into skin until it buckles slightly (monofilament tool)

Charcot's Foot and Ankle (Neuropathic Arthropathy)

Deformity of the foot that is caused by joint and bone dislocation and fractures due to neuropathy and loss of sensation to the foot and ankle. May affect only one foot or both feet. If severe, foot deformity includes collapse of midfoot arch (rocker-bottom foot; Figure 9.1).

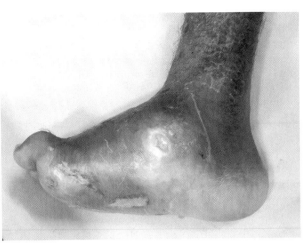

Figure 9.1 Diabetic Charcot foot with characteristic rocker-bottom deformity.
Source: Courtesy of Medicalpal.

Summary of Diabetes-Related Complications

■ Eyes: Cataracts, glaucoma, diabetic retinopathy, blindness
■ Dental: Periodontal disease
■ Cardiovascular: Hyperlipidemia, coronary artery disease, MI, HTN
■ Kidneys: Renal disease
■ Feet: Foot ulcers, skin infections, peripheral neuropathy, amputation
■ Gynecologic/genitourinary: Balanitis (candidal infection of the glans penis), candidal vaginitis

Solving an Insulin-Related Question

The nurse practitioner certification exams are based on the primary care model of care. In general, it is not necessary to memorize specific doses. Keep in mind some broad concepts, such as the peak and duration of each type of insulin. For example:

■ Rapid-acting insulin covers "one meal at a time"
■ Regular insulin lasts "from meal to meal"
■ NPH insulin lasts "from breakfast to dinner"
■ Lantus is "once a day"

Case Scenario

A patient with type 1 DM is prescribed short-acting insulin lispro (Humalog) before meals and insulin glargine (Lantus) once daily. The blood sugar results from the patient's diary (fasting, before lunch, dinner, and bedtime) demonstrate that the lunchtime values are higher than normal. *Which insulin dose should be increased or decreased?*

The short-acting insulin lispro must be increased to compensate for the patient's lunch. The insulin lispro (Humalog) takes about 15 to 30 minutes for onset of action and should cover the patient's carbohydrate intake at meals as a bolus. The duration of action of insulin glargine (Lantus) is about 20 to 24 hours, so that is providing the patient's basal coverage throughout the whole day. If all the patient's mealtime glucoses are high, the basal dose may need to be increased, but since just lunch was higher than normal, the patient likely needs more insulin lispro. The NPH component of the morning dose should be increased. Regular insulin peaks between breakfast and lunch (most of it is gone by lunchtime). In contrast, NPH insulin peaks between 6 and 14 hours. Therefore, it will cover the postprandial spike after lunch.

EXAM TIPS

- Images of funduscopic eye exams may appear on the exam. Review photographs online of diabetic retinopathy. Findings often include cotton-wool spots (soft exudates), neovascularization, microaneurysms with dot, and blot hemorrhages. Hypertensive retinopathy findings are silver wire/copper wire arterioles and arteriovenous nicking.
- Charcot's foot and ankle is more common in people with DM.

HYPOGLYCEMIA

High risk:
- Level 1 hypoglycemia (glucose alert): Blood glucose ≤70 and >54 mg/dL
- Level 2 hypoglycemia: Blood glucose ≤54 mg/dL
- Level 3: Severe event characterized by altered mental and/or physical status requiring assistance for treatment of hypoglycemia
- Look for: Sweaty palms, tiredness, dizziness, rapid pulse, strange behavior, confusion, and weakness; if patient on beta-blockers, the hypoglycemic response can be blunted or blocked.

Treatment Plan
- Glucose (15 g) is preferred treatment for conscious patients. Other options are 4 oz of orange juice, regular soft drink, hard candy. Think of the "15–15 rule": 15 g of carbohydrates to raise blood sugar; recheck in 15 minutes. When blood glucose is normalized, eat a meal or snack afterward (complex carbohydrates, protein).
- Prescribe glucagon for patients at significant risk for severe hypoglycemia. Severe hypoglycemia is defined as blood glucose <54 mg/dL.

PRIMARY HYPERTHYROIDISM (THYROTOXICOSIS)

The classic finding is a very low (or undetectable) TSH with elevations in both serum-free T4 and T3 levels. The most common cause for hyperthyroidism in the United States is a chronic autoimmune disorder, Graves' disease. Hyperthyroidism is more common in females than in males (5:1 ratio).

Graves' Disease

Graves' disease accounts for four out of five cases of hyperthyroidism. An autoimmune disorder causing hyperfunction and production of excess thyroid hormones (T3 and T4). Risk factors include a family history of Graves' disease or Hashimoto's disease, or if the patient has other autoimmune diseases such as rheumatoid arthritis (RA) and type 1 DM.

Classic Case

Middle-aged woman loses a large amount of weight rapidly with anxiety and insomnia. Cardiac symptoms (due to overstimulation) are palpitations, HTN, atrial fibrillation, or premature atrial contractions. Warm and moist skin with increased perspiration. May present with ophthalmopathy and lid lag (Graves' ophthalmopathy). More frequent bowel movements (looser stools). Amenorrhea and heat intolerance. Enlarged thyroid (goiter) and/or thyroid nodules present. May be accompanied by pretibial myxedema (thickening of the skin usually located in the shins and gives an orange-peel appearance).

Objective Findings
- Integumentary: Fine hair, warm skin
- Eyes: Lid lag; exophthalmos in one or both eyes
- Thyroid: Diffusely enlarged gland (goiter), toxic adenoma, or multinodular goiter. May be tender to palpation or asymptomatic
- Cardiac: Tachycardia, atrial fibrillation, CHF, cardiomyopathy
- Respiratory: Dyspnea at rest and on exertion; hypoxemia and hypercapnia; possible tracheal obstruction; exacerbation of asthma if present
- GI: Weight loss, vomiting, abdominal pain, dysphagia, abnormal LFTs
- Genitourinary: Urinary frequency and nocturia
- Extremities: Fine tremors on both hands, sweaty palms, pretibial myxedema
- Neurologic: Brisk deep tendon reflexes
- Psychiatric: Behavioral and personality changes such as psychosis, agitation, and depression

Labs
- Look for very low TSH (<0.05 mU/L) with elevated serum-free T4 and T3. If Graves' disease, will have positive thyrotropin receptor antibodies (TRAb), which are also known as the thyroid-stimulating immunoglobulins (TSIs). The thyroid peroxidase antibody (TPO) is positive with Graves' disease as well as Hashimoto's disease.
- Check TSH. If low, order thyroid panel. Look for very low TSH (<0.05 mU/L) with elevated serum-free T4 and elevated T3. In some patients with very low TSH, only either the serum T4 or the serum T3 will be elevated.
- If thyroid has a single palpable mass/nodule, order thyroid ultrasound. Refer to endocrinologist for management.
- Next step is to order antibody tests to confirm whether Graves' disease is present (TRAb and TPO or TSI).
- In nodular thyroid disease, radioactive iodine uptake (RAIU) and scan to distinguish toxic multinodular goiter and toxic adenoma from Graves' disease; absolute contraindications are pregnancy and breastfeeding.

Treatment Plan

Medications (Thionamides)

- Methimazole (Tapazole): Shrinks thyroid gland/ decreases hormone production.
- Propylthiouracil (PTU): Shrinks thyroid gland/ decreases hormone production. PTU is preferred treatment for moderate to severe hyperthyroidism (can cause liver failure).
- Side effects: Skin rash, granulocytopenia/aplastic anemia, thrombocytopenia (check CBC with platelets), hepatic necrosis (monitor CBC, LFTs).
- Pregnancy: For hyperthyroidism, PTU is preferred treatment during the first trimester, if needed. For high-risk pregnancy, refer to obstetrician.

Adjunctive Treatment

Given to alleviate the symptoms of hyperstimulation (i.e., anxiety, tachycardia, palpitations). Beta-blockers are effective (e.g., propranolol, metoprolol, atenolol).

Radioactive Iodine

Contraindicated during pregnancy or lactation. Permanent destruction of thyroid gland results in hypothyroidism for life (needs thyroid supplementation for life).

Complications

Thyroid storm (thyrotoxicosis): During thyroid storm, an individual's heart rate, BP, and body temperature can elevate rapidly to dangerously high levels. Acute worsening of symptoms due to stress or infection. Look for decreased LOC, fever, abdominal pain. Life-threatening. Immediate hospitalization is necessary.

EXAM TIPS

- If TSH is suppressed (TSH <0.05 mU/L), workup needed for hyperthyroidism.
- Chronic amenorrhea and hypermetabolism result in osteoporosis. Supplement with calcium and with vitamin D 1,200 mg; engage in weight-bearing exercises.

Thyroid Gland Tests

- Thyroid gland ultrasound: Used to detect goiter (generalized enlargement of gland), multinodular goiter, single nodule, and solid versus cystic masses
- Fine-needle biopsy: Used as a diagnostic test for thyroid cancer
- Thyroid scan (24-hour thyroid scan with RAIU): Shows metabolic activity of thyroid gland
  - Cold spot: Not metabolically active (more worrisome; rule out thyroid cancer); fine-needle aspiration biopsy
  - Hot spot: Metabolically active nodule with homogeneous uptake; usually benign; helpful in diagnosing recurrent disease

Laboratory Findings of Thyroid Disease

TSH:
- Normal range is TSH of 0.5 to 5.0 mU/L (third-generation test).
- TSH is used for both screening and monitoring response to treatment.
- Recheck TSH every 6 to 8 weeks. Dose of levothyroxine (Synthroid) is based on the TSH level. Goal is a TSH <5.0 mU/L.
- When TSH is stable, recheck every 6 to 12 months.

Treatment

- Alternative/natural medication (controversial): Armour thyroid is produced from desiccated (dried) pig thyroid glands (contains both T3 and T4).
- Drug-induced thyroid disease: Lithium, amiodarone, high doses of iodine, interferon alfa, dopamine. Monitor TSH.

CLINICAL PEARLS

- People with subclinical and overt hyperthyroidism are at higher risk of bone (osteopenia/osteoporosis) and cardiac (atrial fibrillation) complications. New-onset atrial fibrillation, check TSH.
- Keep TSH between .4 and 4.0 mU/L as goal for thyroid hormone supplementation.

PRIMARY HYPOTHYROIDISM

The classic lab finding for hypothyroidism is a high TSH with low free T4 levels (do not confuse with total T4). Diagnosis is based on the lab findings.

Some of the most common causes are Hashimoto's thyroiditis, postpartum thyroiditis, and thyroid ablation with radioactive iodine (to treat hyperthyroidism). Hashimoto's thyroiditis, chronic autoimmune hypothyroidism, is the most common cause of primary hypothyroidism in iodine-sufficient areas of the world.

EXAM TIP

If patient has elevated TSH (>5.0 mU/L), workup needed for hypothyroidism (e.g., order TSH, free T4).

Hashimoto's Thyroiditis

A chronic autoimmune disorder of the thyroid gland. There is generally no pain with this thyroid swelling. The body produces destructive antibodies (TPOs) against the thyroid gland that gradually destroy it. Almost all patients (90%) with Hashimoto's thyroiditis have elevated TPOs. Most patients have developed a goiter. More common in women with ratio of 8:1.

Subclinical Hypothyroidism (Nonpregnant Adults)

If TSH is >5 mU/L (elevated), but serum-free T4 is within normal range, diagnosis is subclinical hypothyroidism (asymptomatic to mild symptoms of hypothyroidism). Decision to treat with Synthroid should be individualized. Some choose not to treat but recheck same labs again in 12 months.

- Learn to diagnose subclinical hypothyroidism (TSH elevated with normal free T4).
- Patients with normal free T4 but with elevated TSH often do not require treatment (subclinical hypothyroidism). Recheck TSH in about 6 months.

Classic Case

A middle-aged-to-older woman who is overweight complains of fatigue, weight gain, cold intolerance, constipation, and menstrual abnormalities. May complain of dry skin and myalgia. Physical assessment may include goiter, bradycardia, diastolic HTN, and a delayed relaxation of the deep tendon reflexes. Serum cholesterol is elevated. May have a history of another autoimmune disorder (e.g., RA).

Severe hypothyroidism (myxedema coma) is a medical emergency that is rare (mortality rate 30%–50%). Patient presents with cognitive symptoms such as slowed thinking, poor short-term memory, depression (or dementia), hypotension, and hypothermia.

Labs

- Order TSH first (TSH >5.0 mU/L). If elevated, order TSH again with free T4 (free thyroxine). If TSH is high and serum-free T4 is low, the diagnosis is hypothyroidism.
- Next step is to order TPOs (gold-standard test) to confirm Hashimoto's thyroiditis (most common cause of hypothyroidism). If elevated, confirms Hashimoto's thyroiditis.

Table 9.3 Laboratory Results in Thyroid Disease

Condition	TSH	Free T4	T3
Hypothyroidism	>5.0 mU/L	Low	Low
Subclinical hypothyroidism	>5.0 mU/L	Normal	Normal
Hyperthyroidism	<0.05 mU/L	High	High
Subclinical hyperthyroidism	<0.05 mU/L	Normal	Normal

T3, triiodothyronine; T4, thyroxine; TSH, thyroid-stimulating hormone.

- Start older patients at low dose of levothyroxine (Synthroid) (25–50 mcg/day) and gradually increase to avoid adverse cardiac effects from overstimulation (palpitations, angina, MI).
- Check TSH every 6 to 8 weeks to monitor treatment response to thyroid hormone replacement therapy. Aim to keep serum TSH within the normal reference range (about .4 to 4.0 mU/L).

Treatment Plan

- All patients with overt hypothyroidism require treatment (regardless of symptoms).
- Average full replacement dose of synthetic thyroxine (T4, levothyroxine [Synthroid]) in adults is 1.6 mcg/kg body weight per day; dose ranges from 50 to >200 mcg/day.
- Start with lowest dose for older adults or patients with history of heart disease (25 to 50 mcg daily). Watch for angina, acute MI, atrial fibrillation.
- Increase levothyroxine (Synthroid) dose every few weeks until TSH is normalized (<5.0 mU/L).
- Recheck TSH every 6 to 8 weeks until TSH is normalized (TSH <5.0 mU/L). When under control, check TSH every 12 months.
- Advise patient to report if palpitations, nervousness, or tremors because this means that Synthroid dose is too high (decrease dose until symptoms are gone and TSH is in normal range).

- Many patients with subclinical hypothyroidism will eventually develop overt hypothyroidism.
- Advise patient to crush levothyroxine (Synthroid) tablets with teeth before swallowing with water for better absorption. These tablets are synthetic T4.
- Alternative medicine practitioners are more likely to prescribe Armour thyroid tablets (desiccated thyroid glands from pigs), which contain natural T3 and T4 for hypothyroidism.
- All hyperthyroid patients should be referred to an endocrinologist as soon as possible.

KNOWLEDGE CHECK: CHAPTER 9

1. An patient with a body mass index of 33 complains of fatigue and excessive thirst and hunger. The nurse practitioner suspects type 2 diabetes mellitus. Which value during initial testing would confirm the diagnosis?
   A. Fasting plasma glucose level of 105 mg/dL
   B. Glycated hemoglobin level (A1C) of 5.4%
   C. Oral glucose tolerance testing result of 183 mg/dL
   D. Random plasma glucose level of 206 mg/dL

2. A patient presents with an episodic headache, sweating, tachycardia, and hypertension that has been resistant to therapy. The patient also reports self-limited episodes of palpitations, tremor, and diaphoresis. Based on this clinical presentation, which of the following tests would be *most* helpful for diagnosis?
   A. Thyroid panel, including thyroid-stimulating hormone (TSH) and free thyroxine (T4)
   B. Assessment of serum cortisol and adrenocorticotropic hormone (ACTH) levels
   C. 24-hour urine fractionated metanephrines and catecholamines
   D. Assessment of glycosylated hemoglobin

3. On a routine physical exam, a patient is found to have a thyroid nodule. A neck ultrasonography reveals a solid hypoechoic nodule of 2 cm with irregular margins. Laboratory results reveal thyroid-stimulating hormone (TSH) of 6.2 mU/L. Which of the following diagnostic tests is the *next best* step in evaluation?
   A. Fine needle aspiration of thyroid
   B. Assessment of serum antithyroid peroxidase antibodies
   C. Measurement of serum calcitonin concentration
   D. CT scan of the neck

4. The best initial screening test for both hyperthyroidism and hypothyroidism is:
   A. Free T4 (thyroxine)
   B. Thyroid-stimulating hormone (TSH)
   C. Thyroid profile
   D. Palpation of the thyroid gland

5. Which of the following findings is associated with diabetic retinopathy?
   A. Arteriovenous (AV) nicking
   B. Retinal artery narrowing
   C. Papilledema
   D. Microaneurysms

6. Which of the following laboratory results is consistent with a diagnosis of prediabetes according to American Diabetes Association criteria?
   A. Hemoglobin A1C 5.5%
   B. Fasting plasma glucose 128 mg/dL
   C. Hemoglobin A1C 5.9%
   D. Blood glucose 135 mg/dL 2 hours post 75-g oral glucose tolerance test

(See answers next page.)

1. D) Random plasma glucose level of 206 mg/dL

Type 2 diabetes mellitus screening tests include fasting plasma glucose level (>126 mg/dL), random plasma glucose level (>200 mg/dL), and oral glucose tolerance testing (2-hour blood glucose level >200 mg/dL) with a 75-g glucose load. Normal A1C (glycosylated hemoglobin) levels are <6%.

2. C) 24-hour urine fractionated metanephrines and catecholamines

This patient is presenting with the classic triad of episodic headache, sweating, and tachycardia, concerning for a pheochromocytoma. A low risk of suspicion for pheochromocytoma includes those with resistant hypertension and hyperadrenergic spells (e.g., self-limited episodes of palpitations, diaphoresis, tremor), in which case a 24-hour urine fractionated metanephrines and catecholamines test is indicated. A high risk of suspicion for pheochromocytoma includes patients with an incidentally discovered adrenal mass on CT scan, a family history of pheochromocytoma, a genetic syndrome that predisposes to pheochromocytoma, or a history of resected pheochromocytoma. In this case, the first-line test is to measure plasma fractionated metanephrines. While most catecholamine-secreting tumors are sporadic, many are part of a familial disorder, so genetic testing may be indicated during further workup, but usually only after a pathologic diagnosis has been confirmed. A thyroid panel would be helpful in the diagnosis of hypo- or hyperthyroidism. Assessment of serum cortisol and ACTH would aid in the workup of Cushing's or Addison's disease. Assessment of blood glucose would be helpful in this patient presenting with sweating, tremor, and palpitations; however, obtaining a glycosylated hemoglobin would diagnose diabetes and not aid in the diagnosis of a pheochromocytoma.

3. A) Fine needle aspiration of thyroid

Thyroid nodules are often noted by the patient, during routine physical examinations, or when incidentally noted during imaging. Initial evaluation includes a history and physical examination, measurement of serum TSH, and ultrasound to confirm the presence of nodularity and assess the features. If the TSH concentration is normal or high, and the nodule meets sonographic criteria for sampling, the next step is an ultrasound-guided fine needle aspiration biopsy, which is the most accurate method for evaluating thyroid nodules and identifying patients for possible surgery. Fine needle aspiration should be performed in solid and hypoechoic modules if they are ≥1 to 1.5 cm with at least one of the following features: irregular margins, microcalcifications, taller-than-wide shape, macrocalcifications, or peripheral calcifications. A thyroid scintigraphy is indicated if the serum TSH concentration is low (<0.4 mU/L) to determine the functional status of the nodule. The routine measurement of serum calcitonin in patients with nodular thyroid disease is not recommended. While a CT scan may indicate a thyroid nodule during routine imaging, it is not indicated at this time. While measurement of serum antithyroid peroxidase antibodies may be helpful in patients with a high TSH suggestive of chronic autoimmune (Hashimoto's) thyroiditis, it is not necessary, nor does it negate the need for fine needle aspiration biopsy.

4. B) Thyroid-stimulating hormone (TSH)

The best initial screening test for both hypothyroidism and hyperthyroidism is TSH level. A normal TSH rules out primary hypothyroidism in asymptomatic patients. Abnormal TSH should be followed by determination of thyroid hormone levels. Overt hypothyroidism is defined as a clinical syndrome of hypothyroidism associated with elevated TSH and decreased serum levels of T4 or T3 (triiodothyronine). Subclinical hypothyroidism is defined as a condition without typical symptoms of hypothyroidism, elevated TSH (>5 μU/mL), and normal circulating thyroid hormone. Overt thyrotoxicosis is defined as the syndrome of hyperthyroidism associated with suppressed TSH and elevated serum levels of T4 or T3. Subclinical thyrotoxicosis is devoid of symptoms, but TSH is suppressed, although there are normal circulating levels of thyroid hormone.

5. D) Microaneurysms

Diabetic retinopathy is classified as nonproliferative or proliferative based on the absence or presence of abnormal new blood vessels. Nonproliferative retinopathy is characteristic for nerve-fiber layer infarcts (cotton wool spots), intraretinal hemorrhages, hard exudates, and microvascular abnormalities (including microaneurysms, occluded vessels, and dilated or tortuous vessels). AV nicking, retinal arterial narrowing, and papilledema are ocular effects more specific to hypertension.

6. C) Hemoglobin A1C 5.9%

The diagnosis of prediabetes is based on impaired fasting glucose, impaired glucose tolerance, and hemoglobin A1C. A fasting blood glucose of 100 to 125 mg/dL is considered prediabetes. A fasting plasma glucose of ≥126 mg/dL is diagnostic for diabetes. A 2-hour plasma glucose value during a 75-g oral glucose tolerance test between 140 and 199 mg/dL is considered prediabetes. A hemoglobin A1C of 5.7% to <6.5% is prediabetes; a level of ≥6.5% is diagnostic for diabetes.

7. A male patient presents with a waist circumference of 100 cm (about 39 inches), neck circumference of 38 cm (15 inches), blood pressure of 150/90 mmHg, fasting blood glucose of 140 mg/dL, and triglyceride level of 160 mg/dL. The patient has a past medical history of type 2 diabetes, obstructive sleep apnea, chronic kidney disease, and hypertension. The patient meets criteria for metabolic syndrome based on what diagnostic parameters?

   A. Neck circumference, blood pressure, fasting blood glucose
   B. History of type 2 diabetes, blood pressure, triglyceride level
   C. Fasting blood glucose, waist circumference, history of obstructive sleep apnea
   D. Blood pressure, fasting blood glucose, triglyceride level

8. A patient presents complaining of thirst, polyuria, weight loss, and blurry vision. The random plasma blood glucose level is 226 mg/dL. What step is indicated next?

   A. None; diagnosis confirmed based on random blood glucose and symptoms
   B. Repeat plasma blood glucose test on a subsequent day for confirmation of diagnosis
   C. Check of hemoglobin A1C to confirm diagnosis
   D. Performance of an oral glucose tolerance test

9. A patient presents with complaints of fatigue, cold intolerance, weight gain, and constipation. Lab findings are significant for a high thyroid-stimulating hormone (TSH) concentration and low serum-free thyroxine (T4). Based on this clinical presentation, which therapy is indicated?

   A. Methimazole (Tapazole)
   B. Levothyroxine (Synthroid)
   C. Radioiodine ablation
   D. Propylthiouracil (Propacil)

10. A patient presents with symptoms of anxiety, palpitations, fatigue, and insomnia. On physical examination, extremities are warm and moist, periorbital edema is noted, and the patient is tachycardic. There is diffuse thyroid gland enlargement upon palpitation. Which of the following diagnostic laboratory values can be expected in this patient?

   A. High thyroxine (T4) and/or triiodothyronine (T3) concentration, high serum thyroid-stimulating hormone (TSH) concentration
   B. Low T4 and/or T3 concentration, low serum TSH concentration
   C. High T4 and/or T3 concentrations, low serum TSH concentration
   D. Low T4 and/or T3 concentration, high serum TSH concentration

(See answers next page.)

7. D) Blood pressure, fasting blood glucose, triglyceride level

Diagnostic criteria for metabolic syndrome include three or more of the following: fasting blood glucose ≥100 mg/dL or drug treatment for elevated glucose; high-density lipoprotein (HDL) cholesterol <40 mg/dL in men and <50 mg/dL in women or drug treatment for low HDL cholesterol; triglycerides ≥150 mg/dL or drug treatment for elevated triglycerides; a waist circumference ≥102 cm (about 40 inches) in men or ≥88 cm (about 35 inches) in women; and hypertension as defined by blood pressure ≥130/85 mmHg or drug treatment for hypertension. Metabolic syndrome is not defined by neck circumference, history of type 2 diabetes, or obstructive sleep apnea.

8. A) None; diagnosis confirmed based on random blood glucose and symptoms

Diabetes can be diagnosed based on American Diabetes Association criteria. These include hemoglobin A1C ≥6.5%; fasting plasma glucose ≥126 mg/dL; 2-hour plasma glucose ≥200 mg/dL during an oral glucose tolerance test; and random plasma glucose ≥200 mg/dL in a patient with classic symptoms of hyperglycemia. The diagnosis of diabetes mellitus is often made when a patient presents with the classic symptoms of hyperglycemia (e.g., thirst, polyuria, weight loss, blurry vision) in conjunction with a random blood glucose value of 200 mg/dL or higher. No additional tests are required in patients with symptomatic hyperglycemia. In the absence of hyperglycemia symptoms, the diagnosis of diabetes must be confirmed on a subsequent day by repeat measurement for confirmation. If two different tests are concordant for the diagnosis of diabetes, additional testing is not needed. However, if two different tests are conflicting, the test that is diagnostic of diabetes should be repeated to confirm the diagnosis.

9. B) Levothyroxine (Synthroid)

The patient is presenting with overt primary hypothyroidism based on the presenting symptoms and confirmed by the lab values of high TSH value and low serum-free T4 value. Management includes replacement therapy with synthetic thyroxine (levothyroxine [Synthroid]). The treatment of hyperthyroidism in nonpregnant adults includes antithyroid drugs (thionamides such as methimazole [Tapazole] or propylthiouracil [Propacil]), radioiodine, or surgery.

10. C) High T4 and/or T3 concentrations, low serum TSH concentration

Hyperthyroidism causes symptoms of anxiety, emotional lability, weakness, tremor, palpitations, heat intolerance, increased perspiration, and weight loss despite a normal or increased appetite. The skin is usually warm and moist, and hair may be thin and fine. Tachycardia is common, along with atrial fibrillation. Tremors, muscle weakness, and hyperreflexia may be noted. In patients with Graves' disease (an autoimmune disease consisting of hyperthyroidism), exophthalmos, periorbital and conjunctival edema, and a thyroid goiter may be present. Patients with low serum TSH and high free T4 and/or T3 concentrations have primary hyperthyroidism. Patients with hypothyroidism often present with fatigue, cold intolerance, weight gain, constipation, dry skin, myalgia, menstrual irregularities, a goiter, bradycardia, diastolic hypertension, and a delayed relaxation phase of the deep tendon reflexes, among other symptoms. Primary hypothyroidism is characterized by a high serum TSH concentration and a low serum-free T4 concentration. Subclinical hypothyroidism is seen in patients with a high serum TSH concentration and a normal serum-free T4 concentration.

11. A patient presents with decreased mental status, hypothermia, hypotension, and bradycardia. The patient is minimally responsive, and the family reports that the patient takes a medication every day for their thyroid. This clinical presentation suggests which diagnosis requiring emergency resuscitation and support?

A. Diabetic ketoacidosis
B. Hyperosmolar hyperglycemic state
C. Hypoglycemia
D. Myxedema coma

12. Which of the following electrolyte abnormalities may be reflected in a patient with Addison's disease?

A. Hypokalemia
B. Hyperglycemia
C. Hyponatremia
D. Hypocalcemia

13. A patient presents with reports of fatigue, cold intolerance, weight gain, and constipation. Physical examination is notable for bradycardia; coarse, dry skin; and slowed deep tendon reflexes. Which of the following diagnostic laboratory values can be expected in this patient?

A. Low serum thyroid-stimulating hormone (TSH) concentration and a low serum-free thyroxine (T4) concentration
B. High serum TSH concentration and a low serum-free T4 concentration
C. Low serum TSH concentration and a high serum-free T4 concentration
D. High serum TSH concentration and a high serum-free T4 concentration

14. Which of the following hormones stimulates testosterone release by the Leydig cells of the testes?

A. Growth hormone
B. Follicle-stimulating hormone
C. Prolactin
D. Luteinizing hormone

(See answers next page.)

11. D) Myxedema coma

This patient is presenting with signs and symptoms concerning for a myxedema coma, severe hypothyroidism leading to slowing of function in multiple organs. The hallmark presentation includes decreased mental status, hypothermia, hypotension, bradycardia, hyponatremia, hypoglycemia, and hypoventilation. Aggressive treatment is needed for this medical emergency. The diagnosis should be suspected in any patient presenting with these symptoms and with important clues such as the presence of a thyroidectomy scar or a history of radioiodine therapy or hypothyroidism. If suspected, workup for the diagnosis includes measurement of thyroid-stimulating hormone (TSH), free thyroxine (T4), and serum cortisol levels. The serum T4 concentration is usually very low, and the serum TSH concentration may be high (indicating primary hypothyroidism) or low, normal, or slightly high (indicating central hypothyroidism). Both diabetic ketoacidosis (DKA) and hyperosmolar hyperglycemic state (HHS) are characterized by uncontrolled hyperglycemia. In patients with HHS, there is little or no ketoacid accumulation, the serum glucose concentration is usually ≥600 and may often exceed 1,000 mg/dL, the plasma osmolality may reach 380 mosmol/kg, and neurologic abnormalities may be seen. In contrast, patients with DKA present with anion gap metabolic acidosis, ketonemia, and hyperglycemia. However, the serum glucose concentration is usually less than 800 mg/dL and commonly between 350 to 500 mg/dL. Patients with DKA often present with a fruity breath odor and Kussmaul respirations, deep respirations reflecting the compensatory hyperventilation. Hypoglycemia occurs due to low blood glucose resulting in weakness, tremor, palpitations, anxiety, sweating, paresthesias, dizziness, drowsiness, delirium, and confusion.

12. C) Hyponatremia

In the majority of patients (about 70%–80%), hyponatremia is found with adrenal insufficiency (Addison's disease). This electrolyte abnormality is reflective of both sodium loss and volume depletion caused by mineralocorticoid deficiency and increased vasopressin secretion caused by cortisol deficiency. Hyperkalemia, rather than hypokalemia, often occurs due to hypoaldosteronism (since one of the major functions of aldosterone is to promote the urinary excretion of dietary potassium). However, not all patients develop hyperkalemia; patients may have normal potassium levels due to aldosterone-independent regulation of potassium secretion by the distal nephron. Hypoglycemia, rather than hyperglycemia, occurs in adults with adrenal insufficiency secondary to adrenocorticotropic hormone deficiency and in those with type 1 diabetes mellitus who develop adrenal insufficiency. Although rare, hypercalcemia, rather than hypocalcemia, may be associated with acute renal insufficiency.

13. B) High serum TSH concentration and a low serum-free T4 concentration

The patient's clinical manifestations are suggestive of thyroid hormone deficiency. Patients often present with fatigue, cold intolerance, weight gain, constipation, dry skin, myalgia, menstrual irregularities, a goiter, bradycardia, diastolic hypertension, and a delayed relaxation phase of the deep tendon reflexes, among other symptoms. Primary hypothyroidism is characterized by a high serum TSH concentration and a low serum-free T4 concentration. Subclinical hypothyroidism is seen in patients with a high serum TSH concentration and a normal serum-free T4 concentration. Hyperthyroidism causes symptoms of anxiety, emotional lability, weakness, tremor, palpitations, heat intolerance, increased perspiration, and weight loss despite a normal or increased appetite. Hyperthyroidism is characterized by a low TSH concentration and high free T4 and T4 concentration.

14. D) Luteinizing hormone

The luteinizing hormone stimulates testosterone release by the Leydig cells of the testes. It also stimulates steroid release from the ovaries, ovulation, and the release of progesterone after ovulation by the corpus luteum. The growth hormone is responsible for growth regulation during childhood, as well as metabolic functions such as production of insulin-like growth factor-1 and increase in gluconeogenesis. Follicle-stimulating hormone plays a role in estrogen production and follicular development as well as in initiation and maintenance of spermatogenesis. Prolactin has many functions but most notably is responsible for milk production and the development of mammary glands within breast tissues.

15. Which of the following can be used to differentiate primary from secondary adrenal insufficiency?
    A. Adrenocorticotropic hormone (ACTH)
    B. Serum cortisol
    C. Corticotropin-releasing hormone test (CRH)
    D. Insulin-induced hypoglycemia test

16. A patient presents with fatigue, weight loss, nausea, skin hyperpigmentation, and postural hypotension. Laboratory values are significant for serum sodium level of 131 mEq/L, potassium of 5.2 mmol/L, and hemoglobin value of 9.0 g/dL. Diagnostic workup reveals a low cortisol and a very high plasma adrenocorticotropic hormone (ACTH) level. These diagnostic findings are suggestive of which type of adrenal insufficiency?
    A. Secondary adrenal insufficiency
    B. Primary adrenal insufficiency
    C. Adrenal crisis
    D. Tertiary adrenal insufficiency

17. A patient presents with reports of increasing central obesity, resistant hypertension, facial plethora, striae, menstrual irregularities, and hyperglycemia. A high index of suspicion for hypercortisolism is made based on the multiple clinical features. Initial testing for Cushing's syndrome includes which of the following?
    A. Early-morning salivary cortisol
    B. 48-hour urinary free cortisol excretion
    C. Overnight 1 mg dexamethasone suppression test
    D. Late-serum cortisol

18. Which of the following medications may cause weight gain?
    A. Metformin (Fortamet)
    B. Empagliflozin (Jardiance)
    C. Semaglutide (Ozempic)
    D. Glipizide (Glucotrol)

19. A patient with diabetes reports waking up with elevated blood glucose levels. The patient denies evening or night-time snacking and reports following their insulin regimen of basal and bolus insulin. Which of the following can assist with diagnosis and treatment of this patient's fasting hyperglycemia?
    A. Obtaining a blood glucose level prior to eating dinner
    B. Performing an oral glucose tolerance test in the morning
    C. Checking the blood glucose level at 3 a.m.
    D. Assessing the glycosylated hemoglobin (A1C) level

20. Which of the following is the initial medication of choice for hyperglycemia in patients with type 2 diabetes?
    A. Canagliflozin (Invokana)
    B. Exenatide (Byetta)
    C. Glipizide (Glucotrol)
    D. Metformin (Fortamet)

(See answers next page.)

15. A) Adrenocorticotropic hormone (ACTH)

The diagnosis and cause of adrenal insufficiency can be made by measuring and obtaining the results of both serum cortisol and plasma ACTH immediately at the time of patient presentation. Primary adrenal insufficiency is characterized by an inappropriately low serum cortisol and a very high simultaneous plasma ACTH concentration. A patient has secondary (pituitary disease) or tertiary (hypothalamic disease) adrenal insufficiency when both the serum cortisol and the plasma ACTH concentrations are inappropriately low. CRH can be used to differentiate between secondary and tertiary adrenal insufficiency. While valid, the insulin-induced hypoglycemia test is not widely used due to the risks associated with hypoglycemia. It is a rational test of hypothalamic-pituitary-adrenal response to stress; however, there is little reason to perform the test in patients with a suspected recent ACTH deficiency.

16. B) Primary adrenal insufficiency

The patient is likely experiencing primary adrenal insufficiency. While often nonspecific, the presenting clinical manifestations often include fatigue, weight loss, nausea, vomiting, and muscle and joint pain. Hyperpigmentation is the most characteristic physical finding in patients with primary adrenal insufficiency. This finding is not present in patients with secondary or tertiary adrenal insufficiency because corticotropin secretion is not increased. Common laboratory findings include hyponatremia, hyperkalemia, and anemia. In patients with primary adrenal insufficiency, an inappropriately low serum cortisol and a very high simultaneous plasma ACTH concentration can be observed. A patient has secondary (pituitary disease) or tertiary (hypothalamic disease) adrenal insufficiency when both the serum cortisol and the plasma ACTH concentrations are inappropriately low. This patient is not presenting with the predominant manifestation of adrenal crisis, which is shock (e.g., tachycardia, hypotension, cool extremities, dehydration); therefore, this diagnosis is less likely.

17. C) Overnight 1 mg dexamethasone suppression test

Cushing's syndrome includes multiple progressive features, including striae, decreased libido, central obesity/weight gain, menstrual changes, facial plethora/round face, hirsutism, hypertension, ecchymoses, lethargy, dorsal fat pad, and abnormal glucose tolerance. Initial testing includes two or three of the following: late-night salivary cortisol (two measurements), 24-hour urinary free cortisol excretion (two measurements), or the overnight 1 mg dexamethasone suppression test. The low-dose dexamethasone test is a standard screening test used to differentiate patients with Cushing's syndrome of any cause from those who do not have Cushing's syndrome. The late-night serum cortisol relies on the fact that the normal evening nadir in serum cortisol is preserved in patients with central obesity and depression but not in patients with Cushing's syndrome. Because this test is less convenient than the late-night salivary cortisol, it is not routinely used in practice.

18. D) Glipizide (Glucotrol)

Glipizide (Glucotrol) is a sulfonylurea; a side effect of sulfonylureas is modest weight gain. Metformin (Fortamet) (drug class biguanide) is found to promote modest weight reduction (or at least weight stabilization). Empagliflozin (Jardiance) is a SGLT2-inhibitor; semaglutide (Ozempic) is a GLP-1 RA. Both drug classes have been found to cause weight loss.

19. C) Checking the blood glucose level at 3 a.m.

This patient is likely experiencing the "dawn phenomenon," often a cause of the diurnal secretion patterns of hormones. An increased release of the growth hormone at midnight to 2 a.m. can combat the actions of insulin in the early morning hours, increasing blood glucose in the morning. Treatment often includes increasing basal insulin dosing after assessing blood glucose levels beginning at least 3 to 4 hours after the last meal or snack and insulin bolus, as well as at 3 a.m. The patient should already be checking blood glucose prior to dinner to assess bolus dosing of insulin. Performing an oral glucose tolerance test in the morning and obtaining an A1C level would not be helpful in diagnosis to guide treatment.

20. D) Metformin (Fortamet)

Metformin (Fortamet) is recommended as the initial therapy in most patients with type 2 diabetes because of glycemic efficacy, promotion of weight loss, low incidence of hypoglycemia, general tolerability, and favorable cost. Canagliflozin (Invokana) is an SGLT2-inhibitor. Exenatide (Byetta) is a GLP-1 agonist. Glipizide (Glucotrol) is a sulfonylurea. These medications may be prescribed in specific populations or when treatment with metformin is ineffective.

10 GASTROINTESTINAL SYSTEM REVIEW

DANGER SIGNALS

ACUTE APPENDICITIS

Inflammation of the vestigial vermiform appendix. One of the most common causes of acute abdomen and one of the most frequent reasons for emergent abdominal surgery. A young adult complains of acute onset of periumbilical pain that is steadily getting worse. Over a period of 12 to 24 hours, the pain starts to localize at McBurney's point. The patient has no appetite (anorexia). Classic exam findings include low-grade fever and right lower quadrant (RLQ) pain with rebound and guarding. The psoas and obturator signs are often positive. When the appendix ruptures, clinical signs of acute abdomen occur, such as involuntary guarding, rebound, and a board-like abdomen. Refer to ED.

ACUTE CHOLECYSTITIS

Inflammation of the gallbladder. Often occurs as a complication of gallstone disease. Overweight adult patient complains of severe right upper quadrant (RUQ) or epigastric pain that occurs within 1 hour (or more) after eating a fatty meal. Pain may radiate to the right shoulder. Accompanied by nausea/vomiting and anorexia. If left untreated, may develop gangrene of the gallbladder. May require hospitalization.

ACUTE DIVERTICULITIS

Inflammation, often due to perforation of a diverticulum (sac-like protrusion of the colonic wall). Elderly patient with acute onset of high fever, anorexia, nausea/vomiting, and left lower quadrant (LLQ) abdominal pain. Risk factors for acute diverticulitis include increased age, constipation, low dietary fiber intake with high fat and red meat consumption, obesity, lack of exercise, and frequent nonsteroidal anti-inflammatory drug (NSAID) use. Signs of acute abdomen are rebound, positive Rovsing's sign, and a board-like abdomen. Complete blood count (CBC) will often show leukocytosis with neutrophilia and shift to the left. The presence of band forms signals severe bacterial infection (bands are immature neutrophils). Complications include abscess, sepsis, ileus, small-bowel obstruction, hemorrhage, perforation, fistula, and phlegmon stricture. May be life-threatening.

ACUTE PANCREATITIS

Acute inflammatory process of the pancreas. Adult patient complains of acute onset of fever, nausea, and vomiting that is associated with acute onset of abdominal pain that radiates to the epigastric region and left upper quadrant (LUQ). About two thirds of cases are caused by gallstones and chronic alcohol use disorder. Abdominal exam reveals guarding and tenderness over the epigastric area or the upper abdomen that may radiate to the back, as well as positive Cullen's sign (blue discoloration around umbilicus) and Grey Turner's sign (blue discoloration on the flanks). The patient may have an ileus and show signs and symptoms of shock. Refer to ED.

CLOSTRIDIUM DIFFICILE COLITIS

Spore-forming, toxin producing, gram-positive anaerobic bacterium that causes colitis. Can be classified as nonsevere, severe, fulminant, or recurrent. Severe watery diarrhea from 10 to 15 stools a day that is accompanied by lower abdominal pain with cramping and fever. Symptoms usually appear within 5 to 10 days after initiation of antibiotics. Antibiotics, such as clindamycin (Cleocin), fluoroquinolones, cephalosporins, and penicillins, have been implicated as the most likely cause of *C. difficile* infection. Risk factors also include age >65 years and recent hospitalizations.

COLON CANCER

Gradual progression with vague gastrointestinal (GI) symptoms. Tumor may bleed intermittently, and patient may have iron-deficiency anemia. Changes in bowel habits, stool, or bloody stool. Heme-positive stool, dark tarry stool, and mass on abdominal palpation. Males, older patients (>50 years of age), patients with history of multiple polyps or inflammatory bowel disease (IBD) such as Crohn's disease (CD) or ulcerative colitis (UC), and postmenopausal women with iron-deficiency anemia should be referred to GI specialist for colonoscopy and endoscopy. African Americans have the highest incidence of colon cancer in the United States. The U.S. Preventive Services Task Force (USPSTF) recommends screening for colon cancer between ages of 45 and 75 years.

CROHN'S DISEASE

CD is an IBD that may affect any part(s) of the GI tract, from mouth (canker sores), small or large intestine, rectum, and anus. Characterized by transmural inflammation and by skip areas of involvement. If ileum is involved, there is watery diarrhea without blood or mucus. If colon is involved, there is bloody diarrhea with mucus. During relapses, fever, anorexia, weight loss, dehydration, and fatigue with periumbilical to RLQ abdominal pain occur. Fistula formation and anal disease occur only with CD (not UC). May palpate tender abdominal mass. Remissions and relapses are common. Higher risk of toxic megacolon and colon cancer. Risk of development of lymphoma is also increased, especially for patients treated with azathioprine.

ULCERATIVE COLITIS

A form of IBD that is limited to the colon/rectum. Bloody diarrhea with mucus (hematochezia) more common with UC than with CD. Severe "squeezing" cramping pain located on the left side of the abdomen with bloating and gas that is exacerbated by food. Relapses characterized by fever, anorexia, weight loss, and fatigue. Can be accompanied by arthralgias and arthritis that affect large joints, sacrum, and ankylosing spondylitis. May have iron-deficiency anemia or anemia of chronic disease. Disease has remissions and relapses. Increased risk of colon cancer. Risk of toxic megacolon.

ZOLLINGER–ELLISON SYNDROME

A gastrinoma located on the pancreas or the stomach; secretes gastrin, which stimulates high levels of acid production in the stomach. As a result, multiple and severe ulcers in the stomach and duodenum develop. Complaints of epigastric to midabdominal pain. Stools may be a tarry color. Screening by serum fasting gastrin level. Refer to gastroenterologist.

EXAM TIPS

- Classic pain of acute pancreatitis is severe epigastric pain that radiates to LUQ.
- Be aware of presentation of acute appendicitis.

NORMAL FINDINGS

ROUTE OF FOOD OR DRINK FROM THE MOUTH

Esophagus → stomach (hydrochloric acid, intrinsic factor) → duodenum (bile, amylase, lipase) → jejunum → ileum → cecum → ascending colon → transverse colon → descending colon → sigmoid colon → rectum → anus (Figure 10.1).

ABDOMINAL REGIONS

- RUQ: Liver, gallbladder, ascending colon, kidney (right), pancreas (small portion); right kidney is lower than the left because of displacement by the liver
- LUQ: Stomach, pancreas, descending colon, kidney (left)

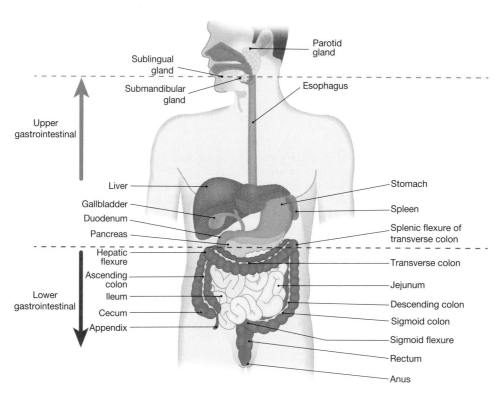

Figure 10.1 Gastrointestinal tract.
Source: Gawlik, K. S., Melnyk, B. M., & Teall, A. M. (Eds.). (2021). (See Resources section for complete source information.)

- RLQ: Appendix, ileum, cecum, ovary (right)
- LLQ: Sigmoid colon, ovary (left)
- Suprapubic area: Bladder, uterus, rectum

ABDOMINAL ASSESSMENTS

Psoas/Iliopsoas Sign

With patient in supine position, have patient raise right leg while applying downward pressure on the leg (Figure 10.2). Positive finding if RLQ abdominal pain occurs with passive right hip extension. Indicates irritation to the iliopsoas group of hip flexors in the abdomen. A positive finding suggests retrocecal appendicitis presentation due to retroperitoneal inflammation.

Obturator Sign

Positive if internal rotation of the hip causes RLQ abdominal pain. Rotate right hip through full range of motion. Positive sign is pain with movement or flexion of the hip. Associated with a pelvic appendix; however, low sensitivity so this assessment is not frequently performed.

EXAM TIP

Know how to perform psoas maneuver. Psoas and obturator signs are positive for acute appendicitis.

Rovsing's Sign

Deep palpation of the LLQ of the abdomen results in referred pain to the RLQ, which is a positive Rovsing's sign (Figure 10.3). While insensitive, Rovsing's sign has good specificity for acute appendicitis. Rule out acute or surgical abdomen. Also called indirect tenderness.

McBurney's Point

Maximal tenderness at 1.5 to 2 inches from the anterior superior iliac spine on a straight line to the umbilicus (in the RLQ). Tenderness or pain is a sign of possible acute appendicitis.

Markle Test (Heel Jar Test)

Instruct patient to raise heels and then drop them suddenly. An alternative is to ask the patient to jump in place.

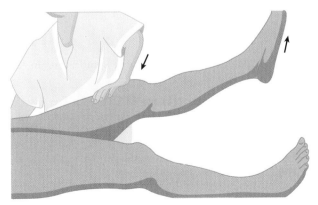

Figure 10.2 Psoas test.

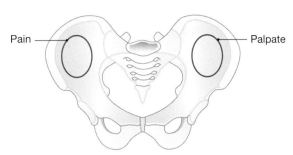

Pain — Palpate

Figure 10.3 Rovsing's sign. Location of the iliac fossa and eliciting the Rovsing's sign.
Source: Gawlik, K. S., Melnyk, B. M., & Teall, A. M. (Eds.). (2021). (See Resources section for complete source information.)

Positive if RLQ pain is elicited or if patient refuses to perform because of pain.

Involuntary Guarding

With abdominal palpation, the abdominal muscles reflexively become tense or board-like. Suspect acute abdomen. Refer to ED.

Rebound Tenderness

Patient complains of worsening abdominal pain when hand is released after palpation of abdomen compared with the pain felt during deep palpation. Suspect acute or surgical abdomen. Refer to ED.

Murphy's Maneuver

Press deeply on the RUQ under the costal border during inspiration (Figure 10.4). Mid-inspiratory arrest and pain in the RUQ is a positive finding (Murphy's sign). Suggestive of cholecystitis or gallbladder disease.

Carnett's Sign

An abdominal maneuver that is used to determine if abdominal pain is from inside the abdomen or if it is located on the abdominal wall. Patient is supine with arms crossed over their chest. Instruct patient to lift shoulders off the table so that the abdominal muscles (rectus abdominus) tighten. Also, can be performed by a straight-leg-raising maneuver. If source of pain is the abdominal wall, it will increase the pain (positive); if the source is likely from an intra-abdominal organ, the pain will decrease.

EXAM TIPS

- Know Cullen's sign (edema and bruising of the subcutaneous tissue around the umbilicus) and Grey Turner's sign (bruising/bluish discoloration of the flank area that may indicate retroperitoneal hemorrhage).
- Know how to perform Rovsing's sign and Markle maneuvers. Positive findings suggest acute appendicitis.

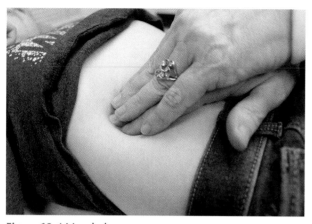

Figure 10.4 Murphy's maneuver.
Source: Gawlik, K. S., Melnyk, B. M., & Teall, A. M. (Eds.). (2021).
(See Resources section for complete source information.)

LABORATORY TESTING

HEPATITIS SEROLOGY

IgM Antibody Hepatitis A Virus (IgM Anti-HAV)

- Acute infection; patient is contagious.
- Hepatitis A virus (HAV) still present (infectious); no immunity yet.
- Screening test for hepatitis A

IgG Antibody Hepatitis A Virus (IgG Anti-HAV)

- Presence means lifelong immunity.
- No virus present and patient is not infectious.
- Can remain detectable for decades.
- History of native hepatitis A infection or vaccination with hepatitis A vaccine (Havrix)

Hepatitis B Surface Antigen (HBsAg)

- Screening test for hepatitis B
- HBsAg is positive when the patient is infected currently or was infected in the past.

Hepatitis B Surface Antigen (HBsAg) and Antibody (Anti-HBs)

- HBsAg is the serologic hallmark of hepatitis B virus (HBV) infection. HBsAg appears weeks after an acute exposure to HBV.
- The disappearance of HBsAg is followed by presence of hepatitis B surface antibody (anti-HBs) conferring antibodies and long-term immunity from reinfection.
- Presence may be due to either a past infection or vaccination with hepatitis B vaccine.

Hepatitis B "e" Antigen (HBeAg)

Marker for actively replicating HBV; highly infectious.

Total Hepatitis B Core Antigen (HBcAg) and Antibody (Anti-HBc)

- Appears at onset of symptoms in acute hepatitis B and persists for life.

- Prescence of IgM anti-HBc indicates acute HBV infection (but may remain detectable up to 2 years after acute infection).
- IgG anti-HBc persists along with anti-HBs in patients who recover from hepatitis B.

Hepatitis C Virus Antibody (Anti-HCV)

- Screening test for hepatitis C
- Unlike hepatitis A and B, a positive anti–hepatitis C virus (HCV; antibody) does not always mean that the patient has recovered from the infection and developed immunity; it may instead indicate current infection because up to 85% of cases become carriers.
- Check HCV RNA (by polymerase chain reaction [PCR]) and HCV antibody. If both are negative, acute HCV is unlikely. If HCV RNA is positive and HCV Ab is positive, patient has HCV infection (either acute or chronic); refer to GI specialist for liver biopsy/treatment.

Antibody Hepatitis D Virus and/or Hepatitis D Virus RNA (HDV RNA)

- Hepatitis D tests by antibody hepatitis D virus (anti-HDV) or HDV RNA test
- Closely associated with HBV infection; presence of HBV is required for complete virion assembly and secretion.
- Infection with both hepatitis B and hepatitis D increases the risk of fulminant hepatitis, cirrhosis, and severe liver damage; low prevalence in the United States
- Transmission by sex, sharing needles, birth to an infected mother, needle sticks, semen, saliva
- Suspect HDV infection in any person with positive hepatitis B antigen (HBsAg) who has severe symptoms of hepatitis or acute exacerbations

EXAM TIPS

- There will be a serology question. You will have to figure out what type of viral hepatitis the patient has (A, B, or C). It is usually hepatitis B.
- HBsAg-positive status always means an infected patient (new infection or chronic).

LIVER FUNCTION TESTS

Aspartate aminotransferase (AST), alanine aminotransferase (ALT), alkaline phosphatase (ALP), and bilirubin are biomarkers of hepatic injury.

Aspartate Aminotransferase (AST)

- Also known as *serum glutamic oxaloacetic transaminase (SGOT)*
- Normal is 0 to 35 U/L
- Present in the liver, as well as the cardiac muscle, skeletal muscle, kidney, and brain
- Elevated in most liver diseases and in those that involve the liver (e.g., hepatitis, cirrhosis, nonalcoholic fatty liver disease [NAFLD], alcohol use disorder, certain drugs, myocardial infarction, mononucleosis).

Alanine Aminotransferase (ALT)

- Also known as *serum glutamic pyruvic transaminase (SGPT)*
- Normal in males is 29 to 33 U/L; in females is 19 to 25 U/L
- Primarily present in liver; more specific biomarker for hepatocellular injury compared with AST.
- Fluctuate with menstrual cycle

Aspartate Aminotransferase/Alanine Aminotransferase Ratio (AST: ALT Ratio)

- A ratio of 2:1 or greater may be indicative of alcohol abuse.

Gamma-Glutamyl Transferase (GGT)

- Normal range is 0 to 30 IU/L.
- GGT is found in many organs of the body but mainly in the liver, kidneys, and pancreas.
- Elevated levels may be an indicator of alcohol abuse or alcoholic liver disease.
- Can also be elevated with medications (phenytoin, barbiturates), biliary disease, liver cancer or metastases, pancreatitis.
- Elevated levels in combination with ALP elevation suggest liver etiology.

EXAM TIP

GGT is elevated in liver disease and biliary obstruction. A "lone" elevation in the GGT is a sensitive indicator of possible alcoholism.

Alkaline Phosphatase (ALP)

- Enzyme derived from bone, liver, gallbladder, kidneys, GI tract, and placenta
- The highest amounts come from the bones and the liver. During the third trimester of pregnancy, elevated levels come from the placenta.
- ALP levels vary with age; in general, higher levels are seen during growth spurts (physiologic osteoblastic activity) in children and teenagers.
- Elevated in biliary obstruction, cholestasis, bone malignancy/metastasis, healing fractures.

EXAM TIPS

- ALP is normally elevated during the teen years due to bone growth. The ALP may also be elevated in bone disorders such as vitamin D deficiency, Paget's disease, and bone cancer. A GGT, which would be elevated with liver disease, may be drawn to differentiate between liver disease and bone disorders.
- ALT is more sensitive to liver damage than AST. AST is also found in other organs such as the heart and skeletal system. Elevated AST and ALT may reflect acute liver injury or inflammation.

DISEASE REVIEW

ACUTE DIVERTICULITIS

- Diverticula are small pouch-like herniations on the external surface of the colon.
- Secondary to a chronic lack of dietary fiber; higher incidence in Western societies. Up to 50% of Americans age 60 years or older have diverticula in their colon.
- In the majority of cases in Western countries, the left colon (descending colon and sigmoid) is involved.
- Diverticulitis occurs when diverticula become infected; high risk of rupture and bleeding; can be life-threatening.
- Hospitalize in moderate-to-severe cases, dehydration, elderly, signs/symptoms of acute abdomen, high fever, comorbidities, or immunocompromise.

Classic Case

Older adult presents with LLQ abdominal pain that is constant and has been present for several days. May present with RLQ or suprapubic pain due to inflamed sigmoid colon or right-sided (cecal) diverticulitis. Associated symptoms include a fever, nausea and vomiting. Reports history of change in bowel habits; up to 50% will have constipation, and some will have diarrhea.

Objective Findings

- Acute diverticulitis: If acute abdomen, positive for rebound, positive Rovsing's sign, and boardlike abdomen, refer to ED.
- Diverticulosis: Physical exam is normal; no palpable mass; no tenderness. Diverticula can be visualized only by colonoscopy.

Labs

- CBC with leukocytosis, neutrophilia >70%, and shift to the left (band forms); the presence of band forms signals severe bacterial infection; bands are immature neutrophils; refer to ED.
- Fecal occult blood test (FOBT) positive if bleeding.
- Reticulocytosis if acute bleeding and low hemoglobin/hematocrit.

Treatment Plan

- Uncomplicated mild cases of diverticulitis can be treated in the outpatient setting. Liquid diet and oral analgesia—reassess in 2 to 3 days and then weekly until resolution of all symptoms.
- Oral antibiotics are not routinely recommended; may be indicated for patients at higher risk of complications (e.g., major comorbidities, immunocompromising conditions).
- Close follow-up needed. If no response in 48 to 72 hours or symptoms worsen (high fever, toxic), refer to ED; moderate-to-severe cases, hospitalize.
- Inpatient treatment recommended for those with abscess, obstruction, fistula, sepsis, severe abdominal pain, perforation, age >70 years, significant comorbidities, immunosuppression, noncompliance, failure of outpatient treatment, or intolerance of oral intake.

Chronic Therapy for Diverticulosis

- High-fiber diet with fiber supplementation such as psyllium (Metamucil) or methylcellulose (Citrucel).
- Tobacco cessation, physical activity, and reduced meat intake.
- Probiotics have been used to prevent recurrences but have limited evidence-based value.
- Colonoscopy for all patients after resolution of symptoms to rule out colon cancer.

Complications

- Perforation, which can cause peritonitis and bleeding
- Abscess
- Obstruction
- Fistula

ACUTE HEPATITIS

An acute liver inflammation with multiple causes, including viral infection, hepatotoxic drugs (e.g., statins), excessive alcohol intake, medications, and toxins.

Classic Case

Adult complains of a new onset of fever, fatigue, anorexia, nausea, malaise, and dark-colored urine for several days. May report sclera have a yellowish tinge (icteric). Skin is jaundiced. May have clay-colored stools. May have RUQ abdominal pain.

Objective Findings

- Skin and sclerae have a yellow tinge (jaundiced or icteric).
- Tenderness over the liver occurs with percussion and deep palpation.

Labs

- ALT and AST levels are often elevated during the acute phase of the illness. Elevations greater than five times the upper limit of normal are suggestive of extensive hepatocellular injury.
- Other liver function tests (LFTs), such as serum bilirubin, ALP, and GGT, may be elevated.
- Elevated ammonia, prothrombin time, and decreased albumin may be observed.

Treatment Plan

Remove and treat the cause (if possible). Treatment is specific to the etiology. Avoid hepatotoxic agents such as alcoholic drinks, acetaminophen, and statins (e.g., pravastatin [Pravachol]). Treatment is supportive. Referral is often indicated for advanced liver disease.

ACUTE PANCREATITIS

- Acute inflammation of the pancreas secondary to many factors, such as alcohol abuse, gallstones (cholelithiasis), elevated triglyceride levels (levels above 1,000 mg/dL), post-endoscopic retrograde cholangiopancreatography (ERCP) (up to 3%), genetics, certain medications, and other rare cases.
- Pancreatic damage and necrosis from activated pancreatic enzymes, microcirculatory impairment, and release of inflammatory mediators.
- Classified as mild acute, moderately severe, and severe acute pancreatitis.

Classic Case

Adult patient complains of nausea and vomiting that is associated with rapid onset of severe epigastric and LUQ abdominal pain. Pain radiates to the back in about half of patients. May have dyspnea, pleural effusions, or acute respiratory distress syndrome. Abdominal exam reveals guarding and tenderness over the epigastric area or the upper abdomen. May have positive Cullen's and Grey Turner's sign. May have ileus and signs and symptoms of shock (e.g., fever, tachypnea, hypoxemia, and hypotension). Refer patient to ED.

Objective Findings

- Cullen's sign, bluish discoloration around umbilicus (hemorrhagic pancreatitis)
- Grey Turner's sign, bluish discoloration on the flank area (hemorrhagic pancreatitis)
- Abdominal distention and hypoactive bowel sounds (suggest ileus)
- May have scleral icterus and jaundice secondary to choledocholithiasis
- Guarding and abdominal rigidity—consider peritonitis

Labs

- Elevated pancreatic enzymes such as serum amylase, lipase, and trypsin
- Elevated AST, ALT, GGT, bilirubin, leukocytosis
- Abdominal ultrasound and CT
- Hypocalcemia

Complications

- Serious complications such as ileus, sepsis, shock, multiorgan failure, death
- Diabetes

CLOSTRIDIUM DIFFICILE–ASSOCIATED DIARRHEA

C. difficile infection is a gram-positive, spore-forming anaerobic bacillus that releases toxins that produce clinical disease. The classic symptom is watery diarrhea a few days after starting antibiotic treatment due to changes in intestinal flora caused by antibiotics. Antibiotics such as clindamycin (Cleocin), fluoroquinolones, cephalosporins, and penicillins are more likely to cause *C. difficile* infection. Most cases occur in hospitalized patients; may also occur in institutionalized patients (nursing facilities). It is spread by fecal–oral contact.

Risk Factors
- Prior or current systemic antibiotic therapy especially with fluoroquinolones, clindamycin, cephalosporins, and penicillins
- Age >65 years
- Recent hospitalization

Classic Case
Adult to older adult patient who is currently on antibiotics or has recently completed a course of antibiotics. History of hospitalization. Acute onset of diarrhea with lower abdominal cramping and pain, anorexia, nausea, and low-grade fever. Non-severe *C. difficile* infection characterized by watery diarrhea (>3 loose stools in 24 hours) with lower abdominal pain and cramping, low-grade fever, and leukocytosis. *C. difficile* colitis has a high recurrence rate, so ask about previous episodes. Suspected patients should be placed on contact precautions.

Labs
- Nucleic acid amplification testing (NAAT) for *C. difficile* of a single stool sample.
- Stool assay (by enzyme-linked immunosorbent assay) for *C. difficile* toxins.
- CBC with leukocytosis (>15,000 cells/μL), basic metabolic panel with serum electrolytes, creatinine, and blood urea nitrogen (BUN).
- Repeat stool testing for test of cure is not recommended. *C. difficile* toxin may persist despite clinical response to treatment. Testing and treatment of asymptomatic patients is not recommended.

Treatment
- Discontinue inciting antibiotic regimen and infection control practices with hand hygiene and contact precautions.
- For initial episode (regardless of severity), fidaxomicin 200 mg PO BID for 10 days or vancomycin 125 mg PO QID × 10 days. Alternative is metronidazole 500 mg PO TID for 10 to 14 days.
- For recurrent episode, treatment with either fidaxomicin or vancomycin in a tapered and pulsed regimen. Adjunctive treatment is bezlotoxumab.
- For third or subsequent recurrent episode, consider fecal microbiota transplant.
- Antimotility agents (loperamide) may be considered in patients with high fluid losses in the absence of ileus or colonic distention.
- Limited evidence of the efficacy of probiotics.
- Supportive care includes rehydration, increasing fluids, managing nutrition and electrolyte imbalances.
- Early oral refeeding is encouraged. Regular, low-residue diet. Restricted diets such as BRAT (bananas, rice, applesauce, toast) not necessary.

CLINICAL PEARL
Handwashing with soap and water is more effective against *C. difficile* than alcohol-based hand wipes.

GASTROENTERITIS

Acute Gastroenteritis
The main symptom of acute gastroenteritis is diarrhea. Diarrhea is defined as loose, watery stools three or more times a day. Acute diarrhea lasts 1 to 2 days; persistent diarrhea lasts 2 to 4 weeks; chronic diarrhea lasts ≥4 weeks. The most common pathogens that cause acute gastroenteritis are viruses (most cases), bacteria, and protozoans.

Viral Gastroenteritis
Acute onset of nausea and vomiting accompanied by watery diarrhea that is not bloody. It is self-limited and of short duration, typically lasting 1 to 3 days. The most common viral pathogen is noroviruses which can cause outbreaks in crowded areas such as nursing homes and cruise ships. Other common pathogens include rotavirus, enteric adenovirus, and astrovirus.

Bacterial Gastroenteritis
Acute onset of high fever, bloody diarrhea, severe abdominal pain with at least six stools in a 24-hour period. Incubation period ranges from 1 to 6 hours if due to contaminated food (enterotoxin) or 1 to 3 days if bacterial infection. Symptoms usually resolve in 1 to 7 days. Antibiotics can reduce the duration of diarrhea but may lead to bacterial resistance and eradication of normal flora. Bacterial pathogens include *Escherichia coli*, *Salmonella*, *Shigella*, *Campylobacter*, *C. difficile* (antibiotic use, recent hospitalization), and *Listeria* (pregnant patients increased risk).

Protozoal Gastroenteritis
Symptoms develop within 7 days of exposure and typically last ≥7 days. It is usually watery diarrhea. Travelers' diarrhea starts within 3 to 7 days after exposure and usually resolves in 5 days. It is usually self-limited. Protozoal pathogens include *Giardia lamblia*, *Entamoeba histolytica*, and *Cryptosporidium*.

Risk Factors
- Travel to developing countries
- Recent antibiotic use
- Immunocompromised state
- Day care or resides in a crowded setting (e.g., nursing homes, institutions)

Preventive Measures
- Drink bottled water during foreign travel; avoid ice cubes
- Food and water precautions when traveling in developing countries
- Wash hands frequently
- Careful food preparation, such as washing vegetables and fruits
- Rotavirus vaccine (infants)

GASTROESOPHAGEAL REFLUX DISEASE

Forty percent of U.S. adults have gastroesophageal reflux disease (GERD). Acidic gastric contents regurgitate from the stomach into the esophagus due to inappropriate relaxation of the lower esophageal sphincter. Diagnosis is based on history and clinical symptoms. Chronic GERD causes damage to squamous epithelium of the lower esophagus, and may result in Barrett's esophagus (a precancer), which increases risk of squamous cell cancer (cancer of the esophagus).

Classic Case

Middle-aged to older adult complains of chronic heartburn of many years' duration. Symptoms associated with large and/or fatty meals that worsen when supine. Long-term history of self-medication with over-the-counter (OTC) antacids and H2 antagonists (H2RAs). Risk factors may include chronic use of NSAIDs, aspirin, or alcohol.

Objective Findings

- Acidic or sour odor to breath
- Reflux of sour acidic stomach contents, especially with overeating
- Thinning tooth enamel (rear molars) due to increased hydrochloric acid
- Chronic sore red throat (not associated with a cold)
- Chronic coughing, hoarseness, wheezing (extraesophageal symptoms)

Treatment Plan

First-line (mild/intermittent GERD) treatment is lifestyle changes. Avoid large and/or high-fat meals, especially 3 to 4 hours before bedtime. Avoid foods or medications that relax the lower esophageal sphincter or foods or medications that irritate the esophagus (Box 10.1). Weight reduction if overweight (body mass index [BMI] >25) or obese. Cease smoking. Smoking increases stomach acid and lowers esophageal sphincter pressure. Combine lifestyle changes with antacids (mild GERD) taken after each meal and at bedtime. If poor response, next step is to prescribe medications and continue with lifestyle modifications.

Medications

H2RAs: First-line treatment for mild-to-moderate symptoms or mild esophagitis. Should be taken at bedtime. Examples: Nizatidine (Axid) 300 mg at bedtime, famotidine 40 mg at bedtime (Pepcid).

- Antacids: Neutralizes gastric pH. Aluminum–magnesium–simethicone (Mylanta, Maalox), calcium carbonate (Tums, Caltrate), aluminum–magnesium (Gaviscon); minerals can bind with certain medications such as tetracycline and levothyroxine (Synthroid).
- Surface agents and alginates: Sucralfate adheres to the mucosal surface, promotes healing, and protects from peptic injury.

Proton pump inhibitors (PPIs): For erosive esophagitis. Refer to gastroenterologist.

- Omeprazole (Prilosec): 20 mg once daily; esomeprazole (Nexium): 40 mg once daily; lansoprazole (Prevacid): 30 mg once daily; pantoprazole (Protonix): 40 mg once daily.
- Dose PPIs: 30 to 60 minutes before meals.
- Long-term use of PPIs: Associated with increased risk of osteoporosis and bone/hip fractures in postmenopausal women (interferes with calcium homeostasis), acute interstitial nephritis, hypomagnesemia, *C. difficile* infection, reduced absorption of iron.

Do not discontinue PPIs abruptly because doing so can cause rebound symptoms (worsens symptoms); taper dose to wean. If no relief after 4 to 8 weeks therapy, if patient is at high risk for Barrett's esophagus, or experiencing worsening symptoms, refer to GI specialist for upper endoscopy/biopsy (gold standard).

EXAM TIPS

- For mild cases of GERD, lifestyle management and antacids or H2RAs. For patients with moderate-to-severe esophagitis, first line is PPIs.
- If patient needs treatment for GERD, start with H2RAs; if poor relief or erosive esophagitis, step up to PPIs.

Box 10.1 Foods and Medications That Can Worsen GERD Symptoms

Foods
- Peppermint or other mint-flavored gum or candy
- Chocolate
- Caffeine
- Alcoholic drinks
- Carbonated beverages
- Tomato sauce
- Citrus drinks (e.g., orange juice)
- Fatty foods

Medications
- Calcium channel blockers
- NSAIDs
- Nitrates
- Opioids
- Anticholinergics
- Iron supplements
- Bisphosphonates
- Tricyclic antidepressants
- Theophylline
- Barbituates

GERD, gastroesophageal reflux disease; NSAIDs, nonsteroidal anti-inflammatory drugs.

Complications

- Barrett's esophagus (a precursor for the development of esophageal cancer)
- Esophageal cancer
- Esophageal stricture/scarring

> **NOTE**
>
> If worrisome or worsening symptoms noticed in patients with GERD—e.g., odynophagia (pain with swallowing), dysphagia (difficulty swallowing), early satiety, weight loss, iron-deficiency anemia (blood loss), or male >50 years—refer to ED and/or gastroenterologist.

CLINICAL PEARLS

- Any patient with a long history of chronic heartburn should be referred to a gastroenterologist for an endoscopy to rule out Barrett's esophagus.
- Patients with Barrett's esophagus have up to 30 times higher risk of cancer of the esophagus (adenocarcinoma type).

EXAM TIPS

- Barrett's esophagus is a precancer (esophageal cancer). Diagnosed by upper endoscopy with biopsy. Worrisome symptoms for esophageal cancer include anorexia, early satiety, anemia, recurrent vomiting, hematemesis, and weight loss.
- Know lifestyle factors to teach patient (e.g., avoid smoking, alcohol, and caffeine).

IRRITABLE BOWEL SYNDROME

Irritable bowel syndrome (IBS) is a chronic functional disorder of the colon (normal colonic tissue) marked by exacerbations and remissions (spontaneous). Commonly exacerbated by excess stress. It may be classified as diarrhea-predominant or constipation-predominant. In some cases, it may alternate between the two.

Classic Case

Young adult to middle-aged female complains of intermittent episodes of moderate-to-severe cramping pain in the lower abdomen, especially in the LLQ. Bloating with flatulence. Relief obtained after defecation. Stools range from diarrhea to constipation or both types with increased frequency of bowel movements.

Objective Findings

- Complete physical exam: Should be performed to exclude other causes.
- Vital signs: Typically normal.
- Abdominal exam: Tenderness in lower quadrants during an exacerbation. Otherwise, the physical exam is normal.
- Rectal exam: Stool is normal with no blood or pus. Stools are heme negative.

Treatment Plan

Lifestyle modifications for initial management: Increase dietary fiber. Supplement fiber with psyllium (Metamucil or Konsyl), methylcellulose (Citrucel), wheat dextrin (Benefiber). Start at low dose (causes gas).

- Avoid gas-producing foods: Beans, onions, cabbage, high-fructose corn syrup. If poor response, use a trial diet of lactose avoidance or gluten avoidance.
- Low FODMAP diet: Diet low in fermentable oligo-, di-, and monosaccharides and polyols in patients with abdominal bloating or pain (e.g., foods that contain fructose, including honey, high-fructose corn syrup, certain fruits) under guidance of registered dietician.
- Decrease life stress: Address anxiety/stress with patient and offer treatment strategies.
- Antispasmodics for abdominal pain: Administer dicyclomine (Bentyl) or hyoscyamine as needed.
- IBS with constipation: Begin a trial of fiber supplements, then trial polyethylene glycol (osmotic laxative).
- Severe constipation: Prescribe lubiprostone or linaclotide (contraindicated in pediatric patients <6 years, has caused death from dehydration).
- IBS with diarrhea: Take loperamide (Imodium) before regularly scheduled meals. Bile acid sequestrants (e.g., cholestyramine) as second-line therapy.
- Severe diarrhea–predominant IBS: 5-hydroxytryptamine (serotonin) 3 receptor antagonist (e.g., alosetron) can be used in female patients who have failed to respond to all other conventional treatments. (Warning: Ischemic colitis, which can be fatal).
- Rule out: Amoebic, parasitic, or bacterial infections; Inflammatory disease of the GI tract. Check stool for ova and parasites (especially diarrheal stools) with culture.

CLINICAL PEARL

Do not give antidiarrheal medications if patient has acute onset of bloody diarrhea, fever, abdominal pain, or pain that worsens with defecation because it may be caused by *Escherichia coli* O157:H7 (a shiga toxin–producing *E. coli* [STEC]), amebiasis, *Salmonella*, *Shigella*, or other pathogens. May need to go to ED.

NONALCOHOLIC FATTY LIVER DISEASE

NAFLD is caused by triglyceride fat deposits (steatosis) in the hepatocytes of the liver. NAFLD can be categorized into nonalcoholic fatty liver (NAFL) and nonalcoholic steatohepatitis (NASH). NAFL is characterized by hepatic steatosis without evidence of significant inflammation whereas hepatic inflammation is present in NASH. NAFLD is more common in Western industrialized countries. Major risk factors include central obesity, type 2 diabetes, metabolic syndrome, and dyslipidemia.

Classic Case

Most patients are asymptomatic. Some patients may have hepatomegaly. Lab findings often show mild-to-moderate elevations of ALT and AST. If symptomatic, complaints of fatigue and malaise with vague RUQ pain.

Labs and Diagnostic Evaluation

- LFTs; ALT and AST may be slightly elevated from two to five times the upper limit of normal; normal transaminase levels do not exclude NAFLD.
- Fasting lipid levels, glucose, A1C.
- Hepatitis A, B, and C serology markers.
- Initial imaging test is liver ultrasound; CT and MRI can also detect hepatic steatosis.
- Liver biopsy is the gold standard for diagnosis.
- NAFLD fibrosis score is used to grade disease activity.

Treatment Plan

- Lose weight, exercise, and watch diet.
- Discontinue alcohol intake permanently.
- Avoid hepatotoxic drugs (e.g., acetaminophen, isoniazid, statins).
- Recommend vaccination for hepatitis A and B and annual flu vaccine.
- Refer to GI specialist.

Patient Education

- All patients with overweight or obesity should be advised to lose weight (especially those with diabetes).
- Lifestyle changes are important (diet, nutrition, exercise).
- Daily aerobic exercise (e.g., walking, swimming, biking) for 30 to 45 minutes is recommended.

PEPTIC ULCER DISEASE

Peptic ulcers are defined as disruptions in the gastric or duodenal mucosal surface, extending beyond the superficial layer. Two major risk factors are associated with peptic ulcer disease (PUD), *Helicobacter pylori* infection and use of NSAIDs. Other risk factors include smoking, alcohol, and genetic and dietary factors. Duodenal and gastric ulcer incidence increases with age. Incidence increases in countries where infection with *H. pylori* exists. Most patients (up to 70%) are asymptomatic.

Etiology

- *H. pylori* (gram-negative bacteria) infection is a major factor associated with PUD.
- Chronic NSAID and aspirin use, which disrupts prostaglandin production, results in reduction of GI blood flow with reduction of protective mucus layer. It inhibits cyclooxygenase (COX 1 and COX 2) enzyme, which reduces production of prostaglandin.
- Cigarette smoking and/or alcohol use.
- Drug-induced PUD can result from bisphosphonates, clopidogrel, anticoagulants, potassium supplements, corticosteroids, chemotherapeutic drugs, illicit drugs (crack cocaine).
- Hormonal or mediator-induced (e.g., gastrinoma)
- Postsurgical or radiation therapy
- Mechanical (e.g., duodenal obstruction)
- Infiltrating disease (e.g., sarcoidosis, Crohn diease)

Classic Case

Adult complains of recurrent epigastric pain, burning/gnawing pain, or ache. Pain relieved by food and/

or antacids with recurrence shortly after meals (gastric ulcer) and 2 to 4 hours after a meal (duodenal ulcer). Pain also recurs when hungry or stomach is empty. Self-medicating with OTC antacid, H2 blocker, and/or PPI. May be taking NSAIDs or aspirin for chronic pain or prophylaxis against heart disease or stroke. Black or tarry stools (melena), red/maroon blood in stool (hematochezia), coffee-ground emesis, or iron-deficiency anemia indicates GI bleeding. If signs of shock (hemorrhage) are present with board-like abdomen and rebound tenderness, call 911. Worrisome symptoms include early satiety, anorexia, anemia (bleeding), recurrent vomiting, hematemesis, and weight loss.

Objective Findings

- Abdominal exam: Normal or mildly tender epigastric area during flare-ups.
- Hemoccult: Can be positive if actively bleeding.

Labs

- CBC (iron-deficiency anemia means bleeding) and FOBT are needed (can be negative if no active bleeding).
- All patients diagnosed with PUD should be tested for *H. pylori* infection.
- Urea breath test is indicative of active *H. pylori* infection and is commonly used to document eradication of *H. pylori* after treatment. Use of PPIs within 2 weeks of the test can interfere with results.
- Stool antigen can be used to confirm infection and post treatment to document eradication.
- With serology (titers), *H. pylori* immunoglobulin (IgG) levels are elevated. Presence of antibodies does not necessarily indicate current infection. *H. pylori* antibodies can be elevated for months to years. Urea breath test and stool/fecal antigen test are more sensitive for active infection than serology/titers.
- Gold standard is upper endoscopy and biopsy of gastric and/or duodenal tissue.
- If multiple severe ulcers or unresponsive to treatment, use fasting gastrin levels to rule out Zollinger–Ellison syndrome as needed.
- Gastric ulcers require an endoscopy to rule out gastric cancer and document healing of ulcer.

Treatment Plan

Treatment for H. pylori–Negative Ulcers

- Stop use of NSAIDs. If a patient needs long-term NSAIDs, ulcer formation risk can be decreased if combined with a PPI or misoprostol.
- Encourage smoking cessation. Stop drinking alcohol.
- Combine lifestyle changes with PPIs or H2RAs (no antibiotics). Duration of therapy is from 4 to 8 weeks. If recurrent ulcers, poor response after 4 to 8 weeks of therapy, or suspect bleeding ulcer, refer to GI.
- H2RAs are nizatidine (Axid) 150 mg twice a day or 300 mg at bedtime; or famotidine (Pepcid) 40 mg at bedtime.
- PPIs are omeprazole (Prilosec) 20 mg daily; esomeprazole (Nexium) 40 mg daily; or lansoprazole (Prevacid) 15 to 30 mg daily.

Treatment for H. pylori–Positive Ulcers

Triple therapy:

- Clarithromycin (Biaxin) 500 mg twice a day *PLUS* amoxicillin 1 g twice a day *OR* metronidazole (Flagyl) 500 mg twice a day if allergic to amoxicillin × 14 days *PLUS*
- Standard-dose PPI orally twice a day × 14 days

Quadruple therapy:

- Bismuth subsalicylate tab 600 mg four times a day *PLUS*
- Metronidazole tab 250 mg four times a day *PLUS*
- Tetracycline cap 500 mg four times a day × 2 weeks *PLUS*
- Standard-dose PPI orally twice a day × 14 days

Sequential therapy, salvage therapy, and other treatment regimens for *H. pylori*: Available for clinical use, but not necessary information for the exam.

EXAM TIPS

- Determine whether question is about *H. pylori*–negative ulcers or *H. pylori*–positive ulcers.
- *H. pylori*–positive ulcers require antibiotics for 14 days *PLUS* PPI orally twice a day.

CLINICAL PEARLS

- About 5% to 30% of peptic ulcers recur within the first year.
- Avoid using clarithromycin therapy if there is high resistance in your area. In the United States, it is generally assumed clarithromycin resistance rates are greater than 15% unless local data suggest differently. The choice of eradication regimens is ultimately decided by local surveillance data.
- PPIs facilitate ulcer healing better than H2RAs.

VIRAL HEPATITIS

Hepatitis A Virus

- Self-limiting infection caused by hepatitis A virus (HAV); does not become chronic. Infection grants life-long immunity. Preventable by vaccination.
- Transmitted via fecal and oral route from contaminated food or drink, or person-to-person contact.
- Risk factors include residence in or travel to areas with poor sanitation, household or sexual contact with another infected person, exposure to daycare centers and residential institutions, and IV drug use.
- Symptoms include acute onset of fever, headache, malaise, anorexia, nausea, vomiting, diarrhea, abdominal pain, dark urine, jaundice.
- Labs include IgM anti–HAV detectable at time of symptom onset, peak of disease, and detectable for 3 to 6 months. IgG antibodies remain detectable for decades and are associated with lifelong protective immunity. Elevations of serum aminotransferases, bilirubin, and ALP.
- Treatment is supportive care.

- Primary prevention is immunization with single-antigen inactivated hepatitis A vaccine (Havrix) for individuals at increased risk (e.g., travelers to areas where hepatitis A is endemic, men who have sex with men, those with occupational risk exposure).
- Hepatitis A is reportable to the public health department.
- Advise patients to avoid drugs and foods that can damage the liver, such as acetaminophen, alcohol/ethanol, statins, isoniazid, and some herbal teas.

Hepatitis B Virus

- Hepatitis B virus (HBV) infection can either be acute and self-limiting, or it can be chronic.
- Horizontal transmission via sexual activity (semen, vaginal secretions, and saliva), blood, blood products, organs. Vertical transmission occurs from mother to infant. Percutaneous transmission (e.g., IV drug use).
- Symptoms vary for acute and chronic disease, anorexia, nausea, jaundice, RUQ discomfort, fatigue. Many chronic patients are asymptomatic (unless they have decompensated cirrhosis or extrahepatic complications).
- Vaccination is three total doses given during infancy (at birth, 1 to 2 months, and 6 to 18 months); various options are available for adults who are at high risk. The dose and schedule depend on the type of vaccine and patient population.
- Treatment of acute HBV mainly involves supportive care (risk of liver failure less than 1%); consider antiviral therapy if indicated (e.g., patients with a severe or protracted course). Preventive measures to all household and sexual contacts who are not immune.
- For treatment of chronic HBV, referral is often indicated as management is complex and depends on multiple factors (comorbidities, viral load, immunologic response). Antiviral agents include pegylated interferon alfa (PEG-IFN-a) or nucleos(t)ide analogs (e.g., entecavir and tenofovir).

Hepatitis C Virus

- Hepatitis C virus can cause both acute and chronic hepatitis. Approximately 14% to 50% of patients spontaneously clear the virus; the rest develop chronic infection. Chronic HCV infection can cause cirrhosis, hepatocellular carcinoma, and require the need for a liver transplant.
- Transmitted via sharing needles, blood transfusions (rare since routine testing of blood supply), mother to infant (vertical transmission), and needlestick injuries in healthcare settings. Less common, spread by sexual contact, sharing personal items (razors or toothbrushes).
- Most are asymptomatic; symptoms of an acute hepatitis syndrome occur 7 to 8 weeks after infection.
- High-risk groups include intravenous drug users, incarcerated or unstably housed populations, people with HIV, men who have sex with men, dialysis patients, healthcare providers, individuals with alcohol use disorder, and perinatally exposed children.

- The USPSTF recommends routine one-time HCV screening for *all* adults ages 18 to 79 years.
- Acute HCV infection is HCV RNA detectable by PCR in the setting of undetectable anti-HCV antibodies that become detectable within 12 weeks.
- Report acute cases of hepatitis C to the health department.
- Recommend the same antiviral treatment (e.g., sofosbuvir-velpatasivr for 12 weeks or glecaprevir-pibrentasvir for 8 weeks) for acute and chronic infection. Refer to GI specialist.
- Advise patient not to share razors, toothbrushes, and nail clippers and to cover cuts and sores. Do not donate blood. Counseling for substance abuse disorder and safe needle handling if indicated.

CASE STUDIES FOR VIRAL HEPATITIS

PATIENT A
- HBsAg: Negative
- Anti-HBs: Positive
- Anti-HBc: Positive
- Results: Immune to hepatitis B due to natural infection.

PATIENT B
- HBsAg: Positive
- IgM anti-HBc: Positive
- Anti-HBs: Negative
- Anti-HBc: Positive
- Results: Patient is acutely infected with hepatitis B infection.

EXAM TIPS

- Hepatitis C has highest risk of cirrhosis and liver cancer.
- Screening test for hepatitis C virus is called the HCV antibody (anti-HCV). If positive, next step is to order HCV RNA test. If positive, patient has hepatitis C.

KNOWLEDGE CHECK: CHAPTER 10

1. Which physical assessment has good specificity for acute appendicitis?
   A. Murphy's sign
   B. Halo sign
   C. Carnett's sign
   D. Rovsing's sign

2. Both hepatitis A and hepatitis B can be transmitted by which of the following modes?
   A. Sneezing and coughing
   B. Maternal–fetal transmission
   C. Consumption of contaminated food or water
   D. Sexual transmission

3. A patient presents with generalized fatigue and concern for hepatitis B virus (HBV) infection. Serology testing is significant for positive HBsAg and IgM anti-HBc. This suggests that the patient:
   A. Was previously infected
   B. Is immune due to vaccination
   C. Is chronically infected
   D. Is acutely infected

4. Patients with hepatitis D are always dually infected with hepatitis:
   A. B
   B. A
   C. C
   D. E

5. A patient presents with left upper quadrant pain. This area of abdominal pain suggests which of the following disease processes?
   A. Acute pancreatitis
   B. Acute cholecystitis
   C. Hepatitis
   D. Splenomegaly

6. A patient presents with right lower quadrant abdominal pain, anorexia, nausea, and vomiting. During the physical assessment, the psoas sign is positive. This suggests which of the following acute processes?
   A. Cholecystitis
   B. Pancreatitis
   C. Appendicitis
   D. Diverticulitis

7. An older adult patient was recently hospitalized and prescribed antibiotics for community-acquired pneumonia. The patient presents with complaints of severe watery diarrhea, lower abdominal pain, and cramping. The patient denies both a history of previous episodes of diarrhea and recent travel. Which of the following regimens is indicated for initial management?
   A. Metronidazole
   B. Fecal transplant
   C. Probiotics
   D. Fidaxomicin

8. A patient undergoes an upper endoscopy for peptic ulcer disease; the gastric mucosal biopsy is positive for *Helicobacter pylori*. The patient has recently been treated with azithromycin for a sinus infection. Which of the following antibiotic regimens is appropriate for this patient?
   A. Bismuth, metronidazole, tetracycline, and a proton pump inhibitor (PPI)
   B. Clarithromycin, amoxicillin, and a PPI
   C. Clarithromycin, metronidazole, and a PPI
   D. Clarithromycin, metronidazole, amoxicillin, and a PPI

(See answers next page.)

1. D) Rovsing's sign
Although they are insensitive tests, the psoas, obturator, and Rovsing's signs have good specificity for acute appendicitis. Murphy's sign is suggestive of cholecystitis or gallbladder disease. Halo sign is suggestive of the presence of cerebrospinal fluid in drainage from a head injury. Carnett's sign distinguishes abdominal wall pain from visceral pain.

2. D) Sexual transmission
Hepatitis A virus is transmitted via the fecal–oral route, via person-to-person contact (e.g., transmission within households, sexual transmission, residential institution or daycare center transmission), contact with contaminated food or water (e.g., consumption of raw or undercooked food or contaminated foods), blood transfusion, or illicit drug use. Maternal–fetal transmission has not been described. Hepatitis B is transmitted through activities that involve percutaneous (e.g., puncture through skin) or mucosal contact with infectious blood or body fluids (e.g., semen, saliva). This includes mother-to-child transmission, blood transfusion, sexual transmission, intravenous drug use, nosocomial infection (e.g., via contaminated instruments or an accidental needlestick), transplant recipients, and blood exposure to minor breaks in the skin or mucous membranes. There is no firm evidence of hepatitis B transmission via body fluids other than blood or semen.

3. D) Is acutely infected
Acute hepatitis B is diagnosed based on the detection of hepatitis B surface antigen (HBsAg) and IgM hepatitis B core antibody (IgM anti-HBc). Markers of HBV replication, hepatitis B e antigen (HBeAg) and HBV DNA are also present in the initial phase of infection. Recovery is indicated by the disappearance of HBV DNA, HBeAg to hepatitis B e antibody (anti-HBe) seroconversion, and HBsAG to hepatitis B surface antibody (anti-HBs) seroconversion. Previous infection is characterized by the presence of anti-HBs and IgG anti-HBc. Immunity after vaccination is indicated by the presence of anti-HBs only. Chronic HBV infection is diagnosed by the persistence of HBsAg for more than 6 months.

4. A) B
Hepatitis D is closely associated with hepatitis B virus (HBV) infection. The presence of HBV is required for complete virion assembly and secretion. Therefore, patients with hepatitis D are always dually infected with HBV.

5. D) Splenomegaly
Left upper quadrant pain is often related to disorders of the spleen (e.g., splenomegaly, splenic infarct, splenic abscess or rupture). Right upper quadrant pain is often due to biliary disorders (e.g., gallstones, acute cholecystitis, acute cholangitis) and hepatic etiologies (e.g., hepatitis, liver abscess). Epigastric pain is often a result of pancreatic and gastric etiologies (e.g., peptic ulcer disease, gastritis).

6. C) Appendicitis
The classic symptoms of appendicitis include right lower quadrant abdominal pain, anorexia, nausea, and vomiting. The psoas sign is associated with a retrocecal appendix. It is considered positive if right lower quadrant abdominal pain occurs with passive right hip extension. The patient draws up the right knee to shorten the muscle because the inflamed appendix may lie against the right psoas muscle. Cholecystitis is associated with a positive Murphy sign. Diverticulitis often presents with pain in the left lower quadrant. Pancreatitis often presents with severe epigastric and left upper quadrant pain.

7. D) Fidaxomicin
The patient is presenting with risk factors and clinical manifestations suggestive of *Clostridium difficile* infection. It should be suspected in patients with acute diarrhea (more than three loose stools in 24 hours) with associated risk factors (e.g., recent antibiotic use, hospitalization, older age). The initial episode of non-severe *C. difficile* infection should be treated with either oral fidaxomicin or oral vancomycin for 10 days. An alternative option is metronidazole; however, it is less effective for treatment of non-severe *C. difficile* infection. Fecal transplant may be indicated in patients with severe and fulminant colitis. Probiotics are not recommended treatment for this patient.

8. A) Bismuth, metronidazole, tetracycline, and a proton pump inhibitor (PPI)
Treatment regimens for *H. pylori* are based on the presence of risk factors for macrolide resistance and the presence of a penicillin allergy. Bismuth quadruple therapy is recommended for patients with any prior exposure to macrolides for any reason and in areas of local clarithromycin resistance rates >15% or eradication rates with clarithromycin triple therapy <85%. Clarithromycin-based triple therapy is used in patients without risk factors. Metronidazole can be used instead of amoxicillin in patients who are allergic to penicillin.

9. A patient presents with dyspepsia and upper abdominal discomfort that radiates to the epigastric area. The patient reports that the pain improves after meals but worsens 2 to 5 hours after a meal. The patient also reports bloating and weight gain. This presentation suggests the presence of which of the following?
   A. Gastric ulcer
   B. Gastroesophageal reflux disease
   C. Duodenal ulcer
   D. Pancreatitis

10. Which of the following is the serologic hallmark of hepatitis B virus infection?
    A. Anti-HBs
    B. HBcAg
    C. Anti-HBc
    D. HBsAg

11. A patient presents with upper abdominal pain and discomfort. The patient also reports bloating, abdominal fullness, nausea, and pain that worsens immediately after eating. The patient reports a history of daily use of nonsteroidal anti-inflammatory drugs (NSAIDs) for chronic back pain. Based on the patient's presentation, which of the following is the *most* accurate diagnostic test?
    A. Abdominal CT scan
    B. Upper endoscopy
    C. Abdominal ultrasound
    D. Urea breath test

12. Which of the following is considered a marker of hepatitis B replication and infectivity?
    A. HBeAg
    B. IgM anti-HBc
    C. HBsAg
    D. Anti-HBs

13. A patient presents for routine laboratory work. An elevated alkaline phosphatase level is noted. In order to confirm that this elevation is due to a liver source, which of the following laboratory tests should be checked next?
    A. Lactate dehydrogenase
    B. Alanine aminotransferase (ALT)
    C. Gamma-glutamyl transpeptidase (GGT)
    D. Aspartate aminotransferase (AST)

14. A healthcare worker is concerned that they may have been infected with hepatitis B due to an accidental needlestick from an infected patient. Serology testing is significant for negative HBsAg and anti-HBc and positive anti-HBs. This suggests that the patient is:
    A. Immune due to natural infection
    B. Immune due to hepatitis B vaccination
    C. Chronically infected
    D. Acutely infected

15. A 30-year-old patient presents with mild-to-moderate lower left quadrant (LLQ) abdominal pain, constipation, and mild abdominal tenderness. Routine laboratory work is significant for elevated C-reactive protein and leukocytosis. Abdominal CT scan is pending to confirm diagnosis. The patient's vital signs are stable, and they are able to tolerate oral intake. Based on this presentation, first-line treatment for most patients includes:
    A. Intravenous antibiotics
    B. Nothing by mouth for complete bowel rest
    C. Oral antibiotics
    D. Pain control with oral analgesics and a liquid diet

16. A patient presents with a long history of crampy abdominal pain, diarrhea, fatigue, and weight loss. Endoscopic findings are significant for transmural inflammation, esophageal ulceration, cobblestone mucosal appearance, and skip lesions with areas of normal-appearing bowel interrupted by large areas of disease along the length of the intestine. These findings are suggestive of what disease?
    A. Ulcerative colitis
    B. Crohn's disease
    C. Irritable bowel syndrome
    D. Gastritis

(See answers next page.)

9. C) Duodenal ulcer

The patient is presenting with symptoms consistent with peptic ulcer disease and, more specifically, a duodenal ulcer. Upper abdominal pain or discomfort is the most common symptom seen with peptic ulcers; about 80% report epigastric pain. The pain of duodenal ulcers is often improved with eating but worsens 2 to 5 hours after a meal, when acid is secreted in the absence of a food buffer, and at night (11 p.m. to 2 a.m.) when the circadian pattern of acid secretion is highest. The pain associated with gastric ulcers generally worsens while eating. Epigastric pain can also be caused by pancreatic etiologies; however, the patient's other symptoms are more specific for peptic ulcer disease. The patient does not report feelings of heartburn or regurgitation, so gastroesophageal reflux disease is less likely.

10. D) HBsAg

Hepatitis B surface antigen (HBsAg) is the serologic hallmark of hepatitis B virus infection; it can be detected in high levels during acute or chronic infection. Hepatitis B core antibody (anti-HBc) appears at onset and can be detected through the course of hepatitis B virus infection. Hepatitis B core antigen (HBcAg) is an intracellular antigen expressed in infected hepatocytes and is usually not detectable. Hepatitis V surface antibody (Anti-HBs) persists for life in most patients, conferring lifelong immunity from reinfection. Immunity after vaccination is indicated by the presence of anti-HBs.

11. B) Upper endoscopy

The patient is presenting with signs and symptoms of peptic ulcer disease (e.g., abdominal pain/discomfort, dyspepsia). Pain that worsens with eating is suggestive of a gastric ulcer. The most accurate diagnostic test for peptic ulcer disease is an endoscopy (sensitivity is about 90%). Additional imaging studies such as CT scan and ultrasound can be used during the initial evaluation; however, they are less sensitive for peptic ulcer disease. Urea breath test is used to exclude *Helicobacter pylori* infection but is not diagnostic for peptic ulcer disease.

12. A) HBeAg

Hepatitis B e antigen (HBeAg) represents hepatitis B virus replication and infectivity; its presence denotes high levels of hepatitis B virus DNA in serum and high rates of transmission. IgM antibody to hepatitis B core antigen (IgM anti-HBc) indicates acute infection with HBV. Hepatitis B surface antigen (HBsAg) is the serologic hallmark of hepatitis B virus infection; it can be detected in high levels during acute or chronic infection. Anti-HBs persists for life in most patients, conferring lifelong immunity from reinfection. Immunity after vaccination is indicated by the presence of anti-HBs.

13. C) Gamma-glutamyl transpeptidase (GGT)

Isolated elevation of alkaline phosphatase requires the confirmation that it is of hepatic origin since it can also come from other sources, such as bone and placenta. A GGT or serum 5'-nucleotidase level should be obtained to confirm that the elevation of alkaline phosphatase is secondary to the liver. These tests, along with liver enzymes, AST, ALT, and lactate dehydrogenase, are elevated in liver disorders but are not increased in bone disorders.

14. B) Immune due to hepatitis B vaccination

Hepatitis B surface antigen is the hallmark of hepatitis B virus (HBV) infection; it can be detected in high levels during acute or chronic infection. Hepatitis B core antibody (anti-HBc) appears at onset of symptoms and persists for life, suggesting previous or ongoing infection with HBV. Since this patient is negative for both HBsAg and anti-HBc, acute or chronic infection is unlikely. The presence of anti-HBs suggests recovery and immunity from HBV infection. Immunity after successful vaccination is indicated by the presence of anti-HBs.

15. D) Pain control with oral analgesics and a liquid diet

Acute diverticulitis should be suspected in patients with LLQ abdominal pain, abdominal tenderness, and leukocytosis. The diagnosis is confirmed based on an abdominal CT scan with contrast. Most uncomplicated cases can be treated outpatient; inpatient treatment is indicated for those with complications (e.g., sepsis, perforation, older age, significant comorbidities). Initial outpatient treatment consists of pain control with oral analgesics and a liquid diet. Patients should be reassessed until resolution of symptoms. Oral antibiotics are often not indicated initially. Inpatient treatment often requires intravenous antibiotics and further management of complications.

16. B) Crohn's disease

The hallmark symptoms of Crohn's disease include crampy abdominal pain, chronic intermittent diarrhea, fatigue, and weight loss. Crohn's disease and ulcerative colitis are subtypes of inflammatory bowel disease. Findings specific to Crohn's disease are transmural inflammation and involvement of any portion of the gastrointestinal tract, whereas ulcerative colitis affects only the colon. Endoscopic findings of Crohn's disease include cobblestone mucosal appearance, skip areas, pseudopolyps, granulomas, esophageal/duodenal ulceration, and gastric inflammation. Patients with irritable bowel syndrome do not have mucosal inflammation on ileocolonscopy. Gastritis refers to inflammation of the lining of the stomach.

17. A patient with irritable bowel syndrome (IBS) presents with intermittent abdominal bloating and mild discomfort despite exclusion of gas-producing foods. Which of the following initial therapies can be recommended next?
    A. Polyethylene glycol
    B. Bile acid sequestrant
    C. Probiotics
    D. Low FODMAP diet

18. A patient with irritable bowel syndrome (IBS) reports increased flatulence and discomfort despite dietary modifications. When asked about their 24-hour diet recall, the patient reports eating eggs and sausage with herbal tea for breakfast, a turkey sandwich with cole-slaw for lunch, and baked chicken with carrots and rice for dinner, with ice cream for dessert. The patient needs further education about the exclusion of which foods?
    A. Coleslaw, ice cream
    B. Eggs, chicken
    C. Turkey, rice
    D. Carrots, herbal tea

19. Ulcerative colitis differs from Crohn's disease in that it:
    A. Can involve any portion of the gastrointestinal tract
    B. Is characterized by transmural inflammation
    C. Affects only the colon and rectum
    D. Presents with diarrhea and abdominal pain

20. Which of the following best describes Cullen's sign?
    A. Cessation of inspiration upon deep palpation of the right upper quadrant of the abdomen
    B. Bruising around the periumbilical area of the abdomen
    C. Deep palpation of the left lower quadrant of the abdomen that causes pain to radiate to the right lower quadrant
    D. Blue–black discoloration that is located on the right flank of the trunk

21. Which of the following is the screening test for hepatitis C virus (HCV)?
    A. Anti-HCV
    B. HBsAg
    C. Anti-HAV
    D. HCV RNA polymerase chain reaction (PCR)

22. Which of the following suggests gallbladder inflammation?
    A. Rovsing's maneuver
    B. Rebound tenderness
    C. Murphy's maneuver
    D. McMurray's maneuver

23. A 45-year-old female patient complains of inter-mittent, burning epigastric pain over the past few months. It is worse at night, especially after a heavy or spicy meal. She goes to sleep about 2 hours after eating. The pain is not, or is only partially, relieved by antacids. The patient is not a smoker and denies radiation of pain to neck, arms, or jaw; diaphoresis; and dyspnea. What is the best next step?
    A. Order a 12-lead EKG
    B. Prescribe a proton pump inhibitor
    C. Instruct patient to stop eating at least 4 hours before bedtime and avoid spicy or heavy meals at night
    D. Schedule a fasting lipid profile, including cho-lesterol, low-density lipoprotein, high-density lipoprotein, and triglycerides

24. A 60-year-old male patient reports a poor appetite and abdominal pain. He states that the middle of his stomach around the umbilicus hurts and that the pain then moved to the right lower side of his abdo-men. Temperature is 100.8°F, pulse is 90 beats/min, respiratory rate is 20 breaths/min, and blood pressure is 110/64 mmHg. During the abdominal exam, the patient has right lower quadrant abdominal tenderness without rebound. Which of the following is the most helpful clue when considering differential diagnoses?
    A. The location of the pain
    B. The patient's vital signs
    C. The patient's poor appetite
    D. The age of the patient

(See answers next page.)

17. D) Low FODMAP diet

Patients with mild and intermittent symptoms should be treated with nonpharmacologic therapies for initial management. Lifestyle and dietary modifications should be started first, such as exclusion of gas-producing foods and a diet low in fermentable oligo-, di-, and monosaccharides and polyols (FODMAPS). Patients may also benefit from lactose and/or gluten avoidance, as well as consumption of soluble fiber (e.g., psyllium) and physical activity. Patients with moderate to severe symptoms can be transitioned to pharmacologic agents. For patients with IBS-related constipation who have failed a trial with soluble fiber, polyethylene glycol can be started. For patients with IBS-related diarrhea, antidiarrheals (e.g., loperamide) are indicated initially with bile acid sequestrants as second-line therapy. Probiotics are not recommended in patients with IBS.

18. A) Coleslaw, ice cream

Patients with IBS should avoid foods that increase flatulence. These include wheat germ, pretzels, bagels, certain dairy products (e.g., milk, ice cream, cheese), some vegetables (e.g., cabbage, Brussels sprouts, cauliflower, broccoli, onions), certain fruits (e.g., prunes, apples, pears, raisins, cherries), legumes (e.g., beans, peas, baked beans, soybeans), fatty and fried foods, high-fructose corn syrup, carbonated beverages, alcohol, caffeine, and artificial sweeteners. This patient should be advised to avoid some of their recent food choices, including the ice cream and the coleslaw (which contains cabbage). Although regular tea, which contains caffeine, could be a concern, most herbal teas are free of caffeine.

19. C) Affects only the colon and rectum

Ulcerative colitis and Crohn's disease are subtypes of inflammatory bowel disease. Ulcerative colitis is an inflammatory condition characterized by diffuse mucosal inflammation of the colon. Crohn's disease is characterized by transmural inflammation and may involve any portion of the gastrointestinal tract (oral cavity to perianal area). Both Crohn's disease and ulcerative colitis can cause crampy abdominal pain and diarrhea.

20. B) Bruising around the periumbilical area of the abdomen

Cullen's sign is bruising around the periumbilical area of the abdomen that is associated with pancreatitis. The color can range from blue–black to purple, and then the color changes as the bruise resolves. It is caused by retroperitoneal bleeding, when the blood migrates to the subcutaneous tissue in the periumbilical area (Cullen's sign) or flank (Grey-Turner sign). It may also be present in other conditions such as splenic rupture, ruptured aortic aneurysm, rectus sheath hematoma, perforated duodenal ulcer, ruptured ectopic pregnancy, and hepatocellular cancer. It occurs in only 3% of patients with acute pancreatitis but suggests the presence of retroperitoneal bleeding in the setting of pancreatic necrosis.

21. A) Anti-HCV

The screening test for hepatitis C is the anti-HCV. The next step is to order the HCV RNA. The screening test for hepatitis B is the hepatitis B surface antigen (HBsAg). The screening test for hepatitis A is the hepatitis A antibody (anti-HAV).

22. C) Murphy's maneuver

Gallbladder inflammation is also known as cholecystitis. If Murphy's maneuver is performed with the patient supine, the palpating hand is placed just below the right costal margin midclavicular area. The patient is instructed to exhale. Then the patient is instructed to inhale and the clinician presses down, palpating the hand over the liver. The result is positive if the patient stops midinhalation due to the pain.

23. C) Instruct patient to stop eating at least 4 hours before bedtime and avoid spicy or heavy meals at night

Lifestyle changes are the first-line treatment for gastroesophageal reflux disease. Patients should stop eating (especially heavy or spicy meals) at least 4 hours before bedtime and avoid caffeine and mint. The patient does not need laboratory testing or a 12-lead EKG due to the negative symptoms of radiating pain, diaphoresis, and dyspnea. Prescribing a proton-pump inhibitor may be indicated, but nonpharmacologic modifications should be trialed first before initiating pharmacologic therapy.

24. A) The location of the pain

When considering differential diagnoses for abdominal conditions, it is important to be mindful of the location of the reported pain. Appendicitis presents with classic symptoms of right lower quadrant pain, which is initially periumbilical in nature and then migrates to the right lower quadrant as the inflammation progresses. While a patient with appendicitis may present with a fever, anorexia, nausea, and vomiting, these are more nonspecific findings that may occur with other abdominal processes. Appendicitis is most common in the second and third decades of life (highest incidence ages 10 to 19 years), so the age of this patient is not suggestive of acute appendicitis.

25. The best test of cure after treating a patient with *Helicobacter pylori* infection is:
   A. Complete blood count with white blood cell differential
   B. Stool guaiac test
   C. *H. pylori* IgM and IgG serology
   D. Urea breath test

26. Which of the following physical exam findings suggests the presence of choledocholithiasis in a patient with acute pancreatitis?
   A. Guarding and abdominal rigidity
   B. Positive Cullen's sign
   C. Positive Grey Turner's sign
   D. Scleral icterus and jaundice

27. A patient with a history of smoking presents for routine follow-up 8 weeks after resolution of acute symptoms involving left lower quadrant abdominal pain, along with nausea, vomiting, constipation, and abdominal tenderness. Previously, the patient reported a diet low in fiber and high in dietary fat. After lifestyle changes and medical management, the patient reports resolution of symptoms. Which of the following is indicated for the patient at this time?
   A. Complete blood count (CBC)
   B. Abdominal CT scan with oral and intravenous contrast
   C. Colonoscopy
   D. Abdominal x-ray

28. According to the U.S. Preventive Services Task Force (USPSTF), at which age (in years) should screening for colorectal cancer be initiated?
   A. 45
   B. 50
   C. 55
   D. 60

29. Which of the following is indicated in the medical management of gastroesophageal reflux disease (GERD) in patients with erosive esophagitis?
   A. Pantoprazole
   B. Famotidine
   C. Sucralfate
   D. Antacid

30. Which of the following *best* describes McBurney's point?
   A. Mild tenderness at 2.5 to 4 inches from the anterior superior iliac spine
   B. Maximal tenderness at 2.5 to 4 inches from the anterior superior iliac spine
   C. Maximal tenderness at 1.5 to 2 inches from the anterior superior iliac spine
   D. Area free from tenderness at 1.5 to 2 inches from the anterior superior iliac spine

(See answers next page.)

25. D) Urea breath test

The urea breath test is a specific (>95%) and sensitive (>88%) test for detecting active *H. pylori* infection in patients with peptic ulcer disease. *H. pylori* serology is not as sensitive or specific as the urea breath test; it can remain positive even if there is no infection. Stool antigen assay can be used to establish the initial diagnosis of *H. pylori* and confirm eradication, but a stool guaiac test determines the presence of blood in the stool. A complete blood count may indicate leukocytosis in a patient with *H. pylori* infection but is not a specific test for identification of a specific infection.

26. D) Scleral icterus and jaundice

Patients with acute pancreatitis may present with scleral icterus due to obstructive jaundice secondary to choledocholithiasis or edema of the head of the pancreas. Patients with concern for a perforation may present with sudden-onset abdominal pain with guarding, rigidity, and rebound tenderness concerning for peritonitis. Cullen's sign (ecchymotic discoloration in the periumbilical region) and Grey Turner's sign (ecchymosis along the flank) may be noted in some patients with acute pancreatitis, suggesting the presence of retroperitoneal bleeding in the setting of pancreatic necrosis.

27. C) Colonoscopy

The patient is presenting with risk factors and a clinical presentation suggestive of diverticular disease. A diet high in total fat and low in dietary fiber is associated with an increased risk, as is a history of smoking. Left-sided abdominal pain is present in 85% of patients; associated symptoms include nausea, vomiting, constipation, and diarrhea. After resolution of symptoms (in about 6 to 8 weeks), a colonoscopy should be performed to assess the extent of the patient's diverticular disease and exclude colon cancer (unless it has already been performed within the previous year). Abdominal imaging is required to establish the diagnosis and may be required in patients with clinical deterioration and in those who fail to improve after medical therapy. An abdominal CT scan can look for new complications that may require further intervention in patients with disease progression. A CT is preferred over abdominal radiographs, which indicate nonspecific abnormalities in 30% to 50% of patients with acute diverticulitis. A CBC is not indicated if the patient has resolution of symptoms; it may indicate an improvement in leukocytosis but is not specific or sensitive to acute diverticulitis.

28. A) 45

According to the USPSTF, it is recommended that adults age 45 to 75 years be screened for colorectal cancer.

29. A) Pantoprazole

In patients with erosive esophagitis, proton pump inhibitors (PPIs) are recommended for treatment in addition to lifestyle and dietary modifications. PPIs have stronger acid suppression, allowing faster control and more effective relief of symptoms compared with histamine 2 receptor antagonists (H2RAs) (e.g., famotidine). H2RAs have limited efficacy in patients with erosive esophagitis. Antacids (e.g., Mylanta) and surface agents and alginates (e.g., sucralfate) are indicated for patients with mild to intermittent symptoms. Antacids do not prevent GERD but are indicated for relief of mild symptoms. Sucralfate adheres to the mucosal surface and promotes healing; however, it has limited efficacy when compared with PPIs.

30. C) Maximal tenderness at 1.5 to 2 inches from the anterior superior iliac spine

McBurney's point is characterized as maximal tenderness at 1.5 to 2 inches from the anterior superior iliac spine on a straight line to the umbilicus (in the right lower quadrant). Tenderness or pain suggests acute appendicitis.

ACUTE KIDNEY INJURY (ACUTE RENAL FAILURE)

Patient presents with sudden onset of oliguria, edema, and weight gain (fluid retention) and complains of lethargy, nausea, and loss of appetite. The condition is characterized by rapid decrease in renal function and elevated serum creatinine. During early stages, serum creatinine and the estimated glomerular filtration rate (eGFR) may not accurately reflect true renal function. Most cases of acute kidney injury (AKI; acute decline of GFR) are usually reversible when the offending substance is stopped. Some of the most common causes of drug-induced AKI are aminoglycosides, contrast agents, nonsteroidal anti-inflammatory drugs (NSAIDs), angiotensin-converting enzyme (ACE) inhibitors, and protease inhibitors.

ACUTE PYELONEPHRITIS

Patient presents with acute onset of high fever, chills, nausea/vomiting, dysuria, frequent urination, and unilateral flank pain. The flank pain is described as a deep ache. May complain of nausea (with/without vomiting) and may have a recent history of urinary tract infection (UTI). Indications for hospitalization include inability to maintain oral hydration, persistently high fever (>101.0°F/>38.4°C), toxic appearance, immune compromise, or suspicion of sepsis or noncompliance to treatment.

BLADDER CANCER

Elderly patient (median age at diagnosis is 69 years in males and 71 years in females) who smokes presents with painless hematuria. The hematuria can be microscopic or gross (pink- to reddish-color urine). The hematuria may only appear at the end of voiding. May have irritative voiding symptoms (dysuria, frequent urination, nocturia) that are not related to a UTI. Patients who have advanced disease with metastases may complain of lower abdominal or pelvic pain, perineal pain, low-back pain, or bone pain. Order a urinalysis (UA), urine culture and sensitivity (C&S), and urine for cytology.

RHABDOMYOLYSIS

Patient complains of an acute onset of muscle pain (not related to physical exertion), muscle weakness, and dark urine (myoglobinuria) (classic triad). Muscle tenderness and swelling may be seen, which rules out compartment syndrome. Myoglobins released from damaged muscle result in reddish-brown or tea-colored urine. Damage to the kidneys can result in AKI, a common complication of rhabdomyolysis. Serum creatine kinase levels are markedly elevated (five times normal value or higher). Blood chemistry abnormalities, elevated aldolase, lactate dehydrogenase, electrolyte abnormalities, and disseminated intravascular coagulation (DIC) can complicate the condition. Ask patient if they have a history of severe exercise, crush injury, high fever, or high-dose statin use. Refer to ED.

KIDNEYS

The kidneys are located in the retroperitoneal area. The right kidney is lower than the left kidney because of displacement by the liver. The basic functional units of the kidney are the nephrons, which contain the glomeruli. The kidneys regulate the body's electrolytes and fluids, which affects blood pressure. Water is reabsorbed back into the body by the action of antidiuretic hormone and aldosterone. The kidneys excrete water-soluble waste products of metabolism (e.g., creatinine, urea, uric acid) into the urine. They secrete several hormones such as erythropoietin (red blood cell [RBC] production), renin and bradykinin (blood pressure), prostaglandins (renal perfusion), and calcitriol/vitamin D_3 (bone). The average daily urine output is 1,500 mL. *Oliguria* is defined as a urinary output of <400 to 500 mL/day (adults).

Right kidney sits lower than left kidney because of displacement by the liver.

SERUM CREATININE

Creatinine is the product of creatine metabolism in skeletal muscle; it also is derived from dietary meat intake. Normal creatinine values differ between males and females due to differences in muscle mass; normal value for males is 0.7 to 1.3 mg/dL, and normal value for females is 0.6 to 1.1 mg/dL. When renal function decreases, the creatinine level often increases. Serum creatinine may be falsely decreased in people with low muscle volume (older adults). Elevated values are seen with kidney damage or renal failure, use of nephrotoxic drugs, and other factors. Serum creatinine levels vary inversely with the glomerular filtration rate (GFR); they increase as the GFR falls.

CREATININE CLEARANCE (24-HOUR URINE)

This test is ordered to evaluate patients with proteinuria, albuminuria, and microalbuminuria. It is a more sensitive test than serum creatinine alone because it reflects the renal function within a 24-hour period. Creatinine clearance is relatively constant and is not affected by fluid status, diet, or exercise. Creatinine clearance is doubled for every 50% reduction of the GFR. Ideally, exercise should be avoided immediately prior to and during the period of specimen collection.

ESTIMATED GLOMERULAR FILTRATION RATE

The eGFR is the best test to measure kidney function. It is used to determine chronic kidney disease (CKD) stages (Table 11.1). A normal eGFR result is >90 mL/min; a result of <60 mL/min for at least 3 months indicates CKD. The eGFR is calculated using serum creatinine, age, and sex. Two estimation equations, the Modification of Diet in Renal Disease and the 2009 Chronic Kidney Disease Epidemiology Collaboration (CKD-EPI), were used to calculate the eGFR, but the 2021 CKD-EPI creatinine equation was developed without a coefficient for race and is now the recommended equation to estimate the GFR.

The GFR is the amount of fluid filtered by the glomerulus within a certain unit of time. The more damaged the kidneys, the lower the eGFR. The GFR is affected by age (it decreases with age), sex (males tend to have more muscle mass), and body size. Some patients with underlying kidney disease may have a normal eGFR, and eGFR is less reliable in pregnancy, muscle wasting, elderly patients, and lower-extremity amputee patients.

EXAM TIPS

- eGFR is considered the best overall measure of renal function in primary care.
- Serum creatinine is a better measure of renal function than blood urea nitrogen (BUN) or BUN to creatinine (BUN:Cr) ratio.

Table 11.1 Chronic Kidney Disease Stages

Stage	GFR	Type of Kidney Damage
Stage 1	≥90 mL/min	Kidney damage with normal or high kidney function
Stage 2	60 to 89 mL/min	Mild loss of kidney function
Stage 3a	45 to 59 mL/min	Mild-to-moderate loss of kidney function
Stage 3b	30 to 44 mL/min	Moderate-to-severe loss of kidney function
Stage 4	15 to 29 mL/min	Severe loss of kidney function
Stage 5	<15 mL/min	Kidney failure

GFR, glomerular filtration rate.

BLOOD UREA NITROGEN

The liver breaks down amino acids into ammonia and then converts it into urea. BUN is a measure of the kidneys' ability to excrete urea (waste product of protein metabolism). If the kidneys are damaged or the renal blood flow is decreased, the urea level becomes elevated. BUN is not as sensitive as serum creatinine or the eGFR; BUN can change independently of the GFR. Urea production is not at a constant rate and may increase with a high-protein diet and enhanced tissue breakdown due to hemorrhage, trauma, or glucocorticoid therapy. A low-protein diet or liver disease can lower BUN without affecting the GFR. Among patients with heart failure, a lower GFR with higher BUN is associated with higher mortality. Among critically ill patients in the ICU, elevation of BUN is independently associated with mortality.

BUN-TO-CREATININE RATIO

A decrease in the blood flow of the kidneys will increase the BUN:Cr ratio. It is used to help evaluate dehydration, hypovolemia, and acute kidney failure. This ratio is useful for classifying the type of failure (renal, infrarenal, or postrenal). A rise in BUN:Cr ratio is suggestive of decreased kidney perfusion (prerenal disease).

URINALYSIS (WITH MICROSCOPIC EXAM)

A complete UA consists of three components (gross evaluation, dipstick analysis, and microscopic exam of urine sediment). It should be performed in a patient with acute or chronic reduction in GFR or unexplained albuminuria or in a patient with suspected kidney disease.

Epithelial Cells

- Large amounts of squamous epithelial cells in a urine sample indicate contamination.
- A few epithelial cells are considered normal. (Squamous epithelial cells are associated with the external urethra and transitional epithelial cells with the bladder.)

White Blood Cells (Leukocytes)

- Normal white blood cells (WBCs) in urine: ≤2 to 5 WBCs/hpf (high-power field)
- Leukocyte esterase: Marker for the presence of WBCs
- Prescence of neutrophils: Commonly associated with bacteria
- Leukocytes in urine (pyuria): Almost always present in males with acute cystitis

Red Blood Cells

- Few RBCs (<3 cells) is considered normal.
- Microscopic hematuria refers to RBCs that are visible only by microscopy.
- Gross hematuria means you can see blood in the urine. Color ranges from pink or red to cola or brown. The bleeding may come from the urethra (urethritis), bladder (cystitis, bladder cancer), or kidneys (kidney stones, pyelonephritis, polycystic kidneys, cancer).
- Can be contaminated by menses, vaginal discharge, semen, hemorrhoids, rectal bleeding.

Protein

- Suggests chronic kidney damage if persistent. Evaluate the serum creatinine and eGFR and send midstream urine for microscopic exam.
- Proteinuria without abnormalities in the urinary sediment and normal kidney function is referred to as *isolated proteinuria*.
- Transient proteinuria is common, especially in patients 18 years or younger and among young adults. Diagnosed if a repeat test is no longer positive for proteinuria.
- Benign causes of proteinuria include fever, intense physical activity, acute illness, dehydration, and emotional stress.
- May be present in acute pyelonephritis (resolves after treatment); recheck urine after treatment.
- Urine dipsticks are sensitive to albumin.
- False-positive results with urinary dipstick testing may be seen with alkaline urine (pH >7.5), if dipstick is immersed too long, highly concentrated urine, gross hematuria, presence of semen, or vaginal secretions.
- To quantify proteinuria, order 24-hour urine for protein-to-creatinine ratio (UPr/Cr).

Nitrites

- Increase due to breakdown of urea into nitrite by bacteria
- Positive result is highly indicative of a UTI.

Casts

- Casts are shaped like cylinders because they are formed in the renal tubules.
- Hyaline casts are nonspecific; can be seen in small volumes in concentrated urine or with diuretic therapy.
- WBC casts may be seen with infections (pyelonephritis) or inflammation (interstitial nephritis).
- RBC casts are caused by microscopic bleeding in the glomeruli; suspect glomerulonephritis (accompanied by edema, weight gain, dark cola-colored urine, or hypertension).

pH

Reference range is 4.5 to 8.0. Useful in the evaluation of kidney stones and infections. Citrus and low-carbohydrate diet are associated with lower acidity, and high-protein diet is associated with higher acidity.

URINE FOR CULTURE AND SENSITIVITY

- Confirms presence of bacteriuria and identifies antibiotic susceptibility on the causative organism
- Obtained by clean-catch voided urine specimen in patients with suspected UTI
- Positive culture is $\geq 10^5$ colony-forming units (CFU)/mL of one dominant bacteria.
- If multiple bacteria are present, may be a contaminated sample.
- Lower values may still be indicative of bacteriuria.

- Understand how to interpret UA results in a patient with a UTI.
- WBC casts with proteinuria and hematuria are associated with pyelonephritis.

ACUTE KIDNEY INJURY

Previously called *acute renal failure*. It is abrupt reduction in GFR and decline in kidney function, causing retention of waste products and dysregulation of volume status and electrolytes. In the majority of cases, prerenal causes and acute tubular necrosis (ATN) are the most common cause. It typically lasts about 7 to 21 days. Some patients recover in a few days, and some require dialysis for several months. Patients with acute kidney injury should be sent to the ED for assessment.

- The Kidney Disease: Improving Global Outcomes (KDIGO) organization has a staging system for AKI. Their guidelines define AKI as:
  - Increase in serum creatinine by ≥ 0.3 mg/dL within 48 hours
  - Increase in serum creatinine ≥ 1.5 mg/dL from baseline (known or presumed in prior 7 days)
- Urine volume <0.5 mL/kg/hr for 6 hours:
  - Prerenal: Usually due to hypoperfusion of the kidneys. Etiologies are listed in Table 11.2.
  - Intrinsic: Caused by damage to the tissues of the kidney or renal tubule, involving pathology of the vessels, glomeruli, or tubules-interstitial. ATN causes 90% of cases, and, generally it is often a reversible injury. See Table 11.2 for etiologies and Box 11.1 for drugs that exert a toxic effect on the kidneys.
  - Postrenal: Usually due to the obstruction of the flow of urine in the renal tubular system to the urethra. To produce AKI, the urethral obstruction is often bilateral or occurs in a patient with only one functioning kidney. Renal parenchyma is not affected. Etiologies are listed in Table 11.2.

General Management of Acute Kidney Injury

- Often involves referral to the ED
- Management also should include referral to a nephrologist

Box 11.1 Nephrotoxic Drugs

- Acyclovir
- Allopurinol (Zyloprim)
- Aminoglycosides (vancomycin)
- Antiretrovirals (adefovir, cidofovir, tenofovir, indinavir)
- Beta-lactams (penicillins, cephalosporins)
- Chemotherapeutics
- Contrast dyes
- Diuretics (thiazides, loop, triamterene)
- Drugs of abuse (cocaine, heroin, ketamine, amphetamines)
- Lithium
- NSAIDs and analgesics (ibuprofen)
- Proton pump inhibitors (lansoprazole, omeprazole, pantoprazole)
- Quinolones (ciprofloxacin)
- Sulfonamides

NSAID, nonsteroidal anti-inflammatory drug.

Table 11.2 Acute Kidney Injury: Causes

Condition	Causes
	Prerenal Causes
Hypovolemia	Blood loss, vomiting, diarrhea, diuretics
Decreased cardiac output	Heart failure, MI, pulmonary edema, pulmonary emboli, tamponade, shock
Third space sequestration	Sepsis, anaphylaxis, pancreatitis, hypoalbuminemic states
Medications that limit GFR	ACE-I, ARB, NSAID
	Postrenal Causes
Bladder obstruction	BPH, prostate cancer, bladder cancer, blood clot
Urethral/renal obstruction	Stones, strictures, blood clots, cancer
Neurogenic bladder	Spinal cord injury, diabetes, drugs
	Intrinsic Causes
Acute tubular necrosis	Ischemia, prolonged hypoperfusion, sepsis, hemorrhage, nephrotoxins
Nephrotoxins	Aminoglycosides, contrast media, heavy metals, IV immunoglobulins
Acute interstitial nephritis related to drugs	NSAIDs, diuretics, penicillins, cephalosporins, sulfa drugs, allopurinol, anticoagulants
Glomerular disease	Poststreptococcal infection (more common in children), IgA nephropathy, others
Thrombosis	Renal artery, renal vein

ACEI, angiotensin-converting enzyme inhibitor; ARB, angiotensin receptor blocker; BPH, benign prostatic hyperplasia; GFR, glomerular filtration rate; IV, intravenous; MI, myocardial infarction; NSAID, nonsteroidal anti-inflammatory drug.

- Emergency dialysis should be performed in patients with hypervolemia with pulmonary edema, severe hyperkalemia, life-threatening uremic symptoms, exposure to certain toxins.
- Initial management includes eliminate any additional insults (e.g., nephrotoxic agents), treat hypovolemic (if present), correct electrolyte imbalances and acidosis, and provide for nutrition management (e.g., dietary restrictions on potassium, phosphorous, fluid intake).

ACUTE PYELONEPHRITIS

Acute bacterial infection of the kidney(s) is most commonly due to gram-negative Enterobacteriaceae such as *Escherichia coli* (75%–95%), *Proteus*, and *Klebsiella*. Outpatient treatment is only for compliant, healthy patients with milder infections that are uncomplicated (immunocompetent adult female with normal urinary/renal systems without comorbidities). Complicated pyelonephritis present if underlying renal disease, male sex, kidney stone, anatomic urinary tract abnormality, or immunosuppression; refer for hospitalization.

Classic Case

Adult patient presents with acute onset of high fever, chills, anorexia, nausea/vomiting, and one-sided flank pain. Some patients may also have symptoms of cystitis, such as dysuria, frequency, and urgency.

Physical Exam and Diagnostic Tests

- Temperature: ≥100.4°F (38.0°C)
- Costovertebral angle tenderness
- UA: Presence of leukocytes, hematuria, +/ nitrites, and mild proteinuria

- Urinary casts (tubular-shaped structures): WBC casts (seen in microscopic exam of urine sediment)
- Urine C&S: Presence of 10^5 CFU/mL of one organism
- Complete blood count (CBC): Leukocytosis (WBC >11,000/mcL), neutrophilia (>80%) with shift to the left (presence of bands [immature neutrophils] suggesting an infection)
- Chemistry profile: Serum creatinine, others

Treatment Plan

May treat mild uncomplicated cases as outpatients with close follow-up. For moderate-to-severe cases or patient with coexisting conditions that compromise immune system, hospitalization is often required for rehydration and management of complications or additional symptoms. Empiric therapy depends on severity of illness:

- Outpatients without risk for resistance: Oral fluoroquinolone (e.g., levofloxacin or ciprofloxacin) for 5 to 7 days
- Outpatients with risk for resistance: Ertapenem or fluoroquinolone

Close follow-up needed for 12 to 24 hours. Complications include bacteremia, sepsis, multiple organ dysfunction, shock, and/or acute renal failure. Pregnant patients, children/elderly, male patients, kidney stones, anatomic abnormalities, diabetes, and immunocompromise should be referred to a specialist for treatment.

EXAM TIP

Recognize classic case of acute simple cystitis versus acute pyelonephritis; be able to distinguish between the two.

ASYMPTOMATIC BACTERIURIA

Asymptomatic bacteriuria (ASB) is defined as the presence of one or more species of bacteria growing in the urine ($\geq 10^5$ CFU/mL) in the absence of UTI symptoms.

- Prevalence among healthy females increases with age from 1% to >20% after 80 years; correlates with sexual activity
- Prevalence among females with diabetes ranges from 8% to 14%.
- Prevalence among males older than 75 years ranges from 6% to 15%

Treatment

Indications for screening and antibiotic therapy for ASB include pregnancy, patients undergoing urologic intervention, and renal transplant recipients. Not recommended to screen or treat in older patients, patients with diabetes mellitus, patients with indwelling bladder catheter, or patients undergoing non-urologic surgery.

CHRONIC KIDNEY DISEASE

CKD is the presence of kidney damage (as defined by structural or functional abnormalities) or decreased GFR (<60 mL/min/1.73 m^2) for 3 or more months, regardless of cause. Staging is based on the GFR (see Table 11.1). More frequent in females than in males. Most often caused by poorly controlled diabetes mellitus and hypertension.

Classic Case

Patient presents with symptoms secondary to diminished kidney function, including edema secondary to fluid overload or hypertension. Elevated serum creatinine, reduced GFR, and abnormal UA. Patient reports nonspecific symptoms such as fatigue, weakness, anorexia, vomiting, and pruritis. Patient in advanced stage may present with encephalopathy and seizures.

Physical Exam

- Signs of volume overload such as weight gain, noticeable edema in extremities, shortness of breath
- Signs of volume depletion such as fatigue, postural dizziness, tachycardia, decreased skin turgor
- Rashes, skin lesions, or skin thickening
- Abnormal bruit or distal pulses in patients with renal artery stenosis
- Palpable, enlarged kidneys (suggest polycystic kidney disease)
- Peripheral neuropathy may be associated with diabetic microvascular disease

Labs

- Basic metabolic panel: Serum creatinine and BUN often are increased
- Urine studies: May show proteinuria (or albuminuria) and/or abnormal RBCs or WBCs on urine microscopy
- Quantification of urine protein and albumin: By random protein-to-creatinine ratio and albumin-to-creatinine ratio

- Other common lab abnormalities: Anemia, hyperphosphatemia, hyperkalemia, metabolic acidosis, hypocalcemia, and elevated parathyroid hormone. Degree of abnormalities depends on severity of CKD and if there is an acute-on-chronic kidney injury.
- CBC: With white cell differential
- Kidney ultrasound: To assess for abnormalities in the kidney, which may warrant further evaluation
- Vascular duplex ultrasound: To evaluate for renal artery stenosis

Treatment

- Patients may or may not require dialysis. It is necessary to establish duration and trajectory of disease.
- Nephrology consult may be necessary for patients with eGFR <30 mL/min/1.73 m^2, persistent protein-to-creatine ratio >500 mg/g, and albumin-to-creatine ratio >300 mg/g; abnormal urine microscopy; history of systemic autoimmune disease or multiple myeloma; or pregnancy.
- Education on nutritional support varies depending on the eGFR, type of kidney disease, and presence of comorbidities. For most patients, optimal diet is similar to the Dietary Approaches to Stop Hypertension (DASH) diet.

HEMATURIA

There are two types of hematuria: microscopic and gross. It can be either transient or persistent. The blood may come from the urethra (urethritis), bladder (cystitis, bladder cancer), prostate (prostatitis), or kidneys (pyelonephritis, polycystic kidneys, cancer). Microscopic hematuria is revealed by a microscopic UA (presence of ≥ 3 RBCs/hpf).

- If infection is suspected (e.g., urethritis, cystitis, pyelonephritis), the UA will often indicate WBCs (with or without nitrites). Often accompanied by symptoms (e.g., dysuria, frequency, urgency, nocturia). Order UA with urine C&S. The infection should be treated, and the UA should be repeated about 6 weeks after completion of antibiotic therapy to ensure resolution of hematuria.
- Suspect gross (or visible) hematuria if color of urine is pink, red, or brown or blood clots are present. If there are visible blood clots in the urine, imaging should be performed, and the patient should be evaluated for cystoscopy. Glomerular bleeding may be suggested if there is gross hematuria without visible blood clots. Refer to a nephrologist.
- New onset of dark reddish-brown urine, edema, proteinuria, fatigue, and decreased urine output after a recent strep throat, scarlet fever, or impetigo infection raises the possibility of poststreptococcal glomerulonephritis, an immune reaction from the infection. It can occur 10 days following the infection and up to 3 weeks after. It is a rare complication that is more common in children.
- If malignancy is suspected, send urine for cytology, and refer to a nephrologist. Risk factors for urothelial or renal malignancy are age older than 50 years, male, smoker, and gross hematuria.

- In a female with a history of recent sexual activity or exercise, stop exercise and repeat UA in 4 to 6 weeks; with menses, repeat UA about 1 week after last day of menses; repeat the UA with microscopic exam.
- Urine may turn a red or orange color due to some medications (e.g., rifampin, phenytoin) and ingestion of certain foods (e.g., beets, rhubarb, senna, food dyes).

NEPHROLITHIASIS (RENAL CALCULI)

The majority of kidney stones are made up of calcium oxalate (70%–80%) and calcium phosphate (15%). Other types of stones include struvite (1%), uric acid (8%), and cystine (1%–2%). More common in males. Prevalence increases with age. Location and size of the stone determine the pain, which can range from a mild ache to severe pain. For example, stones located in the upper urethra or renal pelvis cause flank pain and tenderness, whereas stones on the lower urethra cause pain that radiates to the testicle or the labia of the vagina. Both can cause abdominal pain.

Risk Factors (Calcium Stones)

- Urinary: Lower volume, higher calcium, higher oxalate, lower citrate, higher pH
- Anatomic: Medullary sponge kidney, horseshoe kidney
- Diet: High dietary intake of calcium, vitamin C, oxalate foods, sodium, protein, lower fluid intake, intake of foods high in sucrose and fructose
- Other medical conditions: Obesity, diabetes, gout, inflammatory bowel disease, malabsorptive bariatric surgery
- Non-modifiable: Positive family history, genetic factors, White race

Classic Case

Adult male with acute onset of severe colicky flank pain (renal colic) on one side that comes in waves. When the pain is most severe, the patient cannot stay still and may walk/pace in the exam room. The pain builds in intensity, then lessens and disappears (until the stone moves again). Painful episodes may last 20 to 60 minutes. For some, the pain can be extreme and associated with nausea and vomiting. Majority have gross or microscopic hematuria. Majority will pass stone within 48 hours. Patient should be asked about history of previous episodes, high-protein diet, gout, gastric bypass, calcium intake, high-dose vitamin C, fluid intake, and intake of certain drugs (see the preceding risk factors).

Labs

- UA will often show hematuria in majority of patients. Hematuria is present in about 95% of patients on day 1 and from 65% to 68% on days 3 and 4.
- CT of the abdomen and pelvis without contrast is the preferred imaging method. If CT is not available or patient is pregnant, an alternative test is ultrasound of the kidneys and bladder.

Treatment

- Management depends on stone size. Most patients can be managed conservatively with pain medication and hydration until the stone passes in the outpatient setting as long as tolerating oral medications and fluids.
- For stones that are ≤5 mm, most will pass the stone spontaneously. Instruct patient to strain urine for several days and bring kidney stone to office (if passed) for stone analysis by laboratory.
- For stones >5 and ≤10 mm in diameter, treatment includes tamsulosin for up to 4 weeks to facilitate stone passage. If tamsulosin is not available, can use another alpha-blocker or calcium channel blocker to facilitate stone passage (relaxes smooth muscles of ureters).
- For pain control, NSAIDs (e.g., indomethacin, ketorolac) and opioids (alone or combined with an NSAID) can be used for pain control in acute renal colic. NSAIDs can also decrease ureteral smooth muscle tone (may help relieve ureteral spasms). Note: NSAIDs can induce AKI in patients with preexisting kidney disease or dehydration.
- Urology consult for stones >10 mm; stones >5 mm in diameter if patients have failed to pass the stone after a 4-week trial of an alpha blocker; patients with a UTI, AKI, anuria, and/or unyielding pain, nausea, or vomiting.
- Refer to ED if high fever (possible urosepsis), extreme pain, acute renal failure, large stone, inability to pass stone, inability to tolerate oral medications and fluids, severe nausea, and vomiting.
- For larger stones, methods used to break the stone and remove it include extracorporeal shock wave lithotripsy (ESWL).

Diet

- Increase fluid intake up to 2 to 3 L/day; if calcium oxalate stones, dietary modifications should be advised.
- Avoid high-oxalate foods such as rhubarb, spinach, okra, nuts, beets, chocolate, tea, and meats.

PROTEINURIA

Proteinuria is defined as the excretion of >150 mg/day of protein. Patients with persistent proteinuria should be evaluated to find the cause. The gold-standard test for measuring protein excretion of the kidneys is the 24-hour urine collection. There are four types of proteinuria: glomerular, tubular, overflow, and postrenal.

- The urine dipstick test cannot detect low levels of albumin excretion, and patients with moderately increased albuminuria (previously known as microalbuminuria) may not be detected unless the urine is concentrated.
- Transient proteinuria: Often, caused by fever, intense physical activity, acute illness, dehydration, and emotional stress.
- Serious causes of proteinuria, which is a sign of damaged kidneys, include diabetic nephropathy, hypertensive nephropathy, polycystic kidney disease, sarcoidosis, lupus, rhabdomyolysis, preeclampsia, and eclampsia.

URINARY TRACT INFECTIONS

Cystitis (urinary bladder inflammation) can be uncomplicated, recurrent, a reinfection, or relapse. The majority of infections are caused by Enterobacteriaceae (E. coli, Klebsiella). Other causal agents are Staphylococcus saprophyticus, enterococci, and Pseudomonas aeruginosa. UTIs in children younger than age 3 and pregnant women are more likely to progress to pyelonephritis.

- Infants: UTIs are common in boys in the first 6 months of life (due to anatomic abnormality).
- Children: UTIs in children need further evaluation. About 2.5% of all children will get a UTI. May indicate vesicoureteral reflux or even possible sexual abuse.
- Females: Highest incidence is during the reproductive-age years.
- Older females: Symptoms can be subtle, but onset of new incontinence can be a sign of a UTI.

Risk Factors
- Female sex
- Pregnancy
- History of a recent UTI or history of recurrent infections
- Diabetes mellitus (or immunocompromised status)
- Failure to void after sex or recent sexual intercourse (i.e., honeymoon bladder)
- Spermicide (nonoxynol-9) use can irritate genital tissue (increases risk of HIV and other STIs)
- Other risk factors include infected renal calculi, low fluid intake, poor hygiene, catheterization

Classic Case
A sexually active female complains of new onset of dysuria, frequency, frequent urge to urinate, and nocturia. May also complain of suprapubic discomfort. Not associated with fever. Urine dipstick will show a moderate-to-large number of leukocytes and will be positive for nitrites.

Labs
- UA dipstick (midstream sample): Leukocyte positive (WBCs ≥10/mcL)
- Nitrites: Negative or positive (indicative of Enterobacteriaceae)
- Hematuria (>5 RBCs): May be observed
- Urine C&S (clean voided sample)
  - Generally unnecessary in females with acute simple cystitis.
  - In UTI infection, 100,000 CFU/mL (or 10^5 CFU/mL) of a single organism or 100,000 CFU/mL of one organism and growth of a second organism ≥50,000 CFU/mL
  - Multiple bacteria likely indicates a contaminated sample (growth of >2 organisms)
  - Bacteriuria (with or without indwelling catheter) indicated by >100,000 CFU/Ml

EXAM TIP
Large numbers of squamous epithelial cells in the urine sample may mean contamination.

Treatment
Uncomplicated UTIs (Acute Simple Cystitis in Healthy Adult Females)
- For most healthy females with suspected acute simple cystitis (dysuria, frequency, nocturia), no additional testing is needed beyond the UA. But if fever >99.9°F,

chills, significant fatigue or malaise, flank pain, or CVA tenderness, rule out acute pyelonephritis.

- First-line medications for patients without risk factors for multidrug-resistant infections include nitrofurantoin (Macrobid) 100 mg BID × 5 days, or trimethoprim–sulfamethoxazole (Bactrim, Septra) 160/800 mg BID × 3 days, or fosfomycin (Monurol) 3 g × 1 dose
- For patients with risk factors for bacterial resistance, medications include nitrofurantoin (Macrobid) BID × 5 days, or fosfomycin (Monurol) 3 g × one dose, or pivmecillinam (400 mg orally TID for 3–5 days).
- Alternatives include ciprofloxacin (Cipro) BID or levofloxacin (Levaquin) daily (age 18 years or older) × 3 days
- The urinary analgesic phenazopyridine (Pyridium) by mouth BID × 2 days PRN (as Uristat, AZO); Pyridium will turn urine an orange-yellow color; will stain contact lenses; avoid if liver or renal disease, glucose-6-phosphate dehydrogenase (G6PD) anemia
- Increase fluid intake to 2 to 3 L/day (except if heart failure); restrict dietary oxalate (e.g., beans, spinach, beets, potato chips, french fries, nuts, tea)

> **NOTE**
> If clinical symptoms persist 48 to 72 hours after initiating antibiotics, order urine C&S. Rule out pyelonephritis. Consider switching to another antibiotic drug class and treat for 7 to 10 days.

Recurrent UTIs in Females
- Three or more UTIs (culture positive) in 1 year or two UTIs within 6 months
- Antibiotic prophylaxis should not be first-line therapy.
- For postcoital UTIs (single dose immediately after intercourse), nitrofurantoin (Macrobid) 100 mg, Bactrim DS one tablet, trimethoprim 100 mg, cephalexin (Keflex) 250 mg
- Increase fluid intake (2–3 L/day) especially before and after sex, avoid spermicide (nonoxynol 9)
- If sulfa allergy, cephalexin (Keflex), ciprofloxacin (if >18 years)
- In postmenopausal women, topical vaginal estrogen (Estriol cream), increase fluids (1.5 L/day), postcoital antibiotics (as previously described)
- Strategies with no demonstrated efficacy to prevent UTI in women include cranberry products and oral probiotics
- Rule out urologic abnormality such as infected stones, reflux, fistulas, ureteral stenosis, and other anatomical abnormalities

EXAM TIPS
- Memorize diagnostic characteristic of UTI (>100,000 CFU/mL of one organism).
- Use of the spermicide nonoxynol-9 can increase the risk of UTIs in females.

Acute Simple Cystitis in Adult Males
- Occurs in a small number of males between 15 and 50 years of age. Underlying structural issues (urethral

stricture, benign prostatic hyperplasia [BPH], calculi, uncircumcised) should be considered.

- Symptoms include dysuria, frequency, hesitancy, slow urinary stream, nocturia, and urgency; some have suprapubic pain. If sexually active, rule out gonorrhea and chlamydia infection (use nucleic acid amplification test [NAAT]).
- Diagnosed by classical clinical manifestations and pyuria and bacteriuria on UA and urine C&S.
- Treat with the antibiotics nitrofurantoin, trimethoprim-sulfamethoxazole, or fosfomycin.
- If recurrent infection, rule out ureteral stricture, infected kidney stones, anatomic abnormality, acute prostatitis, sexually transmitted diseases, and so forth. Requires further evaluation; refer to urologist.

NOTE

Long-term use of nitrofurantoin is associated with lung problems, chronic hepatitis, and neuropathy. Nitrofurantoin is contraindicated with renal insufficiency. Baseline chest x-ray, liver function tests, and neurologic exam should be obtained, and patients monitored closely.

CLINICAL PEARLS

- It is not recommended to screen or treat for ASB; this includes older patients, patients with diabetes mellitus, patients with indwelling bladder catheter, and patients undergoing non-urologic surgery.
- Avoid long-term use of nitrofurantoin, if possible. Complications with use include lung problems, chronic hepatitis, and neuropathy.
- Serum potassium should be monitored upon initiation of ACE inhibitor or angiotensin receptor blocker therapy if the patient has kidney disease. Potassium levels may initially rise. Continued monitoring of serum electrolytes is recommended.
- Patients with preexisting kidney disease and/or diabetes are at higher risk of kidney damage from contrast media. Contrast-associated AKI refers to a rise in serum creatinine occurring shortly after administration of iodinated contrast (usually 24 to 48 hours).
- Imaging test with the highest sensitivity/specificity for kidney stones is noncontrast CT scan (initial imaging is renal ultrasonography).

KNOWLEDGE CHECK: CHAPTER 11

1. The nurse practitioner is providing education to a female patient on avoiding urinary tract infection (UTI). The patient requires additional education if they identify what factor as a risk factor for UTI?
   A. Recent sexual intercourse
   B. Previous pregnancy
   C. Low fluid intake
   D. Spermicide use

2. Which of the following symptoms prompts further evaluation in a patient with chronic kidney disease?
   A. Edema
   B. Hypertension
   C. Weakness/fatigue
   D. New-onset oliguria

3. The most frequent cause of acute complicated urinary tract infection (UTI) is:
   A. *Escherichia coli*
   B. *Klebsiella*
   C. Methicillin-sensitive *Staphylococcus aureus* (MSSA)
   D. Methicillin-resistant *Staphylococcus aureus* (MRSA)

4. A patient presents complaining of edema and decreased urine output after taking a prescribed aminoglycoside as an antibacterial agent for a complicated urinary tract infection (UTI) for the past 3 weeks. The nurse practitioner is concerned for which type of kidney injury?
   A. Prerenal
   B. Chronic kidney disease stage 1
   C. Postrenal
   D. Acute tubular necrosis

5. A patient presents with acute renal colic pain, hematuria, nausea, and vomiting. Based on these symptoms, which of the following tests is the preferred imaging to confirm the diagnosis?
   A. Ultrasound of the kidneys and bladder
   B. Abdominal radiography
   C. CT of the abdomen and pelvis without contrast
   D. Intravenous pyelography

6. Which of the following is a cause of prerenal disease in acute kidney injury?
   A. Nephrotoxic agents
   B. Dehydration
   C. Renal calculi
   D. Benign prostatic hypertrophy

7. A patient presents with acute renal colic pain and hematuria. The patient denies nausea, vomiting, and dysuria. Serum creatinine level is 0.8 mg/dL. The patient is afebrile, and urinalysis is unremarkable. Imaging indicates a stone of 5 mm. What is the priority intervention for management of this patient?
   A. Analgesia and hydration
   B. Urologic consultation
   C. Administration of tamsulosin 0.4 mg once daily
   D. Initiation of antibiotics

(See answers next page.)

1. B) Previous pregnancy

While current pregnancy can elevate the risk for UTI, previous pregnancy does not. Other risk factors include recent sexual intercourse, failure to void after intercourse, spermicide use, low fluid intake, female sex assigned at birth, history of recent UTI or recurrent UTIs, diabetes mellitus, and poor hygiene.

2. D) New-onset oliguria

Patients with chronic kidney disease often present with signs and symptoms as a result of diminished kidney function (such as edema or hypertension) or of prolonged kidney failure (such as weakness, fatigability, anorexia, vomiting, pruritis, and even encephalopathy and seizures in advanced stages). However, new onset of an abnormally reduced urine output (seen with oliguria or anuria) is not a common presentation with chronic kidney disease alone. Often, it indicates some component of acute kidney injury superimposed on the chronic disease and requires further evaluation.

3. A) *Escherichia coli*

The most frequent cause of acute complicated UTI is *E. coli*. Other uropathogens include Enterobacterales *(e.g., Klebsiella* and *Proteus* species), *Pseudomonas*, enterococci, and staphylocci (both MSSA and MRSA). It is important to note that the prevalence of a particular pathogen over another depends on the host.

4. D) Acute tubular necrosis

Aminoglycoside is an antibacterial agent that is frequently used in combination with other agents for treatment of septicemia, nosocomial respiratory tract infections, complicated UTIs, complicated intra-abdominal infections, and osteomyelitis. However, aminoglycosides are considered nephrotoxic and can contribute to acute tubular necrosis. Patients with acute kidney injury may present with symptoms of diminished kidney function (e.g., edema, hypertension, decreased urine output). Prerenal disease is often a consequence of volume depletion in the setting of hypovolemia caused by dehydration, hemorrhage, or renal (diuretics) or gastrointestinal (vomiting, diarrhea) fluid loss. Chronic kidney disease is the presence of kidney damage or decreased kidney function for 3 or more months, irrespective of the cause. Postrenal acute kidney injury (often referred to as obstructive nephropathy) is often a result of prostatic disease (hyperplasia or cancer), renal calculi, clots, neurogenic bladder, or medications that cause urinary retention.

5. C) CT of the abdomen and pelvis without contrast

CT of the abdomen and pelvis without contrast is the preferred diagnostic test for nephrolithiasis and reliably detects hydronephrosis. Ultrasound of the kidneys and bladder detects hydronephrosis and can be used as a reasonable alternative to a CT scan, especially for pregnant patients to avoid ionizing radiation and when CT is not available. However, ultrasound is less accurate and has greater variability than CT for diagnosis. Abdominal radiography, intravenous pyelography, and MRI are used as adjunct or follow-up examinations and are rarely used in the initial diagnosis of nephrolithiasis. Abdominal radiography does not detect hydronephrosis and is less accurate than CT for stone detection. Intravenous pyelography detects hydronephrosis but is less sensitive and specific compared with CT for the detection of stones.

6. B) Dehydration

Prerenal disease is often a consequence of true volume depletion in the setting of hypovolemia caused by dehydration, hemorrhage, or renal (diuretics) or gastrointestinal (vomiting, diarrhea) fluid loss. Nephrotoxins are a common cause of acute tubular necrosis, a form of intrarenal acute kidney injury. Postrenal acute kidney injury (often referred to as obstructive nephropathy) is often a result of prostatic disease (hyperplasia or cancer), renal calculi, clots, neurogenic bladder, and medications that cause urinary retention.

7. A) Analgesia and hydration

This patient is presenting with nephrolithiasis. Most patients with a stone ≤5 mm can be treated conservatively at home with pain medication and hydration until the stone passes as long as they are able to tolerate adequate oral intake. The patient's urine should be strained, and any stone that passes should be submitted for analysis. If patients experience uncontrollable pain or fever, hospitalization is often necessary. A urologic consultation is indicated for patients presenting with a stone >10 mm, urinary tract infection, acute kidney injury, anuria, and/or severe pain, nausea, or vomiting. A urinary tract infection is unlikely given that the patient is afebrile, and the urinalysis is unremarkable, so initiation of antibiotics is not indicated at this time. Tamsulosin, an alpha blocker, is indicated for patients with urethral stones >5 mm and ≤10 mm in diameter to facilitate stone passage.

8. An adult nonpregnant female patient presents with complaints of dysuria, urinary frequency, and urgency. Urinalysis is significant for pyuria and bacteriuria. Urine culture and susceptibility testing are pending. The patient's vital signs are otherwise stable, and she denies chills, fever, or flank pain. The patient denies a history of any recent broad-spectrum antimicrobial use, travel, or healthcare exposures. Based on this presentation, which of the following antimicrobial regimens is indicated?

A. No antibiotics are indicated, only symptom management

B. Meropenem 1 g IV every 8 hours plus vancomycin 15 mg/kg IV every 12 hours

C. Trimethoprim-sulfamethoxazole (Bactrim) 160/800 mg PO BID for 3 days

D. Ceftriaxone 1 g IV once daily

9. Which of the following is considered the *best* overall measure of kidney function and is used to stage chronic kidney disease?

A. Creatinine clearance

B. Glomerular filtration rate (GFR)

C. Blood urea nitrogen (BUN)

D. Serum creatinine

10. Which of the following presentations warrants a nephrology consultation in a patient with newly identified chronic kidney disease (CKD)?

A. Pregnant adult female patient with no comorbidities

B. Patient with hypertension that is reactive to treatment therapy

C. Patient with diabetes mellitus and hemoglobin A1C of 6%

D. Patient with family history of systemic autoimmune disease

11. Among patients with nephrolithiasis, what is the most common type of kidney stone?

A. Struvite

B. Cystine

C. Calcium oxalate

D. Uric acid

12. A 55-year-old female patient presents with symptoms of a urinary tract infection (UTI). A clean catch midstream urine specimen is obtained and sent to the laboratory for culture and sensitivity (C&S) testing. Which of the following results is indicative of an uncomplicated UTI?

A. 10^5 CFU/mL of one organism

B. 10^5 CFU/mL of one or more organisms

C. 10^3 CFU/mL of Enterobacteriaceae

D. 10^3 CFU/mL of gram-negative Enterobacteriaceae

13. What sign or symptom suggests the possibility of an uncomplicated urinary tract infection (UTI)?

A. Fever

B. Flank pain

C. Costovertebral angle tenderness

D. Dysuria

14. A new patient, a 54-year-old male athlete with a history of hyperlipidemia, is seen for new onset of generalized myalgia, muscle weakness, oliguria, and tea-colored urine for the past 24 hours. He recently completed running a marathon. He is on a statin and reports taking ibuprofen several times to treat the muscle pain. Which diagnosis is *most* likely?

A. Hyperthyroidism

B. Rhabdomyolysis

C. Pyelonephritis

D. Viral influenza

15. Which of the following conditions would *most* likely contribute to acute tubular necrosis (ATN)?

A. Neurogenic bladder from spinal cord injury

B. Urethral stricture

C. Benign prostatic hyperplasia

D. Sepsis

(See answers next page.)

8. C) Trimethoprim-sulfamethoxazole (Bactrim) 160/800 mg PO BID for 3 days

The patient is presenting with symptoms of acute simple cystitis, an acute infection that is confined to the bladder with no signs of systemic infection (e.g., chills, rigors, fatigue, flank pain, costovertebral angle tenderness). Often, diagnosis can be made based on the classic symptoms in adult nonpregnant female patients; however, a urinalysis and urine culture can confirm the presence of pyuria and bacteriuria. Initial empiric antimicrobial agents without risk factors for multidrug–resistant infection include: nitrofurantoin, trimethoprim-sulfamethoxazole, fosfomycin, and pivmecillinam. Of note, multidrug–resistant gram-negative urinary tract infections should be suspected in any patient with a history of a previous multidrug–resistant isolate; previous use of a fluoroquinolone, trimethoprim-sulfamethoxazole, or broad-spectrum beta-lactam; previous inpatient stay at a healthcare facility; and/or travel to areas with high rates of multidrug–resistant organisms. Antimicrobials are not indicated for patients presenting with bacteriuria without consistent urinary symptoms (asymptomatic bacteriuria). For hospitalized patients who are not critically ill or at risk for an infection with a multidrug–resistant gram-negative organism, ceftriaxone 1 g IV once daily is recommended. For critically ill patients or those with a urinary tract obstruction, meropenem plus vancomycin is recommended.

9. B) Glomerular filtration rate (GFR)

In general, GFR is considered the best index of overall kidney function; declining GFR is the hallmark of progressive kidney disease. Chronic kidney disease is staged according to cause of disease, GFR, and albuminuria. Creatinine clearance is used to estimate the GFR and is determined from a 24-hour urine collection. BUN is a measure of the kidney's ability to excrete urea (waste product of protein metabolism). Creatinine is the product of creatine metabolism in skeletal muscle; it also is derived from dietary meat intake. Normal creatinine values differ between males and females due to differences in muscle mass. When renal function decreases, the creatinine level often increases.

10. A) Pregnant adult female patient with no comorbidities

Indications for a nephrology consult for patients with newly identified CKD include patients with an estimated glomerular filtration rate <30 mL/min/1.73 m², persistent protein-to-creatinine ratio ≥500 mg/g and albumin-to-creatinine ratio ≥300 mg/g, abnormal urine microscopy, personal history of systemic autoimmune disease or known history of multiple myeloma, large cystic kidneys, evidence of rapid loss of kidney function, single kidney with glomerular filtration rate <60 mL/min/m², inability to identify cause of CKD or manage electrolyte abnormalities, resistant hypertension, recurrent nephrolithiasis, pregnancy, hereditary kidney disease, or inability to manage complications of various medications (e.g., chemotherapy agents).

11. C) Calcium oxalate

The majority of kidney stones are made up of calcium oxalate (70%–80%). The other types of stones are calcium phosphate (15%), struvite (1%), uric acid (8%), and cystine (1%–2%).

12. A) 10^5 CFU/mL of one organism

A UTI is diagnosed with a urine C&S result of 10^5 CFU/mL of one organism and is accompanied by symptoms such as dysuria, urgency, frequency, nocturia, and suprapubic discomfort. Do not let the word *uncomplicated* distract you; the numbers are the same with complicated and uncomplicated UTIs.

13. D) Dysuria

An acute uncomplicated UTI is confined to the bladder and may involve dysuria, urinary frequency, or nocturia. An acute complicated UTI refers to any infection that extends beyond the bladder. Complicated UTIs may involve fever (not well-defined but often >99.9°F/37.7°C), flank pain, costovertebral angle tenderness, pelvic or perineal pain in men, and other signs of systemic illness (e.g., chills, rigors, fatigue).

14. B) Rhabdomyolysis

The patient's signs and symptoms along with a history of extreme exercise (running a marathon), taking statins, and taking high-dose nonsteroidal anti-inflammatory drugs (NSAIDs) for muscle pain are highly suggestive of rhabdomyolysis, which is a serious and sometimes fatal syndrome. Acute kidney failure is a common complication of rhabdomyolysis secondary to myoglobins damaging the kidneys. NSAIDs with dehydration can cause or worsen acute kidney injury. Myoglobins released from damaged muscle result in reddish-brown or tea-colored urine. Serum creatine kinase levels are markedly elevated (five times normal value or higher). Blood chemistry abnormalities, elevated aldolase, lactate dehydrogenase, electrolyte abnormalities, and disseminated intravascular coagulation can complicate the condition.

15. D) Sepsis

The three major causes of ATN are kidney ischemia (e.g., all causes of severe prerenal disease), sepsis (often associated with prerenal factors such as decreased kidney perfusion and hypotension), and nephrotoxins (e.g., vancomycin, aminoglycosides, cisplatin, radiocontrast media). Postrenal acute kidney injury (often referred to as obstructive nephropathy) is often a result of prostatic disease (hyperplasia or cancer), renal calculi, clots, urethral strictures, neurogenic bladder, or medications that cause urinary retention.

DANGER SIGNALS

ACUTE BACTERIAL MENINGITIS

Neonates, infants, and older patients are at highest risk for this life-threatening infection. Community-acquired bacterial meningitis is most commonly due to *Streptococcus pneumoniae* (50%) and *Neisseria meningitidis* (30%). Acute onset of high fever, severe headache, and stiff neck (nuchal rigidity) with altered mental status. Meningococcal disease (see "Danger Signals" in Chapter 6). Classic purple petechial rashes appear. Accompanied by nausea, vomiting, and photophobia. Rapid worsening of symptoms progressing to lethargy, confusion, and finally coma. If not treated, fatal. Bacterial meningitis is a medical emergency. Call 911.

ACUTE STROKE (CEREBROVASCULAR ACCIDENT)

Classified as either ischemic (about 80%) or hemorrhagic (20%). Ischemic stroke subtypes: thrombosis, embolism, and systemic hypoperfusion. Presents with acute onset of stuttering/speech disturbance, one-sided facial weakness, and one-sided weakness of the arms and/or legs (hemiparesis). Patient describes a thunderclap-type acute headache. Patients who have hemorrhagic stroke often have poorly controlled hypertension and present with the abrupt onset of a severe headache, nausea/vomiting, and nuchal rigidity (subarachnoid hemorrhage [SAH]). Call 911.

CHRONIC SUBDURAL HEMATOMA

Bleeding between the dura and subarachnoid membranes of the brain. Chronic subdural hematoma (SDH) presents gradually, and symptoms may not show until a few weeks after the injury. Patient with a history of head trauma (falls, accidents) presents with a history of headaches and gradual cognitive impairment (apathy, somnolence, confusion). More common in those with alcohol use disorder, older adults, and those who are on anticoagulation or aspirin therapy.

DANGEROUS HEADACHES

- Thunderclap headache (very severe headache that reaches maximum intensity in 1 minute or less)
- "Worst headache of my life"
- First onset of headache at age 50 years or older
- Sudden onset of headache after coughing, exertion, straining, or sex (exertional headache)
- Sudden change in level of consciousness (LOC)
- Focal neurologic signs (e.g., unequal pupil size, hemiparesis, loss of function, poor gag reflex, difficulty swallowing, aphasia, sudden vision loss, visual field defect)
- Headache with paplledema (increased intracranial pressure [ICP] secondary to any of those listed here)
- "Worst-case" scenario of headaches (rule out) includes the following:
- SAH or acute subdural hemorrhage
- Leaking aneurysm or arteriovenous malformation (AVM)
- Bacterial meningitis
- Increased ICP
- Brain abscess
- Brain tumor

GIANT CELL ARTERITIS

Giant cell arteritis (GCA; also known as temporal arteritis) should be considered in any patient older than 50 years who presents with new headache or change in preexisting headache, abrupt visual disturbances or vision loss, jaw claudication, unexplained fever, and signs/symptoms of vascular abnormalities. Some will complain of excruciating burning pain over the affected temporal artery instead of a headache. The affected temple has an indurated, reddened, and cord-like temporal artery (tender and warm to the touch) that is accompanied by scalp tenderness. Markedly elevated erythrocyte sedimentation rate (ESR) and C-reactive protein (CRP); however, these are nonspecific for GCA. Polymyalgia rheumatica (PMR) is associated with GCA, occurring in about 40% to 50% of patients with GCA. If untreated, GCA can lead to permanent blindness.

MULTIPLE SCLEROSIS

Adult female patient complains of episodic visual loss or diplopia (double vision), problems with balance and walking, and numbness and paresthesia on one side of the face. Accompanied by urinary incontinence (75%) and/or bowel dysfunction (50%). Reports that when bending neck forward/flexion, an electric shock-like sensation runs down the back (Lhermitte sign). Not emergent, but recognition of presenting signs and symptoms is important for diagnosis and treatment.

SUBARACHNOID HEMORRHAGE

Sudden and rapid onset of severe headache described as "the worst headache of my life" accompanied by nausea/vomiting, neck pain or stiffness (positive Brudzinski and/or Kernig signs), photophobia, and visual changes (diplopia, visual loss) with a rapid decline in LOC. The headache may be nonlocalized or localized in the occipital area and neck. May have seizures during the acute phase. Vital signs reveal blood pressure (BP) elevation, temperature elevation, and tachycardia. Depending on the source of the bleed, may have focal neurologic signs or no signs. Usually caused by ruptured cerebral aneurysm or AVM. A "sentinel headache" (sudden intense headache) can precede a spontaneous SAH by days to weeks. An non-contrast CT scan can detect an SAH in approximately 95% of patients within first 24 hours. Associated with a high early mortality rate; some patients die suddenly before hospital evaluation. A medical emergency. Call 911.

NEUROLOGIC TESTING

NEUROLOGIC EXAM

Neurologic testing includes mental status; cranial nerves (CNs); and motor, reflex, and sensory examination.

Folstein Mini-Mental State Exam

See Chapter 25 for a detailed review of the Folstein Mini-Mental State Exam (MMSE).

Cerebellar Testing

The cerebellum coordinates unconscious regulation of balance, muscle tone, and voluntary movements.
- Gait: Tell patient to walk to the other side of room and back. If walking aid (e.g., cane, walker) is used, test patient with the walking aid. Observe gait. Is patient shuffling, scissoring, waddling, or swinging? If acute cerebellar ataxia, patient will have a wide-based staggering gait.
- Tandem gait: Tell patient to walk a straight line in normal gait, then instruct patient to walk in a straight line with one foot in front of the other. Test is positive if patient is unable to perform tandem walking, loses balance, and falls.
- Rapid alternating movements: Tell patient to place hands on top of each thigh and move them (alternating between supination and pronation) as fast as possible. Test is positive if patient is unable to or has problems with performing rapid alternating movements (dysdiadochokinesia).
- Heel-to-shin testing: Patient is in a supine position with extended legs. Tell patient to place the left heel on the right knee and then move it down the shin (repeat with right heel on left knee). Test is positive if patient is unable to keep their foot on the shin.
- Finger-to-nose and finger-to-finger test: Tell patient to fully extend arm, then touch their nose, or ask them to touch their nose, then extend arms and touch your finger. Test is positive if patient is unable to touch or misses touching nose and/or finger to nose (dysmetria).

Proprioception: Romberg Test

Tell patient to stand with arms/hands straight on each side and feet together with eyes open and observe. Next, instruct patient to close both eyes while standing in the same position and observe. Test is positive if patient with eyes closed sways excessively, falls down, or has to keep feet wide apart to maintain balance. Patient unable to remain steady with eyes closed suggests cerebellar ataxia/dysfunction or sensory loss.

CLINICAL PEARL

Acute onset of cerebellar ataxia is considered a medical emergency as it may represent an acute vascular event. Neuroimaging and screening for causative drugs and toxins should be part of the comprehensive assessment.

EXAM TIPS

- Herpes zoster infection (shingles) of CN V ophthalmic branch can result in corneal blindness.
- If rash at tip of nose and the temple area, rule out shingles infection of the trigeminal nerve involving the ophthalmic branch (V1).

Cranial Nerve Testing

Use the mnemonic, "On Old Olympus Towering Tops, A Finn And German Viewed Some Hops." The first letter stands for the names of the CNs. The word order corresponds to the sequential numbering of the CNs. To remember the function (sensory, motor, or both), use the mnemonic, "Some Say Marry Money, But My Brother Says Big Brains Matter Most." The order corresponds to the number of CNs; S corresponds to sensory, M refers to motor function, and B refers to both sensory and motor function.
- CN I: Olfactory (On). Use familiar scent (e.g., coffee, peppermint). Block one nostril at a time.
- CN II: Optic (Old). For visual field testing, patient stands about 2 feet in front of examiner and covers their left (or right) eye. Stretch arm so that it is in the peripheral visual field, and ask patient if they see one, two, or three fingers (all four quadrants). Stare straight ahead at about the same level as the patient (examiner serves as the "control"). Check central distance vision using Snellen chart (patient stands 20 feet away from chart).
- CN III: Oculomotor (Olympus). CN III, CN IV, and CN VI are usually tested together; they control the extraocular muscles (EOM). First look for ptosis. Stand about 2 feet in front of patient as they fixate gaze on the fingers of examiner's hand. Instruct patient to "follow my fingers," while observing for nystagmus (horizontal quick movements of eye in one direction alternate with

slower movements of eyes in opposite direction). Test pupillary function.

- CN IV: Trochlear (Towering). Down and inward eye movement. CN III, CN IV, and CN VI are usually tested together; see CN III.
- CN V: Trigeminal (Tops). Muscles of mastication. Provides the sensory nerves to the face, scalp, cornea, mucous membranes, and nose. Test sensation by lightly touching the forehead area, cheek, and chin. Trigeminal nerve has three branches: the ophthalmic (V1), cheek (V2), and jaw area (V3) (Figure 12.1). Tell patient to close eyes when testing; ask if they can feel the sensation.
- CN VI: Abducens (A). Lateral eye movement. CN III, CN IV, and CN VI are usually tested together; see CN III.
- CN VII: Facial (Finn). Controls the facial muscles that enable facial expressions. Tell patient to close eyelids tightly; try to open eyelids manually. Tell patient to look up and wrinkle forehead, then tell patient to smile. Look for asymmetry and muscle atrophy. Bell's palsy is due to inflammation of the facial nerve (motor portion). The affected side of face will not move, and eyelid may not fully close.
- CN VIII: Acoustic (And). The hearing exam can be done by rubbing patient's hair in front of the ear. Alternative is to hold hand up as a sound screen, then whisper a few numbers, and ask the patient if they heard the words.
- CN IX: Glossopharyngeal (German). Both CN IX and CN X control the palate. They are usually tested together. Tell patient to open mouth and then yawn. Observe for asymmetry; uvula should be midline. Gag reflex can be tested by using tongue blade and lightly touching the back of the throat. Assess voice clarity (rule out dysarthria).

- CN X: Vagus (Viewed). Talking, swallowing, general sensation from the carotid body, carotid reflex. CN IX and CN X are usually tested together; see CN IX.
- CN XI: Spinal accessory (Some). Controls shoulder shrug and head rotation. Tell patient to shrug both shoulders; should be the same level. Then tell patient to rotate head to the left. Place hand on the patient's left cheek and instruct to push against it. Tell patient to turn head to the right side, then follow same procedure. Check sternocleidomastoid muscle for atrophy or asymmetry.
- CN XII: Hypoglossal (Hops). Controls tongue movement. Tell patient to stick out their tongue and move it from side to side. Look for atrophy and asymmetry.

EXAM TIPS

- CN IX: Innervates movement of soft palate (ask patient to yawn or say "aah" to check voice clarity).
- CN XI: The number reminds you of the shoulders shrugging together.

Sensory System

Tell patient to close their eyes for these tests.
- Monofilament testing: Randomly place a monofilament on several different sites of the plantar surface of each foot and one side of the dorsal surface. Place enough pressure so the filament bends.
- Vibration sense: Use 128-Hz tuning fork and tap lightly, then place one end into the distal joint of each thumb. Patient should have eyes closed. For testing feet, place tuning fork on tips of toes and several areas on the soles of the feet (Figure 12.2). Go back and forth to compare one foot with the other. Check for numbness

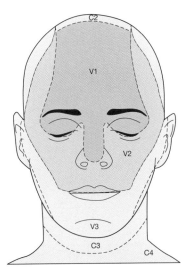

Figure 12.1 Trigeminal V1, V2, and V3 dermatomal divisions of cranial nerve V.
Source: Adapted from Armitage, A. (2015). (See Resources section for complete source information.)

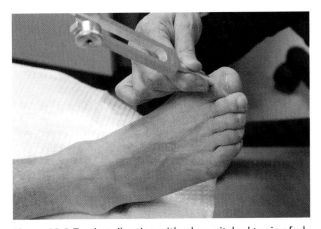

Figure 12.2 Testing vibration with a low-pitched tuning fork.
Source: Gawlik, K. S., Melnyk, B. M., & Teall, A. M. (Eds.). (2021). (See Resources section for complete source information.)

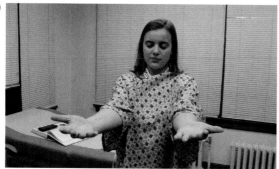
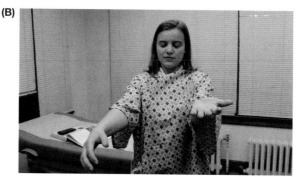

Figure 12.3 Testing for pronator drift. (A) Patient stands with eyes closed and arms straight forward with palms up. (B) Arms drifting sideward or upward after a brisk tap indicate a positive test.

Source: Gawlik, K. S., Melnyk, B. M., & Teall, A. M. (2021). (See Resources section for complete source information.)

or decreased vibration sense. Patient should have eyes closed. Important test for assessing severity of diabetic peripheral neuropathy.

- Sharp–dull touch: Use the sharp end of a safety pin or toothpick for sharp touch testing. For testing for dull sensation, use the head of the safety pin or the eraser end of a pencil.
- Temperature: Test the ability to differentiate hot or cold.
- Positive results: Patient unable to feel the monofilament, discriminate sharp from dull sensation, feel hot and cold temperatures, or sense vibration. Vibration sense is often the earliest to be affected in disease such as peripheral neuropathy (polyneuropathy), which can be caused by diabetes and vitamin B_{12} deficiency anemia.

Stereognosis (Ability to Recognize Familiar Object Through Sense of Touch Only)

Place a familiar object (e.g., coin, key, pen) on the patient's palm and tell the patient to identify the object with eyes closed.

Graphesthesia (Ability to Identify Figures "Written" on Skin)

"Write" a large letter or number on the patient's palms using fingers (patient's eyes are closed).

Motor Exam

- Upper extremities: Tell patient to raise both arms in front of them, then pronate and supinate. Tell patient to bend and extend forearms, then push against resistance provided by examiner.
- Hands: Perform full range of motion with hands and fingers, without and with resistance (by examiner). The dominant hand will be slightly larger due to more muscle development.
- Lower extremities: While supine, tell patient to flex each hip, then raise each leg separately while the examiner provides resistance. Compare legs.
- Feet: Perform full range of motion on toes and ankles; examiner provides resistance.
- Pronator drift test: Have patient stretch out the arms with palms facing up, with eyes open. Tell patient to close eyes. Wait for 20 to 30 seconds, then tap the arms

briskly downward. If positive, one arm goes downward or drifts (Figure 12.3). Positive result occurs in upper motor neuron diseases (stroke, amyotrophic lateral sclerosis [ALS], polio).

- Lower motor neuron lesions (neuropathy, polio, nerve root compression/radiculopathy): Look for muscle weakness, muscle wasting/atrophy, and fasciculations.
- Gross examination (legs) and fine motor movements (hands): Test walking, using hands for manipulation/pincer grasp, jumping, and so forth.

Reflexes

- Both sides should be compared with each other and should be equal.
- There are 31 pairs of spinal nerve roots, named for their associated vertebral body. Each pair of nerve roots exits at the corresponding level, innervating distinct dermatomal distributions (Figure 12.4).

Grading Reflexes

0   No response
1+   Low response
2+   Normal or average response
3+   Brisker than average response
4+   Very brisk response (sustained clonus)

Reflex Testing

- Quadriceps reflex (knee-jerk response): Reflex center at L2 to L4. Tap patellar tendon briskly on each side.

Table 12.1 Deep Tendon Reflexes

Reflex	Affected Nerve Root
Biceps and brachioradialis	C5-6
Triceps	C6-7
Hip flexion Hip extension	L2-3 L4-5
Knee extension (knee jerk) Knee flexion	L3-4 L5-S1
Achilles (ankle jerk)	S1

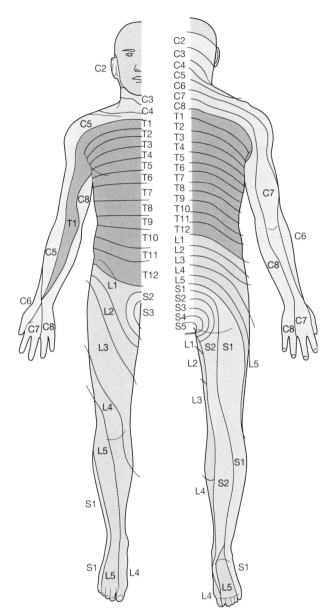

Figure 12.4 Dermatome distribution.
Source: Adapted from Armitage, A. (2015). (See Resources section for complete source information.)

- Achilles reflex (ankle-jerk response): Reflex center at L5 to S2 (tibial nerve). With patient's legs dangling off the exam table, hold the foot in slight dorsiflexion and briskly tap the Achilles tendon. Weak to no response with peripheral neuropathy (diabetes, vitamin B_{12} deficiency anemia).
- Plantar reflex (Babinski's sign): Reflex center L4 to S2. Stroke plantar surface of foot on the lateral border from heel toward the big toe (plantar flexion is normal response). Babinski's sign is positive if toes spread like a fan. Adults should have a negative Babinski's sign. For young infants, Babinski's sign is considered normal finding.

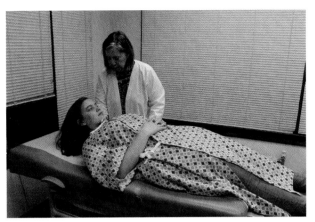

Figure 12.5 Brudzinski's sign test.
Source: Gawlik, K. S., Melnyk, B. M., & Teall, A. M. (Eds.). (2021). (See Resources section for complete source information.)

NEUROLOGIC MANEUVERS

These tests are used to assess for meningeal irritation (suggestive of meningitis or SAH). All are done with the patient in a supine position. In general, these are more sensitive tests in children compared with adults.

Kernig's Sign

Flex patient's hips one at a time, then attempt to straighten the leg while keeping the hip flexed at 90 degrees. Test is positive if there is resistance to leg straightening because of painful hamstrings (due to inflammation on lumbar nerve roots) and/or complaints of back pain.

Brudzinski's Sign

Passively flex/bend the patient's neck toward the chest (Figure 12.5). Test is positive if patient reflexively flexes the hips and knee to relieve pressure and pain (due to inflammation of lumbar nerve roots).

Nuchal Rigidity

Tell patient to touch chest with the chin. Inability to touch the chest secondary to pain is a positive finding.

DISEASE REVIEW

ACUTE BACTERIAL MENINGITIS

A serious acute bacterial infection of the leptomeninges that cover the brain and spinal cord. The most common pathogens in adults are *Streptococcus pneumoniae*, *N. meningitidis*, and *Haemophilus influenzae* (the latter two are gram negative). Bacterial meningitis is a reportable disease (local health department).

Classic Case

Acute onset of fever >100.4°F (38°C), severe headache, stiff neck (nuchal rigidity), and rapid changes in mental status and LOC (confusion, lethargy, stupor). Photophobia and nausea/vomiting.

Labs

- Obtain complete blood count (CBC) with differential, complete metabolic panel, coagulation studies, and blood cultures × 2.
- Perform CT scan of the head *before* lumbar puncture (LP) in patients with one or more of the following risk factors: Papilledema, focal neurologic deficit, abnormal LOC, new-onset seizure (within 1 week of presentation), history of central nervous system (CNS) disease (stroke, mass) or immunocompromise (HIV, immunosuppressive therapy, solid organ or bone marrow transplant).
- Perform LP (elevated opening pressure): Cerebrospinal fluid (CSF) contains large numbers of white blood cells (WBCs) and is cloudy. Definitive diagnosis made from bacteria isolated from the CSF, with presence of elevated protein and low glucose levels in the CSF.
- Do not delay antimicrobial therapy if LP is delayed by imaging studies. Obtain blood cultures and start empiric antibiotics as soon as possible.
- Gram stain and culture and sensitivity (C&S) of CSF and blood are needed; isolation of a bacterial pathogen confirms the diagnosis.

Treatment Plan

- For adults, third-generation intravenous (IV) cephalosporin (e.g., cefotaxime and ceftriaxone) *PLUS* vancomycin *PLUS* ampicillin (for adults >50 years).
- In addition to antimicrobial therapy, dexamethasone is recommended for adults with suspected bacterial meningitis.
- Supportive care with fluid management, reduction of ICP, and prevention of neurologic complications.

Complications

- Patients who recover usually have some degree of permanent neurologic sequelae.
- Older patients have a higher mortality rate due to the presence of comorbid conditions.

ACUTE MILD TRAUMATIC BRAIN INJURY (CONCUSSION)

Early symptoms of acute mild traumatic brain injury (TBI) include confusion, headache, dizziness or vertigo, poor balance, and nausea and vomiting. Most do not lose consciousness. Antegrade and retrograde amnesia are common after the injury. Mild TBI is defined as a Glasgow Coma Scale (GCS) score of 13 to 15 (measured 30 minutes after injury). Most patients are male (2:1). TBI is usually the result of acceleration/deceleration forces on the brain tissue.

Common causes of TBI include motor vehicle collisions, falls, occupational accidents, recreational accidents, and assaults. Sports with the highest rates of TBI include American football, ice hockey, soccer, boxing, and rugby. Mild TBI is a common wartime injury for soldiers who participated in combat.

Treatment Plan

- Ask patient about details of the accident, such as events leading up to the injury and during the episode and events that followed after the concussion.

- Check medication history, inquire if on anticoagulation, chronic acetylsalicylic acid (ASA) therapy, or nonsteroidal anti-inflammatory drugs (NSAIDs) (higher risk of brain hemorrhage).
- Evaluate mental status, including short-term memory and attention span. Perform a neurologic assessment and CN examination; pay attention to vision (CN II), pupil exam, extraocular movements (CN II, IV, VI), and facial movements (CN VII).
- Refer patient to the ED if suspected head trauma; may need a CT scan of head (without contrast).
- Indications for hospital admission
  - GCS score <15
  - Seizures or other neurologic deficit(s)
  - Recurrent vomiting
  - Abnormal head CT (e.g., midline shift, hemorrhage, ischemia, mass effect)
  - Abnormal bleeding

BELL'S PALSY

Abrupt onset of unilateral facial paralysis due to dysfunction of the motor branch of the facial nerve (CN VII). Facial paralysis can progress rapidly within 24 hours. Skin sensation remains intact, but tear production on the affected side may stop. Most cases resolve spontaneously. Herpes simplex virus activation is suspected to be the most likely cause in many cases.

Classic Case

An older adult reports waking up that morning with one side of his face paralyzed. Complains of difficulty chewing and swallowing food on the same side. Unable to fully close eyelid on affected side.

Treatment Plan

- Early treatment with high-dose oral glucocorticoids (prednisone 60–80 mg/day) for 1 week.
- For patients with severe palsy, coadministration with antiviral therapy is recommended: valacyclovir (1,000 mg three times a day) *OR* acyclovir (400 mg five times daily) × 7 days.
- Best if treatment started as soon as possible, within 3 days of onset.
- Protect cornea from drying and ulceration by applying artificial tears (liquid, gel) every hour while patient is awake. Use protective glasses or goggles. At night, use ointment (containing mineral oil and white petrolatum) and cover with eye patch.

Complications

Can cause corneal ulceration. Recurrent attacks happen in 7% to 15% of cases.

CARPAL TUNNEL SYNDROME

Compression of the median nerve (Figure 12.6) as it travels through the carpal tunnel. Commonly caused by activities that require repetitive wrist/hand motion. Both hands affected in 50% of patients. Other factors

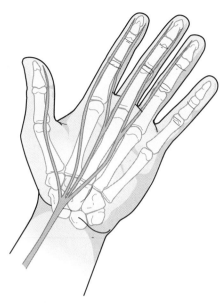

Figure 12.6 Median nerve.

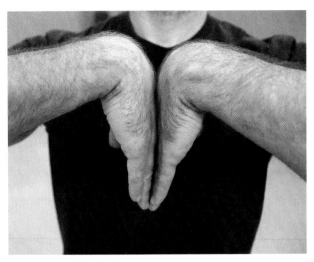

Figure 12.7 Phalen's sign.
Source: Myrick, K. M., & Karosas, L. M. (Eds.). (2021). (See Resources section for complete source information.)

that increase risk are genetic predisposition, diabetes mellitus, thyroid disease, pregnancy, osteoarthritis and rheumatoid arthritis, trauma to the wrist, and obesity. More common in women (3:1).

Classic Case

An adult female patient complains of gradual onset (over weeks to months) of numbness and tingling (paresthesia) in the median nerve territory (i.e., the thumb, index finger, and middle finger areas). Hand grip of affected hand is weaker. Complains of problems lifting heavy objects with the affected hand. Symptoms are worsened by repetitive actions of the hand or wrist and are worse at night, awakening patient from sleep. Chronic severe cases involve atrophy of the thenar eminence (the group of muscles on the palm of the hand at the base of the thumb), which is a late sign. History of an occupation or hobby that involves frequent wrist/hand movements.

Tinel's Sign

Identifies compression of the ulnar nerve. With the elbow relaxed, tap anterior wrist briskly. Positive sign is "pins and needles" sensation of the median nerve over the hand after lightly percussing the wrist.

Phalen's Sign

Identifies median nerve pathology. Engage in full flexion of wrist for 60 seconds (Figure 12.7). Positive sign is numbness or tingling sensation of the median nerve over the hand evoked by passive flexion of the wrist for 1 minute.

EXAM TIPS

- Recognize both Tinel's and Phalen's signs (tests for carpal tunnel syndrome [CTS]) or compression of median nerve).
- CTS refers to the signs and symptoms caused by compression of the median nerve.

CEREBROVASCULAR ACCIDENT OR STROKE

A stroke is classified by either ischemia or hemorrhage. Ischemia can be caused by emboli (secondary to a cardiac, aortic, arterial, or unknown source), thrombosis (either large or small vessel disease), or systemic hypoperfusion. There are two types of brain hemorrhage: intracerebral (bleed directly into the brain) and subarachnoid (bleeding into subarachnoid space and CSF). The obstruction or bleeding causes permanent damage to the brain. Major modifiable risk factors for ischemic stroke are hypertension, dyslipidemia, diabetes, smoking, and physical inactivity. Major risk factors for hemorrhagic strokes include older age, hypertension, cigarette smoking, family history, alcohol use, sympathomimetic drug use, and use of antithrombotic therapy (e.g., antiplatelet and anticoagulant). Most SAHs are due to the rupture of intracranial aneurysms.

Black and Hispanic Americans have an increased stroke risk compared with White Americans. The "stroke belt" refers to the southeastern United States, an area that has a higher regional incidence, prevalence, and mortality rate of strokes.

Classic Case

A patient with embolic stroke presents with the abrupt onset of difficulty speaking, unilateral hemiparesis, and weakness of the arms or legs (or both). Patient with hemorrhagic stroke often initially presents with severe headache, nausea/vomiting, photophobia, and nuchal rigidity that is accompanied by hemiparesis and difficulty speaking.

Hemorrhagic Stroke

- SAH: Sudden onset of severe "thunderclap headache" that is described as "the worst headache of my life." The pain from the headache may radiate and cause neck pain or stiffness (meningismus). The headache may or may not be associated with a rapid decrease in or loss of consciousness (coma, death), seizures, nausea, vomiting, and/or focal neurologic deficit. SAH usually begins abruptly compared with more gradual intracranial hemorrhage (ICH).

- Sentinel headache (a sudden and severe headache): May precede a major SAH a few days to weeks prior to aneurysm rupture.
- ICH: Depending on location and size of hemorrhage, signs and symptoms may vary and may be gradual and progress over minutes or a few hours. Clinical presentation often includes acute onset of focal neurologic deficit such as hemiparesis, aphasia, or visual impairment. If the hemorrhage is large, headache, vomiting, and a decrease in or loss of consciousness may develop.
- Hemorrhagic stroke: May be precipitated by sex or other physical activity.

Acute Ischemic Stroke

- Signs and symptoms: Dependent on the affected brain region and may include a sudden, severe headache, abrupt onset of hemiparesis, visual field deficits, facial droop, ataxia, nystagmus, aphasia, sudden numbness or weakness of the face or extremity, and abrupt decrease in LOC. Middle cerebral artery is the largest cerebral artery and most commonly affected. For example:
  - Left middle cerebral artery occlusion of the superior branch: Right side of face, right arm, right leg weakness, hemianopia, with expressive aphasia (Broca's area)
  - Right middle cerebral artery: Left side of face, left arm, left leg with hemineglect and possible hemianopia
  - Embolic strokes: Sudden onset; deficits indicate focal loss of brain function. Can result when getting up at night to urinate or suddenly coughing or sneezing.
  - Thrombotic strokes: Progression fluctuates with periods of improvement. Patients may have a neck bruit.
  - Systemic hypoperfusion: Reduced perfusion from cardiac pump failure or reduced cardiac output related to other causes. Generalized hypoxemia and hypoperfusion cause decreased oxygen-carrying capacity to the brain.

Treatment Plan

- Call 911.
- Assess the ABCs (airway, breathing, circulation) as soon as possible. Check for airway patency, chest movement, breath sounds from both lungs, and circulation.
- Check and stabilize vital signs and assess neurologic status.

Emergency Department Management

- Assess the ABCs and stabilize patient.
- Determine if ICH is present and decide if reperfusion therapy with IV thrombolysis or mechanical thrombectomy is warranted for patients with ischemic stroke.

- Initial imaging study in the ED is CT scan (without contrast) and then an MRI study if indicated.
- Time is critical. IV thrombolytic therapy with alteplase improves outcomes in patients with acute ischemic stroke with an onset of symptoms ≤4.5 hours earlier.
- Cardiac monitoring for at least first 24 hours after stroke.
- Tests include CBC, coagulation panel, serum electrolytes and creatinine, fasting blood glucose, lipid panel, hemoglobin A1C, ESR, and CRP.
- In hemorrhagic stroke, evaluate for bleeding disorder.

Screening for Visual Field Loss

- Homonymous hemianopia: Visual field loss involving either the two left halves (or the two right halves) of the visual field. Most common cause is stroke. There are many types of hemianopia.
- Screening test: Visual fields by confrontation.

Example: Left-Sided Homonymous Hemianopia

	Left Eye	Right Eye
The diagram at right shows the intact and missing visual fields of a person who has left-sided homonymous hemianopia. The "x" signifies the missing visual fields, and the "==" are the intact visual fields.	xxxxx==== xxxxx==== xxxxx====	xxxx==== xxxx==== xxxx====

Complications of Stroke

- Cardiac complications of myocardial infarction (MI), arrythmias, neurogenic cardiac damage
- Psychiatric complications of depression, fatigue
- Dysphagia, a risk factor for developing aspiration pneumonia
- Falls and bone fractures
- Infection such as pneumonia, urinary tract infection
- Neurologic complications
  - Apraxia, in which patient has difficulty performing purposeful movements.
  - Broca's aphasia, also known as "expressive aphasia." Patient comprehends speech relatively well (and can read) but has extreme difficulty with the motor aspects of speech. Speech length is usually less than four words. Localized to lesions affecting the frontal lobe.
  - Wernicke's aphasia, also known as "receptive aphasia." Patient has difficulty with comprehension but has no problem with producing speech. Reading and writing can be markedly impaired.
  - Intracranial complications, such as cerebral edema, symptomatic hemorrhagic transformation of ischemic stroke, elevated ICP, and hydrocephalus
  - Early neurologic deterioration and seizures
- Pulmonary complications such as neurogenic pulmonary edema, abnormal respiratory patterns, sleep-related breathing disorders
- Gastrointestinal bleeding
- Urinary incontinence
- Venous thromboembolism and pulmonary embolism

Long-Term Management

- BP management
- Management of cholesterol with low-density lipoprotein cholesterol (LDL-C)–lowering therapy
- For ischemic strokes, antithrombotic therapy
- For hemorrhagic strokes, discussion of risks and benefits of antiplatelet therapy and anticoagulation
- Glycemic control for patients with diabetes
- Lifestyle and dietary changes to help reduce risk of stroke
- Rehabilitation such as physical therapy, occupational therapy, speech therapy
- Follow-up imaging as clinically indicated

GIANT CELL ARTERITIS

GCA is also known as Horton disease, cranial arteritis, and temporal arteritis. A systemic inflammatory disorder of the medium and large arteries (vasculitis) of the body. Acute onset of a unilateral headache that is located on the temple and associated with temporal artery inflammation. Visual loss is not uncommon (despite availability of steroids). Peak incidence is between ages 70 and 79 years.

Classic Case

An older male patient complains of headache on his temple along with marked scalp tenderness on the same side. Presence of an indurated cord-like temporal artery that is warm and tender. Sometimes accompanied by jaw claudication (pain with chewing that is relieved when chewing is stopped). Complains of visual symptoms such as amaurosis fugax (transient monocular loss of vision or partial visual field defect) or blindness. Can be accompanied by systemic symptoms such as low-grade fever and fatigue. ESR and CRP levels are markedly elevated but nonspecific for GCA (Table 12.2).

EXAM TIP

GCA is indurated temporal artery, pain felt behind eye/scalp. Treated with high-dose steroids. Untreated may lead to permanent blindness.

Labs

- CBC, complete metabolic panel (including serum creatinine, liver function tests, glucose)
- ESR and CRP levels
- Urine dipstick analysis
- Serum protein electrophoresis
- Bone profile panel (including calcium, phosphorus, albumin, total protein, alkaline phosphatase, 25-hydroxyvitamin D)

Treatment Plan

- Refer to ophthalmologist or rheumatologist, or refer to ED *stat*.
- Temporal artery biopsy is a definitive test for diagnosis and can be done in an outpatient setting using only local anesthesia. Temporal artery color Doppler ultrasound is an alternative diagnostic tool.
- High-dose system glucocorticoids are part of first-line treatment to preserve treatment (prednisone 40–60 mg PO daily or methylprednisolone 500–1,000 mg IV daily).

Table 12.2 Headaches: Classic Signs and Symptoms

Headache	Symptoms	At-Risk Patients	Aggravating Factors
Migraine without aura	Throbbing pain behind one eye Photophobia, phonophobia Nausea/vomiting	Adult females	Stress, menstruation, visual stimuli, weather changes, nitrates, fasting, wine, sleep disturbances, and aspartame
Migraine with aura	Preceding symptoms plus scotoma, scintillating lights, halos, tingling sensation down one limb, dysphasia, motor weakness (hemiplegic migraine)	Adult females	Same as "Migraine without aura"
Trigeminal neuralgia (CN V)	Intense and very brief, sudden, usually unilateral; sharp stabbing pain in one or more branches of CN V (trigeminal)	Older adults and elderly	Cold food, cold air, talking, touch, chewing
Cluster	Severe "ice-pick" piercing, pain behind one eye, with tearing, eye redness, rhinorrhea, ptosis, and miosis on one side (Horner's syndrome)	Middle-aged males	Occurs at same time daily in clusters for weeks to months, usually at night; alcohol consumption
Giant cell arteritis	Unilateral pain, temporal area with scalp tenderness; skin over artery is indurated, tender, warm, and reddened; amaurosis fugax (temporary blindness) may occur	Older adults and elderly	Various genetic and environmental factors contribute
Tension type	Bilateral "band-like" pain, vise-like or tight in quality, continuous dull pain usually generalized, may last several hours; may be accompanied by spasms of the trapezius muscles	Adults	Emotional or physical stress and mental tension, head and neck movements

CN, cranial nerve.

■ Subsequent management includes glucocorticoid tapering, monitoring of disease activity, and imaging surveillance for those with large vessel involvement.

Complications

Permanent blindness may occur if not diagnosed early (ischemic optic neuropathy).

MEDICATION OVERUSE HEADACHE (REBOUND HEADACHE)

Defined as headache occurring 15 or more days per month due to overuse of acute headache medications for >3 months. More common in women. Patients with migraine who are depressed or anxious may be at risk. Patient complains of daily or almost-daily headaches. May be accompanied by irritability, depression, and insomnia. Caused by overuse of abortive medicines such as analgesics, NSAIDs, aspirin, combination NSAID or acetaminophen with caffeine, butalbital, barbiturates, ergots, triptans, or opioids.

Highest risk with opioids, butalbital-containing combination analgesics, and acetaminophen-aspirin-caffeine combinations. Treatment is to discontinue the medicine immediately (if not contraindicated) or gradually taper the dose and/or reduce frequency. A bridge therapy can be used in patients with severe and/or frequent headaches (e.g., NSAIDs). To avoid relapse, limit triptan, ergotamine-dihydroergotamine, or combination analgesic to ≤9 days a month and NSAIDs to ≤14 or fewer days per month.

MULTIPLE SCLEROSIS

Autoimmune disease in which antibodies attack the myelin sheath, leading to demyelination. Peak incidence at 15 to 45 years of age. More common in women (2.3:1) and White people. Multiple sclerosis (MS) tends to affect the optic nerves (CN II), spinal cord, brainstem, cerebellum, and white matter. Four subtypes: Relapsing-remitting MS (85%–90% of cases), primary progressive MS (10%), secondary progressive MS, and clinically isolated syndrome (thought to be a precursor to MS).

Classic Case

Young adult female patient complains of episodes of visual loss, diplopia (double vision), nystagmus, vertigo, problems with balance and walking, foot drop, and numbness and paresthesia on one side of the face. Bowel dysfunction (50%) and/or urinary incontinence (75%). Reports that when bending neck forward/flexion, an electric shock–like sensation runs down the back (Lhermitte sign).

Diagnosis

■ Primarily a clinical diagnosis; history and physical examination are fundamental for diagnosis.
■ MRI of brain and spinal cord is the imaging test of choice to assess for MS lesions.
■ Assess CSF for oligoclonal bands and/or an increased immunoglobulin G index.

Treatment Plan

Refer to neurologist for management.

POLYMYALGIA RHEUMATICA

PMR is an inflammatory condition seen almost exclusively in people age 50 years or older. Peak incidence is between ages 70 and 80 years. It is more common in female patients. The cause is unknown.

■ The ESR is elevated mildly to severely (20% sedimentation rate 104 mm/hr); CRP is also elevated.
■ PMR patients are at a high risk (roughly 5%–30%) of developing GCA. Educate patients diagnosed with PMR on how to recognize symptoms of GCA.
■ Signs/symptoms include bilateral joint stiffness and aching (lasting 30 minutes or longer, commonly in the morning hours) located in the posterior neck, shoulders, upper arms, and hips (pelvic girdle). Pelvic girdle symptoms include groin pain and pain at lateral aspects of the hips, which may radiate to the posterior thigh area. Patient has difficulty putting on clothes, hooking bra in the back, or getting up out of bed or a chair.
■ Severe morning stiffness (gel phenomenon—"gelling," or stiffness, with inactivity) and pain can last until the afternoon if untreated. Symptoms usually respond quickly to oral steroids (e.g., prednisone daily).

PRIMARY HEADACHE
Cluster Headache

An idiopathic and severe one-sided headache that is marked by recurrent episodes of severe and stabbing pain located behind one eye that is accompanied by lacrimation, nasal congestion, and clear rhinitis with conjunctival injection (red eyes), ptosis (drooping eyelid), and miosis (constriction of pupil) on the ipsilateral side (same side as headache). History of head trauma, tobacco use, or a familial history of cluster headache will increase risk (see Table 12.2).

■ Abrupt onset; patient may get agitated during a headache episode.
■ Episodic cluster bouts can happen several times a day (cluster) or recur daily for several weeks; alternating periods of attacks and remission

- Can also have chronic cluster bouts with continual attacks or brief remission of less than 3 months
- Rhythmicity of the relatively short-lived attacks (15 minutes to 3 hours)
- Resolves spontaneously but often return in the future in some patients
- More common in adult male patients; typical onset is between 20 and 40 years of age
- Can be debilitating; increased risk of suicide if it persists (due to severe intensity of pain)

Classic Case

A 35-year-old male patient complains of the abrupt onset of recurrent episodes of brief, "ice-pick," severe, lacerating periorbital pain above the eye/brow area or temporal area that is accompanied by autonomic symptoms such as tearing and clear nasal discharge (rhinitis). Some may have drooping eyelid (ptosis). May be pacing the floor during an acute attack.

Treatment Plan

For initial diagnosis, an MRI scan is recommended to exclude abnormalities in the brain and pituitary gland (e.g., aneurysms, AVM, pituitary macroadenoma, meningiomas). Acute treatment is as follows:

- High-dose oxygen: May relieve headache (100% oxygen at least 12 L/min by mask); continue oxygen treatment for 15 minutes. Avoid in patients with severe chronic obstructive pulmonary disease (COPD) due to the risk of developing severe hypercapnia and carbon dioxide narcosis.
- Triptans: Administer sumatriptan (Imitrex) 6 mg by subcutaneous injection or intranasal route as initial therapy or combination with high-dose oxygen. Intranasal zolmitriptan is another effective option.
- Alternative acute therapies: Intranasal lidocaine, oral ergotamine, and subcutaneous octreotide.

Prophylaxis is as follows:

- If frequent attacks: The calcium channel blocker (CCB) verapamil is the drug of choice of episodic and chronic cluster headache (initial total daily dose of 240 mg oral). Avoid grapefruit juice. If dose >400 mg, EKG monitoring due to risk of bradycardia, right bundle branch block (RBBB), or complete heart block.
- Patients with infrequent attacks can be started on preventive therapy with glucocorticoids alone.
- Alternative preventive therapies include galcanezumab, lithium, topiramate, greater occipital nerve blocks, pizotifen, valproate, capsaicin, triptans, ergotamine, melatonin, and indomethacin.

Complications

Higher risk of suicide (in male patients) compared with other types of chronic headaches.

Migraine Headaches

Migraine is a severe headache generally associated with nausea and/or light and sound sensitivity. A migraine is a disorder of recurrent attacks that often progress through four phases: the prodrome (affective or vegetative symptoms 24 to 48 hours prior to the onset of the headache [occurs in 77% of patients]); the aura (focal neurologic symptoms such as visual, sensory, language, and motor disturbances [occurs in 25% of patients]); the headache (often unilateral with associated photophobia or phonophobia); and the postdrome (symptoms of fatigue and exhaustion once the headache resolves). More frequent in female (17%) than in male (6%) patients. Migraine without aura is the most common type (75%). In children, migraine headaches can present as abdominal pain.

EXAM TIPS

- Migraines can last from 3 hours to 72 hours.
- Cluster headaches are accompanied by eye redness and rhinorrhea; severe periorbital pain. Can occur several times a day. Spontaneously resolves. Common in middle-aged male patients. Treated with high-dose oxygen (caution in patients with COPD).

Classic Case

An adult woman complains of the gradual onset of a throbbing headache behind one eye that gradually worsens over several hours. Reports sensitivity to bright light (photophobia) and noise (phonophobia). Frequently accompanied by nausea and/or vomiting, which can be severe. Migraines can last from 3 to 72 hours; many attacks resolve during sleep (see Table 12.2).

Treatment Plan

Nonpharmacologic Interventions

- Acupuncture
- Rest in a quiet and darkened room with an ice pack to forehead.
- For nausea, drink ginger ale or cola; chew dry toast or saltine crackers.
- Aerobic exercise
- Transcutaneous electrical nerve stimulation
- As much as possible, avoid precipitating foods and activities, such as
  - Nitrates/nitrites found in hot dogs, luncheon meat, and sausage
  - Alcohol and caffeine
  - Sleep changes, stress, and barometric weather changes
  - Odor triggers such as tobacco smoke, perfumes, and other strong odors
  - Visual triggers such as strobe lights, sunlight, and glares
  - Emotional or physical stress

Pharmacologic Options

- Mild-to-moderate attacks: Analgesics (e.g., acetaminophen or NSAIDs alone or in combination) can be effective and considered as first line. If migraine headache with nausea or vomiting, also prescribe antiemetic drug. Educate patient that it is best to take pain medication as soon as pain starts.

- Moderate-to-severe attacks: Oral triptans or combination sumatriptan–NSAID/naproxen (Treximet). If associated with severe nausea or vomiting, non-oral agents such as subcutaneous sumatriptan (Imitrex), nasal sumatriptan, and zolmitriptan (Zomig) with antiemetic drug.
  - Triptans should be avoided in patients with history of ischemic heart disease, Prinzmetal's angina, ischemic stroke, uncontrolled hypertension, hemiplegic or basilar migraine and pregnancy.
  - Warn patient of possible flushing, tingling, chest/neck/sinus/jaw discomfort.
  - Supervise first dose, especially if patient has risk factors for cardiovascular disease (e.g., diabetes, obesity, male >40 years, high lipids). Give first dose in office (theoretical risk of an acute MI).
  - Consider EKG monitoring if patient is at high risk for heart disease.
  - Higher risk of serotonin syndrome if combined with selective serotonin reuptake inhibitors (SSRIs) or serotonin norepinephrine reuptake inhibitors (SNRIs; duloxetine [Cymbalta], venlafaxine [Effexor]). Do not combine or start within 2 weeks of monoamine oxidase inhibitor (MAOI) use.
  - Do not combine with ergots or within 24 hours of ergot use (e.g., ergotamine/caffeine [Cafergot]).
- Calcitonin gene-related peptide (CGRP) antagonists: Rimegepant (Nurtec), ubrogepant (Ubrelvy). Do not mix with ketoconazole, itraconazole, or clarithromycin. Do not mix with grapefruit juice or St. John's wort. Has numerous major drug interactions.
- Serotonin 5-HT-1F receptor agonist: Lasmiditan (Reyvow). Can be used for patients with relative contraindication to triptan due to cardiovascular risk factors. Do not use within 8 hours of driving or operating heavy machinery (causes dizziness).
- Ergots: Ergotamine preparations, alone and in combination with caffeine and other analgesics, can be used for the abortive treatment of migraines (e.g., dihydroergotamine [Migranal]).
  - Ergot alkaloids are potent vasoconstrictors.
  - Do not mix with other vasoconstrictors (e.g., triptans, decongestants).
  - Common side effect is nausea.
  - Ergots and triptans should not be given within 14 days of an MAOI.
- Antiemetics
  - Prochlorperazine: IM, IV, suppository, PO.
  - Trimethobenzamide (Tigan): IM, suppository, PO.
  - Ondansetron (Zofran): IM, IV, PO. Appear to be effective but not considered first-line treatment.

Prophylactic Treatment

Indicated if the headaches are frequent or long lasting or account for a significant amount of total disability.

- Beta-blockers: Propranolol (Inderal), metoprolol (Lopressor), nadolol (Corgard), atenolol (Tenormin)
- CCBs: Verapamil (Verelan), flunarizine (Sibelium), nifedipine (e.g., Adalat) can be used for migraine prevention (although efficacy of CCBs is weak overall)
- Angiotensin-converting enzyme (ACE) inhibitors/angiotensin receptor blockers (ARBs): Lisinopril (Zestril) and candesartan (Amias) have been shown to be effective in smaller studies
- Tricyclic antidepressants (TCAs): Amitriptyline (Elavil), nortriptyline (Pamelor)
- Selective norepinephrine reuptake inhibitor: Venlafaxine (Effexor)
- Anticonvulsants: Valproate (Depacon), topiramate (Topamax), gabapentin (Neurontin)

Migraine With Brainstem Aura

Rare subset of migraine with aura, previously called basilar migraine. Brainstem symptoms such as dysarthria, vertigo, or ataxia, without evidence of motor weakness. Symptoms resemble a stroke, except it is not accompanied by hemiplegia. Focal neurologic findings such as tinnitus, diplopia, bilateral visual symptoms, and bilateral paresthesia. These symptoms are part of the aura; then it is followed by a throbbing occipital headache and nausea. About 77% can have impairment in or loss of consciousness that can last 2 to 30 minutes. Treatment is similar to that for migraine headache with aura.

EXAM TIPS

- Distinguish the drugs used for abortive treatment versus chronic prophylaxis.
- Answer options may list the drug class instead of the generic name.

Tension-Type Headache

Bilateral, non-throbbing headache of mild to moderate intensity, typically without other features. Most prevalent headache. Three main subtypes: infrequent episodic (episodes less than 1 day a month), frequent episodic (1 to 14 days a month), and chronic (15 or more days per month). Influenced by environment, genetic factors, heightened sensitivity of pain pathways in the CNS (and likely the peripheral nervous system), and muscular factors.

Classic Case

An adult patient complains of a headache that is "band-like" and feels like "someone is squeezing my head." Pain is described as dull and constant, and is accompanied by tensing of the neck muscles (see Table 12.2). Patient reports recent increased life stressors. Headache lasts several days.

Treatment Plan

- NSAIDs such as naproxen sodium BID or ibuprofen QID or aspirin every 4 to 6 hours. Acetaminophen is an option if patient is unable to tolerate NSAIDs. If the patient has a poor response to NSAIDs, diclofenac TID can be used as an alternative. During pregnancy, acetaminophen is preferred.
- Combination drugs such as ibuprofen or aspirin with caffeine are an option for patients who do not get satisfactory pain relief from a single agent.
- Diagnosis should be reevaluated in patients who do not respond to initial treatment options to assess for other conditions.
- Limit butalbital use to three times or less per month. Current guidelines do not recommend the use of opioids or butalbital as initial therapy for tension-type headache. Muscle relaxants are not recommended due to lack of efficacy.
- For stress reduction and relaxation, have the patient try yoga, tai chi; exercise several times per week; gradually reduce and stop caffeine intake; follow regular eating/sleep schedule; pursue counseling with a therapist.

EXAM TIPS

- With the exception of tension headaches, most of the other types of headaches that may be seen on the exam cause unilateral pain.
- Muscle tension causes vise-like or tight in quality pain; may last for days.

COMMON DRUGS: HEADACHE TREATMENT

Acute Treatment (As Needed Only)
Nonsteroidal Anti-Inflammatory Drugs
- Naproxen sodium (Naprosyn, Aleve) BID or ibuprofen (Advil, Motrin) TID to QID
- Side effects include GI pain/bleeding/ulceration, renal damage, increased BP in hypertension

Triptans
- Administer sumatriptan succinate (Imitrex) injection, inhalant, PO tablets, or sublingual tablets. For acute pain, give injection subcutaneously (onset 10 minutes).
- Side effects include nausea; dizziness; vertigo; drowsiness; discomfort of throat, nose, and/or tongue.
- Contraindicated for patients with cardiovascular comorbidities, since it causes vasoconstriction (coronary artery spasm, MI, transient myocardial ischemia), arrythmias (atrial fibrillation, ventricular fibrillation, ventricular tachycardia).
- Triptans should not be given within 24 hours of an ergot.
- Do not give within 14 days of an MAOI.

Analgesics
- Acetaminophen (Tylenol) QID as needed
- Side effects include hepatic damage
- Prophylaxis (must be taken daily to be effective)

Prophylaxis
Tricyclic Antidepressants
- Amitriptyline (Elavil), nortriptyline, doxepin, or imipramine
- Side effects include sedation, dry mouth, confusion in older adults

Table 12.3 Treatment of Headaches

Headache	Acute Treatment	Prophylaxis/Other
Migraine	Ice pack on forehead; rest in quiet and darkened room Analgesic taken right away may provide some relief Sumatriptan SC injection; use injection or nasal spray formulation if severe nausea Antiemetics (e.g., prochlorperazine) for nausea	Antihypertensives: Beta-blockers (propranolol, metoprolol, nadolol, atenolol); calcium channel blockers (verapamil, nifidipine); ACE-inhibitors/ARBs (lisinopril, candesartan) Antidepressants: SNRI (venlafaxine) and amitriptyline (TCA) Anticonvulsants: Topiramate, valproate, gabapentin
Giant cell arteritis	High-dose glucocorticoids	Requires routine monitoring of disease activity to evaluate patient's response to therapy
Cluster	Inhalation of 100% oxygen at 12 L/min for 15 minutes Triptans sumatriptan, zolmitriptan Alternatives include: intranasal lidocaine, oral ergotamine, and IV dihydroergotamine	Initial preventative therapy with verapamil (for those with frequent attacks) or glucocorticoids (for those with less frequent attacks)
Trigeminal neuralgia	Initial therapy: Carbamazepine (Tegretol) or oxcarbazepine Alternatives and adjuncts: gabapentin, lamotrigine, phenytoin, or baclofen	Continue medical therapy before attempting a gradual wean (goal for a sustained pain-free interval of at least 6 to 8 weeks); watch for drug interactions
Muscle tension	OTC analgesics (e.g., NSAIDs, acetaminophen), warm bath/shower, massage	Stress reduction, yoga, relaxation, biofeedback

ACE, angiotensin-converting enzymes; ARBs, angiotensin receptor blockers; IM, intramuscular; NSAIDs, nonsteroidal anti-inflammatory drugs; OTC, over the counter; SC, subcutaneous; SNRI, serotonin–norepinephrine reuptake inhibitor; TCAs, tricyclic antidepressants.

Beta-Blockers
- Propranolol (Inderal LA) or atenolol (Tenormin) daily. Careful with older patients.
- Contraindications include second- or third-degree atrioventricular (AV) block, asthma, COPD, bradycardia

Selective Norepinephrine and Serotonin Inhibitors
Venlafaxine (Effexor) daily at bedtime. Consider if patient has both migraine and depression, generalized anxiety disorder, panic disorder, chronic anxiety.

Antiseizure Medications
- Topiramate (Topamax)
- If discontinuing drug, withdraw gradually over a few weeks to minimize risk of seizures or withdrawal symptoms

SEIZURES
Affect 8% to 10% of the population. Intermittent, usually self-limiting. Acute symptomatic seizure occurs at the time of systemic insult or in close association with a documented brain insult. Unprovoked seizures occur in relation to a preexisting brain lesion or progressive nervous system disorder. Seizures can be categorized as focal, generalized, or unknown (if onset is missed or obscured). Epilepsy is characterized by recurrent, unprovoked seizures; epileptic seizures can be focal or generalized.

Focal Seizures
- Focal seizure with retained awareness: Previously called simple partial seizure; symptoms vary depending on which part of the cortex is disrupted.
- Focal seizure with impaired awareness: Previously called complex partial seizure; most common type in adults with epilepsy. Patient appears awake but is not in contact with others in their environment.

Generalized Seizures
- Generalized tonic-clonic seizure: Also called grand mal seizure, major motor seizure, or convulsions; most common type of generalized seizure. Begins with abrupt loss of consciousness; extremities become stiff, and patient may appear cyanotic. Muscles begin to jerk and twitch. Tongue may be bitten.
- Absence seizure: Previously called petit mal; common in childhood; usually lasts 5 to 10 seconds; onset marked by behavioral arrest
- Atypical absence seizure: Often longer, slower onset and offset; blank staring with impaired consciousness, change in muscle tone and movement, repetitive blinking
- Clonic seizure: Rhythmic jerking muscle contractions usually involving arms, neck, and face
- Myoclonic seizure: Sudden, brief muscle contractions alone or in clusters; arms typically involved
- Tonic seizure: Causes sudden muscle stiffening, often with impaired consciousness and falling
- Atonic seizure: Also called drop seizure. Sudden loss of muscle control, usually in legs, that causes collapse to the ground

Classic Case
Adult patient presents after abrupt onset of a generalized tonic-clonic seizure witnessed by their significant other. The patient experienced loss of consciousness, loss of posture, and muscle stiffness of the arms and legs and then the chest and back. This was followed by brief, violent, generalized contractions with progressively longer muscle relaxation, foamy salivation, and biting of the tongue. The patient presents with confusion and suppressed alertness. The spouse describes the seizure because the patient is not able to remember it.

Treatment Plan
- Airway assessment and stabilization of vital signs and airway, followed by obtaining a detailed description of the seizure and the events immediately before it
- Tests including CBC, serum electrolytes, blood glucose, calcium, magnesium, renal function, liver functions, UA, toxicology screen
- Electroencephalogram (EEG) is essential for diagnosis of epileptic seizure
- LP if concern for acute infectious process
- MRI (preferred over CT due to superior sensitivity in detecting causes of seizure and epilepsy)
- Initiation of antiseizure medications (see "Pharmacotherapy," below); not always indicated after a first unprovoked seizure
- Referral to a neurologist
- Indications for hospitalization include first seizure with prolonged postictal state, incomplete recovery after seizure, serious seizure-related injury, status epilepticus, presence of neurologic or systemic illness requiring further attention

Pharmacotherapy
- Antiseizure medication should be initiated in patients with two or more unprovoked seizures.
- Choosing initial therapy involves weighing risks and benefits based on patient-specific data, along with consideration of seizure type, other prescribed medications, and comorbidities.
- More than 25 approved antiseizure medications for adults and/or children include carbamazepine, clobazam, gabapentin, lamotrigine, levetiracetam, phenobarbital, phenytoin, topiramate, valproate.

Seizure Precautions
- Avoid common triggers or precipitating factors such as sleep deprivation, alcohol use, infection, and certain medications
- Avoid unsupervised activities that could be dangerous with sudden loss of consciousness (e.g., bathing, swimming alone, working at heights, operating heavy machinery)
- Patients should be counseled about driving restrictions and understand specific driving limitations

TRANSIENT ISCHEMIC ATTACK
A transient ischemic attack (TIA) is a transient episode of neurologic dysfunction caused by focal ischemia (brain,

spinal cord, or retinal ischemia) without acute infarction of the brain as seen in stroke. The "time-based" definition, which considered timing of 24 hours for resolution, has been replaced by the "tissue-based" definition. It is now more widely understood that permanent neurologic damage can occur with even relatively brief ischemia. TIA is a neurologic emergency and major warning sign. A patient who has a TIA is at higher risk for a subsequent stroke and needs urgent evaluation and treatment.

Depending on severity of the TIA, the signs and symptoms can be subtle to severe. The longer the episode of the TIA, the higher the risk of ischemic brain damage. Typical TIAs cause transient, focal neurologic symptoms that can be located to a single vascular territory in the brain, including transient monocular blindness, aphasia or dysarthria, hemianopia, hemiparesis, and/or hemisensory loss. Atypical TIAs present a loss of some neurologic function.

The ABCD^2 score (*Age, Blood* pressure, *Clinical* features, *Duration* of symptoms, and *Diabetes*) is a clinical prediction tool that helps to predict who is at high risk for suffering a subsequent stroke after a TIA within the first 7 days (Table 12.4).

> **NOTE**
>
> While it can be used to stratify patients according to stroke risk and identify those who need emergency evaluation, the ABCD^2 score predictive performance is not satisfactory. The combination of the ABCD^2 score along with other risk stratification models, brain and vascular imaging, and patient-specific TIA etiology may improve the accuracy of stroke risk prediction after TIA.

Classic Case

Older adult patient reports acute onset of one-sided weakness of the right arm and right leg accompanied by dizziness, vertigo, and poor balance. The patient is difficult to understand because speech is slurred (dysphasia). When patient is instructed to smile and grimace, the right side of the face has no movement and is lopsided. Patient is accompanied by a significant other who reports that the patient has a history of hypertension, atrial fibrillation, hyperlipidemia, and type 2 diabetes. The signs and symptoms eventually resolve, but the patient remains at higher risk of a future stroke.

Risk Factors for Recurrent Ischemic Stroke After Transient Ischemic Attack

- Age ≥60 years
- History of TIA or ischemic stroke within 30 days of index event
- History of diabetes
- Systolic BP ≥140 mmHg OR diastolic BP ≥90 mmHg
- Unilateral weakness
- Isolated speech disturbance
- TIA duration >10 minutes
- Prescence of vascular pathologies (e.g., large artery atherosclerosis, small vessel disease)
- Prescence of acute infarction on MRI or acute or chronic ischemic lesions on CT

"FAST" Mnemonic for Recognizing Stroke

F Face drooping (Instruct patient to smile. Is face lopsided?)
A Arm weakness (Instruct patient to raise both arms. Does one arm drift downward?)
S Speech difficulty (Instruct patient to say, "The sky is blue.")
T Time to call 911 (Even if symptoms go away, call 911.)

Hospitalization Criteria

Hospitalization is recommended for patients with a first TIA (within the past 72 hours) if any of the following conditions are met:

- Presence of known cardiac, arterial, or systemic etiology of brain ischemia that is amenable to treatment
- Acute infarction noted on MRI imaging
- Concurrent serious acute medical issues
- Uncertainty that diagnostic workup can be completed within 24 to 48 hours in the outpatient setting

Treatment Plan

- Refer patient to outpatient specialty TIA clinics or the ED for further evaluation. Find out cause of TIA (or stroke), such as atrial fibrillation, carotid/vertebral atherosclerosis, hypercoagulable state, cocaine use, hypertension. Perform workup to find the extent of brain damage.
- Schedule CT and/or MRI scan as soon as possible (within first 24 hours of the episode). While MRI with diffusion-weighted imaging is considered superior and more specific, noncontrast CT of the head is the standard imaging study for early acute stroke evaluation due to its widespread availability, rapid scan times, and sensitivity for ICH.

Table 12.4 ABCD^2 Score

Risk Factor	Points	Score
Age >65 years	1	
BP when first assessed after TIA: ■ Systolic ≥140 mmHg or diastolic ≥90 mmHg	1	
Clinical features of TIA (choose one only): ■ Unilateral weakness with/without speech impairment ■ Speech impairment without unilateral weakness	2 1	
Duration: ■ TIA duration >60 minutes ■ TIA duration 10–59 minutes	2 1	
Diabetes	1	
Total ABCD^2 score	**(0–7)**	

BP, blood pressure; TIA, transient ischemic attack.

- Start immediate antiplatelet therapy for patients with TIA who do not have a known cardioembolic source at presentation. Exceptions include patients on oral anticoagulation or with a clear new indication for anticoagulation.
  - Low-risk TIA, ABCD^2 score <4: aspirin alone (162 to 325 mg/day).
  - High-risk TIA (ABCD^2 score ≥4): Initiate dual antiplatelet therapy (DAPT) using aspirin (160 to 325 mg loading dose, followed by 50 to 100 mg daily) plus clopidogrel (300 to 600 mg loading dose, followed by 75 mg daily) for the first 21 days. Alternative: Aspirin (300 to 325 mg loading dose, followed by 75 to 100 mg daily) plus ticagrelor (180 mg loading dose followed by 90 mg twice daily)
  - For cardiac evaluation, perform EKG, continuous cardiac monitoring, echocardiography to evaluate for cardioembolic source
  - Tests include CBC, coagulation panel, serum electrolytes and creatinine, fasting blood glucose, lipid panel, hemoglobin A1C, ESR, and CRP
  - For intensive risk factor management, maintain BP <140/90 mmHg; LDL-C lowering with high-intensity statin therapy; glucose control; physical activity; smoking cessation; weight reduction, adequate nutrition; and alcohol reduction.

TRIGEMINAL NEURALGIA (TIC DOULOUREUX)

The trigeminal nerve (CN V) has three divisions: the ophthalmic (V1), maxillary (V2), and mandibular (V3) branches. Most cases are caused by compression of the nerve root by an artery, vein, or tumor, causing a unilateral electric shock–like facial pain that follows one of the branches of the trigeminal nerve. The pain is usually located close to the nasal border and cheeks, but it can move to other areas of the face. There are three types: classic, secondary (underlying disease), and idiopathic.

More common in women; most idiopathic and classic cases start after age 50 years (see Table 12.2).

Classic Case

An older adult complains of the sudden onset of severe and sharp, shooting pains on one side of the face or around the nose that are triggered by chewing, eating cold foods, and cold air. The severe lacerating pain (piercing knifelike pain) lasts a few seconds to 2 minutes. Pain is precipitated by a stimulus on any area of the trigeminal nerve. The patient may stop chewing or speaking momentarily (few seconds) if it causes the pain. Has recurrent paroxysms of unilateral facial pain that follow the distribution of the trigeminal nerve (CN V).

EXAM TIP

Trigeminal neuralgia (tic douloureux) is pain on one side of face/cheek, precipitated by talking, chewing, cold food, or cold air on affected area.

Treatment Plan

- First-line treatment is carbamazepine (Tegretol) or oxcarbazepine (Trileptal).
- Alternatives and/or adjuncts to first-line therapy include gabapentin (Neurontin), lamotrigine (Lamictal), or baclofen.
- Rescue therapy for analgesia while oral medications are titrated includes IV lidocaine, phenytoin, or fosphenytoin, or subcutaneous injections of sumatriptan.
- Obtain MRI or CT scan to rule out a tumor/artery pressing on a nerve or MS. Surgery may be indicated for medically refractory cases (e.g., microvascular decompression, rhizotomy, radiofrequency, nerve block).

KNOWLEDGE CHECK: CHAPTER 12

1. A patient is asked to stand with feet together and arms at their sides and to close their eyes for 30 to 60 seconds without support. The clinician notices that the patient loses their balance. The clinician then whispers a few numbers and asks the patient to repeat what they've heard. Which cranial nerve is being tested?
   A. VIII
   B. X
   C. V
   D. VII

2. The knee-jerk reflex is affected by which of the following nerve roots?
   A. C5-6
   B. C6-7
   C. L2-4
   D. S1

3. A patient presents with a temperature of 100.94°F (38.3°C), nuchal rigidity, and a change in mental status. The patient has a decreased level of consciousness and a history of a recent seizure within a week of initiation of symptoms. Blood glucose is 101 mg/dL. A complete blood count (CBC) and serum electrolytes are pending, but blood cultures have not yet been obtained. Which of the following is the next priority intervention?
   A. Lumbar puncture
   B. Head CT scan
   C. Administration of acetaminophen for the fever
   D. Initiation of antimicrobial therapy

4. A patient presents following a focal motor seizure. The family is concerned that the patient may be experiencing another seizure because the patient is still confused. Physical assessment findings are significant for weakness of the right arm and an altered level of consciousness. These findings likely represent which of the following?
   A. Generalized status epilepticus
   B. Aura
   C. Postictal period
   D. Myoclonic seizure

5. Which of the following disease states has been found to be associated with giant cell arteritis?
   A. Polymyalgia rheumatica
   B. Trigeminal neuralgia
   C. Bell's palsy
   D. Multiple sclerosis

6. Which of the following is a risk factor for a recurrent ischemic stroke after a transient ischemic attack (TIA)?
   A. Age 50 years
   B. Past medical history of hyperlipidemia
   C. Initial blood pressure of 160/90 mmHg after TIA
   D. Duration of TIA symptoms >8 minutes

7. A patient presents with a throbbing headache with visual disturbances. The patient reports seeing a bright spot with an area of visual loss. Which of the following precipitating factors may have exacerbated this type of headache?
   A. Drinking wine
   B. Overeating
   C. Consuming monosodium glutamate
   D. Chewing

8. A 23-year-old female patient is seen in the office by the nurse practitioner for complaints of weakness, poor balance, and problems with walking. She states, "I am so clumsy. Sometimes I fall when I walk." She reports new-onset vision loss and bladder incontinence. Each episode lasts a few days; she has had several in the past 6 months. When she bends her head forward to tie her shoes, she reports a sharp shooting sensation from the upper to lower back. She is anxious and crying. What is the most likely diagnosis for this patient?
   A. Vitamin B_{12} deficiency
   B. Trigeminal neuralgia
   C. Multiple sclerosis
   D. Myasthenia gravis

(See answers next page.)

1. A) VIII

Cranial nerve VIII (the vestibulocochlear nerve) is responsible for both hearing and vestibular function. Hearing is often assessed via the whispered voice test by asking if the patient can repeat whispered words. Vestibular function is tested with the Romberg test, which tests position sense and balance. Loss of balance is a positive sign, which can indicate cerebellar ataxia/dysfunction or sensory loss. Cranial nerve X, vagus, is often assessed by asking the patient to say "Ah" and observing whether the two sides of the palate move fully and symmetrically. Injury to cranial nerve V, trigeminal, would be indicated by dysfunction in facial sensation or facial strength. Cranial nerve VII, facial, can be assessed by asking the patient to form specific facial expressions to assess for facial symmetry.

2. C) L2-4

The affected nerve roots for the commonly tested deep tendon reflexes are as follows: the biceps and brachioradialis reflexes: C5-6, the triceps reflex: C6-7, the patellar reflex: L2-4, and the Achilles reflex: S1 root.

3. B) Head CT scan

The patient is presenting with the classic triad of bacterial meningitis: fever, nuchal rigidity, and a change in mental status. A head CT should be performed before a lumbar puncture if the following risk factors are present: papilledema, focal neurologic deficit, abnormal level of consciousness, new-onset seizure (within 1 week of presentation), history of central nervous system disease (stroke, mass), or immunocompromise (HIV, immunosuppressive therapy, solid organ or bone marrow transplant). While initial laboratory tests, such as a CBC, serum electrolytes, glucose, and coagulation studies, are necessary, the priority is to obtain two aerobic blood cultures and obtain a CT scan prior to the lumbar puncture. Antimicrobial therapy should be initiated as soon as possible after obtaining two aerobic blood cultures.

4. C) Postictal period

After a seizure, the postictal period is the transition from the ictal state back to the patient's baseline level. It is not uncommon for patients to remain confused and have suppressed alertness. Focal neurologic deficits may be present, such as weakness of a hand, arm, or leg that appears following a focal motor seizure involving one side of the body. The postictal state may last only seconds or up to a few hours depending on the part of the brain affected, length of the seizure, medications received, and patient age. An aura is often described as the warning symptom that the patient experiences at the beginning of a seizure. While auras are focal seizures that can cause symptoms, they do not interfere with consciousness. Generalized status epilepticus is less likely because the clinical manifestations are confined to focal movement to one arm, rather than generalized bilateral tonic-clonic movements. A myoclonic seizure is a type of generalized seizure, characterized by sudden, brief muscle contractions that may occur singly or in clusters; impaired consciousness is not common.

5. A) Polymyalgia rheumatica

There is a frequent clinical association between polymyalgia rheumatica and giant cell arteritis. Polymyalgia rheumatica occurs in approximately 50% of patients with giant cell arteritis. About 5% to 30% of patients with polymyalgia rheumatica experience giant cell arteritis. Polymyalgia rheumatica can precede, accompany, or occur after giant cell arteritis. Trigeminal neuralgia, Bell's palsy, and multiple sclerosis have not been found to be associated with giant cell arteritis.

6. C) Initial blood pressure of 160/90 mmHg after TIA

Risk factors for recurrent ischemic stroke after a TIA include age 60 years or older; history of TIA or ischemic stroke within 30 days of index event (1.5%–3.5% in the first 48 hours); history of diabetes; systolic BP ≥140 mmHg or diastolic BP ≥90 mmHg; unilateral weakness; isolated speech disturbance; TIA duration greater than 10 minutes; presence of vascular pathologies (e.g., large artery atherosclerosis, small vessel disease); and presence of acute infarction on MRI or acute or chronic ischemic lesions on CT.

7. A) Drinking wine

Based on the patient's symptoms, the patient is likely presenting with a migraine with an aura, which often involves visual disturbances. An evidence-based review found that stress, menstruation, visual stimuli, weather changes, consuming nitrates, fasting (not overeating, unless it involves specific triggering foods), drinking wine, sleep disturbances, and consuming aspartame are migraine trigger factors. While consuming monosodium glutamate was found to be a general headache trigger, it was unproven as a migraine trigger. Chewing is an aggravating factor for trigeminal neuralgia.

8. C) Multiple sclerosis

The patient's symptoms are highly suggestive of multiple sclerosis, an autoimmune disease that affects the spine and brain. The peak incidence is from age 15 to 45 years. To confirm the diagnosis, an MRI of the spinal cord and brain is necessary. Lhermitte sign is the sharp, shooting, electric-shock sensation from upper to lower spine with neck flexion.

9. The nurse practitioner is instructing the patient to flex both wrists at 90 degrees for 1 minute. A positive test suggests which of the following?
   A. Median nerve inflammation
   B. Meningeal irritation
   C. Appropriate brachioradialis reflex
   D. Scaphoid bone fracture

10. Which of the following is a contraindication for prescribing the "triptan" drug class?
   A. Peptic ulcer disease
   B. Ischemic heart disease
   C. Acute kidney injury
   D. Hepatic impairment

11. Which cranial nerve(s) (CN) is(are) responsible for tongue movement?
   A. VIII
   B. IX and X
   C. XI
   D. XII

12. The clinician places a coin in the patient's palm and asks the patient to identify the object with their eyes closed. This is an example of which test of cortical sensory function?
   A. Graphesthesia
   B. Two-point discrimination
   C. Stereognosis
   D. Light touch

13. When testing the patellar reflex, a brisker-than-average response is observed. This is indicated by which grade of the deep tendon reflex grading scale?
   A. 0
   B. 2+
   C. 1+
   D. 3+

14. The clinician assesses for facial symmetry when asking the patient to raise their eyebrows, squeeze their eyes shut, frown, smile, and puff their cheeks out. Which cranial nerve (CN) is being evaluated?
   A. II
   B. VII
   C. VI
   D. VIII

15. A patient presents with a fever, nuchal rigidity, and altered mental status. During the assessment, the clinician gently raises the patient's head and notices spontaneous flexion of the patient's hips and knees. Based on this finding, which of the following tests should also be performed?
   A. Brudzinski sign
   B. Lachman test
   C. Valgus stress test
   D. Kernig sign

16. An older adult patient presents after a few days of generalized fatigue with a headache over the temple region. The patient reports a low-grade fever, jaw claudication, and transient monocular visual loss. Based on this clinical presentation, which of the following is indicated for diagnosis?
   A. Temporal artery biopsy
   B. Erythrocyte sedimentation rate
   C. C-reactive protein
   D. CT scan

17. Bell's palsy is associated with dysfunction of which cranial nerve (CN)?
   A. III
   B. VII
   C. VIII
   D. XI

(See answers next page.)

9. A) Median nerve inflammation

The test being performed is Phalen's test; it is positive when the patient reports that their fingers (including the thumb) feel numb or tingle. Inflammation of the median nerve is called carpal tunnel syndrome. Kernig's sign (pain with knee extension) and Brudzinski's sign (patient bends hips and knees in response to neck flexion) are special tests for when meningeal irritation is suspected. The brachioradialis reflex is elicited when the nurse practitioner strikes the brachioradial tendon 1 to 2 inches above the wrist, causing forearm pronation and elbow flexion. A scaphoid fracture is a break in one of the small bones of the wrist.

10. B) Ischemic heart disease

Due to limited evidence, it is recommended that triptans be avoided in patients with hemiplegic or basilar migraine, ischemic stroke, ischemic heart disease, Prinzmetal's angina, uncontrolled hypertension, and pregnancy. While a systematic review found no association between triptan use and risk of cardiovascular events, only four relevant studies were identified. Of note, all triptans should be limited to less than 10 days of use per month to avoid medication overuse headache.

11. D) XII

CN XII is responsible for tongue movement. The patient should be told to stick out their tongue; it should be midline. The nurse practitioner should be told to look for atrophy and fasciculations (small, involuntary, flicker-like movements of the tongue).

12. C) Stereognosis

Stereognosis tests the patient's ability to identify a familiar object by touch. Graphesthesia involves writing a number or shape on the palm of the patient's hand and asking the patient to identify what was drawn. Two-point discrimination involves using two ends of a cotton swab and touching the patient's skin at various locations. The patient should be able to identify one- or two-point touch. Light touch tests primary sensory functions and involves lightly touching the skin and asking the patient to respond when and where the sensation was felt.

13. D) 3+

The deep tendon reflex grading scale is used when assessing the biceps, brachioradialis, triceps, patellar, and Achilles reflexes. Grade 0 is no response; Grade 1+ is sluggish or diminished response; Grade 2+ is active or expected response (normal); Grade 3+ is brisker-than-average/slightly hyperactive; and Grade 4+ is brisk/hyperactive.

14. B) VII

CN VII, the facial nerve, can be assessed by asking the patient to form specific facial expressions to assess for facial symmetry. The optic nerve (CN II) can be assessed via distant and near vision tests, ophthalmoscopic examination, and testing for visual fields by confrontation and extinction. The abducens nerve, CN VI, can be evaluated by lateral eye movement. The acoustic nerve, CN VIII, can be evaluated by the whisper test.

15. D) Kernig sign

The patient is presenting with the classic triad of acute bacterial meningitis symptoms: fever, nuchal rigidity, and change in mental status. Specific tests (the Brudzinki sign and Kernig sign) are used when meningeal irritation is suspected, which can occur with meningitis or subarachnoid hemorrhage. The Brudzinski sign refers to spontaneous flexion of the hips during passive flexion of the neck. The Kernig sign is often performed in conjunction with this positive finding and refers to the inability to allow full extension of the knee when the hip is flexed 90 degrees. The Lachman and valgus stress tests are also assessments for the knee but are not specific to an examination for meningeal irritation. The valgus stress test helps to identify injury to the medial collateral ligament. The Lachman test is used to identify a tear to the anterior cruciate ligament.

16. A) Temporal artery biopsy

The patient is presenting with symptoms suggestive of giant cell arteritis (GCA). It should be considered in any patient older than 50 years who presents with a new headache, abrupt onset of visual disturbances, jaw claudication, unexplained fever, and signs/symptoms of vascular abnormalities. While laboratory data can aid in the evaluation of GCA, they are not specific and cannot be relied on as evidence to support a definitive diagnosis. Diagnosis of GCA should be confirmed by temporal artery biopsy or temporal artery color Doppler ultrasound. Imaging with MRI with MR angiography can be useful for diagnosis, but PET, CT, and CT with angiography lack ability to visualize the temporal artery.

17. B) VII

Bell's palsy refers to isolated peripheral facial paralysis (CN VII). Inflammation of the facial nerve causes weakness of the upper and lower portions of the face. The facial nerve allows for facial expression, taste, lacrimation, salivation, and ear sensation. CN III is the oculomotor nerve; CN VIII is the acoustic nerve; and CN XI refers to the spinal accessory.

18. A patient presents with a severe, unilateral, stabbing headache. The patient reports that the pain is localized in the periorbital region and also reports rhinorrhea. Upon physical assessment, ptosis and conjunctival injection are noted. Based on this clinical presentation, which of the following is indicated for initial acute therapy?
    A. Ibuprofen (Motrin) 400 mg
    B. Acetaminophen (Tylenol) 1,000 mg
    C. Oxygen therapy at 12 L/min for 15 minutes
    D. Propranolol (Inderal) 40 mg daily

19. Which of the following tests evaluates cerebellar function?
    A. Pronator drift
    B. Stereognosis
    C. Vibration test
    D. Finger-to-nose test

20. A patient presents with unilateral burning and stabbing facial pain. During assessment, the clinician notices that the pain is localized to the cheek and chin area and worsens while the patient is talking and swallowing. The pain lasts for less than 2 minutes, and the patient reports an electric shock–like pain quality. Based on this clinical presentation, *first-line* pharmacotherapy includes which of the following?
    A. Gabapentin (Neurontin)
    B. Carbamazepine (Tegretol)
    C. Baclofen (Lioresal)
    D. Lamotrigine (Lamictal)

21. A patient presents following a seizure. A family member reports that the patient suddenly lost control of their leg muscles and fell to the ground. This finding suggests which type of generalized seizure?
    A. Atonic
    B. Absence
    C. Clonic
    D. Tonic

22. A ruptured intracranial aneurysm is often the cause of which type of stroke?
    A. Embolic
    B. Intracerebral hemorrhage
    C. Subarachnoid hemorrhage
    D. Thrombotic

23. Which of the following is an indication for hospital admission for a patient with a mild traumatic brain injury?
    A. Glasgow Coma Scale score of 15
    B. No intracranial abnormalities noted on head CT
    C. Headache
    D. Recurrent vomiting

24. Which medication is indicated for acute treatment of a moderate-to-severe migraine attack?
    A. Sumatriptan (Imitrex)
    B. Metoprolol (Lopressor)
    C. Amitriptyline (Elavil)
    D. Topiramate (Topamax)

25. A patient presents with an acute sudden onset of altered mental status. The patient states that they got up to urinate during the night and developed sudden weakness of their face and arm. During the assessment, the clinician notes a facial droop, ataxia, nystagmus, and right-sided weakness. Cardiac auscultation reveals a fast-paced irregular rhythm with a murmur. Based on these physical exam findings, the clinician is concerned for which of the following stroke types?
    A. Intracerebral hemorrhage
    B. Thrombotic
    C. Subarachnoid hemorrhage
    D. Embolic

(See answers next page.)

18. C) Oxygen therapy at 12 L/min for 15 minutes

The patient is presenting with clinical features suggestive of a cluster headache. Clinical features include severe, unilateral, sharp or stabbing pain, with autonomic symptoms ipsilateral to the headache such as ptosis, miosis, lacrimation, conjunctival injection, rhinorrhea, and/or nasal congestion. Initial acute therapy includes either oxygen inhalation or pharmacotherapy with triptans (e.g., subcutaneous sumatriptan) for treatment of an acute cluster headache attack. The acute treatment of a tension-type headache and mild-to-moderate migraine attacks includes simple analgesics such as ibuprofen (Motrin) or acetaminophen (Tylenol). Propranolol (Inderal) has been established as an effective treatment option for migraine prevention.

19. D) Finger-to-nose test

The finger-to-nose test allows the clinician to test the accuracy of movements to assess for cerebellar function. Other coordination tests include rapid alternating movements, finger tapping, and heel-to-shin testing. Pronator drift is also a motor examination but assesses an upper motor neuron pattern of weakness that causes the arm to pronate and drift downward when the patient is asked to hold it extended with palms up. Stereognosis is a test of cortical sensory function; it assesses for the ability to identify a familiar object by touch (such as a key or a coin in the patient's hand). The vibration test is used to test the sensory system by asking the patient to identify where the buzzing sensation is felt when placing a low-pitched tuning fork on various bony prominences.

20. B) Carbamazepine (Tegretol)

The patient is presenting with symptoms consistent with trigeminal neuralgia. Initial pharmacotherapy treatment includes carbamazepine (Tegretol) or oxcarbazepine (Trileptal). Alternatives and adjuncts to first-line therapy include baclofen (Lioresal), lamotrigine (Lamictal), and gabapentin (Neurontin) for patients who are intolerant or have contraindications to carbamazepine (Tegretol) or oxcarbazepine (Trileptal).

21. A) Atonic

Subtypes of generalized seizures include absence (more common in childhood), clonic, myoclonic, tonic, and atonic seizures. Atonic seizures (also known as drop seizures) are characterized by a sudden loss of control of the muscles (usually the legs), which causes the patient to fall to the ground. Absence seizures are characterized by behavioral arrest along with staring and a blank facial expression. Clonic seizures cause rhythmic, jerking muscle contractions. Tonic seizures cause muscle stiffening along with impaired consciousness.

22. C) Subarachnoid hemorrhage

Most spontaneous subarachnoid hemorrhagic strokes are caused by ruptured intracranial aneurysms. Embolic and thrombotic strokes are both ischemic, often caused by an obstruction or blocked arterial access in a particular brain region. An intracerebral hemorrhage is often the cause of hypertension, amyloid angiopathy, and ruptured vascular malformation.

23. D) Recurrent vomiting

Hospital admission is recommended for patients at risk for immediate complications after a mild traumatic brain injury, including those with a Glasgow Coma Scale score of less than 15, seizures or other neurologic deficit(s), recurrent vomiting, abnormal head CT (e.g., midline shift, hemorrhage, ischemia, mass effect), and abnormal bleeding parameters or oral anticoagulation.

24. A) Sumatriptan (Imitrex)

Sumatriptan (Imitrex) is indicated for the acute treatment of a moderate-to-severe migraine attack. Pharmacologic options for prophylactic treatment of migraines include beta-blockers such as metoprolol (Lopressor) and propranolol (Inderal), antidepressants such as amitriptyline (Elavil) and venlafaxine (Effexor), and anticonvulsants such as valproate (Depakote) and topiramate (Topamax). Prophylactic treatment of migraines is indicated for patients with frequent (e.g., four or more headaches per month) or long-lasting (e.g., 12 hours or more) migraines or those that cause significant disability or reduce quality of life.

25. D) Embolic

Embolic strokes often arise from a source in the heart, aorta, or large vessels. Symptoms have a sudden onset but may improve quickly. Cardiac findings, especially atrial fibrillation, murmurs, and cardiac enlargement, suggest a cardiac-origin embolism. Embolic strokes can be precipitated by getting up at night to urinate or by sudden coughing or sneezing. A thrombotic stroke is less likely because thrombotic strokes often present with fluctuating symptoms, varying between normal and abnormal, progressing in a stepwise fashion with some periods of improvement. A subarachnoid hemorrhage is less likely because the patient does not report a headache (which is an invariable symptom). An intracerebral hemorrhage is less likely because in contrast to brain embolism and subarachnoid hemorrhage, the neurologic symptoms for an intracerebral hemorrhage do not begin abruptly and are not maximal at onset.

26. A patient who recently had an ischemic stroke presents with speech difficulties. The family reports that the patient seems to understand what they are saying, but their responses seem unusual. For example, the patient states, "Walk dog," when they mean to say, "I'm taking the dog for a walk." This suggests which complication following a stroke?
    A. Homonymous hemianopia
    B. Broca's aphasia
    C. Apraxia
    D. Wernicke's aphasia

27. A patient presents with acute right-sided weakness, aphasia, and a facial droop. Based on this clinical presentation, which of the following diagnostic tests is the priority to obtain *first* to guide further treatment decisions?
    A. MRI brain without contrast
    B. CT angiography
    C. MRI brain with contrast
    D. CT head without contrast

28. A patient presents with complaints of a severe, unilateral, pulsating headache. The patient also reports nausea and increased sensitivity to light. Based on this clinical presentation, which of the following pharmacotherapy options would be appropriate for acute treatment?
    A. Supplemental oxygen therapy
    B. Sumatriptan (Imitrex)
    C. Propranolol (Inderal)
    D. High-dose steroids

29. A 60-year-old patient presents with a high fever, severe headache, stiff neck, and acute mental status changes. A head CT confirms no acute intracranial abnormalities. The patient has no known immune deficiency. After obtaining blood cultures and performing a lumbar puncture, which of the following antimicrobial regimens is indicated based on this patient presentation?
    A. Vancomycin (Vancocin), ampicillin (Omnipen), cefepime (Maxipime)
    B. Vancomycin (Vancocin), ampicillin (Omnipen), meropenem (Merrem)
    C. Vancomycin (Vancocin), moxifloxacin (Vigamox)
    D. Vancomycin (Vancocin), ceftriaxone (Rocephin), ampicillin (Omnipen)

30. A 54-year-old female patient complains of being "stressed out" at her new job. She reports daily headaches for several months and takes acetaminophen (Tylenol) to self-treat twice a day. She describes the headache as being band-like and dull and accompanied by tight neck muscles bilaterally. She denies nausea, vomiting, visual changes, and photophobia. Which of the following is appropriate management of this patient?
    A. Advise the patient to slowly taper acetaminophen (Tylenol) doses to avoid withdrawal
    B. Discontinue acetaminophen (Tylenol) and encourage stress reduction measures such as exercise and yoga
    C. Advise the patient to increase the acetaminophen (Tylenol) dosage frequency
    D. Start the patient on butalbital and discontinue acetaminophen (Tylenol)

(See answers next page.)

26. B) Broca's aphasia

Broca's aphasia is characterized by non-fluency with sparse output and incorrect grammar. Damage is usually to the frontal lobe. Patients may understand speech and know what they want to say, but they frequently speak in short phrases. Wernicke's aphasia is fluent aphasia with impaired comprehension and is associated with lesions in the posterior superior temporal gyrus. Patients with Wernicke's aphasia may speak in long, complete sentences that have no meaning; they also have difficulty understanding speech. Homonymous hemianopia (often caused by cerebral infarction and intracranial hemorrhage) is a visual field impairment involving the two right or the two left halves of the visual fields of both eyes. Apraxia, or dyspraxia, involves difficulty performing learned motor tasks.

27. D) CT head without contrast

Non-contrast head CT is the preferred imaging study for early and initial acute stroke evaluation due to its availability, rapid scan times, and sensitivity for intracranial hemorrhage or mass lesion. An initial non-contrast CT scan can confirm the ability to proceed with administration of tissue plasminogen activator, if indicated. Further work-up, including CT angiography or MRI, may be subsequently performed, but a non-contrast head CT is the priority due to its speed of acquisition and increased access. MRI reliably detects intracranial hemorrhage and is superior for the detection of acute ischemic stroke, but it is not as readily available and is more limited by patient contraindications or intolerance. A CT angiography is often performed during further evaluation to detect intracranial large vessel stenosis and occlusions.

28. B) Sumatriptan (Imitrex)

The patient is presenting with symptoms consistent with a migraine. Treatment for mild attacks includes simple analgesics (e.g., nonsteroidal anti-inflammatory drugs [NSAIDs], acetaminophen). Treatment for moderate-to-severe attacks includes triptans (e.g., sumatriptan [Imitrex]). Oxygen therapy is a treatment option for cluster headaches. Propranolol (Inderal) is indicated for the prophylactic treatment of migraines. Steroids are not indicated for the acute treatment of migraines.

29. D) Vancomycin (Vancocin), ceftriaxone (Rocephin), ampicillin (Omnipen)

The patient is presenting with symptoms concerning for bacterial meningitis, a medical emergency. Initial management is prompt initiation of empiric antimicrobial therapy after a lumbar puncture and head CT and immediately after blood cultures are obtained. Patients with no known immune deficiency with adequate renal function should be started on ceftriaxone (Rocephin) or cefotaxime (Claforan) plus vancomycin (Vancocin) plus ampicillin (Omnipen) (in patients older than 50 years). Immunocompromised patients (e.g., those with AIDS or lymphoma) need expanded gram-negative coverage. An appropriate regimen includes vancomycin (Vancocin) plus ampicillin (Omnipen) plus either cefepime (Maxipime) or meropenem (Merrem). Antimicrobial therapy should be tailored after culture and susceptibility data are available. Moxifloxacin (Vigamox) is an ophthalmic solution used to treat bacterial infections of the eye; it would not be an appropriate component of therapy for meningitis.

30. B) Discontinue the acetaminophen (Tylenol) and encourage stress reduction measures such as exercise and yoga

Common pain relievers such as acetaminophen (Tylenol) may contribute to medication overuse headaches. Discontinuation of the overused medication is appropriate management. The patient should stop the overused medication and start preventive therapy using an alternative strategy (e.g., stress reduction). Acetaminophen (Tylenol) can be stopped abruptly. In contrast, do not abruptly discontinue opioids, barbiturates (e.g., butalbital), and benzodiazepines; decrease the dose gradually over a slow taper to avoid withdrawal symptoms and seizures. Butalbital is a barbiturate, which can also contribute to medication overuse headaches. Nonpharmacologic therapies should be initiated first, before starting additional pharmacotherapy.

13 | HEMATOPOIETIC SYSTEM REVIEW

ACUTE BLOOD LOSS

Identify and manage the specific site of bleeding. When analyzing the complete blood count (CBC), be aware that the initial hemoglobin and hematocrit (during active bleeding) may be in the normal range if it is checked immediately. It may take several hours for the blood loss to show up in the CBC and the platelet count. The reticulocyte count (0.5%–2%) will increase within a few days. Reticulocytosis is a normal response in acute blood loss.

With acute blood loss of up to 15% of blood volume (class I hemorrhage), there is minimal increase in heart rate with no changes in blood pressure (BP) and respiratory rate. Acute blood loss of 15% to 30% of blood volume (class II hemorrhage) will cause tachycardia (heart rate 100–120 beats/minute), tachypnea (respiratory rate 20–24), and decrease in pulse pressure.

Significant drop in BP usually does not manifest until about 30% to 40% blood loss (severe hemorrhage). Tachycardia (pulse >120 beats/minute) and a weaker pulse, elevated respiratory rate, and diminished urine output and mental status changes will occur. Look for signs and symptoms of shock.

HEMOPHILIA A

The most common type of hemophilia in the United States is hemophilia A. An X-linked recessive disease that predominantly affects males who have only one X chromosome. Hemophilia A is caused by factor VIII deficiency.

Signs and symptoms include easy bruising, excessive bruising, bleeding into joints (hemarthrosis), delayed bleeding or bleeding for several hours to days (circumcision, dental extractions), severe bleeding with minor trauma, heavy menses, and hematuria. Medicines that increase bleeding, such as anticoagulants, aspirin, and nonsteroidal anti-inflammatory drugs (NSAIDs), should usually be avoided. The activated partial thromboplastin time (aPTT) is often prolonged, and the prothrombin time (PT), fibrinogen, and platelets are normal.

HODGKIN'S LYMPHOMA

A cancer of the beta lymphocytes (B cells). Night sweats, fevers, and pain with ingestion of alcoholic drinks. Generalized pruritus with painless enlarged lymph nodes (neck). Anorexia and weight loss. Higher incidence among young adults (20–40 years) or older adults (>60 years), males, and White and Black Americans; median age at diagnosis is

39 years in the United States Identified by the presence of Reed–Sternberg cells.

MULTIPLE MYELOMA

A cancer of the plasma cells. Symptoms of fatigue, weakness, and bone pain that is usually located in the back or chest. Causes proteinuria with Bence–Jones proteins, hypercalcemia, and normocytic anemia. More common in older adults; median age at diagnosis is 65 to 74 years.

NEUTROPENIA

The most common causes of neutropenia (often defined as an absolute neutrophil count [ANC] <1,500 cells/mcL) in adults are inherited disorders and drug-induced neutropenia. Many types of medications may cause neutropenia, such as psychotropics, antivirals, antibiotics, NSAIDs, antithyroids, angiotensin-converting enzyme inhibitors (ACEIs; enalapril, captopril), and propranolol. Initial evaluation includes a CBC with differential, blood smear, health history, medications (including over the counter [OTC]), and physical examination. If the patient is febrile and you suspect bacterial infection, urgent evaluation is important, since the patient is at high risk for bacteremia or sepsis. African Americans may have a slightly lower ANC (benign ethnic neutropenia).

NON-HODGKIN'S LYMPHOMA

A group of metalogic malignancies that are derived from B cell progenitors, T cell progenitors, mature B cells, mature T cells, or natural killer cells. Usually occurs in the older adult (>65 years) and presents with night sweats, fever, weight loss, generalized lymphadenopathy (painless). The prognosis is poor.

THROMBOCYTOPENIA

Thrombocytopenia is defined as a platelet count of <150,000/mcL. Normal platelet count ranges from 150,000 to 450,000/mcL. Symptoms usually do not show until the platelet count is <100,000/mcL. Look for easy bruising (ecchymosis, petechiae), bleeding gums, spontaneous nosebleeds, and hematuria.

VITAMIN B$_{12}$ DEFICIENCY

Gradual onset of symmetric peripheral neuropathy starting in the feet and/or arms. Other neurologic signs are numbness, ataxia (positive Romberg test), loss of vibration and position sense, impaired memory, and dementia (severe cases). Peripheral smear shows macro-ovalocytes, some megaloblasts, and multisegmented neutrophils (>five or six lobes). The mean corpuscular volume (MCV) is >100 fL (macrocytosis).

LABORATORY TESTING

LABORATORY NORMS

Hemoglobin

- Reported as concentration of hemoglobin in whole blood
- 13.6 to 16.9 g/dL in males
- 11.9 to 14.8 g/dL in females
- Vigorous physical activity, pregnancy, older age cause lower values
- Smoking, certain medications, dehydration or hypovolemia, high altitude cause higher values

Hematocrit

- The proportion of red blood cells (RBCs) in 1 mL of plasma
- 40% to 50% in males
- 5% to 43% in females

Mean Corpuscular Volume

A measure of the average size of the RBCs in a sample of blood. Normal value is 82.5 to 98 fL (femtoliter).

- MCV <80 fL with microcytic anemia
- MCV between 80 and 100 fL with normocytic anemia
- MCV >100 fL with macrocytic anemias

Mean Corpuscular Hemoglobin Concentration

- A measure of the average hemoglobin concentration per RBC
- Decreased in iron-deficiency anemia (IDA) and thalassemia (hypochromic); normal in macrocytic and normocytic anemias; very high reflects spherocytosis or RBC agglutination
- Normal value is 32.5 to 35.2 g/dL

Mean Corpuscular Hemoglobin

- Average hemoglobin content in an RBC
- Decreased values mean pale or hypochromic RBCs. Mean corpuscular hemoglobin (MCH) is decreased in IDA and thalassemia. Normal with macrocytic anemias.
- Normal value is 25.0 to 35.0 pg/cell

EXAM TIPS

RBC size is described in many ways, such as:

- MCV <80 fL: Microcytic and hypochromic RBCs, small and pale RBCs
- MCV >100 fL: Macrocytes or macro-ovalocytes, larger than normal RBCs, or RBCs with enlarged cytoplasms

Total Iron-Binding Capacity

- A measure of available transferrin that is left unbound (to iron). Transferrin is used to transport iron in the body. The transferrin concentration can be converted to the total iron-binding capacity (TIBC) by multiplying by 1.389.
- TIBC is elevated if there is not enough iron to transport (as seen with IDA). Normal TIBC is seen with thalassemia, vitamin B_{12} deficiency, and folate-deficiency anemia (because iron levels are normal).
- Normal value is 300 to 360 mcg/dL

Serum Ferritin

- The stored form of iron. Produced in the intestines. Stored in body tissue such as the spleen, liver, and bone marrow. Correlates with iron storage status in a healthy adult. Most sensitive test for IDA.
- Also an acute phase reactant that can increase independent of iron status due to inflammation, infection, or other disorders.
- Serum ferritin is decreased in IDA.
- With thalassemia trait, levels are normal to high. May be high if patient was misdiagnosed with IDA and erroneously given iron supplementation. Avoid iron supplements before testing serum ferritin level.
- Normal value is 40 to 200 ng/mL.

Serum Iron

- Decreased in IDA. Normal to high in thalassemia and macrocytic anemias.
- Value alone is not diagnostic of any condition. Affected by recent blood transfusions and dietary or pharmacologic iron.
- Normal value is 60 to 150 mcg/dL.

Red Cell Distribution Width

A measure of the variability of the size of RBCs in a given sample. Elevated in IDA, vitamin B_{12} or folate deficiency, and myelodysplastic syndrome.

Reticulocytes

- Immature RBCs that still have their nuclei; reflects the rate of RBC production.
- Reticulocytes are slightly larger than RBCs. After 24 hours in circulation, reticulocytes lose their nuclei and mature into RBCs (no nuclei). The bone marrow normally will release small amounts to replace damaged RBCs. RBCs survive for 120 days before being sequestered by the spleen and broken down by the liver into iron and globulin (recycled) and bilirubin (bile).
- 16 to 130 ($\times 10^3$/mcL or $\times 10^9$/L) in males
- 16 to 98 ($\times 10^3$/mcL or $\times 10^9$/L) in females

Reticulocytosis (More Than 2.5% of Total Red Blood Cell Count)

- An elevation of reticulocytes is seen when the bone marrow is stimulated into producing RBCs. It is elevated within a few days with supplementation of iron, folate, or vitamin B_{12} (after deficiency); after acute bleeding episodes, hemolysis, and leukemia; and with erythropoietin (EPO) treatment. Chronic bleeding does not cause elevation of reticulocytes due to compensation.
- If no reticulocytosis after an acute bleeding episode (after 3–4 days), after appropriate supplementation of

deficient mineral (iron, folate, or vitamin B_{12}) or with EPO, rule out bone marrow failure (i.e., aplastic anemia). Diagnosed by bone marrow biopsy.

Poikilocytosis (Peripheral Smear)
- RBCs abnormal with variable shapes seen in the peripheral smear.
- Large oval-shaped cells (macroovalocytes) suggest megaloblastic process (e.g., deficiency of vitamin B_{12} or folic acid).

Serum Folate and Vitamin B_{12}
- Low values if deficiency exists. Deficiency will cause a macrocytic anemia.
- Folate level above 4 ng/mL is normal; 2 to 4 ng/mL is borderline; a level below 2 ng/mL is consistent with folate deficiency.
- Vitamin B_{12} level normal range is above 300 pg/mL; borderline deficiency is 200 to 300 pg/mL; a level below 200 pg/mL is low and consistent with deficiency.

EXAM TIPS
- Order both vitamin B_{12} and folate levels when evaluating MCV >100 fL.
- Learn food groups for both folate and vitamin B_{12}.

White Blood Cells With Differential
- Percentage of each type of leukocyte in a sample of blood. The differential for each type of white blood cell (WBC) should add up to a total of 100%.
- If WBC is elevated (leukocytosis) or decreased (leukopenia), obtain a WBC differential and the peripheral blood smear to examine which cell type is decreased.
- Normal WBC count for adults is 3.8 to 10.4×10^3 mcL
  - Neutrophils or segs (segmented neutrophils): 55% to 70%
  - Band forms (immature neutrophils): 0% to 5%
  - Lymphocytes: 20% to 40%
  - Monocytes: 2% to 8%
  - Eosinophils: 1% to 4%
  - Basophils: 0.5% to 1%

Platelets
- Blood components that form clots and stop or prevent bleeding.
- An elevated platelet count (thrombocytosis) may be reactive or due to a neoplastic condition; a low count (thrombocytopenia) may reflect platelet destruction, sequestration, or ineffective thrombopoiesis.
- 152 to 324×10^3 mcL in males
- 153 to 361×10^3 mcL in females

Hemoglobin Electrophoresis
The gold-standard (definitive) test to diagnose hemoglobinopathies such as sickle cell anemia, thalassemia, and many others. Normal hemoglobin contains two alpha and two beta chains. Adult norms are hemoglobin A (HbA) 97% and hemoglobin A2 (HbA2) 2.5%. An extremely small amount (<1%) of total hemoglobin is fetal hemoglobin (HbF), which is a normal finding.

DISEASE REVIEW

ANEMIAS
Anemia is simply defined as a decrease in the hemoglobin/hematocrit value or reduction in the volume of RBCs below the norm for the patient's age and gender caused by a variety of factors such as blood loss, bone marrow failure, impaired production or hemolysis/destruction of RBCs. See Table 13.1 for a comparison of laboratory characteristics.

Iron-Deficiency Anemia
Microcytic and hypochromic anemia (small and pale RBCs) are caused by IDA or thalassemia trait/minor. IDA is the most common type of anemia in the world, affecting >12% of the world's population.

EXAM TIPS
Learn to differentiate the lab results of thalassemia from IDA:
- If the serum iron and ferritin levels are low with a high TIBC, the patient has IDA.
- If the TIBC and ferritin levels are normal, the patient has thalassemia.

Etiology
Most common cause is blood loss (overt or occult). In adults, blood loss from the gastrointestinal (GI) tract caused by peptic ulcer disease (PUD), NSAID use, or cancer is most likely. Reproductive-aged females (heavy periods, pregnancy), poor diet, post-gastrectomy, and increased physiologic requirement are risk factors.
- Children: Low dietary intake, diet deficient in iron
- Infants: Rule out chronic intake of cow's milk before 12 months of age (causes GI bleeding) in anemic infants

Classic Case
Most are asymptomatic if mild. Moderate-to-severe cases may have pallor of the skin, conjunctivae, and nail beds. Complaints of daily fatigue and exertional dyspnea. May have glossitis (sore and shiny red tongue) and angular cheilitis (irritated skin or fissures at the corners of the mouth). Cravings for nonfood items such as ice or dirt (pica). Severe anemia may cause spoon-shaped nails (koilonychia), systolic murmurs, tachycardia, or heart failure.

Labs
During the early phase of IDA or acute blood loss, the MCV (size) and the mean corpuscular hemoglobin concentration (MCHC) (color) can still be in the normal range, and the RBCs will likely be normocytic and normochromic. The CBC may even be relatively normal in individuals in high-resource settings.

Table 13.1 Comparison of the Laboratory Findings of Common Anemias

Type of Anemia	Diagnostic Tests*	Red Blood Cell Changes
Iron deficiency	*Ferritin/serum iron* ↓ TIBC ↑ RDW ↑	MCV <80 fL (microcytic) MCHC ↓ (hypochromic) Poikilocytosis (variable shapes) Anisocytosis (variable sizes)
Thalassemia	Hemoglobin analysis or genetic testing	MCV <80 fL (microcytic) MCHC ↓ (hypochromic)
Vitamin B_{12} deficiency/ pernicious anemia	*Vitamin B_{12} level* ↓ Hypersegmented neutrophils (>five or six lobes) Autoantibodies to intrinsic factor	MCV >100 fL (macrocytic) Megaloblastic RBCs Normal color (normochromic)
Folate deficiency	*Folate level* ↓ Homocysteine ↑	MCV >100 fL (macrocytic) Megaloblastic RBCs Normal color (normochromic)
Anemia of chronic disease	*MCV 80–100 fL* History of chronic or inflammatory disease	MCV 80–100 fL (normal-sized RBCs) Normochromic RBCs

Sickle cell anemia	*Hemoglobin electrophoresis*
	HbS and HbF ↑
	Reticulocytosis
	A hemolytic anemia
		Sickle-shaped RBCs with shortened life
		  span of 10–20 days (norm is 120 days)
		Howell–Jolly bodies and target cells
		  (peripheral smear)
		Normocytic/normochromic

*Italicized lab tests are diagnostic or the gold standard for the exams.

HbF, fetal hemoglobin; HbS, hemoglobin S; MCHC, mean corpuscular hemoglobin concentration; MCV, mean corpuscular volume; RBC, red blood cell; RDW, red blood cell distribution width; TIBC, total iron-binding capacity.

Decreased
- Hemoglobin and hematocrit
- MCV <80 fL (microcytic RBCs)
- MCHC (hypochromic or pale RBCs)
- Ferritin and iron level
- Reticulocyte count

Increased
- TIBC
- Platelet count

Peripheral Smear

Anisocytosis (variations in size) and poikilocytosis (variations in shape).

Treatment Plan
- Identify cause of anemia and correct cause (if possible). Rule out GI malignancy in older patients.
- Ferrous sulfate 325 mg PO TID between meals (take with vitamin C or orange juice for better absorption). It is absorbed better in an empty stomach, but it is usually taken with meals because it causes lower GI distress.
- The hemoglobin and hematocrit will often normalize in 6 to 8 weeks; continue therapy until the ferritin level increases to normal levels (can take 3–6 months to replace).
- Patients with severe and symptomatic anemia should be treated with RBC transfusion.
- Use of cast-iron cookware can help increase iron source for vegans and vegetarians.

- Increase fiber and fluids. Consider fiber supplements (psyllium, guar gum) for constipation.
- Iron-rich foods are red meat, some beans (e.g., black beans), and green leafy vegetables.
- Common side effects of iron include constipation and black-colored stools; stomach upset may occur. Docusate sodium (Colace) can be used as a stool softener (not a laxative).
- Avoid taking iron supplements at the same time as antacids, dairy products, quinolones, or tetracyclines (iron binds with these substances and is inactivated).
- A modest reticulocytosis will be seen in about 7 to 10 days in patients with moderate or severe anemia. Patients with mild anemia may have little or no reticulocytosis.

Thalassemia

Thalassemia refers to inherited hemoglobinopathies that began in certain regions of sub-Saharan Africa, the Asian-Indian subcontinent, Southeast Asia, and Mediterranean region. Thalassemias are very common (second to sickle cell disease). Thalassemias are categorized by a decreased production of the alpha or beta chains that form on the hemoglobin molecule (alpha and beta thalassemias). Results in a microcytic/hypochromic anemia.
- Alpha thalassemia is more common in southern China, Malaysia, and Thailand. Mild forms can be seen in patients with African ancestry.
- Beta thalassemia is prevalent in Africa.

Classic Case

Vast majority of individuals are asymptomatic. Discovered incidentally because of abnormal CBC results, which reveal microcytic and hypochromic RBCs. Total RBC count may be mildly elevated. Ask about family history of thalassemia.

Labs
- Hemoglobin analysis or genetic testing determines the type of thalassemia. For alpha thalassemia, Hb Barts (gamma chain tetramers) or Hb H (beta chain tetramers); DNA-based testing is required for alpha thalassemia minor or minima. For beta-thalassemia, elevated HbA2 and HbF
- Microcytic anemia, increased RBC count, and nonimmune hemolysis
- Blood smear for poikilocytosis, target cells, teardrop cells, and cell fragments
- Serum ferritin and iron level will be normal (but low in IDA); used to rule out iron deficiency

Treatment Plan
- Treatment is individualized; some may require transfusions for anemia to reduce symptoms or during periods of stress.
- Thalassemia minor often does not need treatment when anemia is very mild.
- Genetic testing and reproductive counseling; educate about the possibility of having a child with the disease if partner also has trait; routine for all individuals with thalassemia.

EXAM TIPS
- Hemoglobin analysis and/or genetic testing is required to confirm the diagnosis of thalassemia.
- The ethnic background may not be "revealed" in a question about thalassemia.

Anemia of Chronic Disease
Also referred to as anemia of inflammation or hypoferremia of inflammation; it is the second most common cause of anemia worldwide.
- Autoimmune diseases (e.g., rheumatoid arthritis [RA], lupus) or chronic inflammatory disorders increase cytokine production and hepcidin, which sequesters iron, making it unavailable to develop RBCs.
- Presents as a mild to moderate anemia with normochromic, normocytic (MCV 80–100 fL) RBCs. The erythrocyte sedimentation rate (ESR or sed rate) or C-reactive protein (CRP) is often elevated.
- Treatment of underlying autoimmune disease can help reduce systemic inflammation, allowing bone marrow to recover.

Anemia in Chronic Kidney Disease
Anemia is common among patients with chronic kidney disease (CKD); the prevalence increases as the glomerular filtration rates decline.
- Defined as hemoglobin concentration <13 g/dL for adult males and postmenopausal women and a hemoglobin <12 g/dL for premenopausal women

- Presents as a hypoproliferative, normocytic, and normochromic anemia.
- Occurs due to the decrease in renal EPO production secondary to the CKD, which reduces the production of reticulocyte and RBCs and causes worsening anemia. In addition, patients may also have functional iron deficiency and/or acute and chronic inflammatory conditions.
- For initial testing, obtain CBC, serum ferritin, serum transferrin saturation, vitamin B_{12}, folate, and reticulocyte count.

Treatment Plan
- The anemia should be treated using conventional methods. If not improving, then erythropoiesis-stimulating agents can be used; recommended when the hemoglobin level is <10 g/dL.
- Iron therapy (PO or IV) may also be used. PO iron may be used for patients not treated with dialysis.
- IV iron is used for hemodialysis patients with severe iron deficiency, severe anemia, risk of ongoing blood loss, and history of side effects or intolerance to oral iron.

CLINICAL PEARLS
- Best absorbed form of iron supplementation (and cheapest) is ferrous sulfate (available OTC). Many oral iron formulations are available; in general, they are all equally effective and relatively inexpensive.
- If patients took an antacid, ask them to wait about 4 hours before taking an iron pill (minimizes binding).
- Iron interacts with tetracycline antibiotics, levothyroxine, and bisphosphonates (decreases effectiveness). To avoid, take iron 2 hours before or after an antibiotic.
- Failure to respond (if treatment compliant) may be a sign of continuing blood loss, misdiagnosis, or malabsorption (e.g., celiac disease).
- Iron poisoning in children (especially if age <6 years) may cause death. Advise patients to store iron supplements in an area that is not accessible to children (or grandchildren).
- Medications reported to lower hemoglobin levels and worsen anemia include angiotensin receptor blockers (ARBs) and ACEIs in patients of chronic diseases (CKD, diabetes, chronic HF, hypertension).

Macrocytic/Megaloblastic Anemias
Vitamin B_{12}–Deficiency Anemia
Caused by a deficiency in vitamin B_{12}, which is necessary for the health of neurons and the brain and normal DNA production of RBCs. Total body supply of vitamin B_{12} lasts 3 to 4 years. Common causes of vitamin B_{12}–deficiency anemia include malabsorption (due to pernicious anemia, gastric disease/infections, or medications such as antacids, H2-receptor antagonists, proton pump inhibitors [PPIs],

and metformin). Chronic vitamin B_{12} deficiency causes nerve damage (peripheral neuropathy, paraplegia) and brain damage (dementia if severe). Neurologic damage may not be reversible. Highest incidence in older women. Most common cause is pernicious anemia.

Pernicious Anemia

A type of vitamin B_{12} anemia. Pernicious anemia is an autoimmune disorder caused by the destruction of parietal cells in the fundus (by antiparietal antibodies), resulting in cessation of intrinsic factor production. Intrinsic factor is necessary to absorb vitamin B_{12} from the small intestine.

EXAM TIPS

- Pernicious anemia is a macrocytic, normochromic anemia due to deficiency of intrinsic factor, which results in malabsorption of B_{12}. It can cause neurologic symptoms.
- A vitamin B_{12} level below 200 pg/mL is consistent with deficiency.

Cobalamin (vitamin B_{12}) deficiency may result from dietary insufficiency. May occur in patients with stomach, small bowel, and pancreatic disorders; infections; and severe dietary deficiencies of meats and milk, as seen in strict vegetarians. Dietary deficiency may take more than 5 years to occur. Iron deficiency commonly coexists with pernicious anemia. Patients with pernicious anemia have a two- to threefold increase in incidence of gastric carcinoma.

- Other causes: Alterations in gastric anatomy (e.g., bariatric surgery, gastrectomy), strict vegans, alcoholics, small bowel disease
- Vitamin B_{12} sources: All foods of animal origin (meat, poultry, eggs, milk, cheese)

Classic Case

Older adult presents with yellowed skin (caused by combined anemia and jaundice) and other signs of anemia (e.g., fatigue, shortness of breath). Vitamin B_{12} deficiency can cause glossitis and loss of papillae and/or hyperpigmentation of the tongue. Neuropathic symptoms may include any of the following:

- Tingling/numbness (paresthesia) of hands and feet
- Neuropathy starts in peripheral nerves and migrates centrally
- Difficulty walking (gross motor)
- Difficulty in performing fine motor skills (hands)
- Depression or cognitive slowing

Objective Findings

Decreased reflexes in affected extremity. If the legs are involved, the ankle jerk (Achilles reflex) may be reduced ("+1" is sluggish, and "0" is none). Normal reflex is grade "+2."

- Motor tests for weak hand grip, decreased vibration sense, abnormal Romberg
- Inflamed tongue and glossitis (not a specific finding)

Warning

Always check both serum B_{12} and serum folate levels in macrocytic anemias. A patient can be deficient in both B_{12} and folate. Consider omitting the folate level in patients with a folate-enriched diet without GI disorders. Untreated B_{12} deficiency anemia results in permanent neurologic sequelae (neuropathy, brain damage).

Labs

- Vitamin B_{12} level: Normal range is >300 pg/mL; borderline deficiency is 200 to 300 pg/mL; a level <200 pg/mL is low and consistent with deficiency
- CBC: Decreased hemoglobin and hematocrit, macrocytic RBCs (MCV>100 fL), mild leukopenia, thrombocytopenia, low reticulocyte count
- Antibody tests: Antiparietal and autoantibodies to intrinsic factor
- Metabolite testing (MMA) and homocysteine level: Elevated (but does not eliminate possibility of folate deficiency)
- Schilling test: Not commonly used now; positive if vitamin B_{12} (radioactive) excretion is normal after administration of intrinsic factor (but has poor excretion when given vitamin B_{12} alone)
- Peripheral blood smear: Macrocytosis, hypersegmented neutrophils (>five or six lobes), evidence of defective erythropoiesis
- Check reticulocyte count and CBC: Approximately 2 weeks after starting supplementation to check for treatment response

Treatment

- Parenteral: Vitamin B_{12} subcutaneous or intramuscular injections 1,000 mcg (1 mg) once weekly for 1 month followed by 1,000 mcg once per month. Parenteral replacement should be used for patients with neurologic changes and/or concerns regarding gastric absorption of vitamin B_{12}.
- Oral: Vitamin B_{12} (1,000–2,000 mcg) by mouth daily if adherence is not a concern. Oral vitamin B_{12} replacement may be as effective as parenteral vitamin B_{12}.

EXAM TIPS

- The screening test for all anemias is the CBC (specifically evaluate the hemoglobin/hematocrit).
- Patients with chronic illness and/or autoimmune disease have higher risk of normocytic anemia.

Folic Acid–Deficiency Anemia

Deficiency in folate (vitamin B_9) results in damage to the DNA of RBCs, which causes macrocytosis (MCV >100 fL). The body's supply of folate lasts 2 to 3 months.

- Most common cause: Inadequate dietary intake (elderly, infants, alcoholics, overcooking vegetables, low citrus intake). Chronic alcoholism and poor nutrition (lack of folate-rich foods such as fresh vegetables and fortified grains) contribute to a decrease in the amount of vitamin B_{12} released from dietary proteins.
- Other causes: Increased physiologic need (e.g., pregnancy) and malabsorption (e.g., gluten enteropathy, gastric bypass) cause folic acid–deficiency anemia.
- Drugs (long term) that interfere with folate absorption: Phenytoin (Dilantin), trimethoprim–sulfa, metformin, methotrexate, sulfasalazine, zidovudine (Retrovir, azidothymidine), and others

Classic Case
Older patient and/or patient with alcoholism complains of anemia signs/symptoms (tiredness, fatigue, pallor or jaundice, and a reddened and sore tongue, or glossitis). If anemia is severe (applies to all anemias), may have tachycardia, palpitations, angina, or shortness of breath. While neurologic deficits are more common to vitamin B_{12} deficiency, they have been reported in folate deficiency, as well. Assess for progressive weakness, ataxia, and paresthesias.

Labs
- CBC: Decreased hemoglobin and hematocrit, macrocytic RBCs (MCV>100 fL), mild leukopenia, thrombocytopenia, low reticulocyte count
- Peripheral smear: Macro-ovalocytes, hypersegmented neutrophils (>five or six lobes)
- Folate level: Above 4 ng/mL is normal; between 2 to 4 ng/mL is borderline; a level below 2 ng/mL is consistent with folate deficiency
- MMA normal, homocysteine elevated: Consistent with deficiency of folate

Medications
- Prevention: Individuals at risk (e.g., malnutrition, chronic alcohol use) should prevent folate deficiency with folic acid supplementation.
- Treatment: Correct primary cause. Administer folic acid PO 1 to 5 mg/day. Treat for 1 to 4 months or until RBC indicators and anemia are normal; some with chronic cause of folate deficiency may require indefinite treatment.
- Women of childbearing age: It is recommended that all women who may become pregnant take a folic acid supplement, 400 mcg daily, at least 1 month (or longer) prior to conception to enhance normal fetal development and decrease the incidence of neural tube defects. Women who have had a previous child born with a neural tube defect require higher doses of folic acid, 4 mg daily.

APLASTIC ANEMIA
Aplastic anemia is caused by destruction of the pluripotent stem cells inside the bone marrow and has multiple causes (e.g., radiation, adverse effects of a drug, viral infection). Bone marrow production slows or stops—all cell lines are affected. The result is pancytopenia (leukopenia, anemia, thrombocytopenia).

Classic Case
Patient with severe case of anemia presents with fatigue and weakness. Skin and mucosa are a pale color. Tachycardia and systolic flow murmur are present. Neutropenia results in bacterial and fungal infections. Thrombocytopenia results in large bruises from trauma and bleeding. Signs and symptoms depend on the severity of blood counts. Some patients are initially asymptomatic. Somatic abnormalities (e.g., skeletal anomalies, short stature) may be present in patients with inherited forms.

Labs
- CBC with differential: RBCs are generally normocytic or macrocytic; few mature neutorphils, most WBCs are lymphocytes, platelets are decreased, low reticulocyte count
- Blood smear: Generally normal, except for cytopenias, no blasts are seen
- Bone marrow biopsy: Required for diagnosis

Treatment Plan
Refer to hematologist as soon as possible. If septic, refer to the ED.

ERYTHROCYTOSIS
Erythrocytosis (polycythemia) refers to an abnormal elevation of hemoglobin and/or hematocrit. Absolute polycythemia can be categorized as primary or secondary polycythemia. An increase of RBC mass caused by a mutation (either acquired or inherited) is categorized as primary polycythemia. Chronic smokers and individuals with long-term chronic obstructive pulmonary disease (COPD), who are long-time residents at high altitudes, or who had EPO treatment have a higher incidence of secondary polycythemia. Relative polycythemia refers to hemoconcentration, or an elevation of hemoglobin or hematocrit due to a decrease in plasma volume alone.

Polycythemia is defined as:
- Hematocrit in adults of more than 48% in women and more than 49% in men
- Hemoglobin in adults of more than 16.0 g/dL in women and more than 16.5 g/dL in men

HEMOCHROMATOSIS
Hereditary hemochromatosis is a genetic disorder in which the intestinal absorption of iron increases, leading to total-body iron overload. It takes decades for significant iron deposition to occur. Symptoms include chronic fatigue, skin hyperpigmentation (bronze), swelling of the second and third metacarpal phalangeal joints (fingers), and generalized joint stiffness. Iron overload damages the organs, including the liver (fibrosis, cirrhosis, and liver cancer), the heart (cardiomyopathy, heart failure, arrhythmias, and death), and other organs. Abnormal lab results include elevation of aspartate aminotransferase (AST) and alanine aminotransferase (ALT), high serum ferritin (>500 ng/dL), and high transferrin saturation. The main treatment for symptomatic patients with very high ferritin levels is therapeutic phlebotomy.

- In a person with normal bone marrow, supplementing the deficient substance (iron, B_{12}, folate) will increase the hemoglobin/hematocrit in about 1 to 2 weeks and will normalize within 4 to 8 weeks.
- Serum vitamin B_{12} levels may be normal in patients with vitamin B_{12} deficiency. Do not rely on vitamin B_{12} levels alone. Also check antibodies, MMA, and other lab tests.
- Untreated vitamin B_{12} deficiency can result in irreversible neurologic damage.
- Any patient complaining of neuropathy or who has altered mental status should have vitamin B_{12} levels checked.

HEMOLYTIC ANEMIAS

A group of genetic diseases that decrease RBC life span with increased lysis. For the exam, there are two: sickle cell trait and glucose-6-phosphate dehydrogenase deficiency (G6PD) anemia. Acute hemolysis of RBCs causes a drop in the hemoglobin and hematocrit, reticulocytosis, and elevation of indirect bilirubin (causes jaundice).

Glucose-6-Phosphate Dehydrogenase Deficiency Anemia

An X-linked recessive genetic disease that is more common in males (XY chromosome, only one X chromosome) that is usually asymptomatic, unless hemolysis occurs. G6PD protects RBCs against oxidative damage. There are five variants of G6PD, a type of hemolytic anemia. It is the most common inherited RBC enzyme abnormality. It occurs most often in the tropical and subtropical zones of the eastern hemisphere (e.g., Africa, Europe, Asia) and is common among Kurdish Jews. Most females with G6PD are unaffected carriers. Infants are at higher risk of neonatal jaundice.

- Hemolysis can be triggered by some drugs (e.g., primaquine, hydroxychloroquine, sulfa drugs, acetazolamide, dapsone), fava beans, red Egyptian and black henna, fever, acute infections, stress, others.
- About 2 to 4 days after drug ingestion, will have hemolytic episode with acute onset of jaundice, yellow sclerae, pallor, fatigue, shortness of breath, tachycardia, and dark urine (abrupt fall of hemoglobin by 3–4 g/dL).
- Check the CBC and peripheral blood smear. Hemolysis can be mild and self-limiting in some, and severe and life-threatening in others.

Genetics Review: X-Linked Recessive

- Father (has G6PD) and mother (unaffected) = daughters (100% carriers), sons (100% not affected)
- Father (unaffected) and mother (carrier) = daughters (50% unaffected; 50% carrier), sons (50% unaffected; 50% have G6PD)

Sickle Cell Anemia

In the United States, sickle cell disease affects about 100,000 Americans. A study of U.S. adult patients found the median survival for Hb SS was 58 years. Higher prevalence in people from Africa, the Mediterranean, the Middle East, and some areas of India.

Complications of sickle cell disease include acute chest syndrome, anemia, avascular necrosis, blood clots, dactylitis (hand–foot syndrome), fever, infection, kidney and liver issues, leg ulcers, pain, priapism, pulmonary hypertension, sleep-disordered breathing, splenic sequestration, stroke, and vision loss.

- All U.S. states and territories and the District of Columbia require that every newborn be tested for sickle cell disease as part of the newborn screening test after birth.
- Approximately one out of every 365 African Americans births in the United States has sickle cell disease.

Classic Case

Most patients with sickle cell trait are asymptomatic. Patients who have full-blown sickle cell disease may present in an aplastic crisis (acute drop in hemoglobin), have frequent sickling episodes (causing vessel obstruction), and have painful vaso-occlusive episodes (due to tissue ischemia and blood hypervisocity). Patient may present with sudden onset of severe pain in extremities, back, chest, or abdomen. Patient may have aching joint pain, weakness, and dsypnea. Factors which precipitate sickling include hypoxia, infections, high altitudes, dehydration, physical or emotional stress, surgery, blood loss, and acidosis. Acute manifestations are related to renal and/or liver dysfunction, priapism, hemolytic episodes, hyposplenism, and frequent infections.

Labs

- CBC: Mild to moderate anemia
- Peripheral blood smear: Classic distorted sickle-shaped RBCs
- Diagnosis of sickle cell disorder can be made by high performance liquid chromatography (HPLC), isoelectric focusing (IEF), or gel electrophoresis techniques. The combination of HPLC and IEF allows for a definitive diagnosis in older children and adults.

Treatment Plan

- Sickle cell is an autosomal recessive pattern genetic disease. Genetic counseling is needed if both partners are at risk. If each parent has the sickle cell trait, one child out of four (25%) will have the disease. Prenatal screening is available as early as 8 to 10 weeks' gestation via chorionic villus sampling or amniocentesis.
- Patients with family history of sickle cell disease or trait, patients with signs and symptoms suggestive of sickle cell disease (aseptic necrosis of the femoral head, unexplained bone pain, hemolysis), or Black patients with normocytic anemia should be screened with peripheral smear, hemoglobin solubility testing, and hemoglobin electrophoresis.
- Patients with sickle cell disease are managed by hematologists for both acute and chronic complications of the disease.

EXAM TIP

The combination of HPLC and IEF provides for a definitive diagnosis of a sickle cell disorder in older children and adults.

High-Altitude Stress

Lower barometric pressure causes a reduction in the arterial PO_2. Patients with coronary artery disease (CAD), congestive heart failure (CHF), or sickle cell anemia are at higher risk of complications. Patients with sickle cell disease should avoid being in an area that is 7,000-ft elevation or higher.

SUMMARY: MICROCYTIC ANEMIAS

IRON-DEFICIENCY ANEMIA VERSUS THALASSEMIA TRAIT

Ferritin Level

- Low in iron deficiency
- Normal in thalassemia trait

Serum Iron

- Decreased in iron deficiency
- Normal in thalassemia trait

Total Iron-Binding Capacity

- Elevated in iron deficiency
- Normal in thalassemia trait

Mean Corpuscular Hemoglobin Concentration

- A measure of RBC color
- Decreased in iron deficiency
- Decreased in thalassemia

Hemoglobin Electrophoresis

- Normal in iron deficiency
- Abnormal in beta thalassemia

Ethnic Background

- IDA is the most common anemia overall.
- Alpha thalassemia is more common in southern China, Malaysia, and Thailand. Mild forms can be seen in patients with African ancestry.
- Beta thalassemia is present in Africa.

KNOWLEDGE CHECK: CHAPTER 13

1. Which of the following can cause a *decrease* in hemoglobin concentration?
   A. Smoking
   B. Pregnancy
   C. Dehydration
   D. High altitude

2. A patient presents with fatigue, symmetric paresthesias, numbness, and gait problems. Past medical history is significant for diabetes mellitus, for which the patient has been prescribed metformin for the past 5 years. Laboratory studies are significant for a macrocytic anemia with mild pancytopenia. Serum level vitamin B_{12} is 150 pg/mL, and folate is 5 ng/mL. These findings are suggestive of which type of anemia?
   A. Vitamin B_{12} deficiency
   B. Thalassemia
   C. Iron-deficiency anemia
   D. Folic acid deficiency

3. Characteristic Reed-Sternberg cells are the hallmark tumor cells for which malignant disorder?
   A. Multiple myeloma
   B. Non-Hodgkin's lymphoma
   C. Chronic myeloid leukemia
   D. Classic Hodgkin's disease

4. A male patient presents for annual lab work. Laboratory results are significant for hemoglobin 10 g/dL, hematocrit 30%, mean corpuscular volume (MCV) 72 fL, and mean corpuscular hemoglobin concentration (MCHC) 28%. Based on these lab values, this anemia is classified as:
   A. Microcytic, hyperchromic
   B. Microcytic, hypochromic
   C. Macrocytic, normochromic
   D. Macrocytic, hypochromic

5. Which of the following laboratory results is consistent with a diagnosis of thalassemia anemia?
   A. Microcytic, hypochromic anemia, normal ferritin
   B. Macrocytic, normochromic anemia, normal total iron-binding capacity
   C. Microcytic, hyperchromic anemia, decreased alpha and/or beta globin chains
   D. Microcytic, hypochromic anemia, low serum ferritin

6. A patient with a past medical history significant for alcohol use disorder presents with fatigue, dyspnea, and jaundice. The patient denies paresthesia, numbness, or gait problems. Laboratory studies are significant for macrocytic anemia. Serum level B_{12} is 315 pg/mL, and folate is 1.5 ng/mL. These findings are suggestive of which type of anemia?
   A. Thalassemia
   B. Iron-deficiency anemia
   C. Vitamin B_{12} deficiency
   D. Folic acid deficiency

7. The inheritance pattern for sickle cell anemia is described as:
   A. Autosomal recessive
   B. X-linked dominant
   C. Autosomal dominant
   D. X-linked recessive

(See answers next page.)

1. B) Pregnancy

During a healthy pregnancy, the maternal red cell mass increases and the plasma volume also increases, leading to a relative decrease in hemoglobin and hematocrit. Intense physical activity and older age can also lower values. Smoking, certain medications (e.g., androgens, sodium-glucose co-transporter 2 [SGLT2] inhibitors), hemoconcentration (as seen with dehydration or hypovolemia), and high altitude can cause higher values and occasionally mask underlying anemia.

2. A) Vitamin B_{12} deficiency

Vitamin B_{12} and folic acid deficiency should be suspected in a patient presenting with macrocytic anemia with mild pancytopenia, hypersegmented neutrophils, and an underlying condition or diet associated with deficiency. Neuropsychiatric symptoms can be seen in both vitamin B_{12} and folate deficiencies. A normal value for vitamin B_{12} is >300 pg/mL, whereas a normal folate level is >4 ng/mL. A vitamin B_{12} level below 200 pg/mL is consistent with deficiency. An adverse effect of long-term use of metformin (and other biguanides) is reduced absorption of vitamin B_{12} secondary to altered calcium hemostasis. In as early as 3 to 4 months after starting treatment with metformin, low serum vitamin B_{12} levels can be seen; however, symptomatic deficiency is likely to present after 5 to 10 years of therapy. For patients receiving metformin, it is recommended to undergo annual monitoring for vitamin B_{12} deficiency. A microcytic (not macrocytic), hypochromic anemia is seen in iron-deficiency anemia and thalassemia.

3. D) Classic Hodgkin's disease

Hodgkin lymphomas are lymphoid neoplasms in which malignant Hodgkin/Reed-Sternberg cells are mixed with a heterogeneous population of nonneoplastic inflammatory cells. The presence of characteristic Reed-Sternberg cells differentiates Hodgkin's disease from non-Hodgkin's disease. Multiple myeloma is characterized by ≥10% clonal plasma cells in the bone marrow or biopsy-proven bony or soft tissue plasmacytoma plus organ or tissue impairment or a biomarker associated with near inevitable progression to end-organ damage. The diagnosis of chronic myeloid lymphoma is suspected by the typical findings in the blood and bone marrow and confirmed by the demonstration of the Philadelphia chromosome, the *BCR::ABL1* fusion gene, or the BCR::ABL1 fusion mRNA.

4. B) Microcytic, hypochromic

The patient is experiencing a microcytic, hypochromic anemia seen in iron-deficiency anemia and thalassemia. The patient's hemoglobin and hematocrit values are low, indicating an anemia (normal range for hemoglobin in males is 13.6 to 16.9 g/dL and for hematocrit in males is 40% to 50%). The normal range for MCV, the average volume size of the red blood cell, is 80 to 100 fL. A level of 72 fL indicates a decreased MCV or microcytosis. Macrocytosis would be seen if the value was >100 fL. The normal range for MCHC, the average hemoglobin concentration per red blood cell, is 32% to 36%; therefore, a level of 28% indicates a decreased MCHC, indicating that this anemia is hypochromic. Hyperchromic would be indicated by a value >36%.

5. A) Microcytic, hypochromic anemia, normal ferritin

In all thalassemia syndromes (except asymptomatic carriers), microcytic hypochromic anemia is present. Alpha and beta thalassemia are hemoglobinopathies caused by a reduction of alpha globin chains or beta globin chains, leading to an imbalance in the alpha to beta ratio. Iron-deficiency anemia is also characterized by a microcytic, hypochromic anemia. However, the ferritin is low and total iron-binding capacity is high in iron-deficiency anemia, whereas these levels are often normal in thalassemia.

6. D) Folic acid deficiency

Vitamin B_{12} and folic acid deficiency should be suspected in a patient presenting with macrocytic anemia with mild pancytopenia, hypersegmented neutrophils, and an underlying condition or diet associated with deficiency. A normal value for vitamin B_{12} is >300 pg/mL, whereas a normal folate level is >4 ng/mL. A folate level <2 ng/mL is considered deficient. Folate deficiency is often a consequence of nutritional deficiency, as seen frequently in patients with alcoholism, substance use disorder, or poor dietary intake of folate-rich foods such as fresh vegetables and grains, as well as malabsorption (e.g., celiac disease, inflammatory bowel disease), certain medications (e.g., methotrexate, sulfasalazine), and increased requirement states (e.g., pregnancy). While neurologic deficits can occur in both vitamin B_{12} and folic acid deficiency, they are more common in patients presenting with vitamin B_{12} deficiency. A microcytic, hypochromic anemia is seen in iron-deficiency anemia and thalassemia.

7. A) Autosomal recessive

The five patterns of Mendelian inheritance are autosomal dominant, autosomal recessive, X-linked dominant, X-linked recessive, and Y-linked. Sickle cell anemia is an autosomal recessive trait. Glucose-6-phosphate dehydrogenase deficiency anemia is an X-linked recessive genetic disease.

8. A male patient presents after a routine physical and annual lab work. Laboratory results are significant for hemoglobin 10 g/dL, hematocrit 30%, mean corpuscular volume (MCV) 74 fL, and mean corpuscular hemoglobin concentration (MCHC) 30%. The patient reports recent fatigue, restless legs syndrome, generalized weakness, and an unusual craving for ice. Treatment for this anemia includes which of the following?
A. Vitamin B_{12} injection
B. Blood transfusion
C. Ferrous sulfate
D. Folic acid

9. An affected man with glucose-6-phosphate dehydrogenase (G6PD) deficiency and an unaffected woman undergo genetic counseling to determine genetic inheritance. Which of the following is *true* if they have one son and one daughter together?
A. The son will be affected.
B. The son will not be affected.
C. The son will be a carrier.
D. The daughter will not be a carrier.

10. Which of the following is the recommended treatment for hereditary hemochromatosis?
A. Genetic counseling
B. Ferrous sulfate supplementation
C. Phlebotomy
D. Dialysis

11. What is the *most common* type of hemophilia in the United States?
A. Hemophilia B
B. Hemophilia C
C. Von Willebrand disease
D. Factor VIII deficiency

12. An older adult male patient visits the nurse practitioner in November for an annual physical exam and laboratory tests. Complete blood count (CBC) results are hemoglobin of 12 g/dL, hematocrit of 36%, and mean corpuscular volume (MCV) of 76 fL. The patient has a history of arthritis and reports taking a nonsteroidal anti-inflammatory drug (NSAID) every day for pain. The patient reports melena and dark stools as well as a craving for ice. Which of the following laboratory tests is the next step in this patient's evaluation?
A. Total iron-binding capacity, ferritin level, iron
B. Homocysteine, folate level
C. Vitamin B_{12} level, folate level
D. Hemoglobin electrophoresis

13. After the initial stages of iron-deficiency anemia (IDA), the patient's red blood cells (RBCs) are:
A. Microcytic
B. Normocytic
C. Macrocytic
D. Hyperchromic

(See answers next page.)

8. C) Ferrous sulfate

Iron-deficiency anemia (IDA) is significant for low hemo-globin and hematocrit, low red blood cell count, low absolute reticulocyte count, low MCV, and low MCHC. The patient's hemoglobin and hematocrit values are below the normal range for males (hemoglobin 13.6 to 16.9 g/dL and hematocrit 40% to 50%). The MCV is 74, which is below the normal range of 80 to 100 fL, indicating microcytic anemia. The MCHC is also below the normal range of 32% to 36%; a level of 30% indicates that this anemia is hypochromic. Pagophagia (pica for ice) is considered a specific finding for iron deficiency; fatigue and weakness may be seen in anemic patients, and restless leg syndrome may also be associated with IDA. All patients with IDA should be treated with iron supplementation (e.g., ferrous sulfate). Thalassemia is also characterized by microcytic, hypochromic anemia, but pica is not generally seen. Folic acid deficiency is characterized by macrocytic and normochromic anemia, whereas macrocytosis is often seen with pernicious anemia, along with decreased serum B_{12} levels. Folic acid supplementation would be recommended with a folic acid deficiency; vitamin B_{12} injection would be appropriate for patients with vitamin B_{12} deficiency with severe anemia and neuropsychiatric findings. A blood transfusion would be indicated for severe and symptomatic anemia.

9. B) The son will not be affected.

G6PD deficiency is an X-linked recessive genetic disease and the most common inherited red blood cell (RBC) enzyme abnormality. In males (who only have one X chromosome), a mutation on the single X chromosome causes the condition. Females must have a mutation on both X chromosomes to be affected with the condition. If only the father has the mutated X-linked gene, the daughter becomes an unaffected carrier because one of their X chromosomes has the mutation while the other is normal. Females with a heterozygous G6PD mutation usually do not have severe hemolytic anemia since half of the RBCs express the normal allele. If sons inherit a mutated X-linked gene from their mother, they will be affected. Fathers cannot pass X-linked recessive conditions to their sons.

10. C) Phlebotomy

Therapeutic phlebotomy is the mainstay of treatment for hereditary hemochromatosis, which causes iron overload deposition in many organs, including the liver and the heart. Chronic iron overload over decades damages the organs. Ferrous sulfate supplementation is the appropriate treatment for iron-deficiency anemia. Genetic counseling is recommended for patients with inherited disorders such as thalassemia, sickle cell anemia, and glucose-6-phosphate dehydrogenase deficiency.

11. D) Factor VIII deficiency

Factor VIII deficiency (hemophilia A) is a genetic disorder that is X-linked recessive. It is the most common type of hemophilia in the United States. Hemophilia B is an inherited deficiency of factor IX, also called Christmas disease. Also an X-linked recessive disorder, it is less common than hemophilia A. Hemophilia C is an inherited deficiency of factor XI, also called Rosenthal syndrome. It is an autosomal recessive disorder.

12. A) Total iron-binding capacity, ferritin level, iron

A male patient with a hemoglobin of 12 g/dL and a hematocrit of 36% has anemia. The MCV of 76 fL indicates microcytic anemia. The most common type of microcytic anemia is iron-deficiency anemia (IDA), which is evaluated by checking the total iron-binding capacity, ferritin level, and iron. In resource-rich countries, the major cause of IDA is blood loss, and gastrointestinal sources are common. The patient is at increased risk for gastrointestinal bleeding with the daily use of NSAIDs; the reported history of melena and ice craving increases suspicion. While the other lab tests may be helpful, evaluation for IDA is a priority given the patient's history.

13. B) Microcytic

During the early stages of IDA, the size (mean corpuscular volume) of the RBCs is often still normal (normocytic). However, when iron stores become depleted, the size, color, and shape of the RBCs will become abnormal. IDA and thalassemia are characterized by microcytic, hypochromic anemia. Folic acid deficiency and pernicious anemia are characterized by macrocytic, normochromic anemia. Anemia of chronic disease is associated with chronic normocytic, normochromic anemia.

14. A Black adult male patient presents with new onset of jaundice, dark urine, fatigue, and anorexia. He was seen a few days previously and treated for a possible urinary tract infection. He is on the third day of nitro-furantoin (Macrobid) 100 mg by mouth (PO) twice a day (BID) x 7 days. Hemoglobin is 11 g/dL, and hema-tocrit is 34%. The mean corpuscular volume (MCV) is 84 fL. The serum indirect bilirubin is elevated. The patient reports a family history of "a blood disease" but cannot remember the name of the disease. Which of the following conditions is most likely?

A. Glucose-6-phosphate dehydrogenase (G6PD) anemia
B. Folic acid deficiency
C. Iron-deficiency anemia (IDA)
D. Pernicious anemia

15. The mean corpuscular hemoglobin (MCH) is:

A. A measure of the average size of the red blood cells in a sample of blood
B. The average hemoglobin content in a red blood cell
C. A measure of the average hemoglobin concentration per red blood cell
D. The average volume (size) of the red blood cells

(See answers next page.)

14. A) Glucose-6-phosphate dehydrogenase (G6PD) anemia

The patient probably has G6PD anemia, a type of hemolytic anemia and the most common inherited red blood cell (RBC) enzyme abnormality. Exposure to certain drugs (e.g., sulfa drugs, acetazolamide, dapsone) or foods (e.g., fava beans) can cause acute hemolysis because these substances cause oxidative damage to the RBC. In the United States, it is seen mostly in Black males or males of African descent. The elevation in the indirect bilirubin levels is caused by hemolysis of RBCs. While rare genetic disorders can be associated with folic acid deficiency, IDA, and pernicious anemia, the use of nitrofurantoin (Macrobid) is less likely to contribute to these types of anemias. Vitamin B_{12} deficiency may be associated with medications such as metformin, histamine receptor antagonists, proton pump inhibitors, and nitrous oxide. Folate deficiency is associated with drugs that interfere with metabolism (e.g., methotrexate, sulfasalazine). Medications that reduce gastric acidity (e.g., proton pump inhibitors, antacids, histamine receptor blockers) may reduce iron absorption.

15. B) The average hemoglobin content in a red blood cell

The MCH is the average hemoglobin content in a red blood cell. The mean corpuscular volume (MCV) is the average volume (size) of the red blood cells. Mean corpuscular hemoglobin concentration (MCHC) is the average hemoglobin concentration per red blood cell. Red cell distribution width (RDW) is a measure of the variation in red blood cell size.

MUSCULOSKELETAL SYSTEM REVIEW

DANGER SIGNALS

ACUTE OSTEOMYELITIS

Patient complains of localized bone pain, swelling, redness, and tenderness of affected area and fever. If on leg or hip, may refuse to walk and bear weight. An acute infection of the bone that causes inflammation and destruction, which can be caused by bacteria, mycobacteria, and fungi. Most cases are due to contiguous spread from a nearby infected wound to the bone. For example, an infected pressure sore on the heel can cause osteomyelitis of the calcaneus (via nonhematogenous spread). Hematogenous spread is seeding of the bone from an infection in the bloodstream (bacteremia). For example, a patient with bacteremia complains of refractory vertebral pain and tenderness (hematogenous osteomyelitis). Direct trauma to the bone can also result in infection. Among the most common bacteria that can cause osteomyelitis is *Staphylococcus aureus* (including methicillin-resistant *S. aureus* or MRSA). An MRI can show changes to the bone and bone marrow before plain x-ray or radiograph. White blood cell (WBC) count, erythrocyte sedimentation rate (ESR; sed rate), and C-reactive protein (CRP) are often elevated. Blood cultures may be positive. Antibiotic treatment is based on culture and sensitivity (C&S) results. May need surgical debridement, amputation, and bone grafts.

BONE METASTASES

Bone pain can feel achy, sharp, and well localized, or it can feel like neuropathic pain (burning shooting pain). It can be severe with night pain and/or pain with weight bearing. It may be accompanied by night sweats, malaise, fever, and weight loss. It can be constant or intermittent and can be exacerbated with movement of the joint or bone. Pathologic fractures may occur. Bone is one of the most common sites of distant metastases. Routine labs may show elevated levels of alkaline phosphatase and/or serum calcium (hypercalcemia). Cancers of the prostate, breast, lung, thyroid, and kidney make up the majority (80%) of cases of bone metastases. A radiograph (x-ray) has poor sensitivity, but it can show bony lesions and may show early lesions. In general, MRI is the most sensitive and specific imaging test.

CAUDA EQUINA SYNDROME

Acute onset of low back pain accompanied by pain radiating down one or both legs, saddle anesthesia and sensory loss of the affected nerve roots, bladder incontinence (or retention of urine), and fecal incontinence. Accompanied by bilateral lower extremity numbness and weakness. Occurs when there is dysfunction or damage to the lumbar and sacral nerve roots of the cauda equina (e.g., disc herniation, epidural abscess, or tumor, etc.). The term *cauda equina* is Latin for "horse's tails," which describes the collection of nerve roots at the end of the spinal cord. A surgical emergency. Needs spinal decompression. Refer to ED.

COLLES FRACTURE

Fracture of the distal radius (with or without ulnar fracture) of the forearm along with dorsal displacement of wrist. History of falling onto outstretched hand, or "FOOSH," (as in navicular fracture). This fracture is also known as the "dinner fork" fracture because of the appearance of arm and wrist after the fracture. It is a common type of wrist fracture.

HIP FRACTURE

Patient has a history of slipping or falling. Sudden onset of one-sided hip pain. Unable to walk and bear weight on affected hip. If mild fracture, may bear weight on affected hip. If displaced fracture, presence of severe hip pain with external rotation of the hip/leg (abduction) and leg shortening. More common in older adults. One-year mortality rate for older adults is approximately 21% secondary to complications of immobility, such as pneumonia and deep vein thrombophlebitis.

PELVIC FRACTURE

History of significant or high-energy trauma such as a motor vehicle or motorcycle accident. Signs and symptoms depend on degree of injury to the pelvic bones and other pelvic structures such as nerves, blood vessels, and pelvic organs. Assess for ecchymosis and swelling in the lower abdomen, hips, groin, and/or scrotum. May have bladder and/or fecal incontinence, vaginal or rectal bleeding, hematuria, numbness. May cause internal hemorrhage, which can be life-threatening. Check airway, breathing, and circulation first (the ABCs).

SCAPHOID (NAVICULAR) FRACTURE

Wrist pain on palpation of the anatomic snuffbox (Figure 14.1). Pain on axial loading of the thumb. History of falling forward with outstretched hand (hyperextension of the wrist) to break the fall. Initial x-ray of the wrist often normal, but a repeat x-ray in 2 weeks will show the scaphoid fracture (due to callus bone formation). High risk of avascular necrosis and nonunion. Place into a thumb spica splint and refer to an orthopedist.

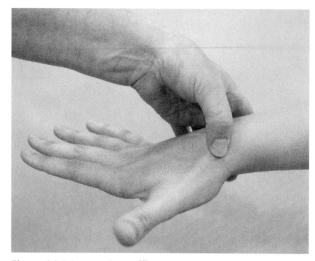

Figure 14.1 Anatomic snuffbox.
Source: Myrick, K. M., & Karosas, L. M. (Eds.). (2021). (See Resources section for complete source information.)

NORMAL FINDINGS

JOINT ANATOMY

- Synovial fluid: Thick serous clear fluid (sterile) that provides lubrication for the joint. Cloudy synovial fluid can be indicative of infection; order C&S
- Synovial space: Space between two bones in a synovial joint filled with synovial fluid
- Articular cartilage: The cartilage lining the open surfaces of bones in a joint
- Meniscus or menisci (plural): Crescent-shaped cartilage located in each knee; two menisci in each knee; aid in dissipating loading forces placed on the knee, stabilization during rotation, and lubricating the knee joint
- Tendon: Connects muscle to the bone (partial or complete tear of tendon or muscle is a strain)
- Ligament: Connects bone to bone (partial or complete tear of a ligament is a sprain)
- Bursae: Saclike structures located on the anterior and posterior areas of a joint that act as padding; filled with synovial fluid when inflamed (bursitis). Cloudy fluid is abnormal and suggestive of infection.

ORTHOPEDIC TERMINOLOGY

Types of Movement
- Abduction: Movement going away from the body
- Adduction: Movement going toward the body

- Flexion: Decreases the angle between two bones; bending
- Extension: Increases the angle and straightens the joint

Hands and Feet
- Metacarpals: Bones of the hands
- Carpals: Bones of the wrist. There are a total of eight wrist bones.
- Phalanges: Fingers and the toes; singular form of the term is *phalanx*.
- Metatarsals: Bones of the feet
- Talus: Ankle bone
- Calcaneus: Heel bone

Proximal and Distal
- Proximal: Body part located closer to the body (compared with distal)
- Distal: Body part farther away from the center of the body

BENIGN VARIANTS
- Genu recurvatum: Hyperextension or backward curvature of the knees
- Genu valgum: Knock-knees
- Genu varum: Bowlegs

EXERCISE AND INJURIES
Within the first 48 hours of an injury:
- Avoid vigorous or strenuous exercise and exacerbating activities; rest is key to reduce risk of increased inflammation and damage to the affected joints
- Engage in gentle range-of-motion (ROM) exercises

RICE Mnemonic
Within the first 48 hours after musculoskeletal trauma, follow these rules:
- **R**est: Avoid using injured joint or limb.
- **I**ce: Apply cold packs on injured area (e.g., 20 minutes on, 20 minutes off) for first 24 to 48 hours.
- **C**ompression: Use an elastic bandage wrap over joints (e.g., ankles, knees) to decrease swelling and provide support.
- **E**levation: This prevents or decreases swelling. Avoid bearing weight on affected joint.

Exercise
- Adults: 150 minutes weekly of moderate-intensity aerobic activity or 75 minutes per week of vigorous aerobic activity or a combination of both; add muscle strengthening exercise at least 2 days a week. In hypertensive adults, aerobic exercise has been found to lower resting systolic/diastolic BP.

- Children and teens (6 to 17 years): 60 minutes daily of moderate-to-vigorous physical activity (mostly aerobic); include muscle-strengthening and bone strengthening activity three times per week
- Non–weight-bearing exercise: Isometric exercises are non-weight-bearing exercises that are performed in a fixed state in which the muscle is flexed against a stationary object. An example is pushing one fist against the palm of the other hand, which is stationary. Biking and swimming are aerobic exercises, which are non–weight-bearing (do not strengthen bones).
- Weight-bearing exercise: In weight-bearing exercises, the bones/muscles are forced against gravity. Weight-bearing exercise is recommended for treating osteopenia and osteoporosis to help strengthen bone durability. Examples include dancing, high-impact aerobics, hiking, jogging/running, jumping rope, stair climbing, and tennis.

ORTHOPEDIC MANEUVERS

Test both extremities. Use the normal limb as the baseline for comparison.

Finkelstein's Test

De Quervain's tenosynovitis is caused by an inflammation of the tendon sheath, which is located at the base of the thumb. The screening test is Finkelstein's (Figure 14.2), which is positive if there is pain and tenderness on the wrist on the thumb side (abductor pollicis longus and extensor pollicis brevis tendons).

Procedure

Tell patient to flex thumb toward the palm, then make a fist by folding remaining fingers over the thumb, then tell patient to ulnarly deviate their wrist. Positive test if patient complains that the tendon (on the side of the thumb) hurts with ulnar deviation.

Drawer Sign

Drawer sign (Figure 14.3) is a test for knee stability. Excessive laxity of affected knee is suggestive of a torn ligament.

Anterior Drawer Sign

Patient lies on examination table (supine). The hip is flexed to 45 degrees, and the knee is bent to 90 degrees.

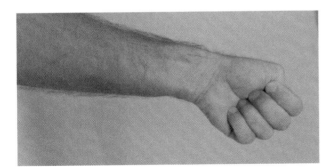

Figure 14.2 Finkelstein's test.
Source: Gawlik, K. S., Melnyk, B. M., & Teall, A. M. (Eds.). (2021). (See Resources section for complete source information.)

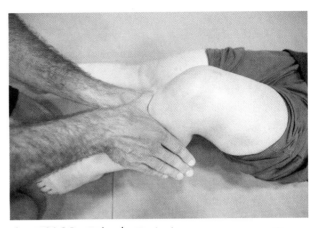

Figure 14.3 Posterior drawer test.
Source: Myrick, K. M., & Karosas, L. M. (Eds.). (2021). (See Resources section for complete source information.)

The examiner sits on the forefoot/toes to stabilize the knee joint. Then examiner grasps the lower leg by the joint line and pulls the tibia anteriorly (like opening a drawer). A positive anterior drawer sign is indicative of a damaged or torn anterior cruciate ligament (ACL).

Posterior Drawer Sign

Patient lies on examination table (supine). The hip is flexed to 45 degrees, and the knee is bent to 90 degrees. The examiner sits on the forefoot/toes to stabilize the knee joint. Then examiner grasps the lower leg by the joint line and pushes it posteriorly (like closing a drawer; see Figure 14.3). A positive posterior drawer sign is indicative of a damaged or torn posterior cruciate ligament (PCL). Sensitivity is 90%, and specificity is 99%.

Lachman's Sign

With the patient's knee in 30 degrees of flexion, the femur is stabilized with one hand, and the other hand is used to apply force to the tibia to displace the tibia forward on the femur (Figure 14.4). Positive result is suggestive of a tear to the ACL.

Collateral Ligaments (Knees)

Positive finding is an increase in laxity of the damaged knee (ligament tear).
- Valgus stress test of the knee: Test for the medial collateral ligament (MCL)
- Varus stress test of the knee: Test for the lateral collateral ligament (LCL)

JOINT INJECTIONS

Administering intra-articular/periarticular joint injections with steroids (e.g., triamcinolone) is indicated for inflammatory arthritis (in patients that have long periods of near remission) as well as soft tissue structures (such as the subdeltoid bursa and tendon sheathing). The use of injections should be limited for any given indication; there is no absolute number but varies with each disease and patient

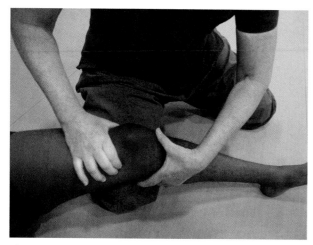

Figure 14.4 Lachman's test.
Source: Myrick, K. M., & Karosas, L. M. (Eds.). (2021). (See Resources section for complete source information.)

specifics. If high resistance is felt when pushing syringe, do not force. Withdraw needle slightly (do not remove from joint) and redirect.

Complications include tendon rupture, nerve damage, infection, bleeding, hypothalamic–pituitary–adrenal (HPA) suppression, others. Joint injections are generally safe in patients who are on anticoagulation therapy; evidence has shown no significant difference in bleeding.

IMAGING

- Plain x-ray films (radiographs): Show bone fractures, osteoarthritis (OA; joint space narrowing, osteophyte formation), damaged bone (osteomyelitis, metastases), metal and other dense objects. Not recommended for soft tissue structures such as menisci, tendons, and ligaments. Often used as the initial imaging modality.
- CT: Combines x-rays (gamma radiation) that are rotating in a continuous circle around the patient with computer software to show slices of three-dimensional images. Can be done with or without contrast. Detects bleeding, aneurysms, masses, pelvic and bone trauma, fractures.
- MRI: Often, the gold standard for injuries of the cartilage, menisci, tendons, ligaments, or joints. MRI uses a magnetic field and radio waves, not radiation (compared with x-rays and CT scans). Can be done without or with contrast. Contraindicated in metal implants, certain cardiovascular (CV) implantable devices, cardiac valves, aneurysm clips, drug infusion pumps, "triggerfish" contact lens, cochlear implant, neurostimulators, electrodes for deep brain stimulation, and bullets, shrapnel, and other metal fragments.

CLINICAL PEARLS

- MRI: Best for soft tissue, joints, and occult fractures.
- X-rays (radiographs): Best for bone injuries such as fractures. Some radiographs are normal for the first 2 to 3 weeks after onset of injury (e.g., stress fractures).

DISEASE REVIEW

ACUTE MUSCULOSKELETAL INJURIES

Treatment: RICE (Rest, Ice, Compression, Elevation)

- Ice is best during first 48 hours postinjury; 15 to 20 minutes per hour several times/day (frequency varies).
- Rest and elevate affected joint to help decrease swelling.
- Compress joints as needed. Use elastic bandage wrap; helps with swelling and provides stability.
- Administer nonsteroidal anti-inflammatory drugs (NSAIDs) (naproxen BID, ibuprofen QID) for pain and swelling PRN.

ANKYLOSING SPONDYLITIS

Chronic inflammatory disorder (seronegative arthritis) that affects mainly the spine (axial skeleton) and the sacroiliac joints (axial spondylarthritis). Other joints affected include the shoulders, hips, knees, and sternoclavicular joints. A few develop diffuse swelling of the fingers (dactylitis).

Classic Case

Young adult male complains of a chronic case of back pain (>3 months) that started at the neck and progressed down to the spine. Neck pain is an early symptom. Reports that the pain gradually progressed from the neck to the upper back (thoracic spine) and then the lower back. Impaired spinal mobility. Joint pain keeps him awake at night. Associated with generalized symptoms such as low-grade fever and fatigue. May have chest pain with respiration (costochondritis) and costovertebral tenderness. Long-term stiffness improves with activity. Some may have mid-buttock pain (sciatica indicates sacroiliac spine is involved). Pain is diminished with exercise and is not relieved by rest. Insidious onset.

Objective Findings

- Causes a marked loss of ROM of the spine such as forward bending, rotation, and lateral bending.
- Decreased respiratory excursion down to <2.5 cm (normal 5 cm). Some have lordosis. Hyperkyphosis (hunchback) occurs after 10 years or more with disease.
- Uveitis occurs in 25% to 35% of patients. Complaints of eye irritation, photosensitivity, and eye pain. Scleral injection and blurred vision occur. Unilateral eye involvement is common. Refer to ophthalmologist as soon as possible (treated with steroids).

Labs

- ESR and CRP: Slightly elevated; rheumatoid factor (RF) is negative.
- Spinal radiograph: Classic "bamboo spine" in late ankylosing spondylitis (resembles bamboo; Figure 14.5).

Treatment Plan

- Refer to rheumatologist.
- If smoker, advise smoking cessation. Screen for anxiety and depression. Refer for physical therapy for initial evaluation and training, including postural training, ROM, stretching.

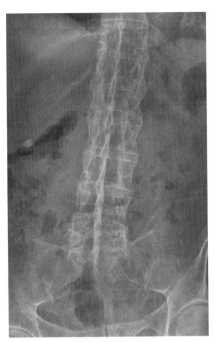

Figure 14.5 Ankylosing spondylitis. Radiograph of characteristic "bamboo" spine.

- Exercise therapy combined with hydrotherapy is more effective than exercise alone.
- Advise patient to buy a mattress with good support.
- First-line initial treatment is NSAIDs such as naproxen up to 500 mg twice a day or ibuprofen (up to 800 mg TID). Any NSAID may be effective; usually the maximum dose is needed to control pain.
- If high risk of bleeding, consider gastro-prophylaxis with a proton-pump inhibitor (PPI) in patients taking NSAIDs long term.
- For severe cases, treatment options are tumor necrosis factor (TNF) inhibitors, biologics (e.g., etanercept), disease-modifying antirheumatic drugs (DMARDS; methotrexate), spinal fusion.

Complications
- Anterior uveitis
- Osteopenia, vertebral and nonvertebral fractures
- Neurologic manifestations: Spinal cord injury, atlanto-axial subluxation, cauda equina syndrome
- Renal and pulmonary disease
- Possible pregnancy complications
- CV disease: Hypertension, heart failure, acute coronary syndromes, strokes, venous thromboembolism, conduction abnormalities, aortic disease

EXAM TIPS
- Ankylosing spondylitis: Know signs and symptoms so you are able to diagnose it on the exam. Bamboo spine is pathognomonic for ankylosing spondylitis.

- Uveitis: Swelling of the uvea, the middle layer of the eye that supplies blood to the retina (refer to ophthalmologist). Initial treatment includes topical steroids. Oral glucocorticoids are recommended for those resistant to initial therapy. Higher risk of uveitis with inflammatory disease (e.g., ankylosing spondylitis, sarcoidosis, inflammatory bowel disease).

ELBOW TENDINOPATHY
Represents a chronic tendinosis at the origin of the wrist flexors or extensors. Common cause of elbow pain. Lateral epicondyle tendon pain (tennis elbow) or medial epicondyle tendon pain (golfer's elbow). Usually caused by overuse injury. Risk factors: increased age, repetitive wrist movement, forceful activity, and poor stroke mechanics among tennis and golf players.

Lateral Epicondylitis (Tennis Elbow)
Classic Case
Gradual onset of pain on the outside of the elbow that sometimes radiates to the forearms. Pain worse with twisting or grasping movements (opening jars, shaking hands). Physical exam will show local tenderness over the lateral epicondyle.

Medial Epicondylitis (Golfer's Elbow)
Classic Case
Gradual onset of aching pain on the medial area of the elbow (the side of the elbow that is touching the body), which can last a few weeks to months. Pain can be mild to severe. More common in women age 45 to 64 years. Occurs over the medial aspect of the elbow (ulnar nerve). Physical exam will show localized tenderness over the medial epicondyle.

Complications
Ulnar nerve neuropathy and/or palsy (long-term pressure/damage). Complaint of numbness/tingling on the little finger and the lateral side of the ring finger and weakness of the hand. Worst-case scenario is development of a permanent deformity called "claw hand." Refer to neurologist if suspect ulnar nerve palsy.

GOUT
Deposits of uric acid crystals (monosodium urate) inside joints and tendons due to genetic excess production or low excretion of purine crystals (by-product of protein metabolism). High levels of uric acid can crystallize in the peripheral joints such as the first joint of large toe (metatarsophalangeal [MTP] joint), ankles, hands, and wrists. More common in middle-aged males older than 30 years of age.

The gold standard for diagnosing gout is performed by joint aspiration of the synovial fluid of the joint. Microscopy exam using a polarized light is used to identify uric acid crystals in the synovial fluid to diagnose gout. Recurrent flares that are accompanied by an elevated serum uric acid (>6.8 mg/dL) level is the most common way to diagnose gout.

Classic Case
Middle-aged man presents with painful, hot, red, and swollen MTP joint of great toe (podagra). Patient is limping due to severe pain from weight bearing on affected joint.

Reports onset is more often at night. History of previous attacks at same site. Precipitated by ingestion of alcohol, meats, or seafood. Chronic gout has tophi (small white nodules full of urates on ears and joints). History of recurrent inflammatory arthritis (gout flare).

Labs

Uric acid level is elevated (>6.8 mg/dL). Treatment target is <6 mg/dL.

- During the acute phase, uric acid level is normal; uric acid level does not begin to rise until after the acute phase.
- An elevated urate level can support diagnosis but is not diagnostic.
- Most accurate time to assess for serum urate is 2 weeks or more after a gout flare subsides.
- Other conditions that increase serum uric acid include chemotherapy and radiation therapy.
- Medications that increase uric acid include hydrochlorothiazide and furosemide.
- WBC is often elevated.
- ESR is elevated.
- CRP is elevated.

Treatment Plan

Gout Flare

- First goal is to provide pain relief. Treatment for gout flare should be started as soon as possible for best results. Medications used are oral steroids, NSAIDs, or colchicine.
- During flares, if patient is taking daily urate-lowering therapy (ULT; e.g., allopurinol, probenecid, febuxostat, lesinurad, pegloticase), do not discontinue it. Can continue taking these meds with gout flare meds.
- Glucocorticoids such as prednisone or prednisolone 30 to 40 mg given once a day PO or divided into BID dosing; taper the dose over the next 7 to 10 days. Shorter duration (5 days) or tapered packs (Medrol Dosepak) are also available. May be given IV if unable to tolerate oral medications.
- NSAIDs can be used as alternative therapy if patient has contraindications to steroids (and does not have renal, CV, or active GI disease); indomethacin BID, naproxen sodium BID, diclofenac BID, celecoxib BID, or ibuprofen (800 mg TID). Do not use narcotics (not effective for gout pain). Can discontinue NSAIDs after 2 to 3 days of complete resolution.

EXAM TIPS

- NSAIDs injure the GI tract by blocking cyclooxygenase-1 (COX-1) and cyclooxygenase-2 (COX-2), resulting in lower levels of systemic prostaglandins.
- Aspirin (acetylsalicylic acid) is a type of NSAID. It affects platelets and clotting permanently, but it will resolve once the affected platelets (life span about 10 days) resolve (if not on chronic NSAIDs).

- Colchicine:
  - Two tablets (1.2 mg) at the onset of pain and then one tablet (0.6 mg) in 1 hour. Total dose on day 1 not to exceed 1.8 mg. Advise to avoid eating grapefruit or drinking grapefruit juice with colchicine.
  - Common side effects include diarrhea, abdominal pain, cramps, nausea, and vomiting.
  - Drug interactions are macrolides, azole antifungals, some antivirals, calcium channel blockers (CCBs), cyclosporine, tacrolimus, others.
  - Contraindications include moderate to severe renal or hepatic impairment.
  - Serious and life-threatening effects are blood cytopenias, rhabdomyolysis, liver failure, neuropathy.
- Joint injection for patients unable to take oral medications with actively inflamed joints and no infection.

Maintenance

- In general, wait several weeks after acute gout flare before starting on ULT. However, in select patients, a reasonable alternative is to initiate ULT during a flare.
- Indications for ULT are frequent or disabling gout flares, clinical or radiographic signs of chronic gouty arthritis, tophaceous deposits, and high risk of future severe gout flares.
- Titrate ULT medication to achieve a serum urate in the range <6 mg/dL. Serum urate levels should be monitored to assure concentrations stay within the goal range.

Urate-Lowering Medications

- Xanthine oxidase inhibitors (XOI): Allopurinol (Zyloprim), febuxostat (Uloric)
  - Boxed warning for febuxostat (Uloric); gout patients with heart disease treated with febuxostat have a higher rate of CV death compared with those treated with allopurinol.
  - Allopurinol (Zyloprim) initial dose is 100 mg daily; increase dose until serum uric level is <6 mg/dL. Check CBC (affects bone marrow), renal function, liver function at baseline, then periodically. Preferred urate-lowering agent and generally well tolerated.
- Uricosoric agents: Probenecid, lesinurad (Zurampic)
- Uricase: Pegloticase IV can cause anaphylaxis and infusion reactions; premedicate with antihistamines and corticosteroids

Allopurinol Hypersensitivity

- If renal disease, at higher risk. Manifests as fever, rash (toxic epidermal necrolysis), and hepatitis. Stop allopurinol immediately if it occurs and refer.
- Consider febuxostat (Uloric) if allergic to allopurinol. Alternative med is probenecid.

Lifestyle Modifications

Lifestyle changes and dietary education are an important part of treatment.

- Patients should be instructed to avoid/minimize alcohol (<2 servings for males/<1 serving for females).
- Avoid fructose- or corn syrup–sweetened beverages, which increase uric acid. Remain well hydrated.

- Recommend Dietary Approaches to Stop Hypertension (DASH) or Mediterranean diet. Advise dietary moderation in purine intake.
- Potential benefit in consumption of cherries, vitamin C, fish, and omega-3 fatty acids.

Complications
Joint destruction, joint deformity, tophi

HAMSTRING MUSCLE INJURY
The hamstring is composed of three muscles and is located in the posterior thigh. The hamstring muscles are used for knee flexion and hip extension. If a complete tear is suspected, refer patients to orthopedic specialist.

Classic Case
Most hamstring injuries are acute. The patient will report hearing a popping noise accompanied by the sudden onset of posterior thigh pain while performing activities such as sprinting. On physical exam, there may be swelling, bruising, warmth, and tenderness on the posterior thigh. A muscular mass might be palpable.

Imaging
Musculoskeletal ultrasonography and MRI are the best methods of assessing hamstring injuries.

LOW-BACK PAIN
Very common disorder. Usually due to soft-tissue inflammation, sciatica, sprains, muscle spasms, or herniated discs (usually on L5–S1). The majority of patients seen in primary care have nonspecific low-back pain, which is usually self-limited. Rule out fracture and other serious etiology.
- Acute back pain: Up to 4 weeks
- Subacute back pain: 4 to 12 weeks
- Chronic back pain: Persists for 12 weeks or longer
- Risk factors: Age, smoking, anxiety, depression, psychologically strenuous work, physically strenuous or sedentary work, obesity

Indications for Further Evaluation
- History of significant trauma
- Suspect cancer metastases
- Suspect infection (osteomyelitis)
- Suspect spinal/vertebral fracture (older adult with osteopenia/osteoporosis, chronic steroid use)
- Patient age older than 50 with new onset of back pain (rule out cancer) or pain that wakes patient from sleep
- Suspect spinal stenosis (rule out ankylosing spondylitis)
- Suspect cauda equina or spinal cord compression
- Suspect radiculopathy (spinal nerve root inflammation such as sciatica)
- Suspect ankylosing spondylitis
- Fevers, night sweats, weight loss, or signs of systemic illness
- Symptoms worsening despite usual treatment
- Common site for herniated disc with symptoms is at L5 to S1 (buttock/leg pain)

Labs
- MRI is best method for diagnosing a herniated disc. Bone scan may be helpful in identifying occult, lytic lesions.
- Imaging for low-back pain without other symptoms increases risk of additional or invasive procedures.

Treatment Plan
- Treatment depends on etiology. For uncomplicated back pain, use NSAIDs (naproxen sodium); apply warm packs if muscle spasms.
- Muscle relaxants if associated with muscle spasms (causes drowsiness; warn patient)
- Abdominal and core-strengthening exercises after acute phase
- Consider chiropractor for uncomplicated low-back pain

> **NOTE**
>
> Complete bedrest is usually not recommended except in severe cases of low-back pain because it will cause deconditioning (loss of muscle tone and endurance) and increased risk of complications from immobility.

Complications
Cauda Equina Syndrome
Acute pressure on a sacral nerve root results in inflammatory and ischemic changes to the nerve. Sacral nerves innervate pelvic structures such as the sphincters (anal and bladder). Considered a surgical emergency. Needs spinal and/or nerve root decompression. Refer to ED.

EXAM TIPS

- Learn how to treat gout flare-up.
- Learn signs/symptoms of cauda equina. If suspected, refer to ED.

Red Flags
- Bladder and bowel incontinence
- Sensory loss in the distribution of the affected nerve roots; may cause saddle anesthesia
- Low back pain accompanied by pain radiating into one or both legs
- Bilateral leg weakness

MEDIAL TIBIA STRESS SYNDROME (SHIN SPLINTS) AND STRESS FRACTURES OF THE TIBIA AND FIBULA
Lower extremity injury caused by overuse, resulting in microtears and inflammation of the muscles and tendons of the tibia. Most athletes with a stress fracture of the tibia or fibula may resemble medial tibial stress syndrome (MTSS), often referred to as "shin splints." Both are common in runners (higher incidence in females) and people with flat feet. Females are at higher risk of stress fracture, especially those with relative energy deficiency syndrome (REDS)—amenorrhea in females, eating disorder, osteoporosis. Onset precipitated or worsened with intensification of activity (increased mileage and/or frequency of training).

Recognize signs and symptoms of a medial tibial stress fracture.

Classic Case

Runner reports increased frequency/distance running and complains of recent onset of pain on the inner edge of the tibia. Pain may be sharp and stabbing or dull and throbbing. Aggravated during and after exercise. Complains of a sore spot on the inside of the lower leg or the shin (tibia). Some patients may have pain on the anterior aspect of the shin. Focal area is tender when touched. Tenderness is much more diffuse and there is no discrete palpable lesion in those with MTSS.

Treatment Plan

- Follow RICE (rest, ice, compression, elevation) mnemonic. Periods of rest are recommended.
- Apply cold packs during acute exacerbation, for 20 minutes at a time, several times a day for first 24 to 48 hours and then as needed.
- Take NSAIDs as needed.
- Compression bandage or sleeve may help decrease swelling. Using cushioned shoes (sneakers) for daily activity helps decrease tibial stress.
- When pain is gone, wait about 2 weeks before resuming exercise. Avoid hills and very hard surfaces until the shin splints have resolved.
- If stress fracture is suspected, recommend lower-impact exercises (e.g., swimming, stationary bike, elliptical trainer).
- Stretch before exercise and start at lower intensity. Wear supportive sneakers.
- If suspect stress fracture, plain radiographs are often the first imaging study; however, they are often normal initially. MRI is highly sensitive and specific. Refer to orthopedic specialist.

MENISCUS TEAR (KNEES)

The two menisci are crescent-shaped pads of fibrocartilage located within the knee joint. Tears in the meniscus result from trauma and/or overuse. Sports with higher risk are soccer, basketball, and football.

Classic Case

Patient may complain of clicking, locking, or buckling of the knee(s). Some patients are unable to fully extend affected knee. Patient may limp. Complains of knee pain and difficulty walking and bending the knee. Some complain of joint line pain. Decreased ROM. Certain movements aggravate symptoms.

Physical Examination

Assess for joint line tenderness and knee ROM. Look for locking or inability to fully extend or straighten the leg, squat, or kneel. Will be unable to squat or kneel. Knee may be swollen (joint effusion). Observe patient's gait.

- Steinman's test: Flex the knee joint and palpate the joint line. Pain over the posterior joint line with flexion is positive for meniscus tear.
- Apley's test: Patient is prone with affected knee flexed at 90 degrees. Stabilize patient's thigh (with examiner's knee or hand). Press the patient's heel downward (push heel toward the floor) while the foot is internally and externally rotated. The examiner is compressing the meniscus between the tibia and femur while twisting the foot. Positive sign is pain elicited with compression of the knee.

Treatment Plan

- Follow the RICE (rest, ice, compression, elevation) rules. Rest the knee and avoid or minimize positions that overstress the knees, such as squatting, kneeling, climbing stairs.
- Apply ice/cold pack for 20 minutes every 4 to 6 hours, elevate the limb. Many need crutches.
- When the pain and swelling are resolved, start quadriceps-strengthening exercises. The quadriceps are the largest muscles of the body; they will help to stabilize the knees. Swimming, water aerobics, and light jogging are possible exercises. NSAIDs or acetaminophen for pain as needed. Locking or unstable knees should be referred to orthopedist; many need arthroscopy to repair menisci.
- Most sensitive imaging for detecting meniscal tear is MRI.

MORTON'S NEUROMA

Inflammation of the digital nerve of the foot between the third and fourth metatarsals. Increased risk with high-heeled shoes, tight shoes, obesity, dancers, runners.

Classic Case

Middle-aged woman complains of many weeks of foot pain that is worsened by walking, especially while wearing high heels or tight narrow shoes. The pain is described as burning and/or numbness, and it is located on the space between the third and fourth toes (metatarsals) on the forefoot. Physical exam of the foot may reveal a small nodule on the space between the third and fourth toes. Some patients palpate the same nodule and report it as "pebble-like."

Mulder Test

This test for Morton's neuroma is done by grasping the first and fifth metatarsals and squeezing the forefoot (Figure 14.6). Positive test is hearing a click along with a patient report of pain during compression. Pain is relieved when the compression is stopped.

Treatment Plan

- Avoid wearing tight, narrow shoes and high heels. Use forefoot pad. Wear well-padded shoes.
- Diagnosed by clinical presentation and history. Refer to podiatrist.

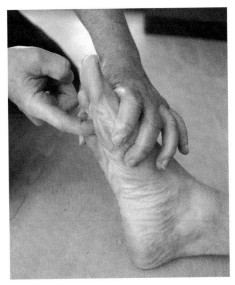

Figure 14.6 Mulder test.
Source: Myrick, K. M., & Karosas, L. M. (Eds.). (2021). (See Resources section for complete source information.)

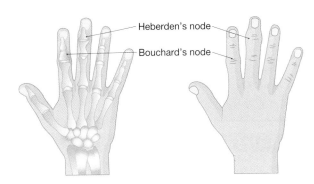

Figure 14.7 Bouchard's and Heberden's nodes.

OSTEOARTHRITIS

OA is often misnamed as degenerative joint disease (DJD) because it was formerly considered a simply degenerative "wear and tear" process. However, the pathogenesis is more complex and involves an inflammatory process with altered joint function that is associated with characteristic pathologic changes in the joint tissue and destruction of the articular cartilage. Large weight-bearing joints (hips and knees) and the hands (Bouchard's and Heberden's nodes) are most commonly affected. It can affect one side or bilaterally. Risk factors include older age, overuse of joints, and positive family history.

Goal of Treatment
- Relieve pain.
- Preserve joint mobility and function.
- Minimize disability and protect joint.

Classic Case
Insidious onset (slow progression over years). Middle-aged or older adult complaining of early-morning joint pain and stiffness with inactivity and motor restriction. Shorter duration of joint stiffness (<30 minutes) compared with rheumatoid arthritis (RA). Pain aggravated by overuse of joint. During exacerbations, involved joint may be swollen and tender to palpation (absence of warmth). May be one-sided (e.g., right hip only). Absence of systemic symptoms (compared to RA). Deformities such as Heberden's and/or Bouchard's nodes may be noted (Figure 14.7). Crepitus and reduced ROM may be noted on exam.
- Heberden's nodes: Bony nodules on the distal interphalangeal (DIP) joints
- Bouchard's nodes: Bony nodules on the proximal interphalangeal (PIP) joints

Nonpharmacologic Management
- Exercise (with caution) at least three times a week. Lose weight. Stop smoking.
- Do isometric exercises to strengthen quadriceps muscles (knee OA).
- Engage in weight-bearing exercise (walking, lifting weights), resistance-band exercises.
- Avoid aggravating activities. Use cold or warm packs and ultrasound treatment.
- Use walking aids. Patellar taping by physical therapist can reduce load on knees.
- Consider the use of glucosamine supplements (limited evidence of benefit), transcutaneous nerve stimulation, tai chi exercises, acupuncture.

Treatment Plan
- In patients with one or a few joints affected, start with topical NSAIDs.
- Oral NSAIDs recommended in patients with inadequate relief with topical NSAIDs or those with symptomatic OA in multiple joints. Use lowest dose of oral NSAIDs such as ibuprofen (Advil), one to two tablets every 4 to 6 hours; naproxen (Aleve) BID; or Anaprox DS one tablet every 12 hours PRN.
  - Use caution or avoid oral NSAIDs in patients with kidney dysfunction, CV disease, peptic ulcer disease (PUD), and those with high bleeding risk (especially those taking anticoagulants).

- All NSAIDs have a boxed warning for risk of CV thrombotic events including MI and stroke; risk is higher for COX-2-selective NSAIDs (e.g., celecoxib). If patient is at high risk for both GI bleeding and CV side effects, avoid NSAIDs.
- GI bleed risk factors include history of uncomplicated ulcer, warfarin (Coumadin), PUD, and platelet disorder

EXAM TIPS

- Ketorolac (Toradol) is limited to 5 days of use. The first dose is given intramuscular or IV.
- Types of treatment methods used for OA: NSAIDs (oral and topical), steroid injection on inflamed joints (not routinely recommended), surgery (e.g., joint replacement).

- Duloxetine is recommended for patients with OA in multiple joints and contraindications to oral NSAIDs.
- Topical capsaicin is recommended when a few joints are involved, and other interventions are contraindicated.
- Intraarticular glucocorticoid injections are not routinely used due to short duration of its effects.
- Acetaminophen is no longer recommended given safety concerns and nonclinically significant effects on pain.
- Opioid analgesics should be avoided if possible given side effects (e.g., nausea, dizziness, drowsiness).
- Rule out osteoporosis and order bone mineral density test (postmenopausal females, chronic steroid treatment males/females).

Topical Medicine

- Diclofenac gel (Voltaren gel) (NSAID); apply to painful area and massage well into skin QID.
- Capsaicin cream applied to painful area QID. Avoid contact with eyes/mucous membranes. Capsaicin comes from chili peppers. Also used to treat neuropathic pain (e.g., post shingles).
- Do not use on wounds/abraded skin. Avoid bathing/showering afterward (so that it is not washed off).

Nonsteroidal Anti-Inflammatory Drug Risk

- High risk of GI bleeding: ketorolac (Toradol)
- Low risk of GI bleeding: Celecoxib (Celebrex)
- High risk of CV events: Diclofenac
- Low risk of CV events: High-dose naproxen

EXAM TIPS

- Do not confuse the treatment options for OA with those for RA.
- Bouchard's nodes (located on PIP) and Heberden's nodes (located on DIP) are seen with OA.

PIRIFORMIS SYNDROME

The piriformis muscle, located in the buttocks, can compress, irritate, and entrap the sciatic nerve between its muscle layers. May account for 0.3% to 6% of sciatic-like syndromes.

Classic Case

Patient complains of sciatica symptoms. Sciatica symptoms may include pain and numbness of the buttocks, which may radiate down the leg. Reports that the pain is worsened by prolonged sitting, driving. Pain can be episodic. History of running, lifting heavy objects, falls, or excessive stair climbing. There are maneuvers that can be done to irritate the piriformis muscle, such as FAIR (flexion, adduction, internal rotation) maneuvers.

Objective Findings

- Obtain history of injury. Perform physical examination of the hip and groin, which includes inspection, palpation, ROM testing, pulses, deep tendon reflexes, and strength testing.
- Freiburg test is positive when pain or sciatic symptoms are caused by placing the hip in extension and internal rotation, and then resisting external rotation.
- Pace sign is pain elicited when the seated patient resists abduction and external rotation.

Imaging

- Radiograph (x-ray): Consider if limited hip ROM or chronic groin pain. Can help diagnose OA of hip.
- Ultrasound: Can help diagnose tendon and soft-tissue injury around the hip and groin.
- MRI: Can help diagnose sciatic nerve compression, stress fracture of femoral neck, cartilage tears, tendon ruptures.

Treatment Plan

- Avoid positions that trigger pain. Follow RICE (rest, ice, compression, elevation) guide; cold packs or heat can be used.
- Warm up and stretch before sports or exercises. Rest, cold packs, and heat may help symptoms.
- NSAIDs and muscle relaxants are the most common method of treatment.
- Refer for physical therapy for stretching and exercises.

Muscle Relaxants

Centrally active skeletal muscle relaxants include:
- Cyclobenzaprine (Flexeril)
- Metaxalone (Skelaxin)
- Tizanidine (Zanaflex)
- Baclofen (Gablofen)
- Carisoprodol (Soma) can be addicting; it is a U.S. Food and Drug Administration (FDA) schedule IV substance.

Side effects include drowsiness, dizziness, nervousness, reddish-purple urine, hypotension; do not mix muscle relaxants with sedating drugs or alcohol

CLINICAL PEARLS

- Naproxen is the NSAID with the fewest CV effects, but it has the same GI adverse effects as other NSAIDs. It can, however, increase BP, so this should be monitored.
- The innervation of the bladder and anal sphincter comes from the sacral nerves and, with cauda equina, symptoms include new-onset incontinence of urine (and/or bowel), saddle-pattern paresthesia, sciatica.

PLANTAR FASCIITIS

Acute or recurrent pain in the plantar region of the foot that is aggravated by walking. Caused by microtears in the plantar fascia due to tightness of the Achilles tendon. Higher risk with body mass index (BMI) >30, diabetes, aerobic exercise, flat feet, prolonged standing.

Classic Case

Middle-aged adult complains of plantar foot pain (either on one or on both feet) that is worsened by walking and weight bearing. Complains that foot pain is worse during the first few steps in the morning and continues to worsen with prolonged walking.

Treatment Plan

- NSAIDs: Naproxen (Aleve) orally twice a day, ibuprofen (Advil) orally every 4 to 6 hours.
- Topical NSAID: Diclofenac gel (Voltaren gel) applied to soles of feet twice a day.
- Orthotic foot appliance: Used at night for a few weeks; it will help to stretch the Achilles tendon.
- Stretching and massaging of the foot: Roll a golf ball with sole of foot several times a day.
- Lose weight: If overweight.
- Shoes: Well-padded soles and/or a heel cup on affected foot.

POPLITEAL (BAKER'S) CYST

A Baker's cyst is a type of bursitis that is located behind the knee (popliteal fossa). The bursae are protective, fluid-filled synovial sacs located on the joints that act as a cushion and protect the bones, tendons, joints, and muscles. Sometimes when a joint is damaged and/or inflamed, synovial fluid production increases, causing the bursa to enlarge. Risk factors include history of trauma, coexistent joint disease; most common include OA, RA, and meniscal tears.

Classic Case

Adult patient with history of OA complains of ball-like mass behind one knee that is soft and smooth. The mass will soften when the knee is bent at 45 degrees (Foucher's sign) because there is less tension. Asymptomatic or will have symptoms such as pressure sensation, posterior knee pain, and stiffness. If cyst ruptures, will complain of severe calf pain, erythema, distal edema, and a positive Homan's sign (resembling venous thrombosis).

Imaging

- Diagnosed by clinical presentation and history. If imaging is desired or the diagnosis is in question, initial test is ultrasound and plain radiography of the knee and calf. MRI if diagnosis is uncertain.
- If patients with concern for thrombophlebitis or vascular compromise, ultrasound can be used to identify the enlarged or ruptured cyst and exclude a deep vein thrombosis (DVT).
- Rule out plain bursitis from bursitis with infection ("septic joint").

Treatment Plan

- Follow RICE (rest, ice, compression, elevation) procedures. Gentle compression with elastic bandage wrap.

- Administer NSAIDs as needed.
- Large bursa can be drained with syringe using 18-gauge needle if causing pain. Synovial fluid is a clear, golden color. If cloudy synovial fluid is present and the joint is red, swollen, and hot, order a C&S to rule out a septic joint infection. After it is drained, an intraarticular injection of a glucocorticoid (triamcinolone acetonide) can decrease inflammation.
- Warn patient that the cyst can recur in the future. Most popliteal cysts are asymptomatic and do not require intervention.

EXAM TIPS

- Recognize Baker's cyst presentation.
- Plain radiograph of a joint (such as x-ray of knee) will show bony changes or narrowing of joint space (OA), but not soft tissue such as the meniscus or ligaments. The best imaging test for cartilage, meniscus, or tendon damage is MRI. The gold-standard test for assessing any joint damage is MRI.

CLINICAL PEARLS

- Do not forget that NSAIDs increase CV risk, renal damage, and GI bleeding.
- The best imaging test for suspected stress fractures is MRI. Plain radiographs do not show stress fractures initially after injury.

RHEUMATOID ARTHRITIS

Chronic, systemic autoimmune and inflammatory disorder that is more common in women (nearly twice as high as in males). Mainly manifested through systemic inflammation of multiple joints and other parts (skin, heart, blood vessels, kidneys, GI, brain/nerves, eyes). The goal of treatment is to prevent joint and organ damage. Patients are at higher risk for other autoimmune disorders, including Graves' disease and pernicious anemia.

Classic Case

Adult, commonly middle-aged, woman complains of gradual onset of symptoms over months with daily fatigue, low-grade fever, generalized body aches, and myalgia. Complains of generalized joint pain, stiffness, and swelling, which usually involves multiple joints bilaterally. It usually starts on the fingers/hands (PIP and metacarpophalangeal [MCP] joints) and the wrists. Commonly reports early-morning stiffness/pain and warm, tender, and swollen fingers in the DIP/PIP joints (also called "sausage joints"). It eventually involves the majority of joints in the body bilaterally.

Objective Findings

- Joint involvement is symmetric with more joints involved compared with DJD.
- Joint may feel "boggy" due to synovial thickening.
- Most common joints affected are hands, wrist, elbows, ankles, feet, and shoulders.
- "Sausage joints"

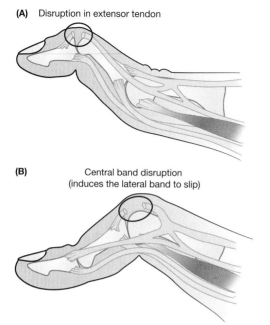

(A) Disruption in extensor tendon

(B) Central band disruption
(induces the lateral band to slip)

Figure 14.8 **(A)** Swan neck and **(B)** boutonniere deformity seen in late/severe cases of rheumatoid arthritis.

- Morning stiffness occurs for at least 1 hour and has been present for >6 weeks.
- Rheumatoid nodules present (chronic disease)
- Ulnar deviation or "ulnar drift"
- Swan neck deformity is flexion of the DIP joint with hyperextension of the PIP joint (Figure 14.8A).
- Boutonniere deformity is hyperextension of the DIP with flexion of the PIP joint (Figure 14.8B).

Labs

- ESR and CRP: Elevated
- CBC: Mild microcytic or normocytic anemia common, may show thrombocytosis and a mild leukocytosis
- RF: Positive in 75% to 80% of patients
- Radiographs: Bony erosions, joint space narrowing, subluxations (or dislocation)
- Serology/antibodies: Anticyclic citrullinated peptide/protein antibodies (ACPA), others

Treatment Plan

- Refer to rheumatologist for early aggressive management to minimize joint damage.
- Nonpharmacologic management includes physical and occupational therapy.

- Joint replacement (hip, knees) ameliorates RA
- Careful assessment is necessary. Never prescribe a biologic or anti-tumor necrosis factor (anti-TNF) medication if signs and symptoms of infection (e.g., fever, sore throat) are present. Tuberculosis (TB) testing should be ordered prior to start of anti-TNF therapy.

Medications

DMARDs are recommended as soon as possible following diagnosis, rather than using anti-inflammatory drugs alone.
- Nonbiologic DMARDs: Methotrexate, sulfasalazine, hydroxychloroquine
- Biologic DMARDs: TNF-alpha inhibitors such as adalimumab (Humira), etanercept (Enbrel), and infliximab (Remicade). Warning—anti-TNFs increase risk of infections, squamous cell skin cancer, and lymphoma.
- Targeted synthetic DMARDs: JAK inhibitors such as tofacitinib and baricitinib

Adjuncts include NSAIDs (e.g., ibuprofen, naproxen sodium) and glucocorticoids to relieve inflammation and pain. Glucocorticoid therapy may be used during the treatment of a flare. Steroid joint injections (synovial space) may be used to reduce synovitis in inflamed joints during a flare.

Complications

- RA increases risk of certain malignancies, such as lymphoma.
- Bone loss, muscle weakness, changes in body compositions.
- Pulmonary and cardiac involvement with pleurisy, parenchymal lung diseases, pericarditis, and myocarditis
- Neurologic complications such as carpel tunnel syndrome, myelopathy, or radiculopathy

Ocular Complications

- Inflammation of the uvea (middle layer eyeball). Sudden onset of eye redness, pain, blurred vision. Can cause vision loss (rare). Refer to ophthalmologist *stat*. Initial treatment includes topical steroids.
- RA increases risk of Sjogren's syndrome, scleritis, and episcleritis.
- When prescribing hydroxychloroquine (Plaquenil), all patients must have an eye exam prior to starting the medication. Frequent eye-exam monitoring should be performed every 6 months or as recommended by the ophthalmologist to assess and prevent retinal damage, which can lead to blindness.

SPRAINS

Sprains are overstretching or tearing of a ligament. Ankle sprains are usually due to sports participation. The most common sports that cause ankle injuries are basketball, indoor volleyball, and soccer. Ankle sprains are caused by overstretching of the joint, partial rupture, or complete rupture of a ligament. Lateral ankle sprains are the most common type.

- Lateral ankle sprain: The most common mechanism of injury is inversion of the plantar-flexed foot.
- Medial ankle sprain: Infrequently injured in isolation. The most common cause is forced eversion of the ankle; it can cause an avulsion fracture of the medial malleolus due to pulling by the ruptured deltoid ligament.

Ottawa Rules (of the Ankle)

- Ottawa rules are used to determine whether a patient needs radiographs of the injured ankle in the ED.
- The Ottawa ankle rules are highly sensitive (96.4%–99.6%) for excluding ankle fracture.
- Plain radiographs of the ankle are only indicated if there is pain in the malleolar zone *and*
  - Bone tenderness over the posterior edge or tip of the medial or lateral malleolus (Figure 14.9) *or*
  - Inability to bear weight both immediately after the injury and for four steps into the ED or provider's office.
- Plain radiographs of the foot are only indicated if there is pain in the midfoot zone *and*
  - Bone tenderness at the base of the fifth metatarsal or at the navicular *or*
  - Inability to bear weight both immediately after the injury and for four steps into the ED or doctor's office.
- In regard to the Ottawa ankle rules:
  - Bearing weight includes the ability to transfer weight twice to each foot (even if limping).
  - Assess for bone tenderness by palpating the distal 6 cm of the posterior edge of the fibula.

Grading of Sprains

Grade I Sprain
Mild sprain (slight stretching and some damage to ligament fibers); patient is able to bear weight and ambulate. There is no joint instability present during the ankle evaluation.

Grade II Sprain
Moderate sprain (partial tearing of ligament); ecchymoses, moderate swelling, and pain are present. Joint tender to palpation. Ambulation and weight bearing are painful. Mild-to-moderate joint instability occurs. Consider x-ray, referral.

Grade III (Complete Rupture of Ligaments)
Severe pain, swelling, tenderness, and ecchymosis. Significant mechanical ankle instability and significant loss of function and motion. Unable to bear weight or ambulate. Refer to ED for ankle fracture.

Physical Examination
First, ask about the mechanics of the injury along with symptoms. Look for swelling and ecchymosis. Palpate the entire ankle (lateral side and medial side), Achilles tendon, and the foot. Check for weight bearing, ROM, ability to ambulate, pedal and posterior tibial pulses. Grade the sprain.

Treatment Plan
- Grade the sprain and determine if ankle x-ray series is needed or refer to an orthopedic specialist if concern for severe sprain, unstable fracture, tendon rupture, or uncertain diagnosis.
- In mild-to-moderate sprains during acute phase, use RICE and elastic bandage wrap.
- NSAIDs (oral) and topical NSAIDs (e.g., Voltaren gel, diclofenac patches) can be used to treat pain and swelling. Can use combination topical and PO NSAIDs.
- Follow the RICE guide (rest, ice, compression, elevation).
- Grade I sprains (mild sprains) do not require immobilization. Use elastic wrap (ACE bandage) for a few days.
- Grade II sprains (moderate sprain) may need more support. Use ACE and an Aircast or similar splint for a few weeks. May require brief period of immobilization and non-weight bearing.

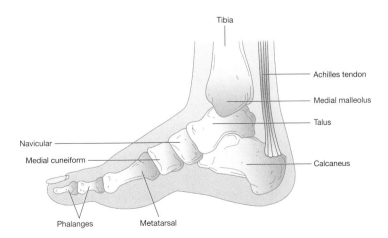

Figure 14.9 Bones and ligaments of the medial ankle.
Source: Myrick, K. M., & Karosas, L. M. (Eds.). (2021). (See Resources section for complete source information.)

- Grade III sprains are often managed by an orthopedic or sports specialist. Non-weight bearing and immobilization for brief period (about 10 days). May require surgery and functional rehabilitation.
- Early rehabilitation is important. Refer for physical therapy after initial swelling and pain have decreased so that the patient can tolerate simple exercises.

SYSTEMIC LUPUS ERYTHEMATOSUS

A multisystem autoimmune disease that is more common in women (9:1 ratio). Characterized by remissions and exacerbations. More common in African American and Hispanic women. Organ systems affected are the skin, kidneys, heart, and blood vessels. Milder form of lupus is called *cutaneous lupus erythematosus.*

Classic Case

Typical patient is a woman between age 16 and 55 years who presents with symptoms such as fever, fatigue, weight loss, and arthralgias. Classic rash is the maculopapular butterfly-shaped rash on the middle of the face (malar rash). May have nonpruritic thick scaly red rashes on sun-exposed areas (discoid rash). Photosensitivity, ocular manifestations, abdominal pains, and joint symptoms. May have cardiac symptoms, vascular abnormalities (e.g., Raynaud's phenomenon), pleuritis, pulmonary hypertension, cognitive dysfunction, anemia, and leukopenia. Urinalysis (UA) may be positive for proteinuria with kidney involvement. Antinuclear antibodies (ANA) are positive in virtually all patients.

Treatment Plan

- Refer to rheumatologist (NSAIDs, analgesics, steroids, antimalarial [Plaquenil], immune modulators [methotrexate, biologics], monoclonal antibodies).
- For mild symptoms: Bedrest, naps, avoidance of fatigue

Patient Education

- Avoid sun between 10 a.m. and 4 p.m. (causes rashes to break out).
- Cover skin with high sun protection factor (SPF; UVA and UVB) sunblock.
- Wear sun-protective clothing, such as hats with wide brims and long-sleeved shirts.
- Use nonfluorescent light bulbs (more sensitive to indoor fluorescent lighting).

TENDINITIS (ALL CASES)

Inflammation of a tendon, resulting in pain. Usually due to repetitive microtrauma, overuse, or strain. Gradual onset. Follow RICE mnemonic for acute injuries.

Rotator Cuff Injury

Rotator cuff injury usually involves damage to the supraspinatus tendon, which helps move the shoulder during abduction and external rotation. Caused by inflammation of the supraspinatus tendon. Jobs or sports with repetitive overhead activity, such as swimming, tennis, golf, weightlifting, gymnastics, and volleyball, increase risk for injury.

Classic Case

Patient with history of repetitive overhead activity (sport or job). Complains of shoulder pain with overhead movements such as brushing hair or putting on a shirt. There is local point tenderness over the tendon located on the anterior area of the shoulder. May have pain at night when sleeping on the side of the affected shoulder.

Maneuvers

- Painful arc test (Figure 14.10): Pain with shoulder ROM; >90 degrees of adduction or pain with internal rotation is suggestive of rotator cuff tendinopathy. Positive

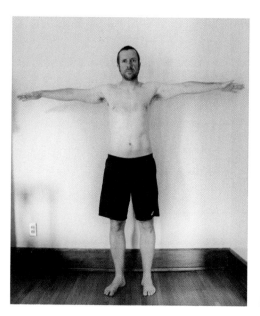
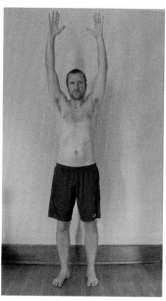

Figure 14.10 Painful arc test.
Source: Gawlik, K. S., Melnyk, B. M., & Teall, A. M. (Eds.). (2021). (See Resources section for complete source information.)

result is shoulder pain that occurs between 60 and 120 degrees of active abduction

- Jobe's test (empty can test; Figure 14.11): Test for the strength of the supraspinatus muscle. Instruct patient to straighten arm at 90 degrees of abduction with 30 degrees of forward flexion, then internally rotate the shoulder. Tell patient to resist when examiner attempts to adduct the arm. Positive result is shoulder pain without weakness (tendinopathy); shoulder pain with weakness suggests tendon tear.

Imaging

- MRI can identify rotator cuff tear(s).

Treatment

- For initial treatment, rest affected shoulder and apply cold packs (20 minutes cold pack, repeated about two to four times per day), especially during acute phase for 24 to 48 hours.
- NSAIDs for pain as needed.
- Physical therapy to rehabilitate shoulder.
- Refer to orthopedic specialist if inadequate or poor response to conservative management.

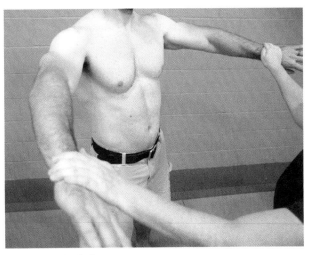

Figure 14.11 Jobe's test.

Source: Myrick, K. M., & Karosas, L. M. (Eds.). (2021). (See Resources section for complete source information.)

KNOWLEDGE CHECK: CHAPTER 14

1. An 18-year-old female patient complains of right ankle pain. She reports twisting her ankle by stepping on a rock while jogging the previous day. She states that she "rolled inward" on her ankle. During the physical exam, the nurse practitioner notes severe swelling and ecchymosis. There is tenderness on the tip of the lateral malleolus. The joint is tender on palpation. The patient is unable to bear weight or ambulate and has significant motor and function loss. Which grade of sprain does this patient have?
   A. I
   B. II
   C. III
   D. IV

2. A 37-year-old male patient complains of an acute onset of pain and redness of his left wrist. He denies trauma or injury to the wrist. He reports that the condition has occurred on the same wrist before. The symptoms started at night after drinking a few glasses of wine. During the physical exam, the left wrist is red, swollen, and tender to palpation. The skin is intact but feels warm to the touch. What is the *most likely* diagnosis?
   A. Wrist sprain
   B. Gout
   C. Osteoarthritis
   D. Cellulitis

3. Regarding the previous case, which of the following is recommended for the initial treatment of this flare?
   A. Interleukin-1 inhibitor
   B. Oral glucocorticoids
   C. Aspirin
   D. Intraarticular glucocorticoids

4. An adolescent female patient reports a sudden onset of posterior right thigh pain. The injury occurred while she was running during a soccer game. She denies falling. She is limping and walking slowly. On physical examination, the midportion of the right hamstring muscle is tender to palpation with some bruising noted. Which of the following conditions is *most likely* in this patient?
   A. Hamstring muscle strain
   B. Baker's cyst
   C. Quadriceps muscle strain
   D. Piriformis syndrome

5. Which organ system is *least* affected by chronic use of nonsteroidal anti-inflammatory drugs (NSAIDs)?
   A. Cardiovascular
   B. Renal
   C. Immune
   D. Gastrointestinal

6. When is the *most accurate* time to assess serum urate in a patient with gout?
   A. During the first 24 hours of a gout flare
   B. One week after a gout flare
   C. No preferred time
   D. Two weeks or more after a gout flare subsides

7. A patient presents with complaints of low back pain that radiates down both legs and difficulty voiding. During the neurologic assessment, the nurse practitioner notes bilateral lower extremity motor weakness with diminished sensation. There is no motor dysfunction in the upper extremities. The nurse practitioner should be concerned for which of the following conditions?
   A. Piriformis syndrome
   B. Cauda equina syndrome
   C. Ankylosing spondylitis
   D. Osteomyelitis

(See answers next page.)

1. C) III

This patient has a grade III sprain, which means that there may be a complete rupture of some of the ligaments. The patient has severe pain and swelling and is unable to bear weight and ambulate, and the ankle has severe ecchymosis with malleolar tenderness. There is significant function and motor loss. This patient requires an ankle x-ray series and imaging (ultrasound and/or MRI). She may need surgical repair and/or casting and should be referred to the ED. Grade I is a mild sprain (slight stretching and some damage to ligament fibers); patient is able to bear weight and ambulate. There is no joint instability present during the ankle evaluation. A grade II sprain is a moderate sprain (partial tearing of ligament); patient presents with ecchymoses, moderate swelling, and pain. There is mild to moderate joint instability on exam with some restriction of range of motion. Ambulation and weight bearing are painful. Ankle sprains are classified from grade I to grade III.

2. B) Gout

The patient is presenting with signs and symptoms of gout of the left wrist. A typical gout flare includes severe pain, redness, warmth, swelling, and disability. The onset is more often at night and can be provoked by alcohol consumption. He has had the same episodes on the same location before (which is a clue; recurrent flares are common). Gout can occur in the peripheral joints, such as the toes, foot, ankle, hand, or wrist. A wrist sprain is unlikely as the patient has denied injury or trauma to the extremity. Osteoarthritis often presents with joint pain stiffness and motor restriction. A gout flare may resemble cellulitis with erythema and swelling; however, cellulitis often does not focus on a joint and is associated with systemic systems such as fever and chills.

3. B) Oral glucocorticoids

Oral glucocorticoids (e.g., prednisone), nonsteroidal anti-inflammatory drugs (NSAIDs) (e.g., naproxen, indomethacin), or colchicine can be used to treat a gout flare. Aspirin is not used because of the paradoxical effects of salicylates on serum urate. Intraarticular glucocorticoids are indicated if the patient is unable to tolerate oral medications. Interleukin-1 inhibitors (e.g., anakinra, canakinumab) are indicated for patients who are unresponsive or have contraindications to initial therapy.

4. A) Hamstring muscle strain

The patient has a hamstring muscle strain that is caused by sprinting during a soccer game. A strain is overstretching of a muscle or tendon. A sprain can range from microtears to complete rupture of the muscle or tendon.

The quadriceps muscle is located on the anterior thigh. Piriformis syndrome can entrap the sciatic nerve, causing sciatica, and will present with symptoms of sciatica. Baker's cyst is located on the posterior knee; it is a type of bursitis. A quadriceps strain is less likely as the patient presents with posterior pain and the quadriceps are located anteriorly on the thigh.

5. C) Immune

Although NSAIDs have been found to have some immune-modifying properties, use of nonselective NSAIDs has clinically important gastrointestinal, renal, and cardiovascular effects. Nonselective NSAIDs have adverse effects on the cardiovascular system (myocardial infarction, stroke, exacerbation of heart failure), renal system (kidney damage), and the gastrointestinal system (dyspepsia, peptic ulcer disease, and bleeding). Other effects include hepatic effects (acute liver injury; uncommon), pulmonary effects (relatively uncommon), hematologic effects, central nervous system side effects, and dermatologic reactions.

6. D) Two weeks or more after a gout flare subsides

During a gout flare, serum levels can be difficult to interpret. Shortly after initiation of urate-lowering therapy, serum urate levels are often normal or even low during an acute gout flare. The most accurate time to assess serum urate level and establish a baseline value is 2 weeks or more after a gout flare completely subsides.

7. B) Cauda equina syndrome

Cauda equina syndrome results from compression and disruption to the lumbosacral nerve roots within the spinal canal. Symptoms include low back pain accompanied by pain radiating into one or both legs, motor weakness of the lower extremities, bladder and rectal sphincter paralysis (leading to problems with bladder and bowel control), and sensory loss of the affected nerve roots. The patient requires prompt neurosurgic or orthopedic consultation. Piriformis syndrome most commonly presents with buttock pain of gradual onset that increases with sitting. Paresthesias may develop, but bladder and bowel issues are uncommon. The predominant symptom in ankylosing spondylitis is chronic back and neck pain and impaired spinal mobility. Osteomyelitis may present with local findings (tenderness, warmth, erythema, and swelling) and systemic symptoms (fever, chills). Patient often presents with new or worsening musculoskeletal pain near soft tissue or surgical wounds.

8. A soccer player presents at an urgent care clinic complaining of swelling and pain on the medial aspect of the right knee. The patient reports twisting the knee when quickly changing directions while running. On physical examination, the knee is swollen with joint tenderness on the medial side of the knee. The patient is unable to squat, kneel, or fully extend the knee. Based on this presentation, the orthopedic maneuver that the nurse practitioner should use to assess for possible injury is known as which test?
A. Flexion pinch
B. Anterior drawer
C. Lachman
D. Empty can

9. Which of the following is the *most sensitive* imaging modality for detecting a meniscal tear?
A. X-ray
B. Ultrasound
C. MRI
D. CT scan

10. A figure skater lands incorrectly after a jump and injures the right ankle. The patient is unable to bear weight immediately after the injury but is able to limp into the clinic. The patient reports pain in the malleolar zone. On physical examination, there is significant swelling, but a palpable dorsalis pedis and posterior tibialis pulse are present. Based on the Ottawa ankle rules, is a radiograph necessary?
A. Yes, the patient reports pain in the malleolar zone.
B. No, there are palpable distal pulses with no concern for neurovascular compromise.
C. Yes, the patient is unable to bear weight immediately after the injury.
D. No, the patient is able to limp into the clinic, so they are considered able to bear weight.

11. A young female patient presents with fatigue, arthralgia, and weight loss. Physical examination is notable for blood pressure of 175/90 mmHg, a pleural friction rub on pulmonary auscultation, and several tender and swollen joints. Lab testing reveals anemia, proteinuria, and positive antinuclear antibodies (ANAs). The patient also reports that her skin feels sensitive to the sun and that she has a new malar rash over her cheeks and nose. Based on this presentation, the nurse practitioner suspects which of the following?
A. Rheumatoid arthritis
B. Systemic lupus erythematosus
C. Ankylosing spondylitis
D. Osteoarthritis

12. Which of the following connects muscle to bone?
A. Tendon
B. Ligament
C. Joints
D. Articular cartilage

13. During the musculoskeletal physical examination, the nurse practitioner asks the patient to spread their fingers. This refers to which type of movement?
A. Flexion
B. Extension
C. Abduction
D. Adduction

14. A patient presents complaining of a burning pain located in the space between the third and fourth toes. The patient reports that the pain is aggravated by walking, especially when wearing high-heeled shoes. Direct palpation reveals tenderness. Based on this presentation, which of the following tests is indicated?
A. Painful arc
B. Apley's
C. Finkelstein's
D. Mulder's

15. An adolescent patient presents with an angular deformity in which the knees point toward the midline. The nurse practitioner refers to this condition as:
A. Genu varum
B. Genu valgum
C. Tibial stress fracture
D. Meniscal injury

(See answers next page.)

8. A) Flexion pinch

Acute meniscal tears often occur when a person changes direction in a way that involves rotating or twisting the knee, usually while playing sports. Patients with meniscal injury often present with joint line tenderness, abnormal knee motion, inability to squat or kneel, joint effusion, and inability to fully extend the knee or loss of smooth passive motion. The flexion pinch test involves flexing the knee and palpating the lateral and medial posterior joint lines for tenderness. A positive finding suggests injury to the meniscus of the knee. The anterior drawer and Lachman tests are used to evaluate an injury to the anterior cruciate ligament. The empty can test can be used to assess supraspinatus function when performing a physical examination of the shoulder.

9. C) MRI

MRI is the most sensitive imaging modality for detecting the extent and type of meniscal tear. However, unless surgery is being considered, plain radiographs can be appropriate for some patients with suspected meniscal tear. Ultrasound can also be used as a safe and inexpensive test to examine the knee, but is not very specific and depends heavily on the examiner. CT scan can also be considered in some patients.

10. D) No, the patient is able to limp into the clinic, so they are considered able to bear weight.

According to the Ottawa ankle rules, plain radiographs of the ankle are indicated only if there is pain in the malleolar zone *and* bony tenderness over the posterior edge or tip of the medial or lateral malleolus or inability to bear weight *both* immediately after the injury and for four steps into the ED or doctor's office. The patient is considered able to bear weight if they can transfer weight twice to each foot (four steps), even if they limp.

11. B) Systemic lupus erythematosus

Systemic lupus erythematosus is an autoimmune disease with a wide range of clinical and serologic manifestations, involving almost every organ system. Patients often present with constitutional symptoms (fatigue, fever, and weight loss) as well as arthralgias. The classic butterfly rash presents over the cheeks and nose after sun exposure. Patients present with symptoms involving the cardiovascular, kidney, gastrointestinal, pulmonary, hematologic, and neurologic systems. It should be suspected when a young female patient presents with fatigue and is found to have hypertension, a malar rash, pleural friction rub, peripheral edema, swollen joints, and associated lab abnormalities (positive ANAs). Rheumatoid arthritis can present with fatigue and joint swelling but often presents with classic features of swan neck deformities and ulnar deviation. The predominant symptom in ankylosing spondylitis is chronic back and neck pain and impaired spinal mobility. Osteoarthritis also presents with joint pain but is often seen in middle-aged or older adults and presents with morning stiffness and classic features such as Heberden's nodes and Bouchard's nodes.

12. A) Tendon

Tendons are connective tissues that connect the muscles to other body structures, typically bones. Bones come together at joints, which are held together by ligaments that hold bone to bone. Articular cartilage provides a smooth surface at the ends of bones to allow for the free, smooth movement of the joint.

13. C) Abduction

Abduction refers to moving the limb or hand laterally away from the body. Spreading the fingers moves away from the midline of the hand. Adduction involves moving the limb or hand toward or across the midline (or bringing the fingers together toward the midline, or the middle digit). Flexion is a joint movement that decreases the angle between two bones. Extension is a joint movement that increases the angle and straightens the joint.

14. D) Mulder's

This patient is presenting with symptoms suggestive of Morton's neuroma. Most patients present complaining of burning pain in the third intermetatarsal space (between the third and fourth distal metatarsals). Overpronation and tight shoes are associated with this condition. Mulder's sign refers to a clicking sensation that occurs when palpating the involved interspace while simultaneously squeezing the metatarsal joints. Finkelstein's test is used to assess for de Quervain's tendosynovitis. The painful arc test is used when evaluating a shoulder injury. Apley's test is used to assess for meniscal injury.

15. B) Genu valgum

Genu valgum ("knock knees") refers to an angular deformity in which the knees point toward the midline. Genu varum (bow-legs) refers to an angular deformity in which the knees point away from midline. A tibial stress fracture presents with localized pain, swelling, tenderness, and inability to hop on the symptomatic leg. Patients with meniscal injury often present with joint line tenderness, abnormal knee motion, inability to squat or kneel, joint effusion, and inability to fully extend the knee or loss of smooth passive motion.

16. A patient presents with pain, stiffness, and swelling of many joints, especially the metacarpophalangeal (MCP) and proximal interphalangeal (PIP) joints of the fingers. Physical examination reveals swelling and edema with redness and warmth noted to the inflamed joints. Swan neck and Boutonniere deformities are noted on the fingers. Based on this presentation, which medication therapy should be started soon after diagnosis?
    A. Disease-modifying antirheumatic drugs (DMARDs)
    B. Nonsteroidal anti-inflammatory drugs (NSAIDs)
    C. Glucocorticoids
    D. Allopurinol

17. Varus stress applied to the knee assesses for which type of injury?
    A. Posterior cruciate ligament
    B. Medial collateral ligament
    C. Anterior cruciate ligament
    D. Lateral collateral ligament

18. A football player presents to the clinic with knee pain. The patient reports a direct blow to the lateral aspect of the knee during a tackle. A plain radiograph is negative for an acute fracture. On exam, there is knee swelling, ecchymosis, and tenderness to palpation. The valgus stress test reveals laxity at about 30 degrees of flexion. Based on this presentation, the nurse practitioner suggests which of the following?
    A. Medial meniscus tear
    B. Medial collateral ligament injury
    C. Lateral collateral ligament injury
    D. Hamstring injury

19. Which of the following nonsteroidal anti-inflammatory drugs (NSAIDs) is associated with a high risk of major cardiovascular events?
    A. Diclofenac
    B. Celecoxib
    C. Ibuprofen
    D. Naproxen

20. A male patient presents with knee pain and stiffness after falling while skiing last week. He notes a popping sensation when he bends his knee and that his knee feels like it "gives out." On examination, there is tenderness over the medial joint line of the knee. Marked flexion and extension of the knee are painful. McMurray's sign is positive. What is the *most likely* diagnosis?
    A. Cauda equina
    B. Hamstring injury
    C. Meniscal injury
    D. Ruptured Baker's cyst

21. A 35-year-old patient presents with chronic back pain that is associated with morning stiffness. The patient reports that the pain started in their neck with an insidious onset and then progressed. The pain improves with exercise, but not with rest, and is worse at night. A radiography reveals a bamboo spine. Based on this presentation, initial treatment therapy includes which of the following?
    A. Disease-modifying antirheumatic drugs (DMARDs)
    B. Tumor necrosis factor (TNF) inhibitor
    C. Janus kinase (JAK) inhibitor
    D. Nonsteroidal anti-inflammatory drugs (NSAIDs)

22. Heberden's nodes and Bouchard's nodes are classic features of which condition?
    A. Rheumatoid arthritis
    B. Osteoarthritis
    C. Ankylosing spondylitis
    D. Acute cutaneous lupus erythema

(See answers next page.)

16. A) Disease-modifying antirheumatic drugs (DMARDs)

This patient is presenting with signs and symptoms suggestive of rheumatoid arthritis (RA). Typical features include pain, stiffness, and swelling of many joints. Often, the MCP and PIP joints of the fingers, the joints of the thumbs and wrists, and the metatarsophalangeal joints of the toes are affected. Characteristic joint deformities of chronic RA include MCP subluxation, ulnar deviation or "ulnar drift," swan neck and Boutonniere deformities of the fingers, and the "bow string" sign (prominent tendons in the hands). All patients with RA should be started on DMARD therapy as soon as possible after diagnosis rather than using anti-inflammatory agents, such as NSAIDs and glucocorticoids, alone. Allopurinol is used in the treatment of gout.

17. D) Lateral collateral ligament

The varus stress test identifies an injury to the lateral collateral ligament. The valgus stress test identifies an injury to the medial collateral ligament. The anterior drawer test helps to identify an injury to the anterior cruciate ligament. The posterior drawer test looks to identify an injury to the posterior cruciate ligament.

18. B) Medial collateral ligament injury

The patient is presenting with concern for an injury to the medial collateral ligament, which is often injured through stress from a direct blow to the lateral aspect of the knee. The valgus stress test is used to identify an injury to the medial collateral ligament; pain or laxity while the knee is flexed at about 30 degrees suggests a positive finding. The varus stress test is used to identify an injury to the lateral collateral ligament. McMurray's test is used to assess for a meniscal injury. Patients with meniscal injury often present with joint line tenderness, abnormal knee motion, inability to squat or kneel, joint effusion, and inability to fully extend the knee or loss of smooth passive motion. A hamstring injury often presents with posterior thigh pain with focal warmth and tenderness.

19. A) Diclofenac

Multiple studies have demonstrated a consistently higher risk of cardiovascular events for diclofenac compared with other NSAIDs. Data from the Coxib and Traditional NSAID Trialists' (CNT) Collaboration analysis suggest that high-dose naproxen may have the best cardiovascular risk profile. Of note, in the Precision trial (2016), naproxen, ibuprofen, and celecoxib were compared, and no significant difference in cardiovascular safety was found.

20. C) Meniscal injury

This patient is likely presenting with a meniscal injury, which occurs when a person changes direction or the knee is twisted while flexed and the corresponding foot is planted. Patients with untreated meniscal tears can present weeks after injury complaining of popping, locking, catching, and the knee "giving out." Provocative maneuvers used to assess for injury include the Thessaly test, McMurray test, and Apley test. Cauda equina is unlikely as the patient does not complain of back pain accompanied by pain radiating into one or both legs; motor weakness of the lower extremities; bladder and rectal sphincter paralysis; or sensory loss of the affected nerve roots. While a popping noise may be heard with a hamstring injury, swelling and bruising would be located on the posterior thigh. A ruptured Baker's cyst is less likely as a ball-like mass is not palpated behind the knee.

21. D) Nonsteroidal anti-inflammatory drugs (NSAIDs)

The patient is presenting with concern for ankylosing spondylitis. Neck pain is often the initial feature, age of onset is usually younger than 40 years, and the pain has an insidious onset, improves with exercise, and is worse at rest and at night. For most patients, initial therapy includes NSAIDs. The addition of DMARDs is typically not indicated. For those with an inadequate response to initial therapy, TNF inhibitor agents can be trialed, along with interleukin 17 inhibitors and JAK inhibitors.

22. B) Osteoarthritis

Heberden's nodes (bony nodules on the distal interphalangeal joints) and Bouchard's nodes (bony nodules on the proximal interphalangeal joints) are characteristic of osteoarthritis. Characteristic joint deformities of chronic rheumatoid arthritis include metacarpophalangeal subluxation, ulnar deviation or "ulnar drift," swan neck and Boutonniere deformities of the fingers, and the "bow string" sign (prominent tendons in the hand). The classic feature of acute cutaneous lupus erythema is the "butterfly rash," a malar distribution over the cheeks and nose that appears after sun exposure. Classic features of ankylosing spondylitis are low back and neck pain, impaired spinal mobility, and postural abnormalities.

23. An older adult patient with osteoarthritis of the knee presents with persistent joint pain, stiffness, and motor restriction. The patient has engaged in physical therapy and weight management strategies with little relief of symptoms. The patient has a history of hypertension and peptic ulcer disease. Which of the following treatment regimens should be trialed *first* in this patient?
    A. Topical diclofenac
    B. Oxycodone
    C. Duloxetine
    D. Acetaminophen

24. A patient with ankylosing spondylitis presents with acute unilateral eye pain, photophobia, and blurring of vision. Initial treatment recommendations include which of the following?
    A. Observation
    B. Oral steroids
    C. Referral to ophthalmologist
    D. Topical antibiotics

25. A patient with an intolerance to glucocorticoids and nonsteroidal anti-inflammatory drugs (NSAIDs) presents with a gout flare. The patient reports intense joint pain, redness, and swelling, which are preventing them from participating in activities of daily living (ADLs). Which of the following is the recommended standard dosing of colchicine for this patient?
    A. Initial dose of 0.2, followed 1 hour later by another 1.6 mg
    B. Initial dose of 1.2, followed 24 hours later by another 0.6 mg
    C. Initial dose of 2.0, followed 4 hours later by another 0.8 mg
    D. Initial dose of 1.2 mg, followed 1 hour later by another 0.6 mg

26. In a patient with osteoarthritis without known cardiovascular disease who is at increased risk of gastrointestinal (GI) bleeding, which of the following analgesics is preferred?
    A. Naproxen
    B. Celecoxib
    C. Ibuprofen
    D. Acetaminophen

27. A patient presents with frequent painful and disabling gout flares. Further education is needed when the patient reports:
    A. "I like to drink soda or juice with meals."
    B. "I eat cherries at least twice per week."
    C. "I like to have one or two glasses of wine on the weekend."
    D. "I eat purine and protein in moderation."

28. A 60-year-old patient presents with shoulder pain after performing construction work. The pain is worse when the patient lifts something above their head. The patient reports waking up during the night in pain while lying on that shoulder. On physical examination, weakness is noted in the affected extremity in external rotation. Based on this presentation, which of the following tests can be used for diagnosis?
    A. Apley's
    B. Mulder
    C. Painful arc
    D. McMurray's

29. Which of the following laboratory findings is present in most patients with *systemic lupus erythematosus* (SLE) and can be used for diagnosis?
    A. Rheumatoid factor (RF)
    B. Uric acid level
    C. Anti-cyclic citrullinated peptide (CCP) antibodies
    D. Antinuclear antibodies (ANA)

30. A 25-year-old patient complains of knee pain and instability after a soccer game injury 2 days ago. Physical examination reveals mild swelling and tenderness along the medial aspect of the knee. While performing the anterior drawer test, the nurse practitioner notes a pronounced anterior translation of the tibia relative to the femur. Based on these findings, which of the following is the most likely diagnosis?
    A. Meniscal tear
    B. Medial collateral ligament (MCL) sprain
    C. Patellar dislocation
    D. Anterior cruciate ligament (ACL) tear

(See answers next page.)

23. A) Topical diclofenac

Nonpharmacologic therapy is recommended first in patients with knee osteoarthritis. For those who have not responded adequately to initial interventions, pharmacologic therapies can be used when symptoms are present. Topical nonsteroidal anti-inflammatory drugs (NSAIDs) are recommended for knee osteoarthritis due to their greater safety. The risk of gastrointestinal, renal, and cardiovascular toxicity is much lower with topical NSAIDs compared with oral formulations. Opioids should be avoided due to their adverse effects for long-term use in the older adult population. Acetaminophen is no longer recommended given safety concerns and nonclinically significant effects on pain. Duloxetine may be used for patients with knee osteoarthritis who have not responded to other initial treatments.

24. C) Referral to ophthalmologist

Acute anterior uveitis is common in patients with ankylosing spondylitis (25%–35%). Uveitis presents as acute unilateral pain, photophobia, and blurring of vision. Treatment requires consultation with an ophthalmologist; therapy should be initiated within 24 hours. Anterior uveitis not due to infection is treated with topical glucocorticoids (not topical antibiotics). Oral glucocorticoids are recommended for patients who are resistant to topical therapy.

25. D) Initial dose of 1.2 mg, followed 1 hour later by another 0.6 mg

For patients who are intolerant to glucocorticoids and NSAIDs, colchicine can be used to treat a gout flare. Colchicine is most effective when taken within 24 hours of onset of a gout flare and should be administered in a total dose on day 1 not to exceed 1.8 mg. The standard initial dose is 1.2 mg, followed 1 hour later by another 0.6 mg.

26. B) Celecoxib

Celecoxib is preferred in patients without known cardiovascular disease who are at increased risk of GI bleeding due to its greater long-term GI safety profile compared with naproxen and ibuprofen. Acetaminophen is no longer recommended for the treatment of osteoarthritis given safety concerns and nonclinically significant effects on pain.

27. A) "I like to drink soda or juice with meals."

Patients with gout should be educated to avoid or replace sugar-sweetened juices and beverages containing high-fructose corn syrup. Patients should be instructed that chronic intake or acute excess of beer, spirits, or wine can increase gout flares and should be educated on reduction of alcohol intake. Low-risk or small-moderate amounts (e.g., one or two drinks daily) are unlikely to trigger flares. Severely purine- or protein-restricted diets are not recommended to prevent or treat gout. Dietary moderation in purine intake may help mitigate triggering flares. Cherries have been found to have potential beneficial effects in patients with gout.

28. C) Painful arc

The patient is presenting with symptoms suggestive of a rotator cuff injury. Patients often complain of shoulder pain with overhead activity. Pain is often worse at night, especially when lying on the affected shoulder. Painful arc test, drop arm sign, and weakness on external rotation can diagnose full-thickness rotator cuff tears in patients older than 60 years. McMurray's and Apley's tests are used to assess for a meniscus injury. The Mulder test is used to assess for Morton's neuroma.

29. D) Antinuclear antibodies (ANA)

In nearly all patients with SLE, the ANA test is positive at some point during their disease course. An elevated uric acid level is seen in a patient with gout. RF and CCP antibodies may help exclude a diagnosis of rheumatoid arthritis (RA) in patients with SLE and predominant arthralgias. Anti-CCP antibodies have a higher specificity for RA and are more useful to distinguish arthritis associated with RA. About 20% to 30% of patients with SLE have a positive RF, so it has less diagnostic yield.

30. D) Anterior cruciate ligament (ACL) tear

The anterior drawer test is a clinical test used to assess the integrity of the ACL. A positive test, indicated by a pronounced anterior movement of the tibia relative to the femur, suggests a tear of the ACL. A meniscal tear may also result from twisting injuries, but it usually presents with joint line tenderness and a positive Apley's test; that is, pain is elicited with compression of the knee while the patient is prone with the knee flexed at 90 degrees. An MCL sprain would present with pain and tenderness on the medial side of the knee and laxity with a valgus stress test. A patellar dislocation would manifest as a palpable deformity with the patella displaced laterally. This is not indicated by the anterior drawer test.

31. A male patient presents with buttock pain that increases while sitting. The patient is a runner and reports running downhill recently. The patient reports noticing the pain when he could no longer sit on his wallet in his back pocket without having symptoms. Which of the following is *most likely* with this presentation?
    A. Piriformis syndrome
    B. Ankylosing spondylitis
    C. Hamstring injury
    D. Morton's neuroma

32. A female runner presents with shin pain. She reports increasing her mileage recently and that the pain increases with impact. On physical examination, a focal palpable area of tenderness is present. The patient is unable to hop on the symptomatic leg without excessive pain. Management of this injury includes which of the following?
    A. Reduction in the number of miles run
    B. Opioids for pain management
    C. Avoidance of running in favor of non-impact activities while the injury heals
    D. Waiting to establish a treatment plan until plain radiographs confirm the injury.

33. Which of the following terms refers to the bones of the hands?
    A. Carpals
    B. Phalanges
    C. Metatarsals
    D. Metacarpals

34. A patient presents with acute wrist pain following a fall. The patient reports trying to break the fall by stretching out their hand. The patient denies hitting their head or any other acute injury. The pain is localized to the radial aspect of the wrist. Focal tenderness is present in the anatomic snuff box. The patient can lift overhead without pain. This presentation is concerning for which of the following injuries?
    A. Rotator cuff injury
    B. Scaphoid fracture
    C. Colles fracture
    D. Osteoarthritis

35. A patient with a history of posterior knee pain and stiffness presents with new calf pain and swelling. Upon physical examination, a mass is palpated behind the knee that is more prominent at full extension and softens on flexion to 45 degrees. Homans' sign is positive, and distal edema is noted. Which of the following is the *preferred* initial imaging modality based on this presentation?
    A. Ultrasound
    B. X-ray
    C. MRI
    D. CT scan

(See answers next page.)

31. A) Piriformis syndrome

The patient is presenting with signs and symptoms suggestive of piriformis syndrome, or entrapment neuropathy of the sciatic nerve. Some runners develop this condition with downhill running because the piriformis muscle undergoes eccentric contraction. The most common presenting symptom is buttock pain of gradual onset that increases while sitting ("wallet sign"). Morton's neuroma is inflammation of the digital nerve of the foot between the third and fourth metatarsals. A hamstring injury often presents with posterior thigh pain with focal warmth and tenderness. Classic features of ankylosing spondylitis are low back and neck pain, impaired spinal mobility, and postural abnormalities.

32. C) Avoidance of running in favor of non-impact activities while the injury heals

The patient is presenting with signs and symptoms concerning for a stress fracture of the tibia and fibula, which is common among runners and usually results from increased training. The pain is exacerbated by running or jumping, and there is focal tenderness and swelling around the fracture sign. While plain radiographs are the initial studies to assess suspected fractures, the presentation of symptoms usually occurs before the appearance on radiographs by weeks. A negative plain radiograph cannot rule out such a stress fracture. Medial tibial stress syndrome (MTSS) is on the differential; however, tenderness is more diffuse, and there are no discrete palpable lesions in those with MTSS. A runner with MTSS can continue running but reduce the total mileage. A runner with a stress fracture requires rest from any inciting activity and stabilization, a short period of non–weight-bearing status, and non-impact activities (e.g., swimming). Over-the-counter analgesics (e.g., acetaminophen) are usually adequate to relieve pain; patients may require opioids if there is inadequate response to other medications, but opoids should be avoided if possible to reduce the risk of side effects.

33. D) Metacarpals

Metacarpals refers to the bones of the hands. *Carpals* refers to the bones of the wrist. *Phalanges* refers to the bones that make up the fingers and toes. *Metatarsals* refers to bones of the feet.

34. B) Scaphoid fracture

Scaphoid fractures often occur from a fall onto an outstretched hand with the wrist in dorsiflexion. Patients typically complain of pain localized to the radial aspect of the wrist. Focal tenderness present in the anatomic snuff box is the most sensitive finding. A rotator cuff injury is unlikely as the patient can lift their arm above their head without pain. Osteoarthritis is less likely as the pain is acute and sustained after a known injury. A Colles fracture involves dorsal displacement of the distal radius fragment. While also associated with a fall onto an outstretched hand, Colles fracture often presents with the classic "dinner-fork" deformity.

35. A) Ultrasound

This patient is presenting with concern for a popliteal cyst. Some patients may experience knee pain and stiffness, while for some patients a swelling or mass behind the knee is incidentally noted. The mass is usually felt with the knee at full extension and may soften or disappear on flexion to 45 degrees (Foucher's sign). A tender cyst enlarging into the calf (a dissecting cyst) can result in erythema, distal edema, and a positive Homan's sign, similar to a deep vein thrombosis. Ultrasound is preferred in patients with possible thrombophlebitis or cyst-related "pseudothrombophlebitis" syndrome because it can detect the enlarged, dissected, or ruptured cyst and the venous circulation. A plain radiograph of the knee can demonstrate joint or bone abnormalities, but it has limited benefit for viewing the cyst. MRI is recommended when there is concern for worsening internal damage, when considering surgery, or when the diagnosis is uncertain after ultrasound. A CT scan is not routinely used because the other imaging techniques are preferred.

ACUTE SEROTONIN SYNDROME (SEROTONIN TOXICITY)

Occurs from high levels of serotonin accumulating in the body due to the introduction of a new drug (drug interaction) or an increase in the dose. Has acute onset (60% of cases occur within 6 hours of change in dose or overdose) with rapid progression. According to the Hunter Toxicity Criteria Decision Rules, a patient must have taken a serotonergic agent and meet one of the following conditions: change in mental state, spontaneous clonus, inducible clonus plus agitation and diaphoresis, ocular clonus plus agitation or diaphoresis, tremor plus hyperreflexia, or hypertonia plus temperature >100.4°F (38°C) plus ocular clonus or inducible clonus.

Look for dilated pupils (mydriasis). Higher risk if combining two drugs that both block serotonin (i.e., selective serotonin reuptake inhibitors [SSRIs], serotonin-norepinephrine reuptake inhibitors [SNRIs], monoamine oxidase inhibitors [MAOIs], tricyclic antidepressants [TCAs], opioid analgesics, over-the counter cough medicines, triptans, tryptophan). If switching to another drug affecting serotonin, wait a minimum of 2 weeks for a washout time. Acute serotonin syndrome is a potentially life-threatening reaction. Refer to ED.

MALIGNANT NEUROLEPTIC SYNDROME

Rare life-threatening idiopathic reaction from typical and atypical antipsychotics. It is most often seen with high-potency, first-generation antipsychotics (e.g., chlorpromazine, haloperidol). Mortality rate of 10% to 20%. It can also be seen in Parkinson disease (parkinsonism hyperpyrexia syndrome) due to withdrawal of L-dopa or dopamine agonist therapy, dose reduction, or switching medications. Syndrome usually develops within 1 to 3 days following initiation or a rapid increase in dose.

Signs and symptoms are sudden onset of high fever, muscular rigidity, bradykinesia, mental status changes, dysautonomia (fluctuating blood pressure [BP]), and urinary incontinence. Look for a history of mental illness and prescription of an antipsychotic(s). This is a potentially life-threatening reaction. Refer to ED or call 911.

SUICIDE RISK FACTORS

- Older people who have recently lost a spouse (due to death or divorce)
- Plan involving a gun or other lethal weapon; access to weapons
- History of attempted suicide and/or family history of suicide
- Mental illness such as depression, bipolar disorder, personality disorders, psychotic disorders, posttraumatic stress disorder (PTSD)
- History of traumatic brain injury
- History of sexual, emotional, and/or physical abuse
- Terminal illness, chronic illness, chronic pain
- Alcohol use disorder, substance use disorder
- Age 15 to 24 years or over age 60 years
- Significant loss (divorce, breakup with boyfriend/girlfriend, job loss, death of a loved one)
- Females make more attempts compared with males, but males are more likely to die by suicide
- Older adult males who recently lost a partner are at highest risk of suicide

AT-RISK PATIENTS

The Baker Act

The Baker Act (i.e., involuntary commitment legislation; name may differ by state) allows 72 hours (3 days) of involuntary detention for evaluation and treatment of persons who are considered at very high risk for suicide and/or hurting others.

Common Mental Health Questionnaires

- Beck Depression Inventory-II: A multiple-choice self-report inventory for evaluating depression. Based on the theory that negative cognitions about the self and world in general can cause depression.
- *Diagnostic and Statistical Manual of Mental Disorders Fifth Edition-Text Revision* (*DSM-5-TR*): The diagnostic manual for mental and emotional disorders created and used by the American Psychological Association (APA).
- Folstein Mini-Mental State Exam (MMSE): A questionnaire used to evaluate an individual for confusion and dementia (e.g., Alzheimer's, stroke); see Table 15.1.
- Geriatric Depression Scale (GDS): A 30-item (yes/no response) questionnaire. Shorter version contains 15 items. Used to assess depression in older adults. Self-assessment format.
- Generalized Anxiety Disorder 7-Item (GAD 7) Scale: A seven-item screening tool for helping to identify patients with anxiety. The GAD 7 is a valid and efficient tool (89% sensitivity and 82% specificity). The higher the score, the higher the anxiety level. Severe anxiety (15 or higher), moderate anxiety (10 points), and mild anxiety (5 points).

Table 15.1 Folstein Mini-Mental State Exam

Cognitive Skill	Action Required
Orientation	What is the date today? (current day, month, year) Location? (name of the city, county, state)
Immediate Recall ■ Recall three objects	Instruct patient that you will be testing their memory; say three unrelated words (pencil, apple, ball); ask patient to repeat words.
Attention and Calculation ■ Counting backward ■ Backward spelling	Say "Starting at 100, count backward and keep subtracting 7." Say "Spell the word *world* backward."
Writing and Copying ■ Writing a sentence ■ Copying a figure	Give person one blank piece of paper and ask them to write a sentence. Draw intersecting pentagons; ask patient to copy the pentagons.
Scoring	Maximum score is 30 correctly done; a score of <19 indicates impairment.

Source: Adapted from Folstein, M. F., Folstein, S. E., & McHugh, P. R. (1975). (See Resources section for complete source information.)

■ Patient Health Questionnaire–9 (PHQ-9): A self-administered questionnaire for depression that scores nine *DSM-5* criteria on a scale of 0 (not at all) to 3 (nearly every day).

EXAM TIP

A question on the MMSE (or the MME) will describe an action (such as asking a patient to spell *world* backward) and ask you to indicate the name of the tool that is being used.

PSYCHOTROPIC DRUGS

SELECTIVE SEROTONIN REUPTAKE INHIBITORS

First-line treatment for:
- Major depression, obsessive-compulsive disorder (OCD)
- Generalized anxiety disorder, panic disorder, social anxiety disorder
- Premenstrual dysphoric disorder
- PTSD

Common Selective Serotonin Reuptake Inhibitors

- Fluoxetine (Prozac): Longest half-life of all SSRIs and the first SSRI (useful for noncompliant patients)
- Paroxetine (Paxil): Shortest half-life
- Citalopram (Celexa): Has fewer drug interactions compared with other SSRIs
- Escitalopram (Lexapro): Compound derived from citalopram (Celexa)
- Other SSRIs: Sertraline (Zoloft), fluvoxamine (Luvox)

EXAM TIPS

- Learn how medication use should be monitored (see Table 15.2).
- Know U.S. Food and Drug Administration (FDA) boxed warnings for SSRIs and antipsychotics.

Side Effects

- Causes loss of libido in men and women, erectile dysfunction, anorexia, insomnia.
- Avoid with anorexic patients and undernourished older adults (depresses appetite more).
- Paroxetine (Paxil): Common side effect is erectile dysfunction.
- Taper SSRIs over 2 to 4 weeks prior to discontinuation. Paroxetine is the most likely to cause symptoms and may need to be discontinued for a period of 3 to 4 weeks or longer.
- Fluoxetine is least likely to cause discontinuation syndrome because of its long elimination half-life; it can be tapered over 1 to 2 weeks.
- Abrupt discontinuation may precipitate dysphoria, fatigue, chills, myalgias, headache, dizziness, gastrointestinal distress. Discontinuation syndrome occurs in 20% to 30%.

EXAM TIPS

- Paroxetine (Paxil) and venlafaxine (Effexor) have short half-lives (compared with other SSRIs), and patients need to be weaned. Do not discontinue abruptly; will cause withdrawal symptoms.
- Of all the SSRIs, paroxetine (Paxil) is most likely to cause erectile dysfunction.

Contraindications

- Avoid SSRIs within 14 days of taking an MAOI (serotonin syndrome).
- Can induce mania with bipolar patients.

TRICYCLIC ANTIDEPRESSANTS

- Not considered first-line treatment for depression.
- Other uses: Postherpetic neuralgia (chronic pain), urinary incontinence.
- Avoid if patient at high risk for suicide because they may hoard pills and overdose (suicide attempt).

Table 15.2 Monitoring of Psychiatric Medications

Drug Class/Drugs	Adverse Effects	Monitor
Atypical Antipsychotics ■ Olanzapine (Zyprexa) ■ Risperidone (Risperdal) ■ Quetiapine (Seroquel)	Obesity Diabetes type 2	All can cause weight gain Check BMI Check weight every 3 months EKG annually for QTC changes
Typical Antipsychotics ■ Haloperidol (Haldol), chlorpromazine	Elevates lipids/triglycerides Extrapyramidal effects Tardive dyskinesia QT prolongation Sudden death Malignant neuroleptic syndrome (rare)	Labs: Fasting blood glucose and lipid profile Boxed warning: Frail elderly are at higher risk of death from antipsychotics Look for extrapyramidal symptoms such as dystonia, parkinsonism, akathisia (inability to stay still), tardive dyskinesia EKG annually for QTC changes
Anticonvulsants ■ Lamotrigine (Lamictal) ■ Carbamazepine (Tegretol) ■ Valproate (Depakote)	Stevens–Johnson syndrome (Lamictal)	Advise patient to report rashes (Stevens–Johnson); some anticonvulsants are also used as a mood stabilizer for bipolar disorder Monitor serum carbamezapine concentration Check serum valproic acid concentration
SSRIs ■ Sertraline (Zoloft) ■ Paroxetine (Paxil) ■ Citalopram (Celexa)* ■ Escitalopram (Lexapro)*	All SSRIs can cause sexual dysfunction Highest risk of erectile dysfunction Older adults on multiple drugs, less risk of drug interactions	Boxed warning: All SSRIs may cause suicidal ideation/plans (<24 years of age) Do not discontinue Paxil abruptly; wean gradually
Atypical Antidepressants ■ Bupropion (Wellbutrin) ■ Bupropion (Zyban)	Seizures	Contraindicated with seizures disorder, eating disorders (e.g., anorexia, bulimia) For smoking cessation
SNRIs ■ Venlafaxine (Effexor) ■ Duloxetine (Cymbalta**)	Can precipitate acute narrow-angle glaucoma Bioavailability reduced by 33% in smokers Venlafaxine: Avoid abrupt discontinuation due to withdrawal symptoms	Avoid with uncontrolled narrow-angle glaucoma Do not take 5 days before or 14 days after MAOI, linezolid, selegiline, IV methylene blue
TCAs ■ Amitriptyline (Elavil) ■ Nortriptyline (Pamelor) ■ Doxepin (Sinequan)	Anticholinergic effects Category X	Do not combine with SSRIs or MAOIs, as they will increase risk of serotonin syndrome EKG annually for QTC changes
Lithium ■ Lithium carbonate (Eskalith)	Contraindicated if sodium depletion, dehydration, significant renal or cardiovascular disease	Used for bipolar disorder; "Ebstein's anomaly" is congenital heart defect caused by lithium Check TSH annually Check serum concentration (narrow therapeutic window of 0.6 to 1.2 mmol/L) Check serum trough level (12 hours after last dose)

BMI, body mass index; IV, intravenous; MAOI, monoamine oxidase inhibitor; SNRI, serotonin-norepinephrine reuptake inhibitor; SSRI, selective serotonin reuptake inhibitor; TCA, tricyclic antidepressant; TSH, thyroid-stimulating hormone.
*Lowest number of drug interactions compared with other SSRIs.
**Cymbalta also used for diabetic peripheral neuropathy.

- Overdose will cause fatal cardiac (ventricular arrhythmia) and neurologic effects (seizures).
- Examples: Doxepin (Sinequan), imipramine (Tofranil), amitriptyline (Elavil), nortriptyline (Pamelor)

EXAM TIP

TCAs are used for herpetic neuralgia and for migraine headache prophylaxis (not acute treatment).

SEROTONIN-NOREPINEPHRINE REUPTAKE INHIBITORS

- Increased available serotonin and norepinephrine in the brain
- Duloxetine (Cymbalta): Can treat generalized anxiety disorder, fibromyalgia, depression, and diabetic peripheral neuropathy; smoking reduces bioavailability by 33%
- Venlafaxine (Effexor): Taper over 2 to 3 weeks to avoid discontinuation syndrome
- Desvenlafaxine (Pristiq)

MONOAMINE OXIDASE INHIBITORS

- Rarely used due to serious food (high tyramine content) and drug interactions
- Phenelzine (Nardil), tranylcypromine (Parnate)
- Do not combine with SSRIs, TCAs, monoamine oxidase B (MAO-B; selegiline [Eldepryl]), serotonin receptor agonists (e.g., sumatriptan [Imitrex], zolmitriptan [Zomig]).

Contraindications

- Do not combine MAOI with SSRI/SNRI or TCA.
- Wait at least 2 weeks before initiating SSRI or TCA (high risk of serotonin syndrome).

High-Tyramine Foods and Monoamine Oxidase Inhibitors

- The combination can cause the tyramine pressor response (elevates BP, risk of stroke); avoid combining with fermented foods such as beer, Chianti wine, some aged cheeses, fava beans.
- High-tyramine foods can also cause migraine headache in susceptible persons.

EXAM TIP

Know MAOI and high-tyramine foods to avoid.

BENZODIAZEPINES (TRANQUILIZERS)

- Benzodiazepines are indicated for anxiety disorders, panic disorder, and insomnia (not first line).
- Diazepam (Valium) and chlordiazepoxide (Librium) are also used for severe alcohol withdrawal and seizures.
- Do not discontinue abruptly because it increases risk of seizures; wean slowly.
- Examples include:
  - Ultra–short acting: Midazolam IV only (Versed), triazolam (Halcion)
  - Medium acting: Alprazolam (Xanax), lorazepam (Ativan)
  - Long acting: Diazepam (Valium), chlordiazepoxide (Librium), temazepam (Restoril), and clonazepam (Klonopin)

DISEASE REVIEW

ABUSE: ALL TYPES

Abusive behaviors are multifactorial. They may include physical, emotional, and sexual abuse and/or neglect, as well as economic abuse or material exploitation. Abuse can happen at any age and during pregnancy (higher risk).

Upon presentation to the ED, for example, the pattern of the injuries is inconsistent with the history given. Older adults who are most likely to be abused are those >80 years old and/or who are frail. Children with mental, physical, or other disabilities and stepchildren are more likely to be abused.

Types of abuse are physical abuse, sexual abuse, emotional/psychologic abuse, and financial abuse, and neglect. A common finding is a delay in seeking medical treatment for the injury. Intimate partner violence (IPV) is defined as intentional control or victimization performed by a person to another with whom the person has an intimate or spousal relationship. The most significant reason for missing the diagnosis of IPV or other abuse is failure to ask.

EXAM TIPS

- There will always be a few questions on abuse. The questions may address physical abuse, child abuse, sexual abuse, and/or elder abuse.
- The abuser is described as a person who does not want the abused person out of sight or interviewed alone.

Risk Factors That Increase Likelihood of Abuse (All Types)

- Increased stress (partner/parent/caregiver)
- Alcohol/drug use disorder
- Personal history of abuse, positive family history of abuse
- Major loss (e.g., financial, job loss)
- Social isolation
- Pregnancy (domestic abuse)
- Elder abuse: Frail elderly and those with dementia are more likely to be abused; about two thirds of all elder abuse is perpetrated by family members (usually an adult child or a spouse); most abused older adults also suffer economic abuse.
- Only certain states have mandatory reporting of partner abuse; be mindful of institutional abuse of older adults, children, and the disabled.

Physical Exam: Abuse (All Types)

- Another health provider (witness) should be in the same room during the exam.
- Interview victim without abuser in the same room.
- Collect visual evidence of trauma via camera to document all injuries. Keep all evidence in a safe place. Use a ruler to

identify and document the size of the injuries. Document direct "quotes" in the patient's history.

- Use the abuse assessment screening tool with a body map to document assessment findings.
- Look for spiral fractures, multiple healing fractures (especially in rib area), burn marks with pattern, welts, and so forth.
- Look for signs of neglect (e.g., dirty clothes, inappropriately dressed for the weather).
- For partner abuse, focus on developing a plan for safety with the patient when appropriate. Give the patient the phone number of a crisis center and/or safe place.
- Sexually transmitted infection (STI) testing:
  - Chlamydial and gonorrheal cultures (must use cultures in addition to the Gen-Probe)
  - HIV, hepatitis B, syphilis, herpes type 2
  - Genital, throat, and anal area culture and testing must be done.
- Abused patient is very fearful and quiet when with the abuser.

EXAM TIPS

- The abuser typically answers all the questions for the patient and will exhibit "controlling" behaviors toward the abused patient.
- Abuse cases: Interview together and then separately.

Treatment Plan

- Provide prophylactic treatment against several STIs (with parental consent for minors).
- Teach the patient the cycle of abuse; educate the patient regarding safety issues and having an escape plan ready for use.
- Healthcare professionals must report actual or suspected child abuse.
- Be aware of individual state guidelines on reporting suspicion of elder abuse.
- Abuse of a disabled person must be reported to the Disabled Person Protective Commission; contact adult protective services or law enforcement agencies with concerns regarding self-neglect.

Good Communication Concepts

- State things objectively; do not be judgmental. Example: Say: "You have bright-red stripes on your back" instead of "It looks as if you have been whipped on your back."
- Open-ended questions are preferred. Example: Say: "What happened to your back?" instead of "What type of object was used to hurt your back?"
- Do not reassure patients (this stops the patient from talking more about their problems). Example: Say: "We will make sure you get help" instead of "Don't worry, everything will be fine."
- Let the patient vent their feelings. Do not discourage patient from talking. Example: Say: "Please tell me why you feel so sad."
- Validate feelings. Example: Say: "Yes, I understand your anger when someone hits you."

EXAM TIPS

- Delaying an action (e.g., waiting until the patient feels better) is always wrong.
- Any answer choice that reassures patients is usually wrong.

ALCOHOL USE DISORDER

Alcohol use disorder is a compulsive desire to drink alcohol despite personal, financial, and social consequences. It may be mild, moderate, or severe per *DSM-5-TR* criteria. Individuals have a strong craving for alcohol and are unable to limit drinking. With alcohol dependence, a patient experiences cognitive, behavioral, and physiologic symptoms that are generated from persistent and chronic use. Abrupt cessation causes withdrawal symptoms. Alcohol abuse occurs when a maladaptive behavior pattern appears from repeated alcohol use.

Definitions

- Elevated blood alcohol level >0.08% is illegal for driving (blood alcohol or breathalyzer) in all U.S. states.
- Standard drink sizes in the United States (considered "one drink"; Figure 15.1):
  - Beer: 12 oz
  - Malt liquor: 8 to 9 oz
  - Wine: 5 oz
  - Liquor/spirits: 1.5 oz or a "shot" of 80-proof gin, vodka, rum, whiskey, or tequila

Dietary Guidelines for Americans (Ethyl Alcohol or Ethanol)

- Women: One drink per day
- Men: Two drinks per day
- Binge drinking: A pattern of alcohol consumption that brings the blood alcohol level to ≥0.08% on one occasion (generally within 2 hours)
  - Males: ≥five drinks in a single occasion
  - Women: ≥four drinks in a single occasion
- Metabolism: Women metabolize alcohol (50%) more slowly than do men and are more susceptible to alcohol-related liver damage.
- Excessive alcohol consumption: Third-leading preventable cause of death in the United States.

EXAM TIPS

- Questions may be asked about who is most likely (or least likely) to become an alcoholic.
- Women are allowed one drink/day, and men are allowed two drinks/day.

People Who Should Abstain From Alcohol

- People who are pregnant (or suspect they are pregnant) or breastfeeding
- People in recovery from alcohol use disorder or people who cannot control the amount they drink

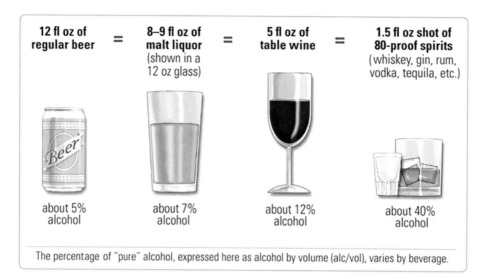

Figure 15.1 U.S. standard drink sizes for alcoholic beverages.
Source: National Institute for Alcohol Abuse and Alcoholism. (n.d.). (See Resources section for complete source information.)

- People with jobs that require alertness and coordination (e.g., pilots, truck drivers)
- People taking medication that interacts with alcohol (Table 15.3)

Labs

Gamma-Glutamyl Transferase

Elevation of gamma glutamyl transaminase (GGT) (with/without alanine aminotransferase [ALT] and aspartate aminotransferase [AST]) is a possible sign of occult alcohol abuse.

Aspartate Aminotransferase/Alanine Aminotransferase Ratio (Liver Transaminases)

- Both AST and ALT are usually elevated (with or without elevated GGT) in alcoholism.
- Ratio of 2:1 with AST/ALT (AST level is double the level of ALT) is associated with alcohol abuse (alcoholic hepatitis).
- ALT is more specific for the liver than AST because AST is also found in the liver, cardiac and skeletal muscle, kidneys, and lungs.

Mean Corpuscular Volume

- Red blood cells (RBCs): May be larger size (mean corpuscular volume [MCV] >100 fL) due to folate deficiency that resembles mild macrocytic anemia.
- Platelets: Chronic alcohol use affects the production and function of platelets in the body. Alcoholism can cause thrombocytopenia; it increases bleeding risk such as stroke.
- Triglycerides: Alcohol affects the synthesis of lipids in the liver. The effect is attributed to the inhibition of lipoprotein lipase activity. Very high levels of triglycerides can increase the risk of acute pancreatitis.

Carbohydrate-Deficient Transferrin

- Biomarker test for chronic alcohol abuse (2–3 weeks or longer). An elevated level is highly suggestive of recent high alcohol consumption, especially if abnormal ALT and/or AST. It can detect binge drinking or daily heavy drinking (≥4 drinks a day). It can also be used to detect a relapse.
- It has been proved to be superior to the GGT or MCV as an indicator of chronic alcohol (ethanol) abuse and hepatitis that is caused by alcohol abuse (with elevated AST and ALT).

EXAM TIPS

- GGT elevation can be a sign of occult alcohol abuse.
- AST/ALT ratio of 2.0 or higher is more likely in alcoholism.

Quick Screening Tests for Identification of Alcohol Abuse/Alcoholism

CAGE Test

- Positive finding of at least two (out of four) is highly suggestive of alcohol abuse:
  - **C:** Do you feel the need to *cut down*?
  - **A:** Are you *annoyed* when your spouse/friend comments about your drinking?
  - **G:** Do you feel *guilty* about your drinking?
  - **E:** Do you need to drink *early* in the morning (an *eye-opener*)?
- Examples of some quotations using CAGE:
  - **C:** "I would like to drink less on the weekends." "I only drink a lot on weekends."
  - **A:** "My spouse nags me about my drinking." "My best friend thinks I drink too much."
  - **G:** "I feel bad that I don't spend enough time with the kids because of my drinking."
  - **E:** "I need a drink to feel better when I wake up in the morning."

Table 15.3 Drugs That Interact With Alcohol (Ethanol)

Drug Class	Drug Examples*	Side Effects/Adverse Effects
Benzodiazepines	Lorazepam (Ativan), clonazepam (Klonopin), alprazolam (Xanax), diazepam (Valium)	Drowsiness, impaired motor control, dizziness, respiratory depression, overdose risk
Hypnotics	Zolpidem (Ambien), eszopiclone (Lunesta), temazepam (Restoril), doxylamine (Unisom)	Drowsiness, dizziness, impaired motor control, memory issues
Opioids	Meperidine (Demerol), oxycodone (Percocet), hydrocodone (Vicodin)	Drowsiness, impaired motor control, respiratory depression
Antidiabetics	Glipizide (Glucotrol), glyburide (DiaBeta), metformin (Glucophage)	Hypoglycemia, flushing, headache, vomiting, palpitations
Statins	Atorvastatin (Lipitor), simvastatin (Zocor)	Liver damage
Herbs	Kava-kava, kratom	Increased sedation, liver damage
Antiseizures	Phenytoin (Dilantin), topiramate (Topamax), gabapentin (Neurontin)	Increased risk of seizures, drowsiness, unusual behavior
Muscle relaxants	Cyclobenzaprine (Flexeril), carisoprodol (Soma)	Drowsiness, increased risk of overdose, impaired motor control
Antipsychotics	Haloperidol (Haldol), olanzapine (Zyprexa), risperidone (Risperdal)	Drowsiness, respiratory depression, impaired motor control, hypotension, seizures
Antihistamines	Diphenhydramine (Benadryl), loratadine (Claritin), cetirizine (Zyrtec)	Drowsiness, dizziness, increased risk of overdose
Hypertensives	Verapamil (Calan), benazepril (Lotensin), losartan (Cozaar), hydrochlorothiazide, clonidine (Catapres), terazosin (Hytrin), doxazosin (Cardura)	Dizziness, drowsiness, fainting, hypotension, arrhythmia

*Not an all-inclusive list.

T-ACE Test

Similar to the CAGE test, except for the first question. The last three questions are from the CAGE test. A positive finding of at least two (out of four) is highly suggestive of alcohol abuse.

- **T:** Does it *take more than three drinks* to make you feel high?
- **A:** Have you ever been *annoyed* by people's criticism of your drinking?
- **C:** Are you trying to *cut down* on drinking?
- **E:** Have you ever used alcohol as an *eye-opener* in the morning (having a drink when you wake up to treat a hangover)?

Short Michigan Alcoholism Screening Test Questionnaire

- A 13-item questionnaire that is a shorter version of the original Michigan Alcoholism Screening Test (MAST) Questionnaire (contains 24 items).
- It can be used in adults and adolescents.
- A disadvantage is time required to take and score it.

Alcohol Use Disorders Identification Test

- A 10-question tool that is used with women, minorities, and adolescents.
- Unlike other alcohol screening tests, the Alcohol Use Disorders Identification Test (AUDIT) has proved to be accurate across all populations. It is one of the most accurate alcohol screening tests (92%).
- AUDIT-C is a shortened, three-question version of AUDIT.

Treatment Plan

- Benzodiazepines (Librium, Valium), antipsychotics if needed (e.g., Haldol)
- Vitamins such as thiamine 100 mg IV, folate 1 mg orally/IV daily, and multivitamins with high-calorie diet
- Refer to the 12-step program at Alcoholics Anonymous (AA), a therapist, and/or a recovery program
- Avoid prescribing a recovering alcoholic/addict drugs with abuse potential such as narcotics or any medication that contains alcohol (e.g., cough syrup)

Medications

- Disulfiram (Antabuse): Causes severe nausea/vomiting, headache, other unpleasant effects
- Naltrexone (Vivitrol): Decreases alcohol cravings

Alcoholics Anonymous

- One of the most successful methods for recovering alcoholics. Founded by Bill Wilson and Dr. Robert Smith.
- Patient is paired with a mentor (a recovered alcoholic); believes in a "higher power."
- Must follow a 12-step program and attend AA meetings (uses "chip" reward).
- Support group for family members and friends is called Al-Anon (Al-Anon Family Groups).
- Support group for teen children of alcoholics is called Alateen.

Acute Delirium Tremens

- Characterized by a sudden onset of confusion; delusions; transient auditory, tactile, or visual hallucinations; tachycardia; hypertension; hand tremors; disturbed psychomotor behavior (picking at clothes); and grand mal seizures.
- Associated with major alcohol withdrawal
- Considered a medical emergency so refer to ED.

Korsakoff's Syndrome (Wernicke–Korsakoff Syndrome)

A complication from chronic alcohol abuse. A neurologic disorder with symptoms that include hypotension, visual impairment, and coma. Signs include mental confusion, ataxia, stupor, coma, and hypotension. Treated with high-dose parenteral vitamins, especially thiamine (vitamin B_1).

Korsakoff's Amnesic Syndrome

A type of amnesia caused by chronic thiamine deficiency due to chronic alcohol abuse. Problems with acquiring (and learning) new information (antegrade amnesia) and retrieving older information (retrograde amnesia). Symptoms include confabulation, disorientation, attention deficits, and visual impairment. Chronic thiamine deficiency damages the brain permanently.

EXAM TIPS

- Recognize Korsakoff's syndrome and that it is caused by chronic thiamine deficiency.
- Al-Anon is the support group for an alcoholic's family and friends.

ANOREXIA NERVOSA

Onset is usually during adolescence. Mortality rate is 5%; the death rate of anorexics is 5 to 10 times greater than that of the general population. It is an irrational preoccupation with an intense fear of gaining weight along with distorted perception of body shape and weight. Patients tend to be secretive, perfectionistic, and self-absorbed. Characterized by severe restriction of food intake, marked weight loss (BMI <18.5), lanugo (face, back, and shoulders), and amenorrhea for 3 months or longer. If purging, loss of dental enamel may be present. Anorexics engage in severe food restriction or cycles of binge eating and purging. Some examples of purging are use of laxatives, vomiting. Excessive daily exercise is common.

EXAM TIPS

- Recognize how anorexic patients present: lanugo, peripheral edema, amenorrhea, BMI <18.5.
- Bupropion (Wellbutrin) is contraindicated for patients with eating disorders. It decreases the seizure threshold.

Complications

- Osteopenia/osteoporosis is due to prolonged estrogen depletion (from amenorrhea) and low calcium intake; higher risk of stress fractures.
- Relative energy deficiency syndrome (REDS) is seen in physically active slender males and females. Females may present with amenorrhea; both males and females exhibit premature osteopenia/osteoporosis and disordered eating.
- Peripheral edema may occur (low albumin from low protein intake).
- Cardiac complications are the most common cause of death (e.g., arrhythmias, cardiomyopathy, atrophy of heart muscles, bradycardia). Hypotension is common with BP <90/50 mmHg.

EXAM TIPS

- REDS is amenorrhea in females, low bone mass, low BMI.
- Patients with anorexia are at higher risk for osteopenia/osteoporosis.

Treatment Plan

Refer to eating disorders therapist or inpatient hospitalization in eating disorder unit.

BIPOLAR DISORDER

Bipolar disorder is characterized by mood instability, alternating cycles of mania and depression. Peak incidence of onset is in the 20s (ranges from age 14 to 30 years). There are two types: bipolar type 1 and bipolar type 2 (hypomania instead of mania). Bipolar patients are at higher risk of suicide; 10% to 15% die by suicide. Manic symptoms are increased energy/activity, grandiosity, less need for sleep, disinhibition, talkativeness, and euphoric mood. The depressive symptoms are similar to major depression. At higher risk of suicide during the depressive phase of the illness. Look for signs and symptoms of depression and suicide warning signs.

- May have psychotic episodes (delusions, hallucinations).
- Bipolar patients have higher rates of substance abuse (40%–60%) and other comorbidities (attention deficit hyperactivity disorder [ADHD], anxiety, OCD, eating disorders).
- Refer to psychiatrist or psychiatric-mental health nurse practitioner (PMHNP) for management.

Medications

Lithium salts (adversely affect kidney and thyroid gland), anticonvulsants (divalproex [Depakote], lamotrigine [Lamictal], carbamazepine [Tegretol]), and second-generation antipsychotics (aripiprazole [Abilify], risperidone [Risperdal], quetiapine [Seroquel], olanzapine [Zyprexa]).

EXAM TIPS

- Differentiate presentations for bipolar disorder and depression.
- Antipsychotics lead to an increased risk of obesity, type 2 diabetes, hyperlipidemia, metabolic syndrome, and hypothyroidism.

INSOMNIA (SLEEP DISORDER)

It is thought that 7 to 8 hours of sleep is the ideal amount. About 40 to 70 million Americans (20% of the population) suffer from either transient (<1 week), short-term (1–3 months), or chronic (>3 months) insomnia. Insomnia can manifest either as difficulty falling asleep (sleep-onset insomnia) or falling asleep but waking up during the night or too early and being unable to go back to sleep. Can cause daytime drowsiness, fatigue, tension headache, irritability, and difficulty concentrating/focusing on tasks. Insomnia is a clinical diagnosis.

Patient self-medicating using alcohol to facilitate sleep may indicate a coexistent alcohol/drug-dependence problem. Abrupt cessation of these agents may cause increased insomnia and/or anxiety.

Risk Factors

Depression, severe anxiety, gastroesophageal reflux disease (GERD), female sex, illicit drug use, musculoskeletal illness, pain, chronic health problems, shift work, alcohol, caffeine, and nicotine. Certain medications (e.g., SSRIs; cardiac, BP, and allergy meds; steroids; angiotensin-converting enzyme inhibitors [ACEIs]; angiotensin receptor blockers [ARBs]) can cause insomnia.

Etiology

- Circadian rhythm disorders, psychic issues, mental illness, environmental factors, certain medications, jet lag, noise, idiopathic causes
- Medical conditions such as obstructive sleep apnea, restless legs syndrome, chronic fatigue syndrome, bipolar disorder, GERD, Alzheimer's disease, Parkinson's disease, arthritis pain, stroke

Classification

- Primary insomnia (25%): Not caused by disease, mental illness, or environmental factors
- Insomnia with medical condition: Caused by disease (physical, emotional, mental) or environmental factors
- Episodic insomnia: Duration of at least 1 month and up to 3 months
- Short-term insomnia: Also known as acute insomnia; duration of <3 months; caused by pain, stress, grief, or other factors; expected to resolve when stressor is gone or when patient has adjusted
- Persistent insomnia: Presence of symptoms for ≥3 months, occurs at least 3 nights per week; it can be primary insomnia or insomnia with medical condition

Treatment Plan

- Sleep hygiene is first-line treatment.
- Improve sleep hygiene (maintain regular sleeping time, nighttime ritual, avoid caffeine/tobacco/heavy meals before bedtime, get out of bed in 30 minutes if not asleep, use bed only for sleep and sex).
- Avoid using media with screens (smartphones, TV, computers) when in bed; the blue light can disrupt melatonin secretion by the pineal gland.
- Cognitive behavioral therapy for insomnia (CBT-I) is recommended for chronic insomnia in most patients, alone or in combination with medications.

- Refer to sleep lab (polysomnography). It is the gold-standard test for sleep apnea; after diagnosis, refer to otolaryngologist.

Medications

Diphenhydramine (Benadryl), an over-the-counter antihistamine, can cause excess sedation and confusion in older adults. It is the most sedating antihistamine. Avoid with the older adults.

Benzodiazepines/Hypnotics (See "Psychotropic Drugs")

Some benzodiazepines are more sedating and are used as hypnotics. This includes triazolam (Halcion) and temazepam (Restoril).

Hypnotics and "sleeping pills" are ideally used for a short duration. But many insomniacs continue using sleeping pills daily to help them sleep. Physical dependence may develop with long-term use. If a patient has been on a benzodiazepine for a long time, do not discontinue abruptly (will increase risk of seizures). Wean off slowly and gradually.

- Short acting (half-life <5 hours): Alprazolam (Xanax), triazolam (Halcion), midazolam (Versed)
- Intermediate acting (half-life 5–24 hours): Lorazepam (Ativan), temazepam (Restoril), clonazepam (Klonopin)
- Long acting (half-life >24 hours): Diazepam (Valium), chlordiazepoxide (Librium)

Nonbenzodiazepine Hypnotics

These drugs have quick onset (15–30 minutes) and lower risk of tolerance and dependence. Do not take if unable to get 7 to 8 hours of sleep. Adverse effects include agitation, hallucinations, nightmares, and suicidal ideation. There have been cases in which a person wakes up and does their normal routine (sleep driving, eating, working) but is unable to recall the incident.

- Zolpidem (Ambien) and eszopiclone (Lunesta) for sleep onset or inability to stay asleep
- Ramelteon (Rozerem) for sleep-onset insomnia (melatonin agonist)
- Temazepam (Restoril), lorazepam (Ativan) for sleep-onset insomnia and sleep maintenance insomnia

EXAM TIP

Buspirone (BuSpar), a nonbenzodiazepine drug for chronic anxiety, is taken twice a day; it is not an as-needed drug like benzodiazepines.

Complementary/Alternative Treatments

- Avoid kava-kava or kava-containing supplements. FDA Consumer Advisory issued; they are associated with liver injury (hepatitis, cirrhosis, fulminant liver failure).
- Valerian root (sedating, also used for anxiety)
- Melatonin (also for circadian rhythm disorders such as shift work, jet lag)
- Chamomile tea
- Meditation, yoga, tai chi, acupuncture, regular exercise (avoid 4 hours before bedtime)

- Valerian root is a natural supplement used for insomnia and anxiety. Do not mix with benzodiazepines, hypnotics, or central nervous system (CNS) depressants.
- In general, there are now more questions on alternative treatments.

MAJOR AND MINOR DEPRESSION

Also known as *unipolar depression* (vs. bipolar depression). Major depressive disorder (MDD) is differentiated as mild, moderate, or severe based on the number and severity of symptoms. Attributed to dysfunction of the neurotransmitters serotonin and norepinephrine. Has a strong genetic component.

Symptoms

- Mood: Depressed mood most of the time; may become tearful
- Anhedonia: Diminished interest or pleasure in all or most activities
- Energy: Fatigued or loss of energy, decreased libido
- Sleep: Insomnia or hypersomnia
- Guilt: Feelings of worthlessness and inappropriate guilt
- Concentration: Diminished concentration and difficulty making decisions
- Suicide: Recurrent/obsessive thoughts of death and suicidal ideation
- Weight: Weight loss (>5% body weight) or weight gain
- Agitation: Psychomotor agitation or retardation

EXAM TIPS

- SIG-E-CAPS mnemonic for remembering signs and symptoms of depression:
  - *Sleep*
  - *Interest*
  - *Guilt*
  - *Energy*
  - *Concentration*
  - *Appetite*
  - *Psychomotor*
  - *Suicide*
- Know degree of functional impairment related to mild, moderate, and severe depression.

Immediate Goal: Assess for Suicidal and/or Homicidal Ideation or Plan

If patient is considered to be a real and present threat of harm to self or others:

- Refer to a psychiatric hospital. Patient must be driven by a family member or friend.
- If none are available, call 911 for police. The police can "Baker Act" the patient. A Baker Act (involuntary commitment) proceeding is a means of providing emergency services for mental health treatment (72 hours) on a voluntary or involuntary basis.

Differential Diagnosis

Rule out organic causes, such as hypothyroidism, anemia, autoimmune disorders, vitamin B_{12} deficiency.

Screening Tools

- Beck Depression Inventory: Contains 21 items
- Beck Depression Inventory for Primary Care (99% specificity): Contains seven items
- Two-item question (PHQ-2): Ask the following two questions. If patient answers yes to either question (or both), it is a positive finding: **(1)** During the past month, have you felt down, depressed, or hopeless? (2) During the past month, have you felt little interest or pleasure doing things?

Labs

- Complete blood count (CBC), chemistry profile, thyroid-stimulating hormone (TSH), folate and vitamin B_{12} levels, urinalysis (UA)
- Rule out organic causes; toxicology screen to rule out illicit drug use if at risk

Treatment Plan

- Rule out diseases such as anemia, diabetes, hypothyroid (TSH/thyroid panel), chemistry panel (high potassium for Addison's disease), and vitamin B_{12} anemia.
- Refer for psychotherapy. Cognitive behavioral therapy (CBT) can reduce symptoms (comparable to an antidepressant medication) and is usually effective; if necessary, refer to psychiatrist or PMHNP. If psychotic, refer to the ED.
- Psychotherapy plus antidepressants work better than either method alone.

Medications

First-line medication is SSRIs. Advise patients that antidepressant effect may take from 4 to 8 weeks (up to 12 weeks) to manifest. SSRIs are also first-line therapy for older adult patients because they have fewer side effects.

- Initiation of medications for older adult patients and patients diagnosed with renal or hepatic disorders should begin at a low dose and increased slowly and gradually as tolerated.
- After initiation, follow up in 2 weeks to check for compliance and side effects.
- Continue SSRI therapy for at least 4 to 9 months after symptoms have resolved (usually on first episode); frequent relapse means patient may need lifetime treatment.

EXAM TIP

SSRIs are also indicated for chronic anxiety disorders (social anxiety disorder, panic disorder).

Other antidepressants include SNRIs (duloxetine [Cymbalta], venlafaxine [Effexor]),TCAs (amitriptyline [Elavil], nortriptyline [Pamelor]).

- Prefer bedtime dosing for TCAs due to sedation. Other uses are postherpetic neuralgia, chronic pain, stress urinary incontinence.

- Avoid TCAs with suicidal patients, because they may hoard the pills and take an overdose (causes fatal arrhythmia).
- Boxed warning for increased risk of death in older adults (with dementia) on antipsychotic drugs such as haloperidol (Haldol) and chlorpromazine (Thorazine).

Selective Serotonin Reuptake Inhibitors: Special Considerations

- Boxed warning: Increased risk of suicidal thinking and behavior in children, adolescents, and young adults; the risk of suicidality is increased in young adults age 18 to 24 years during initial treatment (first 1–2 months).
- Older adult patients: Consider using citalopram (Celexa) and escitalopram (Lexapro). These drugs cause fewer drug interactions than other SSRIs; may prolong QT interval.
- Patients with sexual dysfunction caused by an SSRI: Consider adding bupropion (Wellbutrin) to the SSRI prescription. Another option is to switch to an SNRI or atypical antidepressant.
- Patient with depression who wants to quit smoking: Consider bupropion (Zyban). Can be combined with nicotine-avoidance products (e.g., patches, gum).
- Patient with depression with peripheral neuropathy and chronic pain: Consider duloxetine (Cymbalta), which is also indicated for neuropathic pain.
- Patient with depression with postherpetic neuralgia and chronic pain: Consider TCAs.
- Patient with depression with stress urinary incontinence: Consider TCAs.

Antipsychotics: Adverse Effects

- Pill rolling, shuffling gait, and bradykinesia caused by chronic use of antipsychotics.
- Extrapyramidal symptoms (EPS):
  - Akinesia: Inability to initiate movement
  - Akathisia: A strong inner feeling to move, unable to stay still
  - Bradykinesia: Slowness in movement when initiating activities or actions that require successive steps such as buttoning a shirt
  - Tardive dyskinesia: Chronic condition involving involuntary movements of the lips (smacking), tongue, face, trunk, and extremities (more common in schizophrenia); can be acute as EPS

Anticholinergics: Side Effects

- Many drug classes have strong anticholinergic effects, including antipsychotics, TCAs, decongestants, and antihistamines (e.g., pseudoephedrine).
- Use caution with benign prostatic hyperplasia (BPH; urinary retention), narrow-angle glaucoma, and preexisting heart disease.
- Use the SAD CUB mnemonic to help remember anticholinergic side effects:
  - **S**edation
  - **A**norexia
  - **D**ry mouth
  - **C**onfusion and constipation
  - **U**rinary retention
  - **B**PH

EXAM TIP

Anticholinergics: Use caution with BPH (urinary retention), narrow-angle glaucoma, preexisting heart disease. Antipsychotics (both classic and new generation) have strong anticholinergic effects.

Complementary/Alternative Treatments

Complementary treatments for depression include various herbs and supplements, guided imagery, and lifestyle measures such as exercise and yoga (Table 15.4). Be aware of herb–drug interactions.

EXAM TIP

St. John's wort is used for depression, menopausal symptoms, and other conditions. Herb–drug interactions of St. John's wort include indinavir (protease inhibitor), cyclosporine, oral contraceptives, SSRIs, TCAs.

CLINICAL PEARLS

- Patients starting to recover from depression may commit suicide (from increase in psychic energy). Monitor closely.
- If potentially suicidal, be careful when refilling or prescribing certain medications that may be fatal if patient overdoses (e.g., benzodiazepines, hypnotics, narcotics, amphetamines, TCAs). Give the smallest amount and lowest dose possible, with close follow-up.

MUNCHAUSEN SYNDROME

Also known as "factitious disorder imposed on self." Patient falsifies symptoms of factitious disorders (e.g., abdominal pain, chest pain, seizures) and/or injures self and seeks medical treatment, including multiple surgeries. Munchausen by proxy, a related disorder, refers to a parent using a child (and making the child sick) to obtain medical care. These are rare conditions (1%) that are hard to diagnose.

POSTTRAUMATIC STRESS DISORDER

Characterized by flashbacks, nightmares, intrusive thoughts, avoidance of reminders of trauma, sleep disturbance, and hypervigilance. Causes include being in combat/war, sexual assault (12%), myocardial infarction (MI), stroke, ICU stay (20%). Comorbidity, such as depression, anxiety, antisocial disorder, and substance abuse, is higher in PTSD. Assessment tools include the PTSD Checklist (PCL-5), a 20-item self-report measure (for screening and for monitoring symptoms over time).

Treatment Plan

- The first-line treatment is trauma-focused psychotherapy (exposure therapy, CBT, or eye movement desensitization and reprocessing [EMDR]).
- Medication can be used alone or with psychotherapy. SSRIs are the preferred drug class to treat PTSD.

Table 15.4 Complementary/Alternative Treatments for Depression

Name	Drug Interactions	Adverse Effects/Notes
St. John's wort (*Hypericum perforatum*)	SSRIs (e.g., citalopram [Celexa], paroxetine [Paxil]) Tricyclics (e.g., amitriptyline [Elavil], imipramine [Tofranil]) MAOIs, alprazolam (Xanax), protease inhibitors (indinavir), and many others	Decreases digoxin effectiveness Causes breakthrough bleeding that decreases effectiveness of birth control pills Serotonin syndrome
Amino acid supplements such as 5-HTP, l-tryptophan	SSRIs and MAOIs Dextromethorphan Triptans (e.g., Imitrex, Zomig)	Serotonin syndrome
Omega-3 fatty acids (cold-water fish oil such as from salmon) Folate and vitamin B$_6$ (pyridoxine)	No major drug interactions	High doses of omega-3 fish oil may increase risk of bleeding Supplements are usually stopped about 1 week before surgery
Exercise, yoga, massage, guided imagery, acupuncture, light therapy, mindfulness	—	Exercise is just as effective in treating depression as some drugs

5-HTP, 5-hydroxytryptophan; MAOIs, monoamine oxidase inhibitors; SSRIs, selective serotonin reuptake inhibitors.

SCHIZOPHRENIA

- Psychotic symptoms include delusions and paranoia (disorganized speech and behavior).
- Hallucinations are common (usually auditory) with loss of ego boundaries; flat and restricted affect with poor social skills; executive function is very poor (ability to plan and organize day-to-day activities).
- Onset is usually around the second decade; peak incidence is between 16 and 30 years of age.
- Refer patients to a psychiatrist or PMHNP for management.

Medications

Safety Issues

- Typical antipsychotics: Increases the risk of sudden death among older adults who are in long-term care.
- All antipsychotics: Can prolong QT intervals and cause a fatal arrythmia called *torsade de pointes*, including clozapine (Clozaril), thioridazine (Mellaril), ziprasidone (Geodon), haloperidol (Haldol), quetiapine (Seroquel).
- All medications: Pregnancy testing
- Lithium: Serum creatinine, estimated glomerular filtration rate (eGFR), TSH, chemistry profile, electrocardiogram (EKG; if cardiac risk factors)
- Antipsychotics: A1C, lipid profile, EKG (baseline and annually if older than 40 years)
- Divalproex (Depakote): CBC, comprehensive metabolic profile, valproic acid levels after 2 weeks

SMOKING CESSATION

Tobacco use is the most common cause of preventable death. Discuss smoking cessation at every visit with patients who are smokers.

- With nicotine gum use, follow "chew and park" pattern. Chew gum slowly until the nicotine taste appears, then "park" next to the cheeks (buccal mucosa) until the taste disappears. Repeat pattern several times and discard nicotine gum after 30 minutes of use.

- Patient cannot smoke while on nicotine patches. Do not use with other nicotine products (e.g., gum, inhaler); patient will overdose on nicotine. Nicotine overdose can cause acute MI, hypertension, and agitation in susceptible patients. Nicotine products can be used with bupropion (Zyban).
- Bupropion (Zyban) decreases cravings to smoke. Patients can still smoke while on bupropion; can be combined with nicotine products. Individual eventually loses desire to smoke and finally quits. Contraindications include seizure disorder, history of anorexia/bulimia, abrupt cessation of ethanol, benzodiazepines, antiseizure drugs, severe stroke, and brain tumor. Be careful with depressed patients; may increase risk of suicidal thoughts and behavior.
- Prescribe varenicline (Chantix) therapy for 12 weeks (or longer). Even if not ready to quit, initiating drug will reduce cravings for tobacco use and facilitate quitting; may be combined with nicotine patch (increases risk of adverse effects). Take a careful psychiatric history and avoid prescribing to mentally unstable patients or those with a history of recent suicidal ideation. Adverse effects include neuropsychiatric symptoms; may impair ability to drive or operate heavy machinery. (The Federal Aviation Administration [FAA] prohibits pilots and air traffic controllers from taking the drug.)

EXAM TIPS

- Do not mix nicotine patches with nicotine gum. Do not smoke while on patches.
- Bupropion (Zyban) is for smoking cessation. Patients can smoke while on Zyban.

Electronic Cigarettes

E-cigarettes (e-cigs, vapes, vaping, vape pens, e-hookahs) are devices that heat a liquid into aerosol (vapor), which is inhaled by the user. The liquid contains nicotine, flavoring, and other additives. Vitamin E acetate, used as a diluent, can cause serious lung damage; the diagnosis is called e-cigarette, or vaping, product use–associated lung injury (EVALI). Tetrahydrocannabinol (THC) vapes are also associated with EVALI. More than 2,800 cases of EVALI have been reported to the Centers for Disease Control and Prevention, with 60 deaths.

Flavored vapes (e.g., cotton candy, mint, grape) are very popular with teens. The newer vapes are smaller, easier to hide, and resemble USB flash drives. In 2022, 1 in 10 middle and high school students reported vaping. According to the CDC and FDA, e-cigarettes are not safe for youth, young adults, and pregnant patients.

Symptoms of possible lung damage due to vaping:
- Difficulty breathing, shortness of breath, and/or chest pain
- Mild-to-moderate gastrointestinal (GI) symptoms such as vomiting and diarrhea
- Fevers and fatigue

EVALI should be suspected in younger patients with a history of vaping (or other e-cigarette products) with pneumonia-like symptoms, progressive dyspnea, and/or worsening hypoxemia. Some have a history of asthma, which can become exacerbated with vaping.

EXAM TIPS

- Discuss smoking cessation with patients (who are smokers) at every visit.
- Bupropion (Zyban) is used to treat major depression, seasonal affective disorder, and smoking cessation. It increases risk of seizures; avoid if patient at higher risk of seizures (during abrupt discontinuation of ethanol, benzodiazepines).

MOTIVATIONAL INTERVIEWING

A counseling method used to help an individual resolve a state of indecision (ambivalence) into finding the internal motivation (motivational enhancement) to make positive and healthier behaviors. Recent meta-analyses have shown that motivation interviewing is effective in decreasing drug and alcohol use in adolescents and adults. This method is used for substance use disorder, smoking cessation, alcohol abuse, losing weight, reducing sexual risk behaviors, and other types of unhealthy behaviors.

FIVE PRINCIPLES OF MOTIVATIONAL INTERVIEWING

1. Express and listen with empathy about patient's issues (through reflective listening).
2. Understand the patient's own motivations.
3. Avoid argument (or direct confrontation).
4. Adjust to the patient (rather than opposing the patient).
5. Support self-efficacy (empower the patient). (Alfred Bandura, a psychologist, defined self-efficacy as one's belief in one's ability to succeed in accomplishing a task.)

KNOWLEDGE CHECK: CHAPTER 15

1. Which statement about nicotine gum is *true*?
   A. The patient chews each piece continuously until the nicotine is depleted.
   B. The gum is most effective when used to supplement the nicotine patch.
   C. Patients with depressive symptoms should avoid the product.
   D. Users will likely require several pieces each day.

2. An older adult male with alcohol use disorder is scheduled for a physical exam and laboratory testing. The patient's laboratory blood test results may show:
   A. Increased serum creatinine levels and estimated glomerular filtration rate (eGFR)
   B. Decreased number of platelets and increased mean corpuscular volume (MCV)
   C. Increased serum potassium and increased triglycerides
   D. Decreased aspartate transaminase (AST) and alanine transaminase (ALT) levels

3. Which of the following is part of the female athlete triad?
   A. Lanugo
   B. Premature osteoporosis
   C. Self-absorbed behavior
   D. Insulin resistance

4. Which of the following individuals is at highest risk for suicide?
   A. White female teenager who fails an exam in high school
   B. Black middle-aged female who is newly diagnosed with type 2 diabetes
   C. Older adult White male whose spouse of 40 years recently died
   D. Asian adult whose parent has a chronic illness

5. Which of the following medications is *most likely* to cause erectile dysfunction?
   A. Levothyroxine
   B. Paroxetine
   C. Penicillin
   D. Digoxin

6. An older adult female patient with peripheral neuropathy due to diabetes mellitus is recently diagnosed with major depression. The patient refuses psychotherapy and wants medication. She denies suicidal and homicidal ideation. Which of the following pharmacologic agents is the *best* choice for this patient?
   A. Quetiapine (Seroquel)
   B. Duloxetine (Cymbalta)
   C. Escitalopram (Lexapro)
   D. Olanzapine (Zyprexa)

7. A patient with depression is taking citalopram (Celexa) daily. They inform the nurse practitioner that they recently started taking St. John's wort as a supplement to improve their depression. What recommendation is *most* appropriate?
   A. "Call if you think you are experiencing any reactions to the combination."
   B. "You should stop taking the St. John's wort."
   C. "You may need to adjust your citalopram dosage."
   D. "You should consider taking a different herbal supplement."

8. A male patient's history indicates that they are prescribed phenelzine (Nardil) for depression and anxiety. What information revealed during the patient interview would be the *most urgent* for the nurse practitioner to address with the patient?
   A. Drinks one to two beers each week
   B. Smokes three to four cigarettes daily
   C. Has occasional difficulty sleeping
   D. Reports poor appetite recently

9. A patient reports concern about the amount of alcohol they consume. Which screening tool should the nurse practitioner consider adminstering?
   A. AUDIT
   B. PCL-5
   C. PHQ-2
   D. GAD-7

(See answers next page.)

1. D) Users will likely require several pieces each day.

Nicotine gum aids in smoking cessation by providing an alternative source of nicotine. Each piece provides nicotine for approximately 30 minutes, and users will likely require several pieces each day early in their cessation effort. The patient chews each piece briefly to release the nicotine but then "parks" the gum next to the buccal mucosa until it is depleted. To avoid the risk of nicotine overdose, patients should be cautioned against combining nicotine gum with other sources of nicotine, such as the patch. Patients with depressive symptoms or recent suicidal thoughts should avoid some medications used in cessation—specifically buproprion and varenicline—but no such caution exists for nicotine gum.

2. B) Decreased number of platelets and increased mean corpuscular volume (MCV)

Chronic alcohol use affects the MCV because of reduction of folate levels from dietary deficiency and/or impaired absorption due to excessive use of alcohol. Alcohol also interferes with the production and function of white blood cells. Alcohol interferes with platelet production, with diminished fibrinolysis resulting in thrombocytopenia. Patients with alcoholism are at higher risk for bleeding. Alcoholism can increase AST and ALT because of liver inflammation. Alcohol affects lipid metabolism in the liver, resulting in hypertriglyceridemia.

3. B) Premature osteoporosis

The female athlete triad consists of amenorrhea, premature osteopenia/osteoporosis, and disordered eating. Lanugo and self-absorbed behavior, like the female athlete triad, are often seen with anorexia nervosa, but they are not part of the triad. Insulin resistance is part of metabolic syndrome.

4. C) Older adult White male whose spouse of 40 years recently died

Older adult males who recently lost a partner are at highest risk of suicide.

5. B) Paroxetine

Paroxetine is most likely to cause erectile dysfunction. It can also affect female orgasm. Levothyroxine, penicillin, and digoxin usually do not cause erectile dysfunction.

6. B) Duloxetine (Cymbalta)

Duloxetine (Cymbalta) is a selective norepinephrine reuptake inhibitor (SNRI) that is used for depression, chronic anxiety, and the management of diabetic peripheral neuropathy. Quetiapine (Seroquel) and olanzapine (Zyprexa) are atypical antipsychotics. Escitalopram (Lexapro) is a selective serotonin reuptake inhibitor (SSRI) that is used for depression and generalized anxiety disorder, but it does not have an indication for peripheral neuropathy.

7. B) "You should stop taking the St. John's wort."

Concurrent use of St. John's wort with a selective serotonin reuptake inhibitor (SSRI) such as citalopram can result in drug interactions, reducing the effectiveness of the medication. For this reason, patients taking SSRIs (and many other medications) should be instructed to avoid the supplement. Suggesting that the patient should continue use with caution or adjust the citalopram dosage to accommodate supplementation is unsafe. Similarly, it would be inappropriate to suggest that taking a different supplement may be safe without knowing enough detail to research potential interactions.

8. A) Drinks one to two beers each week

Patients who are prescribed a monoamine oxidase inhibitor (MAOI) such as phenelzine (Nardil) should be advised to avoid alcohol because it contains tyramine. The consumption of tyramine while taking an MAOI can result in severely elevated blood pressure and increased risk for stroke. While the nurse practitioner should discuss smoking cessation, this is less urgent than explaining the dangerous food–drug interaction. Insomnia and anorexia are common side effects of selective serotonin reuptake inhibitors, but reports of occasional difficulty sleeping and recent poor appetite do not suggest any imminent risk for this patient.

9. A) AUDIT

The Alcohol Use Disorders Identification Test (AUDIT) is a highly accurate tool used to screen for potential alcohol use disorder. The PCL-5 (PTSD Checklist) is used to screen for posttraumatic stress disorder. PHQ-2 (Patient Health Questionnaire-2) is a screening tool for depression. GAD-7 is the Generalized Anxiety Disorder 7-Item Scale.

10. The nurse practitioner is conducting the Mini-Mental State Exam (MMSE) on a patient. Which result indicates impairment?
    A. Inability to copy an image of intersecting pentagons
    B. Inability to recall today's date
    C. At least two positive findings
    D. A score of 20

11. The nurse practitioner has finished conducting the CAGE questionnaire with a patient. The patient responded "Yes" when asked if they felt the need to cut down on their drinking and if they felt guilty about their drinking. The patient responded "No" to the other two questions. What is the appropriate next step?
    A. Prescribe disulfiram
    B. Ask the patient to complete the T-ACE questionnaire to obtain more information
    C. Discuss the possibility of alcohol misuse with the patient
    D. Document the results as normal findings

12. A patient who has been prescribed lamotrigine (Lamictal) for bipolar disorder calls the clinic to report a rash. Which syndrome does the nurse practitioner suspect?
    A. Malignant neuroleptic
    B. Acute serotonin
    C. Stevens-Johnson
    D. Korsakoff's

13. Which of the following would best support a diagnosis of "factitious disorder imposed on self"?
    A. Reporting symptoms that cannot be definitively attributed to a health disorder
    B. Denying symptoms that are consistent with a diagnosed disorder
    C. Falsifying symptoms to obtain medical treatment
    D. Intentionally harming another to obtain medical treatment

14. A patient diagnosed with insomnia has expressed a preference for alternative treatment instead of medication. What option should the nurse practitioner suggest?
    A. Kava kava
    B. Melatonin
    C. Diphenhydramine (Benadryl)
    D. St. John's wort

15. While examining an 80-year-old patient who lives with an adult caregiver, the nurse practitioner observes burn marks on the patient's back. The patient appears quiet and fearful in the caregiver's presence. What initial action should the nurse practitioner take?
    A. Report suspected elder abuse to the appropriate state agency
    B. Ask the caregiver to explain the injuries
    C. Have the caregiver wait in a different room
    D. Tell the patient, "You have some burn-like marks on your back."

(See answers next page.)

10. D) A score of 20

The MMSE is used to evaluate an individual for confusion and dementia. Using the exam as an outline, the nurse practitioner asks the patient to recall certain facts or perform certain tasks and then assigns a score based on the patient's response. A maximum of 30 points are assigned, and any score above 19 indicates impairment. Although the MMSE asks the patient to copy an image of intersecting pentagons and to recall the current date, the inability to do either is by itself insufficient to establish impairment. Two or more positive findings in the CAGE or T-ACE exam indicates likelihood of alcohol use disorder.

11. C) Discuss the possibility of alcohol misuse with the patient.

The CAGE questionnaire is a four-question tool used to screen for alcohol misuse. Affirmative responses to two or more questions is highly suggestive of misuse, so the nurse practitioner should inform the patient of this possibility and explore it further. Although disulfiram can be prescribed in confirmed cases of alcohol use disorder, a positive finding on the CAGE questionnaire is an insufficient basis upon which to order the medication. The T-ACE questionnaire is nearly identical to the CAGE test in design and content, so conducting it would not reveal additional information.

12. C) Stevens-Johnson

Stevens-Johnson syndrome—a rare but serious disorder that appears as a skin rash—is a potential adverse effect of lamotrigine (Lamictal), an anticonvulsant sometimes prescribed for treatment of bipolar disorder. Malignant neuroleptic syndrome is associated with the use of antipsychotic medications, and signs include fever, muscle rigidity, mental status changes, and dysautonomia. Acute serotonin syndrome is associated with medications that block serotonin (selective serotonin reuptake inhibitors [SSRIs], monoamine oxidase inhibitors [MAOIs], tricyclic antidepressants [TCAs], triptans, tryptophan). Affected patients exhibit spontaneous clonus; inducible clonus plus agitation and diaphoresis; ocular clonus plus agitation or diaphoresis; tremor plus hyperreflexia; or hypertonia and temperature >100.4°F (38°C) plus ocular clonus or inducible clonus. Korsakoff's syndrome is a neurologic complication of chronic alcohol use disorder, and signs include mental confusion, ataxia, stupor, coma, and hypotension.

13. C) Falsifying symptoms to obtain medical treatment

Factitious disorder imposed on self, or Munchausen syndrome, involves the patient falsifying symptoms of a disorder or inflicting self-harm to obtain medical care. While reporting symptoms that the provider cannot definitively link to a health disorder is possible in Munchausen syndrome, it can also result from other issues, such as limitations of diagnostic measures (e.g., low sensitivity). Denial of symptoms is not characteristic of the disorder, and intentionally harming others to gain access to medical treatment is exhibited in Munchausen by proxy.

14. B) Melatonin

Melatonin is an alternative treatment used for insomnia and other sleep disorders. Nurse practitioners should discourage use of kava kava and kava-containing supplements, which are associated with liver injury. Although diphenhydramine (Benadryl) is available without a prescription, it is not considered an alternative treatment. Some patients may explore St. John's wort as an alternative treatment for depressive symptoms, but it is not known to be effective for sleep disorders.

15. C) Have the caregiver wait in a different room

In cases of possible abuse, the nurse practitioner should attempt to interview the patient without the suspected abuser present. Otherwise, the patient's fear of the abuser may interfere with the examination. Reporting elder abuse is mandatory in some states, but the nurse practitioner should attempt to gather more information about the injuries and the patient's safety before deciding that reporting is appropriate. Asking the caregiver to explain the injuries is confrontational, which may increase risk to the patient if abuse is occurring and could be unfair to the caregiver if it is not. The nurse practitioner should instead try to elicit information from the patient. Although objectively describing the injuries to the patient is an appropriate communication technique, the nurse practitioner should be sure the suspected abuser is out of the room before drawing attention to the injuries.

16. Which of the following is a principle of motivational interviewing?
- **A.** Providing the patient with reasons to change their behavior
- **B.** Emphasizing the need to rely on a support network
- **C.** Confronting the patient for their ambivalence
- **D.** Rolling with the patient's resistance

17. A 20-year-old female patient with co-occurring bulimia nervosa presents to the clinic for treatment of major depressive disorder. Which medication is *contraindicated* for this patient?
- **A.** Paroxetine (Paxil)
- **B.** Fluoxetine (Prozac)
- **C.** Bupropion (Wellbutrin)
- **D.** Duloxetine (Cymbalta)

18. Sexual side effects resulting from use of a selective serotonin reuptake inhibitor (SSRI) can be treated with the adjunctive medication:
- **A.** Buspirone (Buspar)
- **B.** Bupropion (Wellbutrin)
- **C.** Paroxetine (Paxil)
- **D.** Sertraline (Zoloft)

19. A patient who has been successfully treating depressive symptoms with a prescribed selective serotonin reuptake inhibitor (SSRI) expresses interest in taking omega-3 fatty acids as complementary therapy. How should the nurse practitioner advise the patient?
- **A.** Point out that complementary and alternative therapies are ineffective for mood disorders
- **B.** Inform the patient that it may trigger a dangerous interaction with the prescribed medication
- **C.** Suggest tryptophan as a safer alternative
- **D.** Help the patient identify an appropriate dosage

20. A patient accompanied by a family member presents with mental confusion, ataxia, and hypotension. The family member indicates the patient has a history of alcohol use disorder. Which of the following is *most likely* to be included in the treatment plan?
- **A.** Vitamin B_1 (thiamine)
- **B.** Bupropion (Wellbutrin)
- **C.** Paroxetine (Paxil)
- **D.** Triazolam (Halcion)

(See answers next page.)

16. D) Rolling with the patient's resistance

Motivational interviewing is a counseling technique used to help a patient find their internal motivation to make changes to improve their health. The five principles of motivational interviewing are expressing empathy, understanding the patient's motivation, avoiding confrontation, rolling with resistance, and supporting self-efficacy. The nurse practitioner should help the patient identify their own motivation rather than prescribe reasons for changing behavior. Although a support network can be helpful, reliance on that network may run counter to the development of self-efficacy. The nurse practitioner should avoid argument or direct confrontation.

17. C) Bupropion (Wellbutrin)

Bupropion (Wellbutrin), an atypical antidepressant, is contraindicated in patients with anorexia nervosa or bulimia nervosa because it lowers the seizure threshold. Paroxetine (Paxil), fluoxetine (Prozac), and duloxetine (Cymbalta) can all be considered.

18. B) Bupropion (Wellbutrin)

Bupropion (Wellbutrin), an atypical antidepressant, can be prescribed off label for treatment of SSRI-induced sexual side effects. Buspirone (BuSpar) is prescribed for treatment of anxiety. Paroxetine (Paxil) and sertraline (Zoloft) are both SSRIs and can contribute to sexual dysfunction.

19. D) Help the patient identify an appropriate dosage

Omega-3 is one of many options that patients can explore as complementary therapy for mood disorders. High intake can increase bleeding risk, so the nurse practitioner should help the patient identify an appropriate dosage and point out the need to discontinue use ahead of any scheduled surgery. Omega-3 fatty acids are not associated wih any major drug interactions. Tryptophan, on the other hand, can interact with a number of psychotropic medications, including SSRIs.

20. A) Vitamin B_1 (thiamine)

The patient's signs and history are consistent with Korsakoff's syndrome, which is caused by chronic deficiency of vitamin B_1 (thiamine) resulting from chronic alcohol use disorder. Immediate treatment involves administration of high-dose parenteral vitamins, especially vitamin B_1. Bupropion (Wellbutrin) is for depression and smoking cessation. Paroxetine (Paxil) is used for treatment of depression and other mood disorders. Triazolam (Halcion) is given for anxiety or sleep disorders.

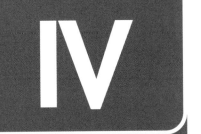

REPRODUCTIVE
REVIEW

16 MALE REPRODUCTIVE SYSTEM REVIEW

DANGER SIGNALS

FOURNIER'S GANGRENE

A rare, rapidly progressing polymicrobial necrotizing fasciitis of the external genitalia and the perineum. Diabetes, trauma to the urethral/penile area, and the use of sodium-glucose cotransporter-2 (SGLT2) inhibitors (canagliflozin, dapagliflozin, empagliflozin) increase risk for this infection. Patient will complain of abrupt onset of severe pain, redness, and swelling of the skin in the perineum, as well as systemic findings such as fever, tachycardia, and hypotension. It spreads rapidly, and the skin often turns black (gangrene). Can include the scrotum and penis. Considered a surgical emergency; requires surgical debridement and IV antibiotics. Refer to ED.

PARAPHIMOSIS

Paraphimosis is when the foreskin cannot be returned back to its original position because of swelling of the head (glans) of the penis. The glans is swollen, reddened, and painful. The highest incidence is among uncircumcised infants and toddlers. If the glans becomes red, swollen, and painful, it may not return back to its original state. It requires emergency treatment because it may cause ischemic changes. A small slit in the foreskin (with topical anesthesia) can help relieve the pressure. In severe cases, a circumcision may be needed. Paraphimosis is considered a urologic emergency. Predisposing factor for paraphimosis is phimosis, a tight foreskin that cannot be retracted to expose the glans penis. Refer to ED.

PRIAPISM

Male complains of a prolonged and painful erection for several hours (≥2–4 hours) that is not associated with sexual stimulation or desire. Patient may awaken with an erection. There are two types of priapism: ischemic and nonischemic. It has a bimodal distribution with peak incidence in children age 5 to 10 years and adults age 20 to 50 years. Priapism can be idiopathic or caused by certain medications and disease states (secondary priapism). The most common cause in adults is medications, such as intracavernosal injections to treat erectile dysfunction. Males with sickle cell disease are at very high risk of ischemic priapism. Other risk factors include high doses of erectile dysfunction drugs, cocaine, and quadriplegia. Ischemic priapism is considered a urologic emergency.

PROSTATE CANCER

Older to elderly man complains of a new onset of low-back pain and rectal area/perineal pain or discomfort accompanied by obstructive voiding symptoms such as weaker stream and nocturia. May be asymptomatic. More common in older men (>50 years), African Americans, and those with obesity, as well as men with a family history of prostate cancer.

TESTICULAR CANCER

Most common solid malignancy affecting males between the ages of 15 and 35 years. Teenage to young adult male complains of nodule, sensation of heaviness or aching, one larger testicle, and/or tenderness in one testicle. Testicular cancer can present as a new onset of a hydrocele (from tumor pressing on vessels). Usually painless and asymptomatic until metastasis. One of the most curable of solid neoplasms with 5-year survival rates of approximately 95%.

TESTICULAR TORSION

A male (usually adolescent) reports waking up in the middle of the night or in the morning with abrupt onset of an extremely painful and swollen, occasionally red scrotum, usually <12 hours in duration. Some have inguinal pain or lower abdominal pain as presenting complaint, frequently accompanied by nausea and vomiting. Affected testicle/scrotum is located higher and closer to the body than the unaffected testicle. Negative cremasteric reflex. Urologic emergency that is more common in neonates and boys post-puberty but can occur at any age. Refer to ED.

TORSION OF THE APPENDIX TESTIS

School-age boy complains of an abrupt onset of a blue-colored round mass located on the testicular surface. The mass resembles a "blue dot." The appendix testis is a round, small (0.03 cm), pedunculated polyp-like structure that is attached to the testicular surface (on the anterior superior area). The blue dot is caused by infarction and necrosis of the appendix testis due to torsion. Cremasteric reflex is present. Torsion of the appendix testes rarely happens in adults. Most cases occur in children aged 7 to 14 years (mean age is approximately 10.5 years).

NORMAL FINDINGS

SPERMATOGENESIS (SPERMARCHE)

- Ideal temperature (for sperm production) is 1°C to 2°C (33.8°F–35.6°F) lower than core body temperature.
- Sperm production begins in late puberty (Tanner stage IV) and continues for the entire lifetime.
- Sperms are produced in seminiferous tubules of the testes.
- Sperms require 64 days (about 3 months) to mature.

TESTES

- Cryptorchidism (undescended testes) increases risk of testicular cancer.
- Production of testosterone/androgens is stimulated by the release of luteinizing hormone.
- Spermatogenesis is stimulated by both testosterone and follicle-stimulating hormone.
- The left testicle usually hangs lower than the right.

PROSTATE GLAND

- Heart-shaped gland that grows throughout the life cycle of the male
- Produces prostate-specific antigen (PSA) and prostatic fluid
- Prostatic fluid (alkaline pH) helps the sperm survive in the vagina (acidic pH).
- The prostate grows throughout a male's life.
- Up to 60% of 60-year-old men have benign prostatic hyperplasia (BPH), proliferation of glandular epithelial tissue, smooth muscle, and connective tissue within the prostatic transition zone. BPH can lead to prostate enlargement and result in lower urinary tract symptoms.

EPIDIDYMIS

Coiled tubular organ that is located at the posterior aspect of the testis. It is the storage area for immature sperm (sperm takes 3 months to mature). Resembles a "beret" on the upper pole of the testes (Figure 16.1).

VAS DEFERENS (DUCTUS DEFERENS)

Tubular structures that transport sperm from the epididymis toward the urethra in preparation for ejaculation. These tubes are cut/clipped during a vasectomy procedure.

CREMASTERIC REFLEX

- The testicle is elevated toward the body in response to stroking or lightly pinching the ipsilateral inner thigh (or the thigh on the same side as the testicle).
- The cremasteric reflex is absent with testicular torsion.

TRANSILLUMINATION: SCROTUM

- Transillumination is useful for evaluating for undescended testicle (cryptorchidism), hydrocele, spermatocele, and other types of scrotal mass.
- Direct a beam of light behind one scrotum (turn off room light); hydrocele will transilluminate (serous fluid inside scrotum) and will have a larger glow than unaffected side.
- Testicular tumor will not transilluminate (solid tumor blocks light).
- Varicocele ("bag of worms") will not transilluminate.

DISEASE REVIEW

ACUTE BACTERIAL PROSTATITIS

Acute infection of the prostate, usually caused by gram-negative organisms. Infection ascends via the urethra with often concomitant infection of the bladder or epididymis. Tends to occur in young and middle-aged men. Most common cause is *Enterobacteriaceae* (*Escherichia coli, Proteus*). If condition occurs in a male <35 years of age, it is treated like gonococcal or chlamydial urethritis.

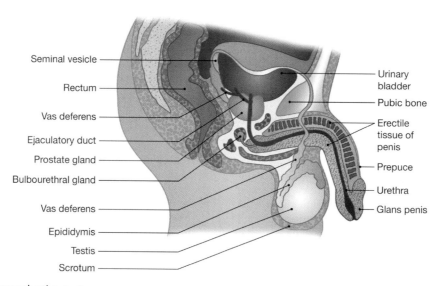

Figure 16.1 Male reproductive system.
Source: Gawlik, K. S., Melnyk, B. M., & Teall, A. M. (Eds.). (2021). (See Resources section for complete source information.)

Classic Case

Male patient complains of sudden onset of fever and chills with suprapubic and/or perineal pain and discomfort. Pain sometimes radiates to back or rectum. Accompanied by urinary tract infection (UTI) symptoms such as dysuria, frequency, and nocturia with cloudy urine. Digital rectal exam (DRE) reveals extremely tender prostate that is warm and boggy. The patient may have an accompanying infection of the bladder (cystitis) or epididymitis.

Objective Findings

- Gently examine prostate: It will be firm, edematous, and noticeably tender.
- Warning: Vigorous palpation and massage of an infected prostate can cause bacteremia.

Labs

- Complete blood count (CBC): Leukocytosis with shift to the left (presence of band cells)
- Urinalysis (UA): Large amount of white blood cells (pyuria), hematuria, bacteriuria
- Urine culture and sensitivity (C&S): If possible, obtain urine after gentle prostatic massage.
- Diagnosis: Based on symptoms and finding of an edematous and tender prostate on exam

Treatment

- Outpatient empiric therapy is fluoroquinolone (e.g., ciprofloxacin 500 mg PO BID) or trimethoprim-sulfamethoxazole (one double-strength tablet PO BID).
- Narrow antibiotic once culture has identified class of organism.
- Prolonged antibiotic course to ensure eradication of infection.
- Men younger than 35 years who are sexually active and men older than 35 years who engage in high-risk sexual behavior should be treated with regimens that cover gonorrhea and chlamydia.
- Antipyretics, stool softener without laxative (Colace), sitz baths, hydration.
- Patient should be hospitalized if septic or toxic.

ACUTE EPIDIDYMITIS

Acute epididymitis is the most common cause of scrotal pain in the adult outpatient setting. Most common due to infection but can also occur from noninfectious causes, such as trauma and autoimmune disease. Rule out testicular torsion (can mimic condition).

- Sexually active males <35 years: More likely to be infected with a sexually transmitted infection (STI) (chlamydia, gonorrhea)
- Males >35 years: Usually due to gram-negative *E. coli*

Classic Case

Adult to older man complains of acute onset of a swollen, red scrotum that hurts. Accompanied by unilateral testicular tenderness with urethral discharge. Scrotum is swollen and erythematous with induration of the posterior epididymis. Sometimes accompanied by a hydrocele and signs and symptoms of UTI. May have systemic symptoms such as fever.

- Positive Prehn's sign: Relief of pain with scrotal elevation
- Cremasteric reflex: Positive

Labs

- CBC for leukocytosis
- UA for leukocytes (pyuria), blood (hematuria), nitrites
- Urine C&S
- Urine nucleic acid amplification test (NAAT) for gonorrhea and chlamydia

Treatment

- For patients at risk of STIs who do not practice anal intercourse, ceftriaxone (500 mg IM × 1 dose) *PLUS* doxycycline PO BID × 10 days; do not forget to treat sex partner.
- For patients at risk of STIs who practice anal intercourse, ceftriaxone (500 mg IM × 1 dose) *PLUS* a fluroquinolone (levofloxacin 500 mg PO daily × 10 days)
- For patients at low risk of STIs, fluoroquinolone (e.g., levofloxacin 500 mg PO daily × 10 days) *OR* trimethoprim-sulfamethoxazole (one double-strength tablet PO BID × 10 days).
- Treat pain with NSAIDs (ibuprofen, naproxen) *OR* acetaminophen with codeine (for severe pain)
- Employ scrotal elevation and scrotal ice packs; bedrest for few days
- Give stool softeners (e.g., docusate sodium [Colace]) if constipated
- Refer to ED if septic, severe intractable pain, abscessed, and so forth

BALANITIS

Candidal infection of the glans penis. When the foreskin (prepuce) is involved, it is called *balanoposthitis*. More common in uncircumcised men and those with diabetes or immune compromise. Use of SGLT2 inhibitors for diabetes management, such as canagliflozin (Invokana), dapagliflozin (Farxiga), and empagliflozin (Jardiance), increases the risk of balanitis and UTI.

Classic Case

Complains of redness, pain, tenderness, or pruritis of the glans and/or foreskin that developed over 3 to 7 days. Physical exam of penis will show redness and shallow ulcers with curd-like discharge on the glans penis. Associated joint inflammation, more sores, and generalized symptoms if balanitis is a manifestation of reactive arthritis.

Treatment

Increase perineal hygiene and bathe affected area with saline solution BID. Additional empiric treatment with topical over-the-counter (OTC) azole creams such as clotrimazole 1% or miconazole 2% BID for 7 to 14 days may be needed. If partner has candidiasis, treat at the same time.

BENIGN PROSTATIC HYPERPLASIA

- Common in the aging male, often starting at age 40 to 45 years, reaching 60% at age 60, and 80% at age 80.
- May be asymptomatic or lead to enlargement of the prostate, causing lower urinary tract symptoms.

- Use the American Urological Association (AUA) urinary symptom score/International Prostate Symptom Score (IPSS) questionnaire to assess the severity of the patient's BPH symptoms.

Classic Case

Older male complains of gradual development (years) of urinary obstructive symptoms such as weak urinary stream, postvoid dribbling, feelings of incomplete emptying, and occasional urinary retention. Nocturia is very common.

Objective Findings

- Perform DRE to estimate prostate size. A normal prostate is about the size of a walnut, firm, and nontender.
- PSA is elevated (norm is 0–4 ng/mL).
- Prostate is symmetrical in texture (rubbery texture) and size is enlarged.

Treatment

- Lifestyle changes may help decrease symptoms and include reduction of caffeine and alcohol intake, avoidance of fluids before bedtime, and avoidance of diuretic medications (if possible).
- Initial treatment is alpha-1 adrenergic antagonist such as tamsulosin (Flomax), terazosin (Hytrin), doxazosin (Cardura).
- For men with concomitant erectile dysfunction, phosphodiesterase type 5 inhibitors (PDE5) are an alternative for initial therapy (e.g., Sildenafil [Viagra])
- For men with low post-void residual urine volumes and overactive bladder symptoms, anticholinergics or beta-3 agonists are a reasonable alternative to first-line therapy. Caution with anticholinergics due to concern for increased risk of urinary retention.
- Therapy to prevent progression includes 5-alpha-reductase inhibitors such as finasteride (Proscar). Duration is usually 6 to 12 months before prostate size is sufficiently reduced to improve symptoms.
- Herbal therapies may include saw palmetto (mild improvement for some); however, insufficient data regarding efficacy and safety, so herbal remedies are not recommended for treatment.
- Combination therapy is indicated for patients with low post-void residual urine volumes and irritative symptoms that persist despite monotherapy.
- Certain drugs may worsen symptoms, such as anticholinergics and sympathomimetics (may cause urinary retention); examples include antihistamines, decongestants, cold medications, caffeine, atropine, antipsychotics, and tricyclic antidepressants (TCAs).

EXAM TIPS

- Finasteride (Proscar) inhibits type II 5-alpha-reductase (it blocks the androgen receptor) and acts directly on the prostate gland to shrink it (temporarily) while on the medication. If patient stops taking Proscar, the size of the prostate gland returns back to its original size.
- The prostate shrinks by 50% while on Proscar (so PSA must be doubled or multiplied by 2).

CHRONIC BACTERIAL PROSTATITIS

Chronic (>6 weeks) or recurrent bacterial infection of the prostate. Some men report a history of acute UTI or acute bacterial prostatitis. Others are asymptomatic. Prostatitis tends to occur in young and middle-aged men. Most commonly caused by *E. coli*. Nonbacterial prostatitis has similar symptoms but is culture negative.

Classic Case

Male presents with a history of several weeks of suprapubic or perineal discomfort that is accompanied by irritative voiding symptoms such as dysuria, nocturia, and frequency. May be accompanied by a low-grade fever. Some men are asymptomatic. Other symptoms include bladder irritation, bladder outlet obstruction, and sometimes blood in the semen.

Objective Findings

Prostate may feel normal, or there may be prostatic hypertrophy, tenderness, edema, and nodularity.

Labs

- UA, urine C&S, PSA
- PSA may be elevated (only about 25% of cases).
- Transurethral ultrasound can measure prostate volume.

Medications

- First-line therapy: Fluoroquinolone such as ciprofloxacin (Cipro) 500 mg PO BID
- Alternatives: Trimethoprim–sulfamethoxazole (Bactrim DS) one tablet PO BID
- Duration: Ranges from 4 to 6 weeks

CRYPTORCHIDISM

Testicle that does not descend spontaneously by age 4 months. Up to 30% premature infants are born with undescended testes. Can affect both or only one testicle. Majority will descend spontaneously by age 12 months. Markedly increases the risk of testicular cancer and sterility. Usually corrected during infancy. Look for empty scrotal sac.

ERECTILE DYSFUNCTION

There are several kinds of male sexual dysfunction, including erectile dysfunction (most common), decreased libido, and ejaculatory disorders. Erectile dysfunction is the inability to produce an erection firm enough to perform sexual intercourse. Sexual dysfunction is common starting in the early 40s and increases with age; erectile dysfunction was reported by 18% of men aged 50 to 59 and 37% of men aged 70 to 79. In men 50 years or older, it is more likely to be related to organic causes. Check medication history; contraindication is nitrates.

- Organic cause: Inability to have a satisfactory erection. Can be caused by aging; neurologic (e.g., Parkinson's disease, Alzheimer disease, stroke, multiple sclerosis [MS], spinal cord damage), vascular (e.g., hypertension, diabetes, smoking), or hormonal (e.g., hypogonadism) factors; or local penile (cavernous) factors (e.g., Peyronie's disease).

- Drug-induced: Antidepressants (e.g., SSRIs (especially paroxetine [Paxil]), antipsychotics, recreational drugs, alcohol, antihypertensives (e.g., beta-blockers, thiazide diuretics).
- Psychogenic cause: Spontaneously has early-morning erection or normal nocturnal tumescence or can achieve a firm erection with masturbation. Can be caused by performance anxiety, depression, relationship issues, and stress.

Labs
Rule out diabetes (fasting blood glucose [FBG], A1C), thyroid disorder (thyroid-stimulating hormone [TSH]), morning serum testosterone.

Treatment
- First-line: Treat with PDE5 inhibitors.
- Other forms of treatment: Vacuum-assisted erection devices, penile self-injection (intracavernosal injection of alprostadil), penile implant, testosterone therapy, and cognitive behavioral therapy (for psychogenic cause).
- Sildenafil citrate (Viagra):
  - 25/50/100 mg; take one dose 30 to 60 minutes before sex; duration of 4 hours; use only one dose every 24 hours.
  - Another use for sildenafil is for pulmonary hypertension (brand name Revatio).
  - Do not combine Viagra with Revatio or guanylate cyclase-C medications such as riociguat (Adempas); it can cause severe hypotension.
  - Careful with alpha-blockers, history of myocardial infarction (MI) in past 6 months, or unstable angina; risk of hypotension.
  - Advise patient to take on an empty stomach; fatty meals and alcohol delay absorption.
  - Do not use with drugs that prolong QT interval (e.g., macrolides).
  - Warning; Viagra can decrease blood flow to the optic nerve, causing sudden vision loss; it has occurred in patients with diabetes, heart disease, hypertension, or other preexisting eye problems.
- Vardenafil (Levitra): Take one dose 30 to 60 minutes before sex; duration is 4 hours.
- Tadalafil (Cialis): 5 mg to 20 mg; can be taken several hours before sex due to long duration (up to 36 hours); may also be prescribed as a daily dose for combined BPH and erectile dysfunction (5–10 mg). Do not combine with an alpha-1 blocker due to increased risk of adverse effects.
- Contraindications: Concomitant nitrates (increased risk of hypotension). Use caution with alpha-blockers, recent post-MI, post–cerebrovascular accident, major surgery, or any condition in which exertion is contraindicated. Avoid combining with grapefruit juice (may increase serum levels/toxicity) or alcoholic drinks.
- Adverse effects: May cause headache, facial flushing, dizziness, hypotension, nasal congestion, priapism, or changes in vision or loss of hearing.

HYDROCELE
- Serous fluid collects inside the tunica vaginalis. During scrotal exam, hydroceles are located superior and anterior to the testes (Figure 16.2). Most hydroceles are asymptomatic.
- More common in newborns. Most cases resolve spontaneously.
- Will glow with transillumination. The glow is larger on the affected scrotum compared with the unaffected scrotum.
- If complaints of testicular pain and scrotal swelling or new-onset hydrocele in an adult or enlarging hydrocele, order scrotal Doppler ultrasound to rule out tumor, testicular hematoma, rupture, testicular torsion, orchitis, or epididymitis. Refer to urologist.

PEYRONIE'S DISEASE
An inflammatory and localized disorder of the penis that results in fibrotic plaques on the tunica albuginea. Results in penile pain that primarily occurs during erection; palpable nodules and penile deformity (crooked penile erections) occur. May resolve spontaneously in small number of cases, but nearly half of cases worsen over time. There are psychologic issues because it can cause erectile dysfunction. Surgical correction if needed.

Labs
None; clinical diagnosis is used.

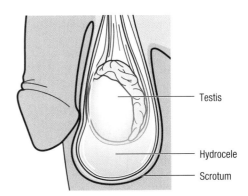

Figure 16.2 Hydrocele.
Source: Myrick, K. M., & Karosas, L. M. (Eds.). (2021). (See Resources section for complete source information.)

Treatment
Refer patient to urologist.

PHIMOSIS AND PARAPHIMOSIS

- Physiologic phimosis is seen in almost all newborn males and is considered normal (Figure 16.3A). The foreskin should not be red or swollen. Avoid forcible retraction, because it can cause tearing, which will cause scarring and development of pathologic phimosis.
- Pathologic phimosis is when the foreskin is truly nonretractable. The foreskin cannot be pushed back from the glans penis because of inflammation. In adults it is due to chronic inflammation and edema of the foreskin. It can complicate sexual function, voiding, and hygiene. Refer to urologist.
- Paraphimosis is when the foreskin cannot be returned back to its original position because of swelling of the head (glans) of the penis (Figure 16.3B). The glans is swollen, reddened, and painful. The highest incidence is among uncircumcised infants and toddlers. Those who have a partial phimosis are often at the greatest risk for developing paraphimosis. If the glans becomes red, swollen, and painful, it may not return back to its original state. It requires emergency treatment because it may cause ischemic changes. A small slit in the foreskin (with topical anesthesia) can help relieve the pressure. In severe cases, a circumcision may be needed. Paraphimosis is considered a urologic emergency. Refer to ED.

PROSTATE CANCER

Most common cancer in men worldwide; in the United States, 11% of males are diagnosed with prostate cancer with the incidence increasing with age. African American males have a higher risk of prostate cancer. Peak diagnosis ranges between 65 and 74 years. Risk factors are age older than 50 years, African American, obesity, and positive family history (first-degree relative increases the risk). For men age 55 to 69 years, prostate cancer screening should be an individualized decision. Studies show that absolute risk reduction of prostate cancer deaths with screening is very small. Individualize management, based on patient's risk factors and age.

Objective Findings

- Painless and hard fixed nodule (or indurated area) on the prostate gland on an older male that is detected by DRE
- Elevated PSA of >4.0 ng/mL
- Screening test not recommended. If patient wants to be tested, order PSA level with DRE; if limited life span (<10 years), not recommended.
- Diagnostic test is biopsy of prostatic tissue (obtained by transurethral ultrasound)

Treatment

- Refer to urologist if PSA >4.0 ng/mL; suspect prostate cancer.
- Individualize screening based on risk factors; discuss risks (bleeding, infection, impotence, procedures, and psychologic trauma) versus benefits.
- Most cancers are not aggressive and are slow growing; watchful waiting/monitoring by urologist is common.
- If symptomatic (nocturia, weak stream, hesitancy, dribbling), alpha-blockers (terazosin [Hytrin]) are first-line therapy. Initiate drug therapy with antiandrogens (Proscar), hormone blockers (e.g., Lupron), and others.

SPERMATOCELE

- A spermatocele (or epididymal cyst) is a fluid-filled cyst that contains nonviable sperm (Figure 16.4). It will transilluminate because it is filled with fluid.
- It can be palpated as a separate smooth and firm lump at the head of the epididymis, which lies above and behind each testicle.
- Spermatoceles do not affect fertility. They are treated only if they cause pain, discomfort, or embarrassment (surgical excision). An ultrasound is the imaging test of choice.

TESTICULAR CANCER

Most common solid malignancy in males age 15 to 35 years.

Classic Case

Teenage to young adult male complains of a painless testicular mass, sensation of heaviness or aching, one larger testicle, or tenderness in one testicle. May present as a new

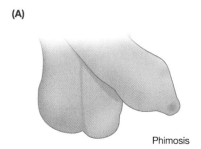

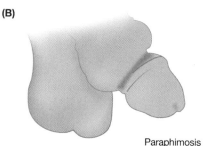

Phimosis

Paraphimosis

Figure 16.3 Phimosis (A) and paraphimosis (B).
Source: Gawlik, K. S., Melnyk, B. M., & Teall, A. M. (Eds.). (2021). (See Resources section for complete source information.)

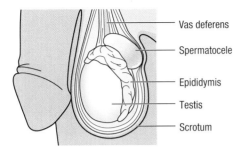

Figure 16.4 Spermatocele.
Source: Myrick, K. M., & Karosas, L. M. (Eds.). (2021). (See Resources section for complete source information.)

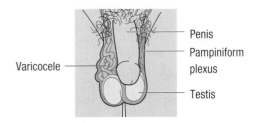

Figure 16.5 Varicocele.
Source: Myrick, K. M., & Karosas, L. M. (Eds.). (2021). (See Resources section for complete source information.)

onset of a hydrocele (from tumor pressing on vessels). Usually painless and asymptomatic until metastasis.

Objective Findings
- Affected testicle feels heavier and more solid
- May palpate a hard, fixed nodule (most common site is the lower pole of the testes)
- A concomitant hydrocele may be present; differentiate with ultrasound.
- Palpate the abdomen for evidence of nodal disease or visceral involvement.

Labs and Treatment
- Ultrasound of the testicle reveals solid mass.
- Gold standard of diagnosis is testicular biopsy.
- Refer to urologist for biopsy and management or surgical removal (orchiectomy).

TESTICULAR TORSION
When the spermatic cord becomes twisted, the testis's blood supply is interrupted. Permanent testicular damage results if not corrected within the first few hours (<6 hours). If not corrected within 24 hours, 100% of testicles become gangrenous and must be surgically removed. More common in males with the "bell clapper deformity," which causes the testicle to lie more sideways than longitudinally. May occur after an inciting event (e.g., trauma, vigorous physical activity) or spontaneously.

Classic Case
An adolescent or adult male reports a sudden onset of severe testicular pain with an extremely swollen red scrotum and diffuse tenderness. Complains of severe nausea and vomiting. The affected testicle is higher than the normal testicle. Cremasteric reflex is absent.

Treatment
- Call 911 as soon as possible.
- Preferred test in the ED is the Doppler ultrasound with color flow study.
- Treatment can be manual reduction or surgery with testicular fixation using sutures.

VARICOCELE
- Varicose veins in scrotal sac (feels like "bag of worms"; Figure 16.5). New-onset varicocele can signal testicular tumor or a mass that is impeding venous drainage. Order an ultrasound of the scrotum. Can contribute to male infertility if large enough (increases temperature of affected testicle). Treatment is surgical removal of varicosities if infertile. Most benign varicoceles are left sided.
- Unilateral right-sided varicoceles are uncommon and may be indicative of a tumor inside the chest, abdomen, or pelvis that is compressing a large vein, such as the vena cava. Another abnormal finding is a varicocele that does not reduce (or drain) in the supine position. Benign varicoceles reduce in volume when the patient is supine due to the blood draining (gravity) from the abnormally dilated scrotal veins.

EXAM TIPS

- In a male with BPH and hypertension, start with alpha-blocker to concomitantly treat blood pressure (e.g., terazosin, doxazosin) first. Works by relaxing smooth muscles on prostate gland and bladder neck.
- Finasteride is a category X drug (teratogenic). Requires special handling. It should not be touched with bare hands by pregnant people.

KNOWLEDGE CHECK: CHAPTER 16

1. A patient with a past medical history of chronic obstructive pulmonary disease (COPD) asks for recommendations on managing his lower urinary tract symptoms secondary to his new diagnosis, benign prostatic hyperplasia (BPH). Which of the following is the *most appropriate* treatment strategy?
   A. Recommend the use of saw palmetto to treat symptoms of BPH
   B. Increase intake of mild diuretics (e.g., caffeine) to ensure adequate urine output
   C. Trial the use of a timed voiding regimen
   D. Reduce fluid intake in the morning

2. Which of the following is *true* regarding prostate-specific antigen (PSA) testing?
   A. A normal PSA result rules out prostate cancer.
   B. There is no single threshold for defining an abnormal PSA value.
   C. Reference ranges are based on height and weight.
   D. Certain medications, such as finasteride, can increase serum PSA levels.

3. A patient presents with penis swelling and severe pain. Upon physical examination, the retracted foreskin cannot be returned to its normal condition. The glans penis and distal foreskin appear swollen, pink, and soft. No blue or black skin discoloration of the glans penis is noted. The patient has been provided pain relief, but manual reduction has failed. Which of the following is indicated to help relieve pressure with this condition?
   A. Advise patient to apply cold packs and to provide updates the following day
   B. Refer patient to ED for invasive reduction in the operating room (OR)
   C. Prepare the patient for emergent circumcision.
   D. Consult urology and prepare for dorsal slit procedure

4. A 13-year-old male patient is brought to an outpatient clinic by his parent with a complaint of a sudden onset of severe left testicular pain. The patient is very nauseous and has already vomited a few times. Physical exam reveals a red, swollen, and tender left scrotum. There is no cremasteric reflex. The abdomen is soft, with no rebound or localized tenderness. Bowel sounds are present. Which of the following is recommended for this patient?
   A. Increased fluid intake and the BRAT diet (bananas, rice, applesauce, and dry toast)
   B. Ordering of ultrasound of the left scrotum
   C. Referral to a urologist by giving the patient's parent the contact information
   D. Referral to the ED

5. Which of the following conditions is a possible effect of the mumps virus, which can affect male fertility?
   A. Salivary gland inflammation
   B. Cryptorchidism
   C. Epididymo-orchitis
   D. Prostatitis

6. What is the *most common* cause of balanitis?
   A. *Pseudomonas*
   B. *Candida albicans*
   C. *Staphylococcus aureus*
   D. *Trichomonas vaginalis*

7. A 37-year-old adult male complains of swelling on the right scrotum that is mildly tender for a few weeks. There is a pressure-like sensation. The right scrotum is larger than the left scrotum. Which of the following tests is an appropriate next step for this patient?
   A. Transillumination
   B. Complete blood count (CBC) with differential
   C. Urology referral
   D. Urinalysis

(See answers next page.)

1. C) Trial the use of a timed voiding regimen

The use of a timed voiding regimen can be helpful in patients who exhibit obstructive complaints or carry a high post-void residual. This technique prompts the patient to empty their bladder based on a time interval (e.g., every 90 to 120 minutes) rather than by the usual sensations, which can be helpful to reduce lower urinary tract symptoms. While herbal remedies may appeal to many patients, there is little data to support their safety and efficacy, and they are not recommended for this patient. Additional lifestyle recommendations include limiting fluid intake before bedtime or prior to travel, limiting intake of mild diuretics (e.g., coffee, alcohol), limiting intake of bladder irritants (e.g., highly seasoned or irritative foods), avoiding constipation, increasing physical activity, practicing Kegel exercises at the time of urinary urgency, and using double-voiding techniques.

2. B) There is no single threshold for defining an abnormal PSA value.

The most commonly used and valuable test for the early detection of prostate cancer is PSA testing. While the likelihood of prostate cancer increases with elevated values, an elevated PSA can also occur in a number of other conditions. Additionally, a PSA result in the normal range does not rule out the possibility of prostate cancer. Certain medications, such as 5-alpha-reductase inhibitors (e.g., finasteride), can reduce PSA levels by about 50% or greater, limiting sensitivity for diagnosing prostate cancer. There is no single threshold for defining an abnormal PSA level; the patient's PSA result should be compared with the age-specific reference range, as well as the prior year's PSA, if available.

3. D) Consult urology and prepare for dorsal slit procedure

This patient is presenting with paraphimosis—a retracted foreskin that cannot be returned to normal position. Patients often present with swelling of the penis and severe penile pain. Management involves *timely* reduction of the foreskin back over the glans penis (the patient should not be sent home). If glans penis necrosis is present (blue/black color and firmness to palpation), emergently consult urology, call 911, and prepare for immediate reduction in the ED or OR. If necrosis is not present (glans penis is pink and soft), provide pain control, ice to reduce swelling, and perform manual reduction (provide manual circumferential compression). If still not reduced (as noted in this patient), provide procedural sedation and advance to a dorsal slit procedure (should consult a urologist or surgeon or have expertise/training to perform this procedure). Injury to the foreskin during manipulation may lead to scarring and phimosis, and ultimately circumcision may be necessary; however, circumcision is not emergently needed at this time.

4. D) Referral to the ED

The sudden onset of testicular pain, with a missing cremasteric reflex accompanied by nausea and vomiting, is highly suggestive of testicular torsion. This is a urologic emergency, so the patient should be referred to the ED. After 6 hours of onset, the risk of ischemia increases. The ED will consult the urology service and obtain an ultrasound of the left scrotum; getting to the ED is the most time-sensitive priority.

5. C) Epididymo-orchitis

Epididymo-orchitis, inflammation of the epididymis and ipsilateral testis, is the most common complication of mumps infection. Among males post puberty who get a mumps infection, 15% to 30% develop epididymo-orchitis. Cryptorchidism is testes/testicle that are/is inside the abdominal cavity, which increases the risk of testicular cancer. Prostatitis and salivary gland inflammation do not increase male infertility.

6. B) *Candida albicans*

Balanitis is inflammation of the glans penis. It can be caused by an infection, an allergic reaction to a soap, or poor hygiene. The most common infectious organism is the yeast *C. albicans*. The glans penis develops erythema, shallow ulcers with a white base, and curd-like discharge. Risk factors include diabetes, obesity, and uncircumcised penis. Less common etiologies include other bacterial infections such as *Gardnerella vaginalis*, group A streptococcus, *S. aureus*, and sexually transmitted pathogens, including *T. vaginalis*. *Pseudomonas* is not associated with balanitis.

7. A) Transillumination

Unilateral scrotal swelling is suggestive of a hydrocele; large ones can cause significant pain due to the accumulation of fluid. Transillumination can be helpful when identifying a hydrocele, which permits the light to shine through while solid lesions will block the light. A urology referral would be appropriate after evaluation if diagnosis remains uncertain and further evaluation and treatment recommendations are needed. A scrotal ultrasound may also be performed if the specific diagnosis is not evident after a physical examination. A urinalysis and CBC with differential are nonspecific in the evaluation of a hydrocele and would not be the appropriate next step unless there was a concern for infection, such as an associated urinary tract infection.

8. Which of the following structures is transected or interrupted during a vasectomy?
   A. Epididymis
   B. Testes
   C. Prostate
   D. Vas deferens

9. A patient with a history of Dupuytren's contracture presents with penile pain, hourglass deformity, and sexual dysfunction. The penile examination reveals a penile plaque and curvature. Based on the history and presentation, this patient is *most likely* presenting with which of the following conditions?
   A. Peyronie's disease
   B. Balanitis
   C. Varicocele
   D. Phimosis

10. A 60-year-old male patient presents with a sudden onset of fever, chills, dysuria, and pelvic pain. On physical examination, the prostate is firm, edematous, and tender. The patient denies high-risk sexual behavior. Based on this presentation, which of the following empiric antimicrobial therapies should be initiated?
    A. Nitrofurantoin
    B. Ceftriaxone
    C. Doxycycline
    D. Ciprofloxacin

11. Which of the following is the *current* recommendation for screening of prostate cancer?
    A. All men age 55 to 69 years should engage in shared decision-making regarding screening.
    B. All men 50 years or older should be screened with a prostate-specific antigen (PSA) test and digital rectal examination.
    C. All men age 55 to 69 years should undergo a digital rectal examination.
    D. All men older than 70 years should be screened due to increased risk of advanced disease.

12. A older adult male patient presents with a unilateral right-sided scrotal mass that feels like a "bag of worms" on physical examination. The patient reports a dull, aching, right-sided scrotal pain. Based on this presentation, which of the following is indicated next?
    A. Transillumination
    B. MRI
    C. CT scan of the abdomen
    D. Biannual semen analysis

13. An adult male patient presents with an acute onset of fever, chills, and fatigue. The patient reports dysuria, frequency, and urgency, along with pelvic pain. Based on this presentation, which of the following is essential in the diagnostic evaluation of this patient?
    A. Blood cultures
    B. Urine culture
    C. Vigorous prostate massage
    D. Complete blood count (CBC) with differential

14. Which of the following increases the risk of testicular cancer?
    A. Peyronie's disease
    B. Phimosis
    C. Balanitis
    D. Cryptorchidism

(See answers next page.)

8. D) Vas deferens

A vasectomy involves the interruption or occlusion of each vas deferens and is the most effective mode (and only method) of permanent male contraception. The epididymis is a highly convoluted duct formed from a singular tubular structure that is estimated to be up to 20 feet in length, which allows space for storage and maturation of sperm. The testes are primarily responsible for testosterone and sperm production. The prostate is a male exocrine accessory gland that consists of exocrine glandular tissue and fibromuscular tissue with the primary function of secretion of fluid that facilitates sperm motility and survival.

9. A) Peyronie's disease

This patient is presenting with Peyronie's disease based on the penile pain, curvature, indentation, hourglass deformity, shortening, and sexual dysfunction. Balanitis is inflammation of the glans penis and presents as pain, tenderness, or pruritis with erythematous lesions. Varicocele describes varicose veins in the scrotal sac and often feels like a "bag of worms." Phimosis is the inability to retract the foreskin.

10. D) Ciprofloxacin

This patient is presenting with symptoms concerning for acute bacterial prostatitis; the patient has a fever, chills, dysuria, and pelvic pain. These patients may also present with perineal pain and cloudy urine. The prostate is often firm, edematous, and tender on exam. Empiric antibiotic therapy should be directed against gram-negative organisms (frequent cause of acute bacterial prostatitis). Unless drug resistance is suspected, empiric treatment often includes a fluroquinolone (e.g., ciprofloxacin, levofloxacin) or trimethoprim-sulfamethoxazole until susceptibility data from the culture results are available. Nitrofurantoin is often avoided in those with prostatitis because of the poor tissue penetration and risk of adverse effects. Sexually active men younger than 35 years and men older than 35 years who engage in high-risk sexual behavior should be treated with regimens that cover *Neisseria gonorrhoeae* (e.g., ceftriaxone) and *Chlamydia trachomatis* (e.g., doxycycline).

11. A) All men age 55 to 69 years should engage in shared decision-making regarding screening.

In 2018, the U.S. Preventive Services Task Force (USPSTF) made the following recommendations: Men who are 55 to 69 years old should engage in shared decision-making about whether they choose to be screened. A deciding factor involves individual patient preferences and health history; the potential benefits must be balanced against the potential harms, including the risks of false-positive tests, prostate biopsy, anxiety, over-diagnosis, and treatment complications. Screening involves a PSA blood test. A digital rectal examination is not recommended as a screening test due to its low sensitivity and specificity for detecting prostate cancer. The USPSTF does not recommend PSA-based screening for prostate cancer in men 70 years and older.

12. C) CT scan of the abdomen

The patient is likely presenting with a varicocele based on the scrotal fullness that has the feel of a "bag of worms" and the dull, aching pain. Usually, varicoceles occur on the left side; unilateral right varicoceles are uncommon and are suspicious for an underlying pathology causing inferior vena cava obstruction. An abdominal and scrotal ultrasound is appropriate, along with a CT of the abdomen with contrast for further workup. An MRI may be indicated after the CT and ultrasound if the diagnosis remains unclear. Most varicoceles do not require intervention; in older men who desire continued fertility, a semen analysis is recommended every 2 years. Transillumination of the scrotum would be helpful to identify a hydrocele.

13. B) Urine culture

Patients with acute bacterial prostatitis are often acutely ill with fever, chills, malaise, irritative urinary symptoms, and pelvic or perineal pain. These classic symptoms of prostatitis often prompt a digital rectal exam, which should be performed gently. Avoid vigorous prostate massage as it is uncomfortable, provides no benefit, and increases the risk of bacteremia. A urine Gram stain and culture should be obtained in all patients with concern for acute prostatitis to establish the microbial etiology. Blood cultures are not routinely recommended or necessary for diagnosis; they may be useful to assess for complications in patients with underlying cardiac valvular disease or concern for sepsis. A CBC with differential may be helpful to identify leukocytosis; however, this finding is nonspecific to the diagnosis. Other common laboratory findings include pyuria and bacteriuria on urinalysis, elevated inflammatory markers, and elevated prostate-specific antigen (PSA) level.

14. D) Cryptorchidism

Males with a history of cryptorchidism are at an increased risk for testicular cancer. Other risk factors include a personal or family history of testicular cancer, infertility or subfertility, genetic disorders, hypospadias, and HIV infection. Peyronie's disease, phimosis, and balanitis have not been shown to increase the risk of testicular cancer.

15. An older adult male patient presents with the inability to sustain an erection for sexual intercourse. The patient has a history of benign prostatic hyperplasia with reports of urgency, nocturia, and hesitancy. Which of the following agents would be helpful for this patient?
    A. Tadalafil
    B. Sildenafil
    C. Avanafil
    D. Vardenafil

16. Which of the following is *contraindicated* while taking a phosphodiesterase type 5 (PDE5) inhibitor?
    A. Alpha-blockers
    B. Beta-blockers
    C. Nitrates
    D. Angiotensin receptor blockers

17. A school-aged male patient presents with an abrupt onset of moderate testicular pain. Physical examination reveals a tender, localized mass that is palpable and appears as a "blue dot" sign. A normal cremasteric reflex is present. This presentation suggests which of the following conditions?
    A. Epididymitis
    B. Torsion of the appendix testis
    C. Acute bacterial prostatitis
    D. Testicular torsion

18. A patient presents with localized testicular pain with tenderness and swelling noted while palpating the epididymis. Scrotal wall erythema is noted, and a positive Prehn sign is seen. The patient denies both a monogamous relationship and anal intercourse. Which of the following treatment regimens is indicated based on this presentation?
    A. Ceftriaxone plus levofloxacin
    B. Levofloxacin
    C. Trimethoprim-sulfamethoxazole
    D. Ceftriaxone plus doxycycline

19. Which of the following anatomical structures provides a space for the storage and maturation of sperm?
    A. Epididymis
    B. Vas deferens
    C. Testis
    D. Prostate gland

20. A male patient with a past medical history of diabetes mellitus presents with severe pain that started on the anterior abdominal wall and migrated to the scrotum and penis. Physical examination reveals tense edema, blisters, and crepitus. The patient has a fever and is tachycardic and hypotensive. This presentation raises concern for which surgical emergency?
    A. Testicular torsion
    B. Torsion of the appendix testes
    C. Fournier's gangrene
    D. Paraphimosis

21. Which of the following is a common complication of sickle cell disease?
    A. Priapism
    B. Testicular cancer
    C. Benign prostatic hyperplasia
    D. Prostate cancer

(See answers next page.)

15. A) Tadalafil

Phosphodiesterase type 5 (PDE5) inhibitors are recommended for initial therapy for men with erectile dysfunction. Sildenafil, vardenafil, tadalafil, and avanafil have similar efficacy; the choice of drug depends on patient's preferences, cost, and adverse effects. However, only tadalafil has been approved for the treatment of lower urinary tract symptoms secondary to benign prostatic hyperplasia.

16. C) Nitrates

PDE5 inhibitors are contraindicated in patients prescribed any form of nitrate therapy due to risk of severe hypotension. Caution should be used when combining alpha-blockers with PDE5 inhibitors. Patients on an alpha-blocker for benign prostatic hyperplasia should be on a stable dose prior to initiating the PDE5 inhibitor, which should be started at the lowest dose due to the risk of hypotension. Beta-blockers and angiotensin II receptor blockers should also be used with caution but are not contraindicated with the use of PDE5 inhibitors. PDE5 inhibitors should be avoided with drugs that are cytochrome P450 3A inhibitors and inducers (e.g., certain antivirals, antifungals, calcium channel blockers, anti-epileptic drugs).

17. B) Torsion of the appendix testis

The patient is presenting with concern for torsion of the appendix testis or appendix epididymis. The pain is of sudden onset, like the pain of testicular torsion, but it is often less severe. The localized pain remains in the area of the appendix testis, and a "blue dot" sign may be apparent due to infarction and necrosis of the appendix testis. A normal cremasteric reflex may be present, whereas the reflex is absent with testicular torsion. Epididymitis presents with an acute onset of pain and swelling localized to the epididymis. Frequency, dysuria, urethral discharge, or fever may be present. Patients with acute bacterial prostatitis are often acutely ill with fever, chills, malaise, irritative urinary symptoms, and pelvic or perineal pain.

18. D) Ceftriaxone plus doxycycline

This patient is presenting with clinical features concerning for acute epididymitis: Localized testicular pain with tenderness and swelling on palpation of the affected epididymis. A positive Prehn sign may be seen (relief of pain with scrotal elevation). For patients at risk for sexually transmitted infections (STIs) who do not practice anal intercourse, treatment should include coverage for *Neisseria gonorrhoeae* and *Chlamydia trachomatis* with ceftriaxone plus doxycycline. For patients at risk of STIs who practice anal intercourse, therapy should include coverage for *N. gonorrhoeae*, *C. trachomatis*, and enteric pathogen infections with ceftriaxone plus a fluroquinolone (e.g., levofloxacin). For patients at low risk of STIs, treatment includes coverage for enteric pathogens with a fluoroquinolone (e.g., levofloxacin) or trimethoprim-sulfamethoxazole.

19. A) Epididymis

The epididymis is a highly convoluted duct formed from a singular tubular structure that is estimated to be up to 20 feet in length, which allows space for storage and maturation of sperm. The testes are primarily responsible for testosterone and sperm production. The prostate is a male exocrine accessory gland that consists of exocrine glandular tissue and fibromuscular tissue, with the primary function of secretion of fluid that facilitates sperm motility and survival. The vas deferens is associated with the arteries, veins, lymphatics, muscle fibers, and nerves to form the spermatic cord; it merges with seminal vesicles to form the ejaculatory duct, which empties into the urethra.

20. C) Fournier's gangrene

Fournier's gangrene is a rare, rapidly progressing polymicrobial necrotizing fasciitis of the external genitalia and the perineum. It is common in patients who are immunocompromised or who have diabetes mellitus, long-standing indwelling catheters, or urethral trauma with associated urinary infection. Clinical features include severe pain that starts on the anterior abdominal wall and migrates to the gluteal muscles, scrotum, and penis. The outside of the involved area may present as tense edema, blisters, crepitus, and subcutaneous gas. Systemic findings such as fever, tachycardia, and hypotension are often present. Testicular torsion, torsion of the appendix testes, and paraphimosis are all concerning for danger signals but do not have this clinical presentation. Torsion of the appendix testes has a sudden onset of pain, like the pain of testicular torsion, but it is often less severe. A "blue dot" sign may be apparent due to infarction and necrosis of the appendix testis. Testicular torsion usually presents with a swollen red scrotum with associated nausea and vomiting. Paraphimosis is when the foreskin cannot be returned to the original position; untreated, it can lead to ischemia.

21. A) Priapism

Priapism (penile erection in the absence of sexual activity or desire) is a common complication in males with sickle cell disease. Most cases are ischemic; over time, recurrent episodes can lead to permanent damage and erectile dysfunction. While there are many complications associated with sickle cell disease, it is not associated with an increased risk for testicular or prostate cancer or benign prostatic hyperplasia.

22. A patient with benign prostatic hyperplasia presents with overactive bladder symptoms such as frequency, urgency, and incontinence. The patient's post-void residual averages more than 300 mL. Which of the following medical therapies would be indicated for symptom relief in this patient?
    A. Phosphodiesterase type 5 (PDE5) inhibitors
    B. Anticholinergics
    C. Beta-3 adrenergic agonists
    D. 5-alpha reductase inhibitors

23. A patient presents with localized testicular pain with tenderness and swelling. Upon physical examination, the scrotum is swollen and erythematous with induration of the posterior epididymis. The patient denies high-risk sexual behavior and reports a monogamous relationship. Which of the following treatment regimens is indicated based on this presentation?
    A. Ceftriaxone plus levofloxacin
    B. Levofloxacin
    C. Azithromycin
    D. Ceftriaxone plus doxycycline

24. Which of the following medications *increases* the risk of erectile dysfunction?
    A. Amoxicillin
    B. Paroxetine
    C. Levothyroxine
    D. Aspirin

25. The physical examination for the patient with benign prostatic hyperplasia (BPH) should include which of the following to estimate prostate size?
    A. Transrectal ultrasound
    B. Digital rectal exam (DRE)
    C. Transillumination
    D. Assessment of cremasteric reflex

(See answers next page.)

22. C) Beta-3 adrenergic agonists

Patients with overactive bladder symptoms (e.g., frequency, urgency, incontinence) may benefit from the use of beta-3 adrenergic agonists or anticholinergics. In particular, beta-3 adrenergic agonists are effective in those with concurrent overactive bladder symptoms secondary to detrusor overactivity to promote relaxation. Anticholinergic agents can be used to treat irritative symptoms due to overactive bladder in patients with benign prostatic hyperplasia who do not have increased post-void residual. Due to the concern for urinary retention, anticholinergics should be avoided when post-void residuals are greater than 300 mL. PDE5 inhibitors can be used as initial therapy in men with BPH and erectile dysfunction. The class, 5-alpha reductase inhibitors, is used to prevent benign prostatic hyperplasia progression rather than treat acute symptoms.

23. B) Levofloxacin

The patient is presenting with clinical features concerning for acute epididymitis: Localized testicular pain with tenderness and swelling on palpation of the affected epididymis. For patients at low risk of sexually transmitted infections (STIs), treatment includes coverage for enteric pathogens with a fluoroquinolone (e.g., levofloxacin) or trimethoprim-sulfamethoxazole. For patients at risk of STIs who do not practice anal intercourse, treatment should include coverage for *Neisseria gonorrhoeae* and *Chlamydia trachomatis* with ceftriaxone plus doxycycline. Alternatively, if the patient is unable to tolerate doxycycline, a single dose of azithromycin can be used. For patients at risk of STIs who practice anal intercourse, therapy should include coverage for *N. gonorrhoeae*, *C. trachomatis*, and enteric pathogen infections with ceftriaxone plus a fluroquinolone (e.g., levofloxacin).

24. B) Paroxetine

Paroxetine (Paxil) is a selective serotonin reuptake inhibitor (SSRI) that can cause erectile dysfunction. Numerous drugs cause erectile dysfunction, including diuretics, angiotensin-converting enzyme inhibitors (ACEIs), calcium channel blockers (CCBs), beta-blockers, SSRIs, benzodiazepines, and antihistamines. Amoxicillin is an antibiotic, levothyroxine is used in the treatment of hypothyroidism, and aspirin is a nonsteroidal anti-inflammatory drug; none of these causes erectile dysfunction.

25. B) Digital rectal exam (DRE)

When evaluating a patient with BPH, the physical examination should include a DRE to estimate prostate size. A normal prostate is about the size of a walnut, firm, and nontender. While not a precise tool, serial DREs are helpful to keep track of prostate size and identify any abnormalities. Transrectal ultrasound is not needed during the physical examination nor for diagnosis; it is only indicated when the treatment option is dependent on total prostate volume or for certain surgical interventions (e.g., prostate biopsy). Transillumination is helpful to differentiate fluid-filled masses (e.g., hydrocele, spermatocel) from solid masses (e.g., torsed testicle). The cremasteric reflex is evaluated by stroking the upper thigh while observing the ipsilateral testis. A normal response is elevation of the testis. The reflex is almost always absent with testicular torsion, which helps to differentiate the diagnosis when evaluating a patient with scrotal pain; however, it is not necessary to assess in patients with BPH, nor can it estimate prostate size.

DANGER SIGNALS

BRCA1- AND *BRCA2*-ASSOCIATED HEREDITARY BREAST AND OVARIAN CANCER

Patients with a personal (or family) history of breast, ovarian, prostate, or pancreatic cancer may benefit from a hereditary cancer risk evaluation (genetic counseling) so that they can find out their risk for these cancers. Breast cancer susceptibility genes (*BRCA1* and *BRCA2*) are inherited in an autosomal dominant pattern. Up to 6% of breast cancer and 20% of ovarian cancer cases are caused by mutations in these genes. Some ethnic groups are at higher risk for *BRCA1* and *BRCA2* mutations. Men with *BRCA* mutations are at higher risk of breast cancer and prostate cancer.

Women who have a high lifetime risk (risk of at least 20%) should undergo annual screening mammogram, annual breast MRI, and clinical breast exam every 6 to 12 months beginning 10 years prior to the age at diagnosis of the youngest affected family member. Ask at what age the family member(s) with breast cancer were diagnosed and screen 10 years earlier. For example, if a sister was age 35 when diagnosed with breast cancer, then screening for breast cancer by MRI can start at the age of 25 years.

DOMINANT BREAST MASS/BREAST CANCER

Adult to older female patient with a dominant mass on one breast that feels hard and is irregular in shape. The mass may be attached to the skin/surrounding breast tissue (or is immobile). Among the most common locations are the upper outer quadrants of the breast (the tail of Spence). Skin changes may be seen, such as the "peau d'orange" (localized area of skin that resembles an orange peel), dimpling, and retraction. Mass is painless or may be accompanied by serous or bloody nipple discharge. The nipple may be displaced or become fixed. Order a diagnostic mammogram with ultrasound and refer the patient to breast surgeon if needed. Be aware that up to 15% of women with breast cancer will have a negative mammogram. An ultrasound can detect the mass. Refer to breast specialist for a diagnostic biopsy. The most common sites for metastatic disease are the bone (e.g., back pain), liver (e.g., jaundice, abdominal pain, anorexia, nausea), lungs (e.g., dyspnea, cough), and brain (e.g., headache).

ECTOPIC PREGNANCY

Reproductive-age sexually active female with pelvic pain that may be diffuse or localized to one side, sometimes accompanied by vaginal bleeding. Pain onset occurs early in the first trimester and may be abrupt or more gradual. Pain can be dull or sharp (but usually not crampy). If intraperitoneal bleeding, the pain may radiate from the middle to the upper abdomen, and/or it may be referred to the shoulder. May shuffle instead of walking normally to decrease jarring of pelvis. Reports amenorrhea to light menses in the previous 6 to 7 weeks. Risk factors include prior ectopic pregnancy, current use of an intrauterine device (IUD), tubal ligation, and in vitro fertilization (IVF). Majority of ectopic pregnancies occur in the fallopian tube. Definite diagnosis is by serum quantitative chorionic gonadotropin level and transvaginal ultrasonography. Leading cause of death for women in the first trimester of pregnancy in the United States. Refer to ED.

INFLAMMATORY BREAST CANCER

Recent or acute onset of a red, swollen, and warm area in the breast of a middle-aged woman (median age 59 years) that is rapidly growing. Symptoms develop quickly. May have breast tenderness or itching. Can mimic mastitis. Often, there is no distinct lump on the affected breast. The skin may be pitted (peau d'orange) or appear bruised. Suspect in women with progressive breast inflammation that does not respond to antibiotics. Most women with inflammatory breast cancer (IBC) have lymph node metastases, and one third have distant metastases when diagnosed. More common in African Americans, who are usually diagnosed at a younger age. A rare but very aggressive form of breast cancer (1%–5%).

OVARIAN CANCER

The typical patient is a middle-aged or older woman with vague symptoms of abdominal bloating or abdominal discomfort, early satiety, gastrointestinal reflux disease-type symptoms, low-back pain, pelvic pain, dyspareunia, and changes in bowel habits. Other symptoms are unusual lower abdominal or lower back pain and/or unusual tiredness or fatigue. Most patients (75%) are diagnosed when it has already spread beyond the ovary, which accounts for the poor overall survival rate. Five-year survival with distant metastases is 25%, but if caught at stage 1 disease, it is >90%. There are currently no laboratory or imaging tests that can detect it at early stages. Annual "CA 125" testing alone lacks sufficient specificity for screening average-risk patients. For women who are at higher risk of ovarian cancer, transvaginal ultrasound was found to perform poorly in detecting early-stage epithelial ovarian cancer.

Look for family history of two or more first- or second-degree (cousins, aunts, uncles) relatives with a history of ovarian, endometrial, or colon cancer or a combination of ovarian and breast cancer. Women with high-risk family history should be referred for genetic counseling and testing (e.g., *BRCA1* and *BRCA2*, Lynch syndrome). Screening can start 10 years before the earliest age of first diagnosis of ovarian cancer in a family member.

PAGET'S DISEASE OF THE BREAST

Older female reports a history of a red-colored rash that is scaly (resembling eczema) and starts on the nipple and spreads to the arcola of one breast. Some women complain of itching, pain, or burning sensation. The skin lesion slowly enlarges and evolves to include crusting, ulceration, and/or bleeding on the nipple. Up to half of women will have a breast mass. Rarely, Paget's disease of the breast (PDB) is found in men.

NORMAL FINDINGS

ANATOMY

Breasts

- Puberty in girls starts with breast buds (Tanner stage II) and ends at stage V.
- During puberty, it is common for both girls and some boys to have tender and asymmetrical breast buds and breasts (gynecomastia). One breast may be larger than the other breast.
- The upper outer quadrant of the breasts (called the "tail of Spence") is where the majority of breast cancer is located.
- Simple breast cysts are benign fluid-filled cysts that are round to oval in shape. The highest prevalence is in women aged 35 to 50 years.
- Fibroadenomas are the most common type of solid breast tumor. They consist of fibrous tissue that can range from a few millimeters to 2.5 centimeters in size. An ultrasound is the imaging test of choice. For some patients, a needle biopsy is needed to confirm the diagnosis. High estrogen levels can make them grow, while low levels (e.g., menopause) can make them shrink. Most fibroadenomas are not associated with an increase in breast cancer, except for complex fibroadenomas.
- Women with *BRCA1* or *BRCA2* gene mutation (or both) have up to a 72% risk of being diagnosed with breast cancer in their lifetime.
- Risk factors for breast cancer in men are cryptorchidism, positive family history, and *BRCA1* and *BRCA2* mutation.
- The diagnostic test for breast cancer (or any type of solid tumor) is the tissue biopsy.

EXAM TIPS

- Palpation of postmenopausal women's breasts will feel softer with less volume and may be pendulous.
- Be familiar with physical breast exam findings (hard irregular mass that is not mobile) and follow-up of breast cancer.

Cervix

- A cervical ectropion looks like bright-red bumpy tissue with an irregular surface on the cervical surface around the os (Figure 17.1). It is a benign finding. It is made up of glandular cells (same cells that are inside the cervical os). It is more friable (bleeds easily) compared with the squamous epithelial cells on the surface of the cervix.
- Some adolescents and adults taking combined hormonal contraceptives and pregnant patients may have large ectropions, and this is considered a normal finding (due to high estrogen). It can change in size (or shape) and will disappear or regress over time.
- If an ectropion is present, it is important to sample the surface of the transformation zone (TZ) area when performing a Pap test. The TZ is the area where the ectropion transitions to the smooth cervical surface of squamous epithelial cells. Abnormal cells are more likely to develop (due to metaplasia) in the TZ.

Cervical and Vaginal Mucus

- Varies from scant ("dry"), thick white, runny white (white and clear mucus), to clear stringy mucus.
- After menses, vaginal discharge is scant. During mid-cycle, a large amount of runny, clear mucus (the mucus plug) is normal, except if the patient is on hormonal contraceptives (which thicken the mucus plug).
- Can be mixed with blood and appear as a red to dark-brownish color during the menstrual cycle.

Uterus

- The uterus includes the uterine corpus and the uterine cervix. The endometrium consists of the glandular epithelium and stroma.
- Fibroids (uterine leiomyoma or myoma) can enlarge the uterus. They can be asymptomatic or may cause heavy menstrual bleeding (menorrhagia), pelvic pain or cramping, and bleeding between periods.

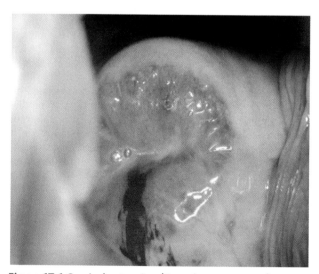

Figure 17.1 Cervical ectropion (6 weeks postpartum).
Source: O'Nell Starkey. Beautiful Cervix Project. (See Resources section for complete source information.)

- Fibroids (uterine leiomyoma or myoma) are usually benign. Can cause urgency if the fibroid is pressing on the bladder.
- On rare occasions, fibroids can be malignant and cause uterine cancer (leiomyosarcoma).

Ovaries
- The ovaries produce estrogen, progesterone, and a small amount of testosterone (androgens).
- Women with polycystic ovary syndrome (PCOS) have multiple cysts on their ovaries, which result in higher estrogen levels and high androgen levels (causes acne, hirsutism, oligomenorrhea, insulin resistance).
- During menopause, the ovaries become atrophied. A palpable ovary in a postmenopausal woman is always abnormal. Rule out ovarian cancer. Order a pelvic/intravaginal ultrasound and refer to a gynecologist.

EXAM TIP

Recognize menopausal female body changes. If palpable ovary (abnormal), rule out ovarian cancer and order an intravaginal ultrasound.

Benign Variants
Supernumerary nipples form a V-shaped line on both sides of the chest down the abdomen and are symmetrically distributed.

MENSTRUAL CYCLE
The following discussion is based on a perfect 28-day menstrual cycle.

Follicular Phase (Days 1–14)
Each month, follicle-stimulating hormone (FSH) is produced by the anterior pituitary. FSH stimulates the maturation of the follicles in a woman's ovary. Estrogen is produced by the developing follicles (or the "eggs"). Estrogen is the predominant hormone during the first 2 weeks of the menstrual cycle. It stimulates the development and growth of the endometrial lining. Also known as the *proliferative phase*.

Ovulatory Phase (Day 14): Midcycle
Luteinizing hormone (LH) is secreted by the anterior pituitary gland, which induces ovulation and the maturation of the dominant follicle on day 14 (of a 28-day cycle). The follicle migrates to the fimbriae of the fallopian tube. It takes about 5 days for the egg to move through the fallopian tube, where conception can take place.

Luteal Phase (Days 14–28)
Progesterone is the predominant hormone during the last 2 weeks of the cycle. It is produced by the corpus luteum and helps to stabilize the endometrial lining.

Menstruation
If not pregnant, both estrogen and progesterone fall drastically, inducing menses. Low hormone levels stimulate the hypothalamus and then the anterior pituitary (FSH), and the cycle starts again.

Menopause
Menopause is defined as the unintentional cessation of menses for 12 consecutive months. The average age of menopause is 51 years. Perimenopause is the time before and immediately after the final menstrual period and can last 10 years. Hormonal fluctuations are common. Premature menopause, or primary ovarian insufficiency, is the unintentional cessation of menses in a patient younger than 40 years.

Patients will often experience significant vasomotor symptoms, and once post menopause, vaginal dryness, decreased lubrication, and changes in libido often occur. If estrogen is not used, patients can experience urinary symptoms as well, such as incontinence.

Women's Health Initiative
- Average age of menopause for women in the United States is 51 years.
- The Women's Health Initiative (WHI) showed that combined estrogen–progestin replacement therapy (ERT) increased the risk of stroke, heart disease, venous thromboembolism (VTE), breast cancer, and pulmonary embolism.
- The U.S. Preventive Services Task Force (USPSTF) does not recommend combined estrogen–progestin or unopposed estrogen for prevention of chronic conditions (heart disease, osteoporosis). But the advice does not apply to women who want hormone therapy for relief of menopausal symptoms. Experts recommend duration of therapy of <5 years because of increased risk of breast cancer. Many experts consider it safe for healthy women within 10 years of menopause (younger than 60 years) with no contraindications for estrogen. Women who have a uterus need both estrogen and progesterone or progestin (decreases risk of endometrial cancer); use unopposed estrogen for women with hysterectomy.
- Estrogen can alleviate dyspareunia and vaginal/urethral atrophy. Estrogen increases the risk of developing or exacerbating systemic lupus erythematosus.

Fertile Time Period
Sexual intercourse 1 to 2 days before ovulation offers the highest chance of pregnancy. This time period is characterized by copious amounts of clear mucus that feels thin and elastic in the vagina. This sign is used in the cervical-mucus method of birth control to indicate the fertile period of the cycle. There are now over-the-counter ovulation kits that can detect urinary LH, which appears within 12 hours after it is in the serum (released by the anterior pituitary). False-positive results are possible with women with PCOS, ovarian insufficiency, and menopause.

Conception
Conception occurs when the sperm fertilizes the egg. As it travels down the fallopian tube into the uterus, the fertilized egg continues to divide until it becomes a blastocyst. The blastocyst implants into the endometrium, where it will become an embryo. It can take 3 to 4 days for the fertilized egg to fully implant in the uterus. The placenta is fully formed by 18 to 20 weeks. Estrogen and progesterone levels increase, along with human chorionic gonadotropin, which is produced by the placenta. Pregnancy lasts 280 days, or 40 weeks.

LABORATORY PROCEDURES

CERVICAL CYTOLOGY

Liquid-based cervical cytology (Pap test) is used to screen for cervical cancer. These tests have a high false-negative rate of 20% to 45%. The liquid-based cervical cytology test ThinPrep, which is read by a computer, is now more popular in the United States than the conventional Pap smear kit. If the cervix bleeds easily when the brush is inserted to obtain the sample, it may be a sign of inflammation. Rule out cervicitis. Some females may have slight spotting after a Pap test.

- Do not perform a Pap test or liquid-based cytology during heavy menstrual bleeding.
- The best time to perform a Pap test is at least 5 days after the period stops.
- Approximately 2 to 3 days before the Pap test, the patient should avoid douching, vaginal foams/medicines, tampon use, and vaginal intercourse.

NOTES

In 2018, both the USPSTF (2018) and the American College of Obstetricians and Gynecologists (ACOG, 2018) provided the following guidelines for cervical cancer screening for average-risk women:

- USPSTF: Does not recommend cervical cytology/Pap tests before age 21 years. Aged 21 to 29 years, screen with cervical cytology alone. Aged 30 to 65 years, can perform Pap test with co-testing (human papillomavirus [HPV] testing). Can space routine Pap tests to every 5 years if co-testing (except if abnormal Pap). See Table 17.1.
- ACOG: HIV-positive women, history of cervical cancer, or diethylstilbestrol (DES) exposure may require more frequent screening and should not follow the routine guidelines.

Liquid-Based Cervical Cytology Test (ThinPrep)

Insert the broom-shaped plastic brush into the cervical os and rotate in the same direction for five turns. If a transformative zone is present, make sure that it is included. Place the brush in the liquid medium and swish gently. Remove brush and cover with the plastic cap. The cervical cytology test is read by a computer, and abnormal results are reviewed by a cytologist and/or pathologist.

Conventional Pap Test

Use wooden spatula to scrape cervical surface (ectocervix). Then insert the brush into the cervical os (endocervix) and twist gently in a circle. Smear the glass slide with both samples. Spray the liquid fixative on the glass slide and label. By sampling the ectocervix first, the chances of bleeding are minimized.

Screening Women Without a Cervix

Stop screening if patient does not have a cervix as a result of a hysterectomy for a benign condition.

THE BETHESDA SYSTEM

The Bethesda System is a standardized system that is used for reporting cervical cytology results. A specimen is satisfactory if both squamous epithelial cells and endocervical cells are present, but the absence of endocervical cells is not unusual. It occurs in approximately 10% to 20% of specimens and is most common in adolescents and postmenopausal women. If a woman is being treated by pelvic radiation or is pregnant, the information should be included in the cytology requisition. Lubricants or excessive blood can interfere with results.

Atypical Squamous Cells of Undetermined Significance

Atypical squamous cells of undetermined significance (ASC-US) is a term used to describe cells that look mildly abnormal but the cause cannot be identified (infection, irritation, or a precancer).

- Age 20 years or younger: Do not perform Pap if younger than 21 years.

Table 17.1 U.S. Preventive Services Task Force Cervical Cancer Screening Guidelines

Age	Screening Exam	Screening Interval
20 years (or younger)	Do not screen (regardless of age of onset of sexual activity)	Do not screen
21–29 years	Liquid-based cytology or conventional Pap test Against routine HPV co-testing if <30 years	Every 3 years
30–65 years	Liquid-based cytology or Conventional Pap smear or Liquid-based cytology plus co-testing (for high-risk HPV)	Every 3 years or Every 5 years (if co-testing) If not co-testing, needs Pap test every 3 years
Older than 65 years	Can stop screening	If not otherwise at high risk for cervical cancer*
Hysterectomy (with cervical removal) not due to cancer	Can stop screening*	If not otherwise at high risk for cervical cancer*

*If no history of CIN stage 2 or 3, AIS, or cervical cancer within previous 20 years.
AIS, adenocarcinoma in situ; CIN, cervical intraepithelial neoplasia; HPV, human papillomavirus.
Source: Data from U.S. Preventive Services Task Force. (2018, August 21). (See Resources section for complete source information.)

- Age 21 to 24 years: Preferred is repeat Pap test in 12 months (acceptable is reflex HPV test).
- Age 25 to 29 years: Preferred is reflex HPV test. Acceptable is repeat Pap test in 12 months.
- Age 30 years or older: Cotesting for high-risk HPV. If HPV positive, refer for colposcopy.

Atypical Squamous Cells and Cannot Exclude a High-Grade Squamous Intraepithelial Lesion

ASC and cannot exclude a high-grade squamous intraepithelial lesion (ASC-H) is a term used to indicate presence of cells that definitely look abnormal. A possible precancer is present and requires more testing and possible treatment. Refer for colposcopy age 21 years or older.

Atypical Glandular Cells

More common in older women (ages 40–69 years). Associated with premalignancy or malignancy in 30% of cases. Risk of cancer goes up with age. There are several subcategories. Follow-up test depends on atypical glandular cell (AGC) subcategory. Follow-up tests include colposcopy, endocervical sampling, and endometrial sampling.

Low-Grade Squamous Intraepithelial Lesions

Cervical cells show changes that are mildly abnormal; usually caused by an HPV infection.

- Age 21 to 24 years: Repeat Pap test in 12 months.
- Age 25 to 29 years: Refer for colposcopy.
- Age 30 years or older: Preferred is repeat Pap test in 12 months; acceptable to refer for colposcopy.

High-Grade Squamous Intraepithelial Lesions

High-grade squamous intraepithelial lesions (HSILs) suggest more serious changes in the cervix than low-grade squamous intraepithelial lesions (LSILs). They are more likely than LSILs to be associated with precancer and cancer.

- Age 21 to 24 years: Refer for colposcopy.
- Age 25 years or older: Refer for immediate excisional treatment or colposcopy. It can be done by LEEP (loop electrosurgical excision procedure) with cervical conization or surgery of the cervix.

Human Papillomavirus DNA Test (Reflex HPV Testing)

- HPV types 16 and 18 cause nearly all cases of cervical cancer. Women are exposed to high-risk HPV through sexual intercourse.
- Gardasil (males or females) is typically given at age 11 or 12 years (but can be given between ages 9 through 26 years). If given before age 15 years, a two-dose series is required. The second dose should be given 6 to 12 months after the first dose (0, 6–12).
- If first dose of Gardasil given at age 15 years or older, a three-dose schedule is recommended (0, 1–2, 6).
- If the vaccine schedule is interrupted, vaccine doses do not have to be repeated (no maximum interval).
- Gardasil is now recommended for those between ages 9 and 45 years.

COLPOSCOPY

A colposcope is a specialized "microscope" used to visualize the cervix, obtain cervical biopsies, and gain access to the cervix during cryotherapy or laser ablative therapy. The diagnostic test for cervical cancer is a biopsy of the cervix, which is obtained during a colposcopy.

- A vaginal speculum is used to expose the cervix.
- After the cervix is visualized, it is washed with acetic acid 3% to 5% (distilled white vinegar), which helps remove mucus and causes the abnormal areas of the cervix to turn a bright-white color that resembles leukoplakia (acetowhitening).
- Biopsy samples are obtained from the acetowhitened areas on the cervix, cervical os (glandular cells), and squamocolumnar junction.
- After a colposcopy, a small amount of cramping and bloody spotting is normal (red, brown, black) in the next few days after the procedure. Nonsteroidal anti-inflammatory drugs (NSAIDs) or analgesics can be used for the pain as needed.

ABLATIVE TREATMENT

Cryotherapy or laser therapy is used to treat abnormal superficial cervical cells.

LOOP ELECTROSURGICAL EXCISION PROCEDURE

The loop electrosurgical instrument is a device that is used like a scalpel to cut through the cervix (conization) to treat cervical cancer and obtain cervical biopsy specimens. Depending on the result of the biopsy (size, depth, and severity), the cancerous cells can be removed by cryotherapy for mild lesions, laser ablation, or surgical conization of the cervix.

POTASSIUM HYDROXIDE SLIDE

Useful for helping with the diagnosis of fungal infections (hair, nails, skin). Potassium hydroxide (KOH) works by causing lysis of the squamous cells, which makes it easier to see hyphae and spores. Vaginal specimens do not require KOH to visualize *Candida*.

WHIFF TEST

A test for bacterial vaginosis (BV). A positive result occurs when a strong, fish-like odor is released after one or two drops of KOH are added to the slide (or a cotton swab soaked with discharge).

TZANCK SMEAR

Used as an adjunct for evaluating herpetic infection (oral, genital, skin). A positive smear will show large abnormal nuclei in squamous epithelial cells. Not commonly used.

EXAM TIPS

- Pap/cytology and HPV testing are not recommended before age 21 years, even if sexually active, or if the person has a sexually transmitted infection (STI), or has multiple sex partners. Can perform bimanual gynecologic exam to check for pelvic inflammatory disease (PID) and test for chlamydia/gonorrhea.
- Do not confuse endometrial biopsy with colposcopy, a test used to visualize the cervix and obtain cervical biopsy.

CLINICAL PEARLS

- Small amount of K-Y Jelly to lubricate tips of the speculum (in patients with atrophic vaginitis to reduce pain and vaginal bleeding) will not affect Pap test results.
- In reproductive-aged females who present with acute abdominal or pelvic pain, always perform a pregnancy test (use good-quality human chorionic gonadotropin [hCG] urine strips).
- Girls and teenagers have larger ectropions. Some adult women on combined hormonal contraceptives may develop ectropion.
- Cervical cancer 5-year survival rates: Localized, 92%; regional spread, 56%; distant metastasis, 17%.

CONTRACEPTION

Infertility is defined as having unprotected sex for 1 year with failure to achieve pregnancy. There is up to an 85% chance of becoming pregnant within 1 year of unprotected sexual intercourse. In the United States, approximately 50% of pregnancies are unplanned. Women seeking to prevent pregnancy can choose from several options with varying degrees of reported effectiveness (Figure 17.2).

MINORS AND CONTRACEPTION

According to the Guttmacher Institute (2023), there are 23 states and the District of Columbia that explicitly allow all individuals to consent to contraceptive services. Some states require a specified age (e.g., age 14 or older) to consent to such care. Married minors or emancipated minors do not need parental consent. A list of state requirements in regard to minors obtaining contraceptive services with/without parental consent is available at https://www.guttmacher.org/state-policy/explore/minors-access-contraceptive-services.

RULE OUT PREGNANCY

According to the Centers for Disease Control and Prevention (CDC) in 2016, a healthcare provider can be reasonably certain that a woman is not pregnant if she has no symptoms or signs of pregnancy and meets the following criteria:

- At least 7 days or less after start of normal menses (or after an induced or spontaneous abortion)
- Has had no sexual intercourse since the start of last normal menses
- Has been correctly and consistently using a reliable method of contraception
- Is within 4 weeks postpartum
- Exclusively breastfeeding or for the vast majority of the time breastfeeds (>85%) and is amenorrhoeic and <6 months postpartum

Check if pregnant with urine pregnancy test before starting hormonal and IUD contraception

COMBINED HORMONAL CONTRACEPTION

Combined hormonal contraception (estrogen and progestin) works in a synergistic manner by stopping ovulation

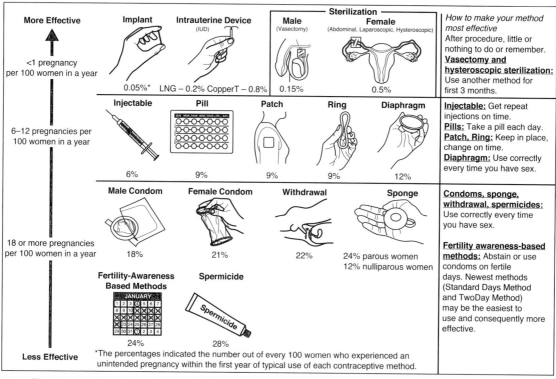

Figure 17.2 Effectiveness of contraceptive methods.

LNG, Levonorgestrel.

Source: Centers for Disease Control and Prevention. (2016). (See Resources section for complete source information.)

(inhibits LH surge) and thickening the cervical mucus plug. There are several types such as oral contraceptives (OCs), transdermal patch, and the vaginal ring.

Combined Oral Contraceptives (9% Typical Use Failure Rate)

Dosed Monophasic Pills

Loestrin FE 1/20: 21 consecutive days of estrogen/progestin (same dose daily). For the last 7 days of the cycle, the placebo pills may contain iron supplementation.

Biphasic Pills

Ortho-Novum 10/11: Contains two different progesterone doses (two phases). The progestin dose increases about halfway through the cycle. Other brands include Mircette and Jenest.

Triphasic Pills

Ortho Tri-Cyclen: Contains 21 days of active pills and 7 days of placebo pills. The dose of hormones varies weekly for 3 weeks ("triphasic"). Progestin used is norgestimate. Indicated for acne. Other brands include Cyclessa, Tri-Norinyl, Tri-Levlen, and Triphasil.

Ethinyl Estradiol and Drospirenone

- 24/4 formulation (24 days hormones/4 days placebo pills)
- Yaz 28 (24 active pills and 4 placebo pills)/Yasmin: Uses drospirenone (a spironolactone analog) as the progestin component. Results in lighter menses and lower rates of unscheduled bleeding. Consider for women with acne, PCOS, hirsutism, or premenstrual dysphoric disorder (PMDD). Higher risk of deep vein thrombosis (DVT) and hyperkalemia.
- Labs: Check the potassium level if patient is on an angiotensin-converting enzyme inhibitor (ACEI), angiotensin receptor blocker (ARB), or potassium-sparing diuretic or has kidney disease.

Extended-Cycle Oral Contraceptive Pills

- 84/7 formulation (84 days hormones/7 days placebo pills)
- Seasonale contains 84 consecutive days (3 months) of estrogen/progesterone with a 7-day pill-free interval; this method typically results in four periods per year, although breakthrough bleeding is not uncommon during the first few months.

EXAM TIPS

- Desogen, Ortho-TriCyclen, and Yaz/Yasmin are all indicated for treatment of acne.
- Women taking Seasonale (84 days hormones/7 days placebo pill) will have only four periods per year.

Non-Oral Forms

Absolute and relative contraindications for non-oral forms of combined estrogen–progesterone method of contraception are the same as OCs.

Cervical Ring (7% Typical Use Failure Rate)

- NuvaRing is a plastic cervical ring that contains etonogestrel and ethinyl estradiol (EE). It is left inside the vagina for 3 weeks (21 days), then removed for 1 week (when woman has her period).
- Educate patient on how to apply (fold in half and insert into vagina). The ring should fit snugly around cervix. To use it continuously, insert a ring every 21 days with no ring-free week in between.
- Do not use NuvaRing if cigarette smoker aged 35 years or older.

Ortho Evra Transdermal Contraceptive Patch (0.7% Typical Use Failure Rate)

- Higher risk of VTE (releases higher levels of estrogen) compared with OC pills. Absolute and relative contraindications for combined estrogen–progesterone method of contraception are the same as OCs.
- Patch can be worn on buttocks, chest (except breast), upper back, arm, or abdomen.
- Wear a new patch 1 week at a time for 3 weeks in a row. During the fourth week, do not wear a patch.

Contraindications to Hormonal Contraceptive Use

Absolute Contraindications

Any condition (past or present) that increases the risk of blood clotting:

- History of thrombophlebitis or thromboembolic disorders (e.g., DVT)
- Genetic coagulation defects, such as factor V Leiden disease
- Major surgery with prolonged immobilization
  Being a smoker older than 35 years, >15 cigarettes per day is also considered a relative contraindication because women <35 years who smoke can take the pill (if no other contraindications exist).
  Any condition that increases the risk of strokes:
- Migraine with aura or focal neurologic symptoms or migraine without aura at age 35 years or older
- History of cerebrovascular accidents (CVAs) and transient ischemic attacks (TIAs)
- Hypertension (if systolic blood pressure [SBP] >160 mmHg or diastolic BP [DBP] >100 mmHg)
  Inflammation and/or acute infections of the liver with elevated liver function tests (LFTs):
- In acute infection or with active liver disease (e.g., mononucleosis) with elevated LFTs, estrogen is contraindicated
- When LFTs are back to normal, can go back on birth control pills
- Hepatocellular adenomas or malignant (hepatoma)
- Cholestatic jaundice of pregnancy
  Known or suspected cardiovascular disease:
- Moderately to severely impaired cardiac function
- Complicated valvular heart disease (risk atrial fibrillation, history of subacute bacterial endocarditis)
- Coronary artery disease (CAD)
- Diabetes with vascular component
- Systemic lupus erythematosus
- Hypertension if SBP is ≥160 or DBP 100 mmHg
- Two or more risk factors for arterial cardiovascular disease (such as older age, smoking, diabetes, hypertension)

Some reproductive system conditions or cancers:
- Known or suspected pregnancy
- Undiagnosed genital bleeding or breast mass
- Breast, endometrial, or ovarian cancer (or any estrogen-dependent cancer)
- <21 days postpartum

Contraindications for drospirenone (Yaz, Yasmin, Slynd) include hyperkalemia, kidney disease or kidney failure, adrenal insufficiency.

Absolute Contraindications Mnemonic: "My CUPLETS"

My Migraines with focal neurologic aura
C   CAD or CVA
U   Undiagnosed genital bleeding
P   Pregnant or suspect pregnancy
L   Liver tumor or active liver disease
E   Estrogen-dependent tumor
T   Thrombus or emboli
S   Smoker aged 35 or older

Relative Contraindications

- Migraine headaches (absolute contraindication in patients >35 years or with focal neurologic findings because of increased risk of stroke)
- Smoker <35 years
- Fracture or cast on lower extremities
- Adequately controlled hypertension

Advantages of the Pill (After 5 or More Years of Use)

Ovarian cancer and endometrial cancers decreased by 40% to 50%

Decreased incidence of:
- Dysmenorrhea and cramps (decrease in prostaglandins)
- Decreased pelvic pain for patients with endometriosis
- Acne and hirsutism (lower levels of androgenic hormones)
- Ovarian cysts (due to suppression of ovulation)
- Heavy and/or irregular periods (due to suppression of ovaries)

New Prescriptions

- Perform thorough health history to find out if patient has a contraindication. Rule out pregnancy.
- Check BP (rule out hypertension). According to the CDC in 2016, a physical examination, Pap test, gynecologic exam, STI testing, and/or laboratory blood testing is not required for initiating contraception in most healthy patients. Exception is pelvic exam before insertion of IUD (to rule out an abnormal uterus or cervicitis) and when fitting a patient for a diaphragm.
- OCs can be started anytime in the menstrual cycle (rule out pregnancy first).
- All patients should be instructed to use "backup" (condoms) in the first week (7 days) during the first pill pack.
  - Quick start: Start taking the pill on the day prescribed (give samples or prescription). Rule out pregnancy first.
  - Day one start: Take the first pill during the first day of the menstrual period. Provides the best protection.
  - Sunday start: Take first pill on the first Sunday after the menstrual period starts. Will avoid having a period on a weekend. Higher chance of ovulation happening.

- Follow-up visit needed within 2 to 3 months to check BP or any side effects and answer patient's questions. Can prescribe up to 12 to 13 months of refills for OCs.

Combined Hormonal Contraceptive Problems

Unscheduled Bleeding (Spotting)

Term used for menstrual bleeding that occurs outside of usual cycle.
- Educate patient that she may have spotting/light bleeding during the first few weeks after starting birth control pills, transdermal patch, or vaginal ring. For most, it will decrease to 10% or less by the third month.
- Discourage patient from switching to another pill brand during the first 3 months because of spotting. Advise patient that most cases resolve spontaneously within a few weeks.
- Patients on OCs with lower estrogen dose (20 mcg EE) have higher rates of unscheduled bleeding, compared with those on OCs with a higher dose of 30 to 35 mcg of EE. If patient still has bleeding after a few weeks, an option is to switch to an OC with 30 mcg of EE (Lo/Ovral, Desogen, Loestrin 2, Nordette). Check if patient is taking pills daily. It takes approximately 3 months for the body to adjust to hormones. Early symptoms can include nausea and breast tenderness a few days after starting hormones. Symptoms usually resolve in 1 month.

Missing Consecutive Days of Oral Contraceptive Pills

- Missed 1 day: Take two pills now and continue with same pill pack ("doubling up"). Continue taking remaining pills at the usual time.
- Missed 2 consecutive days (or >48 hours since last pill should have been taken): Take the most recent missed pill as soon as possible (even if it means taking two pills the same day). Discard any leftover missed pills. Continue taking remaining pills at the usual time.
- Use backup contraception (e.g., condoms) or avoid sex until hormonal pills have been taken for 7 consecutive days.

Pill missed on the last week of hormonal pills (days 15–21 on a 28-day pill pack):
- Omit hormone-free pills (or placebo pills) by finishing the hormonal pills in the current pack and starting a new pill pack the next day.
- Use backup contraception until hormonal pills have been taken for 7 consecutive days. Consider emergency contraception if unprotected sexual intercourse occurred in the previous 5 days.

EXAM TIPS

- Low-dose birth control pills contain 20 mcg to 35 mcg of EE.
- Know what to do if 2 consecutive days of the pill are missed.

Drug Interactions With Oral Contraceptives

These drugs can decrease the efficacy of OCs. Advise patients to use an alternative form of birth control

Table 17.2 Oral Contraceptive Danger Signs

Complaints	Possible Causes
Chest pain (an acute MI)	Blood clot in a coronary artery
Severe headache	Stroke, TIA
Weakness on one side of the body	Ischemic stroke caused by a blood clot in the brain
Visual changes in one eye	Blood clot in the retinal artery of the affected eye
Abdominal pain	Ischemic pain of the mesenteric area caused by a blood clot
Lower leg pain (DVT)	Blood clot on a deep vein of the leg

DVT, deep vein thrombosis; MI, myocardial infarction; TIA, transient ischemic attack.

(condoms) when taking these drugs and for one pill cycle afterward.

- Anticonvulsants: Phenobarbital, phenytoin
- Antifungals (strong CYP3A4 inhibitors): Griseofulvin (Fulvicin), itraconazole (Sporanox), ketoconazole (Nizoral)
- HIV/hepatitis C virus (HCV) protease inhibitors: Indinavir, boceprevir
- Certain antibiotics: Ampicillin, tetracyclines, rifampin, clarithromycin
- St. John's wort: May cause breakthrough bleeding

Pill Danger Signs

Thromboembolic events can happen in any organ of the body. These signs (Table 17.2) indicate a possible thromboembolic event. Advise patient to report these or call 911 if symptoms of ACHES:

   A Abdominal pain
   C Chest pain
   H Headaches
   E Eye problems; change in vision
   S Severe leg pain

Considerations When Choosing an Oral Contraceptive Pill

- Typical use failure rate is 9%.
- Traditional OC pills have 21 days of "active" pills and 7 days of placebo pills. The last 7 days are the "hormone-free" days. The menstrual period usually starts within 2 to 3 days after the last active pill was taken (from very low levels of estrogen/progesterone).
- Some brands of combined hormonal contraceptives (e.g., Loestrin FE) contain iron in the pills taken during the last 7 days of the pill cycle (instead of a placebo pill). The last 7 days (hormone-free) of the pill cycle are there to reinforce the habit of daily pill taking.
- For the *first* pill cycle, advise patient to use "backup" (an alternative form of birth control) for 7 consecutive days. The extended-cycle OCs are another option to consider.
- All the combined oral contraceptives (COCs), the patch, and the NuvaRing contain both estrogen (e.g., EE) and a progestin (e.g., levonorgestrel [LNG], norethindrone, desogestrel).

- The contraceptive patch (e.g., Ortho Evra) results in higher levels of estrogen exposure compared with COCs (higher risk of blood clots, DVT).
- The estrogen in COCs can elevate BP. Patients' BP should be checked within 4 to 8 weeks.
- Breastfeeding women can use the progestin-only pill (POP; "minipill"; e.g., Micronor, Nor-QD) or other progestin-only contraceptives. Barrier methods such as condoms can also be used.

PROGESTIN-ONLY CONTRACEPTION

Depo-Provera (4% Typical Use Failure Rate)

Each dose by injection lasts 3 months. Also known as *depot medroxyprogesterone acetate (DMPA)*. Highly effective. Check for pregnancy before starting dose. Start within first 5 days of cycle (days 1–5) because females are less likely to ovulate at these times. Women on Depo-Provera for at least 1 year (or longer) have amenorrhea because of severe uterine atrophy from lack of estrogen.

- Do not recommend to women who want to become pregnant in 12 months. Causes delayed return of fertility. It takes up to 1 year for most women to start ovulating.
- Boxed warning: Avoid long-term use (more than 2 years). Increases risk of osteopenia or osteoporosis that may not be fully reversible. Using Depo-Provera for more than 2 years is discouraged.

History of Anorexia Nervosa

Avoid using Depo-Provera in this population, because it will further increase their risk of osteopenia/osteoporosis. Consider testing for osteopenia/osteoporosis (dual-energy x-ray absorptiometry [DEXA] scan). Recommend calcium with vitamin D and weight-bearing exercises for patients who are on this medicine.

EXAM TIPS

- Avoid using Depo-Provera in anorexic and/or bulimic patients (very high risk of osteoporosis).
- Some questions will ask for the best birth control method for a case scenario. Remember the contraindications or adverse effects of each method (e.g., Depo-Provera).

Etonogestrel Contraceptive Implant (0.05% Typical Use Failure Rate)

The contraceptive implant contains a long-acting form of progestin (etonogestrel). Initially, unscheduled bleeding is common, but when the endometrial lining atrophies, amenorrhea results. Ovulation may not occur for a few weeks to 12 months after removal.

- Thin plastic rods are inserted on the inner aspect of the upper arm subdermally (nondominant arm). If keloid or heavy scarring occurs, may have problem with removal. Special procedures, including surgery in a hospital, may be needed to remove the implant.
- Norplant II (two rods) is effective up to 5 years. Nexplanon (one rod) is effective for up to 3 years.
- One out of 10 women stop using the implant because of unfavorable changes in menstrual bleeding.

Progestin-Only Pills (7% Typical Use Failure Rate)

- Safe for breastfeeding women, and most effective if woman is exclusively breastfeeding. Also known as the "minipill." Patients with obesity can take POPs.
- It is very important to take the pill at the same time each day. If dose is late (≥3 hours) or a day is missed, the woman should use condoms (backup contraception) or abstain from sexual intercourse for 2 days. There is no placebo week with POPs.
- If vomiting or severe diarrhea occurs within 3 hours after taking a dose, take another pill as soon as possible. Continue taking pills daily at the same time each day. Use backup contraception. Consider use of emergency contraception if unprotected sex.
- For norethindrone 0.35 mg (Micronor), take one pill daily at about the same time each day (each pack contains 28 pills). Start taking pill on day 1 of menstrual cycle or at 6-week postpartum visit when prescribed.
- POPs are slightly less effective than OC pills. An alternative for women who cannot take estrogen, such as breastfeeding mothers, older smokers, and diabetics with microvascular disease.

Emergency Contraception ("Morning-After Pill")

Works best if taken within 72 hours after unprotected sexual intercourse or if 2 consecutive days of birth control pills are skipped. Women and men of all ages can get emergency contraceptive pills (except ulipristal acetate) without a prescription in the United States.

- 89% effective
- For ulipristal acetate (ella), take one pill within 5 days (120 hours) of unprotected sex.
- LNG pills include Plan B One-Step My Way, After Pill, or Next Choice One Dose
- A few birth control pills that contain LNG (e.g., Triphasil) may be used as morning-after pills but are more likely to cause nausea (because of the estrogen).
- Take first dose as soon as possible (up to 72 hours after).
- Take second dose in 12 hours.
- If patient vomits tablet within 1 hour (or less), may need to repeat dose; OTC antiemetics (antihistamine drug class) are dimenhydrinate (Dramamine) and meclizine (Dramamine Less Drowsy).
- Advise patient that if she does not have a normal period in next 3 weeks, she should return for follow-up to rule out pregnancy.

EXAM TIP

Know how to use Plan B (emergency contraception).

OTHER CONTRACEPTIVE METHODS

Intrauterine Device (LNG 0.1%–0.4%/Copper 0.8% Typical Use Failure Rate)

The IUD is the second most commonly used method of contraception in the world (female sterilization is the first). Paragard is copper bearing (effective up to 10 years), and Mirena contains the hormone LNG, which decreases vaginal bleeding. Mirena IUD is effective for up to 5 years and is slightly more effective than copper-bearing IUDs (Cu-IUDs). Copper IUD can cause heavy menstrual bleeding and cramping the first few months of use. IUD can be removed if patient desires pregnancy. Not for women who plan on having a baby within 1 to 2 years. Must be inserted by trained health provider. Rule out pregnancy.

Contraindications

- Active PID or history of PID within the past year
- Suspected or confirmed pregnancy or has STI
- Uterine or cervical abnormality (e.g., bicornuate uterus)
- Undiagnosed vaginal bleeding or uterine/cervical cancer
- History of ectopic pregnancy
- Wilson's disease (for copper IUD)

Increased Risk

- Endometrial and pelvic infections (first few months after insertion only)
- Perforation of the uterus
- Heavy or prolonged menstrual periods (Cu-IUDs)

Education

- With Mirena IUD, approximately 20% of patients will have amenorrhea in 1 year. Some have lighter periods.
- Educate patients to periodically check for missing or shortened string, especially after each menstrual period. If the patient or clinician does not feel the string, order a pelvic ultrasound.

EXAM TIP

Cu-IUD lasts 10 to 12 years. Mirena (progesterone IUD) lasts 5 years.

Barrier Methods

Male Condoms (13% Typical Use Failure Rate)

More effective than the female condom.

Female Condoms (21% Typical Use Failure Rate)

Do not use with any oil-based or silicone oil-based lubricants, creams, and so forth.

Diaphragm With Contraceptive Gel and Cervical Cap (17% Typical Use Failure Rate)

- Not as effective as hormonal forms of contraception. The cervical cap is less effective than a diaphragm. After vaginal birth, the failure rate of the cervical cap increases to 29%.
- The diaphragm must be used with spermicidal gel. After intercourse, leave diaphragm inside vagina for at least 6 to 8 hours (can remain inside vagina up to 24 hours). The cervical cap can be left in the vagina up to 2 days.
- Need additional spermicide application before every act of intercourse. Apply the spermicidal foam/gel inside the vagina without removing the diaphragm.
- The cervical cap (Prentif cap) can be worn up to 48 hours. Compared with the diaphragm, the Prentif cap may cause abnormal cervical cellular change (abnormal Pap).

- Spermicidal gel (nonoxynol-9, or N-9) increases risk of infection with STI, including HIV. It is thought to cause irritation of the cervical surface (breakdown of the skin barrier) after multiple uses.
- Both diaphragm and cervical cap require a prescription and must be fitted.
- Avoid lubricants that contain silicone oil; they can cause deterioration of the silicone diaphragm or cap.
- After each pregnancy by vaginal birth or weight gain (or loss) of 20%, they need to be refitted. The cervical cap and diaphragm cannot be used during menstruation.

Increased Risk
Vaginal and cervical irritation (N-9) increases risk of HIV infection, urinary tract infections (UTIs), and toxic shock syndrome (TSS; rare).

Sponge (Nulliparous 12%/Multiparous 20% Typical Use Failure Rate)
- Available OTC. Made out of soft foam that contains spermicide. It is inserted inside the vagina so that it covers the cervix.
- Can be inserted up to 24 hours before sex, and it should be left in place at least 6 hours after sexual intercourse. The sponge should not be worn for more than 30 total hours.
- Spermicide use (nonoxynol-9) increases risk of HIV infection (see section on diaphragm for rationale).

Increased Risk
- Vaginal and cervical irritation (nonoxynol-9) increases risk of HIV infection.
- TSS is rare.

CLINICAL PEARLS

- Yaz or Yasmin contains estrogen and drospirenone. Has a higher risk of blood clots, stroke, heart attacks, and hyperkalemia.
- Do not recommend Depo-Provera or IUD for women who want **to** become pregnant in 12 to 18 months because it may cause delayed return of fertility. It can take up to 1 year for some women to start ovulating.
- Cu-IUD probably has the broadest indication for use as a contraceptive for women with medical conditions (e.g., diabetics, smoker for more than 35 years, on anticonvulsant or antiretroviral therapy, ovarian cancer, ischemic heart disease, liver tumors).

DISEASE REVIEW

AMENORRHEA
Absence of menses, which can be transient, intermittent, or permanent. Primary amenorrhea is the absence of menarche by age 15 years (or older). The most common cause is hypergonadic hypogonadism (Turner syndrome). Secondary amenorrhea is the absence of menses for more than 3 months in girls/women who previously had regular menstrual cycles, or, if irregular cycles, it is missing menses for 6 months. The most common cause of secondary amenorrhea is pregnancy.

ATROPHIC VAGINITIS (VULVOVAGINAL ATROPHY)
Chronic lack of estrogen in estrogen-dependent tissue of the urogenital tract; results in atrophic changes in the vulva and vagina of postmenopausal women. Estrogen is the most effective treatment for moderate-to-severe vaginal atrophy. Low-dosed topical estrogen therapy is preferred because of low systemic absorption.

Classic Case
Menopausal female complains of vaginal dryness, itching, and pain with sexual intercourse (dyspareunia). Some may have vulvar or vaginal bleeding (fissures) after intercourse. Complains of a great deal of discomfort with speculum examinations (e.g., Pap tests). Pap test result is "abnormal" secondary to atrophic changes. Worsens over time as she gets older. More than half of women do not report symptoms.

Objective Findings
- Atrophic labia with decreased rugae; vulva or vagina may have fissures.
- Dry, pale pink color to vagina

Treatment Plan
- Initial therapy: Nonhormonal vaginal moisturizers and lubricants. Vaginal moisturizers (e.g., Replens) are intended for use 2 to 3 days per week routinely. Lubricants can be water based (e.g., K-Y Jelly), silicone based, or oil based (can break down latex condoms).
- Moderate-to-severe symptoms: Topical conjugated estrogen preferred; it comes in several forms (cream, tablet, capsule, or vaginal ring). Progesterone or progestin supplementation is required (if intact uterus) if using long term to decrease risk of endometrial hyperplasia.
- Tablet or capsule vaginal estradiol inserts: 4 mcg (Imvexxy), 10 mcg (Vagifem, Yuvafem, Imvexxy). Insert into vagina daily for 2 weeks, then use weekly thereafter.
- Ring form of estradiol: Estring designed to release 7.5 mcg of estradiol in the vagina daily. Effective for 90 days only, then replace with new ring.
- If Pap shows atrophy: Needs to be repeated in 3 months because atrophic smears are difficult to analyze and can be misinterpreted. Estrogen can change vaginal cytology back to premenopausal state. Can be used for 2 to 3 months only, then repeat Pap, or it can be used for longer periods for consistent relief of moderate-to-severe vaginal symptoms.

BREAST CANCER
Breast cancer is the most common type of cancer in women, and it is also the second most common cause of death among women in the United States (leading cause of death is heart disease). Most cases of breast cancer in the United States are diagnosed by an abnormal mammogram, but up to 15% of women have a breast mass that is not detected on a mammogram (mammographically occult disease). The gold standard diagnostic is biopsy of the breast/axillary mass.

- Risk factors you cannot change: Older age (50 years or older), genetic mutations (*BRCA1* and *BRCA2*), early menarche (before age 12), late menopause (after age 55), dense breast, personal or family history of breast cancer, radiation therapy to the chest/breast before age 30 (treated for Hodgkin's lymphoma), mother took diethylstilbestrol (DES; 1940–1971).
- Risk factors you can change: Not being physically active, overweight or obese after menopause, hormones (estrogen and progestin) taken during menopause for >5 years, pregnancy at age 30 or older, not breastfeeding, nulliparity, moderate-to-high alcohol intake.
- Breast cancer types: Ductal carcinoma in situ (DCIS), infiltrating lobar carcinoma (CA), infiltrating ductal CA, mixed lobar and ductal CA, PDB, inflammatory breast CA, phyllodes tumor, breast sarcoma (rare).
- Breast cancer receptors: Estrogen receptor (ER), progesterone receptor (PR), HER2 (human epidermal growth factor receptor). Most breast cancers (80%) are hormone-receptor positive (ER and/or PR).

Breast Cancer Screening

USPSTF: Biennial screening mammography for women aged 50 to 74 years. There is insufficient evidence for digital breast tomosynthesis (DBT) as the screening method for breast cancer.

Classic Case

Patient (or clinician) detects a dominant breast mass that is painless. Mass feels hard, has irregular edges, and is not mobile. May have axillary adenopathy, skin changes (dimpling or peau d'orange, thickening), or erythema (IBC). May have nipple discharge (bloody) or erosion. Scaling on the nipple and/or areola is a sign of PDB. Symptoms of metastases include bone (back pain, leg pain), liver (nausea, jaundice, anorexia, pain), lungs (shortness of breath, cough), and/or brain (headache).

Imaging Tests

- Mammogram: Grouped microcalcifications, spiculated high-density mass.
- Breast ultrasound/sonogram: Distinguish if mass is cystic or solid/malignant (e.g., calcifications).
- MRI of the breast (with gondolinium): Used to screen women at high risk of breast cancer. Most invasive breast cancers are enhanced on gondolinium-contrast MRI.

Treatment Plan

- Age 30 years or older with dominant breast mass: Order diagnostic mammogram and breast ultrasound (to determine if cystic or solid). If abnormal mammogram, refer to breast specialist.
- Age 30 years or younger: Order breast ultrasound with/without diagnostic mammogram/breast biopsy. If low clinical suspicion, may observe for one or two menstrual cycles.
- Skin changes (peau d'orange, dimpling): Order diagnostic mammogram with biopsy of underlying mass.
- If family history of breast and/or ovarian cancer (first-degree includes parents/siblings and second-degree relatives are aunts/uncles/cousins): Refer to geneticist.

- Physical exam: Breast examination search for masses and for axillary, supraclavicular, and cervical adenopathy.
- Secondary prevention: Aspirin use at least once per week (associated with up to 50% reduction in death from breast cancer); tamoxifen for certain patients at higher risk at age 35 years or older.

DYSMENORRHEA (MENSTRUAL CRAMPS)

Primary dysmenorrhea refers to the recurrent crampy pain in the pelvic area caused by menstruation that is not caused by disease. Secondary dysmenorrhea refers to the same type of pain caused by a disease such as endometriosis. Endometriosis is associated with heavy menstrual periods (menorrhagia) with severe cramping. The treatment options are NSAIDs, acetaminophen (paracetamol), and/or hormonal methods. All NSAIDs are probably effective.

- Mefenamic acid (Ponstel): 250 mg every 6 hours for pain as needed
- Naproxen sodium (Aleve): 275 mg every 6 to 8 hours as needed
- Ibuprofen (Advil): 400 to 600 mg every 4 to 6 hours as needed
- Ketoprofen (Orudis): 25 to 50 mg every 6 to 8 hours as needed
- Acetaminophen (Tylenol): One to two tablets every 4 to 6 hours as needed (if NSAIDs contraindicated)
- If poor to no relief: Consider extended-cycle OCs such as Yaz (24/4) or extended-cycle OCs (Seasonale). Progestin-only methods may also be effective. Refer to gynecologist to rule out endometriosis or other pathology if severe menstrual cramp pain with heavy menses (can cause iron-deficiency anemia).

EXAM TIP

Mefenamic acid (Ponstel) is an NSAID that is very effective for menstrual pain.

ENDOMETRIOSIS

Pathogenesis not clear; one theory is that it is due to retrograde menstruation where endometrial cells leave the uterus and start growing on the ovaries, pelvis, uterine ligaments, bowel, bladder, or thorax. The lesions are stimulated by estrogen (just like the endometrium where the cells originated). Can result in infertility (25%–35% of women with infertilty have it).

Classic Case

Reproductive-aged woman between 25 and 35 years of age with history of moderate-to-severe pelvic pain during menses, heavy cramping, and dyspareunia. The dysmenorrhea may start approximately 1 to 2 days before menses, during menses, or a few days after menses. Ectopic endometrial tissue (endometriomas) can grow on the pelvis, ovary, peritoneum, bladder, bowel, abdominal wall, or thorax.

Objective Findings

Physical exam findings that suggest endometriosis include nodules in the posterior fornix, adnexal masses, and pain with manipulation of the pelvic organs. Pelvic exam may be normal. Large lesions may show up in pelvic/intravaginal ultrasound. Refer to gynecologist.

Treatment

Estrogen/progesterone contraceptives (birth control pills, patch, or vaginal ring) or progestin-only therapy will suppress the ovary and prevent ovulation and hormonal levels. NSAIDs for dysmenorrhea pain. Gonadotropin-releasing hormone (GnRH) analogues (e.g., leuprolide/Lupron Depot) and aromatase inhibitors for severe cases (anastrozole/Arimidex).

FIBROCYSTIC BREAST CHANGES

Very common condition found in reproductive-aged women between the ages of 30 and 50 years. Previously called *fibrocystic breast disease*. These are nonmalignant breast lesions, which are either nonproliferative (benign) or proliferative (fibroadenomas, fibrosis, papillomas, mild-to-moderate hyperplasia, others). Women with proliferative lesions have a slightly increased risk of breast cancer. Many have cyclic monthly breast changes that occur in the premenstrual period, such as breast engorgement and breast pain (mastodynia), which improve after menses starts.

Classic Case

Woman aged 30 to 50 years complains of the cyclic onset of bilateral breast tenderness and breast lumps that start from a few days (up to 2 weeks) before her period for many years. Once menstruation starts, the tenderness disappears, and the size of breast lumps decreases. May report that the lesion or mass has grown in size. During breast examination, the breast may feel lumpy, nodular, or cystic. If mass present, it is mobile with discrete edge, not attached to the skin, and feels rubbery to firm texture (not hard). Nipples and/or breast may feel tender.

Objective Findings

Multiple mobile and rubbery to firm (not hard) masses on one or both breasts.

Treatment Plan

- Stop caffeine intake. Take vitamin E and evening primrose capsules daily.
- Wear bras with good support.
- Referral needed if dominant mass, skin changes, fixed mass.

LICHEN SCLEROSUS

It is a chronic inflammatory disorder of the skin in the vulva and labia that is seen in children, adolescents, and adults. Can be asymptomatic or cause severe symptoms such as pruritis or skin fissures that are painful. Other lesions can be located in the axillae, inframammary folds, antecubital fossa, waist, and other locations.

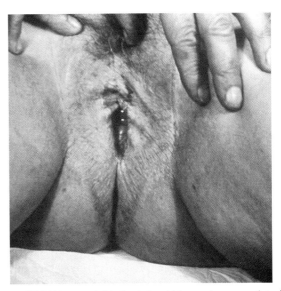

Figure 17.3 Waxy, wrinkled patches/skin erosions associated with lichen sclerosus.
Source: Centers for Disease Control and Prevention/Susan Lindsley. (See Resources section for complete source information.)

Objective Findings

Early skin lesion appears as flat-topped and slightly scaly hypopigmented, white, or mildly red polygonal papules that may coalesce to form larger plaques with peripheral erythema. Over time, when inflammation lessens, the lesion resembles cigarette paper (wrinkled appearance; Figure 17.3).

OVARIAN CANCER

Ovarian cancer is the fifth most common cancer in women in the United States. It is seldom diagnosed during the early stages of the disease. Most often, an older woman complains of vague symptoms, such as abdominal bloating and discomfort, low-back pain, pelvic pain, urinary frequency, and constipation (frequently blamed on benign conditions) for certain women with *BRCA1* and *BRCA2* mutations. By the time the cancer is diagnosed, it has almost always metastasized. Symptoms in patients with metastatic disease depend on area affected and may include bone pain, abdominal pain, headache, blurred vision, and others.

Some experts recommend risk-reducing bilateral salpingo-oophorectomy (BSO) between ages 35 and 40 years (after childbearing is complete) for certain women with *BRCA1* and *BRCA2* mutations. BSO has a significant effect in reducing ovarian cancer risk in this population. Although the USPSTF does not recommend routine screening for ovarian cancer in the general population (Grade D), high-risk women with suspected *BRCA1* and *BRCA2* mutations should be referred for genetic counseling and testing. If ovarian cancer screening is done, a transvaginal ultrasound with serum cancer antigen (CA-125) is ordered. The screening starts at age 30 years (or 5–10 years before earliest age of first diagnosis of ovarian cancer in a family member).

PELVIC ORGAN PROLAPSE IN WOMEN

Herniation of the bladder (cystocele), rectum (rectocele), uterus (uterine prolapse), small bowel (enterocele), or vagina (vaginal vault prolapse; Table 17.3 and Figure 17.4). Caused by weakening of pelvic muscles and supporting ligaments. During early stage, pelvic organ prolapse is usually asymptomatic. Advise the patient to avoid heavy lifting or excessive straining, which can worsen condition, and to avoid chronic constipation, because straining worsens pelvic organ prolapse.

Evaluation

During the gynecologic exam (bimanual exam, speculum exam), instruct the patient to bear down or strain so that herniation becomes more visible and palpable.

POLYCYSTIC OVARY SYNDROME

Hormonal abnormality marked by anovulation or oligo-anovulation (infrequent ovulation), infertility, excessive estrogen, high androgen production (acne, hirsutism), and insulin resistance. These females are at higher risk for type 2 diabetes, dyslipidemia, metabolic syndrome, endometrial hyperplasia, obesity, nonalcoholic fatty liver disease, depression, and obstructive sleep apnea.

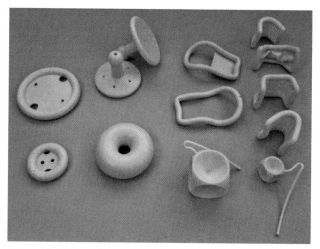

Figure 17.4 Pessaries.

Table 17.3 Pelvic Organ Prolapse

Organ	Description/Treatment Plan
Cystocele (bladder)	Bulging of the anterior vaginal wall; early stage is usually asymptomatic in all types of pelvic organ prolapse. Symptoms: Urinary incontinence and voiding difficulties (e.g., needing to reduce the prolapse using a finger in the vagina for urination or defecation). Plan: Refer for pessary placement, surgical repair.
Rectocele (rectum)	Bulging on the posterior vaginal wall; herniation ranges from mild to rectal prolapse. Symptoms: Feeling of rectal fullness or pressure, sensation that rectum does not completely empty; rectal prolapse can cause fecal incontinence. Plan: Kegel exercises; avoid straining during bowel movement; treat constipation; refer for pessary placement, surgical repair.
Uterine prolapse (uterus)	Cervix descends midline (apical) into vagina; cervix feels firm with pale-pink color and os visible; with third-degree full prolapse, a tubular saclike protrusion is seen outside the vagina. Symptoms: Vaginal discharge or bleeding, sensation of vaginal fullness, feeling that something is falling in the vagina, low-back pain. Plan: Avoid heavy lifting and straining; refer for pessary placement or surgical repair by urogynecologist.
Enterocele (small intestines)	Small bowel slips into the area between the uterus and posterior wall of the vagina, bulging external vagina. Symptoms: Pulling sensation inside pelvis, pelvic pressure or pain, low-back pain, dyspareunia. Plan: Refer for surgical repair.

Classic Case

Teen or young adult with obesity complains of excessive facial and body hair (hirsutism 70%), bad acne, and amenorrhea or infrequent periods (oligomenorrhea). Dark thick hair (terminal hair) is seen on the face, cheek, and beard areas. May have male-pattern baldness when older.

Treatment Plan

- On transvaginal ultrasound, enlarged ovaries seen with multiple small follicles ("ring of pearls" appearance)
- Serum testosterone, dehydroepiandrosterone (DHEA), and androstenedione are elevated. FSH levels are normal or low.
- Fasting blood glucose and 2-hour oral glucose tolerance test (OGTT) are abnormal.

Medications

- OCs are first-line treatment. Use OCs to suppress ovaries.
- Spironolactone is used to decrease and control hirsutism.
- If patient does not want OCs, give medroxyprogesterone tablets (Provera) 5 to 10 mg daily for 10 to 14 days (repeat every 1–2 months to induce menses).
- Metformin (Glucophage) is used to induce ovulation (if desires pregnancy). Warn reproductive-aged diabetic females (who do not want to become pregnant) to use birth control.
- Weight loss reduces androgen and insulin levels.

Complications

PCOS patients are at increased risk for:
- Coronary heart disease (CHD)
- Type 2 diabetes mellitus and metabolic syndrome
- Cancer of the breast and endometrium
- Central obesity
- Infertility
- Nonalcoholic fatty liver disease
- Endometrial hyperplasia

VULVOVAGINAL INFECTIONS

Table 17.4 Vaginal Disorders

Types	Signs/Symptoms	Lab Results
Bacterial vaginosis	"Fish-like" vaginal odor; profuse milk-like discharge that coats the vaginal vault Not itchy/vulva not red; overgrowth of anaerobes	Clue cells; no WBCs Whiff test: positive pH >4.5
Candidal vaginitis	Cheesy or curd-like white discharge Vulvovagina red/irritated	Pseudohyphae, spores, numerous WBCs
Trichomonal vaginitis (trichomoniasis)	"Strawberry cervix" Bubbly discharge Vulvovagina red/irritated	Mobile protozoa with flagella Numerous WBCs
Atrophic vaginitis	Scant to no discharge Fewer rugae, vaginal color pale; dyspareunia (painful intercourse); may bleed slightly during speculum examination (if not on hormones)	Atrophic changes on Pap test Elevated FSH and LH

FSH, follicle-stimulating hormone; LH, luteinizing hormone; WBC, white blood cell.

Bacterial Vaginosis

Caused by an overgrowth of anaerobic bacteria in the vagina. Risk factors include sexual activity, new or multiple sex partners, and douching. Not an STI; therefore, sexual partner does not need treatment. Treatment is especially important for pregnant women. Pregnant women with BV are at higher risk for premature labor or low–birth-weight babies.

Classic Case

Sexually active female complains of an unpleasant and fish-like vaginal odor that is worse after intercourse (if no condom is used). Vaginal discharge is copious and has milk-like consistency. Speculum examination reveals off-white to light-gray discharge coating the vaginal walls. There is no vulvar or vaginal redness or irritation (vaginal anaerobic bacteria do not cause inflammation).

Labs

Wet Smear Microscopy
- Findings: Clue cells and very few white blood cells (WBCs). May see *Mobiluncus* bacteria (82%), a gram-negative anaerobic rod-shaped bacteria.
- Clue cells: Made up of squamous epithelial cells with a large amount of bacteria coating the surface that obliterates the edges of the squamous epithelial cells (Figure 17.5).

Whiff Test
- Apply one drop of KOH to a cotton swab that is soaked with vaginal discharge.
- Positive test occurs when a strong "fishy" odor is released.

Vaginal pH
Alkaline vaginal pH >4.5. Normal vaginal pH is between 4.0 and 4.5 (acidic).

Treatment Plan
- Prescribe metronidazole (Flagyl) twice a day (BID) × 7 days.

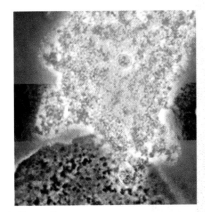

Figure 17.5 Clue cell.
Source: Centers for Disease Control and Prevention (2015).

- Alternative is metronidazole vaginal gel; one applicator at bedtime for 5 days.
- Watch for disulfiram (Antabuse) effect if combined with alcohol (e.g., severe nausea, headache).
- Prescribe clindamycin (Cleocin) cream at site of hidradenitis suppurativa × 7 days (oil based).
- Oil-based creams can weaken condoms.
- Treatment of sex partners is not recommended by the CDC, because BV is not an STI.
- Abstain from sexual intercourse or use condoms until treatment is done (increases cure rate by 50%).

Vulvovaginal Candidiasis

Overgrowth of *Candida albicans* yeast in the vulva/vagina. Considered normal vaginal flora but can also be pathogenic. Diabetics, as well as those who are HIV positive, on antibiotics (e.g., amoxicillin), or have any type of immunosuppression, are at higher risk. (The male penis can also be infected [balanitis].) Asymptomatic women and sexual partners do not need treatment.

Classic Case

Adult female presents with complaints of white cheese-like ("curd-like") vaginal discharge accompanied by severe vulvovaginal pruritus, swelling, and redness (inflammatory reaction). May complain of external pruritus of the vulva and vagina.

Labs

- Wet smear microscopy
- Swipe cotton swab with vaginal discharge in the middle of a glass slide.
- Add a few drops of normal saline (to the discharge).
- Cover the sample with a cover slip and examine it under the microscope (set it at high power).
- Findings are pseudohyphae and spores with a large number of WBCs present (Figure 17.6).

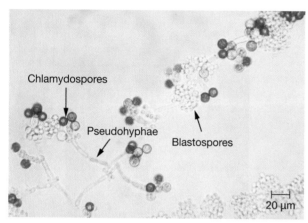

Figure 17.6 Candida blastospores, pseudohyphae, and chlamydospores (micrograph).

Treatment Plan

- Miconazole (Monistat), clotrimazole (Gyne-Lotrimin) × 7 days (OTC)
- Prescription fluconazole (Diflucan) 150 mg tablet × 1 dose, terconazole (Terazol-3) vaginal cream/suppository.
- For severe symptoms or immunocompromised patients, fluconazole (Diflucan) 150 mg in two sequential doses given 3 days apart. Do not use oral fluconazole in pregnancy, since it is teratogenic.
- Lactobacillus (oral or vaginal) does not prevent postantibiotic vulvovaginitis.

Trichomoniasis

Trichomonas vaginalis is a unicellular protozoan parasite with flagella that infects genitourinary tissue (both males and females). Infection causes inflammation (pruritus, burning, and irritation) of vagina/urethra. The most common sites are the urethra (dysuria) and vagina (Figure 17.7). It can also infect the paraurethral glands, Bartholin glands, cervix, bladder, and prostate.

Classic Case

Adult female complains of very pruritic, reddened vulvovaginal area. May complain of dysuria. Copious grayish-green and bubbly vaginal discharge. Male partners may have dysuria and frequency (urethritis) or may be asymptomatic.

Objective Findings

- "Strawberry cervix" from small points of bleeding on cervical surface (punctate hemorrhages) (Figure 17.8)
- Swollen and reddened vulvar and vaginal area; vaginal pH >5.0
- Dysuria (burning) with urination, copious foamy purulent vaginal discharge

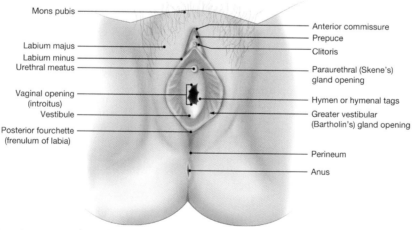

Figure 17.7 External female genitalia (vulva).
Source: Gawlik, K. S., Melnyk, B. M., & Teall, A. M. (Eds.). (2021). (See Resources section for complete source information.)

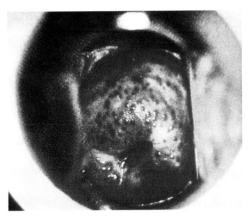

Figure 17.8 *Trichomonas vaginalis* infection.
Source: Centers for Disease Control and Prevention.

Labs

- Microscopy (use low power): Mobile unicellular organisms with flagella (flagellates) and a large amount of WBCs. Trichomonads will remain motile for only 10 to 20 minutes after collection.
- Nucleic acid amplification test (NAAT): For *T. vaginalis* (vaginal samples better than first-voided urine)

Treatment Plan

- Metronidazole (Flagyl) 2 g PO × 1 dose OR 500 mg BID × 7 days
- Tinidazole 2 g PO × 1 dose
- Treat sexual partner because trichomoniasis is considered an STI; avoid sex until both partners complete treatment.

EXAM TIPS

- There will be questions on all the types of vaginitis (BV, trichomonal, candidal, atrophic vaginitis). The questions range from diagnosis, workup, and lab tests to treatment.
- Become familiar with BV. "Clue cells" are squamous epithelial cells that have blurred edges due to the large number of bacteria on the cell's surface (see Figure 17.5).

CLINICAL PEARL

Women who have persistent vaginal infections and UTIs, despite hygiene measures, adequate hydration, and in the absence of sexual exposures from partner(s), should be screened for underlying glucose metabolism disorders and diabetes.

KNOWLEDGE CHECK: CHAPTER 17

1. A 28-year-old female patient presents for contraception. Her past medical history is significant for pelvic inflammatory disease (PID) 6 months ago as well as a seizure disorder, for which she takes phenobarbital. She requests "the pill" because she states she is "already taking a pill every day anyway." Which of the following is the *most appropriate* contraceptive for this patient?
A. Nexplanon
B. Loestrin FE 1/20
C. Seasonale
D. Copper interuterine device (IUD)

2. Which of the following is most strongly associated with the risk of developing breast cancer?
A. Alcohol consumption of more than two to three drinks per week
B. Adherence to a Mediterranean diet
C. Multiparity and breastfeeding
D. First pregnancy at age younger than 25 years

3. A 35-year-old woman smokes approximately 10 cigarettes per day. She started smoking at age 18 years. She has a new male sexual partner and is interested in contraception. She was recently treated for gonorrhea and chlamydia. She is using condoms inconsistently. The urine pregnancy test is negative. She denies a history of hypertension, blood clots, liver disease, heart disease, and diabetes. Her last menstrual period was 5 days ago. Which of the following contraceptive methods is recommended?
A. Oral contraceptive pills
B. Copper intrauterine device (IUD)
C. Etonogestrel implant (Nexplanon)
D. Vaginal ring (NuvaRing)

4. A 22-year-old patient presents for an annual gynecological exam and testing. The Pap test result shows ASC-US. Which of the following is the *best* management for this patient?
A. Check for high-risk human papillomavirus (HPV)
B. Repeat Pap test in 12 months
C. Refer patient for colposcopy
D. Refer patient for endometrial biopsy

5. Which of the following *best* describes primary amenorrhea?
A. Absence of menarche by age 12 years with breast development
B. Absence of menarche by age 15 years with breast development
C. Absence of menses after 3 or more months of regular menses
D. Absence of menses after 6 or more months of irregular menses

6. Which of the following is the *most common* cause of primary amenorrhea?
A. Pregnancy
B. Polycystic ovary syndrome
C. Turner syndrome
D. Hypothyroidism

7. A 27-year-old female patient who has never been pregnant presents with complaints of irregular menses and states that she wants to conceive. She reports that her mast menstrual period was a few months ago and lasted 2 days. Menarche was at 12 years, and her menses used to occur every month, but in the past several years they have occurred only a few times a year. Upon physical examination, hirsutism, acne, and a BMI of 31 are noted. Which of the following is the *most likely* diagnosis?
A. Congenital adrenal hyperplasia
B. 5 alpha-reductase deficiency
C. Turner syndrome
D. Polycystic ovary syndrome

8. A 27-year-old female patient presented at her previous visit with oligomenorrhea for the past year. She is not sexually active with men. Her lab results show the following: elevated HbA1C at 7.1, decreased sex hormone binding globulin (SHBG), elevated serum testosterone, and luteinizing hormone (LH):follicle-stimulating hormone (FSH) ratio elevated at 3:1. Which of the following is the best *next* step in managing this patient?
A. Insert a progestin-secreting intrauterine device
B. Prescribe metformin 500 mg twice daily
C. Prescribe clomiphene citrate
D. Prescribe a combined hormonal oral contraceptive pill

(See answers next page.)

1. A) Nexplanon

Some antiepileptic medications can be teratogenic, so ensuring the best possible efficacy of contraception is important. For this patient, Nexplanon, an etonogestrel contraceptive implant that is effective for up to 3 years, is the best option. Contraindications include pregnancy, liver disease, history of stroke or ischemic heart disease, undiagnosed vaginal bleeding, history of breast cancer, and systemic lupus erythematous with antiphospholipid antibodies. A copper IUD is contraindicated in patients with active PID or a history of PID within the past year. Loestrin FE 1/20 and Seasonale are combined oral contraceptives. Phenobarbital can decrease the efficacy of oral contraceptives, so they would not be the best choice for this patient.

2. A) Alcohol consumption of more than two to three drinks per week

Evidence points to a strong relationship between alcohol consumption and several malignancies, including breast cancer. Diets low in saturated fat, such as the Mediterranean diet, are associated with an overall decreased risk, as is multiparty and breastfeeding. Pregnancy at age 30 years or older is associated with increased risk.

3. C) Etonogestrel implant (Nexplanon)

An etonogestrel implant (Nexplanon) is the best option for this patient. It is a progesterone-only method. The 35-year-old patient is a smoker, so she cannot take oral contraceptives, which contain estrogen/progesterone. An IUD is contraindicated until the patient is retested (4-6 weeks after treatment) to ensure that her gonorrhea and chlamydia infections are gone. The vaginal ring (NuvaRing) contains estrogen and progestin; it is contraindicated for this patient.

4. B) Repeat Pap test in 12 months

The appropriate follow-up for a 22-year-old with a Pap smear result of ASC-US is to perform a repeat Pap test in 12 months. HPV testing is not recommended for this age group with ASC-US. A colposcopy is not recommended for ASC-US, as most cases clear spontaneously in young patients who are not immunocompromised. An endometrial biopsy is not appropriate follow-up for ASC-US, since it does not involve the endometrium.

5. B) Absence of menarche by age 15 years with breast development

Primary amenorrhea is the absence of menarche by age 15 years with breast development. The absence of menses after at least 3 consecutive months is called secondary amenorrhea. All patients with secondary amenorrhea should be ruled out for pregnancy.

6. C) Turner syndrome

Turner syndrome, also called 45,X or monosomy X, is the most common cause of primary amenorrhea in the United States. Pregnancy is the most common cause of secondary amenorrhea. Polycystic ovary disease can cause oligomenorrhea or amenorrhea, but the amenorrhea is usually secondary. Hypothyroidism is more likely to cause secondary amenorrhea.

7. D) Polycystic ovary syndrome

Polycystic ovary syndrome is perhaps the most common endocrinopathy encountered in gynecology settings. It is a multisystem disorder that affects lipids, glucose/insulin, adiposity, cardiovascular health, and reproductive health. Patients with the condition often present with a specific phenotype whereby they have terminal hair on their face and areola, acne, acanthosis nigricans, adiposity, scalp hair thinning, and oligomenorrhea or amenorrhea. These patients must have endometrial protection to avoid the development of endometrial hyperplasia and cancer. Congenital adrenal hyperplasia has different subtypes, but the classical and most common type is due to 21-hydroxylase deficiency. It is part of the newborn screening panel. Turner syndrome is the most common cause of hypergonadic hypogonadism and primary amenorrhea. Patients with Turner syndrome can have a specific phenotype consisting of short stature, webbed neck, low posterior hairline, ovarian dysgenesis, widely spaced nipples, and upper extremity lymphedema.

8. B) Prescribe metformin 500 mg twice daily

The laboratory findings indicate that the patient has polycystic ovary syndrome (PCOS). Because PCOS results in insulin resistance and other endocrine abnormalities, resensitization with metformin is advised. It is important to note that if the patient does not want to conceive, she must be prescribed a contraceptive. Patients who take metformin can have spontaneous resuming of menses and thus can potentially conceive. A progestin-secreting intrauterine device (IUD) offers endometrial protection, which this patient needs to prevent endometrial hyperplasia or cancer. However, prior to placing the IUD, an ultrasound should be performed to rule out preexisting hyperplasia. An oral contraceptive pill could be appropriate, but it will not mitigate the underlying endocrinopathy. Clomiphene citrate was used in the past to induce ovulation, but it would be considered only after an appropriate work-up and if the patient desires conception. However, letrozole is recommended as a first-line ovulation inductor in patients with PCOS.

9. A 50-year-old female patient presents to the clinic with a palpable breast mass. A diagnostic mammogram and ultrasound are ordered. The radiologist states that they see spiculation and a 2-cm poorly defined mass with irregular borders. Which of the following is the most appropriate and evidence-based next step?
   A. Refer to general surgery for a mastectomy consult
   B. Order a core needle biopsy through radiology
   C. Refer the patient to a breast oncologist
   D. Have the patient follow up in 3 months for re-imaging

10. A 19-year-old female patient who has never been pregnant presents with complaints of pelvic pain. Upon further questioning, she states that she has had painful menstrual cycles since menarche at age 12 years. She recently became sexually active and reports considerable pain with deep penetration. She also states that she sometimes has painful bowel movements but denies bright red blood per rectum. A urine human chorionic gonadotropin (HCG) result is negative. Upon physical examination, the cervix is nulliparous without discharge from the os, and there is diffuse tenderness throughout the pelvis without cervical motion tenderness or adnexal masses. Which of the following is the most likely diagnosis?
    A. Endometriosis
    B. Pelvic inflammatory disease
    C. Leiomyoma
    D. Ectopic pregnancy

11. A 23-year-old G1P1 female patient with a last menstrual period about 6 months ago presents with vaginal discharge and odor for 3 days. She is sexually active with her male partner, and she uses a progestin-secreting intrauterine device (IUD) for contraception. She denies fever, chills, or pelvic pain. A urine human chorionic gonadotropin (HCG) result is negative, and a wet mount shows multiple clue cells. Which of the following is the best treatment for this condition?
    A. Remove the IUD and prescribe vaginal metronidazole
    B. Prescribe fluconazole
    C. Prescribe doxycycline
    D. Prescribe oral metronidazole

12. Which of the following is most strongly associated with inflammatory breast cancer?
    A. Dominant mass in the tail of Spence
    B. History of recent mastitis
    C. Peau d'orange appearance of the skin
    D. Galactorrhea

13. Which of the following is the best screening modality for ovarian cancer?
    A. Ultrasound
    B. MRI
    C. CA-125
    D. Genetic testing

14. Which of the following best describes the follicular phase of the menstrual cycle?
    A. It is also known as the proliferative phase.
    B. It is characterized by the shedding of the endometrium.
    C. The dominant hormone is progesterone.
    D. It is also known as the secretive phase.

15. Ovulation typically occurs on what day of the menstrual cycle in a patient who has 28-day menstrual cycles?
    A. 10
    B. 14
    C. 20
    D. 28

16. A 52-year-old female patient presents with a chief complaint of hot flashes. She states that her last normal menstrual period was 10 months ago. She denies using any contraception, and her past medical history is noncontributory. Which of the following is the most likely diagnosis?
    A. Postmenopause
    B. Perimenopause
    C. Hypothyroidism
    D. Polycystic ovary syndrome

17. A 20-year-old female patient presents for a consult for contraception. Which of the following statements is most true about initiating contraception in this patient?
    A. A Pap smear with human papillomavirus (HPV) testing must be done prior to starting contraception.
    B. Patients must have sexually transmitted infection screening before beginning contraception.
    C. A risk/benefit discussion should occur regarding all available contraceptives.
    D. For younger patient, combined hormonal contraceptive pills are preferred.

(See answers next page.)

9. B) Order a core needle biopsy through radiology

Highly suspicious findings for breast malignancy on imaging include speculation, posterior acoustic shadowing, and a poorly defined mass with irregular borders. The most appropriate next step is to order a core needle biopsy. If the biopsy is positive, referral to breast oncology and surgery are appropriate. Abnormal breast imaging without suspicious findings must be followed up with more focused mammographic or ultrasound imaging or a breast MRI.

10. A) Endometriosis

The classic presentation of endometriosis is a younger patient with persistent dysmenorrhea and dyspareunia. Pelvic inflammatory disease should always be considered in a sexually active patient who presents with a more acute onset of pelvic pain, but there would likely be cervical motion tenderness on physical exam. Most patients will also present with a fever, and if an adnexal mass or significant tenderness is palpated, a tubo-ovarian abscess must be ruled out. Leiomyoma rarely presents in such a young patient, but key physical exam findings would be an enlarged uterus, and, depending on where the fibroid was located, the patient might also have abnormal uterine bleeding. An ectopic pregnancy would have a positive HCG result.

11. D) Prescribe oral metronidazole

There is no need to remove an IUD if a patient has vaginitis. Fluconazole is used for yeast infections, and metronidazole is used for bacterial vaginosis. Because this patient has clue cells on her wet mount, bacterial vaginosis can be diagnosed. Either vaginal or oral preparations are indicated.

12. C) Peau d'orange appearance of the skin

Peau d'orange is a classic finding of inflammatory breast cancer. Mastitis is not a precursor for inflammatory breast cancer but can be a misdiagnosis. Galactorrhea is almost always a benign finding.

13. D) Genetic testing

Ultrasound, MRI, and CA-125 have no utility in screening for ovarian cancer. The strongest risk factor for ovarian cancer is a family history and/or a genetic mutation (usually BRCA 1,2 and Lynch syndrome).

14. A) It is also known as the proliferative phase.

The follicular phase is also known as the proliferative phase. Estrogen is the main hormone during this phase.

15. B) 14

Most patients with a 28-day cycle will ovulate around day 14.

16. B) Perimenopause

Perimenopause is the time before and immediately after the final menstrual period. Menopause is defined as the unintentional cessation of menses for at least 12 months.

17. C) A risk/benefit discussion should occur regarding all available contraceptives.

Current guidelines do not recommend Pap/HPV testing in patients younger than 21 years. Even if the patient is of age to receive Pap/HPV testing, it is not required to initiate contraception. Sexually transmitted infection screening is recommended but is not required to initiate contraception. Patients should be educated on all options with a clear risk/benefit discussion.

18. A 24-year-old female patient presents for her annual physical exam and requests a Pap test. She has never had a Pap test and has completed the human papillomavirus (HPV) vaccination series. Which of the following statements is *most* true regarding how best to proceed with this patient?

A. She should receive co-testing with a Pap smear and HPV test.

B. She can defer the Pap smear because she has had the HPV vaccine.

C. She can defer the Pap smear because there is no family history of cervical cancer.

D. She can undergo Pap testing, but HPV testing is needed only if cytology is abnormal.

19. A 25-year-old G1P1 female patient with an last menstrual period about 2 weeks ago presents with vaginal discharge and odor for 3 days. She is sexually active with her male partner, and she uses a progestin subdermal implant for contraception. She denies fever, chills, or pelvic pain. A urine human chorionic gonadotropin (HCG) result is negative, and a wet mount shows multiple flagellated organisms. Which of the following is the *best* treatment for this patient?

A. Fluconazole

B. Metronidazole

C. Doxycycline

D. Ceftriaxone

20. A 39-year-old female patient presents for contraception. She reports smoking "about one pack" of cigarettes per day. Her blood pressure is 130/78 mmHg, and her weight is 212 lb. Which of the following would be the most appropriate contraceptive for this patient?

A. Progestin-secreting intrauterine device

B. Combined hormonal contraceptive pills

C. Combined hormonal transdermal contraception

D. Injectable long-acting progestin

21. A 72-year-old female patient presents for her annual exam. She reports no health issues. She is referred for a baseline Dexa scan, which comes back with a T-score of −2.5 SD. Which of the following is the most appropriate intervention at this time?

A. Swimming or biking at least three times a week

B. Raloxifene (selective estrogen receptor modulator)

C. Alendronate (bisphosphonate)

D. Teriparatide (parathyroid hormone analog)

22. A 68-year-old female patient presents with a chief complaint of vaginal burning and occasional itching. She is not sexually active. She states that she has been treated for yeast infections several times but that the symptoms recur. She is otherwise healthy and takes only paroxetine daily for an anxiety disorder. Upon physical examination, the vulva is atrophic, and the vaginal rugae are pale. Which of the following is the most appropriate *next* step for this patient?

A. Prescribe metronidazole vaginal

B. Prescribe oral fluconazole

C. Prescribe oral estrogen

D. Prescribe vaginal estrogen

23. A 22-year-old G2P2 female patient with a last menstrual period about 2 months ago presents with vaginal discharge, itching, and odor for 3 days. She is sexually active with her male partner and uses a progestin-secreting intrauterine device (IUD) for contraception. She denies fever, chills, or pelvic pain. Upon physical examination, the cervix is erythematous with a strawberry-like appearance. A urine human chorionic gonadotropin (HCG) result is negative, and a wet mount shows motile flagellated organisms. Which of the following statements about the treatment of this condition is *most* true?

A. This is a sexually transmitted infection, so the patient's partner needs treatment as well.

B. Because the patient is currently using an IUD, it needs to be removed.

C. A 5-day course of vaginal metronidazole is indicated.

D. The appropriate treatment is with doxycycline for 7 days.

24. Which assessment finding demonstrates that use of a vaginal dilator for atrophic vaginitis has been effective?

A. Atrophic labia

B. Decreased rugae

C. Narrowing of the vagina

D. Decreased discomfort with sexual activity

25. Which of the following would the nurse practitioner expect to find on a wet-mount slide of a patient diagnosed with bacterial vaginosis?

A. Tzanck cells

B. Large number of leukocytes and squamous epithelial cells

C. Epithelial cells dotted with large numbers of bacteria that obscure cell borders

D. Epithelial cells along with a small amount of blood

(See answers next page.)

18. D) She can undergo Pap testing, but HPV testing is needed only if cytology is abnormal.
Current guidelines state that patients between the ages of 21 and 29 years should not undergo routine co-testing. HPV genotyping should occur if cytology is abnormal. Prior vaccination does not confer immunity to all potential oncogenic strains of HPV. A family history of cervical cancer is irrelevant to screening guidelines.

19. B) Metronidazole
Flagellated organisms indicate that the patient has trichomoniasis, which is a sexually transmitted infection. Thus, the most appropriate treatment for this patient is oral metronidazole, and her partner needs to be treated as well. Fluconazole is used for vaginal candidiasis. Doxycycline is used for chlamydia, and ceftriaxone is used for gonorrhea and pelvic inflammatory disease (with doxycycline and possibly metronidazole).

20. A) Progestin-secreting intrauterine device
The patient has some risk factors for thromboembolic and cardiovascular events, so systemic estrogens and progestins would not be indicated. Patients older than 35 years who smoke should not use systemic estrogen. Patients who weigh >200 lb should not use transdermal contraception. While injectable long-acting progestins can be used, they are associated with weight gain, which the patient may not desire.

21. C) Alendronate (bisphosphonate)
A T-score of -2.5 SD indicates osteoporosis. The first-line treatment is with a bisphosphonate unless there are contraindications. Swimming and biking are not weight-bearing exercises and so would not help a patient strengthen their bones.

22. D) Prescribe vaginal estrogen
The American College of Obstetricians and Gynecologists and the North American Menopause Society both recommend vaginal estrogen for genitourinary atrophy. Systemic estrogen is indicated only for vasomotor symptoms. Fluconazole is used for vaginal candidiasis, and metronidazole is used for bacterial vaginosis.

23. A) This is a sexually transmitted infection, so the patient's partner needs treatment as well.
Motile flagellated organisms indicate trichomoniasis, which is a sexually transmitted infection; thus, the partner needs to be treated as well. Vaginal metronidazole is used for bacterial vaginosis. Trichomonas requires oral treatment. There is no reason to remove an IUD for a trichomonas infection.

24. D) Decreased discomfort with sexual activity
Vaginal atrophy (atrophic vaginitis) is thinning, drying, and inflammation of the vaginal walls that may occur when the body has less estrogen, as with postmenopausal patients. If painful sex is a concern, vaginal dilators may relieve vaginal discomfort by stretching to widen the vaginal canal to assist in reducing discomfort during intercourse. Atrophic labia and decreased rugae are symptoms of atrophic vaginitis and would not indicate effective treatment.

25. C) Epithelial cells dotted with large numbers of bacteria that obscure cell borders
Diagnosis of bacterial vaginosis includes three of four Amsel criteria: (1) white, thick adherent discharge; (2) pH >4.5; (3) positive whiff test (amine odor mixed with 10% potassium hydroxide); and (4) clue cells >20% on a wet mount (large number of squamous epithelial cells whose surfaces and edges are coated with large numbers of bacteria and a few leukocytes).

HELLP (HEMOLYSIS, ELEVATED LIVER ENZYMES, AND LOW PLATELETS) SYNDROME

Serious but rare complication of preeclampsia/eclampsia (15% of cases develop HELLP). Classic patient is a multipara woman older than 25 years of age who is in the third trimester of pregnancy. Presents with the signs and symptoms of preeclampsia accompanied by right upper quadrant (or midepigastric) abdominal pain with nausea/vomiting and malaise (may be mistaken for viral illness). Symptoms can present suddenly. Lab abnormalities are elevation of aspartate aminotransferase (AST), alanine aminotransferase (ALT), total bilirubin (>1.2 mg/dL), and lactate dehydrogenase (LDH) with decreased number of platelets (<100,000 cells/mcL), which may progress to disseminated intravascular coagulation (DIC) in 15% to 38% of patients, peripheral smear with schistocytes and burr cells, and hemoglobin and hematocrit. If severe, right upper quadrant/epigastric pain may have hepatic bleed or swelling, which may be signs of impending hepatic rupture.

PLACENTA PREVIA

The placenta implants too low either on top of the cervix or on the cervical isthmus/neck (Figure 18.1). A multipara woman who is in the late second to third trimester complains of new onset of painless vaginal bleeding that is worsened by intercourse. Blood is bright red in color. From 10% to 20% present with both bleeding and uterine contractions. Uterus is soft and nontender. If cervix is not dilated, treatment is strict bedrest. Administer IV magnesium sulfate if there is uterine cramping. Uterus will usually reimplant itself if mild. Any vaginal or rectal insertion or stimulation is an absolute contraindication (can precipitate severe hemorrhage). Transabdominal ultrasound to diagnose. If cervix is dilated or if hemorrhaging, fetus is delivered by cesarean section (C-section). Severe cases cause hemorrhage; fetus must be delivered to save mother's life. Strong association between placenta previa and amniotic fluid embolism (sudden respiratory distress, hypoxia, and/or seizures followed by DIC during labor or after delivery).

PLACENTAL ABRUPTION (ABRUPTIO PLACENTAE)

Pregnant woman who is in the last few weeks of pregnancy complains of abrupt onset of significant abdominal pain accompanied by a contracted uterus that feels hard (hypertonic); may have uterine contractions. Associated with a sudden onset of dark-red-colored vaginal bleeding. Up to 20% of women do not have vaginal bleeding (blood is trapped between placenta and uterine wall; Figure 18.2). If mild, blood is reabsorbed, and affected area reimplants. Severe cases cause hemorrhage (e.g., DIC); fetus must be delivered to save mother's life. Higher risk in females with history of hypertension, preeclampsia/eclampsia, smoking, trauma, and cocaine use. Strongest risk factor is a history of placenta abruption. Call 911. Requires emergent treatment and C-section. Placenta abruption accounts for 5% to 8% of maternal deaths.

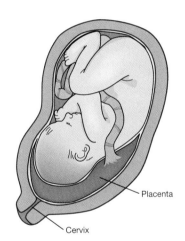

Figure 18.1 Placenta previa.

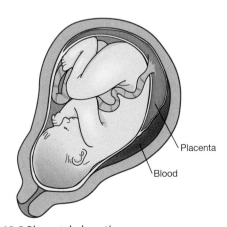

Figure 18.2 Placental abruption.

SEVERE PREECLAMPSIA

A primigravida woman who is in the late third trimester of pregnancy (>34 weeks) complains of a sudden onset of severe recurrent headaches, visual abnormalities (blurred vision, scotomas), and pitting edema. Edema easily seen on the face/eyes and fingers. Sudden rapid weight gain within 1 to 2 days (>2–4 1b/wk). New onset of right upper quadrant abdominal pain. Blood pressure (BP) more than 140/90 mmHg. Urine protein 1+ or higher. Sudden decrease in urine output (oliguria). Visual symptoms, headache, nausea, and vomiting are worrisome signs (encephalopathy). If seizures occur, condition is reclassified as eclampsia. Earliest time period that preeclampsia/eclampsia can occur is at 20 weeks' gestation (and up to 4 weeks postpartum). Hemorrhagic stroke accounts for 36% of pregnancy-associated stroke. Only known "cure" is delivery of fetus or baby. Magnesium sulfate is drug of choice to prevent eclampsia.

EXAM TIPS

- Placenta previa is vaginal bleeding (bright red) without a hypertonic tender uterus.
- Placenta abruptio is vaginal bleeding that is intermittent with hypertonic, hard, and tender uterus.

LABORATORY TESTING

Table 18.1 Laboratory Results During Pregnancy

Test	Elevated	Notes
Liver function	Alkaline phosphatase (2nd to 3rd trimester)	AST, ALT, and GGT no changes
Lipid profile	Total cholesterol, triglycerides, HDL, LDL	Wait 4–6 weeks after pregnancy to check lipids
Thyroid function	Total T3	Free T4, TSH
Complete blood count	WBC Platelet count Sedimentation rate	Hemoglobin and hematocrit are reduced in pregnancy
Renal function	GFR	Lower serum creatinine GFR and renal plasma flow increases

ALT, alanine aminotransferase; AST, aspartate aminotransferase; GFR, glomerular filtration rate; GGT, gamma glutamyl transpeptidase; HDL, high-density lipoprotein; LDL, low-density lipoprotein; T3, triiodothyronine; T4, thyroxine; TSH, thyroid-stimulating hormone; WBC, white blood cell. *Source:* Cunningham, F. G. (2023). (See Resources section for complete source information.)

ALKALINE PHOSPHATASE

Expected to increase during pregnancy due to the growth of the fetal bones. Values higher in multiple gestation pregnancies.

AMNIOCENTESIS AND CHORIONIC VILLUS SAMPLING

- Can be done earlier (10–12 weeks) than the amniocentesis (15–18 weeks). Specimens contain fetal cells.
- Fetal chromosomes/DNA is tested for abnormalities.

BETA HUMAN CHORIONIC GONADOTROPIN

- Manufactured by the chorion (early placenta) by day 8 to day 10.
- High-quality urine home pregnancy tests (e.g., First Response, EPT) can detect pregnancy as early as the first missed period (2 weeks after conception).
- There are higher levels of human chorionic gonadotropin (hCG) with twins/multiple fetuses and with molar pregnancies.

Doubling Time

Doubling time is an important indicator of the viability of a pregnancy. Useful only in the first trimester; thereafter, it loses its predictive value (do not use after week 12).

- Normal finding: hCG doubles every 48 to 72 hours during the first 12 weeks (first trimester) in a normal pregnancy.
- Ectopic pregnancy: The hCG has lower values than normal. Values increase slowly and do not double as expected.
- Inevitable abortion: Values of hCG start decreasing rapidly; there is no doubling. Cervix is dilated.

ERYTHROCYTE SEDIMENTATION RATE

- Increases during pregnancy. By the third trimester, the sedimentation rate ranges from 13 to 70 mm/hr.
- Erythrocyte sedimentation rate (nonpregnant): 0 to 20 mm/hr

HEMOGLOBIN AND HEMATOCRIT

- Both values go down during pregnancy due to hemodilution. The hemoglobin value may be as low as 10.5 g/dL, and the hematocrit value may go down to about 30% (by the third trimester). Called physiologic or dilutional anemia of pregnancy.
- To rule out iron-deficiency anemia, check the mean corpuscular volume (MCV). It is not affected by pregnancy.

LIVER ENZYMES

ALT, AST, bilirubin, and gamma glutamyl transpeptidase (GGT) remain the same in an uncomplicated pregnancy except for alkaline phosphatase.

QUADRUPLE MARKER SCREEN TEST

- Combination of the triple screen hormones plus inhibin-A (hormone released by the placenta). The triple or quadruple screen tests are more sensitive than the alpha-fetoprotein (AFP) alone (but have a higher rate of false positives).
- Gold standard test for genetic disorders is testing of fetal chromosomes/DNA.

SCREENING FOR GENETIC DISORDERS

- Jewish descent (Tay–Sachs disease); this fatal neurologic disease, with no known cure, is more common among Eastern Europeans of Jewish descent
- Whites (cystic fibrosis)
- African Americans (sickle cell anemia)

EXAM TIP

Patients who are European Jewish should be screened for Tay–Sachs disease.

SERUM ALPHA-FETOPROTEIN

- Serum AFP is manufactured by the liver of the fetus and mother. AFP levels are adjusted for weight and race; slightly higher levels are found in Black women and lower levels in Asian women (compared with Whites).
- Majority of maternal AFP comes from the fetus (liver, fetal yolk sac, gastrointestinal [GI] tract).
- It is a biochemical marker used to estimate a pregnant woman's risk of having a fetus/infant with Down syndrome (check between 15 and 18 weeks); also used as an initial screen for open neural tube defects and abdominal wall defects.
- Indications include advanced maternal age and previous births or family history of chromosomal or birth defects (e.g., neural tube defects).

Low Alpha-Fetoprotein

- Mature maternal age is the most common risk factor for Down syndrome (35-year-old or older woman has a 1:350 at term). Women pregnant at age 35 years or older have a "geriatric pregnancy."
- If AFP is low, order the triple screen test (AFP, hCG, and estriol) or the quadruple screen test (AFP, hCG, estriol, inhibin-A) to evaluate for Down syndrome (trisomy 21).

High Alpha-Fetoprotein

- Rule out neural tube defects or multiple gestation. Most common reason for a high AFP is pregnancy dating error.
- If AFP is high (e.g., neural tube defects, omphalocele, gastroschisis), order the triple screen or the quad screen test and sonogram to rule out neural tube abnormalities (higher sensitivity than AFP alone).
- To prevent neural tube defects: Ingest folic acid 400 mcg (0.4 mg) per day (found in leafy green vegetables, fortified cereals). To reduce risk, advise patients to take prenatal vitamins when planning to become pregnant.

SEXUALLY TRANSMITTED INFECTIONS

Screen for hepatitis B surface antigen (HBsAg), HIV, gonorrhea, chlamydia, syphilis, herpesvirus types 1 and 2.

THYROID FUNCTION TESTS

- Total triiodothyronine (T3) is higher during pregnancy because of increased levels of thyroid-binding globulin (TBG).
- Thyroid-stimulating hormone (TSH), free T3, and free thyroxine (T4) results remain unchanged in euthyroid patients.

TITERS

- Check rubella titer.
- Check varicella titers (if no proof of infection).

TRIPLE MARKER SCREEN TEST

- The triple screen test combines the AFP, beta hCG, and estriol serum level values. The hormone level results are used in a formula to figure out the risk for a Down syndrome infant.
- Diagnostic test for genetic anomalies is chromosome testing.

URINALYSIS (DIPSTICK)

Obtain midstream urine before exam (minimizes contamination from vaginal discharge). Check protein, leukocytes, nitrite, blood, glucose.

- Protein: Negative (trace, 1+ to 4+)
- If 20 weeks' gestation or more, rule out preeclampsia if protein 2+ or higher
- If proteinuria present, order urine protein-to-creatinine ratio or 24-hour urine protein

VAGINAL CULTURES

- Group B *Streptococcus* (GBS) is tested for at 35 to 37 weeks. Swab vaginal introitus and rectum (insert up to anal sphincter) for culture and sensitivity (C&S). If positive, administer intrapartum antibiotic prophylaxis with penicillin G 5 million units IV, followed by 2.5 to 3 million units IV every 4 hours until delivery.
- If penicillin allergy, use clindamycin or erythromycin instead.

WHITE BLOOD CELLS

- White blood cell (WBC) count is elevated throughout pregnancy, especially during the third trimester. May climb as high as $16,000$ cells/mm^3 in the third trimester. (WBC in nonpregnant adults: Range is 4,500–10,500 cells/mm^3.)
- Leukocytosis with neutrophilia is "normal" during pregnancy (if it is not accompanied by signs of infection).

DRUGS AND VACCINES DURING PREGNANCY

The new U.S. Food and Drug Administration (FDA) Pregnancy and Lactation Labeling Rule (PLLR) will eventually replace the pregnancy letter categories (A, B, C, D, and X) with new labeling. The new rule is discussed in Chapter 3. Since most of the drugs on the exam were released before the PLLR, the FDA letter categories are still covered in this edition. Most of the drugs used in pregnancy are FDA Category B drugs. Because it is unethical to experiment on pregnant women, a number of drugs used during pregnancy are found to be safe only through many years of use by pregnant women (e.g., penicillins, macrolides).

CATEGORY A DRUGS

Animal and human data show no risk to pregnant women.
- Prenatal vitamins (high-dose multivitamins are not used during pregnancy)
- Insulin
- Thyroid hormone (levothyroxine)
- Folic acid (vitamin B_9), pyridoxine (vitamin B_6)

CATEGORY B DRUGS

- Animal studies show no risk. No human data available.
- Antacids (Tums, Maalox) are safe for pregnant women.
- Docusate sodium (Colace) is a stool softener and is approved for pregnant women. It is not a laxative. Avoid laxatives (e.g., Ex-Lax, Bisacodyl), especially in the third trimester (may induce labor).
- Analgesics (acetaminophen preferred to nonsteroidal anti-inflammatory drugs [NSAIDs] especially in the third trimester); see "Category D Drugs."

Antibiotics for Pregnant Women

- Penicillins: amoxicillin (Amoxil), penicillin, dicloxacillin
- Cephalosporins
  - First generation: cephalexin (Keflex), cefadroxil (Duricef)
  - Second generation: cefuroxime axetil (Ceftin), cefaclor (Ceclor), cefprozil (Cefzil)
  - Third generation: ceftriaxone (Rocephin) injections, cefdinir (Omnicef), cefixime (Suprax)
  - Fourth generation: cefepime (Maxipime) injection/IV (used mainly in hospitals)
- Macrolides
  - Erythromycins
  - Erythromycin ethylsuccinate (E-mycin), erythromycin base, erythromycin stearate, erythromycin estolate (EES)
  - Azithromycin (Zithromax)
  - Clarithromycin (Biaxin) is the only macrolide that is a Category C. Avoid use during pregnancy. Consult with physician before use and discuss risk versus benefits.
- Nitrofurantoin (Furadantin, Macrobid)
  - Do not use with glucose-6-phospate dehydrogenase deficiency (G6PD anemia), because it will cause hemolysis (anemia, jaundice, dark urine).
  - Contraindicated during labor and delivery (or near term) due to increased risk of hemolytic anemia (infant) due to immature erythrocyte enzyme system (glutathione instability).

Antihypertensives for Pregnant Women

Used for women with chronic hypertension or for moderate-to-severe preeclampsia or eclampsia. Use of antihypertensive drugs to control mild hypertension does not alter the course of the disease or diminish perinatal morbidity or mortality of preeclampsia. Refer to obstetrician.
- Methyldopa (Aldomet)
- Calcium channel blockers (Procardia)
- Labetalol (Normodyne)

CATEGORY C DRUGS

Adverse effects seen in animal studies. No human data available.
- Sulfa drugs
  - Considered Category C in third trimester because they can cause hemolytic anemia in the fetus/infant, which results in hyperbilirubinemia. Sulfa drugs displace bilirubin from albumin. High blood levels of unconjugated bilirubin can cross the blood–brain barrier and cause brain damage (kernicterus).
  - Trimethoprim–sulfamethoxazole (e.g., Bactrim DS, Septra)
  - Clarithromycin (Biaxin) is the only Category C macrolide antibiotic. Avoid use in pregnant women. Consult with physician before using Category C drugs during pregnancy.
- Pseudoephedrine (Sudafed): Increases risk of gastroschisis (intestines protrude through abdominal wall defect). Ideally, it should not be used in pregnancy and breastfeeding (repeated doses may interfere with lactation, as it crosses breast milk).

CATEGORY D DRUGS

Evidence of fetal risk. Benefits should outweigh the risk of using the drug.
- Angiotensin-converting enzyme (ACE) inhibitors and angiotensin receptor blockers (ARBs)
  - Cause fetal renal abnormalities, renal failure, and hypotension
  - Captopril (Capoten) and losartan (Hyzaar)
  - Category C in first trimester
  - Category D in second and third trimesters
- Fluoroquinolones
  - Affect fetal cartilage development; a rare side effect is Achilles tendon rupture in athlete; contraindicated in pregnant or lactating women and children younger than 18 years
  - Ciprofloxacin (Cipro)
  - Ofloxacin (Floxin)
  - Gram-positive activity: Levofloxacin (Levaquin), gemifloxacin (Factive), moxifloxacin (Avelox)
- Tetracyclines
  - Stain growing tooth enamel
  - Tetracycline, minocycline (Minocin)
  - Avoid in the third trimester
- NSAIDs
  - Block prostaglandins and may cause premature labor; avoid using especially in the last 2 weeks of pregnancy

- Category D in the third trimester, but Category B during first/second trimester (ibuprofen, naproxen, other NSAIDs)
  - Acetylsalicylic acid (ASA) may be used and is often indicated to prevent preeclampsia in high-risk patients
- Sulfa drugs: Risk of hyperbilirubinemia (neonatal jaundice or kernicterus); sulfa drugs displace bilirubin from albumin; high levels of unconjugated bilirubin will cross the blood–brain barrier and cause brain damage (e.g., mental retardation, seizures, deafness)

CATEGORY X DRUGS

Proven fetal risks outweigh the benefits.
- Isotretinoin, a vitamin A derivative:
  - Used for severe cystic and nodular acne recalcitrant to treatment; it is highly teratogenic.
  - Also avoid vitamin A derivative topicals such as retinol/retinoid, tretinoin (Retin-A), adapalene
- Methotrexate (antimetabolite) and anticancer drugs: Used for some types of autoimmune diseases (psoriasis, rheumatoid arthritis) and certain cancers
- Proscar (antiandrogen): Used for benign prostatic hyperplasia (BPH) and prostate cancer
- Misoprostol (prostaglandin analog): Used as one of the drugs in medical abortions (a component of the "abortion pill")
- Evista and tamoxifen (selective estrogen receptor modulator [SERM]): Use reduces risk of reoccurrence of estrogen receptor–positive breast cancer
- All hormonal drugs (natural or synthetic): Category X in pregnancy—all forms of estrogens, testosterone, finasteride (Proscar), mifepristone (RU-86).
- Any drug that blocks hormone synthesis or binding: Lupron Depot.
- Lupron Depot: Used for infertility, hormone-dependent cancers, and endometriosis.

DRUGS TO AVOID (THIRD TRIMESTER OF PREGNANCY)

- NSAIDs (blocks prostaglandin)
- Aspirin and salicylates (affect platelets). Bismuth subsalicylate (Pepto-Bismol) contains salicylates.
- Sulfa-containing drugs (trimethoprim–sulfamethoxazole, nitrofurantoin) near term. Higher risk of hyperbilirubinemia, jaundice, kernicterus, oligohydramnios, premature closure ductus arteriosus.

VACCINES

- Mumps, measles, and rubella (MMR); oral polio; varicella; and FluMist are contraindicated in pregnancy.
- COVID-19 vaccine is safe and recommended for use in pregnancy.
- One dose of Tdap is recommended during pregnancy; it should not be repeated after 27 weeks' gestation.
- Influenza vaccine is an inactivated virus and is safe to use in pregnant women.

- Recommend for pregnant women, especially if they are pregnant during the fall and winter seasons. Only use the injectable inactivated flu vaccine.
- Live attenuated influenza virus (LAIV) vaccine and flu vaccine via nasal spray (FluMist) are contraindicated.

> **NOTE**
>
> After a live virus vaccine, advise reproductive-aged women not to get pregnant (and use reliable birth control) in the next 4 weeks (MMR) or 3 months (varicella and shingles vaccine). Inactivated flu vaccine and Tdap vaccines are recommended for pregnant women.

TERATOGENS

Agents that can cause structural abnormalities during pregnancy:
- Paroxetine (Paxil): Taking drug during the first trimester increases risk of birth defects, particularly heart defects (others are anencephaly, abdominal wall defects). FDA Category D drug.
- Fluoxetine (Prozac): Heart wall defects and craniosynostosis (premature closure of skull sutures).
- Other SSRIs (citalopram, escitalopram, sertraline): First-trimester exposure may be associated with a low risk of teratogenicity.
- Alcohol: Fetal alcohol syndrome
- Aminoglycosides: Deafness
- Cigarettes: Intrauterine growth restriction (IUGR), prematurity
- Cocaine: Cerebrovascular accidents (CVAs), mental retardation, abruptio placentae
- Isotretinoin: Central nervous system (CNS)/craniofacial/ear/cardiovascular defects
- Lithium: Cardiac defects (Ebstein's anomalies are malformations of tricuspid valve and right atrium that can cause heart failure, sudden death, transient ischemic attack (TIA), stroke; presentation is middle teenager years).
- Chronic hyperglycemia during pregnancy (poorly controlled diabetes or gestational diabetes mellitus [GDM]): Teratogenic state. It increases the risk of neural tube defects and craniofacial defects.

HEALTH EDUCATION

- Take prenatal vitamins with 400 mcg of folic acid daily (start 2–3 months before conception).
- Always wear seatbelt (lap-style seatbelt below uterine fundus).
- Avoid soft cheeses (blue cheese, brie), uncooked meats, raw milk (*Listeria* bacteria).
- Sex is safe except during vaginal bleeding, incompetent cervix, placenta previa, or preterm labor.
- Cat litter or raw/undercooked meat can cause toxoplasmosis (congenital infection).

- Do not eat raw shellfish or raw oysters (*Vibrio vulnificus* infection).
- Be careful with cold cuts, uncooked hot dogs, and "deli" meat (*Listeria* bacteria). Pregnant women are 20 times more likely to become infected and die from *Listeria monocytogenes*.
- Smoking (vasoconstriction causes IUGR) and alcohol (fetal alcohol syndrome) are contraindicated.
- Regular coffee (8 oz/d) is okay. Do not consume an excessive amount of caffeine (premature labor).
- Do not use hot tubs or saunas or expose oneself to excessive heat.

ZIKA VIRUS

Zika infection during pregnancy can cause severe birth defects (e.g., microcephaly) and neurodevelopmental abnormalities. The only way to completely prevent Zika infection during pregnancy is to not travel to areas with Zika outbreak/risk and to use condoms or avoid sex with someone who has recently traveled to a risk area. If travel is necessary, the Centers for Disease Control and Prevention (CDC) recommends the following special precautions for pregnant women and women (and their partners) who are trying to become pregnant (https://www.cdc.gov /pregnancy/zika/index.html).

PREGNANT WOMEN
- Use Environmental Protection Agency (EPA)-registered insect repellents and cover skin.
- Stay in places with air conditioning, screens, and mosquito nets.
- Use condoms or abstain from sex during pregnancy.
- Be alert for symptoms after travel.

WOMEN AND PARTNERS TRYING TO BECOME PREGNANT
Use condoms or abstain from sex according to the following time frames:
- Both partners or only the male partner traveled to an outbreak/risk area: 3 months after return or from the start of symptoms or date of diagnosis
- Only the female partner traveled to an outbreak/risk area: 2 months after return or from the start of symptoms or date of diagnosis

WEIGHT GAIN

- Most weight is gained in third trimester (about 1–2 lb [0.45–0.91 kg] per week).
- Best weight gain is a total gain of 25 to 35 lb (11.3–15.9 kg) if healthy weight before pregnancy (body mass index [BMI] of 18.5–24.9) is ideal.
- Underweight patients (BMI <18.5) to gain a total of 28 to 40 lb (12.7–18.1 kg).
- Obese patients (BMI >30) to gain a total of up to 11 to 20 lb (4.98–9.07 kg).

- After delivery, loss of up to 15 to 20 lb (6.8–9.1 kg) in first few weeks is appropriate.
- For twins, increased weight gain (37–54 lb [16.8–24.5 kg]) is appropriate, but weight gain should not be double that for a single fetus.

ADVANCED MATERNAL AGE

Women who are pregnant at age ≥35 years are considered to be of advanced maternal age and are at higher risk of:
- Chromosomal abnormalities (e.g., Down syndrome), birth defects
- Preeclampsia
- Low–birth-weight infants
- Miscarriage, premature birth
- Complications during delivery (e.g., stillbirth); more likely to have C-section

SIGNS AND CLINICAL METHODS FOR DATING PREGNANCY

Table 18.2 Signs of Pregnancy

Sign	Clinical Finding	Time From Conception
Human chorionic gonadotropin	Amenorrhea; not uncommon to have spotting in first missed menses	Approximately 8–10 days after ovulation (earliest time that it can be detected with standard serum hCG test); serum hCG can detect it earlier
Goodell's sign	Cervical softening	4 weeks
Chadwick's sign	Bluish discoloration of cervix and vagina	6–8 weeks
Hegar's sign	Softening of uterine isthmus	6–8 weeks

hCG, human chorionic gonadotrophin.

POSITIVE SIGNS
- Palpation of fetus by health provider
- Ultrasound and visualization of fetus or embryo
- Fetal heart tones (FHTs) auscultated by health provider: 10 to 12 weeks by Doppler/Doptone; 20 weeks by fetoscope/stethoscope

PROBABLE SIGNS
- Goodell's sign (4 weeks): Cervical softening
- Chadwick's sign (6–8 weeks): Blue coloration of the cervix and vagina
- Hegar's sign (6–8 weeks): Softening uterine isthmus
- Enlarged uterus
- Ballottement (seen in midpregnancy): When the fetus is pushed, it can be felt to bounce back by tapping the palpating fingers inside the vagina
- Urine or blood pregnancy tests (beta HCG)

- The signs with surnames (Goodell, Chadwick, Hegar) are all probable signs.
- To help remember the probable signs of pregnancy, think alphabetically and correlate with where the signs occur, from the outside-in anatomically. Chadwick, vagina. Goodell, cervix. Hegar, uterine isthmus.

- Urine/serum pregnancy tests are considered probable signs (do not confuse them as "positive signs"). Beta hCG also presents in molar pregnancy and ovarian cancer.
- Memorize the three positive signs of pregnancy. This is the shortest list to memorize. By the process of elimination, you can rule out (or in) the correct answer choice.

PRESUMPTIVE SIGNS

The following are the "softest" and least objective signs (from mother). Can be caused by many other conditions besides pregnancy.

- Amenorrhea
- Nausea/vomiting (most common in first trimester in the morning, usually disappears by the second trimester)
- Breast changes (swollen and tender)
- Fatigue
- Urinary frequency
- Slight increase in body temperature
- "Quickening," when mother feels the baby's movements for the first time; starts at 16 weeks

- Palpation of fetal movements by the mother is not considered a positive sign of pregnancy ("quickening"). It is classified as a "presumptive sign."
- Exam questions asking for one of the signs will mix them up (e.g., mix a positive sign with a probable sign). Ensure that the answer option contains the two signs from the same category.

FUNDAL HEIGHTS IN SINGLETON PREGNANCY

12 Weeks (Third Month)
- Uterine fundus first rises above symphysis pubis.
- FHTs are heard by Doppler by 10 to 12 weeks.

16 Weeks (Fourth Month)
Uterine fundus between the symphysis pubis and the umbilicus

20 Weeks (Fifth Month)
- Uterine fundus at level of the umbilicus
- FHTs are heard with fetoscope or stethoscope by 20 weeks.

20 to 35 Weeks
Measure the distance between upper edge of pubic symphysis and the top of the uterine fundus using a paper tape measure. Fundal height in centimeters equals the number of weeks of gestation (±2 cm). For example, a 32-week-gestation fetus should have a fundal height of between 30 and 34 cm.

Fundus at 12 weeks is above symphysis pubis, fundus at 16 weeks is between the symphysis pubis and the umbilicus, and fundus at 20 weeks is at the umbilicus.

NAEGELE'S RULE

- Used to estimate date of delivery (EDD) during the first trimester.
- Assumes regular 28- to 30-day menstrual cycle. Not as useful for irregular menstrual cycles. A full-term pregnancy is 40 weeks (280 days).
- There are two different ways to use Naegele's rule. They are equivalent; pick the one with which you feel most comfortable (LMP = last menstrual period).
  - Method 1: LMP + 9 months + 7 days
  - Method 2: LMP − 3 months + 7 days

Example
A 28-year-old woman who is at 8 weeks' gestation reports that her LMP was on February 20, 2023. Using Naegele's rule, which of the following dates is correct for her expected EDD?
A. November 10, 2023
B. November 27, 2023
C. December 10, 2023
D. December 27, 2023

Solution
Method 1: LMP: 2/20/2023
1. Add 9 months to February: 2 + 9 = 11 (November)
2. Add 7 days to date of the LMP: 20 + 7 = 27
3. EDD = November 27, 2023

Method 2: LMP: 2/20/2023
1. Subtract 3 months from February = November
2. Add 7 days to date of the LMP: 20 + 7 = 27
3. EDD = November 27, 2023

- There is usually one question about the EDD (use Naegele's rule).
- The LMP month on the exam will either be January (01), February (02), or March (03).

If LMP is:	EDD:
January	October
February	November
March	December

SIZE AND DATE DISCREPANCY

The size of the uterus does not match gestational age. Defined as a difference of plus or minus 2 (or +/− 2) from number of weeks of gestation. If the uterine fundus is ≤2 cm (fetus smaller than expected), it can be caused by dating error, IUGR, or other problem. If fundus size is ≥2 cm (fetus larger than expected), it can be due to dating error, macrosomia, or other problem. Order an ultrasound.

PHYSIOLOGIC CHANGES DURING PREGNANCY

CARDIOVASCULAR SYSTEM

Position of the Heart
- Heart is shifted anteriorly toward the left.
- It rotates toward a transverse position as the uterus enlarges.

Heart Rate
Increases during pregnancy by 15 to 20 beats/min. Resting heart rate starts to rise during the first trimester.

Heart Sounds
- Heart sounds are louder in pregnancy.
- The S3 heart sound is common (80%) in pregnant women (but not S4).
- There is wide splitting of S1.
- In the third trimester, splitting of S2 may be heard.

Murmurs
- A systolic ejection murmur (grade II/IV) over the pulmonary and tricuspid areas is common.
- A diastolic murmur is almost always pathologic; refer to cardiology.
- A mammary soufflé (systole or continuous) is heard over the breasts later in pregnancy and during lactation (breastfeeding).

Cardiac Output
- Increases by 30% to 50% and peaks at about 28 to 34 weeks' gestation
- Reduction of systemic vascular resistance and systolic BP

Plasma Volume
- Plasma volume increases by almost 50% by the end of the second trimester.
- Hemodilution results in physiologic anemia of pregnancy (hematocrit and hemoglobin decreased).

Physiologic Anemia of Pregnancy
- Physiologic anemia of pregnancy is most obvious from 6 to 9 months (second and third trimesters).
- Hemoglobin and hematocrit are decreased because of the hemodilution from increased plasma volume. The hemoglobin can decrease to as low as 10.5 g/dL.

Preload and Afterload
- Preload increases because of higher blood volume.
- Afterload goes down because of the decrease in peripheral vascular resistance that occurs during pregnancy.

Blood Pressure
- Systolic and diastolic BP starts to decrease in the first trimester and continues in the second trimester. Many mothers who are hypertensive before pregnancy can be off prescription antihypertensives at this time.
- By the third trimester, BP gradually returns back to pre-pregnancy levels. Antihypertensives used for pregnant women are methyldopa (Aldomet) and labetalol (Normodyne; beta-blocker).

EXAM TIPS

- S3 heart murmur is normal finding in pregnancy.
- Preferred medications for hypertension in pregnancy are methyldopa (Aldomet), labetalol (beta-blocker), hydralazine, and long-acting nifedipine. For methyldopa, check LFTs at baseline and periodically (contraindicated if active hepatic disease). Discontinue if jaundice, abnormal LFTs, or unexplained fever occur.

Vena Cava
- Compression by enlarged uterus (20 weeks' gestation till labor) of the inferior vena cava decreases blood return to the brain, resulting in orthostatic hypotension (postural hypotensive syndrome).
- Advise woman to lie on the left side and change positions slowly.

Coagulation Factors
Pregnancy is a hypercoagulable state (clotting factors go up), especially after labor (puerperium or postpartum period).

Varicose Veins
Varicose veins become more severe during pregnancy.

Edema
Peripheral edema is considered normal in pregnancy. Mild edema of the lower extremities and the feet is most noticeable in the third trimester.

OTHER SYSTEMS

Respiratory System
- Presence of basal rales that disappear with coughing or deep breathing
- Feeling of breathlessness (innocent hyperpnea) and decreased exercise tolerance
- Physiologic dyspnea in pregnancy has a slow onset. Sudden-onset dyspnea is abnormal; rule out pulmonary emboli (pleuritic chest pain, tachypnea, hemoptysis).
- The gravid uterus pushes up the diaphragm as it gets larger; the diameter of the thorax is increased.
- No change in forced expiratory volume in 1 second (FEV1), but total lung capacity drops slightly from 4.2 to 4 L.

Endocrine System

Diffusely enlarged (size up to 15% larger), with higher metabolic activity.

Gastrointestinal System

Decreased peristalsis and decreased lower esophageal pressure from progesterone effects (constipation, heartburn)

Integumentary System (Skin and Hair)

Pigmentary Changes

- Pigmentary changes from increase in melanocyte-stimulating hormone from higher levels of estrogen. Causes the linea nigra (dark pigmented "line" that extends from the mons pubis to the umbilicus located midline).
- The nipples and areola darken.

Chloasma (Melasma)

- Blotchy hyperpigmentation on forehead, cheeks, nose, and upper lip seen in pregnant women and some birth control pill users. Usually gets lighter and regresses within 1 year; however, in some women, hyperpigmentation may be permanent.
- Condition is more common in darker skins (olive skins and darker).

Striae Gravidarum (Stretch Marks)

Most common locations are abdomen, breasts, and thighs. Other less common areas are upper arms, lower back, and buttocks.

Telogen Effluvium (Hair Loss)

During the postpartum period, hair loss may accelerate, but it is temporary.

EXAM TIP

Chloasma/melasma is due to high estrogen level.

Renal System

- Kidney size increases during pregnancy. The ureters and renal pelvis become dilated (physiologic hydronephrosis).
- Glomerular filtration rate (GFR) is much higher in pregnancy because of higher cardiac output and renal blood flow.

Ear, Nose, and Throat

- Some women develop nasal congestion and/or epistaxis due to increased blood flow to the nasopharynx during pregnancy.
- Rule out acute sinusitis if purulent mucus seen in posterior pharynx.

Musculoskeletal System

- Weight gain, enlarged uterus, and hormonal changes contribute to joint ligamentous laxity and exaggerated lordosis of the lumbar spine.
- Up to 60% of pregnant women experience back pain (not related to labor).
- Gait changes to wider stance.

OBSTETRIC HISTORY

Table 18.3 Obstetric History (G-T-P-A-L)

Term	Definition
Gravida or G	Number of pregnancies (twins or multiples counted as one pregnancy)
Term or T	Number of deliveries after 37 weeks
Preterm or P	Number of deliveries after 20 weeks (up to 37 weeks)
Abortion or A	Number of deliveries before 20 weeks (induced or spontaneous)
Living or L	Number of living children

Example: 28-Year-Old G5T3P1A1L5

- G: 5 (five pregnancies total)
- T: 3 (three pregnancies full term)
- P: 1 (one twin pregnancy preterm born at 34 weeks)
- A: 1 (one abortion)
- L: 5 (five living children)

POSTPARTUM (OR PUERPERIUM)

Occurs immediately after delivery and generally lasts about 6 weeks.

BREASTFEEDING

Colostrum and Breast Milk

During the first few days (days 1–2) of breastfeeding, colostrum is produced (thick yellow color), which contains maternal antibodies (passive immunity). By the third to the fourth day, mature breast milk is produced (contains fat, sugar/lactose, water, protein, and antibodies). The full-term healthy infant can be exclusively breastfed for the first 6 months of life, with no supplemental fluids unless ill or dehydrated.

Vitamin D

- All breastfed infants need vitamin D supplementation started within the first few days.
- Formula-fed infants should only be given iron-fortified formula (has vitamin D).

Iron

- All exclusively breastfed infants require iron (ferrous sulfate) supplementation starting at age 4 months at a dose of 1 mg/kg of body weight. Breast milk contains very little iron.
- Most full-term newborns have sufficient iron stores in their bodies for at least 4 months.
- At about 6 months, infants' iron needs can be met through introduction of iron-rich foods, iron-fortified cereals, or iron supplement drops.
- Infants on iron-fortified formula do not need additional iron supplementation.

Breastfeeding Technique

- Breastfeed within the first hour of birth. It provides the baby with colostrum and helps the uterus contract.
- A new mother should be taught proper breastfeeding technique. Refer to lactation specialist if having problems; follow up at home.
- If noisy, assess for improper latch on (check positioning, sucking, clicking noises). Swallowing noises are normal, but not clicking noises.
- For clicking, advise the mother to use her index finger to pull down the baby's chin so that the baby's lower lip will be outside. The baby should have the entire nipple and most of the areola inside its mouth.
- Newborns will nurse about 8 to 12 times per 24 hours.

Steps to a Good Latch

1. Infant's chest and stomach should rest against body; head is straight and not turned to the side.
2. Tickle infant's lips with nipple and aim nipple just above infant's top lip.
3. Ensure nipple and areola are inside the infant's mouth (baby's tongue will cup under the breast with lips turned out; Figure 18.3).
4. May hear/see swallowing, and the infant's ears may wiggle slightly.
5. Breast soreness is normal the first few days of breastfeeding; a proper latch on will help make it more comfortable.
6. If improper latch on, gently place a clean finger in the corner of the infant's mouth to break the seal (suction) and start again.

Sore Nipples

- Advise the mother not to stop breastfeeding. This causes breast engorgement (painful).
- If poor latch, the infant may have to suck harder, which causes pain.
- This results from babies having difficulty "latching on" to an engorged breast.
- Nipple pain is worse during the first week and usually disappears by the second week.

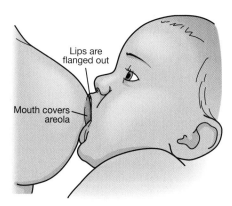

Figure 18.3 Breastfeeding (correct latch-on position).
Source: Adapted from Blausen.com staff. (2014). (See Resources section for complete source information.)

- If nipple pain persists, assess nipples for fissures and infection.
- Start nursing on the less painful breast first.
- Initiate "letdown reflex" of milk by massage/warm shower.
- Apply lanolin or breast milk to nipple after nursing to protect from skin breakdown.
- Avoid using plastic nipple shields, alcohol, and soap. Wear nursing bras with good support.
- May need referral to a lactation specialist (e.g., La Leche League)

Maternal Benefits

- Stimulates uterine contractions (speeds up uterine involution after delivery).
- Increases maternal bonding with infant (oxytocin effect).
- Speeds up weight loss after pregnancy.
- Lowers risk of breast/ovarian cancer.
- Can delay ovulation if mother breastfeeds exclusively.

Fetal Health Benefits

- Lowers risk of infections (necrotizing enterocolitis, acute otitis media).
- Lowers risk of bacterial and viral infections such as otitis media and diarrhea.
- Lower incidence of asthma and allergies in breastfed babies.
- Young infants who are exclusively breastfed get enough fluids and do not need extra water. Juices should be avoided, because they increase the risk of dental caries.
- Lowers risk of sudden infant death syndrome (SIDS) and future obesity.

EXAM TIPS

- Swallowing noises may be heard in breastfeeding, especially in younger babies. If clicking noises are heard during breastfeeding, it is abnormal. Advise the mother to use her index finger to pull down the baby's chin so that the baby's lower lip will latch better onto the areola.
- If a question describes a mother who complains of sore nipples, do not advise her to stop breastfeeding, to supplement with formula, or to use formula at nighttime feedings. The best answer is to advise the mother that it is a common problem during the first 2 weeks and will resolve and to continue breastfeeding.

POSTPARTUM CONTRACEPTION

- Women who exclusively breastfeed (at least every 4 hours daily) with amenorrhea and who are <6 months postpartum are much less likely to ovulate than a woman who does not breastfeed exclusively (lactational amenorrhea method).
- In women who do not breastfeed, ovulation resumes (average) at 39 days postpartum. During the postpartum period and with breastfeeding, combined hormonal contraceptives or any contraceptive method containing estrogen (pregnancy Category X) is contraindicated.

- Postpartum women or women who cannot take estrogens can use methods such as IUDs (copper or levonorgestrel) or progesterone-only contraception such as etonogestrel (Nexplanon), depot medroxyprogesterone (Depo-Provera), progestin-only pills, or barrier methods (condoms, diaphragm, cervical cap).
  - The progestin-only contraceptive pill norethindrone (Micronor) contains 28 active pills that are taken daily (no pill-free week).
  - For maximum effectiveness, pill must be taken at the same time each day (very important). If more than 3 hours late, take dose as soon as possible and use backup (condom) for the next 2 days. Will probably have vaginal spotting for the next few days.

UTERINE INVOLUTION

- It is normal for postpartum women to have uterine contractions (spontaneous or with breastfeeding) during the first 2 to 3 days after giving birth. After delivery, the uterus is the size of a 20-week pregnancy (fundi at the umbilicus).
- A soft boggy uterus accompanied by heavy vaginal bleeding is a sign of atony (inadequate contraction).
- Uterine involution takes about 6 weeks.

DISEASE REVIEW

COMPLETE ABORTION

Vaginal bleeding with cramping occurs. Placenta and fetus are expelled completely. Cervical os will close, and bleeding stops.

GESTATIONAL DIABETES MELLITUS

GDM is diabetes that occurs during pregnancy. GDM mothers are at high risk for type 2 diabetes. GDM has high rates of recurrence (33%–50% chance) in future pregnancies. GDM has concomitant higher rates of neural tube defects (anencephaly, microcephaly), congenital heart disease, birth trauma (shoulder dystocia), preeclampsia, and neonatal hypoglycemia. Risk factors are history of GDM in a previous pregnancy, obesity, ethnicity (Asian, American Indian, Pacific Islander, African American, Hispanic), macrosomic infant (>9 1b), and age (older than 35 years). If there is a history of GDM, check for prediabetes or diabetes at 4 to 12 weeks postpartum and advise lifelong screening at least every 3 years.

Evaluation

- Screen at the first visit if history of GDM and/or presence of risk factors.
- If not high risk for GDM, screen at 24 to 28 weeks' gestation.
- There are two methods of testing for GDM (one-step or two-step strategy).

One-Step Method

- Administer 75-g oral glucose tolerance test (OGTT; check fasting, 1 hour, and 2 hours). Overnight fast of at least 8 hours. Perform test in the morning.

- 2020 diagnostic criteria from the American Diabetes Association (ADA):
  - Fasting: ≥92 mg/dL
  - 1 hour: ≥180 mg/dL
  - 2 hours: ≥153 mg/dL
- The 75-gram OGTT is the preferred test.

Two-Step Method

- Screening: 50-g glucose load (nonfasting), check plasma glucose at 1 hour.
- If ≥140 mg/dL: Rule out GDM. Order 100-g OGTT (fasting, 1 hour, 2 hours, and 3 hours).
- 2020 diagnostic criteria from the ADA:
  - Fasting: ≥95 mg/dL
  - 1 hour: ≥180 mg/dL
  - 2 hours: ≥155 mg/dL
  - 3 hours: ≥140 mg/dL

CLINICAL PEARLS

- GDM is diagnosed in the second to third trimester.
- A woman with diabetes in the first trimester has type 2 diabetes.
- An A1C <6% (second to third trimester) has the lowest risk for large-for-gestational-age infants.

EXAM TIPS

- There are two methods of screening for GDM. One-step method uses the 75-g OGTT (both for screening and diagnosis). Two-step method uses 50-g OGTT test (nonfasting) as the screening test.
- If 50-g OGTT is abnormal (postprandial >140 mg/dL or fasting >95 g/dL), follow-up test is 100-g OGTT (must fast for at least 8 hours).

Treatment Plan

- Glycemic targets in pregnancy are:
  - Preprandial: ≤95 mg/dL
  - 1 hour post meal: ≤140 mg/dL
  - 2 hours post meal: ≤120 mg/dL
  - A1C goal: <6%
- First-line treatment is lifestyle (follow a meal plan and scheduled physical activity):
  - Eat three meals per day plus two or three snacks. Limit carbohydrates.
  - Exercise 30 minutes per day at least 5 days a week (total of 2 hours per week).
  - Low-impact exercises such as walking and swimming are preferred.
- Perform frequent home glucose monitoring (four to six times per day).
- If medication needed, human insulin is the preferred agent. Insulin injections needed if unable to control blood glucose with diet and exercise.

- May need to self-inject insulin from three to six times per day.
- ADA and American Congress of Obstetricians and Gynecologists (ACOG) have endorsed use of oral anti-hyperglycemic drugs glyburide and metformin.
- Check blood glucose at least four times per day (fasting, 1 or 2 hours after the first bite of each meal).

Follow-Up

Test for prediabetes or diabetes at 4 to 12 weeks postpartum and at least every 3 years afterward (future).

NOTE

The lowest rates of adverse fetal outcomes (large-for-gestational age infant, preterm delivery, preeclampsia) occur with an A1C <6% to 6.5%.

EXAM TIPS

- First-line treatment for GDM is lifestyle change (correct diet and scheduled exercises).
- Learn the risk factors for GDM.

INCOMPLETE ABORTION (ABORTION WITH RETAINED PRODUCTS OF CONCEPTION)

Vaginal bleeding with cramping occurs. Placental products remain in the uterus. Cervical os may remain dilated, and bleeding persists; pieces of tissue may be seen at the cervical os. Vaginal discharge may be foul smelling (bacterial vaginosis). Treatment is dilation and curettage (D&C) and antibiotics.

INEVITABLE ABORTION

Cervix is dilated and unable to stop process. Fetus will be aborted.

LACTATIONAL MASTITIS (BREASTFEEDING MASTITIS)

Most common in the first 2 months of breastfeeding. Skin fissures on the nipple(s) allow bacterial entry. Most common organism is *Staphylococcus aureus* (gram positive). Consider methicillin-resistant *S. aureus* (MRSA) bacterial infection (becoming more common). If severe or toxic, refer to ED or admit to the hospital.

Prevention

Frequent and complete emptying of breast and proper breastfeeding technique. Breast engorgement and poor technique increase risk of mastitis.

Classic Case

Patient who is breastfeeding complains of a sudden onset of a red, firm, and tender area (induration) on one breast. May also have fever/chills and malaise (flu-like symptoms). May have adenopathy on the axilla by the affected breast. Most common in the first 3 months of breastfeeding.

Labs

- Usually not needed; this is a clinical diagnosis.
- CBC shows leukocytosis; C&S of milk is usually not required, but it can be useful to guide antibiotic selection, particularly if hospital acquired, severe, or not responding to antibiotic treatment.
- Ultrasound may be useful if mastitis does not respond in 48 to 72 hours.

Treatment Plan

If Low Risk of Methicillin-Resistant Staphylococcus Aureus

- Dicloxacillin 500 mg PO QID or cephalexin (Keflex) 500 mg PO QID for 10 to 14 days.
- Do not use sulfas during the newborn period, due to increased risk of kernicterus.

If High Risk of Methicillin-Resistant Staphylococcus Aureus

- Trimethoprim–sulfamethoxazole (Bactrim) one to two tablets PO BID (can be used if healthy infant is 1 month or older, no jaundice) *or* clindamycin 300 mg PO QID for 10 to 14 days.
- Continue to breastfeed on affected breast during antibiotic treatment. If unable to breastfeed, pump milk from infected breast (and discard) to prevent engorgement. Complete emptying of the breast is important during the infection.
- If breast abscess is suspected, order an ultrasound and refer for incision and drainage.
- NSAID for pain and fever as needed. Apply cold compresses on indurated breast area.
- Refer to lactation consultant if suspect poor breastfeeding technique.

OBSTETRIC COMPLICATIONS

Preeclampsia

Most cases of preeclampsia occur in the late third trimester (34 weeks' gestation or later). It can occur up to 4 weeks after childbirth (postpartum period). Mild cases of preeclampsia may not have symptoms such as headaches, blurred vision, or right upper quadrant abdominal pain.

Can cause multiorgan damage to the brain (stroke); kidneys (acute renal failure); lungs (pulmonary edema); liver (hepatic rupture), as well as DIC and fetal and/or maternal death. Older name is "toxemia." The exact etiology of preeclampsia is unknown. If seizures develop, the woman will be diagnosed with eclampsia.

Risk factors include primigravida, multipara, >35 years of age, obesity, prior history of preeclampsia, hypertension, or kidney disease.

Diagnostic Criteria

Classic triad of hypertension, proteinuria, and edema that occur after 20 weeks' gestation and up to 4 weeks postpartum. Take at least two separate readings (at least 6 hours apart).

- BP: Systolic ≥140 mmHg *OR* diastolic ≥90 mmHg
- Proteinuria: >0.3 g protein in a 24-hour urine specimen. Proteinuria ranges from trace to 1+ to 4+ (severe cases).
- Rapid weight gain of 2 to 5 lb per week: The edema is most obvious in the face, around the eyes, and on the hands.

Treatment Plan

Refer to obstetrician for management. The only definitive "cure" for preeclampsia and eclampsia is delivery of the placenta/fetus.

Preexisting/Chronic Hypertension

Defined as the presence of an elevated BP (>140/90 mmHg) before the 20th week of gestation. Do not confuse this condition with preeclampsia. May be on a prescription. If on an ACE inhibitor or ARB, discontinue as soon as possible and monitor BP closely. Most pregnant women with preexisting hypertension can usually get off their BP medications (temporarily) during the first to second trimester because of the lowering of BP during pregnancy (less peripheral vascular resistance).

Placenta Abruptio (Placental Abruption)

Premature partial to complete separation of a normally implanted placenta from the uterine bed. Rupture of the maternal blood vessels from the decidua basalis. Bleeding ranges from mild to hemorrhage. Controllable risk factors are smoking, cocaine use, hypertension, and encouraged seatbelt use.

Classic Case

Sudden onset of vaginal bleeding (mild to hemorrhage) with abdominal and/or back pain. Painful uterine contractions. Uterus is rigid (hypertonic) and very tender.

Treatment Plan

- Refer to the ED.
- Initial ED labs are CBC, prothrombin time (PT)/partial thromboplastin time (PTT), blood type, cross-match, Rh factor, and so on.
- Abdominal ultrasound and blood transfusion needed.
- If mild contractions, give magnesium sulfate (MgSO$_4$) IV. Strict bedrest is needed.
- Deliver fetus by C-section if mother's life is threatened. Give steroids if fetus is viable.

Placenta Previa

This is an abnormally implanted placenta. The placenta implants too low either on top of the cervix or on the cervical isthmus/neck. Most cases get better spontaneously (will reimplant). Some cases are asymptomatic. Higher risk if previous history of placenta previa or C-section, multipara, older age, smoking, fibroids, or cocaine use.

Classic Case

A multipara woman who is in the late second to third trimester of pregnancy complains of a sudden onset of bright-red vaginal bleeding (light to heavy) accompanied by mild contractions. The uterus feels soft and is not tender.

Treatment Plan

- Refer to ED if bleeding.
- Avoid bimanual examination, because palpation of the uterus may cause severe hemorrhage.
- Use abdominal ultrasound only. No intravaginal ultrasound. No rectal or digital vaginal exams.
- Avoid any vaginal/rectal sexual intercourse.

- Avoid strenuous exercise and lifting of heavy objects. Close fetal and maternal monitoring.
- If contractions, give magnesium sulfate (MgSO$_4$) IV. If mild case, pregnancy can be salvaged, and the placenta will reimplant.

OLIGOHYDRAMNIOS

Amniotic fluid volume is less than expected for gestational age. Usually diagnosed by ultrasound and measured as the amniotic fluid index (AFI <5 cm) or the deepest vertical pocket (DVP). An AFI of 5 to 25 cm is considered normal. The uterus is smaller in size than expected. At higher risk of fetal malformation, pulmonary hypoplasia, umbilical cord compression, and fetal or neonatal death. It may occur in the first, second, or third trimester. Multiple causes; it can be idiopathic or have maternal, fetal, or placental causes. Refer to obstetrician for management.

POLYHYDRAMNIOS

An excessive volume of amniotic fluid (AFI >25 cm) that is more than expected for gestational age. Occurs in approximately 1% of pregnancies. Fetal anomalies (usually associated with genetic abnormality or syndrome) are the most common causes of polyhydramnios. Refer to obstetrician for management.

Rh-INCOMPATIBILITY DISEASE

In Rh-negative mothers with Rh-positive fetuses, the maternal immune system develops antibodies against Rh-positive blood if not given RhoGAM (gamma globulin against Rh factor). Give RhoGAM for all pregnancies of Rh-negative mothers—even if they terminate in miscarriages, abortions, or tubal or ectopic pregnancies.

RhoGAM

Also known as *anti-D immune globulin*. It is made from pooled IgG antibodies against Rh (rhesus) factor. It is an immunoglobulin that helps prevent maternal isoimmunization (self-immunization) or alloimmunization (immunity against another individual of the same species). If RhoGAM is not given to Rh-negative pregnant women, this will result in fetal hemolysis and fetal anemia in her future pregnancies.

- Coombs test detects presence of Rh antibodies in the mother (indirect Coombs test).
- RhoGAM 300 mcg IM first dose is at 28 weeks.
- Give second dose within 72 hours (or sooner) after delivery.
- RhoGAM decreases the risk of isoimmunization of the maternal immune system by destroying fetal Rh-positive red blood cells (RBCs) that have crossed the placenta.

EXAM TIP

Learn action of RhoGAM (Rh antibodies that hemolyze Rh-positive fetal RBCs).

SPONTANEOUS ABORTION

Also known as a *miscarriage*. Spontaneous loss of the fetus before it is viable (<20 weeks).

STILLBIRTH OR FETAL DEATH

Pregnancy loss that occurs at 20 weeks' gestation or later or weight of 350 grams or greater.

THREATENED ABORTION

Vaginal bleeding occurs, but cervical os remains closed. Most of these cases will result in an ongoing pregnancy.

UNCOMPLICATED CHLAMYDIA INFECTION (CERVICITIS, URETHRITIS)

Treating *Chlamydia trachomatis* infection in the mother will help to prevent the transmission (vertical transmission) of the infection to the newborn through the birth canal. Example: Trachoma (or inclusion conjunctivitis of the newborn) and pneumonia

Labs

- Obtain nucleic acid amplification tests (NAATs) such as the Gen-Probe, Amplicor, or ProbeTec.
- Gen-Probe can only be used on the cervix and urethra. Do not use to collect specimens from the eyes.
- Test of cure needed in 3 weeks after completing treatment.

Treatment Plan

- First-line: Azithromycin 1 g orally (single dose)
- Alternative: Amoxicillin 500 mg PO TID × 7 days (lower cure rate than azithromycin)

Sexual Partners

- First-line is azithromycin 1 g orally (single dose)
- Doxycycline 100 mg PO BID × 7 days (do not use if breastfeeding stains tooth enamel, Category D)
- Avoid sexual activity for 7 days; avoid unprotected intercourse until both partners are treated; test for other sexually transmitted infections (e.g., gonorrhea, syphilis, HIV)

URINARY TRACT INFECTIONS

Acute cystitis can occur alone, or it may be complicated by acute pyelonephritis. The most common organism is *Escherichia coli* (75%–95%). Signs and symptoms include dysuria, frequency, urgency, and nocturia. Higher risk of preterm birth and low birth weight is observed.

Asymptomatic Bacteriuria

Pregnant women with asymptomatic bacteriuria are always treated because they are at high risk for acute pyelonephritis and preterm labor. Diagnosis is based on midstream urine C&S results. Obtain specimen before antibiotic treatment and after (to check for eradication of infection). UTIs increase the risk of preterm birth, low birth weight, and perinatal mortality.

Management

- Urine dipstick
  - WBCs (leukocyte esterase): Positive
  - Nitrite: May be positive or negative
- Send midstream urine for urinalysis (UA) and urine C&S.
- Document resolution of infection by ordering post-treatment urine C&S 1 week after completing antibiotic therapy.
- If suspect pyelonephritis, refer to ED.

Medications

- Nitrofurantoin (Macrobid) BID × 5 to 7 days (avoid using during the last trimester). Do not use sulfa drugs (e.g., Bactrim) or nitrofurantoin near term because of the risk of hyperbilirubinemia; causes hemolysis if the mother (or both mother and baby) has G6PD anemia.
- Amoxicillin–clavulanate (Augmentin) BID × 3 to 7 days
- Amoxicillin BID × 3 to 7 days
- Cephalexin BID × 3 to 7 days
- Fosfomycin 3-g single dose

Sulfa Drugs

- Sulfa drugs should be avoided near term (38–42 weeks), during labor, and during delivery. They are also contraindicated in neonates younger than 4 weeks of age.
- These drugs increase the risk of hyperbilirubinemia (bilirubin is toxic to nerves and CNS).
- Complication of hyperbilirubinemia is called "kernicterus" (serious nerve/brain damage).
- Do not use if G6PD anemia is suspected (causes hemolysis).
- Nitrofurantoin causes serious adverse effects, such as pulmonary reactions (interstitial pneumonitis, pulmonary fibrosis), liver damage, neuropathy, and others.

KNOWLEDGE CHECK: CHAPTER 18

1. Hegar's sign is considered a:
   A. Positive sign of pregnancy
   B. Probable sign of pregnancy
   C. Presumptive sign of pregnancy
   D. Problem in pregnancy

2. Which of the following statements is *true* regarding a threatened abortion?
   A. Vaginal bleeding and cramping are present, but the cervix remains closed.
   B. Vaginal bleeding and cramping are present along with a dilated cervix.
   C. The fetus and placenta are both expelled.
   D. The products of conception and the placenta remain inside the uterus along with a dilated cervix.

3. A multigravida patient who is at 28 weeks' gestation has a fundal height of 29 cm. Which of the following is the *best* recommendation for this patient?
   A. Advise the patient that the pregnancy is progressing well
   B. Order an ultrasound of the uterus
   C. Refer the patient to an obstetrician for an amniocentesis
   D. Recommend bedrest with bathroom privileges

4. The nurse practitioner notes the following result on a routine urinalysis of a 37-year-old primigravida patient who is at 30 weeks' gestation: leukocyte = trace, nitrite = negative, protein = 2+, blood = negative. The patient's weight has increased by 5 lb during the past week. Which of the following is *most likely*?
   A. HELLP syndrome
   B. Pregnancy-induced hypertension
   C. Eclampsia of pregnancy
   D. Primary hypertension

5. A 28-year-old multipara patient who is at 32 weeks' gestation presents complaining of a sudden onset of small amounts of bright-red vaginal bleeding. The patient has had several episodes of bleeding and appears anxious. On exam, the uterus is soft to palpation. Which diagnosis is *most likely*?
   A. Placenta abruptio
   B. Placenta previa
   C. Acute cervicitis
   D. Molar pregnancy

6. A 27-year-old patient who is pregnant for the first time presents at 35 weeks' gestation for a prenatal visit. The patient has a history of chronic hypertension and is often unreliable with taking antihypertensive medication. While listening for fetal heart tones, the patient experiences significant acute abdominal pain followed by a gush of vaginal bleeding. Which of the following is the *most important* diagnosis to rule out?
   A. Preterm labor
   B. Placenta previa
   C. Preeclampsia
   D. Placental abruption

7. Magnesium sulfate is used in pregnancy for which of the following?
   A. Severe constipation
   B. Neuroprotection for hypertensive disorders
   C. As an antihypertensive
   D. Preterm labor

8. Which of the following is considered a Category D drug per the U.S. Food and Drug Administration (FDA)?
   A. Nitrofurantoin
   B. Ciprofloxacin
   C. Isotretinoin
   D. Ceftriaxone

9. Which of the following vaccines is contraindicated in pregnancy?
   A. Injected influenza
   B. Measles, mumps, rubella
   C. Tdap
   D. COVID-19

10. A patient presents with a known last menstrual period of January 6. Using Naegele's rule, what would be her estimated due date?
    A. October 13
    B. October 31
    C. September 26
    D. September 30

(See answers next page.)

1. B) Probable sign of pregnancy

Hegar's sign is softening of the lower portion of the uterus and is considered a probable sign of pregnancy. Positive signs include direct visualization (e.g., via ultrasound) or detection (e.g., by fetoscope) of the fetus. Presumptive signs (e.g., amenorrhea, nausea) are the least objective—relying on reports of symptoms from the patient—and may be caused by other conditions.

2. A) Vaginal bleeding and cramping are present, but the cervix remains closed.

Threatened abortion is defined as vaginal bleeding and cramping without the presence of cervical dilation. Bleeding in the presence of dilation may indicate inevitable abortion. Complete abortion involves bleeding accompanied by expulsion of the placenta and fetus. With incomplete abortion, bleeding and dilation occur, but placental products remain in the uterus.

3. A) Advise the patient that the pregnancy is progressing well

Between 20 and 35 weeks, the fundal height is equal to the number of weeks of gestation plus or minus 2 cm. Fundal height is measured as the distance between the pubic bone and the uterine fundus. For example, a patient who is at 30 weeks' gestation who has a fundal height of 29 cm is within normal limits. A fundal height outside these limits requires further assessment; ordering an ultrasound would be the next step. There is no need to recommend bedrest for this patient or to refer them to an obsetrician.

4. B) Pregnancy-induced hypertension

This patient is exhibiting two of the classic triad of symptoms of pregnancy-induced hypertension, or preeclampsia: hypertension, edema (weight gain), and proteinuria. Symptoms of HELLP syndrome include nausea, headache, belly pain, and swelling. Symptoms of eclampsia include upper right abdominal pain, severe headache, and vision and mental status changes.

5. B) Placenta previa

Placenta previa occurs when the placenta implants abnormally, partially, or wholly in the lower segment of the uterus or over the internal os. A classic presentation is painless bright-red vaginal bleeding in the second and/or third trimester. Do not perform digital vaginal or cervical exams in any pregnant patient with bleeding until the location of the placenta is known (abdominal ultrasound). Avoid vaginal exam or rectal exam if placenta previa is suspected, and advise the patient to avoid sexual intercourse. With placenta abruptio, the uterus is hard and tender. In molar pregnancy, bleeding occurs during the first trimester. In acute cervicitis, bleeding occurs between menstrual periods or after intercourse.

6. D) Placental abruption

A placental abruption usually occurs in the later weeks of pregnancy and is characterized by abrupt abdominal pain. There may or may not be vaginal bleeding depending on the location and severity of the abruption. Preterm labor does not cause acute abdominal pain followed by vaginal bleeding. Placental previa does not cause pain. While a patient with underlying hypertension should be followed closely for the development of preeclampsia, this patient's presentation most closely resembles an abruption.

7. B) Neuroprotection for hypertensive disorders

Magnesium sulfate is used when patients are admitted to labor and delivery with a hypertensive disorder in order to help prevent eclampsia. It is not an antihypertensive, and it is not effective for preterm labor. Constipation in pregnancy is often treated with diet and lifestyle changes. Stool softeners can be used as well.

8. B) Ciprofloxacin

Ciprofloxacin is a Category D drug. Nitrofurantoin and ceftriaxone are both Category B drugs. Isotretinoin is a Category X drug.

9. B) Measles, mumps, rubella

The measles, mumps, rubella (MMR) vaccine is a live virus, so it is contraindicated in pregnancy. The American College of Obstetricians and Gynecologists (ACOG) recommends vaccinating pregnant patients with the injectable influenza vaccine, Tdap, and COVID-19.

10. A) October 13

Naegele's rule is last menstrual period + 9 months + 7 days or last menstrual period – 3 months + 7 days.

11. A patient presents for a prenatal exam for a single-ton pregnancy. The patient reports currently feeling well. The fundus is palpated approximately midway between the symphysis pubis and the umbilicus. Based on this information, about how many weeks' gestation would the patient be?
    A. 12
    B. 16
    C. 18
    D. 20

12. A patient presents for a prenatal exam. The patient is G3P1011. Which of the following statements reflects the pregnancy and childbirth history?
    A. This is the third pregnancy. The patient is currently pregnant; has had one live, term birth and one abortion; and has one living child.
    B. The patient has had three pregnancies, with one abortion, one preterm delivery, and one live delivery.
    C. The patient has had two pregnancies: one twin gestation and one abortion.
    D. This is the third pregnancy. The patient has had one live birth and one preterm delivery and is currently pregnant.

13. A 32-year-old G2P1 patient at 31 weeks and 5 days' gestation presents to the clinic with a chief complaint of headache. The patient reports otherwise feeling well and denies any visual changes or nausea. On physical examination, fetal heart tones are auscultated at 160 beats per minute, fundal height is 32 cm, and blood pressure is 162/110 mmHg. Which of the following is the *best* course of action?
    A. Administer nitroglycerin and perform an electrocardiogram
    B. Refer to labor and delivery, order preeclampsia labs, and begin labetalol
    C. Prescribe lisinopril and have the patient return in 24 hours for a blood pressure check
    D. Prescribe labetalol and have the patient return in 2 weeks for a blood pressure check

14. A G2P1 patient presents for an initial prenatal visit at 12 weeks' gestation. The patient's blood type is O negative. Which of the following is the *best* course of action for this patient?
    A. Plan delivery via cesarean section
    B. Check an antibody screen and, if positive, administer RhoGAM
    C. Check an antibody screen and, if negative, recheck at 28 weeks
    D. Plan on administering RhoGAM when the patient is 72 hours post partum

15. A G2P1 patient at 35 weeks' gestation presents for a routine prenatal visit. The patient has no known medical allergies. A Group B *Streptococcus* screen is performed, and the results are positive. Which of the following *best* describes the appropriate course of action?
    A. Treat only if the neonate tests positive after delivery
    B. Prescribe erythromycin 500 mg QID x 7 days
    C. Administer clindamycin 150 mg IV during labor
    D. Administer penicillin G 5 million units IV during labor

(See answers next page.)

11. B) 16

In a singleton pregnancy, if the fundus is palpated midway between the symphysis pubis and umbilicus, it is at approximately 16 weeks' gestation. The level of the umbilicus correlates to 20 weeks' gestation.

12. A) This is the third pregnancy. The patient is currently pregnant; has had one live, term birth and one abortion; and has one living child.

There can be four numbers after the "P" for "para." Para is the total number of pregnancies. The first number after the P is the number of term pregnancies. The second number is how many premature babies were delivered. The third number is how many abortions or miscarriages the patient has had. The fourth number is how many children are alive.

13. B) Refer to labor and delivery, order preeclampsia labs, and begin labetalol

The patient has a hypertensive emergency and must be evaluated in labor and delivery. Outpatient management is not appropriate. Angiotensin-converting enzyme (ACE) inhibitors such as lisinopril should never be used in pregnancy.

14. C) Check an antibody screen and, if negative, recheck at 28 weeks

If the patient is Rh negative, the most appropriate course of action is to check an antibody screen. If the screen is negative, it means there has been no alloimmunization, and RhoGAM can be given in the third trimester. If the antibody screen is positive, alloimmunization has occurred and the patient needs to be referred to maternal–fetal medicine. RhoGAM is given post partum if the neonate is found to be Rh positive.

15. D) Administer penicillin G 5 million units IV during labor

Patients with a positive Group B *Streptococcus* screen are treated during labor and delivery. Unless a true penicillin allergy exists, Pen G is the preferred treatment. Oral treatment during pregnancy is not advised.

ACQUIRED IMMUNODEFICIENCY SYNDROME

Without treatment, people with AIDS typically survive about 2 years, and most patients who receive highly active antiretroviral therapy (HAART) will survive >10 years. Without antiretroviral therapy (ART), HIV infection usually advances to AIDS within 10 years. AIDS is defined by an absolute CD4 cell count of fewer than 200 cells/mm³ along with certain opportunistic infections and malignancies. CD4 levels in healthy people range from 500 to 1,400 cells/mm³. Signs and symptoms that suggest AIDS include those caused by AIDS-defining opportunistic infections such as oral candidiasis, tuberculosis (TB), *Pneumocystis jirovecii* pneumonia, central nervous system (CNS) toxoplasmosis, histoplasmosis, cryptosporidiosis, Kaposi's sarcoma (purple to bluish-red bumps on the skin), and many others. *P. jirovecii* is a leading cause of opportunistic infection in patients with HIV.

ACUTE HIV INFECTION (ACUTE RETROVIRAL SYNDROME)

An estimated 10% to 60% of individuals with early HIV infection may be asymptomatic. It takes approximately 2 to 4 weeks to develop symptoms. The initial immune response may mimic mononucleosis (fever, headache, sore throat, lymphadenopathy, rash, joint ache, myalgia) and may be accompanied by diarrhea and weight loss. May have painful ulcerative lesions in the mouth due to HIV or from coinfection with herpes simplex, syphilis, or chancroid. Very infectious due to extremely high viral load (>100,000 copies/mL) in blood and genital secretions. Most people (97%) develop antibodies within 3 months after exposure. If acute HIV infection is strongly suspected, order the HIV RNA polymerase chain reaction (PCR) test, which can detect infection 7 to 28 days after exposure.

EXAM TIPS

- *Pneumocystis* pneumonia (PCP) prophylaxis is advised when CD4 count is ≤200 cells/mcL.
- Acute retroviral syndrome (or primary HIV infection) with flu-like or mono-like infection is very infectious at this stage. Best if HIV is treated as early as possible.

DISSEMINATED GONOCOCCAL INFECTION

A very small percentage (0.5%–3.0%) of individuals with gonococcal infection may progress to disseminated gonococcal infection (DGI). Two classic forms: One with triad of tenosynovitis (unique to DGI), dermatitis, and polyarthralgia with associated fever, chills, and malaise; other syndrome characterized by purulent arthritis. Consider in sexually active individuals who are younger than 40 years, those who have multiple partners, and in men who have sex with men (MSM) who present with arthralgias or joint pain concerning for septic arthritis. Look for the characteristic skin lesions of DGI (typically, painless and present as pustular or vesiculopustular) (Figure 19.1). May be accompanied by signs of sexually transmitted disease (STD) (e.g., cervicitis, urethritis). Localized infection of the urethra, cervix, rectum, or pharynx often precedes the onset of DGI. Occasionally complicated by perihepatitis (Fitz-Hugh–Curtis syndrome) and rarely endocarditis or meningitis. Refer to infectious disease specialist.

EXAM TIP

If STD symptoms with new onset of swollen red knee on side (or another joint), may be caused by DGI.

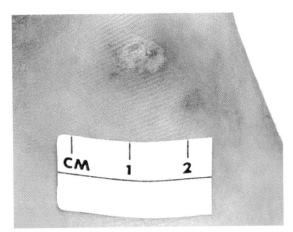

Figure 19.1 Characteristic skin lesion of disseminated gonococcal infection.
Source: Centers for Disease Control and Prevention/Dr. Wiesner.

NORMAL FINDINGS

- Female normal findings are covered in Chapter 17.
- Male normal findings are covered in Chapter 16.

STD SCREENING RECOMMENDED BY THE CENTERS FOR DISEASE CONTROL AND PREVENTION (2022)

- There are approximately 19 million STI incidents each year in the United States; almost half are in young people aged 15 to 24.
- Routine annual screening of all sexually active females aged 25 years or younger for *Chlamydia trachomatis* and gonorrhea. If positive, retest for chlamydia and gonorrhea 3 months after treatment (to check for reinfection, not for test-of-cure).
- Annual testing for syphilis, chlamydia, and gonorrhea in persons with HIV infection.
- Minors do not need parental consent if the clinic visit is related to testing or treating STDs and birth control; no state requires parental consent for STD care.
- STD screening includes obtaining the sexual history and assessment of risk factors for STDs; think of the five Ps (partners, practices, protection, past history of STDs, and prevention of pregnancy).
- Physical exam for STDs includes inspection of the skin, pharynx, lymph nodes, anus, pelvic/genital area, and neurologic system.
- Complications of untreated STD/STI are infertility, ectopic pregnancy, congenital infections, cervical cancer, chronic pelvic pain, chronic hepatitis, chronic syphilis, and HIV/AIDS.

Men Who Have Sex With Men

- Annual screening for chlamydia and gonorrhea at sites of contact (urethra, rectum), regardless of condom use. Screen every 3 to 6 months if at increased risk.
- Annual testing recommended for HIV and syphilis. Retest more frequently if at risk.
- All should undergo hepatitis B screening; consider hepatitis C screening in all adults over the age of 18 unless positivity rate is <0.1%.
- If history of anal-receptive intercourse, a digital anorectal exam can be offered as part of STD care.

Pregnant Patients

- Some STDs such as chlamydia, gonorrhea, and genital herpes can be passed from mother to infant during vaginal delivery. Others, such as HIV, herpes, syphilis, and hepatitis, can cause serious congenital infections in the fetus.
- Screen all pregnant patients for HIV, syphilis, and HBsAg at first prenatal visit.
- Screen all pregnant patients under 25 years of age and those 25 and older if at increased risk for chlamydia and gonorrhea.
- Pregnant patients treated for chlamydia and/or gonorrhea should have a test-of-cure 4 weeks after treatment and be retested within 3 months.
- Retest at 3 months for chlamydia and gonorrhea (check for reinfection, not test-of-cure).
- Consider hepatitis C screening except in settings where positivity rate is <0.1%.

STD RISK FACTORS

- Younger age (females age 15–24 years); sex initiated at a younger age
- Multiple sexual partners; new sexual partner in past 60 days
- Sex with partners recently treated for an STI
- Inconsistent condom use
- Trading sex for money or drugs; sex work
- Use of alcohol or illicit drugs
- Adolescents
- MSM
- History of previous STD
- HIV-positive status
- Pregnant females
- Admission to correctional facility
- Illicit drug use

DISEASE REVIEW

CHLAMYDIA TRACHOMATIS

C. trachomatis is a small gram-negative bacterium that is an obligate intracellular parasite. It is the most common bacterial STD in the United States. Most chlamydial infections are asymptomatic. The highest prevalence is among individuals 14 to 24 years of age.

- Annual screening of all sexually active women younger than 25 years of age is recommended by the CDC, as is screening of older women at increased risk for infection (e.g., those who have a new sexual partner, more than one sexual partner, a sexual partner with concurrent partners, or a sexual partner with an STI).
- During first prenatal visit, screen all pregnant women <25 years and older pregnant women at increased risk. Rescreen younger women <25 years of age in the third trimester.
- Screen young men in high prevalence clinical settings (e.g., correctional facilities, sexual health clinics).
- Annual screening for MSM at sites of contact (urethra, rectum) regardless of condom use, as well as every 3 to 6 months if at increased risk.
- Screen persons with HIV at first HIV evaluation and then at least annually.

Clinical Syndromes and Complications

- Females: Cervicitis (cervix is most commonly infected anatomic site), dysuria-pyuria syndrome due to urethritis, pelvic inflammatory disease (PID), perihepatitis (Fitz-Hugh-Curtis syndrome)
- Males: Urethritis, epididymitis, prostatitis
- All: Conjunctivitis, pharyngitis, proctitis and rectal infection, genital lymphogranuloma venereum, reactive arthritis/reactive arthritis triad
- Complications: PID, complications of pregnancy (e.g., premature rupture of membranes, preterm delivery, low-birth weight, ectopic pregnancy, infertility), upper genital tract infections, chronic pelvic pain, cervical cancer, and chronic infection with hepatitis viruses and HIV

Labs (Both Gonorrhea and Chlamydia)

- Nucleic acid amplification tests (NAATs) are highly sensitive tests for both gonorrhea and chlamydia. Be careful to use the correct NAAT testing kit. Swab samples (vagina, cervix, urethra, rectum, pharynx) or urine specimen can be collected for both males and females.
- Vaginal swab (specimen of choice in females) can be collected by a provider or self-collected in a clinical setting. Self-collected vaginal swab specimens are equivalent in sensitivity and specificity to those collected by a clinician using NAATs.
- Preferred diagnostic test for men is first-catch urine specimen for NAAT. Collect the first part of the urinary stream (15–20 mL) from the first void of the day.
- Rapid NAAT-based tests have been developed (e.g., XPert *C. trachomatis/Neisseria gonorrhoeae* [CT/NG] assay) and can provide results within 90 minutes; use on endocervical or vaginal swabs and urine.
- Tests not routinely recommended include culture, serology, antigen detection, genetic probe methods.
- If male patient shows urethritis symptoms, obtain Gram stain. Polymorphonuclear leukocytes with gram-negative intracellular diplococci can be used for males with gonorrheal urethritis (considered diagnostic). Not commonly used in primary care.

Treatment Plan

Chlamydia

Doxycycline 100 mg BID × 7 days: preferred agent for nonpregnant individuals

- Swallow with large amount of water; doxycycline may cause esophagitis (difficulty and/or pain with swallowing, acute-onset heartburn, nausea/vomiting).
- Nausea, gastrointestinal (GI) upset, photosensitivity (avoid sun or use sunscreen)
- Category D drug; risk of staining tooth enamel and skin hyperpigmentation

Alternative antibiotics

- Azithromycin 1 g PO in a single dose; ideally administered via directly observed therapy; preferred for pregnant individuals
- Fluoroquinolones (e.g., levofloxacin 500 mg once daily for seven days) indicated when coverage is needed for fluoroquinolone-susceptible pathogens (e.g., individual with epididymitis who practice anal sex)

All treated individuals should undergo retesting after 3 months to identify reinfection. Test of cure not routinely recommended but may be indicated at 4 weeks post-treatment for select patients (e.g., pregnancy, persistent symptoms, concern for nonadherence to regimen).

If cervicitis, perform bimanual exam to assess if infection ascended to upper genital tract (rule out PID). Test and treat for other STIs, including HIV and *N. gonorrhoeae*.

EXAM TIPS

- Become familiar with the treatment regimens for chlamydia and gonorrhea.
- If chlamydia, do not give prophylaxis against gonorrhea unless indicated.

Sexual Partners

- Sexual partners should ideally be examined, tested, and presumptively treated, as well as counseled on prevention.
- Expedited partner therapy (EPT) is the practice of treating the sexual partner(s) of a patient diagnosed with an STD without the sexual partner being seen or evaluated by the healthcare provider. EPT is permissible in 46 states, the District of Columbia, and the Commonwealth of the Northern Mariana Islands. EPT is potentially allowable in four states, Puerto Rico, and Guam. Refer to the CDC website to confirm the legal status of your state: www.cdc.gov/std/ept/legal/default.htm.

Pregnant Patients

- Azithromycin 1 g PO in a single dose *or* amoxicillin 500 mg PO TID × 7 days (alternative).
- Test-of-cure recommended 4 weeks after treatment and retest again in the third trimester

Rare Complication: Reactive Arthritis

Formerly called Reiter syndrome. A rare form of arthritis that typically occurs in young males and females following an STI (*C. trachomatis* is the most common inciting pathogen). Spontaneously resolves in 6 months to 1 year. Treatment is supportive (e.g., nonsteroidal anti-inflammatory drugs [NSAIDs]).

Classic Case

A young adult with current chlamydia genital infection complains of red and swollen joints and inflammatory back pain. May have extra-musculoskeletal features such as conjunctivitis, genitourinary tract symptoms, oral mucosal ulcers, and dermatologic manifestations.

EXAM TIP

Azithromycin used for pregnant patients who have chlamydia. Test-of-cure needed 3 to 4 weeks after treatment.

HERPES SIMPLEX VIRUS: HSV-1 AND HSV-2

Asymptomatic shedding (intact skin) occurs intermittently, and patient is still contagious. Becomes latent in the neural ganglia and reactivates on mucosa and skin. Transmission is usually by oral contact with herpetic lesions, mucosal secretions, or direct skin contact. It can be transmitted by oral–oral, oral–genital, and genital-to-genital contact. Other populations at risk are athletes involved in contact sports (especially wrestlers) and teenagers. Children may require hospitalization for dehydration and pain control.

- HSV-1: Usually oral infection, sometimes genital
- HSV-2: Causes most cases of recurrent genital herpes, can be oral

EXAM TIP

HSV-1 infection is more common on oral mucosa, and HSV-2 is more common on the genitals.

Classic Case

HSV-1 lesions are usually located on the lips and mouth (gingivostomatitis), the eyes (herpes keratitis), or the pharynx. HSV-2 lesions are usually located on the genitals. With oral–genital contact, either type of HSV can be located on the face or genitals. Acute onset of small vesicles on a reddened base that rupture easily and become small shallow painful ulcers. Oral ulcers are aggravated by eating/drinking/swallowing acidic foods (e.g., lemons, orange juice, tomato sauce). Primary infection is when the greatest viral shedding occurs (vesicular fluid and crusts are contagious). It is more severe than subsequent recurrences and can last from 2 to 4 weeks. Subsequent recurrences tend to become less severe with time.

Labs

- Diagnostic test: Herpes viral culture or PCR assay for HSV-1 and HSV-2 RNA (more sensitive).
- For all cases of genital ulcers: Rule out syphilis and other STIs.

Tzanck Smear

- Rapid, inexpensive, and simple test that can be performed in the clinic.
- If positive for herpes virus infection (herpes simplex or varicella), it shows multinucleated giant cells. It has poor sensitivity and specificity.

EXAM TIPS

- Tzanck smear shows multinucleated giant cells with herpes virus infection (varicella, herpes simplex).
- Genital herpes treatment duration for 7 to 10 days for treating primary genital herpes infection. For breakouts, duration varies between 2 and 5 days.

Treatment Plan: Genital HSV Infection

First Episode (Primary Genital Herpes)

- Valacyclovir (Valtrex) 1,000 mg PO BID × 7 to 10 days (preferred due to less frequent dosing)
- Acyclovir (Zovirax) 400 mg PO TID × 7 to 10 days
- Famciclovir (Famvir) 250 mg PO TID × 7 to 10 days

Episodic Treatment (Flare-Up)

- Best if treatment started within 24 hours of lesion onset
- Acyclovir 800 mg TID for 2 days or 800 mg BID × 5 days
- Famciclovir (Famvir) 1,000 mg BID × a single duration; or 125 mg BID × 5 days; or 500 mg once, followed by 250 mg BID × 2 days
- Valacyclovir 500 mg BID × 3 days or 1,000 mg once daily × 5 days

Chronic Suppressive Therapy

- Recommended for severe or frequent (six or more per year) recurrences and immunocompetent patients who want to reduce the risk of HSV transmission to an uninfected sexual partner
- Acyclovir (Zovirax) 400 mg PO BID *OR* famciclovir (Famvir) 250 mg PO BID *or* valacyclovir 500 mg once daily or 1,000 mg once daily

Adjunctive Therapy

- Recommend analgesics in severe episodes with multiple painful lesions.
- Sitz bath may be helpful for female patients with dysuria secondary to multiple ulcerations.

EXAM TIPS

- Know first-episode treatment for genital herpes (acyclovir [Zovirax] TID or valacyclovir [Valtrex] BID or famciclovir TID × 7 to 10 days).
- Know flare-up treatment (acyclovir [Zovirax] or valacyclovir [Valtrex] or famciclovir [Famvir] × 2–5 days).

HIV INFECTION

HIV attacks the CD4 T-lymphocytes. HIV is spread by having anal or vaginal sex with someone who has HIV without using a condom; from a mother to baby during pregnancy, birth, or breastfeeding; and by sharing needles, syringes, or other drug infection equipment. HIV super-infection is when a person with HIV gets infected with another strain of the virus. Without treatment, the average patient will progress to AIDS in about 10 years. HIV-1 is the most common strain; HIV-2 accounts for fewer than 0.2% of infections. Currently, there are an estimated 1.2 million people in the United States who have HIV infection. Almost 13% of HIV-infected persons in the United States are unaware of their HIV infection. The CDC recommends that primary care providers conduct routine HIV screening at least once in a lifetime for individuals aged 13 to 64 years.

Risk Factors

- Sexual intercourse with an HIV-infected person; unprotected anal sex conveys greatest probability of HIV transmission
- Received blood products between 1975 and March 1985
- History of injection drug use/partner
- History of other STIs, multiple partners, homeless status, prisoner in jail, and others

Recommendations for Routine HIV Screening (Once a Year)

- Injection drug users and their sex partners
- People who exchange sex for money and drugs
- Sex partners of people with HIV
- Heterosexuals (or their partners) who had one or more sex partners since their most recent HIV test
- People receiving treatment for hepatitis, TB, or an STD
- MSM and bisexuals may benefit from more frequent screening (every 3–6 months)
- Patients should be informed (through practice form/literature/discussion) that an HIV test is included in their standard preventive screening tests and that they may decline the test (opt-out screening); note patient refusal in patient records.

If hairy leukoplakia of tongue, recurrent candidiasis, or thrush, rule out HIV infection.

Diagnostic Tests: Fourth-Generation Testing

Table 19.1 HIV Tests

Type of Test	Rationale
HIV-1/HIV-2 antibody with p24 antigen with reflexes	Also known as the *combination antibody/ antigen assay* (fourth generation). Screening test to diagnose HIV infection. If positive, lab will perform HIV-1/HIV-2 antibody differentiation immunoassay to confirm initial test.
ELISA	Antibody-only tests; can be used as initial test to screen for HIV infection as early as 3 weeks after exposure to the virus. A positive test should be confirmed with either an HIV-1/HIV-2 differentiation assay, or HIV Western blot.
Western blot	Older diagnostic test. Involves following a reactive screening immunoassay with a Western blot test. If positive, next step is HIV RNA PCR test.
Rapid HIV testing kits or point-of-care tests	Also used for screening. Result available in <30 minutes (antibody test). Can be done at home. If positive, follow-up with further testing.
HIV RNA PCR	Tests for HIV virus directly. Used for infants of HIV-positive mothers. Diagnoses acute HIV infection (window stage). Use if indeterminate result on antibody–antigen testing.
CD4 T-cell counts (normally >500 cells/mm³)	Check before starting ART, staging HIV infection, disease progression, and treatment response to ART. If on ART, check at same time as viral load.
Viral load (antigen)	Most sensitive diagnostic test. Monitor treatment response. If on ART, monitor every 1–2 months until nondetectable, then every 3–4 months.

ART, antiretroviral therapy; ELISA, enzyme-linked immunosorbent assay; PCR, polymerase chain reaction.

Step 1: Order HIV-1/HIV-2 antibodies and p24 antigen (fourth-generation antibody/antigen combination assay) with reflexes. ("Reflex" means that if positive, the lab will automatically perform the follow-up test to confirm the result.)
- Detects infection at earlier stages because the p24 antigen is produced before antibodies (window period).
- If negative, no HIV infection.

Step 2: If positive, the lab will perform the confirmatory HIV-1/HIV-2 antibody differentiation immunoassay (to confirm the result of the initial combination assay).
- Detects if infection is from HIV-1, HIV-2, or both viruses.

- If test result is indeterminate, order an HIV RNA test (either qualitative or quantitative).

HIV RNA PCR
- Detects HIV-1 RNA (actual viral presence). Can detect HIV infection as early as 7 to 28 days after exposure.
- Order to test infant if HIV(+) mother or if the HIV-1/HIV-2 antibody differentiation test is indeterminate.
- Suspect HIV infection in someone who is in the window period of HIV seroconversion.
- HIV RNA PCR, CD4 count and percentage, HIV RNA viral load, complete blood count (CBC) with differential, lipids.

Hepatitis A/B/C, syphilis and other STDs, cervical cytology. TB testing by purified protein derivative (PPD) or antibody interferon-Y release assay (IGRA), chest x-ray (CXR) if pulmonary symptoms, HLAB5701 if abacavir treatment, genotypic testing for antiviral resistance.

CD4 T-Cell Counts (Norm 500–1,500 Cells/mL)
- Used to stage HIV infection and determine response to ART.
- If CD4 count goes up (with decrease in viral load), patient is responding to ART (immune system improved).
- Values vary throughout the day. Check at the same time of the day using the same laboratory.

Viral Load
- Number of HIV RNA copies in 1 mL of plasma. Test measures actively replicating HIV virus; progression of disease and response to antiretroviral treatment.
- The best sign of treatment success is an undetectable viral load (<50 copies/mcL).
- If suspect acute or early HIV infection, order fourth-generation combination antibody/antigen immunoassay with viral load test.

If a patient on ART has a CD4 count that increases (from CD4 200 to 400 copies/mL), it suggests that their immune system is getting better.

Prophylaxis for Opportunistic Infections (Primary Prevention)

Pneumocystis Pneumonia
- *P. jirovecii* pneumonia (previously known as *P. carinii* pneumonia).
- CD4 lymphocyte count is <200 cells/mm³
- First line is trimethoprim–sulfamethoxazole (Bactrim DS) one tablet daily. If develops a severe reaction to sulfas, the next step is dapsone plus trimethoprim.
- Alternatives include dapsone, atovaquone, or pentamidine.

NOTE

With dapsone, first check patient for glucose-6-phosphate dehydrogenase (G6PD) anemia due to risk of hemolysis (about 10% of African American males have G6PD).

Toxoplasma gondii *Infections (Protozoa)*

- The most common CNS infection in AIDS patients. CD4 count is ≤100 cells/mm³.
- Infection causes encephalitis/brain abscesses (headaches, blurred vision, confusion).
- First line is to administer trimethoprim–sulfamethoxazole (Bactrim) one tablet BID × 6 weeks.
- Alternative is dapsone plus pyrimethamine and leucovorin.
- Avoid cleaning cat litter boxes and eating undercooked meats.

Monitoring Viral Load: Antiretroviral Therapy

- Best response if HIV infection is treated with ART in early stage. The goal is to decrease the HIV viral load. ART will suppress HIV and increase CD4 counts. Increased CD4 counts indicate that the patient is responding to ART and their immune system is improving.
- Check HIV RNA (viral load) in 2 to 8 weeks after starting therapy, then every 1 to 2 months (or every 4–8 weeks) until the viral load falls to undetectable levels. Monitor viral load, CD4, and CBC every 3 to 4 months the first 2 years of ART.
- Annual cervical cytology (Pap) regardless of age until three negative screens, then every 3 years.

Recommended Vaccines and Screening

- HIV and AIDS patients can receive inactivated vaccines such as hepatitis A vaccine, hepatitis B vaccine, inactivated influenza vaccine, pneumococcal vaccine, Td/Tdap (tetanus diphtheria/tetanus, diphtheria, acellular pertussis) every 10 years, human papillomavirus (HPV) vaccine (until age 26 years), and others as needed.
- Vaccines work best if CD4 counts exceed 200 copies/mm³.
- Cervical cancer screening at time of diagnosis, but no sooner than 21 years of age. Annual cervical cytology (Pap) until three negatives, then every 3 years.

HIV Education

- Do not handle cat litter or eat uncooked or undercooked meat (risk of toxoplasmosis).
- Avoid bird stool, since it contains histoplasmosis spores.
- Turtles, snakes, and other amphibians may be infected with salmonella.
- Use gloves when cleaning animal cages or when handling stool.
- Healthy lifestyle, follow-up visits, and taking ART as directed reduce the risk of infection.

Preventing HIV Transmission

- Use condom every single time you have sex. Genital ulcers increase risk for HIV.
- Do not share needles or syringes if using injectable drugs.
- Do not share any toothbrushes, razors, or other items that may have blood on them.
- Mothers with HIV infection should not breastfeed.
- Limit number of sexual partners.

- Bactrim DS PO is first-line agent for the prophylaxis of PCP; if allergic to sulfa, use dapsone 100 mg PO daily.
- Bactrim DS is used for both prophylaxis and treatment of PCP.

HIV INFECTION: OCCUPATIONALLY ACQUIRED

- Of all healthcare occupations, nurses have the highest rate of occupationally acquired HIV/AIDS.
- Risk of acquisition after needlestick injury is increased with deep injury, device visibly contaminated with patient's blood, needle placement in a vein or artery, and terminal illness in a source patient.
- Infectious fluids include blood, semen/preseminal fluid, vaginal fluids, and breast milk. The fluid must come into contact with mucous membrane or damaged tissue or be directly injected into bloodstream for transmission to occur. Mucous membranes are found inside rectum, vagina, penis, and mouth.

Preexposure Prophylaxis

Preexposure prophylaxis (PrEP) has been shown to reduce HIV transmission by more than 90%.

Daily oral PrEP medications are recommended as a prevention option for sexually active individuals at substantial risk of HIV, such as:

- Anyone with ongoing sexual relationship with an HIV-infected partner with a detectable viral load
- Gay, heterosexual, bisexual, or transgender men who do not use condoms and engage in high-risk sexual behaviors
- Women who have engaged in condomless sex with male partners at high risk
- Individuals who inject drugs and report sharing needles/equipment

Do not confuse with postexposure prophylaxis (PEP). Check for HIV infection before starting medications and check for HIV every 3 months thereafter.

Postexposure Prophylaxis

- The best time to start PEP is as soon as possible. If you think you have been exposed to HIV at work, during sex, through sharing needles, or through sexual assault, go to your health provider or ED right away.
- If source patient HIV status unknown, start PEP while awaiting rapid HIV testing (do not wait for lab results before starting PEP).
- Initial action following exposure is immediate cleansing or irrigation of the exposed site. Small wounds/punctures can also be cleansed with antiseptic or alcohol. Alcohol is virucidal to HIV, hepatitis B virus (HBV), and hepatitis C virus (HCV). For mucosal surfaces, flush exposed mucous membranes with copious amount of water. Irrigate eyes with saline or water.
- Baseline labs include HIV (rapid HIV test and HIV antibody/antigen immunoassay), HCV RNA, HBsAg, and

HBV surface antibody. Consider HIV RNA PCR if acute HIV suspected.

- A minimum of three antiretroviral drugs are used.
- PEP should be started as early as possible. About 72 hours postexposure is the outer limit of effective PEP. Duration should be continued for 4 weeks.

CLINICAL PEARLS

- The HIV antibody/antigen test (fourth generation) can detect infection 18 to 45 days after exposure.
- A nucleic acid test can usually detect HIV about 10 to 33 days after exposure.
- For job-related exposures, contact National Clinician's Postexposure Prophylaxis Hotline (Pipeline) toll free at (888) 448-4911 for advice (11 a.m.–8 p.m. ET, 7 days/week).

HIV INFECTION: PREGNANT PATIENTS

- Fully suppressive ART treatment markedly decreases HIV transmission from mother to infant. It can be given anytime in pregnancy, as early as when pregnancy is diagnosed. Starting earlier in pregnancy is more effective. Prenatal vitamins important. Avoid breastfeeding.
- Preferred ART regimen for those who are treatment naïve is a dual nucleoside reverse transcriptase inhibitor with either dolutegravir or ritonavir-boosted darunavir as a third drug.
- For infants, start prophylaxis with zidovudine (Retrovir) within 8 hours after birth. Recommended for most infants to decrease vertical transmission.

Zidovudine

- Recommended for pregnant women and infants. Check CBC with differential baseline and monitor for bone marrow suppression.
- Reduces rate of perinatal transmission by 70%.
- Start zidovudine (ZDV) as soon as HIV is diagnosed, or if established HIV diagnosis, start as soon as pregnancy is diagnosed.

EXAM TIP

HIV-infected pregnant patients should start AZT as soon as possible.

HUMAN PAPILLOMAVIRUS

Almost all cases of cervical cancer are caused by HPV, which is transmitted through unprotected penile-vaginal contact. Most cases are caused by HPV 16 and HPV 18. Cervical cancer is discussed in Chapter 17. Other HPV types can cause cancer of the oropharynx, anus, vulva/vagina, and penis.

- HPV vaccine (Gardasil 9) can help prevent infections with the oncogenic HPV types.
- The CDC recommends HPV vaccine starting at age 11 to 12 years, or catch-up in older adolescents and young adults (age 13–26 years). Only two doses (0, 6–12 months) are needed if first dose given before age of 15 years. If first dose given at age 15 or older, three doses are needed (0, 1–2, 6 months). Shared decision-making is recommended regarding vaccination for some adults aged 27–45 years.

Condyloma Acuminata (Anogenital Warts)

Manifestation of HPV infection. External anogenital warts that appear as soft white, flesh-colored, erythematous or brown pedunculated, flat, or papular growths. The warts may be flat, cauliflower-shaped, fungating, filiform, smooth, verrucous, or lobulated.

- HPV types 6 and/or 11 are detected in most cases.
- Warts may appear on the vagina, cervix, external genitals, urethra, and anus.
- Other sites are the penis, nasal mucosa, oropharynx, and conjunctiva.
- Biopsy to rule out underlying cancer is not mandatory before initiating therapy, but it is recommended if lesion has suspicious characteristics (fixation, irregular bleeding, ulceration, red/blue/black/brown pigmentation, induration, sudden recent growth) or patient is immunocompromised. Obtain biopsy from the most abnormal area(s) or refer to dermatologist.

EXAM TIPS

- Do not confuse condyloma acuminata (genital warts) with condyloma lata (secondary syphilis).
- HPV strains 16 and 18 are oncogenic/carcinogenic (memorize for exam).

Treatment Plan

Self-Administered Topical Medications (Patient-Applied Methods)

Podophyllotoxin (Condylox) 0.5% gel or cream (antimitotic drug). Contraindicated in pregnancy.

- Apply to external anogenital warts BID x 3 consecutive days (max 0.5 mL/d).
- Hold treatment for 4 days, then repeat this cycle up to four times.

Imiquimod (Aldara) 5% or Zyclara (3.75% imiquimod) is an immune-modulating (or immune response modifier) drug that stimulates the local production of interferon and other cytokines. Contraindicated in pregnancy.

- Apply a thin layer three times per week at bedtime for up to 16 weeks. Do not cover with dressing.
- Leave cream on skin for 6 to 10 hours. Wash off skin with soap and water after.
- Side effects include irritation, ulceration/erosions, hypopigmentation.

Sinecatechins 10% ointment (Veregen). Sinecatechins is a botanical, derived from green tea polyphenols, used for external anogenital warts (not for vagina or anus).

- Apply 0.5-cm strand of ointment on each wart with a finger (use gloves), up to three times per day for up to 16 weeks.
- Wash off skin before sexual contact or before inserting tampon in vagina.
- Can weaken condoms and diaphragms.

Provider-Applied Methods
- Treatment methods include cryotherapy, trichloroacetic acid (TCA), surgical excision, electrosurgery, and carbon dioxide laser therapy.
- Cryotherapy and TCA are best for small warts; surgical excision is beneficial for large warts (>1 cm).

EXAM TIPS

- Imiquimod is an immune-modulator treatment for genital warts, and patient can use at home.
- For pregnant patients, mechanical methods are used to destroy genital warts (e.g., curio, laser, excision). Treatments contraindicated in pregnancy are podophyllotoxin and imiquimod.

NEISSERIA GONORRHOEAE

A gram-negative bacteria that infects the urinary and genital tracts, anorectum, pharynx, and conjunctiva (gonococcal ophthalmia neonatorum). Unlike chlamydia, gonorrhea can become systemic or disseminated if left untreated. Presumptive cotreatment for chlamydia is indicated *only* when chlamydial infection has not been excluded. (Do not cotreat if chlamydial status is confirmed negative.) Women are more likely to be asymptomatic or present with PID. Males are more likely to present with urethritis.

- Screen all sexually active women under 25 years of age. Screen MSM at least annually at sites of contact (urethra, rectum, pharynx) regardless of condom use.
- During first prenatal visit, screen all pregnant women <25 years, and older pregnant women at increased risk. Rescreen again in the third trimester if high risk.
- Screen individuals with HIV at first evaluation and then at least annually.

Classic Case

Sexually active female who is 25 years old with history of a new sexual partner (<3 months) or multiple partners with inconsistent or no condom use. During the speculum examination, cervix can appear normal or with purulent discharge and may bleed easily (friable). Males with urethritis may have penile discharge and dysuria and may report staining of underwear with green purulent discharge. Signs and symptoms depend on the sites infected. Treatment is listed in Table 19.2.

Signs and Symptoms (by Infection Site)
- Cervicitis: Mucopurulent cervix, pain, mild bleeding after intercourse
- Urethritis: Scant to copious purulent discharge, dysuria, frequency, urgency
- Proctitis: Inflammation of the rectum; presents with pruritus, rectal pain, purulent discharge, tenesmus (urge to defecate even if rectum is empty), or avoidance of defecation due to pain
- Pharyngitis: Severe sore throat unresponsive to typical antibiotics, purulent green-colored discharge on the posterior pharynx
- Bartholinitis: Symptomatic involvement of Bartholin's glands, located behind the labia; perilabial pain and discharge, edema and tenderness of the gland
- Endometritis: Menometrorrhagia, or heavy, prolonged menstrual bleeding
- DGI: Results in petechial or pustular skin lesions of the hands/fingers, asymmetric polyarthralgia, tenosynovitis, oligoarticular septic arthritis (arthritis-dermatitis syndrome), or meningitis or endocarditis
- PID signs, symptoms, and treatment discussed in the section "Pelvic Inflammatory Disease"
- Epididymitis and prostatitis discussed in Chapter 16

EXAM TIP

Learn treatment of proctitis.

Labs
- See the "Labs" section for *C. trachomatis*.
- NAAT is the most accurate and preferred diagnostic test for both genital and extragenital infection.
- Another alternative is a gonococcal culture (Thayer–Martin medium) to assess antibiotic susceptibilities of the isolate when resistance is suspected.
- Cotesting for chlamydia (similar clinical syndromes and often coexists).
- Retesting recommended at 3 months after treatment for all patients (due to high rates of reinfection).

Treatment Plan
First-Line Therapy for Uncomplicated Infections
- Ceftriaxone (Rocephin) 500 mg IM × one dose. If weight ≥150 kg (300 lb), ceftriaxone (Rocephin) 1 g IM × one dose.
- If chlamydial infection has not been excluded, cotreat with doxycycline 100 mg PO BID × 7 days. During pregnancy, azithromycin 1 g PO × one dose.
- Do not cotreat for chlamydia if excluded through microbiologic testing.
- A test-of-cure is unnecessary for persons with uncomplicated urogenital or rectal gonorrhea who are treated with any of the recommended or alternative regimens. For persons with pharyngeal gonorrhea, a test-of-cure

is indicated following treatment with culture at 7 days following therapy or by NAAT at 14 days following therapy.

EXAM TIP

Treat uncomplicated gonorrhea with ceftriaxone IM 500 mg × one dose. Cotreat for chlamydia only when chlamydial infection has not been excluded.

Management of Sexual Partners

- EPT is recommended for sex partners of patients with documented gonococcal infection who cannot present for clinical evaluation with a single dose of oral cefixime 800 mg (plus presumptive treatment for chlamydia if indicated).
- Partners of MSM are strongly encouraged to come in for evaluation and management due to the high risk of coexisting infections.
- Avoid sex until both partners finish treatment and no longer have symptoms.

Disseminated Gonococcal Infection

- Ceftriaxone 1 g IV every 24 hours (duration varies between 7 to 14 days)
- Refer to ED for hospitalization and/or infectious disease specialist for appropriate management.

Acute Proctitis

- All patients with proctitis—treatment for gonorrhea and chlamydial infection: Ceftriaxone 500 mg IM as a single dose (1 g if weight ≥150 kg) *plus* doxycycline 100 mg BID for 7 days
- Patients who present with perianal or mucosal ulcers—additional treatment for HSV infection: Valacyclovir 1 g PO BID for 7 to 10 days (alternatives: Famciclovir or acyclovir). If bloody discharge, extend doxycycline course to 3 weeks.

PELVIC INFLAMMATORY DISEASE

An acute, ascending polymicrobial infection of the upper genital tract structures in females. PID can be caused by cervical microorganisms (including *C. trachomatis, N. gonorrhoeae,* and *Mycoplasma genitalium*), as well as the vaginal microflora including other types of anaerobic organisms and bacteria.

Risk Factors for Pelvic Inflammatory Disease

- Sex (primary risk factor)
- History of PID (25% recurrence)
- Multiple partners; STI in the partner
- Age (highest frequency among those 15 to 25 years)
- Inconsistent or incorrect use of condoms
- Complete disruption of vaginal ecosystem (bacterial vaginosis)

Classic Case

Sexually active young woman with acute onset of lower abdominal or pelvic pain that is one-sided or bilateral with new vaginal discharge and/or intermenstrual bleeding. Evidence of cervical motion, uterine, or adnexal tenderness on exam. Reports painful intercourse (dyspareunia). Inflammation of fallopian tubes (salpingitis). May walk in a shuffling gait to avoid jarring pelvis, which is painful. Jumping/running aggravates pelvic pain. Associated fever and chills may occur. Some develop perihepatitis (with right upper quadrant [RUQ] tenderness), peritonitis, and tubo-ovarian pelvic abscess.

CLINICAL PEARLS

- Up to 15% of women with cervicitis due to gonorrhea will develop PID.
- PID is a clinical diagnosis. Even if both gonorrheal and chlamydial tests are negative, treat a sexually active patient who has signs and symptoms of PID combined with a sexual history.
- Better to "overtreat" than to miss treating possible PID infections.
- Adnexal tenderness is the most sensitive physical exam finding for PID (compared with cervical motion tenderness, which may be negative).

Labs

- Rule out pregnancy first in reproductive-age patients.
- NAAT for *C. trachomatis, N. gonorrhoeae,* and *M. genitalium* via vaginal swab (preferred in females) or first-catch urine (preferred in males)
- HIV screening
- Serologic testing for syphilis
- CBC, erythrocyte sedimentation rate (ESR), and C-reactive protein (CRP)

Gram Stain

Useful for gonorrheal urethritis only; look for gram-negative diplococci in clusters inside polymorphonuclear leukocytes.

Treatment Plan

- Antibiotic regimen for outpatients: Ceftriaxone (Rocephin) 500 mg IM (or 1 g for individuals >150 kg) × one dose *PLUS* doxycycline 100 mg PO BID for 14 days *PLUS* metronidazole 500 mg PO BID for 14 days.
- Follow-up: Evaluate for clinical improvement within 72 hours.
- Indications for hospitalization: Severe clinical illness (high fever, nausea/vomiting, severe abdominal pain), suspected pelvic abscess, pregnancy, and possible alternative diagnosis that warrants surgery.
- Counseling: On medication adherence, refraining from sexual activity until treatment completion and symptom resolution, safe sex practices, and screening and prevention of other STIs.

Fitz-Hugh–Curtis Syndrome (Perihepatitis)

Clinical syndrome that occurs in approximately 10% of females with acute PID. Inflammation of the liver capsule and peritoneal surfaces of the anterior RUQ; minimal stromal hepatic involvement. Manifests as a patchy purulent and fibrinous exudate ("violin strings" seen on laparoscopy). Characterized by RUQ abdominal pain and tenderness on palpation with a distinct pleuritic component. The liver function tests are usually normal or slightly elevated.

EXAM TIPS

- Recognize PID symptoms and treatment.
- Learn presentation of Fitz-Hugh–Curtis and Jarisch–Herxheimer syndrome.

SYPHILIS

STI caused by the spirochete *Treponema pallidum*. Majority of patients are male, with most cases occurring among gay, bisexual, and other MSM. If untreated, infection becomes systemic and can progress to cardiovascular, gummatous, and neurologic complications.

Screen for syphilis if HIV infection, MSM, presence of any genital ulcer (especially if painless chancre), previous STD, pregnancy, intravenous drug use, or asymptomatic women at high risk.

Classic Case

Signs and symptoms are dependent on stage of infection.

Primary

- Painless chancre (heals in 6–9 weeks if not treated)
- Chancre has clean base, well demarcated with indurated margins (Figure 19.2)

Secondary

- Systemic illness that develops within weeks to a few months after the chancre develops.
- Secondary syphilis is characterized by a wide variety of signs and symptoms such as generalized symptoms

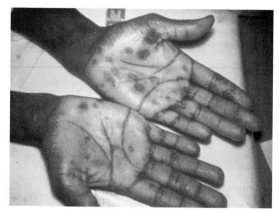

Figure 19.3 Maculopapular rash on palms due to secondary syphilis.
Source: Centers for Disease Control and Prevention.

(e.g., fever, headache, lymph node enlargement), dermatologic findings (e.g., rash, alopecia), GI symptoms, musculoskeletal abnormalities, renal complications, neurologic findings, and visual/auditory symptoms.
- Dermatologic findings
  - Condyloma lata: Infectious white papules [that look like white warts] in warm, moist areas (such as the mouth and perineum)
  - Maculopapular rash (most characteristic finding of secondary syphilis) involving the entire trunk and extremities including the palms and soles that is not pruritic (may be generalized; Figure 19.3)

Latent Stage

Asymptomatic but will have positive titers

Tertiary

- May appear at any time 1 to 30 years after primary infection
- Most common manifestations: Cardiovascular syphilis (especially aortitis), gummatous syphilis (rare granulomatous, nodular lesions), and CNS involvement

Labs

Two types of syphilis serologic tests (treponemal and nontreponemal tests) are required to diagnose syphilis. For those without a prior history of syphilis, note either test can be used as the initial screening test. Confirmatory testing is necessary due to the potential for false-positive screening test results.

- Step 1—Order screening test (nontreponemal tests): Rapid plasma reagin (RPR) or Venereal Disease Research Laboratory (VDRL). If reactive, order confirmatory test.
- Step 2—Order confirmatory test (treponemal tests): Fluorescent treponemal antibody absorption (FTA-ABS), *T. pallidum* particle agglutination assay (TPPA), the *T. pallidum* enzyme immunoassay (TP-EIA), or chemiluminescence immunoassay.

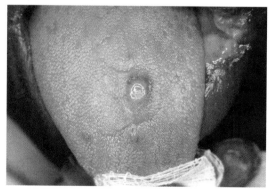

Figure 19.2 Primary syphilitic chancre of the tongue.
Source: Centers for Disease Control and Prevention/Robert E. Sumpter.

- For patients without a history of syphilis: Diagnosis is made when both nontreponemal and treponemal tests are reactive.
- For patients with a history of treated syphilis: The presence of a positive nontreponemal test can indicate a new infection, an evolving response to recent treatment, or treatment failure.
- Note during treatment: If initial test used is RPR, order sequential RPR to document treatment response. If initial test is VDRL, order sequential VDRL. Use the same laboratory to monitor. If RPR or VDRL shows a fourfold or higher (>1:4) decrease in titers, patient is responding to treatment.

EXAM TIPS

- RPR and VDRL are the screening tests for syphilis.
- If positive RPR or VDRL (nontreponemal test), confirm with FTA-ABS (treponemal test). If reactive RPR and reactive FTA-ABS, this is diagnostic for syphilis in patients without a history of prior syphilis.

Treatment Plan

Early Syphilis: Primary, Secondary, or Early Latent Syphilis (<1 year)

Benzathine penicillin G (Bicillin L-A) 2.4 million units IM × one dose

Late Syphilis: Late Latent Syphilis (>1 year) or Tertiary Without Evidence of Neurosyphilis

- Benzathine penicillin G 2.4 million units IM once per week × 3 consecutive weeks
- If penicillin allergy, doxycycline 100 mg PO BID for 28 days or ceftriaxone 2 g IV or IM daily for 10 to 14 days

Neurologic, Ocular, and Otic Syphilis

IV penicillin G 3 to 4 million units IV every 4 hours (or 18 to 24 million units per day by continuous infusion) for 10 to 14 days

Pregnancy

- Same treatment as nonpregnant individuals noted above (penicillin G benzathine therapy).
- For penicillin-allergic patients, refer to allergist for penicillin desensitization.
- Screen all pregnant women at first prenatal visit; repeat at 28 to 32 weeks and at delivery for pregnant women at high risk of infection.

EXAM TIP

Know tertiary syphilis treatment.

Follow-Up

- Recheck RPR or VDRL at 6 and 12 months after treatment (look for at least a fourfold decrease in the pretreatment and posttreatment titers).
- Treat sexual partner(s) from previous 90 days before patient's diagnosis, even if their RPR or VDRL is negative. Test patient and partner(s) for HIV and other STDs.
- Refer to infectious disease specialist for suspected neurosyphilis, poor response to treatment, penicillin allergy, or if primary clinician is not familiar with syphilis management.

Jarisch–Herxheimer Reaction

Acute, self-limited, febrile reaction that occurs within the first 24 hours after the patient receives therapy for any spirochetal infection. Most common after treatment of early syphilis. The symptoms may include fever, chills, headache, myalgia, hypotension, diaphoresis, and worsening rash (if present). There is no way to prevent the reaction; warn patients of the possible signs and symptoms. Treat with general supportive measures such as antipyretics/NSAIDs.

CLINICAL PEARLS

- For chlamydia infections treated with azithromycin 1 g × one dose, instruct patient and partner to abstain from sex for at least 7 days and until symptoms have resolved.
- NAAT can remain positive for 2 to 3 weeks after treatment because of the presence of nonviable organisms.
- False-positive RPR can be caused by pregnancy, Lyme disease, autoimmune diseases, or chronic or acute disease.
- Recheck syphilitic chancre in 3 to 7 days after penicillin injection (should start healing).
- Nontreponemal titers (RPR or VDRL) usually decline after treatment, but in some persons, nontreponemal antibodies can persist for a long time (serofast reaction). Most patients with reactive nontreponemal tests will be reactive for the rest of their lives (low titers), but 15% to 25% revert to being serologically nonreactive in 2 to 3 years.

CDC–RECOMMENDED STI TREATMENT REGIMENS

Table 19.2 Sexually Transmitted Infections: CDC Treatment Guidelines (2020)

Diseases and Organisms	Uncomplicated Infections	Complicated Infections
Chlamydia *Chlamydia trachomatis*	Indications: Chlamydial infection; sexual partner treatment Treatment: Doxycycline 100 mg BID × 7 days Pregnancy: Azithromycin 1 g × one dose	Indications: PID, salpingitis, tubo-ovarian abscess, epididymitis, prostatitis Treatment: Doxycycline 100 mg BID × 14 days
Gonorrhea *Neisseria gonorrhoeae*	Indications: Uncomplicated infection of the cervix, urethra, pharynx, or rectum; sexual partner treatment Treatment: Ceftriaxone 500 mg IM × one dose Weight ≥150 kg (300 lb): Ceftriaxone 1 g IM × one dose *PLUS* cotreatment with doxycycline 100 mg orally BID for 7 days if chlamydial infection has not been excluded	Indications: Disseminated gonococcal infection – gonococcal-related arthritis and arthritis-dermatitis syndrome, gonococcal meningitis and endocarditis Treatment: Ceftriaxone 1–2 g IV or IM every 12–24 hours *PLUS* cotreatment with doxycycline 100 mg orally BID for 7 days if chlamydial infection has not been excluded
Syphilis *Treponema pallidum*	Indications: Primary or secondary syphilis or early latent <1 year, sexual partner treatment Treatment: Benzathine penicillin G 2.4 mU IM × one dose Retreat if clinical signs recur or sustained fourfold titers	Indications: >1-year duration late latent syphilis, tertiary syphillis Treatment: Benzathine penicillin G 2.4 mU IM weekly × 3 consecutive weeks Follow-up of cases is mandatory (any stage of disease); referral often indicated

BID, two times a day; CDC, Centers for Disease Control and Prevention; IM, intramuscular; PID, pelvic inflammatory disease.
Source: Adapted from the Centers for Disease Control and Prevention (2020).

KNOWLEDGE CHECK: CHAPTER 19

1. Which of the following antigens is a component of the HIV 1/2 combination antibody/antigen testing?
   A. p24
   B. p20
   C. p18
   D. p14

2. A sexually active 16-year-old patient with cervicitis is tested for gonorrhea and chlamydia. The nucleic acid amplification test (NAAT) result shows that the patient is positive for gonorrhea. Which of the following is appropriate treatment for this patient?
   A. Cephalosporin
   B. Cephalosporin and macrolide
   C. Tetracycline
   D. Tetracycline and sulfonamide

3. The Jarisch-Herxheimer reaction is a response to treatment of which of the following organisms?
   A. *Neisseria gonorrhoeae*
   B. *Chlamydia trachomatis*
   C. *Treponema pallidum*
   D. *Rickettsia rickettsii*

4. Which of the following has been classified as a nationally notifiable disease by the Centers for Disease Control and Prevention (CDC)?
   A. Gonorrhea
   B. Herpes simplex virus (HSV)
   C. Human papillomavirus (HPV)
   D. Pelvic inflammatory disease (PID)

5. A 30-year-old male patient with a history of HIV infection has been on antiretroviral therapy (ART) since diagnosis at age 28 years. Which of the following indicates that the patient's immune system is responding to ART?
   A. HIV viral load is higher compared with the previous test.
   B. CD4 count is higher compared with the previous test.
   C. Complete blood count (CBC) shows an increase in leukocyte count.
   D. Genetic testing of the patient's HIV strain shows that it is sensitive to current HIV regimen.

6. Which human papillomavirus (HPV) strains are oncogenic and cause the majority of cervical cancer cases?
   A. HPV 6 and HPV 11
   B. HPV 16 and HPV 18
   C. HPV 2 and HPV 4
   D. HPV 40 and HPV 51

7. Which of the following is the *most characteristic* finding of secondary syphilis?
   A. Fever
   B. Adenopathy
   C. Chancre
   D. Rash

8. Which of the following is a risk factor for pelvic inflammatory disease (PID)?
   A. Choice of contraceptive method
   B. Female patient age 40 years
   C. Multiple sexual partners
   D. Family history of PID

(See answers next page.)

1. A) p24

The p24 antigen appears early in HIV infection and enables earlier detection. The preferred test for HIV screening is the fourth-generation HIV 1/2 combination antibody with p24 antigen test. If there is a strong suspicion of HIV infection, also order the HIV RNA polymerase chain reaction (PCR) test, which detects the HIV virus directly. p20, p18, and p14 are not components of the HIV 1/2 combination antibody/antigen testing.

2. A) Cephalosporin

As of December 2020, the Centers for Disease Control and Prevention recommends that patients with gonorrhea-positive testing be treated with a higher dose of cephalosporin than previously recommended. Additionally, the recommendation for cotreatment of chlamydia with positive gonorrhea has been removed, provided chlamydia status is confirmed negative. The first-line treatment for gonorrhea-positive culture is ceftriaxone 500 mg intramuscularly (IM) for patients who weigh ≤150 kg and 1 gram IM for patients who weigh ≥150 kg. If the patient has a cephalosporin allergy, the recommended alternative is 240 mg IM plus azithromycin 2 g orally. Screening for gonorrhea again in 3 months is recommended due to the high rates of reinfection.

3. C) *Treponema pallidum*

The Jarisch-Herxheimer reaction is an immune reaction caused by treatment of the spirochete *T. pallidum* (syphilis) with benzathine penicillin G, given by intramuscular injection. When large amounts of treponema are killed, it releases foreign antigens that the body responds to with symptoms such as fever, chills, headache, myalgia, tachycardia, and increased respiratory rate, all of which occur in the first few hours after treatment and peak in 6 to 8 hours. It is a self-limited reaction. Treatment is corticosteroids, antipyretics, and general supportive measures. Other spirochete bacteria that may elicit this reaction are *Borrelia burgdorferi* (Lyme disease) and *Leptospira leptospirosis*, also known as Weil's disease or swamp fever.

4. A) Gonorrhea

According to the CDC, four sexually transmitted infections are nationally notifiable conditions: chlamydia, gonorrhea, syphilis, and chancroid. To report a disease, contact the local county health department. While a serious infection, PID is not nationally notifiable. HPV infections are not nationally notifiable because most sexually active individuals will acquire at least one type of HPV infection, and most infections will clear and are not associated with clinical disease. HSV infections are not nationally notifiable.

5. B) CD4 count is higher compared with the previous test.

One of the best indicators that the patient is responding to the ART regimen is an increase in the CD4 count. Another indicator is a decrease in the viral load. An increased leukocyte count seen on the CBC may indicate worsening infection, inflammation, or injury. Genetic testing is not used to assess treatment response.

6. B) HPV 16 and HPV 18

Most cases of cervical cancer are caused by HPV. HPV 16 and HPV 18 cause 70% of cervical cancer cases in the United States. There are more than 150 HPV types. HPV can also cause cancer of the vulva, vagina, penis, and anus, as well as oropharyngeal cancers.

7. D) Rash

About 25% of individuals with untreated syphilis develop a systemic illness within weeks to a few months that represents secondary syphilis. Secondary syphilis is characterized by a wide variety of signs and symptoms such as generalized symptoms (e.g., fever, headache, lymph node enlargement), dermatologic findings (e.g., rash, alopecia), gastrointestinal symptoms, musculoskeletal abnormalities, renal complications, neurologic findings, and visual/auditory symptoms. The rash is the most characteristic finding of secondary syphilis—classically diffuse, symmetric macular or papular lesions involving the entire trunk and extremities, including the palms and soles. Primary syphilis is characterized by the presence of a chancre.

8. C) Multiple sexual partners

Risk factors for PID include sex (primary risk factor); multiple sexual partners; sexually transmitted infection in the sexual partner; age (highest frequency among those age 15 to 25 years; incidence in female patients older than 35 years is only one seventh that in younger female patients); a personal previous episode of PID; and other conditions (e.g., complete disruption of the vaginal ecosystem). The choice of contraceptive method does not clearly affect the risk of PID; however, consistent and correct condom use has been found to reduce the risk significantly.

9. A patient reports a history of a painless lesion about a month ago. The patient now presents with a rash, fever, headache, malaise, and complains of anorexia. The patient reports a history of unprotected sexual encounters with multiple partners. The patient denies any allergies. Based on this presentation, which of the following is the appropriate treatment course?
   A. Single dose of penicillin G benzathine 2.4 million units intramuscularly (IM)
   B. Penicillin G benzathine 2.4 million units IM once weekly for 3 weeks
   C. Penicillin G 3 to 4 million units intravenously (IV) every 4 hours for 10 to 14 days
   D. Doxycycline 100 mg orally two times per day for 14 days

10. A patient presents with a painless chancre; this is most characteristic of which stage of syphilis disease?
    A. Late
    B. Primary
    C. Secondary
    D. Tertiary

11. Which of the following includes appropriate screening guidelines for sexually transmitted infections (STIs), according to the Centers for Disease Control and Prevention (CDC)?
    A. Screening for chlamydia is not required for men who have sex with men if they practice consistent condom use.
    B. All pregnant patients should be screened for herpes simplex virus-2 (HSV-2) at their first prenatal visit.
    C. A heterosexual 20-year-old male patient who is in a monogamous relationship should be screened for gonorrhea annually.
    D. A sexually active female patient who is 35 years old and has a history of gonorrhea should be screened for chlamydia.

12. A patient with HIV presents for routine annual lab work. The CD4 count is 175 cells/mcL. The patient denies any allergies. Which of the following prophylactic antimicrobials is indicated based on this CD4 cell count?
    A. Trimethoprim-sulfamethoxazole is indicated to prevent toxoplasmosis.
    B. Metronidazole is indicated to prevent histoplasmosis.
    C. Azithromycin is indicated to prevent cryptococcus.
    D. Trimethoprim-sulfamethoxazole is indicated to prevent pneumocystis pneumonia.

13. A patient presents with painful genital ulcers and generalized symptoms of fever, headache, and fatigue. Upon physical examination, the vesicles are 2 to 4 mm with underlying erythema and are progressing to erosions and ulcerations. The patient denies a history of genital lesions and reports that this is the first occurrence. Based on this presentation, which of the following is the appropriate therapy?
    A. Valacyclovir 1,000 mg orally twice a day for 7 to 10 days
    B. Intravenous acyclovir 5 mg/kg every 8 hours for 5 days
    C. Famciclovir 250 mg orally twice a day for an extended duration with required follow-up
    D. Topical acyclovir applied to the lesions twice a day

14. Which of the following is the specimen of choice when screening male patients using the nucleic acid amplification test (NAAT)?
    A. Urethral swab
    B. First-catch urine
    C. Meatal swab
    D. Rectal swab

(See answers next page.)

9. A) Single dose of penicillin G benzathine 2.4 million units intramuscularly (IM)

The patient is presenting with signs and symptoms consistent with secondary syphilis. Weeks to months after infection, untreated individuals will develop secondary syphilis with systemic symptoms including fever, rash, headache, malaise, fatigue, and lymphadenopathy. Treatment for early syphilis (primary, secondary, and early latent syphilis) includes a single dose of penicillin G benzathine 2.4 million units IM. Treatment for late latent syphilis or tertiary syphilis includes penicillin G benzathine 2.4 million units IM once weekly for 3 weeks. For patients with neurosyphilis, treatment includes penicillin G 3 to 4 million units IV every 4 hours for 10 to 14 days. If patients are allergic to penicillin, doxycycline is an appropriate treatment alternative.

10. B) Primary

The initial clinical manifestation of syphilis infection is a localized skin lesion called a chancre. Secondary syphilis produces a wide variety of symptoms such as a rash, fever, malaise, sore throat, gastrointestinal disturbances, musculoskeletal abnormalities, and neurologic complications. Tertiary syphilis includes patients with late syphilis who have symptomatic presentations involving the cardiovascular system or gummatous syphilis disease.

11. D) A sexually active female patient who is 35 years old and has a history of gonorrhea should be screened for chlamydia.

According to the CDC, all sexually active female patients who are 25 years old should be screened for chlamydia and gonorrhea. Screen sexually active women older than 25 years if they are at increased risk (e.g., previous or coexisting STI, history of exchanging money or drugs for sex). Men who have sex with men should be screened at least annually for chlamydia, gonorrhea, and syphilis regardless of condom use. All pregnant patients younger than 25 years should be screened for chlamydia, gonorrhea, and syphilis; those older than 25 years at increased risk should be screened as well. Routine HSV-2 serologic screening among pregnant patients who are asymptomatic is not recommended. There is insufficient evidence for screening heterosexual men at low risk of infection for chlamydia and gonorrhea.

12. D) Trimethoprim-sulfamethoxazole is indicated to prevent pneumocystis pneumonia.

Antimicrobial therapy is indicated in certain patients with HIV to prevent an opportunistic infection. Trimethoprim-sulfamethoxazole is indicated to prevent pneumocystis pneumonia in patients with a CD4 count ≤200 cells/mcL. Alternative agents include dapsone, atovaquone suspension, or aerosolized pentamidine. For patients with a CD4 count ≤150 cells/mcL, antifungal prophylaxis is not indicated to prevent infection with histoplasmosis due to limited evidence. For patients with CD4 counts ≤100 cells/mcL, trimethoprim-sulfamethoxazole is indicated to prevent reactivation of *Toxoplasma gondii* and a positive *T. gondii* IgG serology. Preventive therapy for cryptococcal disease is not recommended; however, screening may be useful in certain patients.

13. A) Valacyclovir 1,000 mg orally twice a day for 7 to 10 days

This patient is presenting with clinical manifestations consistent with genital herpes simplex virus (HSV) infection; the characteristic lesions of HSV begin as grouped 2- to 4-mm vesicles with underlying erythema that progress to vesicles, pustules, erosions, and ulcerations. Vesicles and pustules may have an umbilicated appearance due to central depression. Systemic symptoms may occur during the first episode, such as fever, headache, malaise, and myalgias. Antiviral therapy is indicated for most patients experiencing a first episode of genital HSV; treatment should be started within 72 hours of lesion appearance. For a first episode, valacyclovir 1,000 mg orally twice daily for 7 to 10 days is recommended along with acyclovir 400 mg three times daily and famciclovir 250 mg three times daily. Parenteral therapy is indicated in patients with a complicated infection (e.g., central nervous system involvement, end-organ disease, disseminated HSV). Chronic suppressive therapy may be indicated for patients with severe or frequent recurrence or for immunocompetent patients. Topical antiviral therapy is not recommended in the treatment of genital herpes.

14. B) First-catch urine

Although NAAT can be performed on urethral, meatal, and rectal swabs, first-catch urine is the specimen of choice when screening male patients for *Chlamydia trachomatis* and *Neisseria gonorrhoeae* infections. The vaginal swab is the specimen of choice for female patients.

15. A young adult patient presents with fever, lower abdominal tenderness, and pelvic discomfort. The patient reports being sexually active. A recent pregnancy test was negative. The physical assessment reveals acute cervical motion, uterine, and adnexal tenderness on bimanual pelvic examination, and mucopurulent vaginal discharge. The patient denies a history of dysuria or urinary frequency. These findings are suggestive of which diagnosis?
A. Ectopic pregnancy
B. Cystitis
C. Pelvic inflammatory disease
D. Appendicitis

16. A female patient presents with cauliflower-shaped, pedunculated, flesh-colored warts that vary in size and are generalized in the vulva and perineum area. The patient reports a history of unprotected sexual activity; a pregnancy test is positive, and the patient indicates an interest in continuing the pregnancy. Based on this presentation, which of the following is the *preferred* treatment option for this patient?
A. Imiquimod cream
B. Podophyllin cream
C. Sinecatchins ointment
D. Trichloroacetic acid

17. A patient presents with a fever and lower abdominal pain with pelvic discomfort. Acute cervical motion, uterine, and adnexal tenderness is noted on bimanual pelvic examination. The patient denies dysuria or other urinary symptoms. Which of the following tests is a *priority* to obtain for this patient?
A. Pregnancy test
B. Hepatitis panel
C. Urinalysis
D. C-reactive protein

18. Routine annual screening for a sexually active 24-year-old female patient is positive for chlamydia via nucleic acid amplification test (NAAT). A pregnancy test is negative. The patient denies any allergies. Which of the following is indicated as first-line treatment?
A. Azithromycin 1 g orally in a single dose
B. Levofloxacin 500 mg orally once daily for 7 days
C. Doxycycline 100 mg orally twice daily for 7 days
D. Amoxicillin 500 mg orally three times daily for 7 days

19. Which of the following is the *most common* pathogen associated with sexually acquired reactive arthritis?
A. *Neisseria gonorrhoeae*
B. *Chlamydia trachomatis*
C. *Treponema pallidum*
D. *Escherichia coli*

20. A female patient comes to the urgent care clinic with complaints of unusual discharge and vaginal pruritis. The patient also reports dysuria and peri-labial pain. The nurse practitioner performs a pelvic examination and notes that the cervical discharge is purulent and yellow/green in color. The cervix is friable and bleeds easily. The symptoms and physical assessment are concerning for cervicitis. What diagnosis does the nurse practitioner suspect?
A. Genital herpes simplex virus infection
B. Fitz-Hugh-Curtis syndrome
C. Primary syphilis
D. Gonorrhea

(See answers next page.)

15. C) Pelvic inflammatory disease

A clinical diagnosis of pelvic inflammatory disease is highly suggested in sexually active young female patients who are at risk for sexually transmitted infections. Often, patient presentation includes pelvic or lower abdominal pain and evidence of cervical motion, uterine, or adnexal tenderness. Additional supportive findings include fever, mucopurulent discharge or cervical friability, presence of white blood cells on microscopy of vaginal secretions, and detection of genital infection with *Neisseria gonorrhoeae*, *Chlamydia trachomatis*, and *Mycoplasma genitalium*. While cervical motion tenderness may be found in other conditions, such as appendicitis and ectopic pregnancy, the patient's pain is not localized to the right iliac fossa, and the patient does not have a positive pregnancy test. Cystitis is also less likely because the patient denies a history of urinary frequency and/or dysuria.

16. D) Trichloroacetic acid

The patient is presenting with clinical manifestations suggestive of condylomata acuminata (anogenital warts). The preferred medical treatment for pregnant patients is trichloroacetic acid because it has no systemic absorption or known fetal effects. Cryoablation is also considered safe and effective for pregnant patients. Podophyllin, podophyllotoxin, and interferons are contraindicated due to the potential for fetal harm. Imiquimod and sinecatechins are not recommended due to limited evidence and potential for fetal harm.

17. A) Pregnancy test

The findings are presumptive of a clinical diagnosis of pelvic inflammatory disease (PID). For all female patients suspected of having PID, the following tests should be obtained: pregnancy test (to rule out ectopic pregnancy and complications of intrauterine pregnancy); microscopy of vaginal discharge (to assess for increased white blood cells); nucleic acid amplification tests (NAATs) for *Neisseria gonorrhoeae*, *Chlamydia trachomatis*, and *Mycoplasma genitalium*; HIV screening; and serologic testing for syphilis (to rule out sexually transmitted infections that share similar risk factors with PID). While an erythrocyte sedimentation rate and C-reactive protein can often be obtained to assess severity, these tests have poor sensitivity and specificity for the diagnosis of PID. A urinalysis should be checked in female patients with urinary symptoms. Hepatitis virus testing may be indicated depending on the patient's risk history, but it is not a priority at this time.

18. C) Doxycycline 100 mg orally twice daily for 7 days

Most chlamydial infections are asymptomatic; annual screening is recommended for all sexually active female patients younger than 25 years and for those older than 25 years if at increased risk for infection. The first-line recommended regimen for chlamydial infection in adolescents and adults is doxycycline 100 mg orally twice daily for 7 days. Alternative regimens include azithromycin and levofloxacin. Azithromycin is the recommended regimen for chlamydial infection during pregnancy; amoxicillin is the alternative regimen during pregnancy.

19. B) *Chlamydia trachomatis*

Reactive arthritis is a rare disease that can occur following a sexually transmitted infection; *C. trachomatis* appears to be the most common pathogen associated with sexually acquired reactive arthritis. Other inciting pathogens include Campylobacter, Salmonella, and Shigella.

20. D) Gonorrhea

Most female patients with genital gonococcal infections are asymptomatic. However, symptomatic cervical infection can present with findings consistent with cervicitis. This includes vaginal pruritis, a mucopurulent cervical discharge, and a friable cervical mucosa. The patient may also have dysuria and peri-labial pain from involvement of the urethra and/or Bartholin's glands. Primary syphilis is characteristic for a chancre. Fitz-Hugh-Curtis syndrome occurs in approximately 10% of female patients with acute pelvic inflammatory disease and causes inflammation of the liver capsule and peritoneal surfaces. The syndrome is characterized by right upper quadrant pain, abdominal pain, and tenderness on palpation with a distinct pleuritic component. Genital herpes simplex virus infection presents with genital lesions that appear as small vesicles with an erythematous base that can rupture easily.

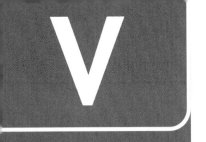

PEDIATRICS AND ADOLESCENTS REVIEW

DANGER SIGNALS

CHLAMYDIAL OPHTHALMIA NEONATORUM (TRACHOMA)

Symptoms will show 5 to 14 days after birth. Eyelids become edematous and red with profuse watery discharge initially that later becomes purulent or bloody. When obtaining a sample, collect conjunctival epithelial cells by swabbing the everted eyelid. Rule out concomitant chlamydial pneumonia, which commonly occurs in infants with trachoma, with nasopharyngeal sampling. Treated with systemic antibiotics such as azithromycin 20 mg/kg daily × 3 days or erythromycin ethylsuccinate four times a day (QID) × 14 days. Use only systemic antibiotics. Topical therapy has a high failure rate and does not eradicate nasopharyngeal infections. Prenatal screening and treatment is recommended for all pregnant patients <25 years old and those >25 years old with risk factors for sexually transmitted infection (STI). Reportable disease.

CHLAMYDIAL PNEUMONIA

In infants with ophthalmia neonatorum, also rule out concomitant chlamydial pneumonia. Obtain nasopharyngeal culture for chlamydia. Infant will present between 2 and 8 weeks with frequent staccato cough with bibasilar rales, tachypnea, hypoxia, hyperinflation, and bilateral, symmetric infiltrates on chest x-ray. Treated with azithromycin 20 mg/kg daily × 3 days or erythromycin QID × 2 weeks. Daily follow-up. Reportable disease.

CRYPTORCHIDISM (UNDESCENDED TESTICLE)

Empty scrotal sac(s) without spontaneous descent of testicle into scrotum by 4 months. Most cases involve undescended testicles. One or both testicles may be missing. Testis does not descend with massage of the inguinal area. Majority of cases of cryptorchidism are associated with patent processus vaginalis. Infant should be sitting, and the exam room should be warm to relax muscles when massaging the inguinal canal. Another option is to examine the child after a warm bath.

Increased risk of testicular cancer if testicles are not removed from the abdomen. Surgical correction (orchiopexy) is typically recommended within the first year of life if testicle does not spontaneously descend by 4 months.

DEHYDRATION

Signs of severe dehydration (>10% weight loss) in an infant are weak and rapid pulse, tachypnea or deep breathing, parched mucous membranes, anterior fontanelle that is markedly sunken, skin turgor showing tenting, cool skin, acrocyanosis, anuria, and change in baseline level of consciousness (LOC; such as obtundation, lethargy, or coma). Refer severely dehydrated infants to the ED for intravenous (IV) hydration. Severe dehydration due to acute gastroenteritis is one of the leading causes of death of infants in the developing world.

DOWN SYNDROME

A genetic defect caused by trisomy of chromosome 21 (three copies instead of two). The most common chromosomal disorder among live births; the average life span is 60 years in the United States.

Affected persons have a round face that presents with decreased anterior–posterior diameter with up-tilted eyes (palpebral fissures) and low-set, small ears. Chronic open mouth caused by enlarged tongue (macroglossia), accompanied by a shorter neck. Short fingers, small palms, and a broad hand with a single transverse palmar crease are additional signs. Newborns have hypotonia and poor Moro reflex. Higher risk of intellectual disability, congenital heart defects, feeding difficulties, congenital hearing loss, thyroid disease, cataracts, sleep apnea, and early onset of Alzheimer's disease (average age 54 years).

Educate parents about importance of cervical spine positioning and monitoring for myelopathic signs and symptoms. Contact sports (football, soccer, gymnastics) may place at higher risk of spinal cord injury due to atlantoaxial instability. Avoid trampoline use unless under professional supervision. Special Olympics requires specific screening for some sports.

EXCESSIVE NEWBORN WEIGHT LOSS (>10%)

Newborns are expected to lose weight during the first few days of life. Weight loss can vary by feeding method and delivery type; infants delivered by cesarean section (C-section) tend to lose a larger percentage of birth weight than their vaginally delivered counterparts. Formula-fed infants may lose up to 5%, and breastfed infants may lose 7% to 10% of their birth weight.

Any loss from birth weight should be regained within 10 to 14 days. Weight loss beyond 10% in neonates is considered abnormal. Assess the infant for dehydration, electrolyte disturbances, and hyperbilirubinemia, and the mother and infant for lactation difficulties.

FETAL ALCOHOL SYNDROME

Also known as fetal alcohol spectrum disorder. Classic fetal alcohol syndrome (FAS) facies is a small head (microcephaly) with shortened palpebral fissures (narrow eyes) with epicanthal folds and a flat nasal bridge. There is a thin upper lip with no vertical groove above the upper lip (smooth philtrum). Ears have an underdeveloped upper curve that is folded over. Can range from neurocognitive and behavioral problems (e.g., attention deficit disorder [ADD]) to more severe intellectual disabilities. There is no safe dose or time for alcohol during pregnancy. Alcohol adversely affects the central nervous system (CNS), somatic growth, and facial structure development.

GONOCOCCAL OPHTHALMIA NEONATORUM

Can be a serious cause of morbidity. Infection can rapidly spread, causing blindness. Symptoms usually show within 2 to 5 days after birth. Do not delay treatment by waiting for culture results. Symptoms include injected (red) conjunctiva with profuse purulent discharge and swollen eyelids. Majority of cases of congenital gonorrhea infection are acquired during delivery (intrapartum). Coinfection with chlamydia is common with gonococcal infection. Any neonates with acute conjunctivitis presenting within 30 days or less from birth should be tested for chlamydia, gonorrhea, herpes simplex, and bacterial infection.

Order Gram stain, gonococcal culture (modified Thayer–Martin media), or polymerase chain reaction (PCR) test for *Neisseria gonorrhoeae*, herpes simplex culture, and PCR for *Chlamydia trachomatis* of eye exudate. Hospitalize and treat with ceftriaxone, 25 to 50 mg/kg body weight IV or IM in a single dose, not to exceed 250 mg. Preferred prophylaxis is with ophthalmic 0.5% erythromycin ointment (1-cm ribbon per eye) immediately after birth. Screen (and treat) mother and sexual partner for STIs.

POOR WEIGHT GAIN (FAILURE TO THRIVE)

Defined as weight for age that falls below second percentile for gestation-corrected age and sex when plotted on appropriate growth chart (on more than one occasion). Also, infants whose rate of weight change decreases over two or more major percentile lines (90th, 75th, 50th, 25th, and 5th) exhibit poor weight gain (failure to thrive) (e.g., child at 50th percentile goes down to 5th percentile over a few months). Use World Health Organization (WHO) growth charts until the age of 2 years, and then Centers for Disease Control and Prevention (CDC) growth charts. In most cases seen in primary care, causes are usually inadequate dietary intake, diarrhea, malabsorption (celiac disease, cystic fibrosis, food allergy), frequent infections, and psychosocial factors such as poverty, family discord, and poor maternal bonding.

SUDDEN INFANT DEATH SYNDROME

A sudden infant death in apparently healthy infants <12 months, which cannot be explained after a thorough case investigation that includes a scene investigation, autopsy, and review of clinical history. Higher risk with prematurity, low birth weight, young maternal age, and maternal smoking and/or drug use. Cause hypothesized to be a multifactorial convergence of intrinsically vulnerable infant (genetic predisposition) during a critical development period with exogenous stressors. To decrease risk, position infants on their backs (supine); use a firm sleep surface; encourage breastfeeding and routine immunizations; room share without bedsharing; offer a pacifier for sleep times; and avoid soft objects and loose bedding in the sleep area, smoke exposure, and overheating infant.

SKIN LESIONS

CAFÉ AU LAIT SPOTS

Flat light-brown to dark-brown spots >5 mm (0.5 cm). If six or more spots larger than 5 mm (0.5 cm) in diameter are seen, rule out neurofibromatosis or von Recklinghausen's disease (e.g., neurologic disorder marked by seizures, learning disorders). Refer to pediatric neurologist if the spots meet the same criteria to rule out neurofibromatosis.

CONGENITAL DERMAL MELANOCYTOSIS

The most common type of pigmented skin lesions in newborns. Formerly called Mongolian spots. Present in almost all Asian neonates and in more than half of American Indian, Hispanic, and Black neonates. Variations on blue-gray patches or stains with ill-defined borders. A common location is the lumbosacral area (but can be located anywhere on the body). May be mistaken for bruising or child abuse. Usually fade by age 2 to 3 years.

ERYTHEMA TOXICUM NEONATORUM

Small pustules (whitish-yellow color) that are 1 to 3 mm in size and surrounded by a red base. Erupt during the second to the third day of life. Located on the face, chest, back, and extremities. Lasts from 1 to 2 weeks and resolves spontaneously.

FAUN TAIL NEVUS

Tufts of hair overlying spinal column usually at lumbosacral area. May be a sign of neural tube defects (spina bifida, spina bifida occulta). Perform neurologic exam focusing on lumbosacral nerves (fecal/urinary incontinence, problems with gait). Order ultrasound of lesion to rule out occult spina bifida.

MILIA, MILIARIA, OR "PRICKLY HEAT"

Most common in neonates. Multiple white 1- to 2-mm papules located mainly on the forehead, cheeks, and nose. Due to retention of sebaceous material and keratin. Resolves spontaneously.

SEBORRHEIC DERMATITIS ("CRADLE CAP")

Excessive thick scaling on the scalp of younger infants; can also be seen on the ears, face, and neck folds. Treated by softening and removal of the thick scales on the scalp after soaking scalp a few hours (to overnight) with vegetable oil or mineral oil. Shampoo scalp and gently scrub scales with soft brush. Prevention is by frequent shampooing with mild baby shampoo and removing scales with soft brush or comb. Self-limited condition that resolves spontaneously within a few months.

VASCULAR LESIONS

Nevus Flammeus (Port-Wine Stain)

Neonates with pink-to-red, flat, stain-like skin lesions located on the upper and lower eyelids or on the V1 and V2 branches of the trigeminal nerve (cranial nerve [CN] V) should be referred to a pediatric ophthalmologist to rule out congenital glaucoma. Blanches to pressure. Irregular in size and shape. Usually unilateral. Large lesions located on half the facial area may be a sign of trigeminal nerve involvement and Sturge–Weber syndrome (rare neurologic disorder). The lesions do not regress and will grow with the child. These lesions can be treated with pulsed-dye laser (PDL) therapy.

Nevus Simplex (Salmon Patches)

Often referred to as "stork bites" or "angel kisses." Flat pink patches found on the forehead, eyelids, and nape of neck (Figure 20.1). Usually appear on both sides of the midline (i.e., on both eyelids or across the entire nape of neck). Blanchable, but color changes with crying, breath holding, and room temperature changes. Consider Beckwith–Wiedemann or FAS if glabellar lesion seen. Typically fade by 18 months.

Superficial Hemangioma (Strawberry Hemangioma)

Not usually seen at birth, but appear in the first few days to months. Raised vascular lesions ranging in size from 0.5 to 4.0 cm that are bright red in color and feel soft to palpation. Usually located on the head or the neck. The lesions often grow rapidly during the first 12 months of life, but the majority will involute gradually over the next 1 to 5 years. Watchful waiting is the usual strategy. Can be treated with PDL therapy. If more than five lesions noted, consider imaging to check for hepatic hemangiomas.

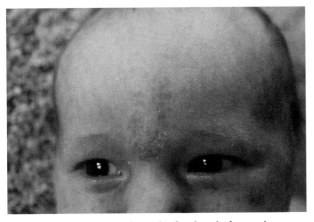

Figure 20.1 Salmon patch on the forehead of a newborn.
Source: Gawlik, K. S., Melnyk, B. M., & Teall, A. M. (Eds.). (2021). (See Resources section for complete source information.)

SCREENING TESTS

VISION SCREENING

Newborn Vision

- Newborns are nearsighted (myopia) and have a vision between 20/200 and 20/400.
- They can focus best at a distance of 8 to 10 inches.
- During the first 2 months, the infant's eyes may appear crossed (or wander) at times (normal finding). If one eye is consistently turned in or turned out, refer to pediatric ophthalmologist.
- Human face is preferred by newborns.
- Newborns do not shed tears, because the lacrimal ducts are not fully mature at birth.
- White neonates are born with blue-gray eyes. It is normal for their eye color to change as they mature.
- Retinas (CN II) are immature at birth and reach maturity at age 6 years.

Infant Screening

- 1 month: Infant can fixate briefly on the mother's face. Prefers to look at the human face.
- 3 months: Infant will hold the hands close to the face to observe them. Hold a bright object or a toy in front of the infant. Watch behavior as the infant fixates and follows the toy for a few seconds. Avoid using objects/toys that make noises when testing vision.
- 6 months: Makes good eye contact. Turns head to scan surroundings with 180-degree visual field.
- 12 months: Makes prolonged eye contact when spoken to. Will actively turn head around 180 degrees to observe people and surroundings for long periods. Recognizes self in a mirror and parents and favorite people from a longer distance.
- Retina and optic disc: Set fundoscope lens at 0 to −2 diopters. Fundus appears dark orange to red (red reflex). The red reflex of both eyes should be symmetrical in shape and color.

Abnormal Findings

Strabismus

- Misalignment of the eye. Horizontal strabismus may be esotropia (inward turning of the eyes) or exotropia (outward turning of the eyes). Vertical strabismus may be hypertropia (one eye deviates upward compared with the other) or hypotropia (one eye deviates downward).
- Uncorrected strabismus can result in permanent visual loss and abnormal vision such as diplopia (double vision). Treatment includes eyeglasses, eye exercises, prism, and/or eye muscle surgery.

Amblyopia ("Lazy Eye")

If corrected early, affected eye can have normal vision.

Esotropia

- Misalignment of one or both eyes ("cross-eyed"). Infants (<20 weeks) may have intermittent esotropia, which usually resolves spontaneously.

- Some infants with obvious epicanthal folds appear "cross-eyed" (pseudostrabismus), but corneal light reflex will be normal. Refer to pediatric ophthalmologist if in doubt.

Red Reflex

Screening test for cataracts and retinoblastoma. Abnormal if there are white-colored opacities (cataracts) or white spots (leukocoria). Determine presence of white reflex, rule out retinoblastoma, and refer infant to pediatric ophthalmologist as soon as possible. Even if the test is normal during the visit, but a parent reports that one eye appears white on a digital photograph, refer. If absence or decreased intensity of red reflex, rule out cataract and refer to pediatric ophthalmologist. Procedure: Perform test in a darkened room. Use a direct ophthalmoscope and shine light about 12 to 18 inches away from the infant. Normal finding is symmetrical and round orange-red glow from each eye.

Congenital Cataracts

Red reflex exam on neonate shows a round, white-colored pupil.

Light Reflex Test or Corneal Light Reflex (Hirschberg Test)

Screening test for strabismus. Abnormal if corneal light reflex is not clear or if it is "off-center." Procedure: Shine light directly in eyes (24 inches away) using a fixation target. Infant or child must look directly forward with both eyes aligned. Observe for the symmetry and brightness of light reflecting from both eyes.

Indications for Referral

- Abnormal red reflex (rule out retinoblastoma, cataract, glaucoma)
- Presence of white reflex (rule out retinoblastoma)
- Strabismus (rule out CN III, IV, and VI abnormalities, retinoblastoma)
- Greater than two-line difference between each eye
- Esodeviation present after 3 to 4 months of age
- Corneal light reflex test with abnormal result
- Shape/appearance of pupils not equal
- New onset of strabismus (e.g., retinoblastoma, brain mass, bleeding, lead poisoning)

HEARING SCREENING FOR NEWBORNS

Universal screening for hearing loss is done while in nursery before discharge. Each state has its own rules about neonatal hearing exams.

Auditory Brainstem Response

Measures the CN VIII by the use of "click" stimuli.

Otoacoustic Emissions

Gross hearing test: As a response to loud noise, look for startle response (neonates), blinking, turning toward sound. Measures the middle ear mobility only. Less sensitive than the auditory brainstem response (ABR).

Mnemonic Device (HEARS) for High-Risk Factors for Hearing Loss

H (hyperbilirubinemia that is severe)
E (ear infections frequently; ear anomalies)
A (Apgar scores low at birth)
R (rubella, cytomegalovirus [CMV], toxoplasmosis infections)
S (seizures)

Premature infants and infants admitted to NICUs have a higher incidence of hearing loss compared with full-term infants.

LABORATORY TESTS

Newborn screening is required by all 50 states and the District of Columbia. Testing varies from state to state. Blood is obtained by heel stick or from cord blood. A spot of blood is blotted into filter paper for stable transport.

HEMOGLOBIN AND HEMATOCRIT

Normal newborns have hemoglobin F (fetal hemoglobin) and hemoglobin A. Healthy term infants have enough iron stores to last up to 6 months. Screening for anemia is done in late infancy (9–12 months) for healthy full-term infants. Not screened at birth, because hemoglobin is elevated from maternal red blood cells (RBCs) mixed with fetal RBCs.

LEAD SCREENING

High-risk children (e.g., children living below poverty level or living in homes built prior to 1978) should be screened at ages 1 and 2 years (12 and 24 months).

PHENYLKETONURIA

Phenylketonuria (PKU) testing is federally mandated. Severe intellectual disability results if not treated early. Disorder is an inability to metabolize phenylalanine to tyrosine because of a defect in the production of the enzyme phenylalanine hydroxylase. Perform test only after infant has protein feeding (breast milk or formula) for at least 48 hours. Higher risk of false negatives if done too early (<48 hours). Treated by following special diet (phenylalanine-free diet).

SICKLE CELL DISEASE

The required test can detect four types of hemoglobin (F, S, A, and C).

THYROID DISEASE

Testing for congenital hypothyroidism is federally mandated. Lack of thyroid hormone results in mental and somatic growth retardation. Treated by thyroid hormone supplementation.

PHYSIOLOGIC CONCERNS IN INFANCY

NUTRITIONAL INTAKE

Breastfeeding is preferred over formula. If formula is used, start with one fortified with iron. See Chapter 18 for breastfeeding concerns in newborns.

Breastfeeding

Give vitamin D drops (400 IU of vitamin D) starting in the first few days of life if breastfeeding because breast milk alone does not provide adequate levels of vitamin D. Infant formula is supplemented with vitamin D, iron, other vitamins, and essential fatty acids.

- Breast milk or formula contains 20 calories per ounce.
- Decreased risk of maternal breast and ovarian cancer, type 2 diabetes, and hypertension; decreased risk of neonatal infections, SIDS, asthma, and obesity later in life.

Colostrum

Sticky and thick, yellowish fluid that comes before breast milk. Secreted first few days after the birth and contains large amounts of maternal antibodies and nutrients.

Cow's Milk

- Avoid cow's milk the first year of life (causes gastrointestinal [GI] bleeding).
- High quantities are a common cause of iron-deficiency anemia in babies and young children.

Solid Foods

- Recommended to wait until about 6 months for complementary foods. Start with a single-grain, iron-fortified baby cereal, mix with four tablespoons of breast milk/formula. Serve once or twice a day after bottle or breastfeeding. Avoid feeding only rice cereal due to possible exposure to heavy metals such as arsenic.
- Introduce one food at a time for 4 to 5 days (if allergic, easier to identify offending food).

EXAM TIPS

- Colostrum (IgG antibodies): Looks like thick, yellowish fluid and is secreted the first few days of breastfeeding before mature milk release.
- Breastfeeding: Supplement with vitamin D the first few days of life. Avoid cow's milk during first 12 months of life (causes GI bleeding, iron-deficiency anemia).

ELIMINATION

Meconium

Thick dark-green to black-colored stool that is odorless. Most full-term neonates pass meconium stool within a few hours of birth. Failure to pass meconium within 48 hours of birth is worrisome and may be a sign of intestinal obstruction, Hirschsprung's disease, hypothyroidism, or cystic fibrosis.

HEAD FINDINGS

Head Circumference

Also known as the *occipitofrontal circumference (OFC)*. Use paper tape (cloth tape stretches) and place above the ear.

- Average head circumference at birth is 13.7 inches (35 cm).
- Head circumference is measured at each wellness visit until age 36 months (3 years).
- In newborns, chest is about 1 to 2 cm smaller in size than the head circumference.
- Head circumference will increase by 12 cm during the first 12 months.
- Fastest rate of head growth is during the first 3 months of life (2 cm per month).

Abnormal Findings

Cephalohematoma

Traumatic subperiosteal hemorrhage that is more common when assisted delivery is needed. Swelling does not cross the midline or suture lines. If significant, can be associated with hyperbilirubinemia.

Caput Succedaneum

Diffused edema of the scalp that crosses the midline. Caused by intrauterine and vaginal pressure from prolonged or difficult vaginal labor. The scalp becomes molded and "cone shaped." Self-limited and resolves spontaneously.

EXAM TIPS

- Head circumference grows by up to 12 cm (first 12 months).
- Caput succedaneum crosses midline, and cephalohematoma does not (blood blocked by skull sutures).

WEIGHT GAIN AND LENGTH

Birth Weight

Neonates lose up to 10% of body weight but should regain it by age 2 weeks. They double their birth weight by 4 to 6 months and triple their birth weight by 12 months.

Infant Weight

- 0 to 6 months: 6 to 8 ounces per week and 1 inch per month
- 6 to 12 months: 3 to 4 ounces per week and 0.5 inch per month

If the child's weight and/or length decelerates across two or more major percentiles, rule out poor weight gain (failure to thrive) (see "Danger Signals"). In addition, any child who is at the third to fifth percentile is considered to have poor weight gain. Of the many causes of poor weight gain, the most common in primary care are undernutrition and malnutrition. Evaluate the child, but do not forget to assess maternal bonding and depression.

Length and Height

Length (linear growth) of infants is measured from birth to about 24 months. Starting at the age of 2 years, measure height (child is standing up) and calculate body mass index (BMI). Plot the measurements on the infant's or child's percentile growth chart.

EXAM TIPS

- Weight loss of 7% to 10% starts after birth, but neonates should regain birth weight in 2 weeks.
- Birth weight doubles at 4 to 6 months and triples at 12 months.

DENTITION

Epstein's pearls are white papules found on the newborn's gum line that resemble an erupting tooth. They typically resolve by a few weeks after birth.

First Teeth (Primary Teeth)

Both left and right teeth erupt bilaterally at the same time (symmetrical). Symptoms are drooling, chewing on objects, irritability, crying, and low-grade fever. Teeth are typically lost in same order that they erupted

- 6 to 10 months: Lower central incisors (lower front teeth)
- 2.5 years: Has complete set of primary teeth (20 teeth)

First Permanent Teeth (Deciduous Teeth)

6 years: Shed primary central incisors; first permanent teeth to erupt are upper and lower first molars and central incisors.

EXAM TIPS

- Epstein's pearls are white papules found on gum line that resemble an erupting tooth.
- Do not confuse questions asking for the "first tooth" with the "first permanent tooth."

GENITOURINARY ANOMALIES

- Hypospadias: Urethral meatus located on the ventral aspect of the penis. Location may be at the glans or shaft. Some have two urethral openings; one opening is normal, and the other opening is lower on the glans or shaft. Refer to pediatric urologist.
- Epispadias: Urethral meatus is located on the dorsal aspect (upper side) of the penis. Refer to pediatric urologist.
- Hydrocele: Presence of fluid inside the scrotum (tunica vaginalis/processus vaginalis) that results in swelling of the affected scrotum. Fairly common in newborn males. Skin is normal color and temperature. Affected testicle(s) will show increased size in the glow of light compared with the normal scrotum (transillumination). Darken the room and place the light source on the scrotal skin. Compare each scrotum.
- Newborn female vagina swollen with small amount of blood-tinged discharge: Caused by withdrawal of maternal hormones and will disappear within a few days.
- Cryptorchidism: Retention of one or both testicles in the abdominal cavity or the inguinal canal. Markedly increases risk of testicular cancer and infertility. Order inguinal and abdominal ultrasound. Typically corrected surgically before age 12 months.

EXAM TIPS

- Cryptorchidism increases risk of testicular cancer. Refer to pediatric urologist for evaluation between 6 and 12 months of age.
- Hydrocele is fluid collection inside the scrotum (tunica vaginalis/processus vaginalis). Scrotal sac will appear "brighter" or will have more light glow compared with scrotum with a testicle (solid objects block light, so less glow of light).

REFLEX TESTING

Anal Wink

Gently stroke the anal region. Look for contraction of the perianal muscle. Absence is abnormal and suggestive of a lesion on the spinal cord (e.g., spina bifida).

Plantar Reflex (Babinski Reflex)

Upward extension of the big toe with fanning of the other toes. Starting on the heel, firmly stroke the outer side of the sole toward the front of the foot (Figure 20.2).

Palmar Reflex (Grasp Reflex)

Place a finger on the infant's open palm. The infant closes its hand around the finger. Pulling away the examiner's finger causes the infant's grip to tighten.

Moro Reflex (Startle Reflex)

Sudden loud noise will cause symmetric abduction and extension of the arms followed by adduction and flexion of the arms over the body. Disappears by 3 to 4 months.

- Absence on one side: Rule out brachial plexus injury, fracture, or shoulder dystocia.
- Absence on both sides: Rule out spinal cord or brain lesion.
- Older infant: Persistence of Moro reflex is abnormal. Rule out brain pathology.

Step Reflex

Hold baby upright and allow the dorsal surface of one foot to touch the edge of a table. Baby will flex the hip and knee and place the stimulated foot on the tabletop (stepping motion). Absent with paresis and breech births. Disappears by 6 weeks.

Blink Reflex

Eyelids will close in response to bright light or touch.

Tonic Neck Reflex (Fencing Reflex)

Turning head to one side with jaw over shoulder causes the arm and leg on the same side to extend. The arm and leg on the opposite side will flex.

Rooting Reflex

Stroking the corner of the mouth causes baby to turn toward stimulus and suck. Disappears by 3 to 4 months.

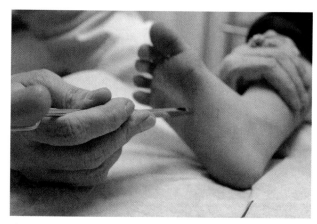

Figure 20.2 Plantar reflex test.
Source: Gawlik, K. S., Melnyk, B. M., & Teall, A. M. (Eds.). (2021). (See Resources section for complete source information.)

A strong Moro reflex in an older infant (age ≥6 months) is abnormal and indicative of brain damage.

IMMUNIZATIONS

MUMPS, MEASLES, AND RUBELLA AND VARICELLA VACCINE

Live attenuated virus vaccine (Table 20.1). Not recommended before age 12 months (not effective due to immaturity of immune system). If dose given before 12 months of age, must be repeated.

- Avoid salicylates for 6 weeks (theoretical risk of Reye's syndrome). Children (age birth to 12 years) should not be given any aspirin or any aspirin products (e.g., Pepto-Bismol, Pamprin, Alka Seltzer, Kaopectate).
- First dose (mumps, measles, and rubella [MMR] and varicella): 12 months
- Second dose (MMR and varicella): 4 to 6 years (preschool age)
- Proof of varicella: Documentation of chickenpox or herpes zoster on the chart by a healthcare provider, record of two doses, or a positive varicella titer

Table 20.1 contains only the childhood vaccines that must be given by a definite age and should not deviate from schedule.

INFLUENZA VACCINE

The CDC recommends use of injectable flu vaccines. The nasal spray form (live attenuated influenza vaccine) is not to be used.

- Do not give influenza vaccines before age 6 months, because they are not effective (immature immune system). It takes 2 weeks to produce antibodies after vaccination.
- Recommended for everyone age 6 months or older (with rare exceptions), but especially for children 6 months to 4 years of age; people with congenital heart disease, asthma, cystic fibrosis, sickle cell anemia, heart disease, and chronic obstructive pulmonary disease (COPD); those who will be pregnant during the influenza season; American Indians/Alaska Natives; healthcare personnel; elderly; and others.
- Administer fall to winter as injection.
- Trivalent inactivated influenza vaccines (protect against three types of influenza virus).
- Quadrivalent influenza vaccines (protect against four types of influenza virus).

Contraindications

Influenza Injection (Trivalent Inactivated Vaccine)

- Age younger than 6 months
- If history of egg allergy (hives only), can receive the flu vaccine injection. But if severe reaction to eggs (hypotension, wheezing, nausea and vomiting) requiring medical treatment or epinephrine, the patient can receive the flu vaccine only in an outpatient or inpatient clinic that has a health provider who can treat anaphylaxis (e.g., epinephrine, intubation, oxygen).

Table 20.1 Immunization Schedule (Birth to 6 Years)

Vaccine	Birth	2 Months	4 Months	6 Months	12 Months - 3 Years	4–6 Years
Hepatitis B (HepB)	#1	#2 at 1–2 mo		#3 at 6–18 mo		
Rotavirus (RV or RV5)		#1	#2	#3*		
Diphtheria, tetanus, acellular pertussis (DTaP)		#1	#2	#3	#4 at 15–18 mo	#5
Haemophilus influenzae type b conjugate vaccine (Hib)		#1	#2	#3**	#3 or #4 at 12–15 mo**	
Pneumococcal conjugate form of vaccine (PCV13 or PCV15)		#1	#2	#3	#4 at 12–15 mo	
Inactivated polio (IPV)		#1	#2	#3 at 6–18 mo		#4
Measles, mumps, rubella (MMR)					#1 (12–15 mo)	#2
Varicella (VAR)					#1 (12–15 mo)	#2
Hepatitis A (HepA)					#1 (12–23 mo with #2 at min 6 mo after #1)	
Influenza (IIV)				#1***		

*Rotarix (RV) requires two doses, and RotaTeq (RV5) requires three doses.
**There are five forms of Hib vaccine that require three or four doses, with varying administration schedules. This dose is not recommended when using the PedvaxHIB vaccine.
***The first time IIV is given, a second dose 4 weeks after the initial dose is recommended. Subsequent IIV vaccination is needed only once annually.
Note: Most vaccines have a range (from 3 to 6 months) when they can be given. For a complete list of all vaccine schedules: www.cdc.gov/vaccines.
Source: Adapted from the Centers for Disease Control and Prevention (2020).

- Moderate-to-severe illness with fever (wait until patient is better)
- History of Guillain–Barré syndrome

DIPHTHERIA, TETANUS, PERTUSSIS VACCINES

Diphtheria, tetanus, acellular pertussis (DTaP) is the form of vaccine used in the United States. It has fewer side effects compared with older DTP form.

- Diphtheria–tetanus (DT): This form is used for infants and children younger than age 7 years unable to tolerate pertussis component.
- Tdap vaccine: For age 7 years and older. At age 11- to 12-year visit, give the Tdap. Or if due for tetanus booster, give Tdap once in a lifetime. Then tetanus diphtheria (Td) or Tdap every 10 years for lifetime.
- Tdap vaccine: Can be given to pregnant and breastfeeding patients. Tdap given to children younger than age 7 years is *not* valid (use DTaP).

Side Effects of DTaP/DT

- Fever (defined as 100.4°F) in up to 50% of patients
- Swelling, pain, and/or redness at injection site in up to 50% of patients
- Irritability in up to 50% of patients
- Acute encephalopathy 1 in 110,000

Contraindications

- Severe allergic reaction
- Encephalopathy (i.e., prolonged seizures, change in LOC) not attributable to another cause within 7 days of administration of the vaccine)

Precautions

- Fever ≥105°F (within 48 hours of dose)
- Seizures (within 3 days or less of dose)
- Collapse or shock-like state within 48 hours after dose

Not Considered Contraindications to DTP/DTaP Vaccination

- Family history of seizures
- Family history of sudden infant death syndrome (SIDS)
- Fever <105°F from prior DTaP vaccination

VACCINE ADVERSE EVENT REPORTING SYSTEM

A national postmarketing vaccine safety surveillance program in the United States managed by both the CDC and the U.S. Food and Drug Administration (FDA). Report vaccine adverse events at www.vaers.hhs.gov.

IMMUNIZATION TIPS

By age 15 to 18 months, the following vaccines are usually completed (for most infants):
- Hepatitis B vaccine (three doses)
- If hepatitis B surface antigen (HBsAg)–positive mother, give neonate hepatitis B immunoglobulin (HBIG) and the hepatitis B vaccine.
- *Haemophilus influenzae* type b (Hib) vaccine (several types of Hib vaccines; may require two, three, or four doses)
- Pneumococcal vaccine (PCV 13 or PCV15; four doses)
- Rotavirus vaccine (two or three doses)
- Hepatitis A (HepA; two doses)

GROWTH AND DEVELOPMENT

NEWBORNS

- Strong primitive reflexes (e.g., Moro, rooting, fencing)
- Head lag
- Grasps finger tightly if placed on the baby's hand (grasp reflex)
- Seedy yellow stool after each feeding (if breastfed)
- Eats every 2 to 3 hours or nurses 8 to 10 times a day
- Does not produce tears when crying; tear ducts are not mature at birth
- Sleeps 16 hours per day
- Report high-pitched cry, "catlike" cry, hypotonic microcephaly (concern for cri du chat syndrome)

2 MONTHS OLD

- Follows objects past midline
- Coos vowels and makes gurgling sounds
- Lifts head 45 degrees when prone
- Smiles in response to another

4 MONTHS OLD

- Smiles spontaneously (social smile)
- Begins to babble

Fine Motor

- Brings hands to mouth
- Can swing at dangling toys

Table 20.2 Growth and Development Milestones: Infancy

Age	Characteristics	Abnormal
Neonate	Strong reflexes. Minimum of six to eight bowel movements per day. Urinates eight times a day.	Jaundice at birth (hemolysis). High-pitched cry. Irritable. "Floppy" (hypotonic). Poor reflexes.
2 months	Smiles. Able to coo. Makes gurgling sounds. Can hold head up. Starts to recognize parents.	Inability to hold head up. Avoids eye contact. Floppy.
6 months	Sits up without support. Rolls in both directions (front to back, back to front). Says single-syllable sounds. Tries to get things out of reach by "raking" (uses palms to reach).	Lack of babbling. Does not laugh. Inability to turn head past midline (180 degrees).
9 months	Pincer grasp (fine motor). Plays pat-a-cake and peek-a-boo. Waves "bye-bye." May be afraid of strangers (can be clingy). Can stand holding on. Crawls.	Infantile reflexes strong. Persistence of primitive reflexes (e.g., startle, fencing). Does not babble. Does not bear weight on legs with support. Unable to sit with help.
1 year (12 months)	Supports own weight. Walks with hands held. Separation anxiety. Can "climb" stairs by crawling up or down. Starts to cruise (moves from one piece of furniture to another for support).	Unable to support own weight. Lack of babbling. No response to smiles, poor eye contact, loss of previously learned skills (autism).

Gross Motor
- Holds head steady and unsupported
- Rolls from front to back (supine to prone)

6 MONTHS OLD
Fine Motor
- Has palmar grasp of objects
- Reaches for toys using palmar grasp
- Brings things to mouth
- Starts to pass things from one hand to the other

Gross Motor
- Begins to sit up independently without support
- Rolls over in both directions (back/supine to stomach and stomach to back/supine)

Language
- Starts to say consonants
- Is very curious and will look around environment

Other
Report failure to follow objects past midline (180 degrees), poor eye contact

9 MONTHS OLD
Fine Motor
- Pincer grasp starts and can pick up things (e.g., food) between thumb and forefinger
- Waves "bye-bye"
- May clap hands and play clapping games such as pat-a-cake

Gross Motor
- Pulls self up to stand
- Crawls and "cruises"
- Bears weight well

Language
- Plays peek-a-boo
- Report absence of babble, inability to sit alone, strong primitive reflexes such as the Moro (startle reflex) or fencing (tonic neck reflex)

Other
"Stranger anxiety" very obvious

12 MONTHS OLD
Fine Motor
Can use "sippy" cup

Gross Motor
- Stands independently
- May walk independently
- Starts to cruise (moves from one piece of furniture to the next for support)

Language
- Can say one to two words other than repetitive sounds (e.g., mama, dada)
- Can say exclamations, such as "Uh-oh!"
- Knows first name
- Follows simple directions, such as "Pick up toy"

Other
- Growth rate slows down
- Report absence of weight bearing, inability to transfer objects hand to hand

SAFETY EDUCATION
- Advise parent to learn infant cardiopulmonary resuscitation (CPR; basic life support [BLS] course).
- Avoid heating formula in the microwave.

- Do not leave a baby on the changing table (e.g., to answer phone).
- Do not position cribs next to strings or cords. When the child is crawling, hide electrical cords. Close toilet seats (safety lock); lock bathroom doors; lock cabinets with cleaning products.
- Turn pot handles away from the edge of stove; use rear burners on the stove.
- Use safety locks for stove handles, low cabinets, and doors.

Choking Prevention

- Remove objects smaller than 2 inches.
- Examples of choking sources are grapes, raw carrots, hot dogs, latex balloons, coins, and buttons. Cut up food into small pieces.
- Avoid giving hard candy to children younger than 6 years.
- Encourage at least one parent to attend infant/child BLS course.

Car Safety

- Infants and toddlers up to the age of 2 years should be in a rear-facing car seat (Table 20.3).
- Safest place in the car for infant or child younger than 13 years is in the back seat.
- Avoid used infant safety seat if its parts are missing or if it is damaged.
- Air bags in cars can cause serious brain injury if they hit the child's head or neck area.
- Turn off the air bag on the front seat if the person who is using the seat is under the weight limit, which is usually set at 100 lb (check car manual).

Toxic Exposures

Chronic exposure to secondhand smoke increases rates of SIDS, otitis media, bronchitis, pneumonia, and wheezing and coughing. It also affects lung development and exacerbates asthma.

DISEASE REVIEW

COARCTATION OF THE AORTA

Congenital narrowing of a portion of the aorta. Most commonly the coarctation is distal to the subclavian artery and is typically noted at the area where the ductus arteriosus attaches. Newborn may be asymptomatic if mild case of patent ductus arteriosus (PDA). Severe cases will have heart failure or shock when PDA closes. Up to 30% of infants with this condition have Turner's syndrome. Female infants noted to have a coarctation should get a karyotype analysis.

Screening

Compare the femoral and brachial pulses simultaneously. Absence or delay of the femoral pulse when it is compared with the brachial pulse is diagnostic. Neonate is pale, irritable, dyspneic, and diaphoretic. If abnormal, order cardiac echocardiogram, EKG, and chest x-ray.

Older Infants

May be asymptomatic. Take blood pressure (BP) measurements of both arms and thighs.

- Normal finding: Systolic BP is higher in legs than in arms.
- Abnormal finding: Systolic BP higher in arms than in thighs. Palpate pulse in all four extremities. There is a delay or change in amplitude of pulses. Bounding radial pulses are compared with femoral pulse.

CONGENITAL LACRIMAL DUCT OBSTRUCTION (DACRYOSTENOSIS)

Also known as *congenital nasolacrimal duct obstruction*. Occurs in approximately 6% of newborns. Usually spontaneously resolves within 6 months in the majority of infants.

Classic Case

An infant's parent reports persistent tearing and eyelash matting in the morning on one or both of the baby's eyes, but no conjunctival erythema. When the lacrimal duct is

Table 20.3 Car Safety Seats

Age Group	Type of Seat	Notes
Infants and toddlers	Rear-facing car seat with harness system until age of 2 years; convertible car seats can be used as rear- and front-facing car seats	Children under age 2 years are 75% less likely to be killed or injured in a car crash if they are in a rear-facing seat
Toddler to preschool	Safest if rear-facing seat up to age of 2 years; forward-facing car seat with harness system Weight limit ranges from 80 to 100 lb (depends on brand)	Children aged 2 years or older (or if over the weight or height limit for rear-facing car seat) until they have reached the weight limit
School age	Booster seats (belt-positioning booster seats)	Use until child has reached 4 feet, 9 inches or is 8–12 years of age; shoulder belt should cross the middle of the child's chest and shoulders
Older child to teenager	Seat belt with lap belt	All children aged 13 years or younger should sit in the back seat and use a seat belt with the lap belt

palpated, reflux of mucoid discharge or tears may be seen. Yellow- to green-colored purulent eye discharge is abnormal in the absence of other signs of infection (rule out acute dacryocystitis), can occur with chronic dacryostenosis, and is suggestive of a bacterial overgrowth in the lacrimal sac. A short course of topical ophthalmic antibiotics can be beneficial if copious or extremely bothersome.

Treatment Plan
Lacrimal sac massage/compression: Place a clean finger on the lacrimal sac and apply moderate downward pressure over the lacrimal sac for 2 to 3 seconds. Perform maneuver two or three times per day.

Complication: Acute Dacryocystitis
Look for redness, warmth, tenderness, and swelling on one of the lacrimal ducts. Occurs commonly with dacryocystoceles. Culture discharge and treat with systemic antibiotics for 7 to 10 days to prevent complications of preseptal or orbital cellulitis. Usually caused by streptococcal or staphylococcal organisms.

DEVELOPMENTAL DYSPLASIA OF THE HIP
Higher risk with breech births, female sex, family history, and oligohydramnios.

Screening
Birth to 3 Months
Look for asymmetry in the creases of the legs. Examine infant front and back without diapers. Check that gluteal, thigh, and popliteal folds match.

Barlow Maneuver/Test
Bend infant's knees to 90 degrees, place index and middle finger over the greater trochanter. Gently push both knees together at midline downward, then pull upward (Figure 20.3A). Will hear "clunk" sound when the trochanter slips back into the acetabulum (reducible dislocated hip).

Ortolani Maneuver/Test
Hold each knee and place your middle finger over the greater trochanter (outer thigh over the hips). Rotate the hips in the frog leg position (abduction with gentle traction anteriorly) (Figure 20.3B,C). During abduction, resistance may be felt at 30 to 40 degrees. Sensation of instability is positive if audible or palpable movement of femoral head over posterior acetabular rim, which allows the hip to "relocate" in the acetabular cavity.

If either screening exam is positive, refer to a pediatric orthopedist. Order an ultrasound of the hips.

Older Infants (≥4 Months)
Continue to perform the Barlow and Ortolani maneuvers until the child is fully weight-bearing/walking.
- Look for leg that is turned outward.
- One femur appears shorter when infant is supine (Galeazzi sign).
- Hip has limited range of motion.
- If preceding findings are present, order a hip ultrasound and refer to orthopedic specialist.

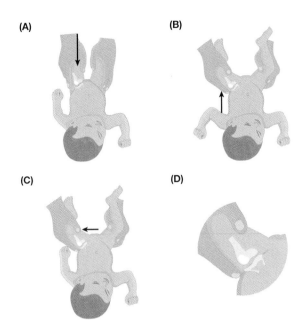

Figure 20.3 Barlow (A) and Ortolani (B, C) maneuvers. Positive testing indicates that the femoral head is partially or completely dislocated from the acetabulum (D).
Source: Gawlik, K. S., Melnyk, B. M., & Teall, A. M. (Eds.). (2021). (See Resources section for complete source information.)

FEVER
Fever is a temperature greater than 100.4°F (38°C). Evaluate using a rectal thermometer in newborns and very young infants, as other measurement methods are less accurate. Evaluation of fever in newborns and young infants is difficult because there are many causes ranging from self-limited to life-threatening. Numerous risk factors increase the possibility of febrile infections, including prematurity, prolonged rupture of membranes during delivery, and maternal Group B *Streptococcus* infection that was inadequately treated during delivery. Risk for fever increases with inadequate/delayed immunizations, daycare attendance, close-contact exposures, and secondhand smoke exposure, and in uncircumcised males younger than 1 year.

Viral illnesses, malignancy, rheumatologic disorders, and bacterial illnesses may cause fever. Serious bacterial illnesses in this age group include meningitis, bacteremia, sepsis, pneumonia, and urinary tract infection.

Classic Case
Previously healthy infant at age 2 months is seen in the ED for fever of 102.5°F (39.2°C) for the last 24 hours. Exclusively breastfed, has had decreased intake at the breast, is more fussy than usual, has had a small decrease in urine output measured by wet diapers, and is not sleeping as usual. No other notable symptoms. Infant has a sibling who attends preschool and has also been febrile with

a cough, runny nose, and eye drainage. Infant's exam is notable for a repeat temperature of 101.7°F (38.7°C) (rectal), oxygenation at 97% on room air, respiratory rate of 40, and slight tachycardia at 150 bmp. Infant is alert and crying but consolable. Exam otherwise negative with no obvious source for the fever.

Treatment Plan

Treatment of fever should be based on accurate evaluation of temperature, so repeating the temperature using an accurate measurement device is critical. Point-of-care testing may be useful when evaluating a febrile infant, as rapid influenza, COVID testing, and urinalysis can help rule out suspected diagnoses. If source of fever is not readily apparent, a complete blood count (CBC), urine sample via catheterization for urine culture, viral respiratory cultures, and stool cultures may all be indicated.

Initial treatment depends on age, appearance (well, ill, or toxic appearing), history, and physical exam. In general, any infant who is toxic appearing should be admitted for further workup including CBC with differential, blood cultures, urinalysis, urine culture, and possibly lumbar puncture. Often, if younger than 90 days or older and ill appearing, child will be started on IV antibiotics while workup is pending.

Older children with fever can be given oral fluids to help prevent dehydration and antipyretics such as acetaminophen or ibuprofen (only older than 6 months) to improve the child's comfort.

Complications

Differentiating serious bacterial illnesses from milder illnesses is key in this age group. Failure to do so puts the child at risk for delayed diagnosis, complications from a serious bacterial illness, and potentially death.

INFANT COLIC (RULE OF 3s)

The goal when evaluating an infant with colic is to rule out conditions causing pain and/or discomfort, infections, environment, and formula "allergy."

- Crying *for no apparent reason* that lasts ≥3 hours a day in an infant younger than 3 months. Crying usually occurs at the same time each day.
- Crying occurs >3 days in a week.
- The excessive crying usually resolves by 3 to 4 months.

JAUNDICE (HYPERBILIRUBINEMIA)

Elevation is due to increased breakdown of fetal RBCs exceeding the infant's liver capacity to conjugate bilirubin. Free, unbound, unconjugated bilirubin (breakdown product from old RBCs) is toxic to cells and can be deposited in tissue, such as the brain and nerve cells, causing necrosis. Elevated conjugated hyperbilirubinemia may indicate an underlying disorder *but* is not toxic to the CNS. White infant's color is yellow or orangish tinge, or the soles of the feet are yellow; jaundice more difficult to detect visually in infants with darker skin, so blood tests should be done.

Pathologic Jaundice

- Jaundice within first 24 hours of life. Always pathologic; evaluate for sepsis, congenital TORCH (toxoplasmosis, others [syphilis, hepatitis B], rubella, cytomegalovirus, and herpes simplex) infections, occult hemorrhage, or erythroblastosis fetalis
- Jaundice of full-term infant after 2 weeks of age. Requires evaluation; consider sepsis, hemolytic disease, metabolic disorders, and intestinal obstruction Bilirubin level increases too rapidly (>5 mg/dL per day). Total bilirubin levels >17 mg/dL

Nonpathologic Jaundice

- Physiologic and breastfeeding jaundice most common
- Consider breast milk jaundice if full-term exclusively breastfed infant with jaundice after 3 weeks of age

Physiologic Jaundice

Also known as *neonatal unconjugated hyperbilirubinemia* or *neonatal icterus*. Jaundice appears when bilirubin level is ≥5 mg/dL. Jaundice first appears on the head/face (sclera is yellow) and progresses downward to the chest, abdomen, legs, and soles of the feet.

Physiologic jaundice starts after 24 hours and will usually clear up within 2 to 3 weeks without intervention other than pushing adequate feedings/intake. The total bilirubin levels in White and African American infants can peak at 7 to 9 mg/dL, but Asian infants have higher peak values (10–14 mg/dL).

Breast Milk Jaundice

Breast milk jaundice usually starts to show after 4 to 5 days of life. It peaks at 7 to 14 days and can take more than 1 month to clear. It is thought to be caused by a substance in breast milk that inhibits hepatic conjugation of bilirubin. Bilirubin levels may exceed 20 mg/dL. Often a brief (12-hour) period of breastfeeding cessation, with pumping to maintain milk supply and fluid and caloric supplementation for the infant, will lower bilirubin levels enough to resume breast milk as the sole nutritional source. Some infants will also need phototherapy.

Breastfeeding Jaundice

In contrast to breast milk jaundice, breastfeeding jaundice is actually a downstream sequalae of poor intake of calories and failure to produce stool. This can also occur in bottle-fed infants with poor intake but is less common.

Treatment Plan

- Check bilirubin level. Use noninvasive methods first (transcutaneous bilirubin testing).
- If suspect pathologic jaundice, order serum fractionated bilirubin level, Coombs test, CBC, reticulocyte count, and peripheral smear.
- Medical intervention is usually not needed unless total bilirubin levels are approaching or exceeding hour-specific values on a risk-based nomogram.
- Keep baby well-hydrated with breast milk or formula. Feed infant every 2 to 3 hours (10–12 times per day).

- First-line treatment is phototherapy. Light used in the blue spectrum is the most effective wavelength. The skin converts bilirubin into a nontoxic water-soluble form so that it is excreted in the urine.
- All newborns should be seen for follow-up within the first 5 days of life to check for jaundice.

Complications

Bilirubin encephalopathy/kernicterus: Neurologic disorder caused by high levels of unbound bilirubin in circulation that damaged the infant's CNS. Associated with severe intellectual disability and seizures.

PHYSIOLOGIC ANEMIA OF INFANCY

Hemoglobin drops at the lowest level in life (nadir) at 8 to 12 weeks of age. Full-term infants' hemoglobin decreases to 9 to 11 g/dL. Number of RBCs declines after birth because of an increase in oxygen availability and a decrease in erythropoietin production by the kidneys. When the hemoglobin level is at its lowest, oxygen needs exceed the body's ability to deliver it, thus stimulating erythropoietin production and RBC production from the bone marrow.

EXAM TIPS

- Asymmetry of thigh/gluteal folds: Rule out congenital hip dysplasia or hip fracture.
- Developmental milestones: Rolls from front to back and back to front at 6 months; plays pat-a-cake and peek-a-boo at 9 months.

KNOWLEDGE CHECK: CHAPTER 20

1. Which of the following statements regarding physiologic jaundice is correct?
   A. It appears when bilirubin levels reach 3 mg/dL.
   B. It first appears on the feet and progresses upward on the body.
   C. It generally clears within 2 to 3 weeks with adequate feedings.
   D. It begins within the first 24 hours of life.

2. A neonate is noted to have shortened palpebral fissures and microcephaly with a small jaw. This infant is *most likely* to be diagnosed with:
   A. Down syndrome
   B. Fetal alcohol syndrome
   C. Growth delay
   D. Hydrocephalus

3. A new parent reports that their 6-month-old infant has a cold and a fever of 99.8°F. The infant is not irritable and is feeding well without problems. The parent wants to know whether it is okay for the infant to be immunized at this time. Which of the following statements is *true*?
   A. The infant should not be immunized until they are afebrile.
   B. An infant with a cold can be immunized at any time.
   C. An infant with a cold can be immunized as long as their temperature is not higher than 100.4°F.
   D. Because immunization is so important, it should be given to the infant as scheduled.

4. An infant is noted to have a strawberry hemangioma. The nurse practitioner knows that further education is needed when the patient's parent states:
   A. "It will most likely disappear by the age of 1 to 5 years."
   B. "We will watch the hemangioma to see what happens."
   C. "It will be treated with laser therapy if it has not resolved in 12 months."
   D. "Strawberry hemangiomas are benign."

5. Which of the following is considered an abnormal finding?
   A. A "clunk" sound heard while performing the Ortolani maneuver
   B. A 6-month-old infant starting to babble
   C. Flat pink patches on the forehead of a 12-month-old infant
   D. A 12-month-old who is "cruising"

6. An infant is being seen for a well-child exam. The infant is able to use a pincer grasp, says "Dada," and balances well on the feet with support. This child is likely what age in months?
   A. 6
   B. 9
   C. 12
   D. 15

7. A newborn infant is seen at a 2-week well-child visit and is noted to have a watery discharge from both eyes. The parent noted some blood in the discharge yesterday. The infant is otherwise well with no respiratory symptoms. Which of the following is the *next best* management step?
   A. Treat empirically with ceftriaxone intramuscularly (Rocephin)
   B. Treat with ophthalmic erythromycin ointment (Ilotycin)
   C. Collect a swab of the inner eyelid
   D. Order a chest x-ray

8. A child is seen for a well visit. Which of the following findings would require a consult or referral for further evaluation?
   A. A 3-day-old with multiple 1- to 2-mm white papules on the forehead and nose
   B. A 4-month-old with thick yellow scale behind the ears and on the eyebrows
   C. A 6-month-old with a round, orange-red glow from each eye on fundoscopic exam
   D. A 9-month-old with a Moro reflex

(See answers next page.)

1. C) It generally clears within 2 to 3 weeks with adequate feedings.

Physiologic jaundice represents a normal transitional state that resolves once the infant's liver can keep up with the demand for bilirubin conjugation. It starts after the first 24 hours of life when the bilirubin level reaches 5 mg/dL or higher. The condition is initially apparent on the newborn's face before it progresses downward on the body. It will usually clear within 2 to 3 weeks without intervention other than adequate feedings.

2. B) Fetal alcohol syndrome

Classic symptoms of fetal alcohol syndrome include small palpebral fissures and microcephaly with a small jaw. Upward deviation of palpebral fissures, macroglossia, and hypotonia are classically found in infants born with trisomy 21, or Down syndrome. Unusually large head size and downward deviation of eyes are characteristic of hydrocephalus.

3. C) An infant with a cold can be immunized as long as their temperature is not higher than 100.4°F.

It is fine for an infant to be vaccinated even if they have a mild illness. A vaccine will not make a mild illness worse. A child can be vaccinated even if they have a low-grade fever, cold, runny nose, cough, otitis media, or mild diarrhea.

4. C) "It will be treated with laser therapy if it has not resolved in 12 months."

True strawberry hemangiomas will eventually resolve by the time the child goes to kindergarten. Most will reduce or disappear in the first 2 years without intervention, so watchful waiting of this benign skin lesion is the most useful strategy. Laser treatment is rarely needed.

5. A) A "clunk" sound heard while performing the Ortolani maneuver

The "clunk" sound during the Ortolani maneuver is a positive finding and signifies a possible hip abnormality (hip dysplasia) in infants. Refer the infant to a pediatric orthopedist. Infants start to babble at 6 months. At 12 months, babies learn to "cruise," or hold onto furniture while walking. Flat pink patches found on the forehead, eyelids, and the nape of the neck of infants are salmon patches, which typically fade by 18 months.

6. B) 9

At 9 months, an infant has a refined pincer grasp, is stringing similar sounds together, and may be pulling to a stand and standing with support. Milestones for a 6-month-old would include babbling, rolling in both directions, and sitting without support. By 12 months, most children are cruising or walking, have one to two words other than "Mama" and "Dada" in their vocabulary, and can use a sippy cup with dexterity. By 15 months, children are walking independently, are using a spoon, and have more than six words in their vocabulary.

7. C) Collect a swab of the inner eyelid

The first step with this patient would be to collect a swab of the inner eyelid to gather a sample of the discharge and also one of the epithelium. Given the presentation, this infant appears to have a chlamydial infection in the eye. As the patient has no respiratory symptoms, a nasopharyngeal swab would be more appropriate than a chest x-ray at this time. Ophthalmic erythromycin (Ilotycin) is used prophylactically for gonorrheal infections of the eye, and ceftriaxone (Rocephin) is the treatment of choice for infants with gonococcal ophthalmia neonatorum.

8. D) A 9-month old with a Moro reflex

Persistence of a Moro reflex after age 4 to 5 months is concerning for underlying brain pathology. A 3-day-old may present with the normal finding of milia, while seborrheic dermatitis is common in infants age 2 to 4 months. A 6-month-old should have a bilateral red reflex; failure to see a red reflex would be concerning.

9. Which of the following in a newborn would be *most concerning* for an associated neurologic disorder?
   A. Erythema toxicum found on the face
   B. Congenital dermal melanocytosis on the sacral area
   C. Café au lait spots (more than five lesions) on the chest
   D. Nevus flammeus on the shoulders and upper chest area

10. Which of the following is *true* regarding a caput succedaneum?
    A. It is commonly associated with assisted deliveries.
    B. It can be associated with jaundice.
    C. It is described as diffuse edema that crosses the suture lines.
    D. It is swelling that is localized to one area of the skull.

11. An infant is being seen for a 4-month well-child visit. The patient is up to date on immunizations at this point. Which of the following is the correct set of immunizations to order?
    A. Hep B, Hib, PCV, IPV, rotavirus, DTaP, influenza
    B. Hep B, Hib, PCV, IPV, rotavirus, DTaP
    C. Hib, PCV, IPV, rotavirus, DTaP
    D. MMR, varicella, Hep A

12. A 12-month-old is seen for routine well care. The patient is found to have weak femoral pulses and has a blood pressure (BP) greater than the 90th percentile for their height. Which of the following would be the *next best* step to determine the diagnosis?
    A. Check BP in the right arm compared with the left
    B. Compare BPs in the upper and lower extremities
    C. Order a chest x-ray
    D. Perform an electrocardiogram (EKG)

13. Which of the following would increase the risk that a child's Barlow or Ortolani test would be positive?
    A. 6-month-old who rolls from front to back and back to front
    B. Male newborn with history of vacuum-assisted delivery
    C. Newborn female with a history of breech delivery
    D. 2-month-old with a negative Galeazzi sign

14. An infant is noted to have upward deviation of palpebral fissures, macroglossia, and hypotonia. Which of the following is *most likely* the infant's underlying issue?
    A. Amblyopia
    B. Down syndrome
    C. Esotropia
    D. Fetal alcohol spectrum disorder

15. Separation anxiety begins for infants at what age in months?
    A. 6
    B. 9
    C. 12
    D. 15

(See answers next page.)

9. C) Café au lait spots (more than five lesions) on the chest

Café au lait spots, particularly when there are more than five lesions, can be associated with neurofibromatosis. While port-wine stains (nevus flammeus) can be associated with neurologic involvement of cranial nerves V1 and V2 if located on the eyelid and with Sturge-Weber disease if found unilaterally over the face, port-wine stains found on other areas of the body are rarely associated with neurologic issues. Erythema toxicum can be a normal finding on the face of a newborn. Congenital dermal melanocytosis is most commonly found on the sacral and medial gluteal area. It is not associated with underlying neurologic issues.

10. C) It is described as diffuse edema that crosses the suture lines.

A caput succedaneum is a diffuse swelling that is secondary to prolonged delivery or pressure on the head as the infant moves through the birth canal. The pressure causes fluid to build up under the scalp. Cephalohematoma is due to periosteal blood vessel rupture over a particular skull bone, usually secondary to an assisted delivery. As the blood is contained in the subperiosteal space, it is localized to one area of the skull and does not spread diffusely. The large collection of blood can increase the bilirubin levels in the infant's bloodstream and put them at risk for jaundice.

11. C) Hib, PCV, IPV, rotavirus, DTaP

If the patient is up to date on immunizations and requires an age-appropriate vaccine series, they would receive rotavirus #2, DTaP #2, Hib #2, pneumococcal #2, and IPV #2 today. The patient is too young for an influenza vaccine, and Hep B #2 should have been given at 1 to 2 months, as the first dose is typically given in the hospital immediately after delivery. MMR and varicella cannot be given until after 12 months. Hep A is typically given between 12 to 23 months.

12. B) Compare BPs in the upper and lower extremities

A brachiofemoral delay is diagnostic for coarctation of the aorta (CoA); however, this is sometimes subtle or hard to determine in this age group, so comparing upper-extremity BP to a lower-extremity measurement can help solidify the diagnosis. In CoA, the BP will be ≥20 mmHg higher in the arms than in the legs/thighs. If the BPs are abnormal, chest x-ray, echocardiogram, and EKG should then be ordered.

13. C) Female newborn with a history of breech delivery

Risk factors for developmental dysplasia of the hip (DDH) include firstborn, female, breech presentation, oligohydramnios, and family history of DDH. Delivery, other than breech presentation, has not been associated with increased risk of DDH. A negative Galeazzi sign is a normal finding and is indicative of equal leg lengths. Rolling front to back and back to front at 6 months is a normal developmental milestone. Some developmental milestones can be delayed if DDH requires bracing or casting.

14. B) Down syndrome

Upward deviation of palpebral fissures, macroglossia, and hypotonia are classically found in infants born with trisomy 21, or Down syndrome. Fetal alcohol spectrum disorder ranges in presentation but most classically will have microcephaly with a flat nasal bridge and a thin lip with a smooth philtrum. Esotropia is the upward deviation of the eye, and amblyopia is a visual disturbance characterized by decreased vision due to abnormal visual development.

15. C) 12

Stranger apprehension is sometimes seen at age 9 months as infants become more cautious of their world; however, separation anxiety, or the fear that a parent will leave and not return, begins at 12 months and can last until a child is 2 to 3 years old. At 15 months, most toddlers are affectionate and will hug, kiss, and cuddle parents and inanimate objects. At 6 months, infants know and like to watch familiar faces.

DANGER SIGNALS

EPIGLOTTITIS

Acute and rapid onset of high fever, chills, and toxicity. Child complains of severe sore throat and drooling saliva. Will not eat or drink; has muffled (hot potato) voice and anxiety. Characteristic tripod sitting posture with hyperextended neck and open-mouth breathing. Stridor, tachycardia, and tachypnea. Usually occurs between ages 2 and 6 years. Before the vaccine was used, most cases were due to *Haemophilus influenzae* type b (Hib). Other pathogens include *Staphylococcus aureus*, *Streptococcus pyogenes*, and fungi. Now rare due to the Hib conjugate vaccine. Prophylaxis with rifampin (duration is 4 days) for close contacts. Reportable disease to the public health department. A medical emergency. Call 911.

NEUROBLASTOMA

Most common presentation is an abdominal (retroperitoneal or hepatic) mass that is fixed, firm, and irregular and frequently crosses the midline. The most common site is the adrenal medulla (sits on top of the kidneys). About half of patients present with metastatic disease. May be accompanied by weight loss, fever, subcutaneous nodules, Horner's syndrome (miosis, ptosis, anhidrosis), periorbital ecchymoses ("racoon eyes"), bone pain, hypertension, and, rarely, opsoclonus myoclonus syndrome. Most are diagnosed in children between the ages of 1 and 4 years. Elevated urinary catecholamines help with diagnosis. After ruling out bowel obstruction, ultrasound is initial imaging choice for abdominal masses. Refer to general pediatric surgeon.

NONACCIDENTAL TRAUMA (CHILD ABUSE)

The majority of perpetrators are parents. About 16% of perpetrators are persons whom the child is exposed to such as day-care staff and unmarried partners. Multiple red flags for nonaccidental trauma (NAT) include posteriomedial rib fractures, spinal fractures, metaphyseal avulsion fractures, bruises or fractures in various stages of healing, delay in seeking medical care, and injuries that are inconsistent with explanation.

Infants and children who are developmentally or physically disabled are at higher risk. Nurses, nurse practitioners, and several other professionals are required to report suspected or actual child abuse to authorities.

ORBITAL CELLULITIS

Young child complains of abrupt onset of deep eye pain that is aggravated by eye movements and is accompanied by a high fever and chills. Affected eye will appear to be bulging (proptosis or exophthalmos). Extraocular eye movements (EOMs) exam will be abnormal because of ophthalmoplegia (limited movement of eyeball) from infection of the ocular fat pads and muscles. More common in younger children. Ethmoid sinusitis is more likely to cause orbital cellulitis compared with frontal/maxillary sinusitis. Can be life-threatening. A serious complication of rhinosinusitis, acute otitis media, or dental infections. Refer to ED for further evaluation, which generally involves a CT scan or MRI.

OSTEOMYELITIS

More common in children. Boys are two times more likely than girls. Infections typically occur at the metaphyses, so the area overlying the metaphysis is often exquisitely tender to the touch. Patient is febrile and toxic appearing and usually will not bear weight or move extremity due to pain. Requires emergent hospitalization, intravenous (IV) antibiotics, and operating room (OR) debridement. Growth plate infection can result in growth stunting of the affected limb.

PRESEPTAL CELLULITIS (PERIORBITAL CELLULITIS)

More common than orbital cellulitis. An infection of the anterior portion of the eyelid that does not involve the orbit/globe or the eyes. Rarely causes serious complications (compared with orbital cellulitis). Younger children are most likely to be affected. Young child complains of a new onset of red, swollen eyelids and eye pain, or sometimes no pain (Figure 21.1). Eye movements do not cause pain, and EOM exam is normal (both are abnormal with orbital cellulitis). No visual impairment. May be hard to distinguish from orbital cellulitis. Refer to ED.

SEPTIC ARTHRITIS

Primarily disease of infants and toddlers. Can occur if osteomyelitis spreads to the joint space but is more commonly from hematogenous spread. *S. aureus* is most common organism. Abrupt onset of unilateral hip or knee pain is the most common presentation. Knee may present with swelling and warmth, but hip rarely presents with palpable findings. If patient tolerates weight bearing, antalgic limp noted. At rest, patient will prefer hip flexion, abduction,

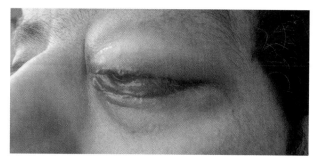

Figure 21.1 Preseptal (periorbital) cellulitis.
Source: Courtesy of Bobjgalindo.

and external rotation or knee in partial flexion. Requires emergent joint aspiration and empiric IV antibiotics.

WILMS' TUMOR (NEPHROBLASTOMA)

Asymptomatic abdominal mass that extends from the flank toward the midline. The nontender and smooth mass rarely crosses the midline (of the abdomen). Some patients have abdominal pain and hematuria. One fourth of patients have hypertension. Higher incidence in African American girls. Peak age is 2 to 3 years. The most common renal malignancy in children. While performing the abdominal exam, palpate gently to avoid rupturing the renal capsule (causes bleeding and seeding of abdomen with cancer cells). Initial imaging test is an abdominal ultrasound. Refer to pediatric cancer center.

EXAM TIPS

- Wilms' tumor is a congenital tumor of the kidneys. More common in African American girls.
- Epiglottitis presentation is sitting posture with hyperextended neck and open-mouth breathing.

GROWTH AND DEVELOPMENT

Table 21.1 summarizes normal and abnormal childhood development from 2 through 5 years of age. See Chapter 20 for corresponding discussion of newborn through 1 year and Chapter 22 for the school-age child.

15 MONTHS
Fine Motor
- Feeds self with spoon
- Can drink from a cup

Gross Motor
Walks independently for longer distances

Language
- Follows commands with gestures
- Vocabulary of four to six words

Table 21.1 Growth and Development Milestones: Age 2 to 5 Years

Age	Characteristics	Abnormal
2 years	Walks. Runs. Climbs stairs up and down on own by holding onto handrails. Speech mostly understood by family. Follows two- or three-step instructions. Copies a line.	Unable to speak meaningful two-word "sentences." Does not understand simple commands. Loss of speech, social skills, or previously learned behaviors and/or does not say words by 16 months (autism).
3 years	Speaks three- to five-word sentences; understood by strangers. Copies a circle with crayon or pencil. Rides tricycle. Builds towers of more than six blocks. Runs and climbs easily.	Speech hard to understand or unclear speech. Unable to understand simple commands. Falls down often. Does not speak in sentences. No eye contact. Loses skills they once had.
4 years	Copies a cross with crayon or pencil. Draws person with three body parts. Plays "Mom" and "Dad." Hops and stands on one foot up to 2 seconds. Cooperates with other children. Names some colors and some numbers.	Unable to speak in full sentences. Inability to skip, run, hop. Cannot put on clothes without help. Unable to play with other kids. Unable to follow three-part commands.
5 years	Can draw a person with six body parts. Counts 10 or more things. Is aware of gender. Speaks clearly.	Unusually withdrawn. Not active. Trouble focusing on one activity for >5 minutes.

Source: Centers for Disease Control and Prevention (2020).

18 MONTHS
Fine Motor
Turns pages of book

Gross Motor
Can walk up steps

Language
- Can point to four body parts
- Vocabulary of 10 to 20 words

2 YEARS
Language
- Speaks in two- or three-word sentences (intelligible mostly by family)
- Follows two-step commands
- Knows common pictures in a book

Fine Motor

- Stacks five or six cubes
- Can copy straight line

Gross Motor

- Goes up stairs using same foot; uses railing for support
- Runs, jumps, and climbs
- Is very active and energetic

Behaviors

- Temper tantrums common at this age
- Easily frustrated and says "no" often; defiant behaviors
- May have a favorite stuffed toy (transitional object)
- Toilet training now in progress
- Report loss of speech, social skills, or previously learned skills; flapping hands; avoidance of social interaction (rule out autism); unsteady walking; inability to speak in two-word sentences.

3 YEARS

Language

- Speaks in sentences using three to five words
- Most speech understood by strangers
- Knows first name and age
- Magical thinking prominent at this age (3 to 5 years); may have an imaginary friend; may believe they have special powers

Fine Motor

- Copies a circle
- Can stack more than six cubes

Gross Motor

- Pedals a tricycle
- Can throw a ball overhand
- Walks up and down stairs with alternating feet

Behaviors

- Freud classified this age as the "Oedipal stage" (phallic stage). The child expresses the desire to marry the parent of the opposite sex; occurs between the ages of 3 and 5 years (preschool).
- Plays with other children (group play) but does not like to share toys or take turns.
- Imagination is becoming more active (pretends that a broom is a "horse").
- Report any regression in previously learned skills, "clumsy" with frequent falls, minimal vocabulary or speech difficult to understand, speech dysfluencies, no or poor eye contact.

EXAM TIPS

- Speech of a 2-year-old includes two-word phrases mostly understood by family members.
- Speech of a 3-year-old includes three- to five-word sentences that can be mostly understood by strangers.

4 YEARS

Fine Motor

- Mature pencil grasp
- Can copy a cross
- Draws a person with two to four body parts

Gross Motor

- Rides a bicycle with training wheels
- Hops on both feet
- Dresses with little assistance

Other

- According to Piaget, 4-year-old children are at the pre-operational stage.
- Ready to learn the alphabet, spell or read short words, and learn basic math concepts

EXAM TIPS

- Three-year-old can ride a tricycle. Child can ride a bicycle with training wheels at the age of 4 to 5 years.
- Three-year-old can copy a circle. (An easy way to memorize this fact is that when you take the "3" and join the two halves, it forms a circle.)

CLINICAL PEARL

Early referral to birth-to-3 programs is important for toddlers and preschool-aged children who are not meeting developmental milestones.

HEALTH EDUCATION, SAFETY, AND SCREENING

U.S. HEALTH STATISTICS: TODDLERS

Top Three Causes of Death (Age 1 to 4 Years)

- Drowning
- Congenital anomalies
- Motor vehicle accidents

Top Three Cancers

- Leukemia
- Brain and nervous system tumors
- Lymphomas

The most common cancer in children is leukemia. The most common type of leukemia in children is acute lymphocytic leukemia (ALL). The remaining cases are due to acute myelogenous leukemia (AML). Medulloblastomas are the most common type of childhood brain cancer (most occur before age 10 years).

NUTRITION

Have regular mealtimes (3 meals/day) and snacks (2 to 3 per day). Preference for the same food, prepared in the same way every day or at every meal, is common. Transition from whole milk to lower-fat milk at age 2 years. Limit fruit juice intake. Cut solid food into bite-size pieces. Avoid hard foods, such as nuts, raw carrots, and hard candies, as well as other choking hazards like gumdrops, jelly beans, and whole grapes (cut in quarters if offering), and whole hot dogs (cut into slices that are then quartered).

TOILET TRAINING

Clues that a child is ready include that the child is walking, can reach potty chair, knows the difference between wet and dry, can communicate when having a bowel movement, can pull down own pants, can stay dry for up to 2 hours at a time, and shows interest in the toilet or potty seat. Make sure that child can understand basic instructions.

Most children are ready for "potty" training at 18 to 24 months. Some children may not be ready until 36 months of age. During toilet training, signs that a child is ready to use the potty are squirming, holding genital area, and squatting.

Most children master daytime bladder and bowel control by age 3 to 4 years. Nighttime control of urine is usually the last toileting skill that is mastered. Complete nighttime control may not happen until child is closer to 5 years of age. Children between 5 and 6 years of age with primary nocturnal enuresis should be evaluated by pediatric urology, and interventions (e.g., behavioral conditioning, bed-wetting alarms, responsibility/reward charts) should be started.

CAR SAFETY

- Toddlers should be placed in the back seat in a forward-facing safety seat with a harness system until they outgrow the height and weight limits of the seat. Make sure anchors and tethers are used correctly.
- Children younger than age 12 years should be restrained in the back seat.

SAFETY EDUCATION

- Child should be supervised at all times.
- Hold child's hand when crossing the street and when shopping.
- Use rear burners on stove. Turn pot handles away from reach.
- Keep tools and sharp objects out of reach. Inspect toys for loose parts or breakage.
- Water safety education needed. Put fences around pools. Never leave child alone in the pool.

DISEASE REVIEW

AUTISM

Signs of autism spectrum disorder may appear in early childhood. Screening starts at age 18 months. Five behaviors to look for:

- Does not point/show/reach (by 12 months)
- No babbling (by 12 months)
- Does not say single words (by 16 months)
- Does not say two-word phrases on their own (by 24 months)
- Loss of language or social skills (at any age)

Classic Case

A 3-year-old boy with autism is enrolled in a preschool program. The child's mother goes inside the school to drop the child off at the classroom. After she gives him a hug, she leaves the room. How would the child react during and after his mother's departure?

- At this age, a 3-year-old boy (who does not have a diagnosis of autism) would most likely cry, protest, and cling to his mother's legs when she tries to leave.
- A child with autism may not protest, cling, or cry when his mother leaves (as would be expected in a child who does not have autism). If the child's mother hugs him, a 3-year-old child may hold his body stiffly and not return the hug. Some may push the mother away because they do not like to be touched.

Diagnosis and Treatment

- Typically diagnosed by a developmental pediatrics clinician using highly specialized diagnostic tools.
- Multimodal interventions are used to ameliorate some of the cognitive and behavioral issues.

EXAM TIPS

- Four-year-old can copy a cross (the number "4" resembles a cross at the center) and draw a "stick person" with three body parts.
- Red flags for autistic behavior are loss of skills at any age; no pointing, showing, reaching, or babbling by 1 year; no words by 16 months; and no two-word phrases by 2 years.

KNOWLEDGE CHECK: CHAPTER 21

1. Which statement about Wilm's tumor is correct?
   A. Palpation causes significant pain in the child.
   B. It is a congenital tumor of the bladder.
   C. Microscopic or gross hematuria is sometimes present.
   D. The tumor commonly crosses the midline of the abdomen when it is discovered.

2. Which of the following is an expected behavior for a 3-year-old child?
   A. Speaks in two- to three-word sentences
   B. Can draw a cross
   C. Can copy a circle
   D. Walks up stairs using the same foot

3. A concerned new parent reports that their son, who is 3 years old, is not toilet trained yet. Which of the following is an appropriate reply?
   A. Recommend a referral to a pediatric urologist
   B. Advise the parent that the child is developing normally
   C. Recommend a bed-wetting alarm
   D. Recommend a voiding cystogram

4. Which motor skill is within the parameters of normal growth and development for a 2-year-old child?
   A. Throws a ball overhand
   B. Pedals a tricycle
   C. Stacks seven or more cubes
   D. Runs, jumps, and climbs

5. Which of the following statements is *true* regarding neuroblastoma?
   A. It is a lateralized, well-demarcated mass.
   B. It involves invasion of the renal capsule.
   C. It can be diagnosed by urinary catecholamine levels.
   D. It rarely presents as metastatic disease.

6. A 3-year-old boy is seen by the primary care provider for a 3-week history of limping. He is noted to be overall well-appearing, is afebrile, and is sitting with his hip and knee flexed. He is tender to palpation over the groin area, but no palpable abnormalities are found. Which of the following is the *most likely* diagnosis?
   A. Developmental dysplasia of the hip
   B. Normal gross motor development
   C. Osteomyelitis
   D. Septic arthritis

7. In the pediatric urgent care clinic, a 2-year-old patient with an unknown previous medical history presents with stridor, fever, a 1-day history of refusing to eat or drink, and drooling. Which of the following is the *next best* step for managing this patient?
   A. Do a trial of oral rehydration therapy in the office
   B. Prescribe rifampin × 4 days
   C. Perform a rapid strep test/throat culture
   D. Call emergency medical service (EMS) for transport to the closest ED

8. A 2-year-old child is seen for a well-child exam. The developmental finding that might warrant further evaluation for autism spectrum disorder would be if the child:
   A. Gets frustrated easily
   B. Is defiant and says "no"
   C. Is very active in the exam room
   D. Has 10 single words in their vocabulary

9. Which of the following findings would be consistent with right knee osteomyelitis?
   A. Erythematous and swollen joint
   B. Knee kept flexed and hip abducted and externally rotated
   C. Exquisite tenderness over the distal femur
   D. Weight bearing with antalgic gait

(See answers next page.)

1. C) Microscopic or gross hematuria is sometimes present

A Wilms' tumor is a congenital tumor of the kidney. It is non-tender and smooth and rarely crosses the midline of the abdomen. Microscopic or gross hematuria may be present. Once diagnosed, it should not be palpated, since doing so increases the risk for rupture of the tumor capsule and spread of the tumor cells.

2. C) Can copy a circle

A 3-year-old child can copy a circle, speak in three- to five-word sentences, and walk up and down stairs using alternating feet. Speaking in shorter sentences and walking up stairs using the same foot are behaviors expected of a 2-year-old. The ability to draw a cross is expected of a 4-year-old.

3. B) Advise the parent that the child is developing normally

Toilet training begins at approximately age 2 years and may take 1 to 2 years to complete. Boys who are not toilet trained by age 3 years may still be developing normally. Referral to pediatric urology and/or behavioral interventions would not be appropriate until age 5 years for daytime wetting accidents. Interventions could be initiated at age 5 to 6 years if the child was struggling with nighttime bedwetting. A voiding cystogram is typically used as a diagnostic tool for recurrent urinary tract infections.

4. D) Runs, jumps, and climbs

A 2-year-old child has the gross motor skills necessary to run, jump, and climb. Throwing a ball overhand, pedaling a tricycle, and stacking seven or more cubes are typical of a 3-year-old child.

5. C) It can be diagnosed by urinary catecholamine levels

Because a neuroblastoma originates from the adrenal gland, it often produces excessive levels of catecholamines, which can be detected in a urinary sample. About half of all patients found to have a neuroblastoma have metastatic lesions. It is often found on abdominal exam with a diffuse, irregular mass that crosses the midline.

6. D) Septic arthritis

A child with septic arthritis at the hip typically will not have any palpable abnormalities due to the deep nature of the hip joint and may look uncomfortable but non-toxic. A child with osteomyelitis will likely be febrile, appear toxic, and have pain at the femoral metaphysis. Developmental dysplasia of the hip at age 3 years would be a missed diagnosis and typically would present with a leg-length difference and gait abnormalities. A limp in a child is not a normal developmental finding.

7. D) Call emergency medical service (EMS) for transport to the closest ED

The child is presenting with signs of possible epiglottitis, so emergent management of the airway should be the primary management decision. While performing a rapid strep test or throat culture is not unreasonable in a child of this age with fever and sore throat, it would not be the next best step if epiglottitis is suspected, as it could exacerbate the child's condition. Oral rehydration therapy could also exacerbate the condition, and likely the child would refuse because they are unable to handle their own secretions at this time. Rifampin therapy is the treatment of choice for the patient's family members, but it would be initiated well after the child is stabilized.

8. D) Has 10 single words in their vocabulary

By age 2 years, neurotypically developing children will have about 20 to 50 single words with several two-word phrases. A limited vocabulary of 10 single words would be seen in a 12- to 15-month-old; in a 2-year-old, it should raise a red flag to investigate for developmental issues. Getting frustrated easily, being defiant, and having excessive energy/activity are all normal developmental findings in a 2-year-old child.

9. C) Exquisite tenderness over the distal femur

Osteomyelitis typically presents with exquisite tenderness over the metaphysis/bone, not usually the joint space. Typically, a child with a lower extremity osteomyelitis will not bear weight due to the pain, although it is possible they may bear weight (but guard in their walking) with a septic knee joint. Septic arthritis presents with true joint swelling and knee flexion with hip abduction and external rotation if the hip joint is involved.

10. A 3-year-old child presents with a red eye. Which of the following exam findings would be *most indicative* of preseptal cellulitis?
    A. Proptosis
    B. Painful extraocular movements
    C. Leukocoria
    D. Eyelid erythema and swelling

11. A child is seen in the ED for not wanting to use their right arm after a fall. The provider is concerned for possible child abuse. Which of the following would *increase* the risk for abuse in this child?
    A. Developmentally appropriate for age
    B. Care sought immediately after fall
    C. History consistent with injury
    D. Metaphyseal avulsion fracture on x-ray

12. A child presents for a well-child visit, and their parent notes that the child plays well with others at daycare but primarily likes to play with an imaginary friend. The child's four- to five-word sentences are somewhat difficult to fully understand, and the child draws a circle during the exam. This child is likely what age in months?
    A. 18
    B. 24
    C. 36
    D. 48

13. Which of the following would be inappropriate anticipatory guidance for parents of a toddler?
    A. "Children at this age need assistance to cross the street."
    B. "Children should be in a car seat in the backseat."
    C. "Choking hazards are less of a concern at this age."
    D. "Water safety and supervision are important."

14. Which of the following is a leading cause of cancer in toddlers?
    A. Leukemia
    B. Lymphoma
    C. Nephroblastoma
    D. Medulloblastoma

15. A toddler who was born prematurely is being assessed for hearing loss. Which assessment finding is a high-risk factor for hearing loss?
    A. Hypobilirubinemia
    B. Low Apgar scores
    C. Single ear infection
    D. Exposure to chlamydia in utero

(See answers next page.)

10. D) Eyelid erythema and swelling

Preseptal cellulitis does not involve the globe or orbit of the eye and is restricted to the eyelid and surrounding soft tissue. Proptosis and painful extraocular movements are hallmark signs of orbital cellulitis, while leukocoria can be found in children with glaucoma, cataracts, or retinoblastoma.

11. D) Metaphyseal avulsion fracture on x-ray

Metaphyseal avulsion fractures are thought to occur due to excessive force from shaking or twisting a limb, so higher suspicion for abuse should occur if these are seen. Children who are developmentally or physically disabled are at higher risk for abuse than their developmentally appropriate peers. Delayed care and an inconsistent history would also raise red flags.

12. C) 36

A 3-year-old child performs interactive play with others, may have magical thinking, has a growing vocabulary with three quarters of the speech understandable, and has fine motor skills that allow drawing of a circle. Children younger than 3 years have significantly fewer words in their vocabulary and are not yet stringing words together in sentences; they have an immature pencil grasp, which makes drawing shapes more difficult; and they may only perform parallel play rather than interactive play. By 4 years old, the child should have completely understandable speech, be riding a bike with training wheels, and be engaging in cooperative/collaborative play with others.

13. C) "Choking hazards are less of a concern at this age."

Choking hazards continue to be a concern during the toddler years, as children still have small airways and tend to put a lot of items into their mouths. Foods should be cut into quarters, and toys should not have small or breakable parts. Toddlers do not have the hearing, eyesight, or depth perception to cross the street alone and should be assisted by an adult. Toddlers through school-aged children should ride in the backseat of the car, as this is the safest location in the case of a crash. Drownings are the leading cause of death in 1- to 4-year-old children, so care should be taken to supervise children around any water sources.

14. A) Leukemia

Leukemias cause 28% of all cancers in the 1- to 4-year-old age range. Medulloblastoma is the leading type of brain tumor, but central nervous system tumors make up only 26% of cancers in this age group. Nephroblastoma is the most common renal tumor, but it is only seen in about 5% of children. Lymphoma is seen in 8% of toddlers.

15. B) Low Apgar scores

The mnemonic for high-risk factors for hearing loss is HEARS: Hyperbilirubinemia; ear infection frequency; low Apgar scores; exposure to rubella, cytomegalovirus, or toxoplasmosis; and seizures. Exposure to chlamydia in utero is not a risk factor for hearing loss.

ABSENCE SEIZURES

Brief episodes during which child suddenly stops whatever they are doing and stares. If in school, teacher may tell parent that child is daydreaming and inattentive. A common type of pediatric seizure. Also called *petit mal seizure*. First-line therapy is ethosuximide. Refer to pediatric neurologist.

DOWN SYNDROME: ATLANTOAXIAL INSTABILITY

Up to 15% of Down syndrome patients have atlantoaxial instability (excessive mobility at the articulation of C1 and C2). Medical clearance is recommended for some sports participation. Children/adolescents (or older) with Down syndrome who want to participate in sports need cervical spine x-rays (including lateral view). Patients with atlantoaxial instability are restricted from playing contact sports (e.g., basketball, tackle football, soccer) and other high-risk activities (e.g., trampoline jumping). Persons with Down syndrome without evidence of atlantoaxial instability may participate in low-impact sports and sports not requiring extreme balance.

KAWASAKI DISEASE/SYNDROME

Onset of high fever (up to 104.0°F) for 5 or more days. Presence of at least four of the following clinical signs: enlarged lymph nodes in the neck, bright-red rash (more obvious on groin area), bilateral conjunctivitis (dry, no discharge), oral mucosal changes (e.g., dry cracked lips, "strawberry tongue"), and swollen hands and feet. After fever subsides, skin peels off hands and feet. Treated with high-dose aspirin and IV gamma globulin.

Most cases (75%) occur in children younger than 5 years. Resolves within 1 to 3 weeks but may have serious sequelae, such as aortic dissection, dilation or aneurysms of the coronary arteries, and hearing loss. Requires close follow-up with pediatric cardiologist for several years because effects may not be apparent until child is older (or an adult).

LEUKEMIA

Complains of extreme fatigue and weakness. Pale skin and easy bruising. May have petechial bleeding (pinpoint to small red spots). May have bleeding gums and nosebleeds. Some have bone or joint pain, lymphadenopathy, or swelling in the abdomen. Leukemias are the most common type of cancer in children and adolescents; the most common type in children is acute lymphocytic leukemia (ALL).

Acute Lymphocytic Leukemia

Most common form of leukemia in childhood (75%). Fast-growing cancer of the lymphoblasts, which are immature lymphocytes. Peak occurrence at 2 to 4 years of age. Almost all patients have neutropenia with varying degrees of anemia and thrombocytopenia. Girls have slightly higher chance of cure compared with boys.

Acute Myelogenous Leukemia

Acute myelogenous leukemia (AML) is a fast-growing cancer of the bone marrow that affects immature or precursor blood cells, such as myeloblasts (WBCs), monoblasts (macrophages, monocytes), erythroblasts (RBCs), and megakaryoblasts (platelets). Children with Down syndrome who have AML tend to have better cure rates, especially if the child is younger than 4 years.

REYE'S SYNDROME

History of febrile viral illness (chickenpox, influenza) and aspirin or salicylate intake (e.g., Pepto-Bismol) in a child. Theoretical risk of Reye's syndrome after varicella immunization. Abrupt onset with quick progression. Death can occur within a few hours to a few days. Mortality rate of up to 52%. Although most cases are in children, disease has been seen in teenagers and adults. This disease is now rare, with fewer than 1,000 cases per year in the United States.

Clinical Staging

Mild to Moderate

- Stage 1: Severe vomiting, lethargic/sleepy, elevated alanine aminotransferase (ALT) and aspartate transaminase (AST)
- Stage 2: Deeply lethargic, restless, confused/delirious/combative, hyperactive reflexes, hyperventilation
- Stage 3: Obtunded or in light coma, decorticate rigidity

Severe

- Stage 4: Coma, seizure, decerebrate rigidity, fixed pupils, loss of reflexes
- Stage 5: Seizures, deep coma, flaccid paralysis, absent deep tendon reflexes (DTRs), respiratory arrest, death

STILL'S MURMUR

A benign systolic murmur that is described as having a vibratory or musical quality. Becomes louder in supine position or with fever. Minimal radiation. Grade I or II intensity. Most common in school-age children. Usually resolves by adolescence.

HEALTH PROMOTION AND SAFETY

MEDICAL CONDITIONS AND ATHLETIC PARTICIPATION

For information about medical conditions and athletic participation, see Table 22.1.

U.S. HEALTH STATISTICS: SCHOOL-AGE CHILDREN

Top Causes of Death: Age 5 to 9 Years (Early School Age)

- Accidents (unintentional injuries)
- Cancer
- Congenital malformations, deformations, and chromosomal abnormalities

IMMUNIZATIONS

Children Age 5 to 6 Years

- If vaccines were not administered at age 4 years, administer measles, mumps, and rubella (MMR); varicella; inactivated poliovirus vaccine (IPV); and diphtheria, tetanus, acellular pertussis (DTaP).
- If history of chickenpox is documented on chart by health provider, do not need varicella.

Table 22.1 Medical Conditions That May Disqualify Youth From Sports Participation*

Condition	Rationale
Hypertrophic cardiomyopathy	Risk of sudden cardiac death with intense exercise
Atlantoaxial instability (Down syndrome, juvenile rheumatoid arthritis)	Instability between C1 and C2 can cause spinal cord compression
Marfan syndrome	Risk of aortic aneurysm and cardiac death, lens eyes displacement, joint hypermobility
Ehlers–Danlos syndrome (vascular form)	Risk of cerebral or cervical artery aneurysm, spondylolisthesis, joint hypermobility
Acute rheumatic fever with carditis	Exercise worsens heart inflammation
Mitral valve prolapse, especially if significant mitral valve pathology	Risk of sudden cardiac death
Fever	Risk of heat illness, hypotension, and increased cardiopulmonary effort
Infectious diarrhea	Risk of dehydration and heat illness; contagious
Pink eye	Contagious
Bleeding disorders (e.g., hemophilia)	Risk for injury and uncontrolled bleeding, especially with contact sports
Solitary kidney (e.g., born with one kidney or has had one kidney removed)	Risk of injury to the one functional kidney is too great, especially in contact sports

*List is not all-inclusive. Individuals with some conditions are approved to play low-contact or noncontact sports.
Source: American Academy of Pediatrics (2008). (See Resources section for complete source information.)

EXAM TIP

Rubeola is measles.

Children Age 7 to 12 Years

- If child is age 7 to 9 years with an incomplete immunization record for DTaP, give Tdap as first catch-up dose, followed by tetanus diphtheria (Td) vaccine.
- Tdap booster should be administered to all 11- to 12-year-olds (regardless of whether it was used in a catch-up schedule).
- Most common "middle school" vaccines at 11 to 12 years of age are Tdap, meningococcal conjugate vaccine (MCV4; Menactra, Menveo, and MenQuadfi), and human papillomavirus (HPV) vaccine (Gardasil or Cervarix).
- HPV vaccine can be administered as young as age 9 years.
- See Table 22.2.

Table 22.2 Routine and Catch-Up Immunizations: Age 7 Years and Older*

Vaccine	Immunizations
Hepatitis B	Total of three doses over 6 months. If missing a booster, give until total of three doses. Do not repeat series.
Measles, mumps, rubella	Give second dose (if needs to catch up). Live virus precautions.
Varicella	Give second dose (if needs to catch up) if no proof of varicella. Live virus precautions.
Tetanus	Give Tdap at age 11–12 years (or older if missed this dose). Replace one Td booster with Tdap.
Hepatitis A	Give second dose (if needs to catch up). Recommended for children with certain health or lifestyle conditions placing them at risk.
Influenza	Needed annually after age 6 months.
Human papillomavirus	Give first dose at age 11–12 years (can start at age 9 years). Initial vaccination at 9–14 years: Two-dose series (6–12 months apart). Initial vaccination at ≥15 years: Three-dose series (give second dose 1–2 months after first; give third dose 6 months after first dose). Gardasil: Can be given up to age 45 years.
Meningococcal	Give first dose at age 11–12 years. Give booster at age 16 years. Meningococcal conjugate vaccine (MCV4) is recommended for all college freshmen living in dormitories.

*This table is a simplified version and is designed for studying for certification exams only. Do not use this table as a guideline for clinical practice.
Source: Adapted from Centers for Disease Control and Prevention (2020).

NOTES

- HPV vaccine is recommended for girls and boys.
- If first dose of HPV given between 9 and 14 years, only two doses are needed; three doses needed if series started at 15 years or older.
- If no history of varicella immunization (or having had the disease), then give the varicella vaccine.
- If child did not complete hepatitis A or B series, administer next dose and resume interval dosing. Do not restart hepatitis A or B series.

Meningococcal Vaccines

There are six types of meningococcal vaccines; only two of them are discussed here:

- MenACWY-D (Menactra) and MenACWY-CRM (Menveo): Administer vaccine first dose at age 11 to 12 years. If missing, catch-up age is 13 to 18 years. If first dose at age 13 to 15 years, need booster (second dose) at age 16 to 18 years.
- Also used for high-risk children with: Asplenia, functional asplenia (sickle cell), splenectomy, HIV infection, and complement deficiencies. Youngest age for Menactra is 9 months, and youngest age for Menveo is 2 months.

EXAM TIPS

- All 11- to 12-year-old children should be vaccinated with single dose of quadrivalent meningococcal vaccine (MenACWY); brand names are Menactra, Menveo, and MenQuadfi.
- Immunizations are needed at age 11 to 12 years (Tdap, HPV, MCV4).

Primary Series of Vaccination: Missing or Not Done

After Seventh Birthday (Never Been Vaccinated)

- Tetanus (three doses) (first dose should be Tdap, and then subsequent two doses should be given as Td; repeat Td every 10 years)
- IPV (three doses)
- Hepatitis B (three doses)
- Hepatitis A (two doses)
- MMR (two doses)
- Varicella (two doses) if no history of chickenpox
- HPV (two or three doses based on age given; administer if younger than 45 years)

EXAM TIPS

- Know that youngest age group for HPV vaccine (Gardasil) is 9 years, and it can be given up to age 45 years.
- HPV may cause cancers of the cervix, vagina, vulva, penis, anus, pharynx, and base of tongue and tonsils (oropharynx).

GROWTH AND DEVELOPMENT

5 YEARS

Fine Motor
- Copies square
- Can draw a person with six body parts
- Begins to print some letters and numbers

Gross Motor
- Can ride a bicycle (use bike helmet)
- Hops on one foot
- Can dress and undress self

Other
Likes to help parents with certain household chores; likes to help adults

6 YEARS

Fine Motor
- Copies a triangle (copies a diamond at age 7 years)
- Ties shoes

Gross Motor
- Climbs trees
- Skips

Other
Begins more formal schooling with instruction in basic math and reading skills

7 TO 10 YEARS OLD

- Freud classified this age group under the "latency stage."
- The major task for this age group is to succeed in school and interact with their peer group. May have a "best" friend(s).
- Some girls may start puberty at age 8 to 9 years.

TV and Electronics Use
Limit to 2 hours a day or less. Use parental-control software.

11 TO 12 YEARS

- Major task at this age is to assert independence.
- This age group is in Piaget's concrete operational stage (Table 22.3).
- Early abstract thinking starts at about 11 years.
- Starts to think of the future.
- Fully immersed in hormonal changes associated with puberty.

DISEASE REVIEW

AUTISM SPECTRUM DISORDER

Autism spectrum disorder (ASD) is a neurodevelopmental disorder that affects the normal development of communication and social skills. The exact cause is unknown. Autism affects more boys than girls. There are several theories about the cause, but they are unproven. Autism is hard to diagnose before the age of 18 months.

Table 22.3 Jean Piaget's Stages of Cognitive Development

Stage	Age	Goal
Sensorimotor	Birth to 2 years old	Object permanence
Preoperational	2–7 years old	Egocentric, pretend play
Concrete operational	7–11 years old	Conservation, math, numbers
Formal operational	12 years to adulthood	Abstract thinking, logic, ethics, morals

Classic Case

Child who is extremely sensitive to noises, touch, smells, and/or textures. Will refuse to wear tight or rough-textured clothes because they feel "itchy." Prefers to be alone. Has poor eye contact. Does not interact with others. Slow-to-poor language development. Has repeated body movements such as flapping arms. Some may appear to be progressing normally but suddenly regress. Language, physical, and social skills disintegrate.

Treatment Plan

- Refer to psychiatrist or psychologist for testing and evaluation.
- Intensive rehabilitation is needed at younger ages (i.e., occupational therapy [OT], physical therapy [PT], speech therapy).
- Risperidone (Risperdal) is an antipsychotic that is prescribed for some older patients.

CHILDHOOD RASHES

Be familiar with the appearance of these rashes for the exam (Table 22.4 and Figures 22.1 through 22.8).

FRAGILE X SYNDROME

Classic Case

Child has macrocephaly (>50th percentile for age/sex) and global developmental delays. Skills and behavior acquisition slow compared with peers. Hyperactive behavior or specific learning disabilities (particularly involving math and problem-solving) can be seen. High correlation with autism and anxiety. Tends to avoid eye contact. Patient has a long face with prominent forehead, jaw, and large or protruding ears. Large body with flexible flat feet.

Treatment Plan

- Refer for genetic testing.
- Refer patient to developmental pediatrician or psychiatrist/psychologist for interdisciplinary evaluation and multimodal interventions.

EXAM TIP

Recognize physical characteristics of fragile X syndrome.

Table 22.4 Childhood Rashes

Condition	Appearance of Rash and Associated Findings
Hand–foot–mouth disease	Multiple small blisters appear on the hands, feet, and around rectum. Small ulcers inside mouth, throat, tonsils, and tongue.
Impetigo	"Honey-colored" crusted lesions. Fragile bullae (bullous type).
Measles (rubeola)	Koplik's spots (small white papules) inside the cheeks (buccal mucosa) by the rear molars. Erythematous maculopapular rash that begins on face and spreads from head to feet but spares palms and soles.
Varicella	Generalized rash in different stages; new lesions appear daily for about 5 days. Papules → vesicles → pustules → crusts. Pruritic. Very contagious.
Scarlet fever	"Sandpaper" rash with sore throat. Strawberry tongue is not specific (also seen in Kawasaki disease).
Pediculosis capitis (head lice)	Ovoid white nits on hair hard to dislodge. Red papules that are very itchy; nits are initially located in the hairline area behind the neck and the ears.
Molluscum contagiosum	Smooth, waxlike, round (dome-shaped) papules ranging in size from a pinhead to the size of a pencil eraser (2–5 mm). Central umbilication with white plug. Caused by the poxvirus.
Scabies	Maculopapular rash located in interdigital webs of hands, feet, waist, axillae, groin. Very pruritic, especially at night. Can resemble pimples, eczema, and insect bites.

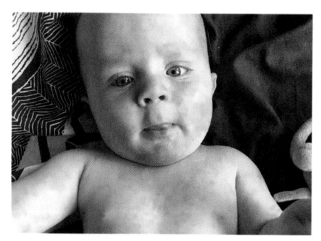

Figure 22.1 Hand–foot–mouth disease.

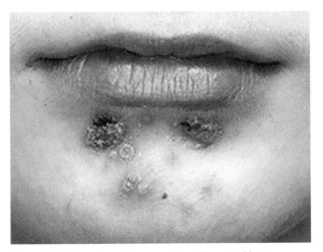

Figure 22.2 Impetigo. "Honey-colored" crusted lesions.

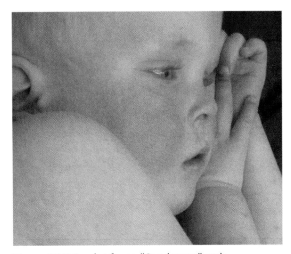

Figure 22.5 Scarlet fever. "Sandpaper" rash.

(A)

(B)

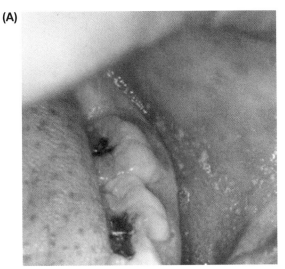

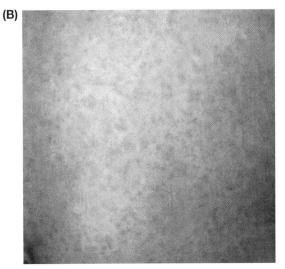

Figure 22.3 Measles (rubeola). (A) Koplik's spots (small white papules) inside the cheeks by rear molars.
(B) Erythematous maculopapular rash.
Source: Centers for Disease Control and Prevention/Heinz F. Eichenwald, MD.

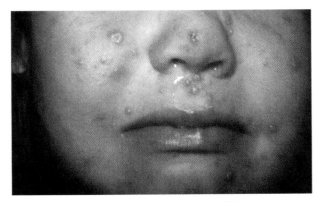

Figure 22.4 Varicella. Generalized rash in different
stages—papules, vesicles, pustules, crusts.

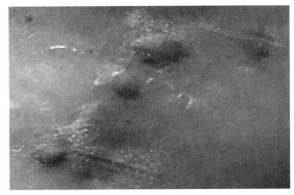

Figure 22.6 *Pediculosis capitis* (head lice). Red papules initially
located in the hairline area behind the neck and the ears.

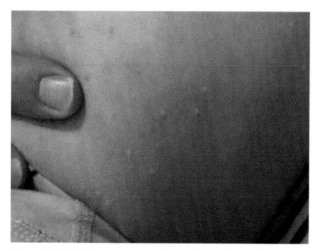

Figure 22.7 Molluscum contagiosum. Smooth waxlike, round (dome-shaped) papules; central umbilication with white plug.

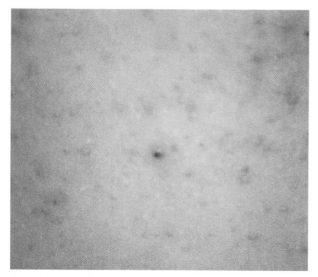

Figure 22.8 Scabies. Maculopapular, pruritic rash that can resemble pimples, eczema, and insect bites.
Source: Centers for Disease Control and Prevention.

FUNCTIONAL CONSTIPATION (ENCOPRESIS)

Rome IV criteria diagnosis of functional constipation in children (age 4 years or older). Up to 80% of children with functional fecal incontinence may also have constipation. Must meet two or more of the following criteria at least once per week (for at least 1 month). Order a plain film (x-ray) of the abdomen to check for retained stool.

- History of withholding of stool
- History of painful or hard bowel movements
- History of large-diameter stools that may obstruct the toilet
- Presence of large fecal mass in rectum
- Two or fewer defecations in toilet per week
- At least one episode of fecal incontinence per week (thin fluid with feces that bypass a large stool mass and leak around it); ask patient if fecal soiling of underwear

HAND–FOOT–MOUTH DISEASE

A common acute viral illness that mainly affects children younger than 10 years of age. Most common cause is the coxsackievirus A16. Spread through direct contact with nasal discharge, saliva, blister fluid, or stool. Patient is most contagious during the first week of the illness.

Classic Case

Acute onset of fever, severe sore throat, headache, and anorexia. Multiple small blisters appear on the hands and feet and around the rectum. Ulcers are present inside the mouth, throat, tonsils, and tongue. Child will complain of sore throat and mouth pain with acidic foods.

Treatment Plan

- Treatment is symptomatic; self-limited illness; complete recovery usually occurs within 5 to 10 days.
- Ibuprofen or acetaminophen for pain and fever every 4 to 6 hours; do not use aspirin.
- Use salt-water gargle (1/2 teaspoon salt in one glass of warm water).
- Drink cold fluids (avoid soda, orange or lemon juice, tomato juice).

EXAM TIPS

- Child at age 11 years is at early abstract thinking stage (Piaget).
- Recognize hand–foot–mouth disease, scabies, impetigo, varicella, and other childhood rashes.

KNOWLEDGE CHECK: CHAPTER 22

1. What is the most common type of cancer in young children?
   A. Acute lymphoblastic leukemia
   B. Multiple myeloma
   C. Aplastic anemia
   D. Non-Hodgkin's lymphoma

2. The parents of a 7-year-old boy tell the family nurse practitioner that his teacher has complained of the child's frequent episodes of daydreaming. The parents report that sometimes when the child is at home, he seems not to hear them, "blanking out" for a short period of time. Which of the following seizures is *most* likely?
   A. Clonic
   B. Absence
   C. Grand mal
   D. Atonic

3. One developmental milestone is the ability to draw a stick figure "person" with six separate body parts. What is the age group that this finding is associated with?
   A. 2 years old
   B. 3 years old
   C. 4 years old
   D. 5 years old

4. A child complains of severe pruritus that is worse at night. Several family members also have the same symptoms. Upon examination, areas of excoriated papules are noted on some of the interdigital webs of both hands and on the axillae. This finding is *most* consistent with:
   A. Contact dermatitis
   B. Impetigo
   C. Larva migrans
   D. Scabies

5. Which statement about the human papillomavirus (HPV) vaccine is true?
   A. Patients as old as 26 years can receive the vaccine.
   B. The Centers for Disease Control and Prevention (CDC) does not recommend the vaccine for males.
   C. For children younger than 16 years, only two doses of the vaccine are needed.
   D. The minimum age at which the vaccine can be given is 9 years.

6. A 5-year-old child is diagnosed with Kawasaki disease after 5 days of high fever. With whom should this child follow up on a routine basis to monitor for sequalae?
   A. Infectious disease
   B. Cardiology
   C. Ophthalmology
   D. Dermatology

7. A child is seen for an annual well-child exam and is noted to be thinking in an abstract manner. This child's age is *most likely* how many years?
   A. 5
   B. 7
   C. 9
   D. 11

8. A 5-year-old child is seen for a routine well visit. The child has been noted by their kindergarten teacher to be struggling to acquire some of the early literacy skills. The child also has difficulty with basic problem solving. Physical exam reveals a tall child with a large head, prominent forehead, and large ears. What is the *most likely* diagnosis?
   A. Autism spectrum disorder
   B. Marfan syndrome
   C. Fragile X syndrome
   D. Fetal alcohol syndrome

9. An 11-year-old girl is seen for a well visit. She has the following immunizations on her shot record: DTaP x 5, IPV x 4, MMR x 2, varicella x 2, Hep B x 3, Hep A x 1, influenza given 2 months ago. What immunizations should she receive today?
   A. DTaP, MCV4, varicella, and Hep A
   B. Tdap, MCV4, HPV, and Hep A
   C. Td, MCV, and Hep A
   D. Hep B, Hep A, HPV, and MCV4

10. A kindergarten-aged child presents with a fever to 102.5°F and has a decreased appetite. The child complains of a sore throat and headache. On exam, ulcers on an erythematous base are noted on the inside of the lower lip and cheeks, and three small blisters are noted on the right hand. Which of the following is appropriate anticipatory guidance for this patient's parents?
    A. Offer the child warm tomato soup
    B. Use a lemon juice and water swish-and-spit solution
    C. Offer aspirin every 4 to 6 hours for pain and fever
    D. Use a salt-water gargle/rinse several times a day

(See answers next page.)

1. A) Acute lymphoblastic leukemia

Acute lymphoblastic leukemia, a malignancy of the bone marrow, is the most common type of cancer in children. It is more common in boys and in children between the ages of 2 and 4 years. Aplastic anemia is bone marrow suppression (not cancer) usually caused by medications or a viral infection. Multiple myeloma and non-Hodgkin's lymphoma are more common in older adults.

2. B) Absence

An absence seizure is a seizure that usually lasts less than 15 seconds. During the seizure, the child may appear not to be listening, to have "blanked out," or to be daydreaming. Clonic seizures are characterized by rhythmic jerking of the muscles in the arms, neck, or face. A grand mal (or generalized tonic-clonic) seizure involves an abrupt loss of consciousness followed by stiffening of the extremeties and muscular twitching. An atonic seizure (or drop seizure) involves a sudden loss of muscle control, typically in the legs, that causes the individual to collapse.

3. D) 5 years old

By 5 years of age, a child can draw a stick person with six body parts and copy a square. Children should be able to copy a straight line or circle at ages 2 and 3, respectively. A 4-year-old child can copy a cross and draw a stick person with three body parts.

4. D) Scabies

Scabies is a parasitic disease (infestation) of the skin caused by the human itch mite *Sarcoptes scabiei*. The rash is generally characterized as red, raised, excoriated papules. The scabies mite is generally transmitted from one person to another by direct contact with the skin of the infested person and can also be acquired by wearing an infested person's clothing (fomites), such as sweaters, coats, or scarves. Following the incubation period, the infested person will complain of pruritus (itching), which intensifies at bedtime under the warmth of the blankets. Common sites of infection are the webs of fingers, wrists, flexors of the arms, axillae, lower abdomen, genitalia, buttocks, and feet.

5. D) The minimum age at which the vaccine can be given is 9 years.

The HPV vaccine can be given to patients as young as 9 years. Although it is not recommended as a routine vaccination for patients over the age of 26, it can be administered in individuals up to age 45 years. It is recommended for both males and females. If it is given before age 14 years, only two doses are required. If the patient is older than 14 years, three doses are required.

6. B) Cardiology

Serious sequelae, such as aortic dissection, coronary artery aneurysms, and dilation, may not appear until the child is older, so routine follow-up with cardiology is recommended. Once the rash and other signs of inflammation resolve, usually in 4 to 8 weeks, the child should not need continued monitoring by dermatology, ophthalmology, or infectious disease.

7. D) 11

According to Piaget, early abstract thinking starts at about 11 years old, while 7- and 9-year-olds are typically concrete operational thinkers. The 5-year-old is still in pretend play and is considered in the preoperational thinking stage.

8. C) Fragile X syndrome

Children with Fragile X syndrome often have developmental delays or specific learning disabilities pertaining to problem solving. These children may struggle with acquiring skills at the same speed as their peers and have a phenotypic presentation of a long, narrow face with a large forehead and large ears, as well as tall stature prior to puberty but potentially impaired height gain during puberty. People with Marfan syndrome are usually tall and thin with long arms, legs, fingers and toes. They are not usually found to have cognitive delays or difficulties with learning. Autism spectrum disorder is a neurodevelopmental issue that typically affects communication and social skills without any specific phenotypic findings. Fetal alcohol syndrome (FAS) is phenotypically described as small eyes, a thin upper lip, a smooth philtrum, and slow growth. Variable degrees of intellectual disability are noted with FAS.

9. B) Tdap, MCV4, HPV, and Hep A

Because the patient is up to date on her infant immunizations, with the exception of the second Hep A, she should receive all of the 11- to 12-year-old vaccines. These include HPV, MCV4, and Tdap. DTaP is not used outside of the toddler and preschool age range, and this patient has a complete varicella schedule. Td might be used if this child required catch-up vaccinations for tetanus and diphtheria, but the first in that catch-up series should be a Tdap to cover for pertussis.

10. D) Use a salt-water gargle/rinse several times a day

This child likely has coxsackie A16 virus (also referred to as hand-foot-mouth disease). A child with this illness will be bothered by warm or hot liquids. Acidic foods such as lemon or tomato juice can irritate the lesions. Aspirin should never be given to kindergarten-aged children.

ACETAMINOPHEN POISONING (INTENTIONAL INGESTION)

Acetaminophen damages the liver, resulting in mild-to-severe fulminant liver failure. Acetaminophen is also known as *paracetamol* and is sold as Tylenol and others.

- Stage I (up to 24 hours after overdose): Patients are usually asymptomatic but may have nausea and vomiting and, with very large doses, lethargy, and malaise.
- Stage II (18–72 hours after overdose): Patients complain of right upper quadrant pain with abdominal pain, nausea, and vomiting; elevated liver function tests (LFTs), prothrombin time, and bilirubin concentrations; possible nephrotoxicity (elevated blood urea nitrogen [BUN], creatinine).
- Stage III (72–96 hours after overdose): Hepatic necrosis presents as jaundice, clotting disorders, hypoglycemia, and hepatic encephalopathy. Acute kidney injury with oliguria may develop. Most deaths from organ failure occur within 72 to 96 hours.
- Stage IV (4 days–3 weeks after overdose): If patient survives, symptoms and signs of organ failure resolve.

With acute overdose, serum acetaminophen concentration should be measured as soon as possible, but at least 4 hours must have passed since ingestion to obtain accurate blood level (if <4 hours, blood level is not accurate). Antidote is N-acetylcysteine given intravenously.

HODGKIN'S LYMPHOMA

Patient presents with enlarged and painless cervical, axillary, groin, or supraclavicular lymphadenopathy associated with fever (Pel-Ebstein sign), fatigue, unexplained weight loss, and night sweats. May report having severe pain on or over malignant areas a few minutes after drinking alcohol.

- Hodgkin lymphoma presents as enlarged lymph nodes with fever, night sweats, and occasionally pain (lymph nodes) after drinking alcohol.
- The most common cancers in teens aged 15 to 19 years are Hodgkin's lymphoma and germ cell tumors such as testicular and ovarian cancer.

TESTICULAR CANCER

Teenage-to-adult male complains of a "heaviness" in scrotum or a hardened mass that is usually painless. Some patients may have testicular discomfort or numbness, but not pain. The affected testicle has a firm texture. More common in males from the age of 15 to 35 years. Cryptorchidism is a strong risk factor.

TESTICULAR TORSION (ACUTE SCROTUM)

Pubertal male awakens with abrupt onset of unilateral testicular pain that increases in severity. Pain may radiate to the lower abdomen and/or groin. Almost all patients (90%) also have nausea and vomiting. Ischemic changes result in severe scrotal edema, redness, and testicular pain. Ipsilateral (same side) cremasteric reflex is absent, and the testicle may be noted to be high riding with a transverse lie. Highest incidence is during adolescence. May be confused with torsion of appendix testis (more common in prepubertal boys, less nausea/vomiting, "blue dot sign"). Urinalysis (UA) is negative for pyuria and bacteriuria. Doppler ultrasound is the initial diagnostic test. Testicle will become nonfunctional if not repaired within 24 hours. Surgical emergency. Refer to ED.

- Antidote of acetaminophen poisoning is oral or IV *N*-acetylcysteine.
- Recognize presentation of testicular torsion and testicular cancer.

ADOLESCENCE

Defined as the onset of puberty until sexual maturity.

PUBERTY

The period in life when secondary sexual characteristics start to develop because of hormonal stimulation. Ovaries start producing estrogen and progesterone. Testes start producing testosterone. All of these changes result in reproductive capability.

- Puberty starts at Tanner stage II in girls (breast bud) or boys (testicular enlargement and scrotal rugation/color starts to become darker). Puberty ends at Tanner stage V (adult stage).
- Tanner stage III in boys is elongation of the penis (testes continue to grow). Only Tanner stages II to IV need to be memorized for the exam.

Girls

- Precocious puberty if puberty starts before age 8 years
- Delayed puberty if no breast development (Tanner stage II) by age 12 years

Growth Spurt

- Majority of physical changes occur between the ages of 10 and 13 years.
- Majority of skeletal growth occurs before menarche. Afterward, growth slows down.
- Girls start their growth spurts approximately 2 years earlier than boys.

Pubertal Timeline

Breast development → peak growth acceleration → menarche. Most of a girl's height is gained before menarche. Skeletal growth in girls is considered complete within 2 years after menarche.

Ovulation Pain (Mittelschmerz)

Unilateral midcycle (about 14 days before the next period) pelvic pain that is caused by an enlarging ovarian follicle or the rupture of the follicle at the time of ovulation. Pain may last a few hours to a few days. May occur intermittently.

Menarche

- Average age is about 12 years in the United States (range is 8–15 years).
- The first 1 to 2 years after the onset of menarche, it is common to have irregular periods because of irregular ovulation (may skip a month or longer intervals, lighter bleeding).
- After Tanner stage II starts (breast bud stage), girls start menses within 2 years.
- Delayed puberty is determined if no breast development by age 13 years or if menarche does not begin by 15 years.

Menstrual Cycle

- Average duration is 28 days. In younger teens, cycles range from 21 to 45 days; in young adults, they can range from 21 to 35 days.
- Average duration of menstrual bleeding is about 3 to 5 days (range 2–7 days).
- Day 1 of the menstrual cycle starts as spotting; then, blood flow becomes heavier for 2 to 3 days, and then bleeding lightens until it stops.
- The most fertile period in the cycle is about 3 days before and during ovulation (days 11–14).

Dysmenorrhea

- Painful periods are due to severe menstrual cramps caused by high levels of prostaglandins.
- Treatment is use of heating pads and nonsteroidal anti-inflammatory drugs (NSAIDs) such as ibuprofen (Advil, Motrin) and naproxen (Aleve).

EXAM TIP

Adolescent health history is obtained from both parent or guardian and child initially; then the adolescent is interviewed alone without the parent.

Boys

- Precocious puberty if starts before age 9 years
- Delayed puberty if no testicular enlargement by age 14 years

Growth Spurt

Boys' growth spurts are approximately 2 years later than girls' (ages 11–15 years).

Spermarche

Average age is 13.3 years.

TANNER STAGES

Table 23.1 Tanner Stages

Stage	Girls: Breasts	Boys: Penis and Testes	Boys/Girls: Pubic Hair
I	Prepuberty	Prepuberty	None
II	Breast bud	Testes enlarge Scrotal rugae	Few straight, fine hairs
III	Breast and areola One mound	Penis lengthens	Darker, coarse Starts to curl
IV	Breast and areola Secondary mound	Penis thickens	Thicker, curly Darker, coarse
V	Adult size	Adult size	Adult pattern Spreads to inner thigh

EXAM TIPS

- There is no need to memorize pubic hair changes. Memorize only the breast changes (girls) and the genital changes (boys).
- There will likely be very few questions about Tanner staging (girl or boy).

HEALTH PROMOTION AND SAFETY

U.S. HEALTH STATISTICS (ADOLESCENTS)

Top Three Causes of Death (15–19 Years Old)

1. Accidents (e.g., motor vehicle crashes)
2. Assault/homicide (e.g., intentional firearm use)
3. Intentional self-harm (suicide)

IMMUNIZATION SCHEDULE FOR ADOLESCENTS

See the immunization schedule in Table 23.2.

EXAM TIPS

- Meningococcal vaccine is recommended for all, starting at age 11 to 12 years (not just for college freshmen living in dormitories).
- Vaccine Adverse Event Reporting System (VAERS) is a government program to report clinically adverse events.

Table 23.2 Immunization Schedule (Ages 11–18 Years)*

Vaccine	Immunization Schedule
Tdap (Boostrix, Adacel)	All 11- or 12-year-olds: Give Tdap as booster and then Td or Tdap every 10 years for lifetime. Age 13 to 14 years (or older): Give Tdap if did not receive it at age 11 to 12 years.
HPV (Gardasil)	Minimum age is 9 years. All 11- or 12-year-olds: Give to girls and boys. Need two doses 6 months apart. Age 15–45 years: Needs three doses at intervals of 0, 1 to 2, and 6 months.
Meningococcal (ACWY-D [Menactra, MenQuadfi], MenACWY-CRM [Menveo], MenB-4C [Bexsero], MenB-FHbp [Trumenba])	All 11- or 12-year-olds: Give single dose of MenACWY, with booster at age 16 years. Catch-up: Age 13–18 years, give MenACWY. If first dose at age 13–15 years, needs booster at age 16–18 years. If first dose at age 16 years, no booster dose is needed. Clinical discretion: Young adults 16–23 years may be vaccinated (if at increased risk for meningococcal disease) with either Bexsero or Trumenba.
Influenza inactivated	Vaccinate everyone from age 6 months and older annually.
Hepatitis B (Recombivax HB)	Catch-up: Give remaining doses if not completed.
Hepatitis A (HAVRIX, VAQTA)	Catch-up: Give second dose if not completed.
MMR	Catch-up: Give the second dose if not completed.
Varicella	If no reliable history of chickenpox (verbal okay). Live virus precautions should be reviewed.

*This table is a simplified version and is designed for studying for the certification exams only. Do not use this table as a guideline for clinical practice.

HPV, human papillomavirus; Tdap, tetanus, diphtheria, and pertussis.

Source: Adapted from CDC (2022).

CLINICAL PEARL

Children and adolescents normally have higher blood levels of alkaline phosphatase compared with adults because of growing bone. It is produced by the osteoblasts.

LEGAL ISSUES

Right to Consent and Confidentiality

- No parental (or guardian) consent is necessary for treatment of sexually transmitted infections (STIs).
- Consent laws vary by state for contraceptive services and prenatal care.

Emancipated Minor Criteria

These minors may give full consent as an adult without parental involvement:
- Legally married
- Active duty in the armed forces
- Living separately from their parents and self-supporting

Confidentiality

Confidentiality can be broken in the following situations:
- Gunshot wounds and stab wounds, which must be reported to the police (regardless of victim's age)
- Child abuse (actual or suspected abuse), which must be reported to the authorities
- Suicidal ideation and/or suicide attempt (discharge to parents/guardians or hospital)
- Homicidal ideation or intent (especially mental health providers)

HEALTH PROMOTION

During a physical examination or wellness visit, assess teenager for high-risk behaviors. Intensive behavior counseling is recommended. The following are high-risk behaviors to screen for:
- Sexual activity: Use of condoms, birth control, intimate partner violence (e.g., sexual coercion, rape), signs/symptoms of STIs
- Safety: Driver safety; seatbelt/helmet use; access to guns/gun safety; smoking, alcohol, and drug use
- Social history: Family, peers, school performance, work
- Mental health: Signs/symptoms of depression and antisocial behaviors (e.g., gangs)

EXAM TIPS

- No parental consent is needed for health services related to STI testing. Consent laws vary by state for contraceptive services and prenatal care. If not related to sexual activity, then need parental consent (dysmenorrhea, headache, upper respiratory infection [URI]).
- Memorize the criteria for an emancipated minor. Do not confuse the right to confidentiality with emancipated minor status.

DISEASE REVIEW

ADOLESCENT IDIOPATHIC SCOLIOSIS

Lateral curvature of the spine that may be accompanied by spinal rotation. More common in girls (80% of patients). Painless and asymptomatic. Scoliosis will most likely worsen (66% of cases) if it starts near the beginning of the growth spurt. Rapid worsening of curvature is indicative of secondary cause (e.g., Marfan or Ehlers–Danlos syndrome, cerebral palsy, myelomeningocele).

Classic Case

Teen complains that one hip, shoulder, breast, or scapula is higher than the other (Figure 23.1). No complaints of pain.

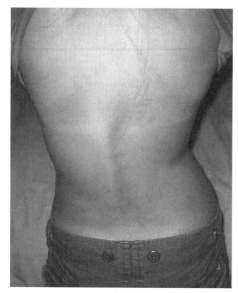

Figure 23.1 Scoliosis (female age 18 years).

Screening Test: Adam's Forward Bend Test

Have patient bend forward with both arms hanging free. Look for asymmetry of spine, scapula, or thorax and lumbar curvature. Check height. Measure the Cobb angle (degree of spinal curvature). Full-spine x-rays are used to measure degree of curvature.

Treatment Parameters

- Curves <20 degrees: Observe and monitor for changes in spinal curvature
- Curves of 20 to 40 degrees: Bracing (e.g., Milwaukee brace)
- Curves >40 degrees: Surgical correction with Harrington rod used on spine and other options

Management

- Check Tanner stage (Tanner stages II–V).
- Order spinal x-ray (posterioanterior [PA] view) to measure Cobb angle.
- Refer all patients with scoliosis to a pediatric orthopedic specialist.

EXAM TIPS

- Scoliosis treatment needed for a ≥20-degree curve; for curves <20 degrees, observe for worsening.
- Screening test for scoliosis is the Adam's forward bend test.

ANOREXIA NERVOSA

- Usual onset is during adolescence. Involves an irrational preoccupation with and intense fear of gaining weight.
- There are two types. Patient engages in restriction (dieting, excessive exercise) or in binge eating and purging.

Some examples of purging are excessive use of laxatives, enemas, diuretics, and vomiting.

Clinical Findings

- Marked weight loss (body mass index [BMI] ≤18.5), bradycardia (40–49 beats/min), vital signs unstable, hypotension
- Lanugo (increased lanugo, especially in the face, back, and shoulders)
- Osteoporosis or osteopenia
- Swollen feet (low albumin), dizziness, abdominal bloating

EXAM TIPS

- Recognize how patients with anorexia nervosa present (i.e., lanugo, peripheral edema, amenorrhea, significant weight loss >10% of body weight). Low albumin level results in peripheral edema.
- Increased risk of stress fractures, osteoporosis, or osteopenia.

DELAYED PUBERTY

Absence of secondary sexual characteristics by the age of 13 years for girls (such as a breast bud) or at the age of 14 years for boys. The child remains in Tanner stage I (prepubertal).

Labs

- Serum pregnancy test.
- Check prolactin level. If prolactin level is elevated, next step is to order a CT scan of the sella turcica (location of pituitary gland inside the skull).
- For primary amenorrhea (no menses by age 15 years), rule out hypogonadism by checking hormone levels (e.g., follicle-stimulating hormone [FSH], luteinizing hormone [LH], thyroid-stimulating hormone [TSH]). Rule out chromosomal disorders, absence of uterus/vagina, and imperforate hymen.
- X-ray of the hand is used for estimating "bone age." When the long-bone epiphyses (growth plates) are fused, skeletal growth is finished. Refer to pediatric endocrinologist if no growth spurt, delayed puberty, others.

GYNECOMASTIA

Excessive growth of breast tissue in males. Can involve one or both breasts. Physiologic gynecomastia is benign and is more common during infancy and adolescence. Normal in up to 40% of pubertal boys (peaks at age 14 years). Most cases resolve spontaneously within 6 months to 2 years.

Classic Case

Adolescent male is brought in by a parent who is concerned about gradual onset of enlarged breasts or asymmetrical breast tissue (one may be larger). Child is embarrassed and scared about breast changes. Affected breast may be tender to palpation.

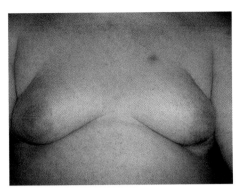

Figure 23.2 Gynecomastia.

Objective Findings

Round, rubbery, and mobile mound (disklike) under the areola of both breasts (Figure 23.2). Skin has no dimpling, redness, or changes. If mass is irregular, fixed, or hard, or if rapid growth in breast size or if secondary cause suspected, refer to specialist.

Treatment Plan

- Evaluate for Tanner stage (check testicular size, pubic hair, axillary hair, body odor).
- Check for drug use of both illicit and prescription (e.g., steroids, cimetidine, antipsychotics).
- Rule out serious etiology (e.g., testicular or adrenal tumors, brain tumor, hypogonadism).
- Recheck patient in 6 months to monitor for changes.

KLINEFELTER SYNDROME

A condition in which males are born with an extra X chromosome (i.e., 47, XXY). Condition occurs approximately one in 1,000 live births. It is one of the causes of primary hypogonadism (deficiency in testosterone). Testicles are small and firm with small penis. Tall stature, wider hips, reduced facial and body hair, and higher risk of osteoporosis (compared with normal males). Treatment includes testosterone replacement and fertility treatment.

OSGOOD–SCHLATTER DISEASE

A common cause of knee pain in young athletes. Caused by overuse of the knee. Repetitive stress on the patellar tendon by the quadriceps, rapid growth of the bones, and lack of flexibility of the soft issues and muscle causes pain, tenderness, and swelling at the tendon's insertion site (the tibial tuberosity). Usually affects one knee but can be bilateral. Most common during rapid growth spurts in teenage males who are physically active and/or play sports that stress the patellar tendon (e.g., basketball, soccer, running). Condition abates when growth stops.

Classic Case

A 14-year-old male athlete undergoing a rapid growth spurt complains of a tender bony mass over the anterior tubercle of one knee. The pain is worsened by some activities (squatting, kneeling, jumping, climbing up stairs). The knee pain improves with rest and avoidance of aggravating activity. Reports the presence of bony mass on the anterior tibial tubercle that is slightly tender. Almost all cases resolve spontaneously within a few weeks to months. Rule out avulsion fracture (tibial tubercle) if acute onset of pain post trauma (order lateral x-ray of knee).

Treatment Plan

Follow RICE: Rest affected knee. Use ice pack three times/day for 10 to 15 minutes. Avoiding aggravating activities or sports will typically reduce or resolve pain. Adolescent may continue to play based on degree of pain after sports participation. Play does not necessarily worsen the condition. Use acetaminophen (Tylenol) or NSAIDs for pain as needed. Quadriceps strengthening and quadriceps/hamstring stretching exercises aimed at stabilizing the knee joint may also be beneficial.

EXAM TIPS

- For Klinefelter syndrome, understand how patient looks.
- Know the Osgood–Schlatter presentation.

PRIMARY AND SECONDARY AMENORRHEA

- Primary amenorrhea: No menarche by the age of 15 years in the presence of normal growth and secondary sex characteristics. Nearly half of cases are caused by chromosomal disorders (43%) such as Turner syndrome.
- Secondary amenorrhea: No menses for more than three cycles or 6 months, if previously had menses. Most common cause is pregnancy. Other causes are ovarian disorders, stress, anorexia, and polycystic ovary syndrome (PCOS).

Secondary Amenorrhea Associated With Exercise and Underweight

- Excessive exercise and/or sports participation has a higher incidence of amenorrhea (and infertility) because of a relative caloric deficiency.
- "Female athlete triad" is anorexia nervosa/restrictive eating, amenorrhea, and osteoporosis.

Labs

- Pregnancy test (serum human chorionic gonadotropin [HCG])
- Serum prolactin level (rule out prolactinoma-induced amenorrhea)
- Serum TSH (rule out thyroid disease); also FSH and LH (rule out premature ovarian failure)
- If amenorrhea for more than 6 months, measure bone density

Treatment Plan

- Educate about increasing caloric intake and decreasing exercise
- Prescribe calcium with vitamin D 1,200 to 1,500 mg daily and vitamin E 400 IU daily

Complications

- Osteopenia/osteoporosis (stress fractures)
- Myocardial atrophy, arrhythmia (sudden death), brady-cardia, hypotension
- Hypoglycemia, dehydration, electrolytes
- Lanugo (fine, downy hair), telogen effluvium (hair loss), xerosis (dry skin), infertility
- Low BMI, cachexia, anemia, respiratory failure

PSEUDOGYNECOMASTIA

Bilateral enlarged breast is due to fatty tissue (adipose tissue). Common in obese boys and men. Both breasts feel soft to touch and are not tender. No breast bud or disklike breast tissue is palpable.

Labs

None. Diagnosed by clinical presentation.

TURNER'S SYNDROME

Females with complete or partial absence of the second sex chromosome (45, X). Occurs in approximately one in 2,500 live-born females. Congenital lymphedema of hands and feet, webbed neck (Figure 23.3), high-arched palate, and short fourth metacarpal. Short stature (height usually below 50th percentile). Ovarian failure, cardiovascular and renal issues, ear malformations, and other health problems, as well as amenorrhea due to premature ovarian failure (infertility).

EXAM TIP

Understand the difference between gynecomastia and pseudogynecomastia.

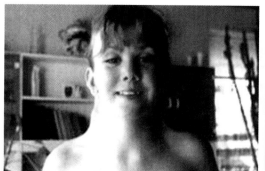
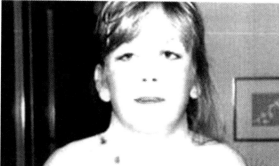

Figure 23.3 Turner's syndrome (before and after surgery to correct neck webbing).
Source: Courtesy of Johannes Nielsen.

KNOWLEDGE CHECK: CHAPTER 23

1. A 16-year-old patient is being seen in the clinic for a health issue. What care can the nurse practitioner provide without first obtaining parental consent?
   A. Rapid throat culture to rule out strep
   B. Varicella vaccine
   C. Intramuscular antibiotics for urinary tract infection
   D. Urine testing for sexually transmitted infections (STIs)

2. Which of the following Tanner stages is associated with penile lengthening?
   A. II
   B. III
   C. IV
   D. V

3. A 14-year-old male patient, who is active in basketball, complains of pain and swelling on both knees. On physical exam, there is tenderness over the tibial tuberosity of both knees. Which of the following is *most* likely?
   A. Chondromalacia patella
   B. Left knee sprain
   C. Osgood-Schlatter disease
   D. Tear of the medial ligament

4. A 14-year-old female patient is worried that she has not started to menstruate. During physical examination, the nurse practitioner tells the patient's parent, who is in the room with the patient, that the patient is starting Tanner stage II. What are the physical exam findings during this stage?
   A. Breast buds and some straight pubic hair
   B. Fully developed breasts and curly pubic hair
   C. Breast tissue with the areola on a separate mound and curly pubic hair
   D. No breast tissue and no pubic hair

5. Which minor is legally recognized as an adult when seeking care?
   A. Unmarried 16-year-old seeking contraception
   B. 15-year-old who thinks they may be pregnant
   C. 17-year-old who is enlisted in the U.S. Army and reports abdominal pain
   D. 14-year-old being treated for a sexually transmitted infection

6. Which of the following is the *most common* cause for secondary amenorrhea?
   A. Polycystic ovaries
   B. Pregnancy
   C. Anorexia nervosa
   D. Physiologic delay of puberty

7. A 14-year-old female patient is seen in the ED with nausea and vomiting and right upper quadrant pain for 2 days. The family reveals that they found an empty Tylenol bottle in the patient's room 2 days ago and that she has been more depressed in the last couple of weeks. If this was intentional ingestion of Tylenol, which of the following would the nurse practitioner expect to see on the labs?
   A. Elevated liver function
   B. Decreased renal function
   C. Elevated glucose level
   D. Decreased bilirubin concentration

8. A 16-year-old male patient presents to the urgent care clinic with acute onset of testicular pain. Which of the following characteristics would be most consistent with testicular torsion?
   A. Loss of cremasteric reflex
   B. Blue dot sign
   C. Palpable scrotal mass
   D. Enlarging testicle

9. Which of the following best describes Klinefelter syndrome?
   A. It is the complete or partial absence of a second sex chromosome.
   B. It is associated with short stature.
   C. It is commonly associated with tibial tuberosity tenderness.
   D. It causes primary hypogonadism.

10. A 15-year-old female patient reports not having started her period. The patient has minimal to no breast development. Her mother started her period when she was 12 years old. The patient has a negative pregnancy test. Which of the following is the next step in her management?
    A. Order a bone age
    B. Order CT of the sella turcica
    C. Draw FSH, LH, and TSH levels
    D. Reassure the patient that she will likely start her period soon

(See answers next page.)

1. D) Urine testing for sexually transmitted infections (STIs)

Minors do not need parental consent for any testing or treatment for STIs, contraception, or diagnosis and management of pregnancy. Performing other testing and giving in-office treatments or vaccines does require a parent (or guardian) to consent to the actions.

2. B) III

In Tanner stage III in males, the penis begins to lengthen. Tanner stages are as follows: I, prepubertal small penis; II, penis length remains unchanged; III, penis begins to lengthen; IV, penis increases in circumference; and V, scrotum and penis are mature size.

3. C) Osgood-Schlatter disease

Osgood-Schlatter disease is characterized by bilateral pain over the tibial tuberosity upon palpation, along with knee pain and edema with exercise.

4. A) Breast buds and some straight pubic hair

Tanner stage II in females is noted for breast and papilla elevated as a small mound and increased areola diameter (breast buds). Tanner II pubic hair for females is sparse, straight hair along the medial border of the labia.

5. C) 17-year-old who is enlisted in the U.S. Army and reports abdominal pain

There are three primary ways for a minor to become emancipated: marriage, court order, and military service. Although minors do not require parental consent to receive contraception, treatment of sexually transmitted infection, or care related to pregnancy, only emancipation allows them to be legally recognized as adults and, therefore, give full consent for any type of treatment.

6. B) Pregnancy

Secondary amenorrhea is defined as no menses for more than three cycles or 6 months in a female patient who already has a menstrual cycle. The *most common* cause is pregnancy. Other less common causes are ovarian disorders, stress, anorexia, and polycystic ovary syndrome. Delayed puberty and menarche are considered primary amenorrhea.

7. A) Elevated liver function

In the initial stage of acute acetaminophen poisoning, patients may be asymptomatic for up to the first 24 hours. In the second stage (hours 18 to 72), patients will typically present with elevated liver function test results, bilirubin, and prothrombin time, and possibly with elevated renal function. Hypoglycemia may be present in the third stage (hours 72 to 96).

8. A) Loss of cremasteric reflex

Testicular torsion is associated with scrotal edema; redness; a high-riding, transverse-lie testicle that is painful; and loss of ipsilateral cremasteric reflex. The blue dot sign is associated with torsion of the appendix testis, while a palpable scrotal mass is more likely to be testicular cancer. An enlarging testicle is a normal Tanner II developmental stage.

9. D) It causes primary hypogonadism.

Klinefelter syndrome is a condition in which males are born with 47XXY. This genetic addition causes primary hypogonadism or a deficiency in testosterone, which then leads to delayed pubertal maturation. Turner syndrome, identified by complete or partial absence of the second sex chromosome 45XO in females, is associated with short stature, webbed neck, a high-arched palate, and primary ovarian failure. Osgood-Schlatter disease is due to repetitive stress on the patellar tendon at the tibial tuberosity, which becomes tender due to the swelling and microtears.

10. C) Draw FSH, LH, and TSH levels

For primary amenorrhea, the first step (after confirming that the patient is not pregnant) is to rule out hypogonadism by evaluating FSH, LH, and TSH. A bone age may be helpful to determine if the patient is a "late bloomer" or has familial constitutional delay (i.e., has skeletal maturity younger than her chronological age). A CT of the sella turcica is only done when/if prolactin levels are elevated. Given that the patient has no signs of puberty, reassurance is not appropriate at this time.

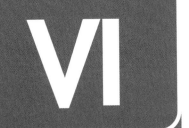

GERONTOLOGY REVIEW

PHYSIOLOGIC CHANGES

Aging affects physiologic rhythms, causing disturbances of body temperature, plasma cortisol (and secretion of other hormones), and sleep patterns. Decreased heart rate, blood pressure (BP) variability, and diminished sensory perception and response to stress occur, along with increased vulnerability to disease due to difficulty maintaining homeostasis. Physiologic reserves are maximized, leading to frailty.

INTEGUMENTARY SYSTEM

With aging, the skin atrophies; the epidermis and dermis thin; and there is less subdermal fat and collagen (less elasticity, causing skin wrinkling). Skin is fragile, more likely to shear from stress, and slower to heal. Oil production is lower and skin is drier (xerosis) due to decreased sebaceous and sweat gland activity. There is a decrease in sensitivity to touch, vibration, and temperature as well as a reduction in vitamin D synthesis. Fewer melanocytes lead to graying of hair.

Seborrheic Keratoses

Soft, wartlike skin lesions that appear "pasted on" (Figure 24.1). Mostly seen on the back and trunk. Benign.

Senile Purpura

Seen in patients older than 65 years. Nonpalpable, purple-colored patches with well-demarcated edges (Figure 24.2). Located on the extensor surfaces of the forearms and hands after a minor trauma. Lesions eventually resolve over several weeks, but residual brown appearance can occur when hemosiderin deposits in the tissue. Benign.

Lentigines

Also known as "liver spots." Tan- to brown-colored macules with a "moth-eaten" border on the dorsum of the hands and forearms caused by sun damage. More common in light-skinned individuals. Benign.

Stasis Dermatitis

Stasis dermatitis, or stasis eczema, affects the lower extremities secondary to impaired venous circulation (from peripheral vascular disease [PVD]). Can appear dry and scaly, ulcerated, neovascularized. Acutely, can appear inflamed with weeping plaques, vesiculation, and crusting. Chronically, often appear hyperpigmented (from hemosiderin deposition).

Actinic Keratosis (Solar Keratosis)

Flat or thickened plaque with color varying from skin-colored to red, white, or yellow (Figure 24.3). May appear scaly or have a horny surface and is found on sun-damaged

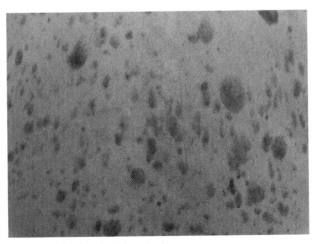

Figure 24.1 Seborrheic keratosis.
Source: James Heilman, MD.

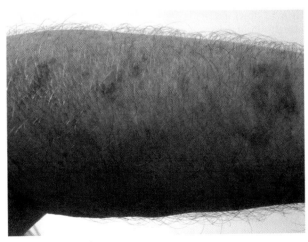

Figure 24.2 Senile purpura.
Source: José Reynaldo da Fonseca.

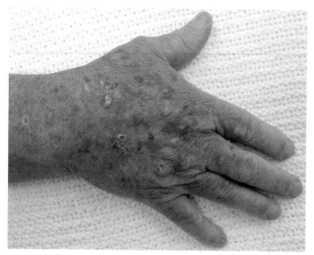

Figure 24.3 Actinic keratosis (solar keratosis).
Source: James Heilman, MD.

skin. Condition is secondary to sun exposure and has the potential for malignancy. It is a precancerous form of squamous cell carcinoma.

Nails

Growth slows and nails become brittle, yellow, and thicker. Longitudinal ridges develop.

EYES

Eye structure changes, causing visual disturbances and slower adaptation to light. Presbyopia is caused by loss of elasticity of the lenses, which makes it difficult to accommodate or focus on close objects. Close vision is markedly affected. Onset is during early to mid-40s. Can be remedied with reading glasses or bifocal lenses. Cornea is less sensitive to touch. Watering eyes are more common. Arcus senilis, cataracts, glaucoma, and macular degeneration are more common.

Arcus Senilis (Corneal Arcus)

Opaque grayish-to-white ring with a sharp outer border and an indistinct central border at the periphery of the cornea. Typically bilateral; unilateral finding associated with contralateral carotid artery disease. Develops gradually and is not associated with visual changes. Caused by deposition of lipids. Incidence increases with age; some evidence that prevalence is nearly 100% by age 80 years. In patients younger than 40 years, can be a sign of cardiovascular disease. Check fasting lipid profile.

Cataracts

Cloudiness and opacity of the lens. Significant cause of blindness. Common in patients older than 60 years. There are three types (nuclear sclerosis, cortical spoking, and posterior capsular haze). Color of the lens is white to gray. Cataracts cause gradual onset of decreased night vision, blurred or distorted vision, sensitivity to glare of car lights (driving at night), halos around lights, and double vision. In mature cataract, the red reflex disappears.

Tests are red reflex (reflection is opaque gray vs. orange-red glow), comprehensive eye exam, and dilated fundus exam to rule out other pathology.

Glaucoma

Normally, the anterior chamber of the eye is modestly pressurized, helping to maintain the eye's shape. Aging is associated with the loss of cells that help with efficient drainage of the anterior chamber. This loss causes increased anterior chamber pressure secondary to a bottleneck at the drainage canal, resulting in angle-closure glaucoma, a medical emergency that must be treated to prevent permanent blindness. Symptoms include decreased vision, halos around lights, headache, severe eye pain, and nausea and vomiting.

Open-angle glaucoma causes progressive peripheral visual field loss followed by central field loss. Patients rarely experience symptoms as long as central vision is preserved.

Tests are dilated fundus examination, visual field testing, measurement of intraocular pressure via tonometry, and gonioscopy for diagnosing angle-closure glaucoma.

Macular Degeneration

Deterioration of the macula, the central portion of the retina. Loss of central visual fields results in loss of visual acuity (wavy or blurred vision). Leading cause of irreversible vision loss in adults older than 60 years. May find drusen bodies. Two types are dry (most common) and wet (can progress more quickly and cause severe vision loss or blindness).

Tests are dilated fundus examination, fluorescein angiography, optical coherence tomography, and Amsler grid to evaluate central-vision changes.

EARS
Presbycusis (Sensorineural Hearing Loss)

Difficulties with high-frequency hearing and impaired speech recognition in noisy environments. Increased risk of cerumen impaction. There are degenerative changes of the ossicles, fewer auditory neurons, and atrophy of the hair cells, resulting in sensorineural hearing loss.

CARDIOVASCULAR SYSTEM

Increased risk for coronary artery disease and hypertension. Left ventricle stiffens and hypertrophies with aging. The mitral and aortic valves may contain calcium deposits. Aorta increases in diameter and stiffness, increasing the load on the heart. Ventricular cardiomyocytes hypertrophy. Greater increase in pulmonary capillary wedge pressure. Thickened intimal layer of arteries and arteriosclerosis result in increased systolic BP because of increased vascular resistance (isolated systolic hypertension).

Baroreceptors are less sensitive to changes in position. There is decreased sensitivity of the autonomic nervous system. BP response is blunted. Intrinsic heart rate decreases by five to six beats per minute each decade. Maximum heart rate decreases. There is higher risk of orthostatic hypotension. S4 heart sound is a normal finding in a patient older than 75 years if not associated with heart disease. The left ventricle hypertrophies with aging (up to 10% increase in thickness).

RESPIRATORY SYSTEM

Total lung capacity remains relatively the same with aging. Forced vital capacity (FVC) and forced expiratory volume in 1 second (FEV1) decrease with age. Residual volume (air left in the lungs at the end of expiration) increases with age because of decrease in lung and chest wall compliance. The chest wall becomes stiffer, and the diaphragm is flatter and less efficient. Full airway expansion occurs only in the standing position.

Mucociliary clearance (fewer cilia) and coughing are less efficient. The smaller airways collapse sooner during expiration. Responses to hypoxia and hypercapnia decrease. Decreased breath sounds and crackles are commonly found in the lung bases of older adult patients without presence of disease. Cough is weaker due to diminished respiratory muscle strength causing impaired clearance from the airways.

RENAL SYSTEM

Renal size and mass decrease by 25% to 30%. The steepest decline in renal mass occurs after age 50 years. Reduction in functional glomeruli is almost 50%. Renal clearance of drugs, concentrating and diluting ability, and response to sodium are less effective. Creatinine clearance decreases with age. The serum creatinine is a less reliable indicator of renal function in the older adults because of the decrease in muscle mass, creatine production, and creatinine clearance. Serum creatinine can be in the normal range, even if renal function is markedly reduced. Risk of kidney damage from insults and nephrotoxic agents such as nonsteroidal anti-inflammatory drugs (NSAIDs) is much higher. Renin and angiotensin II levels are lower in older adults. Fluid and electrolyte balance is relatively maintained, but ability is impaired to retain water, solute, amino acids, and glucose. Hormonal function is affected.

GENITOURINARY SYSTEM
Bladder

The capacity of the bladder decreases with age. Both the compliance of the bladder and the rate of urine flow decrease. These factors contribute to the increased amount of urine that remains in the bladder after urination (residual urine). Prevalence of urinary incontinence increases with age.

Male Reproductive System

Prostatic hypertrophy occurs with age. Gradual decline in male reproductive ability includes greater stimulation needed for an erection, fewer spontaneous erections, and prolonged refractory times between erections. Sperm production decreases. Sperm have an increased frequency of chromosomal abnormalities, impaired motility, and decreased ability to fertilize.

Female Reproductive System

Estrogen and progesterone production decreases significantly. Decline in oocyte numbers and menopause occurs after an average age of 51 years. In postmenopausal women, the urethra becomes thinner and shortens, and the ability of the urinary sphincter to close tightly decreases (because of declining estrogen). Urinary incontinence is two or three times more common in women. The vagina loses elasticity, and dryness and atrophy are common. Vaginal pH often rises, increasing susceptibility to colonization of microflora. Greater stimulation is needed for arousal.

MUSCULOSKELETAL SYSTEM

Muscle mass, strength, and power decrease with age and can contribute to morbidity in older adults. Decline in bone mass is about 0.5% per year in healthy older adults, increasing risk of fractures and osteoporosis. Fracture rate of repair is slowed. Deterioration of articular cartilage is common after age 40 years. Stiffness in the morning that improves with activity is a common symptom of osteoarthritis (degenerative joint disease). Age-related imbalance of bone resorption and bone deposition occurs. Fractures heal more slowly because of decrease in the number of osteoblasts.

As humans age, height declines because of loss of vertebral cartilage and bone; by age 70 years, height has decreased from its peak by 2.5% to 5%; this loss becomes more rapid after age 70 years. Compression fractures of vertebrae are a sign of osteoporosis (kyphosis) and contribute to loss of height. Skeletal muscle loss begins at 50 years and continues because of loss of muscle fiber numbers and size.

GASTROINTESTINAL SYSTEM

Receding gums and dry mouth are common. Decreased sensitivity of the taste buds results in decrease in appetite. Aspiration risk increases because of loss of esophageal muscle compliance, altered food bolus transfer to the pharynx, and decreased strength and coordination of the tongue. Delayed gastric emptying occurs. Higher risk of gastritis and gastrointestinal damage from decreased production of prostaglandins. Decreased efficiency in absorbing some vitamins (e.g., folic acid, vitamin B_{12}) and minerals (e.g., calcium) by the small intestines.

Increased risk of colon cancer between ages 40 and 50 years. Diverticula are common. Large bowel (colon) transit time is slower. Constipation is more common. Laxative abuse is more common. Fecal incontinence may occur because of loss of muscle mass and weakness of external anal sphincter, drug side effects, underlying disease, neurogenic disorders, or a combination of these factors.

Liver

Liver size and mass decrease due to atrophy (20%–40%). Liver blood flow and perfusion decrease (up to 50% in some older adults). Fat (lipofuscin) deposition in the liver is more common. Liver function tests (alanine aminotransferase [ALT], aspartate aminotransferase [AST], alkaline phosphatase) are generally not affected by age, while serum albumin declines slightly with normal aging. Metabolic clearance of drugs is slowed by 20% to 40% because the cytochrome P450 (CYP450) enzyme system is less efficient. Higher serum low-density lipoprotein (LDL) levels are seen, partly due to reduction in LDL receptors.

ENDOCRINE SYSTEM

Minor atrophy of the pancreas occurs. Increased levels of insulin are seen along with mild peripheral insulin resistance. Changes or disorders of circadian rhythm hormonal secretion (growth hormone, melatonin, and other hormones) can cause changes in sleep patterns.

IMMUNE SYSTEM

The immune system is less active, increasing the risk of infection, malignancy, and autoimmune disorders. Older adults are less likely to present with symptoms such as fever during infections. Nonspecific signs of infection include falls, delirium, anorexia, and generalized weakness. Typical body temperature is slightly lower. There is a decreased antibody response to vaccines and a decreased ability to mount inflammatory cytokine responses to infection.

Adaptive immunity is affected more by aging than innate immunity. Adaptive immunity consists of cellular and humoral immune responses. Cellular immunity is affected by a decline in T cell number and reduced T cell expansion, differentiation, and signaling intensity. Humoral immunity is affected by a decrease in B cell precursors in the bone marrow and peripheral B cells. T and B cells are less responsive to stimulation with antigens.

HEMATOLOGIC SYSTEM

There are no changes in red blood cell life span, blood volume, or total number of circulating leukocytes. Bone marrow mass decreases while fat in the bone marrow increases. Hematopoietic functional reserves are decreased. Compensatory response to insults (e.g., phlebotomy, hypoxia) is delayed and weakened. There is a higher risk of thrombi and emboli because of increased platelet responsiveness causing a decrease in bleeding time with age.

NEUROLOGIC SYSTEM

Hallmark of aging is slowed reaction times, decreased proprioception, and increased risk of falls. Cognitive function remains stable if no underlying disease, but ability to solve problems is affected by reaction times. Executive function declines with age, most dramatically in those older than 70 years. Attention span decreases. Cranial nerve testing may show differences in ability to differentiate sensation and motor responses. Deep tendon reflexes may be brisk or absent. Neurologic responses may be impaired by medications, causing slower reaction times.

PHARMACOLOGIC ISSUES

Drug clearance is affected by renal impairment, less efficient liver CYP450 enzyme system, slow gastric emptying, increased gastric pH, decreased serum albumin, and relatively higher ratio of fat to muscle tissue (extends fat-soluble drugs). Older adults have an increased sensitivity to benzodiazepines and anticholinergic drugs such as hypnotics, tricyclic antidepressants, antihistamines, and antipsychotics. Polypharmacy is more common because older adults may have more disease conditions for which therapies are prescribed. This increases the risk of an adverse drug event and decreases physical and cognitive capability. The American Geriatrics Society has made a list of potentially inappropriate medication use in older adults, known as the Beers Criteria® (see Chapter 25).

EXAM TIPS

- Adaptive immunity is affected more by age than innate immunity.
- Anticholinergic drugs cause constipation, urinary retention (especially men with benign prostatic hyperplasia), blurred vision, dry mouth, and orthostatic hypotension.

KNOWLEDGE CHECK: CHAPTER 24

1. Which of the following is a physiologic change that occurs in the aging body?
   A. Increased intrinsic heart rate
   B. Hypertrophied left ventricle
   C. Decreased platelet responsiveness
   D. Increased muscle mass

2. An older patient has been taking digoxin (Lanoxin), metformin (Glucophage), atenolol (Tenormin), and aspirin for several months. During an office visit, the patient reports dark areas in the central vision fields. The patient's digoxin level is 1.3 ng/mL. Which of the following is the most likely cause?
   A. Acute angle-closure glaucoma
   B. Cataracts
   C. Retinal detachment
   D. Age-related macular degeneration

3. Which of the following physiological changes is present in the lungs of older adults?
   A. Increased FEV1
   B. Decreased residual volume (RV)
   C. Increased lung compliance
   D. Earlier airway collapse with shallow breathing

4. Upon examination, the nurse practitioner notes small, verrucous skin lesions on the back of an older patient. These skin lesions have a "stuck-on" appearance. Which of the following is the most likely cause?
   A. Seborrheic keratosis
   B. Senile purpura
   C. Lentigines
   D. Actinic keratosis

5. Which of the following cutaneous lesions can progress to squamous cell carcinoma?
   A. Seborrheic keratosis
   B. Actinic keratosis
   C. Stasis dermatitis
   D. Lentigines

6. An 80-year-old patient presents with a gray-white ring around their corneas seen bilaterally in both eyes. Based on this clinical finding, which of the following is true?
   A. Because the patient is older than 50 years, further work-up is recommended.
   B. This finding may be indicative of advanced carotid vascular disease.
   C. The nurse practitioner should check a fasting lipid profile stat.
   D. This is a clinically insignificant finding with an incidence that increases with age.

7. A patient presents with bilateral, painless progression of blurred vision. The patient complains of difficulty driving at night, especially due to the glare of oncoming headlights. The patient reports more difficulty with distance vision and better near vision. Nondilated fundus examination reveals lens opacity. These findings are suggestive of which of the following conditions?
   A. Cataract
   B. Arcus senilis
   C. Open-angle glaucoma
   D. Macular degeneration

8. Which of the following age-related changes increases an older adult's risk for aspiration?
   A. Gum recession exposing the tooth cementum
   B. Decreased lower esophageal sphincter tone
   C. Decreased food clearance from the pharynx
   D. Delayed gastric emptying

9. A patient presents with decreased vision, halos around lights, a severe headache, and eye pain. Physical assessment reveals conjunctival redness and corneal edema. Emergent ophthalmologic examination is necessary. Based on this clinical presentation, which of the following tests is the *gold standard* for diagnosis?
   A. Dilated fundus examination
   B. Gonioscopy
   C. Visual field testing
   D. Slit-lamp examination

(See answers next page.)

1. B) Hypertrophied left ventricle

Physiologic changes that occur with aging include an increased prevalence of hypertrophy of the left ventricle, with an average increase in wall thickness of about 10%. Increased platelet responsiveness (resulting in a procoagulant state) and decreased intrinsic heart rate and muscle mass are other physiologic changes that occur in the older adult.

2. D) Age-related macular degeneration

The patient is experiencing symptoms of macular degeneration (changes in central vision), which can be attributed to atenolol (Tenormin) use. The patient's digoxin level is within normal range (0.7 to 1.5 ng/mL). Additionally, the patient's vision changes are not typical of digoxin toxicity, which includes yellowish-green halos. Metformin (Glucophage) and aspirin do not cause macular degeneration.

3. D) Earlier airway collapse with shallow breathing

In older adults, airways tend to collapse earlier with shallow breathing than in younger patients, which increases the risk of pneumonia. Lung compliance decreases with older age; therefore, FEV1 also decreases and residual volume increases.

4. A) Seborrheic keratosis

The skin lesions are descriptive of seborrheic keratoses, which are soft, wart-like (verrucous), benign lesions that frequently appear on the back and trunk of older adults. Actinic keratosis is considered the most common precancerous lesion of squamous cell carcinoma in older adults. Actinic keratoses appear as rough, scaly patches on parts of the body exposed over years to the sun. Senile purpura are bright, purple-colored patches located on the forearms and hands and are benign. Lentigines, also known as "liver spots," are brown-colored macules located on the hands and forearms of older adults and are benign.

5. B) Actinic keratosis

Actinic keratoses are common cutaneous lesions that usually present as scaly, erythematous macules or papules on sites of chronic sun exposure. While the risk is low, they may progress to squamous cell carcinoma. Approximately 10% of actinic keratoses progress to cutaneous squamous cell carcinoma.

6. D) This is a clinically insignificant finding with an incidence that increases with age.

This patient is presenting with clinical features suggestive of arcus senilis, which is characterized by a white or gray ring around the cornea. The incidence increases with age, with a prevalence of nearly 100% in individuals older than 80 years. Arcus senilis is usually clinically insignificant and is often a benign finding in older adults. However, in individuals younger than 50 years (especially men), the condition is associated with a greater incidence of underlying atherosclerotic disease requiring further workup and a lipid analysis. This is not necessary for individuals older than 50 years. The presence of arcus senilis seen unliterally is suggestive of advanced carotid vascular disease.

7. A) Cataract

These clinical findings are suggestive of a cataract, which is opacity of the lens of the eye that may cause blurred or distorted vision, glare problems, and blindness. Arcus senilis is characterized by a white or gray ring around the cornea. Macular degeneration causes central vision loss. Open-angle glaucoma is characterized by progressive peripheral visual field loss followed by central field loss.

8. C) Decreased food clearance from the pharynx

In healthy older adults, the strength and coordination of the tongue is impaired, causing less effective mastication. In addition, the transfer of a food bolus to the pharynx is altered, which leads to increased aspiration risk in older adults. The gums recede, exposing the tooth cementum, which puts the older adult patient at risk for decay and root caries. Diminished esophageal contractions and decreased lower esophageal sphincter tone result in increased gastric acid exposure. Delayed gastric emptying may contribute to increased rates of gastritis.

9. B) Gonioscopy

The patient is presenting with signs and symptoms of acute primary angle-closure glaucoma. The clinical presentation often includes decreased vision, halos around lights, headache, severe eye pain, nausea, and vomiting. Clinical signs that suggest a rapid increase in intraocular pressure include conjunctival redness, corneal edema or cloudiness, a shallow anterior chamber, and a mid-dilated pupil (4 to 6 mm) that reacts poorly to light. Diagnosis begins with emergent examination of both eyes by an ophthalmologist, including the following tests: gonioscopy, visual acuity, evaluation of the pupils, measurement of intraocular pressure, slit-lamp examination of the anterior segments, visual field testing, and undilated fundus examination. Gonioscopy is the gold standard in the diagnosis of angle-closure glaucoma.

10. Which of the following is an example of an expected age-related neurological change?
    A. Inability to recall the United States capital
    B. Loss of memory of how to tie one's shoes
    C. Inability to recognize own daughter and son
    D. Difficulty reciting the alphabet while walking around the room

11. Prevention of adverse drug events in the older adult is facilitated by:
    A. Increase in body fat relative to skeletal muscle
    B. Frequent medication reconciliation
    C. Decreased creatinine clearance
    D. Use of herbal supplements

12. An older adult patient reports difficulty hearing a question asked by the clinician. How should the nurse practitioner respond?
    A. Face the patient directly and state the question in a different way
    B. Re-state the question in a louder voice
    C. Exaggerate mouth movements while repeating the question
    D. Ask the question to the patient's family member

13. A patient presents for a routine annual exam. The patient complains of back pain and height loss. A chest x-ray indicates an incidental finding of a vertebral fracture. The patient reports a recent fall from standing height. This fracture is likely the results of:
    A. Osteoarthritis
    B. Rheumatoid arthritis
    C. Osteoporosis
    D. Osteomalacia

14. Applanation tonometry is a diagnostic test used in the evaluation of a patient with open-angle glaucoma in order to:
    A. Examine the fundus
    B. Measure corneal thickness
    C. Test the patient's visual field
    D. Measure intraocular pressure

15. Which statement from a patient about sexuality in the older adult requires further education?
    A. "Erectile dysfunction is common with older age."
    B. "It may take longer to become sexually aroused."
    C. "Older adults are no longer interested in sexuality."
    D. "Condoms should still be used after menopause."

(See answers next page.)

10. D) Difficulty reciting the alphabet while walking around the room

While there are cognitive and behavioral changes associated with normal aging, certain memory performances, like procedural memory (memory of performing different actions or skills such as riding a bike or tying one's shoes) and semantic memory (memory of objects, general facts, and concepts) are well preserved. The ability to recognize familiar objects and faces remains stable over the lifetime. Attention span decreases with simple attentive tasks as a result of aging; there is a decreased ability to focus on a task in a busy environment or perform multiple tasks at one time.

11. B) Frequent medication reconciliation

Caution should be made when prescribing for older adults; their increase in body fat relative to skeletal muscle causes an increased volume of distribution of the drug. The natural decline of renal and hepatic function causes decreased drug clearance and metabolism. The combination of larger drug storage reservoirs and decreased clearance prolongs drug half-lives, which leads to increased plasma drug concentrations. Doses should be properly adjusted for renal insufficiency, which is more common with advancing age. Herbal and dietary supplements may interact with prescribed drug therapies and lead to adverse drug events. It is important to continually review the patient's medication regimen and make changes based on the current clinical status, goals of care, and risks/benefits of each medication.

12. A) Face the patient directly and state the question in a different way

Age-related auditory changes affect high-frequency hearing acuity and impair speech recognition in noisy environments. Older patients cannot decipher many consonant sounds because they are higher in frequency (e.g., t, k, ch). It is often better to rephrase a question rather than to repeat the question in a louder voice, because the pitch frequency is often higher when volume is increased. Older patients often have difficulty distinguishing sounds from background noise, so extraneous noise should be minimized as much as possible during conversation. The nurse practitioner should speak clearly, slowly, distinctly, and naturally without shouting or exaggerating mouth movements. It is important to include the patient in medical decision making, so deferring to a family member is inappropriate.

13. C) Osteoporosis

Osteoporosis is characterized by low bone mass, skeletal fragility, and microarchitectural deterioration that results in decreased bone strength as well as increased risk of fracture. There are no clinical manifestations until there is a fracture, which is most commonly a vertebral fracture. Osteoporosis is often diagnosed as an incidental finding on chest or abdominal radiograph. Symptoms include height loss. Fragility fractures support the clinical diagnosis of osteoporosis; they often occur spontaneously or from minor trauma, such as a fall from standing height. Osteomalacia is characterized by defective mineralization of newly formed osteoid at sites of bone turnover, often caused by severe vitamin D deficiency, lack of sun exposure, or malabsorption. Osteoarthritis causes joint pain, stiffness, and motor restriction. Osteoarthritis can be confused with rheumatoid arthritis when it involves the hand joints. However, rheumatoid arthritis is characterized as a symmetric, inflammatory, peripheral polyarthritis. Osteoarthritis is frequently associated with characteristic Heberden nodes, whereas rheumatoid arthritis targets the metacarpophalangeal and proximal interphalangeal joints.

14. D) Measure intraocular pressure

Intraocular pressure can be measured by applanation tonometry, pneumotonometry, or air-puff tonometry. During applanation tonometry, intraocular pressure is determined from the force required to flatten (applanate) a constant area of the cornea. It is the most accurate method and is subject to less artifact. An ophthalmoscope is used to examine the fundus; cupping seen in the fundus is suspicious for glaucoma. Pachymetry is the measurement of corneal thickness obtained by ultrasound or other devices. Visual field testing can be performed by automated perimetry, which can reliably detect visual field loss in patients with glaucoma.

15. C) "Older adults are no longer interested in sexuality."

Some studies have shown that adults in their 80s can remain sexually active. While greater stimulation is needed to obtain an erection, spontaneous erections occur less often, erections are less firm, and ejaculations are less forceful, sexuality is often not affected by age. Patients should be referred to a urologist for treatment of erectile dysfunction that is not responding to lifestyle changes and/or pharmacotherapy such as phosphodiesterase inhibitors (sildenafil [Viagra], tadalafil [Cialis], vardenafil [Levitra], avanafil [Stendra]). Patients should be advised to use condoms with new sexual partners to protect from sexually transmitted infections, including HIV.

ACTINIC KERATOSIS (PRECURSOR OF SQUAMOUS CELL CARCINOMA)

Small, rough, scaly, pink-to-reddish lesions that enlarge slowly over years. Located in sun-exposed areas such as the cheeks, nose, back of neck, arms, and chest. More common in light-skinned individuals. Squamous cell precancerous skin lesions. Diagnostic method of choice is biopsy. Small number of lesions can be treated with cryotherapy. Larger numbers with wider distribution are treated with 5-fluorouracil cream.

ACUTE ANGLE-CLOSURE GLAUCOMA

Older adult with acute onset of severe eye pain, headache, and nausea and vomiting. Complains of blurred vision and halos around lights. Conjunctival redness, corneal edema or cloudiness, shallow anterior chamber, and mid-dilated pupil that reacts poorly to light. Call 911. Do not delay treatment, as blindness can occur without intervention. Tonometry is done in the ED to quickly measure the intraocular pressure, which will be elevated.

CEREBROVASCULAR ACCIDENT

Cerebrovascular accident (CVA) is a sudden onset of neurologic dysfunction lasting longer than 24 hours. Also called a stroke. Deficits can include changes such as blurred vision, hemianopia (loss of vision in half of the visual field), severe headache, slurred speech, one-sided upper and/or lower extremity numbness or weakness, and confusion. Signs and symptoms are dependent on location of infarct. Two types of CVAs: ischemic and hemorrhagic (e.g., intracerebral and subarachnoid). Ischemic is more common. In comparison, a transient ischemic attack (TIA) is a temporary episode of acute cerebral insufficiency without acute infarction.

COLORECTAL CANCER

Unexplained iron-deficiency anemia, blood on rectum, hematochezia, melena, abdominal pain, and/or change in bowel habits. Asymptomatic patients discovered by routine screening or emergency presentation of intestinal obstruction, perforation, or acute GI bleed. Rectal cancer can present with tenesmus, rectal pain, and diminished-caliber (ribbonlike) stools. Prognosis depends on pathologic stage at presentation. About 20% of cases have distant metastases at time of presentation. Refer to gastroenterologist and oncologist.

ELDER ABUSE

- Screen for abuse, neglect, and financial exploitation
- Presence of bruising, skin tears, lacerations, and fractures that are poorly explained
- Presence of sexually transmitted infection, vaginal and/or rectal bleeding, bruises on breasts are indicators of possible sexual abuse
- Malnutrition, poor hygiene, and pressure injuries

Interview Elder Alone With These Three Questions
- Do you feel safe where you live?
- Who handles your bills and finances?
- Who prepares your meals?

FRACTURES OF THE HIP

Acute onset of limping, guarding, and/or inability or difficulty with bearing weight on the affected side. New onset of hip or groin pain; may be referred to the anterior thigh or knee. Unequal leg length and external rotation of affected leg. May have history of osteoporosis or osteopenia. Fractures of the hip are a major cause of morbidity and mortality in older adults. Up to 20% of older adults with hip fractures die from indirect complications (e.g., pneumonia).

GIANT CELL ARTERITIS

Temporal headache (one-sided) with tenderness or induration over temporal artery; may be accompanied by sudden visual loss in one eye (amaurosis fugax). Scalp tenderness and jaw claudication on affected side. Associated with polymyalgia rheumatica. Initial lab tests include erythrocyte sedimentation rate (ESR) and C-reactive protein (CRP), which are both usually elevated. Temporal artery biopsy is definitive diagnosis. Considered an ophthalmologic emergency (can cause blindness).

- Ribbonlike (low-caliber) stool in older adult with iron-deficiency anemia: Rule out colon cancer.
- In giant cell arteritis, ESR and CRP will both be elevated.

RETINAL DETACHMENT

New onset or sudden increase in number of floaters or specks on the visual field, flashes of light, and the sensation that a curtain is covering part of the visual field. Considered a medical emergency that can lead to blindness if not treated. Risk factors are extreme nearsightedness, history of cataract surgery, and family or personal history of retinal detachment. Treated with laser surgery or cryopexy (freezing).

SEVERE BACTERIAL INFECTIONS

Atypical presentation is common in older patients compared with younger patients. Older adults with severe infections may be afebrile. The white blood cell (WBC) count can be normal. Nonspecific signs include sudden decline in mental status (e.g., delirium, confusion), new onset of urine/bowel incontinence, falls, worsening inability to perform activities of daily living (ADLs), generalized weakness, and/or loss of appetite. Serious infections include pneumonia, pyelonephritis, bacterial endocarditis, sepsis, and others. In adults age 65 years and older, pneumonia and influenza are common causes of death. The most common infection in adults >65 years is urinary tract infection (UTI).

EXAM TIPS

- Know signs and symptoms of acute angle-closure glaucoma, hip fracture, and retinal detachment.
- Actinic keratosis is precancer of squamous cell skin cancer.

TOP THREE LEADING CAUSES OF DEATH (>65 YEARS)

1. Heart disease
2. Cancer
3. COVID-19

CANCER IN OLDER ADULTS

Aging and advancing age are the most common risk factors for cancer. Eighty percent of all cancers occur in people older than 55 years. Cancers among older adults may be caused by gene-related DNA damage, familial genetics, decrease in immunity, decreased healing rates, environment, and hormonal influences.

- Cancer with highest mortality: Lung and bronchial cancer
- Cancer with second-highest mortality: Colorectal cancer
- Median age of diagnosis: Breast cancer, 62 years; prostate cancer, 66 years; colorectal cancer, 67 years; lung cancer, 71 years

LUNG AND BRONCHUS CANCER

The cancer with the highest mortality. More people die of lung cancer each year than of colon, breast, and prostate cancers combined. Most patients with lung cancer are older adults. A very small amount of people diagnosed with lung cancer are younger than 45 years.

- Most common risk factor: Smoking (causes 80% of cases); other risk factors include exposure to radon (second-leading cause of lung cancer), secondhand smoke, and outdoor pollution, as well as occupational exposure to carcinogens.

- Most common type of lung cancer: Non–small cell lung carcinoma (82%)
- Screening: The U.S. Preventive Services Task Force (USPSTF) recommends annual screening for lung cancer in adults (ages 50–80 years) who have at least a 20-pack-year smoking history and currently smoke (or have quit within the past 15 years); screening test is low-dose CT (LDCT). Discontinue annual screening if patient stops smoking for 15 years or longer or develops a health problem that substantially limits life expectancy (or the ability or willingness for curative lung surgery).

Classic Case

An older male smoker (or ex-smoker) presents with a new onset of productive cough with large amounts of thin mucoid phlegm (bronchorrhea) and occasional blood-tinged phlegm. The patient complains of worsening shortness of breath or dyspnea. He reports unexpected weight loss and a persistent, dull, achy chest pain that does not go away.

Treatment Plan

- Order chest radiograph (e.g., nodules, lesions with irregular borders, pleural effusion).
- The next imaging exam needed is contrast-enhanced chest CT scan.
- Tissue biopsy is needed for diagnosis and staging.
- Baseline labs include complete blood count (CBC), chemistry metabolic panel, liver function panel, albumin, and lactate dehydrogenase.
- Refer patient to a pulmonologist for bronchoscopy and tumor biopsy.

COLORECTAL CANCER

The second most leading cause of cancer deaths in the United States. About 20% of cases have distant metastases at time of presentation. It is staged using the tumor-node-metastasis (TNM) staging system (stages I–IV).

- Risk factors: Advancing age (most common). Personal or family history of colorectal cancer or adenomatous polyps, certain genetic syndromes, personal history of chronic inflammatory bowel disease, and type 2 diabetes.
- Lifestyle risk factors: Lack of regular physical activity, high-fat diet, low-fiber diet, long-term smoking, low calcium intake
- Screening: Start screening at age 45 years and continue through age 75 years, with more individualized decision-making from ages 76 to 85 years. Testing includes guaiac-based fecal occult blood test (gFOBT) annually; multi-target stool DNA test every 3 years; flexible sigmoidoscopy every 5 years alone or in combination with gFOBT annually; colonoscopy every 10 years; or CT colonography every 5 years.

Classic Case

An older adult presents with tenesmus, rectal pain, and diminished-caliber (ribbonlike) stools. Patient reports hematochezia, abdominal pain, and anorexia with unintentional weight loss. Patient has unexplained iron-deficiency anemia.

Treatment Plan

- Baseline labs include CBC, chemistry metabolic panel, and urinalysis (UA).
- Check occult blood in stool (e.g., guaiac based, stool DNA).
- Serum carcinoembryonic antigen (CEA) is useful for surgical treatment planning and assessment of prognosis but has low diagnostic ability.
- Colonoscopy is most accurate diagnostic test; lesions can be localized and biopsied, neoplasms detected, and polyps removed.
- Refer to gastroenterologist for colonoscopy and management.

MULTIPLE MYELOMA

Myeloma is a cancer of the bone marrow that affects the plasma cells of the immune system (production of monoclonal immunoglobulins). The highest incidence of myeloma is in African Americans (double or triple that of other races). Multiple myeloma is a cancer found mostly in older adults. Diagnosis requires clonal bone marrow plasma cells >10% or biopsy-proven bony or soft-tissue plasmacytoma plus elevated **C**alcium levels, **R**enal insufficiency, **A**nemia, and **B**one lesions (CRAB).

Classic Case

Older adult with anemia complains of bone pain with generalized fatigue and weakness. The bone pain is located on the central skeleton (chest/back/shoulders/hips/pelvis), worsens with movement, and rarely occurs at night.

Treatment Plan

- Baseline labs include CBC, FOBT, chemistry panel, and UA.
- Serum protein electrophoresis with immunofixation and serum-free light chain assay
- Bone marrow aspiration and biopsy
- Imaging with MRI and/or PET
- Refer patient to hematologist and oncologist

PANCREATIC CANCER

The most lethal cancer in terms of prognosis, with a 5-year survival rate of 11%. More than 90% of cases arise from the exocrine portion of the pancreas. Most patients already have metastases by time of diagnosis. The most common presentation is weakness (asthenia), weight loss, anorexia, abdominal pain, epigastric pain, dark urine, jaundice, and nausea.

Treatment Plan

- Initial labs include aspartate transaminase (AST), alanine transaminase (ALT), alkaline phosphatase, bilirubin, lipase, and CA 19-9 tumor marker (used as a prognostic marker but not a diagnostic test).
- Imaging begins with transabdominal US and/or CT of the abdomen. If a mass is detected, a multiphase, contrast-enhanced helical multidetector row CT (MDCT) is needed to assess disease extent.
- Histologic confirmation is the gold standard for diagnosis.
- Refer to a gastrointestinal (GI) surgeon for Whipple procedure or other interventions.

CLINICAL PEARLS

- Patients with a personal or family history of colorectal cancer or advanced adenomatous polyps and other risk factors are considered at increased risk for colorectal cancer; screening recommendations may be changed to start at an earlier age and/or performed more frequently.
- If the chemistry profile shows marked elevations in the serum calcium and/or alkaline phosphatase, it is suggestive of cancerous metastasis of the bone.

ATYPICAL PRESENTATIONS IN OLDER ADULTS

Atypical disease presentations are more common in this age group. The immune system becomes less robust as people age, and there is increased risk of bacterial and viral infections because of changes in skin and mucosal barriers, decreased cellular and humoral immunity, and impaired cell signaling. Vaccines may not be as effective because of decreased antibody response.

Older adults are more likely to be asymptomatic or present with subtle symptoms. Older adults are less likely to have a high fever during an infection. Instead, they are more likely to suffer low-grade temperature elevations or acute cognitive dysfunction such as confusion, agitation, and delirium. Cognitive dysfunction may also result from use of multiple prescriptions to manage multiple comorbid conditions. Polypharmacy increases the chances of adverse drug reactions and drug–drug interactions.

Atypical presentations of common diseases are detailed below. For management of diseases not included in this chapter, see the other system-review chapters in this book.

DISEASE REVIEW

ACUTE ABDOMEN

Older adult patients may have more subtle symptoms such as the absence of abdominal guarding and other signs of acute abdomen. The abdominal pain may be milder. The WBC count may be only slightly elevated, or it may be normal. Patients may have low-grade fever with anorexia and weakness.

ACUTE MYOCARDIAL INFARCTION

Atypical presentations of acute coronary syndrome are common and occur more often in older adult patients, women, and those with diabetes. Patients may be asymptomatic. Symptoms may consist of dyspnea, weakness, nausea and/or vomiting, epigastric pain or discomfort, palpitations, syncope, or cardiac arrest.

BACTERIAL PNEUMONIA

Fever and chills may be absent or mild (oral temperature >100.0°F [>37.78°C] or rectal temperature >99.5°F [>37.5°C]). Mental status changes may be only present symptom. Tachycardia, tachypnea, hypoxemia, or increased work of breathing may be present. Chest auscultation may reveal crackles (rales) and rhonchi with other signs of consolidation. Patient more likely to become confused and weak with loss of appetite. The WBC count may be normal or mildly elevated. *Streptococcus pneumoniae* is the predominant organism, but polymicrobial infection and gram-negative organisms (e.g., *Haemophilus influenzae*, *Legionella pneumophila*) are becoming more common. Older adults are more vulnerable to aspiration pneumonia, so incorporate interventions to limit aspiration.

CHRONIC CONSTIPATION

There are two types of constipation: Idiopathic and functional. Constipation is the most common GI complaint. Self-treatment is common with over-the-counter (OTC) fiber and laxatives. Constipation has many secondary causes such as prescription and OTC drugs, neurologic disease (Parkinson's disease, dementia), irritable bowel syndrome (IBS), diabetes, and hypothyroidism. Lifestyle factors that contribute to constipation are immobility, low-fiber diet, dehydration, dairy intake, and ignoring the urge to have bowel movement.

Drugs that cause constipation are iron supplements, calcium channel blockers, antihistamines, anticholinergics, antispasmodics, antidepressants, antipsychotics, opiates, and calcium-containing antacids.

Classic Case

Older adult complains of years-long history of constipation. Describes stool as dry and hard, "ball-like" pieces. Reports straining often to pass stool. Accompanied by feelings of fullness and bloating. Patient takes laxatives daily (suggesting laxative abuse). Has noted hemorrhoid that is bleeding (reports bright-red blood on toilet paper and blood streaks on stool surface).

Treatment Plan

- Education and behavior modification (bowel retraining). Teach "toilet" hygiene such as going to the bathroom at the same time each day; advise not to ignore the urge to defecate.
- Dietary changes such as eating dried prunes and/or drinking prune juice. Increased intake of fruit and vegetables.
- Ingesting bulk-forming fiber (25–35 g/day) (Table 25.1) once daily. Do not take with other medication (will absorb drugs and decrease their effectiveness). Take with full glass of water (can cause intestinal obstruction).
- Increase physical activity, especially walking.
- Increase fluid intake to 8 to 10 glasses/day (if no contraindication).
- Consider laxative treatment (see Table 25.1). Avoid daily use of laxatives (except for fiber supplements) and chronic treatment with laxatives.

Table 25.1 Constipation Treatment Options

Type of Laxative	Name	Notes
Bulk-forming	Psyllium (Metamucil) Wheat dextrin (Benefiber) Methylcellulose (Citrucel) Polycarbophil (FiberCon)	Absorb water and increase fecal mass; may be used alone or in combination with increase in dietary fiber.
Stimulants (irritants)	Bisacodyl (Dulcolax), oral and suppository Senna extract (Senokot) Sodium picosulfate (e.g., Dulcolax drops)	Stimulate colon directly, causing contractions. Daily ingestion may be associated with hypokalemia, protein-losing enteropathy, and salt depletion.
Osmotics (hyperosmotic agents)	Lactulose (Enulose) Polyethylene glycol or PEG 3350 (MiraLAX) Saline laxatives: Milk of magnesia, magnesium citrate, magnesium sulfate	Act as hyperosmolar agents to increase water content of stool, making stool softer and easier to pass. Excessive use may result in electrolyte imbalance and volume overload in patients with renal and cardiac dysfunction.
Guanylate cyclase-C receptor agonist	Linaclotide (Linzess) Plecanatide (Trulance)	Stimulate intestinal fluid secretion and transit; for chronic idiopathic constipation. Contraindications include mechanical GI obstruction (known or suspected).
Chloride channel activators	Lubiprostone (Amitiza)	Enhance chloride-rich intestinal fluid secretion; role in treatment of chronic constipation still to be determined. Contraindications include mechanical GI obstruction (known or suspected).
Prostaglandin analog	Misoprostol (Cytotec)	Can be used to treat some patients with severe constipation. Avoid in patients who could become pregnant since it induces labor and can lead to loss of fetus.

(continued)

Table 25.1 Constipation Treatment Options (*continued*)

Type of Laxative	Name	Notes
Antigout agent	Colchicine (Colcrys)	May be effective for the treatment of chronic constipation. Avoid in patients with renal insufficiency. Can induce a myopathy.
5-HT(4) receptor agonists	Prucalopride (Motegrity)	Prokinetic agent used for chronic idiopathic constipation; safe and well tolerated in patients age 65 years or older. Contraindications include intestinal perforation or obstruction, obstructive ileus, severe inflammatory conditions of the GI tract.
Lubricant	Mineral oil	Can be used as an enema to help soften the stool and provide lubrication.
Surfactants	Docusate sodium (Colace)	Stool softener, which lowers surface tension of stool, allowing water to more easily enter the stool. Few side effects, but less effective than other laxatives.

GI, gastrointestinal; IBS, irritable bowel syndrome; PEG, polyethylene glycol.

Bowel Retraining Program

- Choose time of the day patient prefers for bowel movements. Usually in mornings about 20 to 40 minutes after eating breakfast.
- Spend about 10 to 15 minutes on the toilet each day at the same time. Avoid straining.

DEMENTIA AND COGNITIVE IMPAIRMENT

- The most common cause of neurodegenerative dementia in older adults is Alzheimer's disease (60%–80%).
- Vascular dementia (caused by cerebrovascular disease or impaired cerebral blood flow) is the second most common form.
- One of the most helpful methods of diagnosing dementia is by eliciting a thorough history of the changes in the patient's memory, behavior, function, and personality from family members and close contacts of the patient.
- Assessment of functional status and cognitive testing (cognitive performance scales) of the patient is important.
- Rule out secondary causes by ordering lab tests for infectious disease, vitamin B_{12} deficiency, thyroid-stimulating hormone (TSH), syphilis (only if high clinical suspicion based on sexual history or travel).
- MRI is more sensitive than CT when neuroimaging is indicated. Unless contraindications or time/cost constraints, MRI should be performed to assess for underlying etiology.

EXAM TIPS

- Alzheimer's disease is the most common cause of dementia in the United States.
- Vascular dementia is the second most common cause of dementia.

Assessment of Functional Status

Activities of Daily Living

- Self-care activities that are necessary for "independent" living depending on the person's environment (e.g., home, retirement community, nursing home).
- Basic ADLs such as eating (self-feeding), personal hygiene (brushing teeth, bathing), ambulation (walking, wheelchairs), bowel and bladder management
- Instrumental ADLs (IADLs) such as shopping and preparing meals, housework, using electronics (stoves, telephones, TV), managing finances, driving a car
- Advanced ADLs (AADLs) such as fulfilling multiple roles (spouse, parent, caretaker) while also participating in recreational or occupational tasks

Katz Index of Independence in Activities of Daily Living

Measure used to assess older adult's independence, progression of an illness, need for care, or effectiveness of treatment and rehabilitation. Contains six items. Each item is scored a "1" (independence; ability to perform tasks with no supervision, direction, or personal assistance) or "0" (dependence; needs supervision, direction, personal assistance, or total care). The highest possible score is 6 points (independent), and the lowest is 0 points (very dependent). Independence is defined as:

- Bathing: Able to bathe self completely or needs help in bathing only one body part (e.g., back, genitals)
- Dressing: Can get clothes from closet/drawer and put on clothes without help (except tying shoelaces)
- Toileting: Able to get on/off toilet, including pants/underwear, cleans genital area without help
- Transferring: Able to move in/out of bed or chair unassisted; mechanical transfer aids acceptable
- Continence: Has complete control (urination and defecation)
- Feeding: Can get food from plate into mouth; able to feed self (okay if another person prepares food)

Lawton Instrumental Activities of Daily Living Scale

Measure used to assess an older adult's independence. This instrument is most useful for identifying how a person is functioning at the present time and to identify improvement or deterioration over time. Contains eight categories that are considered more complex than the activities measured in the Katz Index. Individuals are scored according to their highest level of functioning in each category. A summary score ranges from 0 (low function, dependent) to 8 (high function, independent). Categories are:

- Ability to use telephone
- Shopping
- Food preparation
- Housekeeping
- Laundry
- Mode of transportation
- Responsibility for own medications
- Ability to handle finances

"Get Up and Go" Test

Best used as a global assessment of an individual's fall risk. Patient is asked to rise from the chair, stand still momentarily, walk a short distance, turn around, walk back to the chair, turn around, and sit down in the chair. Rated on a 1 (normal) to 5 (severely abnormal) scale. Identifies deficits in leg strength, balance, vestibular dysfunction, and gait. Can also be used with a timed performance approach.

Fried Physical Frailty Phenotype

Five criteria used to measure frailty: Weight loss (>10 lb), weakness (grip strength; measure with a digital hand dynamometer), exhaustion (self-report), walking speed (15 feet), and physical activity (kcal/week). An individual who meets one or two of the criteria has "intermediate" frailty; an individual who meets three or more criteria is considered "frail."

Cognitive Performance Scales

Mini-Mental State Examination (MMSE)

A brief screening exam to assess for cognitive impairment. High sensitivity and specificity. Score range is 0 to 10 (severe), 10 to 20 (moderate), 20 to 25 (mild), 25 to 30 (questionable significance; mild deficits). It covers the following elements:

- Orientation to time and place (10 points)
  - Ask about year/season/date/day/month
  - Where are we now? Name state (county, town/city, hospital, floor)
- Short-term memory (3 points)
  - Name three unrelated objects and instruct the patient to recite all three words
  - Instruct patient to remember the words as they will be asked again later
- Attention and calculation (5 points)
  - Serial 7s (ask the patient to count backward from 100 by sevens)
  - As an alternative, instruct the patient to spell *world* backward
- Recall (3 points)
- Say to the patient, "Earlier I told you the names of three things. Can you tell me what they were?"

- Language (8 points)
  - Show the patient two simple objects (e.g., pencil, coin); instruct patient to name them.
  - Instruct the patient to repeat the phrase, "No ifs, ands, or buts."
  - Give the patient a blank piece of paper. Instruct patient, "Take the paper in your right hand, fold it in half, and put it on the floor."
  - Write on the paper, "Close your eyes." Instruct the patient to read it and do what it says.
  - Instruct the patient to make up and write a sentence about anything.
  - Use a questionnaire with a picture of two pentagons that intersect and ask the patient to copy the picture exactly.

Mini-Cog Test

A 3-minute tool to screen for cognitive impairment in older adults in the primary care setting. Reasonable sensitivity but relatively poor specificity. Score range is 0 to 2 (dementia), 3 to 5 (no dementia). Three steps:

- Step 1: Three-word recognition (one point for each word): Instruct the patient to repeat three words. There are six versions of words that can be used (two examples are listed here): banana, sunrise, chair (version 1); leader, season, table (version 2).
- Step 2: Clock drawing (score from 1 to 6, with ≥3 representing cognitive defect): Instruct the patient to draw a clock by putting in the numbers first; indicate a specific time by saying, "Set the hands to 10 past 11," or "Set the hands at 20 minutes after 8."
- Step 3: Three-word recall: Ask the patient to recall the three words stated in Step 1.

Clock drawing test may also be used alone to assess for cognitive impairment due to its convenient administration and scoring; applicability to a wide range of patients of any language, education, and culture background; and high inter-rater reliability, test–test reliability, sensitivity, and specificity.

Addenbrooke's Cognitive Examination III (ACE-III)

Screening test that is composed of tests of attention, orientation, memory, language, visual perceptual, and visuospatial skills. It is useful in the detection of mild cognitive impairment, Alzheimer's disease, and frontotemporal dementia.

Revised Index of Social Engagement (RISE)

Measures social engagement and ease in interactions with others—for example, engaging in planned activities, accepting invitations, pursuing involvement in facility life, initiating interactions, and reacting positively to interactions. Used for patients in long-term care facilities.

Geriatric Depression Scale (Short Form; GDS-SF)
Self-report questionnaire consists of 15 items used to screen for depression in older adults. Takes <10 minutes to complete. It can help the provider quickly determine if further assessment is necessary.

Patient Health Questionnaire-9 (PHQ-9)
A nine-item depression scale to assist in the diagnosis of depression and monitor treatment response. It has demonstrated ease, validity, and reliability and can be used for all patient populations.

Delirium (Acute Confusional State)
A reversible, temporary process. Duration is usually brief (hours to days). Acute and dramatic onset. Patient may be excitable, irritable, and combative, with short attention span, memory loss, and disorientation. Secondary to medical condition, drug, intoxication, adverse reaction to medicine.

Etiology
- Prescription medications (e.g., opioids, sedatives, hypnotics, antipsychotics, polypharmacy)
- Substance use (e.g., alcohol, heroin, hallucinogens), use of plants (e.g., marijuana, jimsonweed, salvia)
- Drug–drug interactions, adverse reactions, psychiatric illness
- Abrupt drug withdrawal (e.g., alcohol, benzodiazepines)
- Preexisting medical conditions (e.g., heart failure, renal failure)

- Infections (e.g., sepsis, UTI, pneumonia)
- Electrolyte imbalance
- ICU patients with sensory overload

Treatment Plan
Remove offending agent and/or treat illness, infection, or metabolic derangement, and delirium resolves.

"Sundowning" Phenomenon
- This condition occurs in both delirium and dementia.
- Starting at dusk/sundown, the patient becomes very agitated, confused, and combative; symptoms resolve in the morning; seen more with dementia; recurs commonly.

Treatment Plan
- Avoid quiet and dark rooms.
- Have well-lit room with a radio, TV, or clock.
- Familiar surroundings are important; do not move furniture or change decor.
- Avoid drugs that affect cognition (e.g., antihistamines, sedatives, hypnotics, narcotics).
- Maintain routines.
- Observe and minimize triggers.
- Use distraction (e.g., watch TV, take a walk, play music, reminisce).

Dementia
An irreversible brain disorder that involves loss of learned cognitive and physical/motor skills. The presentation and the signs and symptoms are determined by the etiology and location of the brain damage (Table 25.2). Gradual and insidious onset except if caused by stroke or acute brain damage.

Table 25.2 Types of Dementia

Disease	Brain Pathology	Presentation
Alzheimer's disease (#1 cause of dementia)	Deposits of beta amyloid protein and neurofibrillary tangles on the frontal and temporal lobes	Most common initial symptom is memory impairment, such as difficulty remembering names and recent events, plus wandering, apathy, apraxia, aphasia, and agnosia. Progression to impaired judgment/problem-solving and executive skills, confusion, visuospatial impairments, and neuropsychiatric symptoms including apathy, social disengagement, and irritability. Terminal stage is characterized by difficulty speaking, swallowing, and walking. Sleep disturbances and seizures are common.
Vascular dementia (#2 cause of dementia)	Any dementia primarily caused by cerebrovascular disease or cerebral blood flow (e.g., multi-infarct/ischemic damage due to atherosclerotic plaques, bleeding, and/or blood clots)	Cognitive decline clinically attributed to a vascular cause. Symptoms of stroke with cognitive symptoms such as memory loss, impaired executive function, impaired judgment, and apathy; location of infarct determines symptoms.
Dementia with Lewy bodies	Aggregated alpha-synuclein protein is a key component of Lewy bodies and Lewy neurites	Core clinical features include cognitive fluctuations, visual hallucinations, REM sleep behavior disorder, and parkinsonism (muscle rigidity, tremors). Executive function is impaired with fluctuations in alertness and cognition; sensitive to adverse effects of neuroleptics.

(continued)

Table 25.2 Types of Dementia (*continued*)

Disease	Brain Pathology	Presentation
Parkinson's disease	Loss of dopamine receptors in the basal ganglia of the substantia nigra	Cardinal features include tremor (pill-rolling), bradykinesia, and rigidity. Causes postural instability, difficulty initiating voluntary movements, masked facies, depression, plus features of DLB (sleep disturbance, visual hallucinations); prevalence of dementia in Parkinson's patients is 40%.
Frontotemporal dementia (Pick's disease)	Symmetric or asymmetric atrophy in the frontal and/or temporal lobes	Causes personality change, social withdrawal, loss of spontaneity, apathy and loss of empathy, loss of motivation/desire to do task (abulia), impulsive, disinhibition; exhibits utilization behavior (e.g., uses and reuses same object, such as using a spoon to eat, comb hair, and gesture).
Mixed dementia	Mixture of two or more types (e.g., Alzheimer's and vascular dementia)	If Alzheimer's and vascular dementia, symptoms of both conditions are present.
Wernicke–Korsakoff syndrome (or Wernicke's encephalopathy)	Chronic thiamine (vitamin B_1) deficiency due to chronic alcohol use disorder, malabsorption, poor dietary intake, increased metabolic requirement, and in dialysis patients	Classic triad includes encephalopathy, oculomotor dysfunction, and gait ataxia. Can cause vestibular dysfunction, horizontal movement nystagmus (both eyes), and peripheral neuropathy; if caught early, treatment with high-dose IV thiamine may reverse some symptoms, but if late, can cause permanent brain damage.
Normal pressure hydrocephalus	Increased amount of cerebrospinal fluid (but with normal intracranial pressure)	Causes gait dysfunction (body bent forward, legs wide apart, slow), impaired thinking, urinary incontinence, impaired executive function, reduced concentration, apathy, changes in personality; treatment involves an implanted ventricular shunt.

DLB, dementia with Lewy bodies; IV, intravenous; REM, rapid eye movement.

Dementia affects executive skills adversely. *Executive function* is defined as self-regulation skills, attention, planning, multitasking, self-control, motivation, and decision-making skills. These higher level cognitive skills are regulated in the frontal lobes of the brain.

Differential Diagnosis
- It is important to obtain a thorough health/medical/drug history.
- The patient should be accompanied by family during the interview. Family members and friends will report patient's signs and symptoms. Refer to neurologist for further assessment.
- Rule out correctable causes such as vitamin B_{12} deficiency, hypothyroidism, psychiatric disorders, infection, adverse/drug interactions, heavy metal poisoning, neurosyphilis, electrolyte imbalances, and others.
- Parkinson's dementia and dementia with Lewy bodies (DLB) may resemble each other.
- Remember that normal pressure hydrocephalus can cause dementia-like symptoms that mimic Alzheimer's disease.
- The preferred imaging test for dementia signs/symptoms is MRI of the brain.

Mild Cognitive Impairment
Mild cognitive impairment (MCI) involves a cognitive change that is unexpected for normal aging but does not meet criteria for dementia. Objective memory impairment but also ability to function in daily life. May progress to dementia, remain stable, or even be temporary with deficits reverting to normal. Cognitive assessments of moderate length (5 to 15 minutes), such as the MMSE, are more sensitive for screening for MCI.

Alzheimer's Disease
Rare before age 60 years. Incidence doubles every 10 years after age 60. Accumulation of neurofibrillary plaques/tangles, extracellular deposits of amyloid beta, and neurofibrillary degeneration. Overproduction and/or decreased clearance of amyloid beta peptides. Average life expectancy after diagnosis is between 8 and 10 years but may range from 3 to 20 years. Seizures occur in 10% to 20% of patients with Alzheimer's disease.
Common *A*s:
- *A*mnesia: Loss of memory; most common initial symptom
- *A*phasia: Difficulty expressing and understanding language
- *A*praxia: Difficulty performing learned motor tasks; loss of ability to carry out skilled movements and gestures
- *A*gnosia: Inability to recognize familiar people or objects

Classic Cases
- Mild: Still functioning independently, but family or friends notice early symptoms.

- Problems coming up with the right word when talking
- Forgetting something that was just read or seen/repeats same questions. Forgetting important dates
- Losing or misplacing important objects; getting lost on familiar routes
- Problems managing personal finances and money; poor judgment
- Becomes withdrawn, anxious, and/or depressed; easily upset; personality changes
- Moderate: Usually the longest stage; requires greater levels of care.
  - Wanders and gets lost
  - Has problems with speech and following instructions
  - Stops paying bills
  - May start a conversation and forget to complete sentences
  - Loses ability to read and write
  - Has problems recognizing familiar people (agnosia) and is unable to recall current or past information about themselves
  - Demonstrates personality and behavior changes like delusions or compulsions
- Severe: Alzheimer's disease progresses inexorably. Symptoms are severe, and the patient requires total care.
  - Unable to feed self
  - Incontinent of bowel and bladder
  - Unable to control movements, so they stop walking and use wheelchair or are bedridden
  - Incoherent or mute and have difficulty communicating pain
  - Apathetic

Treatment Plan

Most patients with Alzheimer's disease are taken care of at home by a family member or caregiver during the early stages of the disease. As disease progresses, many patients are placed in skilled nursing facilities or assisted-living dementia units. In later stages of the disease, families may consider palliative and hospice care.

Medications

- Mild-to-moderate dementia (MMSE 10–26): Begin trial of a cholinesterase inhibitor (increases longevity of acetylcholine), such as donepezil (Aricept) (initial dose 5 mg PO once daily), rivastigmine (Exelon), or galantamine (Razadyne).
- Moderate-to-severe dementia (MMSE ≤18): Add memantine (Namenda) (initial dose 5 mg PO once daily) in combination with a cholinesterase inhibitor, or use memantine (Namenda) alone in patients who do not tolerate or benefit from a cholinesterase inhibitor.
- Severe dementia (MMSE <10): Continue memantine or discontinue drug administration to maximize quality of life.
- Improvement within 3 to 6 months. Stop if no longer effective.

Adjunct Treatment

- Physical activity and exercise have been shown to slow functional decline in patients.
- Maintain adequate nutrition via assisted feeding and oral nutritional supplements.
- Limit alcohol consumption.
- Vitamin E 1,000 IU twice daily for mild-to-moderate Alzheimer's disease. May provide a small benefit, but risks must be discussed.
- Address safety concerns such as preventing falls, wandering, and home safety (e.g., with cooking).

Rehabilitation

- Cognitive rehabilitation: May help during early stages of dementia to maintain memory and compensate for declining function
- Physical and occupational therapy: May improve performance of ADLs.

Driving and Early-Stage or Mild Dementia

- Evaluate for safety and monitor regularly.
- Ask family or close contacts about patient's driving ability, traffic accidents, getting lost, difficulty making decisions, and so forth.

Complications

- Death is often the result of an overwhelming infection such as pneumonia or sepsis.
- Hip fractures are also a common cause of death (from complications).

EXAM TIPS

- Recognize classic presentation of Parkinson's and Alzheimer's diseases.
- Recognize the sundowning phenomenon.

ESSENTIAL TREMOR

The most common type of action or postural tremor. Usually seen in the arms or hands and may progress to include the head. Exact etiology is unknown. Essential tremor can occur in children and adults. It is not curable, but the symptoms can be controlled by medication. In some patients with essential tremor, the tremors can worsen with anxiety and may improve with small amounts of alcohol. Medications can be taken as needed (anxiety) or daily.

Treatment Plan

- Nonselective beta-blocker: Propranolol 60 to 320 mg per day. Long-acting propranolol (Inderal LA) is also effective. Contraindications include uncompensated heart failure, cardiogenic shock, severe sinus bradycardia, sick sinus syndrome, second- or third-degree heart block, bradycardia. Higher risk of bronchospasm (may lead to drug discontinuation in patients with chronic obstructive pulmonary disease or asthma).
- Antiseizure agent: Primidone (Mysoline) 25 to 750 mg per day at bedtime

- Second-line therapies: Propranolol plus primidone, gabapentin (Neurontin), topiramate (Eprontia), and benzodiazepines.
- Referral: To neurologist for evaluation and treatment.

HYPOTHYROIDISM

Very common in patients age 60 years or older. Subtle and insidious symptoms such as sleepiness, severe constipation, weight gain, and dry skin. Problems with memory. If severe, may mimic dementia. Slower movements. Appears apathetic.

NEUROCOGNITIVE FINDINGS

- Abulia: Loss of motivation or desire to do tasks; loss of willpower; indifference to social norms (e.g., urinates in public)
- Akathisia: Intense need to move because of severe feelings of restlessness
- Akinesia: Reduced voluntary muscle movement (e.g., Parkinson's disease)
- Amnesia: Memory loss; anterograde amnesia is memory loss of recent events (occurs during disease), and retrograde amnesia is memory loss of events in the past (before the onset of disease)
- Anomia: Problems recalling words or names
- Aphasia: Difficulty using (speech) and/or understanding language; can include difficulty with speaking, comprehension, and written language
- Apraxia: Difficulty with or inability to remember learned motor skill
- Astereognosis: Inability to recognize familiar objects placed in the palm (place a coin on palm and ask patient to identify object with eyes closed)
- Ataxia: Difficulty coordinating voluntary movement
- Confabulation: Lying or fabrication of events due to inability to remember events
- Dyskinesia: Abnormal involuntary jerky movements
- Dystonia: Abnormal movements and muscle tone (continuous muscle spasms)

OSTEOPOROSIS

The USPSTF (2018) recommends screening women age 65 years or older for osteoporosis. Osteopenia and osteoporosis are caused by a gradual loss of bone density secondary to estrogen deficiency and other metabolic disorders. Most common in older women (White or Asian descent) who are thin with small body frames, especially if positive family history. Treat postmenopausal women (or men age 50 years or older) who have osteoporosis (T-score –2.5 or less) or history of hip or vertebral fracture. Other risk groups include:

- Patients on chronic steroids (e.g., severe asthma, autoimmune disorders) are at high risk for glucocorticoid-induced osteoporosis; rule out osteoporosis in older women (or men) on chronic steroids, especially if accompanied by other risk factors
- Patients who have anorexia nervosa and/or bulimia
- Long-term smokers
- Long-term users of proton pump inhibitors (PPIs), such as omeprazole (Prilosec)
- Gastric bypass, celiac disease, hyperthyroidism, ankylosing spondylitis, rheumatoid arthritis (RA), and others
- The "female athlete triad" is a combination of low weight with history of amenorrhea or menstrual dysfunction and low bone density; at higher risk for osteoporosis

Lifestyle Risk Factors

- Low calcium intake (low intake of dairy), vitamin D deficiency, inadequate physical activity
- Alcohol consumption (three or more drinks per day), high caffeine intake
- Smoking (active or passive)

Bone Density Test Scores

- Use DEXA to measure the bone mineral density (BMD) of the hip and spine; do baseline and repeat in 2 years (if on treatment regimen) to assess the efficacy of the medicine.
- T-score of –2.5 or lower standard deviation (SD) at the lumbar spine, femoral neck, or total hip region indicates osteoporosis
- Pharmacologic therapy if osteoporosis or postmenopausal with history of fragility fracture, history of hip fracture, or recent fracture
- T-scores between –1.5 and –2.4 SD indicate osteopenia

Treatment Plan

- Weight-bearing exercises 30 minutes three times per week. Weight-bearing exercises are walking, jogging, aerobic dance classes, most sports, yoga, tai chi. Swimming, biking, and isometric exercises are not considered weight-bearing exercise.
- 1,200 mg calcium daily with vitamin D 800 IU daily
- Smoking cessation if a smoker (smoking cigarettes accelerates bone loss)
- FRAX (Fracture Risk Assessment Tool) will give the 10-year probability of hip fracture and major osteoporotic fracture (spine/forearm/shoulder). Website is www.sheffield.ac.uk/FRAX.

Medications

Bisphosphonates

- First-line drugs for treating postmenopausal osteoporosis, glucocorticoid-induced osteoporosis (women and men), and osteoporosis in men
- Potent esophageal irritant (advise patients to report sore throat, dysphagia, midsternal pain); may cause esophagitis, esophageal perforation, gastric ulcers, reactivation/bleeding peptic ulcer disease (PUD)
- Increases BMD and inhibits bone resorption
- Fosamax (alendronate) PO daily or weekly

- Actonel (risedronate) PO daily, weekly, or monthly
  - Take immediately upon awakening in morning with full glass (6–8 ounces) of plain water (do not use mineral water).
  - Take tablets sitting or standing and wait at least 30 minutes before lying down.
  - Do not crush, split, or chew tablets; swallow the tablets whole.
  - Never take these drugs with other medications, juice, coffee, antacids, vitamins.
  - Will cause severe esophagitis or esophageal perforation if lodged in the esophagus.
- Consider prophylaxis for high-risk postmenopausal women with osteopenia.
- Repeat DEXA after 2 years of therapy.
- Contraindications include inability to sit upright, esophageal motility disorders, history of PUD or history of GI bleeding, chronic kidney disease, certain types of bariatric surgery (e.g., Roux-en-Y gastric bypass)
- Osteonecrosis of the jaw (mandible or maxilla) more likely if on intravenous or intramuscular bisphosphonates; patient complains of jaw heaviness, pain, swelling, and loose teeth.

Selective Estrogen Receptor Modulator Class
- Raloxifene (Evista) is a Category X drug.
- Does not stimulate endometrium or breast tissue, since it blocks estrogen receptors (ERs).
- Approved for use in postmenopausal women with osteoporosis who are at higher risk for breast cancer.
- Do not use to treat menopausal symptoms (aggravates hot flashes).
- Boxed warning due to increased risk of deep vein thrombosis (DVT), pulmonary embolism, and endometrial/uterine cancers; increased risk of death from stroke (postmenopausal women with history of heart disease).
- These drugs reduce risk of breast cancer (if taken long term up to 5 years).
- Selective estrogen receptor modulators (SERMs) are an option for patients who cannot tolerate or have contraindications to bisphosphonates.
- Used as adjunct treatment for ER-positive breast cancers.

Tamoxifen (Nolvadex)
- Tamoxifen (Nolvadex) is a Category X drug.
- Used for treatment of breast cancer that is hormone-receptor positive and for prophylaxis in women at high risk for breast cancer; can be taken up to 5 years.
- Increased risk of DVT, endometrial cancer, strokes, and pulmonary emboli.
- Causes hot flashes, white or brownish vaginal discharge, weight gain or loss.

Parathyroid Hormone Analog
- Teriparatide (Forteo) injection is recombinant human parathyroid hormone (PHT) for treatment of osteoporosis; it comes as a prefilled injector.
- It increased the incidence of osteosarcoma in rats.

Other: Miacalcin and Calcitriol
- Calcitonin salmon, derived from salmon; weak anti-fracture efficacy compared with bisphosphonates and PTH.
- Calcitriol is a vitamin D analog; must be on a low-calcium diet; monitor patient for hypercalcemia, hypercalciuria, and renal insufficiency; may be effective in preventing glucocorticoid and posttransplant-related bone loss.

PARKINSON'S DISEASE
Progressive neurodegenerative disease with marked decrease in dopamine production. More common after age 50 years. Men are more likely to have Parkinson's disease than women (1.4:1). The classic symptoms are tremor (worse at rest), muscular rigidity, bradykinesia, and postural instability (see Table 25.2). Dementia and depression are common.

Classic Case
An older adult patient complains of a gradual onset of motor symptoms such as pill-rolling tremors of the hands and cogwheel rigidity with difficulty initiating voluntary movement. Walks with slow shuffling gait. Has poor balance and often falls (postural instability). Generalized muscular rigidity with masked facies. Reports depression, excessive daytime sleepiness, and difficulty with executive function (making plans or decisions, performing tasks). Signs and symptoms of dementia. Worsening of seborrheic dermatitis (white scales, erythema).

Treatment Plan
If mild Parkinson's disease symptoms do not markedly interfere with function, it is usually not necessary to prescribe pharmacotherapy immediately after diagnosis. Consider treatment for significant bradykinesia or gait disturbance and moderate-to-severe hand tremors (dominant hand), depending on patient preference and degree to which the tremors interfere with ADLs, work, and social function. Ask the patient about fatigue, which is a common problem. May nap more frequently and experience sleep disorders including insomnia, daytime sleepiness with sleep attacks, restless leg syndrome, and REM sleep behavior disorder.

Medications
- First-line drug: Carbidopa–levodopa (Sinemet) (dopamine precursor)
  - Start at low doses. Carbidopa 25 mg/levodopa 100 mg (half tablet) PO BID to TID with meal or snack to avoid nausea. Titrate up slowly to control symptoms.
  - Adverse effects include motor fluctuations (wearing-off phenomenon). May cause or worsen dyskinesia, dizziness, somnolence, nausea and vomiting, headache, impulse control disorders, orthostatic hypotension, peripheral neuropathy, psychiatric behavior abnormalities. Rare but can cause withdrawal syndrome, with pyrexia, muscle rigidity, reduced level of consciousness, and autonomic instability.

- Dopamine agonists: Ergot types, such as bromocriptine (Parlodel), have limited use in Parkinson's disease; replaced by newer dopamine agonists that are nonergot types, such as pramipexole (Mirapex), ropinirole (Requip), and transdermal rotigotine (Neupro). Effective as monotherapy in patients with early disease.
  - Do not abruptly discontinue dopamine agonists. Dopamine withdrawal syndrome (8%–19%) causes panic attacks, anxiety, craving for drug.
  - Adverse effects include nausea, vomiting, sleepiness, orthostatic hypotension, confusion, and hallucinations. Can cause impulse control disorders (compulsive gambling, sex, or shopping).
- Monoamine oxidase-B (MAO-B) inhibitors: Reasonable alternative to levodopa as first-line therapy. Selegiline (Eldepryl), rasagiline (Azilect), or safinamide (Onstryv)
  - Does not have dietary restrictions like monoamine oxidase inhibitors (MAOIs).
  - Adverse effects include nausea and headache. May cause confusion, insomnia, jitteriness, hallucinations. Do not combine with MAOIs or serotonin antagonists (selective serotonin reuptake inhibitors [SSRIs], triptans).
- Alternative pharmacotherapy:
  - Anticholinergics: Benztropine (Cogentin). Can be useful in younger patients with disturbing tremor; no significant bradykinesia or gait disturbance
  - Dopamine agonist: Amantadine (Gocovri). Alternative to early levodopa in younger patients who are at risk for dyskinesia, particularly when tremor is prominent
- Nonpharmacologic: Exercise, physical therapy, speech therapy, mindfulness, and meditation
- Device assistance or surgery: Consider continuous infusions or deep brain stimulation

Complications
- Acute akinesia (loss of voluntary movement; sudden exacerbation of Parkinson's disease)
- Dementia
- Frequent falls may result in fractures (e.g., hip).
- Drug-related adverse effects such as tardive dyskinesia, dystonia, motor fluctuations

EXAM TIPS

- Wernicke–Korsakoff syndrome is caused by vitamin B_1 (thiamine) deficiency.
- First-line treatment for Parkinson's disease is levodopa (Sinemet) immediate release.

URINARY INCONTINENCE

Should not be considered a normal aspect of aging. Evaluate all cases. May be acute and temporary (e.g., UTI, high intake of caffeinated beverages) or chronic. Two or three times more common in women. Risk factors are obesity, increasing parity, vaginal delivery, menopause, age, smoking, and diabetes. Some foods and drinks worsen urinary incontinence because of their diuretic effect (e.g., caffeinated drinks, alcohol, carbonated drinks, citrus fruits, spicy foods). Some medications (e.g., diuretics) may have a similar effect. Table 25.3 describes the types of urinary incontinence.

Table 25.3 Types of Urinary Incontinence

Type	Description and Treatment Plan
Stress incontinence	Increased intra-abdominal pressure (laughing, sneezing, bending, lifting) causes involuntary leakage of small-to-medium volume of urine. Highest incidence in middle-aged women (peak at 45–49 years). Treatment plan includes lifestyle modification; pelvic floor muscle (Kegel) exercises; bladder training; topical vaginal estrogen; trial of duloxetine (Cymbalta), a serotonin norepinephrine reuptake inhibitor.
Urge incontinence	Sudden and strong urge to void immediately before involuntary leakage of urine. Involuntary loss of urine can range from moderate-to-large volumes. Condition also known as "overactive bladder." Most common type of incontinence among men. Treatment plan includes Kegel exercises, bladder training, addition of pharmacotherapy if initial treatments ineffective.
Overflow incontinence	Frequent dribbling of small amounts of urine from overly full bladder due to bladder outlet obstruction (e.g., benign prostatic hyperplasia [BPH]) or underactive detrusor muscle (e.g., spinal cord injury, multiple sclerosis). Highest incidence in older men. Treatment plan is specific to etiology—for example, BPH treatment (discussed in Chapter 16).
Functional incontinence	Problems with mobility (walking to the toilet) or inability to pull down pants in a timely manner. The impaired mobility may be temporary or permanent. Treatment plan includes bedside commode, raised toilet seats with handles, physical therapy for strengthening and gait.
Mixed incontinence	Symptoms that are a mixture of stress and urge incontinence. Treatment plan includes lifestyle modification and pelvic floor muscle training.

Treatment Plan

- First-line treatment: Lifestyle modifications for all types (stress, urge, mixed), including weight reduction, dietary changes, fluid restriction, caffeine reduction, and smoking cessation.
- Dietary: Avoid certain beverages (e.g., alcohol, coffee, tea, carbonated drinks) and excessive fluid intake (>64 ounces); decrease fluid intake before bedtime.
- Constipation: Treat as indicated to decrease risk of urinary retention and subsequent urge or overflow incontinence.
- Kegel exercises (pelvic floor exercises): All types of urinary incontinence, especially stress incontinence. Kegel exercises also have been found to help with fecal incontinence.
- Moderate to advanced pelvic organ prolapse (cystocele, rectocele, enterocele, uterine prolapse, vaginal eversion): Refer to urologist or gynecologist specializing in urinary incontinence and pelvic organ prolapse repair.

Kegel Exercises

Tell the patient to:

- Identify the muscles used to stop urinating (stop urinating midstream to confirm this). Do not tighten muscles of the abdomen, buttocks, thighs, and legs at the same time.
- Squeeze and hold these muscles and slowly count to five.
- Relax and release these same muscles to a slow count of five.
- Repeat this 10 times. Aim for at least three sets of 10 repetitions three times a day for 15 to 20 weeks.

Behavioral Bladder Training

- Bladder training to delay urination after feeling the urge to urinate. At first, have the patient try holding off urinating for 10 minutes each time. The goal is to lengthen the time between trips to the bathroom to every 2 to 4 hours.
- Double voiding helps to empty the bladder more completely to avoid overflow. Double voiding means urinating and then waiting a few minutes and voiding again.

Medications

Serotonin-Norepinephrine Reuptake Inhibitor

- Duloxetine (Cymbalta): 40 mg PO BID. May be effective for stress incontinence.
- Contraindications: Use of an MAOI concurrently or within 14 days

Anticholinergics

- Oxybutynin (Ditropan): 2.5 to 5 mg PO TID (immediate release); other formulations include extended release, transdermal patch (twice a week), transdermal gel.
- Trospium (Trosec): 20 mg PO BID (immediate release); 60 mg orally once daily in the morning (extended release)
- Darifenacin (Enablex): 7.5 mg PO once daily (dose may be increased to 15 mg once daily)

- Contraindications: Urinary retention, gastric retention, severe decreased motility of GI tract, uncontrolled narrow-angle glaucoma

Beta-3-Adrenergic Agonists

- Mirabegron (Myrbetriq): 25 to 50 mg extended-release tablets; used to treat symptoms of overactive bladder
- Vibegron (Gemtesa): 75 mg oral dose daily
- Contraindications: Hypersensitivity

URINARY TRACT INFECTIONS

UTIs are the most common infection in adults age 65 years and older. Diagnosis can be difficult in this population due to higher prevalence of chronic urinary symptoms and baseline cognitive impairment. Patients usually have no fever or can be asymptomatic. May become acutely confused, delirious, agitated, or even septic. Testing recommended for classic signs and symptoms (e.g., acute dysuria, new or worsening urgency or frequency, new incontinence, gross hematuria, suprapubic or costovertebral angle tenderness) because neither positive UAs nor urine culture results necessarily indicate a true infection.

CLINICAL PEARLS

- Refer patients with suspected Alzheimer's disease or Parkinson's disease to a neurologist for diagnostic evaluation and management.
- UTI is a common cause of acute mental status changes in older adults.
- Idiopathic Parkinson's disease is associated with low serum vitamin B_{12} levels due to levodopa. Check vitamin B_{12} level.
- If the levodopa dose is too high, peak-dose dyskinesia can occur in a patient with Parkinson's disease. Manage by lowering the levodopa dose, shortening the interdose interval, and switching to a longer-acting formulation.
- Cholinesterase inhibitors can be used to treat patients with Parkinson's disease dementia, but there is an increased risk of side effects, including worsened tremor and nausea.

OTHER COMMON GERIATRIC CONDITIONS

These diseases are covered under their respective organ systems:

- Acute diverticulitis (Chapter 10)
- Anemia (Chapter 13)
- Bacterial pneumonia (Chapter 8)
- COPD (Chapter 8)
- Heart failure (Chapter 7)
- Type 2 diabetes mellitus (Chapter 9)
- Glaucoma (Chapter 5)
- Heart disease/murmurs (Chapter 7)
- Hyperlipidemia (Chapter 7)
- Hypertension (Chapter 7)
- Macular degeneration (Chapter 5)
- Menopause/atrophic vaginitis (Chapter 17)
- Temporal arteritis (Chapter 12)

PHARMACOLOGIC ISSUES: OLDER ADULTS

Drug clearance is affected by renal impairment, a less efficient liver cytochrome P450 system, malabsorption, and relatively higher fat-to-muscle tissue ratio (extends half-life, fat-soluble drugs). Older adults have an increased sensitivity to benzodiazepines, hypnotics, tricyclic antidepressants (TCAs), and antipsychotics. The American Geriatrics Society (AGS) provides a Beers Criteria® list of potentially inappropriate medication use in older adults (AGS, 2023). Deprescribing measures should be used when appropriate for older adult patients. Table 25.4 includes an abbreviated summary of potentially inappropriate medications.

GERIATRIC SYNDROMES ASSOCIATED WITH POLYPHARMACY

- Constipation: Anticholinergics, calcium channel blockers, opioids
- Dizziness: Anticholinergics, antihypertensives, sulfonylureas (can cause hypoglycemia)
- Delirium and dementia: Anticholinergics, benzodiazepines, corticosteroids, H2 antagonists, sedative hypnotics
- Falls: Anticonvulsants, antidepressants (SSRIs and TCAs), antihypertensives (e.g., alpha-blockers → orthostatic hypotension), antipsychotics, benzodiazepines, opioids
- Urinary incontinence: Anticholinesterase inhibitors, antidepressants, antihistamines, antihypertensives (specifically calcium channel blockers, diuretics, alpha-1 blockers), antipsychotics, opioids, sedative-hypnotics

EXAM TIP

Selegiline (Eldepryl) is an MAO type B inhibitor. Avoid tyramine-containing foods and caffeine due to risk of hypertensive crisis or serotonin syndrome. Drugs that alter serotonin are SSRIs, serotonin-norepinephrine reuptake inhibitors (SNRIs), TCAs, and MAOIs. Discontinue treatment if any symptoms arise.

Table 25.4 Potentially Inappropriate Medications for Older Adults (Beers Criteria®)*

Drug Class	Drugs to Avoid and Potential Adverse Effects
Alpha-blockers	Terazosin (Hytrin), clonidine (Catapres); high risk of orthostatic hypotension
Antihistamines	Diphenhydramine (Benadryl) and others; newer generation has lower incidence (Claritin); risk of confusion, dry mouth, constipation
Antidepressants (tricyclic)	Amitriptyline (Elavil), imipramine (Tofranil), doxepin (Silenor); highly anticholinergic, sedating, can cause orthostatic hypotension
Atypical antipsychotics	Quetiapine (Seroquel), olanzapine (Zyprexa); boxed warning for higher risk of mortality in older adult patients in nursing homes
Antispasmodics	Dicyclomine (Bentyl), scopolamine (Transderm); highly anticholinergic, uncertain effectiveness
Benzodiazepines: Short–intermediate acting Long-acting	Risk of cognitive impairment, delirium, falls, fractures; older adults have higher sensitivity to benzodiazepines Alprazolam (Xanax), lorazepam (Ativan), triazolam (Halcion) Diazepam (Valium), clonazepam (Klonopin)
Central alpha-agonists	Clonidine (Catapres); high risk of adverse central nervous system effects, may cause bradycardia and orthostatic hypotension Digoxin for first-line treatment of atrial fibrillation
Insulin, sliding scale	Short- or rapid-acting insulin (e.g., lispro [Humalog]); high risk of hypoglycemia without improvement in hyperglycemia management
Lubricant laxatives	Mineral oil (oral); may increase risk of aspiration, safer alternatives available
Nonsteroidal anti-inflammatory drugs	Indomethacin (Indocin), ketorolac (Toradol), others; high risk of gastrointestinal bleeding and peptic ulcer disease, especially age >75 years or taking corticosteroids or anticoagulants
Proton pump inhibitors	Omeprazole (Prilosec), esomeprazole magnesium (Nexium); risk of *Clostridoides difficile* infection, bone loss, and fractures
Prokinetic agent	Metoclopramide (Reglan); can cause extrapyramidal effects, including tardive dyskinesia
Sedative hypnotics	Zolpidem (Ambien), eszopiclone (Lunesta); high risk of delirium, adverse central nervous system effects (e.g., impaired psychomotor function, syncope, falls), minimal improvement in sleep latency
Sulfonylureas (avoid long-acting first generation)	Glyburide (DiaBeta), chlorpropamide (Diabinese); can cause prolonged hypoglycemia and/or syndrome of inappropriate antidiuretic hormone secretion

*List is not all-inclusive.
Source: 2023 American Geriatrics Society Beers Criteria® Update Expert Panel. (2023). (See Resources section for complete source information.)

KNOWLEDGE CHECK: CHAPTER 25

1. A nurse practitioner instructs a patient to spell *world* backward. Which of the following tests is being performed?
   A. MMPI
   B. CAGE
   C. MMSE
   D. PHQ-9

2. When evaluating a case of giant cell arteritis, the erythrocyte sedimentation rate (ESR) is expected to be:
   A. Normal
   B. Lower than normal
   C. Elevated
   D. Indeterminate

3. Which of the following is a cardinal clinical sign in a patient with Parkinson's disease?
   A. Pill-rolling tremors
   B. Inability to recognize familiar people or objects
   C. Wide-based gait
   D. Increased facial movements due to tics

4. A 68-year-old female patient complains of leaking a small amount of urine whenever she sneezes, laughs, and/or strains. The problem has been present for many months. The patient denies dysuria, frequency, and nocturia. The urine dipstick test is negative for white blood cells, red blood cells, ketones, and urobilinogen. This clinical presentation suggests which type of incontinence?
   A. Urge
   B. Overflow
   C. Urinary
   D. Stress

5. Which of the following cancers has the highest rate of mortality?
   A. Lung and bronchus
   B. Colorectal
   C. Pancreatic
   D. Breast

6. A female patient is in the hospital recovering from a motor vehicle collision. The patient sustained a femur fracture and is experiencing urinary incontinence due to impaired mobility that delays access to the bathroom. Which of the following treatment options would be appropriate for this patient?
   A. Pelvic floor muscle (Kegel) exercises
   B. Bedside commode and physical therapy
   C. Duloxetine (Cymbalta), a serotonin-norepinephrine reuptake inhibitor
   D. Bladder training

7. Which of the following is a category in the Katz Index of Independence in Activities of Daily Living?
   A. Housecleaning
   B. Dressing
   C. Preparing meals
   D. Exercising

8. A patient presents with complaints of a bilateral action tremor in the arms and hands. The patient reports that the tremor is activated by voluntary movement, especially drinking from a glass. The tremor is absent when the affected body part is fully relaxed and supported. These symptoms suggest which of the following disease conditions?
   A. Parkinson's disease
   B. Tardive dyskinesia
   C. Acute akinesia
   D. Essential tremor

9. A patient's family member reports that recently the patient has become acutely agitated and confused in the evening hours. The patient's family member is concerned for the patient's safety and asks for treatment recommendations. Which of the following interventions would be helpful for this condition?
   A. Moving the furniture to avoid falls and safety hazards
   B. Using a mechanism of distraction (e.g., playing music) when the patient is agitated
   C. Administering an over-the-counter antihistamine to facilitate sleep
   D. Using a dark room for sleeping to allow the patient proper sleep hygiene

(See answers next page.)

1. C) MMSE

The nurse practitioner is instructing the patient to perform a task in the Mini-Mental State Examination (MMSE), which assesses for cognitive impairment. The Cut, Annoyed, Guilty, Eye (CAGE) questionnaire is used to screen for alcohol use disorder. The Minnesota Multiphasic Personality Inventory (MMPI) is a personality test, and the Patient Health Questionnaire-9 (PHQ-9) is used to screen for depression.

2. C) Elevated

Headache is the most common chief complaint and presents in more than two thirds of patients with giant cell arteritis. The headache tends to be new or different in character from previous headaches and is typically sudden in onset, localizing to the temporal region. Any new headache and fever in patients older than 50 years warrants a consideration of giant cell arteritis. ESR greater than 50 mm/hr is suspect. The normal ESR for male patients is 0 to 15 mm/hr, and for female patients it is 0 to 20 mm/hr. The ESR can be slightly more elevated in older adults.

3. A) Pill-rolling tremors

Clinical signs of Parkinson's disease include pill-rolling tremors, difficulty initiating voluntary movements, and shuffling gait with cogwheel rigidity. Facial movement decreases, resulting in generalized rigidity with masked facies. Inability to recognize familiar people or objects, or agnosia, is a sign of Alzheimer's disease. Wide-based gait is a sign of cerebellar ataxia.

4. D) Stress

The signs and symptoms of stress incontinence occur with increased abdominal pressure caused by sneezing, laughing, and/or straining, which results in the leakage of a small amount of urine through a weakened sphincter. It is more common in women ages 45 to 49 years. The urethra and bladder neck fail to close completely because of loss of connective tissue support.

5. A) Lung and bronchus

Lung and bronchus cancer accounts for the most deaths, with 130,180 people annually expected to die from this type of cancer. Colorectal cancer is the second most common cause of cancer death, followed by pancreatic cancer, which is the third deadliest cancer. Breast cancer mortality has decreased due to increased screening, earlier detection, awareness, and improved treatment.

6. B) Bedside commode and physical therapy

This patient's clinical manifestations suggest functional incontinence, which involves intact urinary storage and emptying functions; the patient has physical problems reaching the bathroom in a timely manner. Treatment options include use of a bedside commode and raised toilet seat with handles and physical therapy for strengthening and gait. Pelvic floor muscle (Kegel) exercises are especially useful for patients experiencing stress urinary incontinence. Bladder training is most effective for female patients with urgency incontinence. Duloxetine (Cymbalta), a serotonin-norepinephrine reuptake inhibitor, may be effective for stress urinary incontinence in some patients.

7. B) Dressing

The Katz Index of Independence in Activities of Daily Living contains six items to assess a patient's independence: bathing, dressing, toileting, transferring, continence, and feeding. The highest possible score is 6 points (independent), and the lowest is 0 points (very dependent).

8. D) Essential tremor

An essential tremor is an action tremor that often affects the hands and arms bilaterally. It can also be seen in the head, voice, and face or trunk (rare). Common daily activities are often affected, such as writing, drinking from a glass, and using utensils. Classically, tremor due to Parkinson's disease is a rest tremor that occurs unilaterally, distinguishing it from an essential tremor. Tardive dyskinesia is a medication-induced hyperkinetic movement disorder that causes oral, facial, and lingual dyskinesia. A sudden exacerbation of Parkinson's disease can cause acute akinesia, which causes an akinetic state (without motion) that can last for several days.

9. B) Using a mechanism of distraction (e.g., playing music) when the patient is agitated

The patient's symptoms suggest the sundowning phenomenon, characterized by behavioral deterioration in the evening hours. Distraction can be helpful during an episode of agitation. The patient should be encouraged to watch television, take a walk, play music, or engage in another familiar hobby. It is important to maintain sleep hygiene; however, an appropriately lit room with a radio, television, or clock can help re-orient the patient. A dark room can be a safety hazard because it impairs visual acuity. It is essential to maintain routine, and familiar surroundings are important, so furniture should not be moved. Drugs that can affect cognition (e.g., sedatives, antihistamines, hypnotics, narcotics) should be avoided because they can worsen cognitive impairment.

10. The clinician asks a patient with Alzheimer's disease to demonstrate how they use a comb. The clinician is assessing for which sign or symptom of the disease?
A. Apraxia
B. Aphasia
C. Amnesia
D. Agnosia

11. Which of the following medications for the treatment of constipation is considered an osmotic agent?
A. Psyllium
B. Docusate
C. Polyethylene glycol
D. Bisacodyl

12. A patient presents with a sudden onset of new flashes of light, floaters, and black dots in their vision. The patient reports a disruption in vision, "like a curtain is being pulled down." These symptoms suggest which medical emergency?
A. Retinal detachment
B. Amaurosis fugax
C. Homonymous hemianopia
D. Acute angle-closure glaucoma

13. A patient presents with one discrete lesion on the side of the head. Assessment reveals an erythematous, scaly macule that is 1 cm in diameter. Which of the following is an appropriate choice of therapy?
A. 5% topical fluorouracil cream
B. Photodynamic therapy
C. No treatment because the lesion is less than 2 cm
D. Liquid nitrogen cryotherapy

14. The acronym CRAB can be used to recall the characteristics of multiple myeloma. Which of the following *correctly* represents the mnemonic?
A. C: Calcium levels low
B. R: Renal insufficiency
C. A: Anorexia
D. B: Bradycardia

15. A patient presents with pill-rolling, generalized slow movement, and increased resistance to passive movement. The patient reports a tendency to fall and a feeling of imbalance. These symptoms are suggestive of which disease pathophysiology?
A. Deposits of beta amyloid beta peptides
B. Ischemic damage due to atherosclerotic plaques
C. Dopamine depletion from the basal ganglia
D. Chronic thiamine deficiency

16. A patient with Alzheimer's disease scores a 15 on the Mini-Mental State Examination (MMSE). Which of the following is an appropriate treatment option for this patient?
A. Initiation of memantine (Namenda) alone
B. Combination therapy of donepezil/memantine (Namzaric)
C. Initiation of donepezil (Aricept) alone
D. Maximizing of quality of life and patient comfort

(See answers next page.)

10. A) Apraxia

Apraxia, or dyspraxia, involves difficulty performing learned motor tasks, which can occur later in the disease progression of Alzheimer's. The patient has the desire and physical ability to perform the tasks but has lost the ability to execute or carry out the skilled movement and gesture. Apraxia can be assessed by asking the patient to perform ideomotor tasks, such as using a comb. Progression of apraxia can cause difficulty with multistep motor activities, then with dressing, using utensils, and other self-care tasks. Aphasia involves language difficulty—the loss of spoken language or speech comprehension. Agnosia involves the inability to recognize and identify objects or persons. Amnesia refers to the loss of memory.

11. C) Polyethylene glycol

Osmotic agents include polyethylene glycol, lactulose, sorbitol, glycerin, magnesium sulfate, and magnesium citrate. Bulk-forming laxatives include psyllium, methylcellulose, polycarbophil, and wheat dextrin. Docusate is a surfactant (softener). Stimulant laxatives include bisacodyl and senna.

12. A) Retinal detachment

Retinal detachment can cause light flashes, floaters, visual disruption (e.g., a dark shadow or "curtain"), and loss of peripheral and/or central vision. A patient with acute angle-closure glaucoma often presents with decreased vision, halos around lights, headache, severe eye pain, and nausea and vomiting. Homonymous hemianopia (often caused by cerebral infarction and intracranial hemorrhage) describes a visual field impairment involving the two right or the two left halves of the visual fields of both eyes. Amaurosis fugax refers to transient vision loss in one or both eyes. Transient vision loss may be seen in patients with giant cell arteritis.

13. D) Liquid nitrogen cryotherapy

The patient is presenting with the classic clinical features consistent with actinic keratosis: an erythematous, scaly macule, papule, or plaque lesion that ranges from a few millimeters to 2 cm in diameter. The choice of therapy depends on number and distribution of lesions, patient preference, side effects, and treatment availability. Liquid nitrogen cryotherapy can be used as treatment for patients with one or a few discrete, isolated lesions. First-line therapy for patients with multiple thin lesions on the face or scalp includes 5% topical fluorouracil cream. While photodynamic therapy is an alternative option for the treatment of multiple lesions, it is not available in all office-based dermatology offices.

14. B) R: Renal insufficiency

The diagnosis of multiple myeloma requires clonal bone marrow plasma cells greater than 10% or biopsy-proven bony or soft-tissue plasmacytoma, plus the presence of related organ or tissue impairment suggested by elevated Calcium levels, Renal insufficiency, Anemia, and Bone lesions (CRAB).

15. C) Dopamine depletion from the basal ganglia

The patient is presenting with clinical features consistent with Parkinson's disease: a rest tremor ("pill-rolling"), generalized slowness of movement (bradykinesia), rigidity, and postural instability causing a feeling of imbalance and an increased risk of falls. The pathophysiology of Parkinson's disease involves the progressive degeneration of dopamine-producing neurons in the basal ganglia, including the substantia nigra in the midbrain. Dopamine depletion causes major disruptions in the connections to the thalamus and motor cortex, leading to the classic presentation of bradykinesia and rigidity. The pathophysiology of Alzheimer's disease involves the overproduction and/or decreased clearance of amyloid beta peptides, a family of proteins. Vascular dementia is caused by cerebrovascular disease or impaired cerebral blood flow. Wernicke's encephalopathy results from thiamine deficiency.

16. C) Initiation of donepezil (Aricept) alone

For patients with mild-to-moderate dementia (MMSE 10–26), it is recommended to begin a trial of a cholinesterase inhibitor (increases longevity of acetylcholine), such as donepezil (Aricept). For patients with moderate-to-severe dementia (MMSE ≤18), it is recommended to add memantine (Namenda) in combination with a cholinesterase inhibitor or use memantine (Namenda) alone in patients who do not tolerate or benefit from a cholinesterase inhibitor. For patients with severe dementia (MMSE <10), memantine (Namenda) can be continued, or all drug administration may be discontinued to maximize quality of life.

17. A 60-year-old male patient had a colonoscopy this year, which was normal. The patient has no personal or family history of colon cancer. He asks when he needs to follow up with additional screening. The clinician recommends:
    A. High-sensitive guaiac-based fecal occult blood test annually
    B. Flexible sigmoidoscopy every 2 years
    C. CT colonography every 3 years
    D. Colonoscopy screening every 5 years

18. An older adult patient with a history of chronic urinary incontinence at baseline presents with a new onset of delirium and falls. Which of the following is an appropriate *next* step for this patient?
    A. Serum creatinine
    B. Urinalysis
    C. Urine culture
    D. Workup for onset of new delirium

19. Screening for lung cancer is recommended for which of the following patients?
    A. 45-year-old with a 10 pack-year smoking history
    B. 55-year-old with a 20 pack-year smoking history who currently smokes
    C. 60-year-old with a 5 pack-year smoking history who currently smokes
    D. 65-year-old with a 15 pack-year smoking history who quit 20 years ago

20. Which of the following findings is a *concern*, rather than an expected finding, in older adults?
    A. Diminished appetite
    B. Decreased visual acuity
    C. Pill-rolling of the fingers
    D. Difficulty staying asleep through the night

(See answers next page.)

17. A) High-sensitive guaiac-based fecal occult blood test annually

According to the U.S. Preventive Services Task Force, it is recommended that adults age 45 to 75 years be screened for colorectal cancer. The recommended intervals for colorectal cancer screening tests for asymptomatic adults who are at average risk of colorectal cancer (i.e., no prior diagnosis of colorectal cancer, adenomatous polyps, or inflammatory bowel disease; no personal diagnosis or family history of known genetic disorders that put them at risk of colorectal cancer) are high-sensitivity guaiac-based fecal occult blood test or fecal immunochemistry testing (FIT) every year, stool DNA-FIT every 1 to 3 years, CT colonography every 5 years, flexible sigmoidoscopy every 5 years, flexible sigmoidoscopy every 10 years + FIT every year, and/or colonoscopy screening every 10 years.

18. D) Workup for onset of new delirium

It is not recommended to perform urine testing based on nonspecific symptoms (such as mental status changes and functional decline) in the absence of findings concerning for systemic infection. In the older adult population, urine testing is indicated in the presence of classic signs and symptoms of urinary tract infection (e.g., acute dysuria, new or worsening urgency or frequency, new incontinence, gross hematuria, suprapubic or costovertebral angle tenderness) or physiologic signs of serious acute illness (e.g., fever, other major vital sign abnormalities, changes in level of consciousness).

19. B) 55-year-old with a 20 pack-year smoking history who currently smokes

The U.S. Preventive Services Task Force recommends annual screening for lung cancer with low-dose CT in adults age 50 to 80 years who have a 20 pack-year smoking history and currently smoke or quit within the past 15 years.

20. C) Pill-rolling of the fingers

The cardinal features of Parkinson's disease are tremor, typically described as pill-rolling, bradykinesia, and rigidity. This is not a common finding seen with aging adults and may require further diagnostic workup. Cerebral neurons decrease with aging, and older adults experience decreased sensory functions of smell, taste, and vision. Nerve impulse conduction decreases, causing delayed responses to stimuli, unsteady gait, sleep disturbances, decreased level of cognition, diminished appetite, and decreased range of motion.

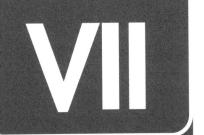

VII

PROFESSIONAL ROLE REVIEW

26 ETHICAL GUIDELINES AND ADVANCED PRACTICE LAW

ETHICAL CONCEPTS

BENEFICENCE

The obligation to help the patient—to remove harm, prevent harm, and promote good ("do no harm"). Acting in the patient's best interest. Compassionate patient care. The core principle in patient advocacy. Examples:

- Educating patient with a new prescription about how to take the medication
- Encouraging a patient to stop smoking and enroll in smoking cessation program
- Prescribing or advocating for effective postoperative pain medication

NONMALEFICENCE

The obligation to avoid harm. Protecting a patient from harm. Example: A patient with osteoporosis wants to be treated with bisphosphonates. The nurse practitioner (NP) advises that the patient is not a good candidate for these drugs because of a past medical history of gastrointestinal (GI) bleeding and peptic ulcer disease (PUD). The NP decides not to prescribe bisphosphonates.

UTILITARIANISM

The obligation to act in a way that is useful to or benefits the majority. The outcome of the action is what matters with utilitarianism. It also means to use a resource (e.g., tax money) for the benefit of most. It may resemble justice (see next definition), but it is not the same concept. Example: The Special Supplemental Nutrition Program for Women, Infants, and Children (WIC) is for only pregnant women and children, not other adults and elderly men. The reason may be that it would cost society more if women (and their fetuses), infants, and children are harmed by inadequate food intake (e.g., affects the brain growth).

JUSTICE

The quality of being fair and acting with a lack of bias. The fair and equitable distribution of societal resources. Example: A man with alcoholism who is homeless and has no health insurance presents to the ED with abdominal pain. The patient is triaged and treated in the same manner as other patients who have health insurance.

DIGNITY

The quality or state of being worthy of ethical and respectful treatment. Respect for human dignity is an important aspect of medical ethics. A person's religious, personal, and cultural beliefs can influence greatly what a person considers "dignified" treatment. Examples:

- Hospital gowns should be secured correctly so that when patients get up to walk, their backs are not visible.
- Foley catheter urine bags should not be visible to visitors so patients are not embarrassed. NPs should move urine bags to the opposite bed rail so that they are not visible to outsiders.

FIDELITY

The obligation to maintain trust in relationships. Dedication and loyalty to one's patients. Keeping one's promise. Example: The relationship between a patient and their healthcare team is important. The primary care NP should try their best to develop a trusting relationship with a patient.

CONFIDENTIALITY

The obligation to protect the patient's identity, personal information, test results, medical records, conversations, and other health information. This "right" is also protected by the Health Insurance Portability and Accountability Act (HIPAA), which restricts release of patient information. Psychiatric and mental health medical records are protected information and require separate consent. Example: The HIPAA Privacy Rule protects most "individually identifiable health information" in any format (oral, paper, electronic). It is known as protected health information (PHI). The PHI includes demographic information (name, address, date of birth, Social Security number) as well as the individual's past, present, or future physical/mental health and provision of care.

AUTONOMY

The obligation to ensure that mentally competent adult patients have the right to make their own health decisions and express treatment preferences. If the patient is mentally incapacitated (dementia, coma), the designated surrogate's choices are respected. (See later discussion on advance healthcare directives.) A mentally competent patient can decline or refuse treatment even if their adult children disagree. Example: An alert older woman who has breast cancer decides to have a lumpectomy after discussing the treatment options with her oncologist. The woman's adult daughter tells the NP that she does not want her mother to have the surgery because she thinks her mother is "too old." The NP has a duty to respect the patient's decision. This case is also a good example of the NP acting as the patient advocate.

ACCOUNTABILITY

Healthcare providers are responsible for their own choices and actions and do not blame others for their mistakes. Example: An NP has an adult male patient with acute bronchitis who complains of acute onset of chest pain. He is diagnosed with pleurisy. The patient goes to the ED and is diagnosed with an acute myocardial infarction (MI). The NP made an error in diagnosis and is held accountable for the decision and actions in a court of law.

> **NOTE**
>
> *Paternalism* describes situations in which one person interferes with or overrules the autonomy of another. In healthcare, it occurs when a provider or family member makes decisions for an elderly patient because they "believe" that it is in the patient's best interest. The opinion (or desire) of the patient is minimized or ignored. The patient is "powerless."

VERACITY

The obligation to present information honestly and truthfully. In order for patients to make an informed and rational decision about their healthcare, pertinent information (including "bad" news) should not be withheld or omitted. Example: The mammogram result of a 64-year-old female patient is highly indicative of breast cancer. The patient's adult son does not want his mother to know about the results. The NP has a duty to discuss the mammogram results with the patient and refer her to a breast surgeon.

EXAM TIP

Become familiar with some of the ethical concepts (e.g., beneficence, veracity, nonmaleficence, justice) and how they are applied (see examples provided in this chapter).

THE AMERICAN NURSES ASSOCIATION CODE OF ETHICS FOR NURSES

The American Nurses Association (ANA) *Code of Ethics for Nurses With Interpretive Statements* (2015) contains "the ethical standard for the profession and provides a guide for nurses to use in ethical analysis and decision-making." According to the ANA, the Code "is a nonnegotiable standard." Each nurse "has an obligation to uphold and adhere to the code of ethics."

For example, under Provision 4.4, "Nurses may not delegate responsibilities such as assessment and evaluation; they may delegate selected interventions according to state nurse practice acts."

LEGAL TERMS

OMBUDSMAN

A person who acts as an intermediary (or as a liaison) between the patient and an organization (long-term care facilities or nursing homes, hospitals, governmental agencies, courts). The ombudsman investigates and mediates the complaint from both sides and attempts to reach a fair conclusion.

GUARDIAN AD LITEM

An individual who is assigned by a court (and has the legal authority) to act in the best interest of the ward. The ward is usually a person who is a child or someone who is frail or vulnerable. Adults who are incompetent may be assigned a guardian ad litem by the court.

ADVANCE HEALTHCARE DIRECTIVES

Living Will

A document that contains the patient's instructions and preferences regarding healthcare if the patient becomes seriously ill or is dying. It contains the patient's preferences (or not) for aggressive life-support measures. Healthcare providers should ensure that there is a copy of the document in the patient's chart.

Healthcare Power of Attorney

The patient designates a person (family member or a close friend) who has the legal authority to make future healthcare decisions for the patient in the event that the patient becomes mentally incompetent or incapacitated (e.g., comatose). Also known as a "healthcare proxy," "durable medical power of attorney," or "healthcare surrogate."

It goes into effect when the patient's doctor has determined that they are physically or mentally unable to communicate in a willful manner. To be legal, it must be signed in the presence of two adult witnesses who must also sign the document (the designated surrogate cannot act as a witness). Power is only for healthcare decisions (not financial assets).

Power of Attorney

A document whereby the patient designates a person (the "agent") who has the legal authority to make all decisions for the incapacitated patient. The document should be signed and notarized. Also known as the "durable power of attorney." This role is broader and encompasses not only healthcare decisions but also other areas of the patient's life, such as those relating to financial affairs.

HEALTH INSURANCE PORTABILITY AND ACCOUNTABILITY ACT

Also known as the "HIPAA Privacy Rule" (or Public Law 104–191). The law was passed by the U.S. Congress and enacted in August 1996. The law provides protections for "the use and disclosure of individuals' health information"—called "protected health information" by organizations subject to the Privacy Rule, which are called "covered entities."

COVERED ENTITIES

All healthcare providers, health insurance companies, healthcare plans, laboratories, hospitals, skilled nursing facilities (SNFs), and third-party administrators (TPAs) who electronically transmit health information must follow the HIPAA regulations.

WHAT IS A THIRD-PARTY ADMINISTRATOR?

A TPA is the organization that does the processing of claims and administrative work for another company (health insurer, health plan, retirement plan).

EXAM TIPS

- Understand the role of an ombudsman, guardian ad litem, and others who act on behalf of a patient.
- A TPA is the organization that does the processing of claims and administrative work for another company (health insurer, health plan, retirement plan).

HIPAA REQUIREMENTS (NOT ALL-INCLUSIVE)

- Health providers are required to provide each patient with a copy of their office's HIPAA policy (patient to sign the form).
- The HIPAA form must be reviewed and signed annually by the patient.
- A mental health provider has the right to refuse patients' requests to view their psychiatric and mental health records.
- When patients request to review their medical records, the health provider has up to 30 days to comply.
- Patients are allowed (under HIPAA) to correct errors in their medical records.
- Providers must keep identifying information (name, date of birth, address, Social Security number) and any diagnosis/disease or health concerns private except under certain conditions (see list that follows).

WHEN PATIENT CONSENT IS NOT REQUIRED

- To contact the health plan/insurance company that is paying for the medical care
- To contact a third party or business associate (e.g., accounting, legal, administrative) that the insurance company or doctor's office hires to assist in payment of their services (e.g., medical billing services)
- To perform certain healthcare operations (medical services review, sale of healthcare plan, audits)
- To contact collection agency for unpaid bills
- To report abuse/neglect or domestic violence
- To consult with other healthcare providers

HIPAA CASE SCENARIOS

- If a staff member (who is not involved in the patient's care) calls the attending NP and wants to discuss a patient's progress, the NP cannot release information to the staff member.
- How to communicate results of lab tests or procedures? The Rule "does not prohibit us from leaving messages for patients on their answering machines"; however, we must "reasonably safeguard" their privacy. It is prudent to avoid leaving messages about lab results, medication names, or types of tests on the patient's voice mail. Leave the clinic name (exceptions exist), your name, and phone number for the patient to contact you.
- See Table 26.1 for examples of HIPAA case scenarios.

HIPAA, PSYCHOTHERAPY, AND MENTAL HEALTH RECORDS

Psychotherapy records made by a mental health professional are treated differently under HIPAA. They should be separated from the patient's other medical records.

Table 26.1 HIPAA and Patient Care

Situation	Description	Notes
Putting patient charts on door box	Place the chart so that the front of the chart is facing the door (so that patient name is hidden).	Limit access to certain areas; ensure area is supervised.
Having sign-in sheets on front desk	This is allowed if it does not list patient's diagnosis.	Attendance list can show names, dates, and time.
Calling a patient in the waiting room to go inside the clinic exam room	Use only first name. If more than one person with same first name, use the first letter of last name.	If you have two patients named Ann (e.g., Ann Lee and Ann Smith), use Ann L. and Ann S.
Leaving messages on voice mail	When calling, first provide your name and contact information. Be concise. Limit to 60 seconds. Maximum of three calls per week. Information that can be given may include appointment reminders, notifications about prescriptions, and preoperative and postoperative instructions.	Avoid leaving messages about lab results, diagnosis, or other sensitive information on the patient's voice mail.
Having a colleague who works in same clinic or hospital call, wanting information about a patient's progress	If staff member is not part of the healthcare team, no patient information can be released to that person.	HIPAA also does not allow such a person to access a friend's or family member's records without permission.

(continued)

Table 26.1 HIPAA and Patient Care (*continued*)

Situation	Description	Notes
Having a family member call, wanting information about a patient's progress	Put on hold and tell patient about the call. If patient gives permission, you can speak with the family member.	If patient does not consent, then advise the family member about the patient's decision. Do not release patient information.
Having inappropriate access of health information on the computer	Viewing the records of your relatives, friends, or coworkers is an HIPAA violation.	Do not allow someone to use your computer password.
Using personal devices (smartphones, laptops, tablets)	Ideally, it is best to avoid using personal devices at work. Requirements: Secure Wi-Fi with passwords, regular encrypted backups, antivirus software, policies, etc.	If you want to use a personal device, discuss it with your manager and/or consult information technology. Best practice is to use the facility's or clinic's devices.
Discussing a patient's drugs and other instructions with a health aide who is with the patient	Discussing information is allowable.	If patient has the capacity to make healthcare decisions, discussing information is allowable.
Discussing patient's treatment in front of a patient's friend who is visiting	Discussing treatment with the patient's friend is allowable if the patient gives consent or requests that the friend come inside the treatment room.	Discussing patient information with others is allowable if patient agrees to it.

HIPAA, Health Insurance Portability and Accountability Act.
Source: HIPAA Journal (2015). (See Resources section for complete source information.)

A separate consent form is needed to release psychotherapy records. The exceptions are mandatory reporting of abuse and "duty to warn" when the patient threatens serious and imminent harm to others. "In situations where the patient is given an opportunity and does not object, HIPAA allows the provider to share or discuss the patient's mental health information with family members or other persons involved in the patient's care or payment for care."

EXAM TIPS

- Become familiar with how HIPAA is applied in real life. Study the HIPAA case scenarios in Table 26.1.
- It is a HIPAA violation to leave any laboratory results on a patient's voice mail.

MINORS

The health records of a minor (by law, an individual younger than 18 years) can be released to parents or legal guardians without the minor's consent. If authorization is needed to release a minor's medical record, the parent or legal guardian must sign for it (except for emancipated minors; emancipated minors can sign their own legal documents).

HEALTH INSURANCE

THE AFFORDABLE CARE ACT (2010)

This national health insurance legislation, officially known as the Patient Protection and Affordable Care Act (ACA) and unofficially nicknamed Obamacare, was signed by President Obama in March 2010 (and upheld by the U.S. Supreme Court in 2012), with the goal of expanding health insurance for the millions of Americans who were then uninsured. It expanded health coverage through various provisions (e.g., allowing adult children younger than age 26 to be insured under their parents' healthcare insurance). This comprehensive reform of U.S. health insurance law prohibits an insurance company from rejecting people with preexisting health conditions. Although increased numbers of Americans gained insurance as a result of the law's passage, many millions more still lack coverage.

CONSOLIDATED OMNIBUS BUDGET RECONCILIATION ACT OF 1985

Also known as "COBRA coverage." Provides for the continuation of coverage of preexisting group health insurance (from the employer) for workers and their families who lose their coverage (between jobs, quit job, or are fired) for a fixed period of time. COBRA coverage is generally offered for 18 months (up to 36 months in some cases).

EXAM TIPS

- COBRA is a law that allows a person to continue group health insurance coverage from a job even if they have quit (the individual has to pay the insurance premiums).
- No separate consent is required for entities that pay or process the patient's health bills, such as health insurance companies, health maintenance organizations (HMOs), medical billers, or collection agencies (or third-party contractors hired by the company to pay or to process claims).

MANAGED CARE
Both HMOs and preferred provider organizations (PPOs) are classified as "managed healthcare plans."

Health Maintenance Organizations
Patients are assigned a primary care provider (PCP), who is the "gatekeeper." The patient has a set "copay" per visit, and the participating physician/health provider is paid a set fee (per patient) monthly. The physician receives a monthly check from the HMO.

- Specialist/consultant: The PCP must first approve the referral. The patient is limited to seeing the physicians/specialists who are enrolled in the HMO's network.
- "Out-of-network physicians" or not referred by the PCP: The visit may not be covered, or it will be reimbursed at a lower rate.

Preferred Provider Organization
The patient can visit any provider in the network without a referral. Not assigned a PCP (as in HMOs). The patient can choose their own PCP. No referral is needed to see a specialist who is part of the PPO panel. PPOs are usually more expensive than HMOs.

CASE MANAGEMENT

Healthcare case managers are usually experienced RNs who act as coordinators for the outpatient management of patients with certain diagnoses, usually chronic, resource-intensive diseases (e.g., asthma [children], chronic obstructive pulmonary disease [COPD], chronic heart failure, diabetes). The process is called *case management*. Case management is mainly done by telephone.

PATIENT-CENTERED MEDICAL HOME

Patient-centered medical home (PCMH) is a healthcare delivery model that is also known as the *primary care medical home*. It is another way to deliver patient-centered primary care. In PCMH, the patient and family are considered important members of the healthcare team. Most of the patient's healthcare needs are taken care of in the home setting. Other team members may include physicians, APRNs, physician assistants (PAs), nurses, pharmacists, nutritionists, social workers, educators, and care coordinators.

Delivery of healthcare is coordinated to ensure smooth transition between home and hospital, home health agency, and community services. The patient and/or family has 24-7 access to a member of the team by phone, video chat, or email.

QUALITY-IMPROVEMENT PROGRAMS

Quality improvement involves monitoring, identifying problems, measuring outcomes, and establishing new parameters for improved performance. The goal of these programs is to improve the quality of care, decrease complications, decrease hospitalizations, lower patient mortality, decrease system errors, and increase patient satisfaction. Patient outcomes are important indicators of a health system's quality. Example: A "problem" is identified (e.g., diabetic complications such as peripheral neuropathy and retinopathy). Then outcome measures are identified (e.g., hemoglobin A1C <6.5%). Be familiar with what a good outcome is for a disease (for diabetics, a good outcome is A1C <6.5%) and what a poor outcome is (A1C >8%).

RISK MANAGEMENT IN HEALTHCARE

Risk management is an important aspect of quality-improvement/quality-assurance programs in the healthcare setting. It is the systematic organizational process used to identify risky practices to minimize adverse patient outcomes and corporate liability. For example, high-risk areas that are usually checked by risk managers are medication errors, hospital-acquired infections, patient identification problems, and falls. Risk management promotes safe and effective patient care practices.

EXAM TIPS

- The "medical home" is a method of primary healthcare delivery. Healthcare providers and therapists (physical, occupational, speech) deliver care in the patient's home, with the family. These patients have chronic long-term illness. To communicate, technology is used, such as phone, video chat, or email.
- Use common sense in answering questions on quality improvement and risk management. Keep in mind the goals of these processes: to improve the quality of care, decrease complications, decrease hospitalizations, lower patient mortality, decrease system errors, and increase patient satisfaction. Look for the answer that fits these goals.

ACCREDITATION

Accreditation is a voluntary process through which a nongovernmental association evaluates and certifies that an organization (e.g., hospital, clinic, nursing program) has met the requirements and excels in its class. For example, the American Nurses Credentialing Center and the National League for Nursing Accrediting Commission are accreditation organizations.

THE JOINT COMMISSION
The Joint Commission (TJC) is an independent, not-for-profit organization that accredits healthcare organizations (hospitals, nursing homes, home care, laboratories) via inspection and evaluation of their facilities (charged a fee). Achieving TJC certification means that a facility has met or

surpassed the organization's strict requirements. The purpose of the accreditation process is to enhance quality of care and patient safety.

SENTINEL EVENT REPORTING

A sentinel event (SE) is a patient safety event (not primarily related to the natural course of the patient's illness or condition) that results in any of the following: death, permanent harm, and/or severe temporary harm with intervention required to sustain life. When an SE occurs, the healthcare organization is expected to conduct a root cause analysis (RCA), make improvements to reduce risk, and monitor effectiveness of the improvements. Accredited organizations are strongly encouraged but are not required to report SEs to the TJC.

Examples of Sentinel Events

- Suicide that occurs while receiving care in a staffed around-the-clock facility or within 72 hours of discharge
- Unanticipated death of an infant or discharge of infant to the wrong family
- Rape or assault of a staff member, visitor, or vendor
- Invasive procedure on the wrong patient, the wrong procedure is done on a patient, or the procedure is done to the wrong limb
- Unintended retention of a foreign object
- Fire, flame, or unanticipated smoke or heat during an episode of patient care

ROOT CAUSE ANALYSIS

RCA is a structured, facilitated team process used in healthcare to identify the contributing factors that result in an error. The TJC has mandated the use of RCA to analyze SEs. The gathered data are analyzed for the root causes (usually a combination of human, environmental, and system factors). The goal is to identify the system breakdowns that resulted in an inadvertent mistake and to propose at least one corrective action to reduce or eliminate each root cause. When an SE occurs, an RCA is recommended. The focus is on the system and not on blaming individuals.

OUTCOMES ANALYSIS

Outcomes analysis refers to analysis and tracking of patient outcomes by using outcome measures such as surveys and questionnaires.

HOSPICE

The majority of hospice care in the United States takes place in patients' homes (59% die in their own homes). The goal is palliative care, not curative care. Ensuring the patient's quality of life and comfort is the ultimate goal of hospice care. Hospice care is available for both pediatric and adult patients.

An interdisciplinary team provides hospice care. This team usually consists of the patient's primary physician, hospice physician, RN, nursing assistants, therapists, social workers/grief counselor, and clergy. Hospice staff are on call 24 hours a day. They provide grief-and-loss counseling for patients and family members.

Hospice is covered under Medicare Part A, Medicaid, and most health insurance plans. Hospice patients are allowed to have physical therapy (PT), occupational therapy (OT), and speech therapy if prescribed (see www.medicare.gov/coverage/hospice-care).

ELIGIBILITY CRITERIA

- The hospice physician and the patient's physician certify that the patient is terminal and has 6 months (or less) to live. The hospice physician approves of admission.
- Patient is rapidly declining or exhibits worsening symptoms.
- Patient needs assistance with two or more activities of daily living (ADLs).
- Patient accepts palliative care, not curative care. If they do not want to be in hospice (even if all criteria are met), then patient is not eligible.

EXAM TIPS

- A patient may meet the criteria for hospice admission, but if the patient refuses hospice care, then the patient is not eligible.
- If the patient meets the criteria for hospice care, Medicare Part A will reimburse hospice.

Examples of Terminal Conditions

- Metastatic cancers (e.g., lung cancer, colon cancer)
- End-stage lung disease (e.g., COPD)
- End-stage heart disease (e.g., congestive heart failure [CHF] class III or IV)
- End-stage liver disease
- HIV/AIDS with comorbidities and refusal/discontinuation of antiretrovirals
- End-stage renal disease with plan to discontinue dialysis
- Amyotrophic lateral sclerosis, Parkinson's disease, stroke, coma
- End-stage dementia (e.g., Alzheimer's disease)

RESPITE CARE

Short-term respite care for the primary caregiver that is reimbursed by Medicare. This gives the primary caregiver a break, even if it is only a few hours. For example, respite care gives the caregiver a chance to go see a movie and to relax and rest.

KNOWLEDGE CHECK: CHAPTER 26

1. Which of the following is an example of how the "utilitarian" principle is applied?
   A. Helping a patient decide among the various types of treatment that are available for their condition
   B. Using limited financial resources for programs that help the most people and have the lowest possible negative outcomes
   C. Minimizing the possible poor outcomes when offering treatment choices to a patient
   D. Being more careful when using healthcare financial resources for any purpose

2. The oncology nurse practitioner (NP) sees a new patient who is 85 years old. The patient is recently diagnosed with stage 4 metastatic cancer and speaks only Farsi. The NP calls for a certified medical Farsi interpreter to interpret during the office visit. The patient's adult child states that the interpreter is not needed and that they are capable of interpreting correctly for their parent. The NP's commitment to using a certified medical translator is *most closely* related to which ethical concept?
   A. Veracity
   B. Nonmaleficence
   C. Beneficence
   D. Justice

3. An 83-year-old patient is newly diagnosed with atrial fibrillation with a CHADSVASc score of 2. The patient has a history of multiple gastrointestinal bleeds requiring transfusions, falls with injury, and reports of 6+ alcoholic drinks per day. The nurse practitioner (NP) will have a discussion with the patient about reducing their high bleeding risk before considering starting anticoagulation for stroke prevention. The NP is demonstrating which ethical concept?
   A. Justice
   B. Nonmaleficence
   C. Utilitarianism
   D. Confidentiality

4. What legal authority does a healthcare power of attorney allow the adult child of a patient?
   A. The adult child may refuse a surgery that a competent patient has consented to.
   B. The adult child can access the patient's bank account to pay the patient's bills if they become incapacitated.
   C. The adult child can make healthcare decisions on behalf of the patient only if they are incapacitated.
   D. Having healthcare power of attorney always allows the adult child to change the patient's living will.

5. A colleague of a nurse practitioner (NP) recommends that the colleague's adult family member establish care with the NP as their primary care provider. After the first visit between the NP and the patient, the colleague asks the NP how the visit went with their family member. Under the Health Insurance Portability and Accountability Act of 1996 (HIPAA), the NP is legally allowed to disclose what information to their colleague?
   A. "The visit went great! We discussed how to lose weight in a healthy manner."
   B. "I will need your family member's permission to say how the visit went."
   C. "I cannot disclose specifics, but their diet has to change."
   D. "You are welcome to look at their chart."

6. What is a required provision of the Health Insurance Portability and Accountability Act (HIPAA) signed into law in the United States in 1996?
   A. Patients are not allowed to request corrections to their medical records.
   B. Healthcare providers have up to 60 days to provide a patient with a copy of their medical records if requested.
   C. Mental health providers can refuse to provide patients with a copy of their medical records.
   D. Patient consent is not required for a new outside medical office to request medical records.

(See answers next page.)

1. B) Using limited financial resources for programs that help the most people and have the lowest possible negative outcomes

Generally, the utilitarian principle refers to societal programs that will affect or benefit the largest number of people in a positive manner. It is not used to refer to an individual person.

2. A) Veracity

The NP has an obligation to use the certified medical translator to ensure that the diagnosis and treatment plan are communicated truthfully to the patient in a manner they can understand. Veracity is the NP's responsibility to present information truthfully and honestly. Nonmaleficence is the obligation to protect the patient from harm. Beneficence is the obligation to promote good and act in the patient's best interest. Justice is the duty to act fairly and without bias.

3. B) Nonmaleficence

Nonmaleficence is the obligation to protect the patient from harm. Starting anticoagulation for stroke prevention in a patient with a high bleeding risk could potentially cause harm. There should be discussion of the risk/benefits with the patient and how to minimize harm before proceeding with anticoagulation. Justice is the duty to act fairly and without bias. Utilitarianism is the obligation to act in a way that benefits the majority. Confidentiality is the obligation to protect the patient's private health information

4. C) The adult child can make healthcare decisions on behalf of the patient only if they are incapacitated.

The healthcare power of attorney allows the adult child to make healthcare decisions only if the patient becomes incapacitated and is no longer able to make competent decisions. It does not allow the adult child to overule the decisions made by a competent patient, nor does it override the patient's living will unless it specifically states so in the healthcare power of attorney. A durable power of attorney is required to make financial decisions for the patient.

5. B) "I will need your family member's permission to say how the visit went."

HIPAA protects the private health information (PHI) of all patients. A disclosure of PHI from one healthcare provider to another is allowed only for consultation. The colleague is not allowed to view their family member's chart or ask for information regarding the care and treatment of the family member. The NP cannot disclose any PHI to the colleague without the patient's permission.

6. C) Mental health providers can refuse to provide patients with a copy of their medical records.

Mental health providers are allowed to refuse a patient access to their medical records, and mental health records require a separate consent form for release of those records. Patients are allowed to correct their medical records, and patient consent is always required to release medical records to a new office. Healthcare providers must provide medical records to the patient within 30 days of the request.

7. A new patient requests that the nurse practitioner (NP) leave the results of their sexually transmitted infection (STI) testing on their voice mail because they typically miss phone calls. The best reply by the NP is:
   A. "Yes, I'll leave a voice mail with the results and any potential treatment too."
   B. "Let's set up your patient portal where I can send encrypted messages with your lab results instead."
   C. "I can leave your results on your voice mail as long as your outgoing message confirms your identity."
   D. "Can a family member stop by the office and pick up your results?"

8. Which of the following statements is *true* regarding The Joint Commission (TJC)?
   A. All healthcare and nursing home facilities are required to be certified by TJC.
   B. The purpose of TJC is to enhance patient safety.
   C. TJC is a division of the Department of Health and Human Services.
   D. TJC's primary mission is to investigate sentinel events at hospitals.

9. An surgical nurse practitioner (NP) was involved in the care of a patient who was found to have a retained surgical sponge after surgery. The sponge was removed during a second procedure, and the patient was safely discharged home without further complications. What is the correct action for the NP to recommend at this time?
   A. This is a sentinel event and a root cause analysis should be performed by the facility.
   B. If the facility is accredited by the Joint Commission, the event must be reported to that organization.
   C. No further action is required as no major complications occurred for the patient.
   D. The NP should recommend discipline for the circulating nurse who is responsible for confirming the count.

10. A patient with progressive chronic heart failure and a history of multiple hospitalizations for heart failure tells the nurse practitioner (NP), "I am tired of going to the hospital; I'm getting worse every time that I am discharged home." Which of the following would be the *most appropriate* statement by the NP regarding hospice care?
   A. "If you transition to hospice care, the staff there will stop all your medications."
   B. "Hospice care can be beneficial for symptom control but is not typically covered by insurance."
   C. "You can enter hospice care as soon as your physician approves your admission."
   D. "Hospice care allows more resources for you and your family if you decide that a curative medical approach is no longer your goal."

(See answers next page.)

7. B) "Let's set up your patient portal where I can send encrypted messages with your lab results instead."
While disclosing private health information (PHI) on a voice mail is not specifically against the rulings of the Health Insurance Portability and Accountability Act (HIPAA), NPs have the obligation to reasonably safeguard a patient's PHI. Voice mail or answering machines are not considered secured for leaving specific and potentially sensitive PHI. It is prudent to leave only a name and a callback number (avoiding the clinic name in some cases if it is potentially sensitive). A password-secured patient portal with the ability to send encrypted messages is a method to communicate securely with patients. A family member cannot pick up a patient's results unless they are specifically indicated on the HIPAA form signed by the patient.

8. B) The purpose of TJC is to enhance patient safety.
The purpose of TJC is to enhance quality care and patient safety through accreditation of healthcare facilities. Accreditation is voluntary, not mandatory, for healthcare facilities in the United States. TJC is a nongovernmental organization. While TJC mandates what procedures accredited facilities must follow in investigating sentinel events, it does not perform the investigations.

9. A) This is a sentinel event and a root cause analysis should be performed by the facility.
A retained object during surgery is considered to be a sentinel event, and a root cause analysis is recommended to be performed by all Joint Commission–accredited facilities. Reporting sentinel events to the Joint Commission is strongly encouraged but not mandatory. Performing no further action prevents the opportunity to correct the mistakes that led to the error. Recommending discipline for a member of the surgical team is inappropriate given that no investigation has yet taken place to determine the root cause of the event.

10. D) "Hospice care allows more resources for you and your family if you decide that a curative medical approach is no longer your goal."
Admission into hospice for patients who are ready for this approach allows the patient and their family access to hospice RNs and social workers, respite care for caregivers, and much more. Hospice care is covered by government and most commercial insurers. While the hospice provider may stop some or all of the patient's medications, generally medications that improve symptoms are continued, and decisions around medication are made jointly with the patient. (For example, typically it is recommended to continue diuretics to improve shortness of breath and edema for a patient with end-stage heart failure.) The hospice physician, not the patient's physician, approves admission.

PROFESSIONAL ROLES AND REIMBURSEMENT REVIEW

THE NURSE PRACTITIONER ROLE

HISTORY
Loretta C. Ford, PhD, RN, FAAN, and Henry K. Silver, MD, started the first nurse practitioner (NP) program at the University of Colorado in 1965. Initially, it was a certificate program and later became a master's program in the 1970s. The first NPs were pediatric NPs who practiced in poor rural areas where there were no physicians (because of a severe shortage of primary care physicians).

REGULATION OF NURSE PRACTITIONERS
Educational Requirements
An NP must meet the minimal educational requirements that are mandated by the nurse practice act of the state (where they plan to practice).

State Nurse Practice Act
The nurse practice act is enacted into law by the state legislature. Therefore, the NP's legal right to practice is derived from the state legislature. Each state has its own nurse practice act that contains regulations that dictate the educational requirements, responsibilities, and scope of practice for NPs and other nurses (e.g., RNs, licensed practical nurses, midwives) who practice in the state. NP practice is not regulated by the federal government, the American Medical Association (AMA), or the U.S. Department of Health and Human Services (DHHS).

State Board of Nursing
The state board of nursing (SBON) is responsible for enforcing the state's nurse practice act. The SBON is a formal governmental agency that has the statutory authority to regulate nursing practice. The SBON has the legal authority to license, monitor, and discipline nurses. The SBON is also authorized to revoke a nurse's license (after formal hearings).

Title Protection
Professional designations, such as RN, NP, or APRN, are protected by law. It is illegal for any person to use these titles without a valid license. Title protection is under mandate by a state's nurse practice act. Title protection protects the public from unlicensed "nurses."

Licensure and Certification
Licensure is a legal requirement to practice as an NP. It is obtained through a governmental entity, the SBON. The NP must meet the minimal educational and clinical requirements in order to become licensed.

Certification is generally a "voluntary" process and is done through a nongovernmental entity such as a professional nursing association or specialty organization. The majority of states in the United States now mandate board certification (or certification) as a condition to obtain licensure.

Standards of Professional Nursing Practice
Standards are authoritative statements of the duties that all RNs, regardless of role, population, or specialty, are expected to perform. According to the American Nurses Association (ANA), these include both the Standards of Practice and the Standards of Professional Performance. They are developed by professional societies (e.g., ANA) as well as specialty organizations; for example, the American Association of Nurse Practitioners (AANP) publishes *Standards of Practice for Nurse Practitioners*.

EXAM TIP

NPs receive their "right to practice" from the state legislature.

Collaborative Practice Agreements
The state practice environment differs for each specific state. Some states allow full practice under the exclusive authority of the SBON, some states allow reduced practice, and some have restricted practice. In these states, the NP must be under the supervision or delegation of an outside health discipline such as the Board of Medicine.

A collaborative practice agreement is a written agreement between a physician and NP outlining the NP's role and responsibility to the clinical practice. A copy of the collaborative practice agreement must be kept at the NP's practice setting and mailed to the SBON. Most states require an annual review of the agreement that contains signatures of the individuals involved and dates.

Agreements With Physicians and Dentists
NPs can sign collaborative practice agreements with physicians (MDs), osteopaths (DOs), and dentists/dental surgeons (DMDs/DDSs). Chiropractors (DCs) and naturopaths (NDs) are not considered physicians under nurse practice acts. In some states, physicians are the only practitioners who can legally sign a death certificate.

Prescription Privileges

The majority of states require NPs to have a written practice protocol with a supervising physician in order to prescribe drugs. The protocol usually contains the list of drugs (by name, class, or condition) that an NP is allowed to prescribe. In the United States, all 50 states grant prescriptive authority to NPs, including the right to prescribe controlled substances (varies by state).

Prescription Pads

The NP's prescription pad or electronic prescribing record should contain the following:

- Practice setting name, NP's name, designation, and license number
- Clinic's name, address, and phone number; if the practice has several locations or sites, the other clinics where the NP practices should also be listed on the pad.
- To reduce fraud, it is best if the Drug Enforcement Administration (DEA) number is not listed (only for controlled substance prescriptions).

Food and Drug Administration–Controlled Substances

- Tamper-resistant prescription pads are required by Medicare and Medicaid, as well as when prescribing U.S. Food and Drug Administration (FDA)–controlled substances.
- A controlled substance prescription can be typed, but it must be signed by the prescribing practitioner the day it is issued.

SCHEDULE II DRUG PRESCRIPTIONS

- Substances in this schedule have a high potential for abuse with severe psychologic or physical dependence.
- These cannot be called in. They must be written on tamper-resistant pads and signed by the prescriber (not stamped).
- There is some variation among the different state laws regarding prescriptions of Schedule II drugs.
- Examples: Codeine, morphine, hydrocodone, oxycodone, opium, fentanyl, methadone, amphetamines.

E-Prescribing (Electronic Prescriptions)

- A method of sending prescriptions electronically directly to the pharmacy
- Preferred method of prescribing by Medicare and Medicaid

NURSING LEADERSHIP STYLES

SITUATIONAL LEADERSHIP

Leader is flexible and can adjust their leadership style to fit the changing needs of an organization. Can establish rapport easily and bring out the best in people. The result is that staff members are engaged with the goals of the organization and are more productive. Situational leadership theory was developed by Ken Blanchard and Paul Hersey.

TRANSFORMATIONAL LEADERSHIP

Leader has the ability to communicate vision to staff members. May have charismatic personality. Good communication skills. Staff members usually have higher job satisfaction with this type of leader.

LAISSEZ-FAIRE LEADERSHIP

Leader engages in minimal supervision and direction of staff members. Prefers "hands-off" approach. May not like to make decisions. This style of leadership works well if workers are experienced, like autonomy, and are self-directed. New or unexperienced staff may feel anxious with this type of authority because of minimal supervision and feedback.

AUTHORITARIAN LEADERSHIP (AUTOCRATIC)

Leader likes control and structure and prefers to give directions. May have many rules. Makes decisions with no (or minimal) staff input. Motivated, independent, and self-directed staff may be unhappy in this type of environment.

DEMOCRATIC LEADERSHIP

Leader may like to have more frequent staff meetings because they value staff members' input and feedback. Team shares in decision-making process, which may be slow due to desire to include all of staff in process. Leader values relationships and staff opinions.

SERVANT LEADERSHIP

Leader likes to work along with others in an effort to share power and encourage others to grow and develop. May assume many roles. Develops relationships with staff members and treats staff as individuals, which results in high job satisfaction for staff. But this type of leader may not like to make decisions that can be controversial.

EXAM TIP

There are various types of nursing leadership.

MALPRACTICE INSURANCE

The two types of malpractice insurance are claims based and occurrence based.

CLAIMS-BASED POLICY

This type of malpractice insurance covers claims only if the incident occurred when the NP paid the premium *and* only if the NP is still enrolled with the same insurance company at the time the claim is filed in court. The claim will not be covered (in the future) if they do not have the same insurance company as when the lawsuit was filed. Buying "tail coverage" can help address this issue.

Tail coverage insurance will cover the NP for malpractice claims that may be filed against them in the future. When an NP with claims-based malpractice insurance retires or changes jobs, it is advisable to buy tail coverage insurance. Example: An NP who has been retired for 2 years has a claim filed against her for an incident that occurred while she was employed and insured. The NP discontinued her claims-based malpractice insurance when she retired.

In this case, the claim will not be covered. But if she had bought tail coverage, then it would be covered.

OCCURRENCE-BASED POLICY

This type of malpractice policy is not affected by job changes or retirement. If a claim is filed against the NP in the future, it is covered if they had an occurrence-based policy at the time the incident occurred. Example: An NP who has been retired for 2 years has a claim filed against her for an incident that occurred while she was employed and insured. Since she carried an occurrence-based policy, the claim will be covered.

EXAM TIPS

- Claims-based malpractice insurance will cover claims only if the NP is still enrolled with the same insurance company at the time the claim is filed in court.
- Occurrence-type malpractice insurance will cover a lawsuit in the future even if the NP no longer carries the policy, as long as the NP had an active policy during the alleged incident.

MALPRACTICE LAWSUITS

- Plaintiff: The patient or whoever is acting on behalf of the patient (e.g., the patient's representative) who files the lawsuit claiming injury and/or damage by another party
- Defendant: The party who responds to the lawsuit filed by another party who claims an injury and/or damage (e.g., NP, hospital)

ELEMENTS OF A CASE

The plaintiff must prove that all of the following occurred:
- A duty is owed (a legal duty exists).
- The duty was breached (e.g., not following standard of care).
- The breach caused an injury (proximate cause).
- Damage occurred.

PHASES OF A MEDICAL MALPRACTICE TRIAL

- A lawsuit is filed in the appropriate court.
- The "discovery" phase (e.g., requesting of medical records, depositions, expert opinions) occurs.
- Plaintiff has the "burden of proof."
- Court trial phase (or settle out of court or arbitration) occurs.
- The judgment is given.
- Either the case is dismissed, or damages are awarded (e.g., physical harm, emotional/mental harm).

EXPERT WITNESSES

Ideally, the NP who will testify as an expert witness should be someone who practices in the same specialty and geographic area as the NP defendant. For example, an NP who practices in Los Angeles, California, may not be the best choice as an expert witness for an NP who is being sued and who is practicing in Miami, Florida.

REIMBURSEMENT

BUDGET RECONCILIATION ACT OF 1989 (HR 3299)

The first law allowing NPs to be reimbursed directly by Medicare. Prior to this act, only certified pediatric and family NPs were allowed to be primary providers as long as they practiced in designated "rural" areas.

BALANCED BUDGET ACT OF 1997

Together with the Primary Care Health Practitioner Incentive Act, this law broadened Medicare coverage of NP and clinical nurse specialist services. The Health Insurance Portability and Accountability Act (HIPAA) of 1996 required health providers to have a National Provider Identifier (NPI) number to bill Medicare and Medicaid. NPs can be reimbursed directly by Medicare Part B, Medicaid, Tricare, and some health insurance plans. Medicare will reimburse NPs at 85% of the Medicare Physician Fee Schedule.

NATIONAL PROVIDER IDENTIFIER NUMBER

The NPI is a unique 10-digit identification number assigned to healthcare providers (or to any entity that bills Medicare/Medicaid). It is issued by the National Plan and Provider Enumeration System (NPPES). All providers who provide services and bill Medicare must have an NPI number. Individual healthcare providers may obtain only one NPI for themselves.

To become a Medicare-approved provider, one must first obtain an NPI number online. An individual provider's NPI identifier lasts for their lifetime. The identifier does not change regardless of state or group affiliations. Medicare requires the NPI number for financial transactions. Electronic claims submission is required by Medicare and Medicaid. Medicare uses electronic fund transfer (EFT) to reimburse providers.

"INCIDENT TO" BILLING AND MEDICARE

"Incident to" billing is a way to bill Medicare for outpatient services rendered by a nonphysician health provider (NP, physician assistant [PA]) and receive the 100% physician fee. The location of the services can be at the physician's office, a separate or satellite office, or an institution or in the patient's home.

During the first visit, the physician must evaluate the patient (and write a care plan). Follow-up visits by the NP can be billed as "incident to" so long as the same health problems are being addressed. The physician's NPI number is used to bill for the service. The "incident to" billing is reimbursed at 100% of the physician rate. But if the same patient is seen for a new problem by the NP (or PA), then the visit is billed under the NP's or PA's NPI number (85% of physician fee).

MEDICAL CODING AND BILLING

Every time an NP bills Medicare, Medicaid, and/or a health insurance plan, they must submit an electronic claim. The claim form, or the "superbill," must contain both the *International Classification of Diseases*, 11th edition (*ICD-11*; World Health Organization [WHO], 2022) code(s) or the diagnosis and the Current Procedural Terminology (CPT) code(s). If a bill is missing the *ICD-11* code or CPT code, the bill will be rejected (not paid) and it has to be resubmitted with the required information. The services rendered must show medical necessity and the appropriateness of diagnostic and/or therapeutic services that were completed.

What Is the *ICD-11* Code?

The *ICD-11* code is used to indicate the patient's diagnosis as determined by the *International Classification of Diseases*, 11th edition (WHO, 2022). Each disease is assigned a specific *ICD-11* code.

EXAM TIPS

- The NPI contains 10 numbers/digits.
- The *ICD-11* is used for diagnosis codes. The CPT code is used to bill for outpatient office procedures and services. Both the *ICD-11* and CPT codes are required for each bill.

What Is the CPT?

The CPT is a five-digit code or alphanumeric code (letter with the digits) that is used to identify medical procedures (suturing, incision and drainage [I&D]) and other medical services. It is owned and maintained by the AMA.

What Are Evaluation and Management Service Codes?

Evaluation and Management Service (E&M) codes are used to bill for patient visits and are part of the CPT. If a bill is missing an E&M code, the healthcare provider will not be reimbursed for the time they spent with the patient. E&M codes are based on the history, examination, and medical decision-making (complexity) that take place. The provider must document that these three components have been met (or exceeded). The complexity and time spent with the patient are assigned codes by the CPT system. Example: A "problem-focused" visit requires documentation of the chief complaint with a brief history of present illness (HPI), but it does not require a review of systems (ROS) or a past, family, and/or social history.

EXAM TIPS

- Identify a problem-focused visit (see example in "What Are Evaluation and Management Service Codes?").
- "Incident to" billing is used for Medicare patients and refers to billing of a follow-up visit performed by a nonphysician provider billed under the physician's NPI number (the nonphysician provider is paid 100% vs. the rate of an NP or PA, who receives only 85%).

MEDICARE AND MEDICAID

Both Medicare and Medicaid programs are under the aegis of the Centers for Medicare & Medicaid Services (CMS). The CMS is one of the agencies under the U.S. Department of Health and Human Services (DHHS).

MEDICARE PART A (INPATIENT HOSPITALIZATION)

"Automatic" at age 65 if the person paid the premiums (automatically deducted from paycheck by the employer). If the person never paid the premiums (e.g., never worked outside the home), the person is not eligible for Medicare coverage. Also covers persons with end-stage renal diseases at any age. Certain religious groups (e.g., Amish, Mennonite) do not participate in Medicare. Medicare Part A will pay for the following "medically necessary" services:

- Inpatient hospitalization (including inpatient psychiatric hospitalization)
- Hospice care
- Home healthcare
- Skilled nursing facility (SNF) care

Medicare Part A will not pay for custodial care (nursing homes, retirement homes).

MEDICARE PART B (OUTPATIENT INSURANCE)

Medicare Part B is a voluntary program with monthly premiums. One must enroll during the "general enrollment period." Medicare Part B will pay for the following "medically necessary" services:

- Outpatient visits (including walk-in clinics, urgent care clinics, ED visits)
- Laboratory and other types of tests (EKsG, x-rays, CT scans)
- Durable medical equipment
- "Second opinions" with another physician (surgery)
- Kidney dialysis (outpatient), self-dialysis equipment/supplies, organ transplants, and many others
- Ambulance service for emergency care or transportation to a hospital or SNF if transport in any other vehicle will endanger patient's health

Medicare Part B does not pay for:

- Most eyeglasses and eye exams (except following cataract surgery that implants an intraocular lens)
- Hearing aids
- Most dentures and dental care
- Cosmetic plastic surgery (unless it is medically necessary)
- Over-the-counter drugs and most prescription drugs

Medicare Part B does pay for some health prevention services:

- Abdominal aortic aneurysm screening
- Influenza shots once a year and Pneumovax and Prevnar 13 (each once in a lifetime)
- Screening mammogram (once every 12 months for women age 40+)
- Hepatitis B vaccine series for individuals at medium or high risk
- Hepatitis C screening if high risk
- Screening colonoscopy or flexible sigmoidoscopy (age 50 years or older) every 10 years if low risk

- Routine Pap smears (once every 2 years or once every 12 months for women at high risk)
- Prostate cancer screening (digital rectal exam [DRE] and prostate specific antigen [PSA] once a year after age 50)
- Bone density testing allowed once every 24 months if at risk for osteoporosis, taking prednisone, or taking bisphosphonate therapy to monitor progress
- HIV screening; sexually transmitted infection screenings covered once every 12 months
- Physical exams (once a year)
- Smoking-cessation counseling and treatment
- Alcohol misuse screening and counseling
- Diabetes screening (twice yearly if at risk)
- Cardiovascular disease screening

MEDICARE ADVANTAGE (MEDICARE PART C)

Medicare Advantage Plans cover both inpatient care (Part A) and outpatient care (Part B), and some plans cover some prescription drugs. They are administered by private health insurance companies approved by Medicare.

MEDICARE PART D

- Also known as the Medicare prescription drug benefit. Only individuals who are enrolled (or eligible) for Medicare Part A and/or Part B are eligible. One type of Part D coverage is called the Medicare Advantage (MA) plan.
- All prescription drug plans have a list of preferred drugs (the formulary). If a nonformulary drug is used, it may not be covered, and the patient has to pay for it "out of pocket."

MEDICAID

Authorized by Title XIX of the Social Security Act. A federal and state matching program. Provides health insurance coverage for low-income individuals and their families who meet the federal poverty-level criteria. Covers children, pregnant women, adults, seniors, and individuals with disabilities (e.g., blindness). Pays for healthcare and prescription drugs.

Currently, Medicaid is the single largest payer for mental health services in the United States. It covers care offered by substance use disorder and family planning services (including contraception) as well as by maternal and infant health programs.

CHILDREN'S HEALTH INSURANCE PROGRAMS

The Children's Health Insurance Program (CHIP) and the Children's Health Insurance Program Reauthorization Act of 2009 (CHIPRA) cover uninsured children (infancy to adolescents) and pregnant women.

HEALTH TECHNOLOGY

TELEHEALTH

Telehealth is a broad term that encompasses a range of services and technologies designed to extend access, capacity, and delivery of healthcare, as well as to improve patient care and outcomes. Services include live videoconferencing (e.g., consultation between patient and provider), patient monitoring (e.g., devices that remotely collect and send patient data to providers or testing facilities), and mobile health (e.g., patient health portals or personal health apps). Telehealth is not restricted to clinical services; it can also include a wide range of nonclinical services such as provider training and continuing education. The full list of services payable under the Medicare Physician Fee Schedule can be found at www.cms.gov/Medicare/Medicare-General-Information/Telehealth/Telehealth-Codes.

Telemedicine, a subset of telehealth, refers to remote clinical services provided via secure audio and video connection. Telemedicine is commonly used for management of chronic conditions, medication management, follow-up visits, and specialist consultation.

HEALTH INFORMATION TECHNOLOGY FOR ECONOMIC AND CLINICAL HEALTH ACT

The Health Information Technology for Economic and Clinical Health Act (HITECH Act) was signed into law in 2009 as an incentive for healthcare providers to adopt the use of electronic health records (EHRs) and supporting technology. The act included incentives for early adoption of those technologies until 2015. After 2015, it began to issue financial penalties (e.g., reductions of Medicare and Medicaid reimbursement) for providers and entities who had not adopted EHR technologies. In addition, it strengthened enforcement of HIPAA security and privacy laws and penalties for breaches.

KNOWLEDGE CHECK: CHAPTER 27

1. A patient whose only source of insurance is Medicare Part A may be responsible for the entire cost of what type of care?
   A. Inpatient hospital care
   B. Inpatient psychiatric hospital care
   C. Custodial care
   D. Skilled nursing facility care

2. The nurse practitioner is discussing Medicare Part B with a patient. The nurse practitioner realizes there is a need for further patient education if the patient states:
   A. "Medicare Part B covers me because I'm older than 65."
   B. "Medicare Part B will cover the cost of my wheelchair."
   C. "Medicare Part B will cover my mammograms since I'm older than 50."
   D. "Medicare Part B will cover the anesthesia I received during my emergency appendectomy."

3. Some nurse practitioners bill directly for their services. Regarding reimbursement, who is considered a third-party payer?
   A. Patient
   B. Healthcare provider
   C. Health insurance company
   D. Federal government

4. Medicare Part D reimburses for which of the following services?
   A. Preventive healthcare such as routine Pap smears and physical exams
   B. Prescription drugs
   C. Alcohol use disorder counseling
   D. Over-the-counter drugs and vitamins

5. Which of the following statements is accurate regarding the HITECH Act?
   A. It required immediate conversion of patient records to electronic format.
   B. It provided insurance coverage for children and pregnant people.
   C. It provided financial incentives for adoption of telehealth technologies.
   D. It encouraged adoption of electronic health records.

6. Nurse practitioners and clinical nurse specialists derive their legal right to practice from:
   A. The nurse practice act in the state where they practice
   B. The laws of the state where they practice
   C. The Medicare statute
   D. The board of nursing in the state where they practice

7. Which is a *true* statement regarding claims-based malpractice insurance policies?
   A. If the insurance company's lawyer finds the nurse practitioner (NP) negligent, it is the NP's responsibility to pay for the claim.
   B. Claims against the NP are covered as long as the NP had an active malpractice policy at the time of the incident.
   C. Claims against the NP are usually paid if the NP is found not to be negligent.
   D. Claims against the NP are covered if both the incident and the claim happen when the policy is still active.

8. Which of the following statements is *correct* regarding certification for nurse practitioners?
   A. Certification is granted by state boards of nursing.
   B. Certification dictates the scope of practice within the United States.
   C. Certification grants the ability to practice within a state.
   D. Certification is obtained through a nongovernmental entity.

9. Which statement is *true* regarding a medical malpractice trial?
   A. The plaintiff claims that injury or damage could have resulted from malpractice.
   B. The discovery phase determines damages after judgment is given.
   C. The defendant has the burden of proof.
   D. The plaintiff must prove that a breach of duty occurred.

10. Which type of leader shares decisions and activities with group participants?
    A. Democratic
    B. Authoritarian
    C. Laissez-faire
    D. Situational

(See answers next page.)

1. C) Custodial care
Medicare Parts A and B do not cover custodial care or nursing home care (help with bathing, dressing, using bathroom, and eating). Medicare Part A coverage includes inpatient hospitalization, inpatient psychiatric hospitalization, and skilled care given in a certified skilled nursing facility.

2. D) "Medicare Part B will cover the anesthesia I received during my emergency appendectomy."
According to the Medicare.gov website, Medicare Part A covers anesthesia that is received while in an inpatient hospital. Medicare Part B covers outpatient care, durable medical equipment (e.g., wheelchair, walker), home health services, and other medical services, including some preventive services such as annual physical exams and mammograms (baseline age 50 years).

3. C) Health insurance company
Third-party payers are health insurance companies, health plans (health maintenance organizations or preferred provider organizations), Medicare, and Medicaid. The "first party" is the patient. The "second party" is the healthcare provider.

4. B) Prescription drugs
Medicare Part D is a voluntary program that charges a premium. Like all Medicare services, patients need to enroll during the "open enrollment" periods during the year (there is a penalty for late enrollment). There is a drug formulary, and not all drugs are available or reimbursed. Use of generic drugs is preferred, as there is a spending limit. Medicare Part B will reimburse for alcohol use disorder counseling and some preventive care. Medicare does not reimburse for vitamins and over-the counter medications.

5. D) It encouraged adoption of electronic health records.
When signed into law in 2009, HITECH provided financial incentives for healthcare providers to adopt electronic health records and strengthened privacy policies related to patient information. After 2015, HITECH began to issue financial penalties (e.g., reductions of Medicare and Medicaid reimbursement) for providers and entities who had not adopted electronic health record technologies. Coverage for uninsured children and pregnant people is provided by the Children's Health Insurance Program (CHIP) and the Children's Health Insurance Program Reauthorization Act of 2009 (CHIPRA). Although telehealth technologies can play an important role in providing care, and some telehealth services are reimbursable under Medicare, the technology was not addressed by HITECH.

6. A) The nurse practice act in the state where they practice
The nurse practice act is a statute enacted by the legislature of each state. The act delineates the legal scope of the practice of nursing within the geographic boundaries of the jurisdiction. The purpose of the act is to protect the public. The state board of nursing is the agency that enforces the nurse practice act. The Medicare statute provides the funds for paying for health services for those age 65 years and older.

7. D) Claims against the NP are covered if both the incident and the claim happen when the policy is still active.
As long as the NP has been paying the premiums to keep a claims-based policy active, the NP will be covered for any incident that occurs during that time. When the NP stops paying the premiums for a claims-based malpractice insurance policy, it is no longer active.

8. D) Certification is obtained through a nongovernmental entity.
Certification is obtained through a nongovernmental entity such as a professional nursing association or specialty organization. State boards of nursing have the power to license and discipline nurses, but not to grant nurse practitioner certifications. While scope of practice is heavily influenced by the specific certification, scope within each state is ultimately dictated by state legislatures through state nurse practice acts. The right to practice is obtained through licensure, not through certification.

9. D) The plaintiff must prove that a breach of duty occurred.
In a malpractice trial, the plaintiff must prove that a breach of duty occurred and that the direct outcome was injury and damage. The potential for injury is insufficient. The discovery phase, which includes the gathering of evidence and expert opinion, occurs after the lawsuit is filed but before the trial. The burden of proof lies with the plaintiff, not with the defendant.

10. A) Democratic
Democratic leadership is characterized by equality among the leader and other participants. Decisions and activities are shared. Authoritarian leadership, also known as autocratic leadership, is a leadership style characterized by individual control over all decisions and little input from group members. Laissez-faire leadership, also known as delegative leadership, is a type of leadership style in which leaders are hands-off and allow group members to make the decisions. Situational leadership is not based on a specific skill of the leader; instead, the leader modifies the style of management to suit the requirements of the organization.

28 NURSING RESEARCH

SOURCES OF DATA

PRIMARY SOURCES (PREFERRED)

In research, primary sources are preferred. They are the research from which the data originated. Primary sources are factual and not subject to interpretation by others.

SECONDARY SOURCES

Secondary sources are created when the original data (primary data) are interpreted or analyzed by another person (not the original researcher). These are "secondhand" accounts.

EXAM TIP

Primary data are the preferred source in research (original study that produced the data).

ETHICAL ISSUES IN NURSING RESEARCH

INSTITUTIONAL REVIEW BOARDS

An important duty of institutional review boards (IRBs) is to ensure the rights, safety, and welfare of human research subjects who are participating in research studies in their institution, hospital, or clinic. According to U.S. Food and Drug Administration (FDA) guidelines, IRBs have the authority to approve or reject research proposals that are submitted to their institution or hospital. If an IRB member has a conflict of interest, they must recuse themselves from deliberation and abstain from voting.

Committee Members

The members of the IRB committee are formally designated to review and monitor research that involves human subjects at their institution. The IRB members are individuals who are affiliated with the institution. Therefore, physicians, clinicians, or retail pharmacists who are not affiliated with the institution are generally not included in an IRB committee (unless they are hired as consultants). In addition, experienced staff members, not recent graduates, are preferred. The size of the IRB and the number of members depend on the type of institution.

EXAM TIP

Know the definition of an IRB. The IRB's most important role is to protect the rights of the human subjects enrolled in a study.

VULNERABLE POPULATIONS

Almost all types of biomedical and behavioral research in the United States require informed consent. "Vulnerable populations" require special protections and consent requirements:
- Infants and children younger than 18 years of age
- Pregnant patients
- Fetuses
- Prisoners
- Refugees, ethnic minorities
- Persons with mental or physical disabilities, visual or hearing impairment
- Persons who are economically disadvantaged

BELMONT REPORT

A report that outlines the important ethical principles that should be followed when performing research that involves human subjects. The Belmont Report was issued by the National Commission for the Protection of Human Subjects of Biomedical and Behavioral Research (1979).

TUSKEGEE SYPHILIS EXPERIMENT

The Tuskegee experiment was an infamous study of 600 African American sharecroppers (1932–1972) in Alabama. The men were all tested for syphilis infection, and those who had positive results were never informed or treated. Because of this study, laws were passed that protect human subjects' rights and mandate informed consent.

INFORMED CONSENT OF HUMAN SUBJECTS

Research subjects must be informed that they have the right to withdraw from the research study at any time without adverse consequences or penalty. There are additional requirements for minors and vulnerable subjects:
- Describe the study. Inform the subject of what they are expected to do (e.g., questionnaires, labs).
- Describe the risk or the discomforts of participating in the study in the present and the future (if applicable).
- Describe the benefits of participating in the study in the present and the future (if applicable).

- Discuss the alternatives to the study. Allow enough time for the subject to ask questions.
- Discuss whether there is any compensation or reward for participation.
- Discuss how confidentiality and data will be secured to protect the subject's identity.
- Give the number and/or email address of the contact for the study so that the subject can contact that person if they have any concerns or problems with the study.

MINORS

Any persons who are younger than 18 years of age.

Emancipated Minor Criteria

- Legal court document declaring that the minor is an "emancipated minor"
- Active duty in the U.S. military
- Legally binding marriage (or divorced from a legally binding marriage)

Consent Versus Assent

Consent may be given only by individuals who are aged 18 years or older. A minor (who is not emancipated) as young as the age of 7 years up to age 17 years can give assent to participate in a research study but cannot give consent legally. The child should be assured that they can withdraw from the study after discussing it with their parents.

The parent or legal guardian must first consent to the minor's participation in the study. In addition, the researcher needs parental permission to speak with the minor in order to obtain assent (the child signs a separate assent form).

EXAM TIPS

- Know which groups are considered vulnerable populations.
- Know the definition of assent. Assent refers to minors because they legally cannot give consent (unless an emancipated minor).

RESEARCH-RELATED TERMS

STATISTICAL SIGNIFICANCE

- α: Also known as the "significance level" or "p-value." It is usually set as either $p <.05$ or $p <.01$.
  - A significance level of $p <.05$ means that there is a 5% probability that study results are due to chance.
  - A significance level of $p <.01$ means that there is only a 1% probability that the study results are due to chance. Therefore, an α of $p <.01$ is "better" than an α of $p <.05$.
- Control group: Subjects in an experiment who do not receive treatment.

- N: This letter indicates the total size of the population.
- n: This letter indicates the number of subjects in the subpopulation.
- Significance level: Also known as the "α" or a "p-value." The p-value is usually set at either $p <.05$ or $p <.01$. See additional explanation under "α."

RESEARCH TERMS

Variables are any attribute or characteristic that varies and is measurable.

- Independent variable: Variable that is being manipulated and is used to influence the dependent variable. In experimental studies, the researcher has control over the independent variable.
- Dependent variable: This is the result of the manipulation of the independent variable. Example: Manipulation by researcher (independent variable) allows a response to manipulation that can be observed and measured (dependent variable).

EXAM TIPS

- Understand the difference between a dependent and an independent variable.
- Know the definition of N (total number of subjects) versus n (subgroup).

- Hypothesis: An idea (or supposition) that can be tested and refuted. When conducting research, an examiner tests a hypothesis (or several hypotheses) and can either accept or refute the hypothesis.
  - Null hypothesis (H_0): This is the opposite of the hypothesis being studied. Example: If the hypothesis is "Corn plants grow faster when exposed to sunlight," the null hypothesis is "Corn plants will not grow faster when exposed to sunlight." If the research data meet the set p-value ($p <.01$), the results are considered significant (not due to random chance), and the null hypothesis can be rejected. If the null hypothesis cannot be rejected, it means that there is no relationship between the variables, and the results are due to chance.
- Normal curve: A bell-shaped curve.
- Measures of distribution:
  - Mean: Also known as the average. Calculated by adding all of the scores together and dividing it by the total number of scores. Example: 5, 5, 5, 10, 10 ($35 \div 5 = 7$, average is "7").
  - Median: The number that is in the middle when values are arranged from lowest to highest (chronological order). Example: 1, 3, 4, **5**, 7, 10, 14 (median value is "5").
  - Mode: The most common value or frequently occurring value in a set of scores. Example: 3, 5, **7, 7, 7**, 8, 9, 10, 10 (mode is "7").
- Range: The difference between the largest and smallest values in a distribution. Example: 2, 3, 5, 7, 10, 15 ($15 - 2 = 13$, range is "13").

RESEARCH DESIGNS

TYPES OF STUDIES

Prospective

Studies done in the present (to the future). Longitudinal studies are a type of prospective study. Data are obtained in the present and then periodically measured in the future.

Retrospective

Studies done on events that have already occurred (e.g., chart reviews, recall of events). Another name for this study design is *ex post facto*.

Longitudinal

Long-term studies that follow the same group of subjects (or cohort) over many years to observe, measure, and compare the same variables over time. These are observational studies (with no manipulation or intervention). For example, the Framingham Heart Study has tracked the same research subjects ($N = 5,029$) from the town of Framingham, Massachusetts. The goal is to study the development and identify the risk factors that are associated with the development of cerebrovascular disease.

Cohort

Cohorts are simply groups of individuals that share some common characteristic (e.g., gender, age, job, ethnicity). Cohort studies are useful for studying the causative factors or risk factors of a disease(s). For example, the Nurses' Health Study is a longitudinal cohort study that examined the effects of oral contraceptive use in nurses over the long term. It has been expanded to study the effect of lifestyle choices on health.

Cross-Sectional

A cross-sectional study compares differences and similarities between two or more groups of people or phenomena and collects data at one point in time.

Case Study

An in-depth investigation of a single person, group, or phenomenon.

Descriptive

In these studies researchers observe and collect pertinent information but do not manipulate or change the environment. Also known as *observational studies*.

Correlational

A type of observational study in which the relationship (interrelationships) between at least two variables is evaluated. There are three types of correlations:

- Positive correlation: Two variables change together in the same direction. For example, when variable A increases, then variable B also increases.
- Negative correlation: An increase in one variable results in a decrease in the other. For example, when variable A increases, this causes variable B to decrease.
- No correlation: The variables are not related. For example, a change in variable A does not affect variable B.

Experimental

An important criterion is the use of random sampling and random assignment of research subjects. There is at least one control group and one (or more) intervention or treatment group (manipulation). Causality can be determined: If A + B occur, this will cause C.

Quasi-Experimental

The design is similar to an experimental study, except there is no randomization of the research subjects. Instead, recruitment of subjects is by convenience sample.

EXAM TIPS

- Experimental studies use randomization with subject selection.
- Correlational studies search for relationships between a minimum of two variables.

DEDUCTIVE VERSUS INDUCTIVE REASONING

Deductive Reasoning

Involves going from more general to more specific findings. Also known as "top-down" logic. In research, this means starting with a theory (generalization) and then narrowing it down by formulating specific hypotheses (deduction). Quantitative studies (Table 28.1) use deductive reasoning.

Inductive Reasoning

The opposite of deductive reasoning. Also known as "bottom-up" logic. Involves going from specific findings to generalizations. One starts with specific observations, and from these, one may detect a pattern that helps to formulate tentative hypotheses, which may help to generate new theory. Qualitative studies (see Table 28.1) use inductive reasoning.

EXAM TIP

Deductive logic is used with quantitative studies, and inductive logic is used in qualitative studies.

RESEARCH PROCESS

The phases of the research process generally can be summarized as follows:

- Phase I—Conception: Formulate research problem or question; review literature; develop hypothesis(es)
- Phase II—Design and Planning: Select research design; identify population/sample; determine protocols, methods, resources required, and ethical considerations; prepare proposal; submit to IRB for approval
- Phase III—Implementation: Recruit participants (obtain consent); implement research design; collect data

Table 28.1 Qualitative Versus Quantitative Studies

Component	Qualitative Studies	Quantitative Studies
Data	Involves words, narratives, subjective opinions	Numerical and measurable data
Number of subjects	Few individuals	May involve large numbers of individuals, databases
Subject recruitment	Small number of subjects, not randomized	Randomization possible if experimental design
Data gathering	In-depth interviews, focus groups, observations; audio or video is recorded, data are transcribed	Questionnaires, instruments, measurements, surveys
Logic	Inductive reasoning, specific data can be generalized	Deductive reasoning
Design	May change and evolve to adapt to situation or subjects	Systematic, design is known before research starts
Statistical testing	Interpretation of common themes and patterns; uses limited statistics such as chi-square	Pearson correlation, paired t-test, simple/multiple regression, analysis of variance (ANOVA), etc.
Notes	Researcher is a participant and also an observer (degree of participation varies)	Researcher is an objective observer, declares bias (funding sources)

- Phase IV—Analysis: Organize, analyze, and interpret data.
- Phase V—Dissemination: Prepare final report; publish and disseminate findings (e.g., journal articles, poster presentations, lectures).

HUMAN GENETIC SYMBOLS

The exam may include questions about genetic symbols (Table 28.2). The symbol for a healthy male is an empty square, and for a diseased/affected male, it is a filled square. The symbol for a healthy female is an empty circle, and for a diseased/affected female, it is a filled circle. A diagonal dash across a symbol means that the person is dead.

Table 28.2 Genetic Symbols

Gender	Symbol	Description
Healthy male	□	Empty square
Diseased male	■	Filled square
Healthy female	○	Empty circle
Diseased female	●	Filled circle
Death	⧄	Diagonal dash across a symbol

KNOWLEDGE CHECK: CHAPTER 28

1. What is the *best* description of a variable?
   A. It is an important part of every research study.
   B. It is the probability that a factor is important for the research data.
   C. It is the value or number that occurs the most frequently.
   D. It is a condition, characteristic, or factor that is being measured.

2. The research symbol that is used to indicate the "total population" in a research study is:
   A. n
   B. N
   C. P
   D. α

3. The *most* important job of an institutional review board (IRB) is to:
   A. Protect the interests of the hospital or research institution
   B. Protect the rights of the human subjects who participate in research done at the institution
   C. Protect the researcher and the research team from litigation
   D. Evaluate research protocols and methodology for appropriateness and safety

4. Which of the following groups is classified as a "vulnerable population" and has additional protections as human subjects?
   A. People who are incarcerated
   B. Parents of young children
   C. Elderly people
   D. Persons younger than 21 years

5. A data set consists of the values 1, 1, 2, 4, and 7. When considering this set, what term describes the number 3?
   A. Mode
   B. Median
   C. Mean
   D. Range

(See answers next page.)

1. D) It is a condition, characteristic, or factor that is being measured.

A variable is a condition, characteristic, or factor that is being measured. An independent variable is the one being manipulated that is not affected by the others. A dependent variable changes depending on the manipulation of the independent variable.

2. B) N

The correct symbol to indicate the total number of subjects in a study (total population) is N. For example, if a research study has a total number of subjects or total population of 100, then N = 100. The lower-case letter n is used to indicate a subpopulation. For example, if a study uses a total population of N = 100 that is divided into two groups of 50 subjects, then n = 50. The letter p is used to indicate p-value. The symbol α denotes the significance level.

3. B) Protect the rights of the human subjects who participate in research done at the institution

Every research institution has an IRB, whose job is to review all of the research that is conducted in that institution. The IRB's most important role is to protect the rights of the human subjects who participate in research done at the institution of which the IRB is a part (e.g., research hospital, university)

4. A) People who are incarcerated

Vulnerable populations, who require special protections and consent requirements in research, include people who are incarcerated, children younger than 18 years, pregnant people and fetuses, refugees, persons with disabilities, and those who are economically disadvantaged. There are no special protections afforded to parents, the elderly, or persons between the ages of 18 and 21.

5. C) Mean

The mean is the average of the set's values. In this case, the values in the set sum to 15; since there are 5 values, the mean is 3. The mode is the value that appears most frequently, which in this set is 1. The median is the value that appears in the middle of the set when its components are arranged from smallest to largest; this set's median is 2. The range is the difference between the smallest and largest values, which is 6 for this set.

EVIDENCE-BASED MEDICINE AND EPIDEMIOLOGY

EVIDENCE-BASED MEDICINE: DEFINITION

Evidence-based medicine (EBM) is "the conscientious, explicit and judicious use of current best evidence in making decisions about the care of individual patients" (www.cochrane.org). It is also known as evidence-based practice. There will be several questions on the American Nurses Credentialing Center (ANCC) exam that will test your ability to sort and rate articles by the level of evidence.

HIERARCHY OF RESEARCH EVIDENCE

- Meta-analysis: This is a statistical method that combines data from multiple studies (systematic review), resulting in higher statistical power and a single conclusion. This method is considered the gold standard for evaluating research evidence for EBM.
- Systematic review: A type of literature review that identifies, selects, and analyzes multiple research articles concerning a health condition, disease, or other

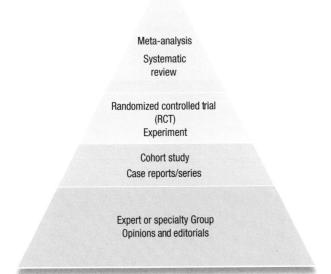

Figure 29.1 Ranking of research evidence.

health-related practice. Follows specific methodology to identify all the relevant studies on a specific topic. Studies to be included must meet explicit criteria. Studies are ranked from grade A (best evidence) to grade D (poor evidence). After a systematic review is done, the acceptable studies are pooled together, and statistical testing of the data (meta-analysis) is performed.

- Randomized controlled trial: Subjects are randomly assigned to either the control group or the treatment group(s). The intervention may be a drug, procedure, or device. Some randomized controlled trials (RCTs) use a double-blind design (the intervention is hidden from the patient, clinician, and/or researchers). RCTs are experimental studies.
- Experimental study: In a nutshell, an experiment involves random subject selection, one placebo or control group, and one or more intervention group(s). An RCT is a type of experimental study.
- Cohort study: A type of research that is used to investigate risk for diseases, risk factors for death, and other conditions. The research subjects are observed for a long period. There is no intervention done (not an experiment). The goal is to identify risk factors and associations (not causation) of a disease(s). Example: The Nurses' Health Study is a large cohort study of female RNs age 30 to 63 years who reside in the state of Massachusetts. A cohort study can be a type of prospective study (present to future).
- Case report: A detailed report of one patient with a disease or an unusual condition that includes demographics, signs and symptoms, diagnosis, response to treatment, and so forth.
- Case series: A series of case reports that involves a series of individuals who are given similar treatment.
- Opinions and editorials: Opinions and editorials can be biased and may not be based on solid evidence. They are the weakest form of evidence.

RESEARCH DATABASES

- Cochrane Reviews: The gold standard database and resource for EBM. These are systematic reviews (Cochrane Database of Systematic Reviews). The organization does not accept commercial or conflicted funding. Also known as the Cochrane Collaboration (www .cochrane.org).

- Medline®: The U.S. National Library of Medicine's (NLM) premier bibliographic database contains more than 26 million journal articles in the life sciences with a concentration in biomedicine. These articles are from 5,200 current biomedical journals published around the world. PubMed® is a component of Medline that contains more than 30 million citations of biomedical, medical, and other life science literature and abstracts.
- Cumulative Index to Nursing and Allied Health Literature (CINAHL): The world's largest source of full-text nursing and allied health journals (>1,300 journals). CINAHL provides indexing of more than 4,000 journals.

GRADES OF RESEARCH EVIDENCE

Research evidence receives a letter grade: A (best evidence), B, C, and D (poor evidence). Well-designed controlled experimental trials (double-blind RCTs) are considered to be grade A (or level 1) evidence.

STATISTICAL TERMS (EVIDENCE-BASED MEDICINE)

- CI: A measure of the degree of certainty in a sampling method. Example: A 95% CI is a range of values that you can be 95% certain contains the true mean of the population.
- Absolute risk reduction (ARR): A measure of the difference between two different treatments in terms of their ability to reduce a particular outcome (e.g., myocardial infarction [MI], stroke).
- Relative risk reduction (RRR): A measure of how much risk is reduced in the experimental group compared with the control group.
- Number needed to treat (NNT): The number of patients you have to treat to avoid one bad outcome (e.g., MI, stroke). Example: An NNT of seven means that it is necessary to treat seven patients to avoid one bad outcome.
- Positive predictive value (PPV): The probability that a person with a positive screening test result has the disease.
- Negative predictive value (NPV): The probability that a person with a negative test result does not have the disease.

EPIDEMIOLOGY TERMS

- Active immunity: Immunity to a disease developed either through vaccination or by infection.
- Passive immunity: Immunity to a disease after receiving antibodies (immunoglobins) from another host. Example: Colostrum from breastfeeding gives the neonate antibodies from the mother.
- Herd immunity: Resistance to a disease in a large number of people in the population, which is usually due to immunization programs.
- Health: A state of complete physical, mental, and social well-being.
- Horizontal transmission: Transmission of an infecting agent from one individual to another. Example: Horizontal transmission of HIV and other sexually transmitted infections occurs through sexual intercourse.
- Vertical transmission: Transmission of an infecting agent from mother to infant. Congenital infections from mother to infant can be passed through vertical transmission. Also, an HIV-positive mother who breastfeeds her infant can infect her infant with HIV through vertical transmission.
- Endemic: A baseline level of a particular disease in a population.
- Epidemic: Rapid increase of a disease in a population that involves a large number of people.
- Pandemic: An epidemic that occurs over a very large area (several countries or continents). It involves a large proportion of the global population.
- Morbidity: An illness or any departure from physical and/or mental health.
- Mortality: Death.
- Infant mortality: Infant deaths per 100,000 live births. The leading cause of death in an infant's first year of life is congenital malformations (including chromosomal abnormalities).
- Sensitivity: Ability of a screening test to correctly identify a person *with* the disease.
- Specificity: Ability of a screening test to correctly identify a person *without* the disease.

EXAM TIPS

- Memorize the definitions of sensitivity and specificity.
- Learn the difference between endemic, epidemic, and pandemic.

KNOWLEDGE CHECK: CHAPTER 29

1. According to evidence-based medicine (EBM) experts, which of the following types of research has the *lowest* ranking?
   A. Randomized controlled trial (RCT)
   B. Experimental study
   C. Cohort study
   D. Editorial

2. Which of the following definitions describes the term specificity?
   A. Ability of a screening test to correctly identify a person with a disease
   B. Probability that a person with a negative test result does not have the disease
   C. Degree of certainty in a sampling method
   D. Ability of a screening test to correctly identify a person without a disease

3. Which type of evidence identifies, selects, and analyzes multiple research articles concerning a health condition, disease, or other health-related topic?
   A. Meta-analysis
   B. Cohort study
   C. Systematic review
   D. Case series

4. Which of the following definitions describes the term "epidemic"?
   A. Rapid increase of a disease in a population that involves a large number of people
   B. Resistance to a disease in a large number of people in a population
   C. Baseline level of a particular disease in a population
   D. Rapid increase of a disease that occurs over a very large area (several countries or continents)

5. According to evidence-based medicine (EBM) experts, which of the following types of research provides the *highest* level of evidence?
   A. Meta-analysis
   B. Randomized controlled trial (RCT)
   C. Cohort study
   D. Expert opinion

(See answers next page.)

1. D) Editorial

Editorials and professional society opinions are considered the lowest level of evidence because they are subjective and not based on research. The ranking of types of research is as follows: (1) RCT, (2) experimental study, (3) cohort study, and (4) editorial.

2. D) Ability of a screening test to correctly identify a person without a disease

Specificity measures the ability of a screening test to correctly identify a person without a disease. It is often confused with sensitivity, which measures the ability of a screening test to correctly identify a person with a disease. Negative predictive value is the probability that a person with a negative test result does not have the disease, and confidence interval measures the degree of certainty in a sampling method.

3. C) Systematic review

A *systematic review* is a literature review that identifies, selects, and analyzes multiple research articles concerning a health condition, disease, or other health-related topic. A *meta-analysis* is a statistical method that combines data from multiple studies (systematic review), resulting in higher statistical power and a single conclusion. A case series is a collection of case reports (a case report is the report of one patient with a disease or an unusual condition) that features multiple individuals who are given similar treatment. A cohort study is used to investigate risk factors and causes of disease. An example of a cohort study is the Framingham Study.

4. A) Rapid increase of a disease in a population that involves a large number of people

Epidemic is the rapid increase of a disease in a population that involves a large number of people. A pandemic is the rapid increase of a disease (epidemic) that occurs over a very large area (several countries or continents). Endemic is the baseline level of a particular disease in a population, and herd immunity is the resistance to a disease in a large number of people in a population.

5. A) Meta-analysis

Meta-analyses and systematic reviews offer the highest level of evidence. The ranking of types of research is as follows: (1) meta-analysis, (2) RCT, (3) cohort study, and (4) expert opinion.

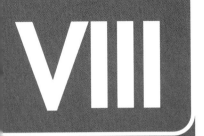

PRACTICE TESTS

30 PRACTICE TEST I

This practice test is based on the blueprint for the American Academy of Nurse Practitioners Certification Board (AANPCB) Family Nurse Practitioner certification exam.*
It includes 150 questions.

1. The nurse practitioner overhears a coworker explaining the Health Insurance Portability and Accountability Act (HIPAA) to a patient. Which statement from the coworker requires correction?
   A. "HIPAA provides federal protections for personal health information."
   B. "HIPAA applies to all healthcare providers and payers who bill electronically and send health information over the internet."
   C. "Patients have the right to view their mental health–related and psychotherapy-related health information."
   D. "HIPAA gives patients the right to view and correct errors in their medical records."

2. A patient who has been prescribed warfarin (Coumadin) is advised to monitor carefully when eating leafy green vegetables for which of the following reasons?
   A. The high vitamin K levels will decrease the international normalized ratio (INR).
   B. The vegetables have too much ascorbic acid, which can interact with the medicine.
   C. The high-fiber content will decrease the absorption of the warfarin (Coumadin).
   D. The vitamins in the vegetables will increase the activity of the warfarin (Coumadin).

3. The parent of an 8-year-old boy reports the presence of a round red rash on the child's left lower leg. It appeared 1 week after the child returned from visiting his grandparents, who live in Massachusetts. During the skin exam, the maculopapular rash is noted to have areas of central clearing, making it resemble a round target. Which condition is most likely?
   A. Erythema migrans
   B. Rocky Mountain spotted fever
   C. Meningococcemia
   D. Larva migrans

4. A 74-year-old male patient presents with an acute-onset unilateral headache with a reddened and indurated temple. The patient is at risk for:
   A. Vertigo
   B. Amaurosis fugax
   C. Ptosis
   D. Cranial nerve (CN) VII paralysis

5. A young adult patient with myasthenia gravis is diagnosed with pertussis. Which antibiotic is considered generally safe in a patient with this condition?
   A. Erythromycin
   B. Trimethoprim-sulfamethoxazole
   C. Clarithromycin
   D. Azithromycin

6. A patient presents with a new onset of jaundiced sclera, right upper quadrant tenderness, and anorexia. The nurse practitioner (NP) draws labs with the following results: aspartate transaminase (AST) = 24 mg/dL; alanine transaminase (ALT) = 13 mg/dL; HbsAg = negative; anti-HBc = negative; anti-HBs = positive. How will the NP interpret these data?
   A. The patient has never been exposed to hepatitis B.
   B. The patient has never been exposed to hepatitis D.
   C. The patient has immunity from hepatitis B vaccinations.
   D. The patient has active hepatitis B.

7. Which of the following laboratory tests is the most sensitive test for evaluating an active *Helicobacter pylori* infection of the stomach or duodenum?
   A. *H. pylori* titer
   B. Fasting gastrin level
   C. Upper gastrointestinal (GI) series
   D. Urea breath test

8. The nurse practitioner (NP) is assessing a 63-year-old male patient who has a history of intravenous drug use as a young adult. He presents with fatigue, nausea, pruritus, and icteric sclera. Which screening will the NP recommend for this patient?
   A. Chest x-ray
   B. Urine specimen
   C. Hepatitis C virus antibody test
   D. Electroencephalogram

---

* AANPCB is the sole owner of its certification programs. It does not endorse this exam preparation resource, nor does it have a proprietary relationship with Springer Publishing.

9. A 10-year-old child presents with external ear pain, swelling, and decreased hearing in the left ear. The child is on a swim team and practices daily. Upon physical examination, the child does not want the left ear touched. There are no other abnormal findings. The nurse practitioner will advise the patient to (Select all that apply.):
   A. Use aluminum acetate solution as needed.
   B. Keep water out of the ear during treatment.
   C. Apply polymyxin B-neomycin-hydrocortisone suspension drops four times a day for 7 days.
   D. Apply steroid nasal spray twice daily for 1 week.
   E. Take levofloxacin for 10 days.

10. An 18-year-old female patient is being followed up for acne by the nurse practitioner (NP). During the facial exam, papules and pustules are noted, mostly on the forehead and the chin areas. The patient has been using over-the-counter (OTC) topical antibiotic gels and medicated soap daily for 6 months without much improvement. The NP will recommend:
    A. Isotretinoin (Amnesteem)
    B. Tetracycline (Sumycin)
    C. Clindamycin topical solution (Cleocin-T)
    D. Minoxidil (Rogaine)

11. During a sports participation exam of a 14-year-old high school athlete, the nurse practitioner notes a split of the S2 component of the heart sound during deep inspiration that disappears upon expiration. The heart rate is regular, and no murmurs are auscultated. Which of the following is a *true* statement regarding this finding?
    A. This is an abnormal finding and should be evaluated further by a cardiologist.
    B. A stress test should be ordered.
    C. This is a normal finding in some young athletes.
    D. An echocardiogram should be ordered.

12. The nurse practitioner (NP) is evaluating a 72-year-old male patient with an acute flare-up of gout. Which medication will the NP prescribe?
    A. Colchicine
    B. Celecoxib (Celebrex)
    C. Calcium gluconate
    D. Steroid injection

13. The nurse practitioner notices a medium-pitched, harsh systolic murmur during an episodic examination of a 37-year-old female patient. It is best heard at the right upper border of the sternum. Which condition is most likely?
    A. Mitral stenosis
    B. Aortic stenosis
    C. Pulmonic stenosis
    D. Tricuspid regurgitation

14. A middle-aged female patient is seen by the nurse practitioner (NP) for a hypertension management follow-up. The patient has been taking chlorthalidone (Hygroton) 12.5 mg daily for 30 days and has a history of smoking, emphysema, and breast cancer. The patient's current blood pressure is 168/92 mmHg. What adjustment will the NP make to the treatment plan?
    A. Add propranolol (Inderal).
    B. Decrease chlorthalidone (Hygroton).
    C. Increase chlorthalidone (Hygroton).
    D. Add captopril (Capoten).

15. The nurse practitioner (NP) is performing a sports participation physical for a male high school student who plays football. His body mass index (BMI) is calculated at 26, and his parent is concerned that it is too high. What educational information should the NP share with the patient and the parent?
    A. BMI is a set parameter used as an indicator for obesity.
    B. BMI can be elevated in people with higher muscle mass.
    C. BMI is not a good tool to use to measure obesity.
    D. BMI varies in individuals of similar stature.

16. Which of the following findings is associated with thyroid hypofunction?
    A. Graves disease
    B. Eye disorder
    C. Thyroid storm
    D. Myxedema coma

17. The nurse practitioner orders a pulmonary function test for a patient exhibiting signs of an obstructive lung disease. Which of the following is a potential diagnosis?
    A. Asthma
    B. Pleural disease
    C. Pulmonary fibrosis
    D. Diaphragm obstruction

18. Which hematologic finding would be expected in an 18-month-old patient diagnosed with beta thalassemia minor?
    A. Decreased hemoglobin A
    B. Normochromic red blood cells (RBCs)
    C. Elevated mean corpuscular volume
    D. Elevated mean corpuscular hemoglobin concentration

19. A 2-day-old full-term infant presents with jaundice symptoms. Which of the following interventions should be implemented first?
    A. Check bilirubin level.
    B. Schedule a follow-up visit.
    C. Advise parent to feed infant five to six times per day.
    D. Prescribe phototherapy.

20. A nurse practitioner sees a fair-skinned patient who is experiencing recurrent small acne-like pustules and papules on the cheeks, nose, and chin, as well as chronic dry eyes. Which diagnosis is most likely?
    A. Rocky Mountain spotted fever
    B. Herpes zoster ophthalmicus
    C. Acne rosacea
    D. Actinic keratosis

21. Which finding will the nurse practitioner expect to see in a 13-year-old male patient with Cushings syndrome?
    A. Excess estrogen
    B. Delayed puberty
    C. Pseudogynecomastia
    D. Accelerated growth in height

22. A recreational soccer player presents with knee pain following a game. On examination, the nurse practitioner notes swelling and joint line tenderness in the knee. McMurray's test is positive, and a Lachman's test is negative. Which diagnosis is most likely?
    A. Anterior cruciate ligament (ACL) tear
    B. Lateral collateral ligament (LCL) tear
    C. Meniscus tear
    D. Traumatic knee sprain

23. Which lifestyle factor is associated with secondary polycythemia vera?
    A. High-fat diet
    B. Smoking
    C. Alcohol use disorder
    D. Sedentary lifestyle

24. An elderly patient presenting with a cough with blood-tinged sputum and fever is diagnosed with pneumonia. Which of the following organisms is most likely to be the cause?
    A. *Haemophilus influenzae*
    B. *Bordetella pertussis*
    C. *Treponema pallidum*
    D. *Streptococcus pneumoniae*

25. Which class of diuretics is contraindicated in patients who are allergic to sulfa products?
    A. Thiazides
    B. Beta-blockers
    C. Direct renin inhibitors
    D. Potassium-sparing diuretics

26. Resonance over the lungs upon percussion may indicate which condition?
    A. Emphysema
    B. None; normal lung tissue
    C. Bacterial pneumonia
    D. Pleural effusion

27. An 82-year-old female patient presents to the nurse practitioner (NP) with fatigue and complaints of watery diarrhea. She states she may have a dozen watery stools per day accompanied by stomach cramps. Upon assessment, the NP notes the patient is currently taking a course of antibiotics for acute bronchitis. Which diagnosis is most likely?
    A. Hepatitis B
    B. *Clostridium difficile* colitis
    C. Allergic reaction to the antibiotics
    D. Acute pancreatitis

28. The nurse practitioner is screening a patient for melanoma using the ABCDE acronym. An abnormal finding is a lesion with a diameter of how many millimeters?
    A. <2 mm
    B. <3 mm
    C. >6 mm
    D. <4 mm

29. A 25-year-old patient with a history of diabetes is positive for serum ketones and has a serum glucose level >300 mg/dL. Which diagnosis is most likely?
    A. Diabetes insipidus
    B. Diabetic ketoacidosis
    C. Hypoglycemia
    D. Somogyi phenomenon

30. A new female patient is 40 years old and works as a postal employee. She is being evaluated for complaints of a new-onset erythematous rash on both cheeks and the bridge of the nose, accompanied by fatigue. She reports a history of Hashimoto thyroiditis and is currently being treated with levothyroxine (Synthroid) 1.25 mg daily. Which of the following conditions is most likely?
    A. Atopic dermatitis
    B. Thyroid disease
    C. Lupus erythematosus
    D. Rosacea

31. A 40-year-old female patient complains of periods of dizziness and palpitations that have a sudden onset. The EKG shows P-waves before each QRS complex and a heart rate of 170 beats/min. A carotid massage decreases the heart rate to 80 beats/min. These findings best describe:
    A. Ventricular tachycardia
    B. Paroxysmal atrial tachycardia
    C. Atrial fibrillation
    D. Ventricular fibrillation

32. Which medication can be prescribed to a patient to manage both hypertension and benign prostatic hyperplasia (BPH)?
    A. Silodosin (Rapaflo)
    B. Terazosin (Hytrin)
    C. Finasteride (Proscar)
    D. Phenoxybenzamine (Dibenzyline)

33. A middle-aged female patient with a history of osteoarthritis and asthma reports to the nurse practitioner that she has been taking ibuprofen twice daily for many years. Which organ systems are at risk of damage from chronic nonsteroidal anti-inflammatory drug (NSAID) use? (Select all that apply.)
A. Endocrine
B. Respiratory
C. Gastrointestinal
D. Renal
E. Cardiovascular

34. A 78-year-old female patient presents with confusion, hallucinations, and seizures. Her spouse reports that she has been taking amitriptyline (Elavil) for 20 years. The nurse practitioner performs an EKG. The EKG reading (which follows) that indicates that the patient may be experiencing an overdose is:

A.
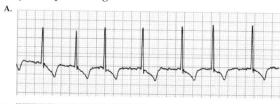

B.
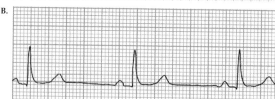

C.
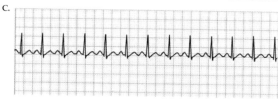

D.
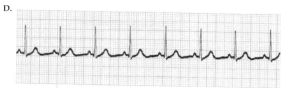

35. Treatment for mild preeclampsia includes which of the following? (Select all that apply.)
A. Bedrest with bathroom privileges
B. Close monitoring of weight and blood pressure
C. Close follow-up of urinary protein, serum creatinine, and platelet count
D. Prescription of methyldopa (Aldomet) to control blood pressure
E. Administration of magnesium sulfate

36. A 19-year-old female patient has recently been diagnosed with acute hepatitis B. She is sexually active and monogamous. She reports that her male partner uses condoms inconsistently. What would the nurse practitioner recommend for her partner who was also tested for hepatitis with the following results: HBsAg (-), anti-HBc (-), anti-HBs (-), anti-HCV (-), anti-HAV (+)?
A. Hepatitis B vaccination
B. Hepatitis B immunoglobulin
C. Hepatitis B vaccination and hepatitis B immunoglobulin
D. No vaccination needed at this time

37. The nurse practitioner sees a 58-year-old female patient who reports abscesses and pustules in the axilla and groin and under the breasts, which burst and drain purulent green discharge. She has a history of smoking and a body mass index (BMI) of 37.1. Which diagnosis is most likely?
A. Impetigo
B. Carbuncles
C. Shingles
D. Hidradenitis suppurativa

38. Which gram-positive pathogen most commonly causes meningitis?
A. *Neisseria meningitidis*
B. *Streptococcus pneumoniae*
C. *Haemophilus influenzae*
D. *Klebsiella pneumoniae*

39. A patient complains of shortness of breath and coughing shortly after starting exercise, as well as during exercise. After asking the patient to run on a treadmill for 5 minutes, the nurse practitioner (NP) auscultates expiratory wheezes in the lower bases. Which drug class will the NP prescribe?
A. Short-acting beta2-agonist (SABA)
B. Combination of inhaled corticosteroid (ICS) with long-acting beta2-agnoist (LABA)
C. Long-acting beta2-agonist (LABA)
D. Inhaled corticosteroid (ICS)

40. Which test will confirm the diagnosis of prostate cancer?
A. Prostate-specific antigen (PSA)
B. Digital rectal exam (DRE)
C. Complete blood count (CBC) with differential
D. Tissue biopsy

41. A 60-year-old female patient who works as a truck driver presents to the outpatient urgent care clinic of a hospital complaining of worsening of her low-back pain the past few days. Pain is accompanied by numbness in the perineal area. She describes the pain as "sharp and burning" and points to the left buttock. She reports that the pain started on the mid-buttock of the left leg and recently started to go down the lateral aspect of the leg toward the top of the foot. During the physical exam, the ankle jerk and the knee jerk reflex are 1+ on the affected leg and 2+ on the other leg. The pedal, posterior tibialis, and popliteal pulses are the same on both legs. Which of the following actions should the nurse practitioner consider first for this patient?
   A. Order an MRI scan of the lumbosacral spine as soon as possible.
   B. Write a prescription for ibuprofen with a muscle relaxant and advise the patient to follow up with her primary care provider within 3 days.
   C. Refer the patient to an orthopedic surgeon.
   D. Refer the patient to physical therapy for 10 to 12 weeks.

42. A 30-year-old female patient reports having had no period for the past 12 weeks. She is sexually active, and her male partner has been using condoms inconsistently. The urine pregnancy test result is positive. Which of the following is a true statement regarding this pregnancy?
   A. The fundus of the uterus should be at the level of the symphysis pubis.
   B. The cervix should be dilated about 0.5 inches at this time of gestation.
   C. "Quickening" starts during this period.
   D. Hegar sign is present during this period of pregnancy.

43. A patient has been managed for Graves' disease for 2 years. During a recent office visit, the patient is found to also have atrial fibrillation. Which new medication will the nurse practitioner add to the treatment regimen?
   A. Furosemide (Lasix)
   B. Warfarin (Coumadin)
   C. Cholestyramine (Prevalite)
   D. Metoprolol (Lopressor)

44. A female patient experiencing frequent urinary tract infections (UTIs) and vaginal infections is being seen in the office for the third time in 7 months with complaints of urinary burning and frequency, vaginal discharge, and severe itching. The nurse practitioner orders testing for which possible underlying condition?
   A. Diabetes insipidus
   B. Anemia
   C. *Helicobacter pylori* infection
   D. Diabetes mellitus

45. A school-age child presents with low-grade fever and suspected hearing loss. Upon examination, the nurse practitioner notes erythema and bullae on the bulging tympanic membrane. There is decreased motility of the tympanic membrane on insufflation. Which diagnosis is most likely?
   A. Otitis externa
   B. Bullous myringitis
   C. Purulent otitis media
   D. Serous otitis media

46. A 49-year-old female patient complains of generalized morning stiffness, especially in both wrists and hands. It is much worse in the morning and lasts for a few hours. She also complains of fatigue and generalized body aches that have been present for the past few months. Which of the following is most likely?
   A. Osteoporosis
   B. Rheumatoid arthritis
   C. Osteoarthritis
   D. Gout

47. What would be included in the initial treatment plan for a patient experiencing a transient ischemic attack (TIA)?
   A. Schedule CT and/or MRI within 48 hours of attack.
   B. Initiate daily aspirin therapy.
   C. Prescribe high-dose steroids.
   D. Maintain blood pressure below 160/90 mmHg

48. A 68-year-old patient arrives at the clinic reporting a sudden, erupting rash on their forehead and temple area, with a swollen eye on the same side. The patient is experiencing photophobia, eye pain, and blurred vision. To which specialist will the nurse practitioner refer the patient?
   A. Neurologist
   B. Dermatologist
   C. Oncologist
   D. Ophthalmologist

49. A 70-year-old patient presents to the urgent care clinic with complaints of a "blinding headache." Vital signs reveal a blood pressure of 200/110 mmHg. The patient notes a 10-year history of taking atenolol (Tenormin) and occasional use of fluticasone (Flovent) over the past 3 years. Which of the following questions should the nurse practitioner ask the patient?
   A. "Do you have a family history of hypertension?"
   B. "Do you have a family history of hypercholesterolemia?"
   C. "Are you currently using fluticasone (Flovent)?"
   D. "Do you have a history of migraine headaches?"

50. Which medication is contraindicated in a 4-year-old child diagnosed with impetigo?
   A. Amoxicillin
   B. Dicloxacillin
   C. Tetracycline
   D. Mupirocin

51. Which condition is a core disorder on the recommended uniform screening panel (RUSP) for newborns?
    A. Hypermethioninemia
    B. Tyrosinemia type II
    C. Galactokinase deficiency
    D. Congenital adrenal hyperplasia

52. The nurse practitioner is educating a patient newly diagnosed with migraines about potential triggers. What statement by the patient suggests that more teaching is required?
    A. "Cigarette smoke could precipitate a migraine."
    B. "I should avoid foods that are high in potassium."
    C. "My sleep patterns should be as consistent as possible."
    D. "Stress reduction techniques could be helpful."

53. A middle-aged male patient presents with right eyelid pain for 24 hours. He denies vision changes or discharge from the eye. Upon physical examination, the nurse practitioner (NP) notes a painful, swollen red abscess on the upper right eyelid. How will the NP document this finding?
    A. Cholesteatoma
    B. Papilledema
    C. Pinguecula
    D. Hordeolum

54. An elderly patient who is in excellent health is concerned about staying healthy in their retirement years. They are unsure of their vaccination history. Which vaccinations will the nurse practitioner recommend? (Select all that apply.)
    A. Shingles/zoster vaccination
    B. Annual influenza vaccination
    C. Pneumococcal vaccine
    D. Human papillomavirus (HPV) vaccination
    E. Measles, mumps, rubella (MMR)

55. A middle-aged male patient with hypertension presents to the public health clinic with complaints of an acute onset of fever, chills, and cough that is productive of rusty-colored sputum. The patient reports episodes of sharp pains on the left side of his back and chest whenever he is coughing. His temperature is 102.2°F, pulse is 100 beats/min, and blood pressure is 130/80 mmHg. Urinalysis does not show leukocytes, nitrites, or blood. These findings are most consistent with:
    A. Atypical pneumonia
    B. Upper urinary tract infection
    C. Bacterial pneumonia
    D. Acute pyelonephritis

56. A 20-year-old pregnant patient has been diagnosed with gonorrhea. The nurse practitioner should test the patient for:
    A. Herpes simplex virus 1 (HSV-1)
    B. Genital warts
    C. Syphilis
    D. Chlamydia

57. Which patient is a potential candidate for oral contraceptive use?
    A. Sexually active patient with amenorrhea
    B. Patient with history of emboli that resolved with heparin therapy 15 years ago
    C. 29-year-old patient who smokes cigarettes
    D. Patient with hepatitis C infection

58. The nurse practitioner would test the obturator and psoas muscles to evaluate for:
    A. Cholecystitis
    B. Acute appendicitis
    C. Inguinal hernia
    D. Gastric ulcer

59. When assessing a patient using a Snellen chart, the nurse practitioner records the visual acuity as 20/80. This assessment means that the patient:
    A. Can see at 20 feet what a person with normal vision sees at 80 feet
    B. Can see at 80 feet what a person with normal vision sees at 20 feet
    C. Has experienced a 20% decrease in acuity in one eye and an 80% decrease in the opposite eye
    D. Has presbyopia

60. Physiologic anemia of pregnancy is caused by:
    A. Increase in the cardiac output at the end of the second trimester
    B. Physiologic decrease in the production of ed blood cells (RBCs) in pregnant patients
    C. Increase of up to 50% of the plasma volume in pregnant patients
    D. Increase in the need for dietary iron in pregnancy

61. A 28-year-old female patient is seen in the office with acne, hirsutism, and oligomenorrhea. Blood is drawn for a free androgen index (FAI), and the results reveal a 9.8 level. The diagnosis is polycystic ovary syndrome (PCOS), which puts the patient at additional risk for which condition(s)? (Select all that apply.)
    A. Congestive heart failure
    B. Metabolic syndrome
    C. Infertility
    D. Type 2 diabetes mellitus
    E. Endometriosis

62. Upon auscultation of a 6-year-old patient, the nurse practitioner (NP) hears a systolic murmur that sounds like a musical vibration and becomes louder in the supine position. The murmur is grade I/II in intensity with minimal radiation. The NP will:
    A. Refer the patient to a pediatric cardiovascular surgeon.
    B. Refer the patient to a pediatric cardiologist.
    C. Note on the record to monitor with an annual physical exam.
    D. Schedule an echocardiogram.

63. During a physical examination, the nurse practitioner palpates the right upper quadrant (RUQ) while the patient takes a deep inspiration. Which diagnostic test is being performed?
    A. Markle test
    B. Rovsing sign
    C. Murphy sign
    D. Psoas test

64. An elderly, fair-skinned male patient presents to the clinic for a routine examination. The nurse practitioner notes a lesion on his nose. The lesion is a small, translucent papule with a central ulceration, telangiectasia, and rolled borders. Which diagnosis is most likely?
    A. Acral lentiginous melanoma
    B. Basal cell carcinoma
    C. Actinic keratosis
    D. Seborrheic keratosis

65. A 14-year-old boy is brought in by his parents, who report that their son has been complaining for several months of recurrent bloating, stomach upset, and occasional loose stools. They report that the patient has difficulty gaining weight and is short for his age. They have noticed that his symptoms are worse after eating large amounts of crackers, cookies, and breads. They deny seeing blood in the patient's stool. Which of the following conditions is most likely?
    A. Amebiasis
    B. Malabsorption
    C. Crohn colitis
    D. Celiac disease

66. A cauliflower-like growth with foul-smelling discharge is seen during an otoscopic exam of the left ear of an 8-year-old boy with a history of chronic otitis media. The tympanic membrane and ossicles are not visible, and the patient seems to have difficulty hearing the nurse practitioner's instructions. Which condition is most likely?
    A. Chronic perforation of the tympanic membrane with secondary bacterial infection
    B. Chronic mastoiditis
    C. Cholesteatoma
    D. Cancer of the middle ear

67. A 67-year-old female patient presents with a 3-day-old cat bite that has become swollen, reddened, and painful to the touch. The nurse practitioner (NP) notes there is purulent discharge at the site of the bite. Which medication will the NP prescribe?
    A. Gentamicin
    B. Tetanus toxoid
    C. Rabies prophylaxis
    D. Amoxicillin-clavulanate (Augmentin)

68. An elderly patient presents with a new onset of sleepiness, weight gain of 10 pounds in a month, xerosis, and anomia. The patient's lab values are free thyroxine (T4) of 0.8 ng/dL, thyroid-stimulating hormone (TSH) of 7.2 mU/L, and a score of 28 on the Mini-Mental State Examination (MMSE). Which medication will the nurse practitioner prescribe?
    A. Levothyroxine (Synthroid)
    B. Propylthiouracil (Tapazole)
    C. Memantine (Namenda)
    D. Carbidopa-levodopa (Sinemet)

69. Heberden nodes are commonly found in which of the following diseases?
    A. Rheumatoid arthritis
    B. Osteoarthritis
    C. Psoriatic arthritis
    D. Septic arthritis

70. Which of the following is a contraindication of the influenza vaccination?
    A. Asthma
    B. Sickle cell anemia
    C. Age younger than 6 months
    D. American Indian heritage

71. A 44-year-old male patient presents with a body mass index (BMI) of 32 and a waist circumference of 41 inches. His lipid panel shows total cholesterol of 198 mg/dL, high-density lipoprotein (HDL) of 31 mg/dL, and triglycerides of 175 mg/dL. His blood pressure is 124/70 mmHg. Which finding indicates elevated risk for cardiovascular disease?
    A. Age
    B. Total cholesterol
    C. HDL
    D. Blood pressure

72. Which of the following selective serotonin reuptake inhibitors (SSRIs) is most likely to cause erectile dysfunction?
    A. Paroxetine (Paxil)
    B. Escitalopram (Lexapro)
    C. Venlafaxine (Effexor)
    D. Amitriptyline (Elavil)

73. A 46-year-old male patient presents at the urgent clinic with a swollen lower right leg that is reddened and tender to the touch. The patient reports no recent injury; however, he notes that yesterday he returned from a cross-country business trip. The nurse practitioner will:
    A. Instruct the patient to apply warm compresses to the area.
    B. Send the patient for a Doppler study and a d-dimer test.
    C. Instruct the patient to elevate the right leg.
    D. Prescribe nonsteroidal anti-inflammatory drugs (NSAIDs).

74. Which condition is associated with the findings in the radiograph that follows?

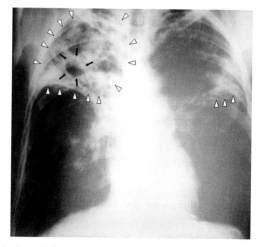

    A. Atypical pneumonia
    B. Tuberculosis (TB)
    C. Bacterial pneumonia
    D. Viral pneumonia

75. A 68-year-old female patient presents to the clinic complaining of increasing mid-back pain. Her past medical history is significant for a vertebral compression fracture at T11 1 year ago. An x-ray obtained during the encounter reveals a new vertebral compression fracture at T12. Lab work reveals elevated serum alkaline phosphatase. The nurse practitioner (NP) notes a 1-inch decrease in the patient's height from the previous year. Which medication will the NP prescribe?
    A. Alendronate (Fosamax)
    B. Colchicine
    C. Allopurinol (Zyloprim)
    D. Ferrous sulfate

76. A 45-year-old patient presents to the clinic with complaints of chills, fever, and malaise. Clinical findings show nontender red spots on the palms of both hands and the soles of the feet. Splinter hemorrhages on the nail beds are also noted. The nurse practitioner suspects which of the following conditions?
    A. Congestive heart failure
    B. Infective endocarditis
    C. Dissecting abdominal aortic aneurysm
    D. Acute myocardial infarction

77. A prostate-specific antigen (PSA) test is most likely to provide accurate results if the patient reports what?
    A. Urinary retention
    B. Urinary tract infection (UTI)
    C. Sexual activity earlier in the day
    D. Vigorous exercise 3 days prior

78. While performing a newborn assessment, the nurse practitioner notes discharge, swelling, and redness on one of the infant's lacrimal ducts. The parent reports crusting on the infant's eyes. Which diagnosis is most likely?
    A. Dacryostenosis
    B. Jaundice
    C. Red reflex abnormality
    D. Myopia

79. During the physical exam of a 60-year-old adult, the nurse practitioner (NP) performs an abdominal exam. The NP is checking the left upper quadrant (LUQ) of the abdomen. During percussion, an area of dullness is noted beneath the lower left ribcage. Which of the following is a true statement regarding the spleen?
    A. The spleen is not palpable in the majority of healthy adults.
    B. The spleen is 8 to 10 cm in the left midaxillary line at its longest axis.
    C. The spleen is 2 to 6 cm between the 9th and 11th ribs on the left midaxillary line.
    D. The splenic size varies depending on the patient's sex.

80. An elderly male resident in a long-term care facility has suddenly developed a fever of 102.3°F (oral) and is complaining of chills and pain that radiates from the perineal area to the rectum and back. The prostate is extremely tender, warm, and boggy upon digital rectal examination (DRE). Urinalysis reveals pyuria and hematuria. What is the initial diagnosis?
    A. Acute prostatitis
    B. Chronic urinary tract infection (UTI)
    C. Kidney stones
    D. Chlamydial urethritis

81. The nurse practitioner who is evaluating a patient with polycystic kidney disease will pay close attention to which area of the kidney?
    A. Loop of Henle
    B. Glomerulus
    C. Renal tubules
    D. Bowman capsule

82. A nurse practitioner (NP) sees a patient for an evaluation of sexually transmitted infections. Assessment reveals Fitz-Hugh-Curtis syndrome. The NP will prescribe:
    A. Benzathine penicillin G 2.4 mU IM weekly for 3 weeks
    B. Doxycycline 100 mg PO twice a day for 14 days
    C. Ceftriaxone 500 mg IM x one dose plus azithromycin 1 g PO x one dose
    D. Ceftriaxone 500 mg IM x one dose plus doxycycline 100 mg twice daily x 14 days plus metronidazole 500 mg twice daily x 14 days

83. A 4-year-old boy diagnosed with acute otitis media returns in 48 hours with a possible rupture of the tympanic membrane (TM) of the right ear. The parent reports seeing pus and a small amount of blood on the pillow that morning. The child states that his ear is no longer painful. During the ear exam, the otoscope is used to visualize the TM, which has a perforation on the lower edge that is draining a small amount of purulent discharge. What type of ear drop will the nurse practitioner most likely prescribe?
    A. Gentamicin
    B. Ofloxacin
    C. Tobramycin
    D. Neomycin sulfate

84. A 14-year-old girl with short stature, swollen hands and feet, and a webbed neck presents to the primary care clinic. Upon assessment, she is found to be at Tanner stage I. Which test will the nurse practitioner order to confirm a diagnosis?
    A. CT scan
    B. Karyotype
    C. Prolactin level
    D. X-ray of the hand

85. A possible side effect of the use of nifedipine (Procardia XL) is:
    A. Hyperuricemia and hypoglycemia
    B. Hyperkalemia and angioedema
    C. Edema of the ankles and headache
    D. Dry hacking cough

86. A 6-year-old child with a history of rheumatic fever is being examined by the nurse practitioner in a follow-up after hospitalization. Auscultation of the heart reveals a loud blowing, high-pitched murmur radiating to the axilla. Which diagnosis is most likely?
    A. Aortic stenosis
    B. Mitral regurgitation
    C. Mitral stenosis
    D. Aortic regurgitation

87. The nurse practitioner (NP) is discussing tetracycline with a young, sexually active female patient being treated for a bacterial sinus infection. The NP will advise the patient to:
    A. Not take birth control pills while on tetracycline
    B. Practice abstinence while on the antibiotic and then resume birth control pills
    C. Not take tetracycline and birth control pills at the same time
    D. Use an additional method of contraception while on the antibiotic and for one pill cycle after treatment is complete

88. A 25-year-old male patient presents to the clinic with a low-grade fever and a single eschar on his back. He complains of burning at the site and states, "The area was white, then red. Now there is a red spot in the center." The patient notes that he recently traveled to the Southeast for a camping trip. Which diagnosis is most likely?
    A. Rocky Mountain spotted fever
    B. Early Lyme disease
    C. Brown recluse spider bite
    D. Melanoma

89. A 67-year-old female patient with a 30-pack-year history of smoking presents for a routine annual physical examination. She complains of being easily short of breath and is frequently fatigued. Physical examination reveals diminished breath sounds, hyperresonance, and hypertrophied respiratory accessory muscles. Her complete blood count (CBC) results reveal that her hematocrit level is elevated. Her pulmonary function test (PFT) results show increased total lung capacity. Which diagnosis is most likely?
    A. Bronchogenic carcinoma
    B. Chronic obstructive pulmonary disease (COPD)
    C. Acute bronchitis
    D. Congestive heart failure (CHF)

90. The nurse practitioner (NP) is evaluating a middle-aged female patient who has experienced gradual weight gain, lack of energy, dry hair, and an irregular period for the past 8 months. Routine annual laboratory testing shows a thyroid-stimulating hormone (TSH) level of 10 mU/L. The NP decides to order a thyroid profile. Results show that TSH is 8.50 mU/L and serum-free thyroxine (T4) is decreased. During the physical exam, the patient's body mass index (BMI) is 28. The heart and lung exams are both normal. Which of the following is the best treatment plan for this patient?
    A. Advise the patient that the decreased TSH level means her thyroid problem has resolved.
    B. Start the patient on levothyroxine (Synthroid) 25 mcg orally daily.
    C. Start the patient on Armour thyroid.
    D. Refer the patient to an endocrinologist.

91. A 56-year-old patient presents to the clinic with reports of right hip pain that worsens after activity, decreased range of motion (ROM) of the right hip, and difficulty getting up after sitting for long periods. The nurse practitioner hears crepitus in the right hip upon movement. Which condition is most likely?
    A. Fracture of the right hip
    B. Rheumatoid arthritis
    C. Medial tibial stress fracture
    D. Osteoarthritis

92. Which of the following requires attention because of the potential to become cancerous?
    A. Lentigo
    B. Seborrheic keratosis
    C. Actinic keratosis
    D. Rosacea

93. Which of the following is a warning sign for scoliosis?
    A. Raised right iliac crest
    B. Thoracic kyphosis
    C. Lumbar lordosis
    D. Osteopenia

94. A male nursing home resident reports that his previous roommate was recently started on tuberculosis (TB) treatment. A Mantoux test and chest x-ray are ordered for the patient. What is the minimum size of induration in millimeters considered positive for this patient?
    A. 3
    B. 5
    C. 10
    D. 15

95. Which skin condition produces "honey-crusted," pruritic vesiculopustules that rupture and crust?
    A. Psoriasis
    B. Scabies
    C. Impetigo
    D. Measles

96. A patient is diagnosed with Bell's palsy and prescribed high-dose steroids for 10 days, with minimal improvement. During a follow-up visit, the nurse practitioner suspects the patient has herpes simplex virus 1 (HSV-1). Which is the most appropriate medication to prescribe?
    A. Acyclovir
    B. Trimethoprim-sulfamethoxazole
    C. Penicillin
    D. Ciprofloxacin

97. A 29-year-old female patient presents to the clinic with complaints of painful sexual intercourse and pain when urinating. The patient's temperature is 100.1°F. Upon physical examination, the nurse practitioner (NP) notes a healthy appearance of the internal and external genitalia. The patient has lower abdominal and cervical motion tenderness in response to palpation. What will the NP order to confirm a diagnosis and determine the appropriate treatment?
    A. Blood cultures
    B. Cervical culture
    C. Vaginal cultures
    D. Ultrasound imaging

98. An elderly female patient is diagnosed with trigeminal neuralgia. Which assessment finding would the nurse practitioner expect?
    A. Bilateral joint stiffness and aching in the shoulders and upper arms
    B. Shooting pain at the base of the head
    C. Shock-like facial pain
    D. Severe pain in or around one eye

99. A 15-year-old male patient presents with lower right-sided abdominal pain, an elevated temperature, and a white blood cell (WBC) count of 17,000. He complains of nausea and vomiting over several days. The nurse practitioner flexes his right leg at his hip and knee, which results in moderate discomfort. Which diagnosis is most likely?
    A. Hepatitis
    B. Appendicitis
    C. Cholecystitis
    D. Nephrolithiasis

100. A 66-year-old female patient's dual-energy x-ray absorptiometry (DEXA) scan reveals early-onset osteoporosis. What will the nurse practitioner recommend to address the condition?
A. Low-protein diet
B. Swimming 3 days each week
C. Daily isometric exercise
D. Minimal caffeine consumption

101. The nurse practitioner (NP) refers a 12-year-old boy with a swollen, red scrotum and ascending testicle to the ED with a diagnosis of testicular torsion. Which additional objective finding led the NP to this diagnosis?
A. Absent cremasteric reflex
B. Present cremasteric reflex
C. Hematuria
D. Pyuria

102. Which hemopoietic disorder will the nurse practitioner assess for in a 3-year-old child with lead poisoning?
A. Iron-deficiency anemia
B. Thalassemia minor
C. Pernicious anemia
D. Normocytic anemia

103. A patient has been taking albuterol via a metered-dose inhaler for a month and remains in the yellow zone. Which of the following statements is true?
A. Medication should be lowered to produce desired effects.
B. The patient is at 50% to 80% of their personal best.
C. The patient is at 80% to 100% of their personal best.
D. Current medication dosage places the patient at risk for hypoxia.

104. The nurse practitioner (NP) is treating an elderly female patient with recurrent depression. The patient refuses to take her medication. The patient's adult child states, "She seems worse than ever. What should we do?" Which of the following is the most appropriate response by the NP?
A. "Let's try a different pharmacotherapeutic regimen."
B. "Can you bring her in for one-on-one counseling sessions?"
C. "I will refer your mother to a psychiatric-mental health NP."
D. "The nurse practice act will not allow me to continue care for your mother."

105. An older adult patient is diagnosed with a urinary tract infection. Which drug class may put this patient at risk for an Achilles tendon rupture?
A. Sulfonamides
B. Quinolones
C. Cephalosporins
D. Penicillins

106. Which statement will the nurse practitioner (NP) make when discussing prostate cancer screening with a 65-year-old African American patient?
A. "I recommend that you have both a blood test and a physical exam to screen for prostate cancer."
B. "You are at increased risk for prostate cancer, so an annual blood test for screening will be of benefit."
C. "Based on your risk factors, you should have a blood test to screen for prostate cancer every 2 years."
D. "Screening has only a small benefit of reducing chance of death from prostate cancer, so you can decide if you want to be screened."

107. A 32-year-old sexually active female patient is diagnosed with bacterial vaginosis based on findings of copious milk-like vaginal discharge. Speculum exam reveals gray/white discharge on the vaginal walls and a fishlike odor based on the whiff test. The patient will be treated with a 5-day course of metronidazole vaginal gel, one application at bedtime, and advised to do which of the following?
A. Douche after intercourse.
B. Ensure that the sexual partner is seen and treated.
C. Abstain from sexual intercourse during treatment.
D. Use a condom during sexual intercourse.

108. An older adult male patient presents to the clinic for a routine examination. The nurse practitioner notes multiple rough, scaly patches on the patient's forearms, face, and back of the ears. Which diagnosis is most likely?
A. Seborrheic keratosis
B. Purpura
C. Lentigines
D. Actinic keratosis

109. Upon examination of a 26-year-old patient, the nurse practitioner (NP) finds elongated papilla of the lateral aspects of the patient's tongue. The patient has been diagnosed with the Epstein-Barr virus (EBV). How will the NP document this finding?
A. Koplik spots
B. Geographic tongue
C. Oral hairy leukoplakia
D. Cheilosis

110. What is the most common pathogen found in community-acquired pneumonia (CAP)?
A. *Chlamydia pneumoniae*
B. *Streptococcus pneumoniae*
C. *Pseudomonas aeruginosa*
D. *Mycoplasma pneumonia*

111. The nurse practitioner will monitor what side effect in a patient taking hydrochlorothiazide?
A. Hypoglycemia
B. Hyperkalemia
C. Hypertriglyceridemia
D. Hypernatremia

112. A male patient presents with reports of urethritis, migratory arthritis in the large joints, and ulcers on the glans penis secondary to a chlamydial infection. What might be included in the treatment plan? (Select all that apply.)
    A. Treat with nonsteroidal anti-inflammatory drugs (NSAIDs).
    B. Prescribe antibiotics to treat infection.
    C. Treat with alpha-linolenic acid (LNA).
    D. Recommend rest and comfort measures.
    E. Prescribe a corticosteroid.

113. A patient uses a sliding scale in conjunction with a long-acting insulin to manage type 1 diabetes. Which insulin should the patient prepare for an elevated blood sugar between breakfast and lunch?
    A. Insulin isophane and insulin regular
    B. Insulin glargine (Lantus)
    C. Insulin lispro (Humalog)
    D. Neutral protamine Hagedorn (NPH)

114. A patient presents to the primary care clinic with complaints of headache, nonproductive cough, and fatigue for the past 2 weeks. The nurse practitioner auscultates crackles and wheezing. A chest x-ray shows patchy infiltrates. The patient does not have comorbidities or recent use of antibiotics. What is the most appropriate treatment for this patient?
    A. Azithromycin (Z-Pak) daily x 5 days
    B. Levofloxacin (Levaquin) 750 mg orally x 5 to 7 days
    C. Amoxicillin-clavulanate (Augmentin) 1,000/62.5 mg orally as needed x 5 to 7 days
    D. Moxifloxacin (Avelox) 400 mg orally daily x 5-7 days

115. The nurse practitioner (NP) has confirmed a diagnosis of acute hepatitis C in a patient. The NP is required to do which of the following?
    A. Isolate the patient for 14 days.
    B. Instruct the patient to wear a mask in public.
    C. Instruct the patient to wear an identification bracelet.
    D. Report the case to the health department.

116. The nurse practitioner is performing a vision screening on a newborn. Which finding would prompt a referral to a pediatric ophthalmologist?
    A. Inability to produce tears
    B. Fixation on mother's face
    C. One eye turned inward
    D. Bluish-gray eyes

117. A male high school football player suffered a deceleration pivoting injury of his left knee during a game. He states that he felt a sudden "pop" with subsequent swelling, and the knee seemed to buckle. Which action by the nurse practitioner is appropriate when examining this patient? (Select all that apply.)
    A. Conduct Lachman's test.
    B. Apply ice to the joint.
    C. Perform isometric exercises.
    D. Support the joint with a compression wrap.
    E. Refer to an orthopedic specialist.

118. The nurse practitioner is performing an assessment of a 6-month-old child. What motor skills are expected at this age? (Select all that apply.)
    A. Palmar grasp of objects
    B. Sitting up
    C. Standing independently
    D. Moving from one piece of furniture to another
    E. Feeding self without assistance

119. A 72-year-old female patient has a complicated urinary tract infection (UTI). The nurse practitioner will prescribe medication treatment for a minimum of how many days?
    A. 3
    B. 7
    C. 10
    D. 14

120. Which mineral lab finding is deficient in a patient presenting with lethargy, weight gain, bradycardia, and a goiter?
    A. Fluoride
    B. Calcium
    C. Sodium
    D. Iodine

121. An underweight 15-year-old female cross-country runner presents with a complaint of progressive bilateral leg pain for 5 to 6 weeks. Upon examination, the nurse practitioner notes inflammation in the left tibial area and that the patient has pes planus. Patient history reveals amenorrhea for 1 year. Which diagnosis is most likely?
    A. Plantar fasciitis
    B. Medial tibial stress syndrome
    C. Morton neuroma
    D. Degenerative joint disease

122. The nurse practitioner (NP) is caring for a 4-year-old patient with sickle cell disease who is experiencing a febrile illness. Which hemopoietic laboratory value will the NP use to evaluate the efficiency of the patient's bone marrow response?
    A. B lymphocyte
    B. C-reactive protein
    C. Prothrombin time
    D. Reticulocyte count

123. When examining a preschool-aged child, the nurse practitioner (NP) notes wheezing and diffused crackles upon auscultation of the lungs. Throat examination appears erythematous without pus or exudate. Respirations are 24 breaths/min, and temperature is 99.2°F. The parent states that the child has been coughing for several weeks. Chest x-ray shows diffuse interstitial infiltrates. What will the NP include in the treatment plan?
A. Azithromycin
B. Fluid restriction
C. Amoxicillin–clavulanate
D. Albuterol nebulizer

124. An adult female patient who was recently diagnosed with lupus complains that her hands and feet always feel cold, even in the summertime. Sometimes her fingertips become numb and turn a blue color. The fingertips eventually turn dark red in color. Which of the following is most likely?
A. Chronic arterial insufficiency
B. Normal reaction when one feels very cold
C. Peripheral vascular disease
D. Raynaud phenomenon

125. A thrill initially presents at which grade level of a heart murmur?
A. V
B. II
C. III
D. IV

126. An older adult patient is diagnosed with herpes zoster opthalmicus. Which cranial nerve is infected with this disorder?
A. VII
B. V
C. III
D. IV

127. The nurse practitioner (NP) is managing a stable 53-year-old patient with emphysema. In addition to reinforcing smoking cessation and medication schedules, which annual intervention will the NP recommend?
A. Pneumococcal polysaccharide vaccine (PPSV23)
B. Live attenuated influenza vaccine (LAIV)
C. Quadrivalent inactivated influenza vaccine (QIV)
D. Pneumococcal conjugate vaccine (PCV13)

128. Following a routine annual exam of a 59-year-old postmenopausal patient, the nurse practitioner refers the patient to a gynecologist, who then orders a pelvic/intravaginal ultrasound. Which finding on the exam most likely prompted the referral and subsequent order?
A. Positive Pap smear
B. External genital warts
C. Vaginal atrophy
D. Palpable ovary

129. Which diagnostic test is used to confirm a diagnosis of vaginal candida infection?
A. pH
B. Whiff test
C. Wet mount
D. Tzanck smear

130. Which of the following is associated with male aging?
A. Increased levels of estrogen
B. Decreased sperm production
C. Increased production of semen
D. Decreased concentration of sperm

131. The nurse practitioner is educating a 72-year-old patient regarding screening for colon cancer. The patient is at average risk. What diagnostic testing should be performed annually for this patient?
A. Flexible sigmoidoscopy
B. Colonoscopy
C. Fecal occult blood test
D. CT colonography

132. What is the priority treatment for a patient who presents with an asthma exacerbation?
A. Prescribe albuterol as needed.
B. Teach patient how to properly use a spacer.
C. Assess asthma triggers.
D. Apply nebulizer treatment.

133. A patient has several well-defined, primary lesions <20 mm over the trunk and extremities. After completing a dermascopic exam, the nurse practitioner (NP) diagnoses Bowen disease. Which treatment will the NP recommend?
A. Moh surgery
B. Radiation therapy
C. Curettage and electrodessication
D. Standard excision

134. The presence of chronic cough might lead the nurse practitioner to rule out what differential diagnosis?
A. Chronic bronchitis
B. Allergic rhinitis
C. Acute viral upper respiratory infection (URI)
D. Gastroesophageal reflux disease (GERD)

135. A 5-year-old child is assessed for dysuria and frequency. Which antibiotic would the nurse practitioner prescribe on finding the urine culture positive for gram-negative bacteria?
A. Ciprofloxacin (Cipro)
B. Trimethoprim-sulfamethoxazole (Bactrim DS)
C. Levofloxacin (Levaquin)
D. Doxycycline

136. A patient presents with a wedge-shaped, superficial, yellow, triangular mass on the nasal side of the left eye. The patient denies pain or vision changes. PERRLA is normal. Which diagnosis is most likely?
    A. Pinguecula
    B. Chalazion
    C. Hordeolum
    D. Pterygium

137. What are U.S. Preventive Services Task Force (USPSTF)–recommended guidelines for breast cancer screening?
    A. Baseline mammogram should start at age 50 years and repeat every 2 years until age 74 years.
    B. Baseline mammogram should start at age 40 years and repeat every 3 years until age 74 years.
    C. Baseline mammogram should start at age 50 years and repeat every year until age 74 years.
    D. Baseline mammogram should start at age 55 years and repeat every 3 years.

138. While reviewing lab results for a patient with suspected recreational drug misuse, the nurse practitioner (NP) notes an elevated blood urea nitrogen (BUN) level. Which additional test will the NP order to confirm or rule out renal failure in this patient?
    A. Serum creatinine
    B. Estimated glomerular filtration rate (eGFR)
    C. Intravenous pyelogram (IVP)
    D. MRI

139. A 44-year-old male patient with Down syndrome begins to develop impaired memory and difficulty with his usual daily routines. He is having problems functioning at the job where he has been employed for the past 10 years. The physical exam and routine labs are all negative. The vital signs are normal. His appetite is normal. The most likely diagnosis is:
    A. Tic douloureux
    B. Stroke
    C. Alzheimer's disease
    D. Delirium

140. The most important job of an institutional review board (IRB) is:
    A. Protecting the interests of the hospital or the research institution
    B. Protecting the rights of the human subjects who participate in research done at the institution
    C. Protecting the researcher and research team from lawsuits
    D. Evaluating research protocols and methodology for appropriateness and safety

141. When considering a data set, what is the median?
    A. It is the value that occurs most frequently.
    B. It is the value that occurs in the middle when the set is arranged from smallest value to largest.
    C. It is the average of all values in the set.
    D. It is the difference between the smallest and greatest values.

142. A 15-year-old female patient who attends a public school is referred to the nurse practitioner (NP) by one of her teachers. The patient's parents are recently divorced. The patient has been missing school and is falling behind in her schoolwork. After closing the exam room door, the NP starts to interview the patient, asking about her moods, her appetite, her sleep, whether she has any plan to hurt herself or others, and other questions. In what type of health prevention activity is the NP engaging?
    A. Primary prevention
    B. Secondary prevention
    C. Tertiary prevention
    D. Dropout prevention program

143. A 14-year-old girl with amenorrhea is tested for pregnancy and has a positive result. The patient tells the nurse practitioner (NP) that she is seriously considering terminating the pregnancy. She tells the NP that she wants to be referred to a Planned Parenthood clinic. The NP's beliefs are anti-abortion. Which of the following is the best action by the NP?
    A. Tell the patient about the NP's beliefs and advise her against getting an abortion.
    B. Advise the patient that a peer who is working with the NP can answer the patient's questions more thoroughly.
    C. Excuse themself from the case entirely.
    D. Refer the patient to an obstetrician.

144. A nurse expert is called to testify in a malpractice lawsuit. What would be the purpose and content of the nurse's testimony?
    A. Testify about the actions she would have taken in a similar situation
    B. Testify about the standards of nursing care as they apply to the facts in the case
    C. Testify about the laws that govern healthcare in the area
    D. Provide an expert opinion of the other nurse's actions

145. A physician is referring a patient to a nurse practitioner (NP). What type of relationship will exist between the physician and the NP?
    A. Consultative
    B. Collaborative
    C. Professional
    D. Advocate

146. What is the pedigree symbol for a male with a disease?
A. Empty square
B. Empty circle
C. Filled-in square
D. Filled-in circle

147. A 13-year-old girl is brought by her mother to the health clinic because the girl is complaining of vaginal discharge and pain. The patient's mother tells the nurse practitioner (NP) that the patient is not sexually active yet. The patient's mother is divorced, lives with a partner, and works full time. During the exam, the NP notes that the vaginal introitus is red, with tears and a torn hymen. The cervix is covered with green discharge. The NP suspects that the child has been sexually abused by the mother's partner. Which is the best action for the NP to take during this visit?
A. Ask the mother questions about her partner's behavior.
B. Advise the mother to watch how her partner interacts with her daughter and to call within 1 week to discuss the partner's behavior.
C. Advise the mother that the NP suspects that her daughter has been sexually abused.
D. Report the child sexual abuse to the department of Child Protective Services (CPS).

148. Which of the following benzodiazepines has the shortest half-life?
A. Lorazepam (Ativan)
B. Alprazolam (Xanax)
C. Triazolam (Halcion)
D. Clonazepam (Klonopin)

149. The nurse practitioner (NP) is evaluating a 16-year-old female patient who complains of fatigue and headaches. The patient is wearing multiple layers of clothing, and her hair is limp and dry. Upon examination, the NP finds the patient's skin to have a yellow cast and notes a fine, downy hair on the patient's body. Which diagnosis is most likely?
A. Alopecia
B. Anorexia nervosa
C. Bulimia
D. Amenorrhea

150. The nurse practitioner (NP) is completing a health assessment on a 15-year-old female patient who is in the office for her annual physical exam. The patient reports feelings of hopelessness and sadness for several months, no history of suicidal ideation, and a struggle with anorexia nervosa. The patient scores an 11 on the Beck Depression Inventory. In addition to cognitive-behavioral therapy and family discussions, which first-line pharmacotherapy agent is indicated?
A. Sertraline (Zoloft)
B. Lithium carbonate (Eskalith)
C. Bupropion (Wellbutrin)
D. Fluoxetine (Prozac)

1. C) "Patients have the right to view their mental health–related and psychotherapy-related health information."

Mental health and psychotherapy/psychiatric records do not have to be released to patients even if they request those records. Otherwise, any type of medical record can be released if requested by the health insurance or health plan for billing purposes and reimbursement. HIPAA applies to all healthcare providers, health plans, health insurance companies, medical clearinghouses, and others who bill electronically and transmit health information over the internet.

2. A) The high vitamin K levels will decrease the international normalized ratio (INR).

Vitamin K and warfarin (Coumadin) have opposing effects. Vitamin K helps to decrease bleeding time; warfarin (Coumadin) helps to increase bleeding time. By interfering with the desired effect of warfarin, a high intake of vitamin K can decrease the INR. Patients do not need to avoid foods high in vitamin K, but they do need to closely monitor their intake for consistent comsumption. Significant changes in consumption can impact the effects of the currently prescribed warfarin dose. Ascorbic acid and fiber will not interfere with warfarin, nor will the vitamins increase the activity of the warfarin.

3. A) Erythema migrans

Erythema migrans is a symptom of early Lyme disease. It is an annular lesion that slowly enlarges with time (days to weeks) and has central clearing. It is caused by a bite from an infected (*Borrelia burgdorferi*) blacklegged tick. If untreated, infection will spread to the joints, nervous system, and heart. Most cases of Lyme disease occur in the Northeast, the mid-Atlantic, Wisconsin, Minnesota, and northern California. Rocky Mountain spotted fever produces a diffuse petechial rash that starts on the extremities and quickly spreads to the trunk. Meningococcemia produces petechial or hemorrhagic lesions to the axillae, ankles, wrists, and flanks. Larva migrans produces a serpiginous patterned rash rather than an annular lesion.

4. B) Amaurosis fugax

The patient is experiencing temporal arteritis (giant cell arteritis), which causes an acute headache in one temple area with an indurated, reddened temporal artery and scalp tenderness. A major complication of this condition is transient blindness (amaurosis fugax) of the affected eye. Vertigo is not a common complication of temporal arteritis, but often occurs with multiple sclerosis. Ptosis is seen frequently with cluster headaches rather than temporal arteritis. CN VII paralysis is often observed with Bell palsy or injury to the specific nerve.

5. B) Trimethoprim-sulfamethoxazole

Macrolides (clarithromycin, azithromycin, erythromycin) are contraindicated in patients with myasthenia gravis because of the risk for respiratory collapse. An antibiotic that is generally considered safe to prescribe for a patient with myasthenia gravis and pertussis is trimethoprim-sulfamethoxazole as a recommended second-line agent for pertussis after a macrolide.

6. C) The patient has immunity from hepatitis B vaccinations.

The hepatitis B vaccination series produced immunity; there was no exposure to hepatitis B. The AST and ALT (liver enzymes) are within normal range. AST ranges from 0 to 45 mg/dL, and ALT ranges from 0 to 40 mg/dL. There are no lab values that indicate that the patient was screened for hepatitis D, as hepatitis B is the precursor. If the patient had active hepatitis B, the results would be as follows: HbsAg +, anti-HBc +, IgM anti-HBc +, and anti-HBs -. If the patient had never been exposed to hepatitis B, the results would be all negative for HbsAg, anti-HBc, and anti-HBs. A patient who was previously vaccinated but never had an infection would have a negative HbsAg and anti-HBc and a positive anti-HBs.

7. D) Urea breath test

The urea breath test is a very sensitive test used to evaluate a patient for an active *H. pylori* infection. It can also be used to document treatment response after a treatment regimen of antibiotics (14 days) and proton-pump inhibitor (PPI) therapy. An *H. pylori* titer cannot distinguish between past exposure and current infection. Fasting gastrin level is used to determine if Zollinger-Ellison syndrome or gastrinoma is the cause of ulcerations. An upper GI x-ray series cannot be used to determine if the cause of an ulcer is specifically due to *H. pylori*.

8. C) Hepatitis C virus antibody test

The Centers for Disease Control and Prevention (CDC) recommends hepatitis C screening in adults born from 1945 through 1965. Hepatitis C is transmitted by sharing needles and can become a chronic infection. Intravenous drug users and persons within this age group are considered high risk for hepatitis C. Given the history, chest x-ray, urinalysis, and electroencephalogram would not be indicated.

9. A, B, C) Use aluminum acetate solution as needed; Keep water out of the ear during treatment; Apply polymyxin B-neomycin-hydrocortisone suspension drops four times a day for 7 days.
The symptoms and history of the patient make otitis externa the most likely diagnosis. Otitis externa, also called swimmer's ear, is inflammation of the ear canal. A recommended treatment plan for moderate disease with intact membrane includes the use of aluminum acetate solution prophylactically and as needed. Aluminum acetate solution provides soothing, effective relief of minor skin irritations and inflammation. The patient should be advised to keep water out of the ear during treatment, so swimming activities should be adjusted. Recommended treatment includes the application of a topical antibiotic and a glucocorticoid such as polymyxin B-neomycin-hydrocortisone suspension drops four times a day for 7 days and/or ofloxacin otic drops twice daily x 7 days. A steroid nasal spray would not be included in the treatment of otitis externa. Levofloxacin may be prescribed for non-intact membrane.

10. B) Tetracycline (Sumycin)
First-line treatment for acne vulgaris includes OTC medicated soap and water with topical antibiotic gels. The next step in treatment would be the initiation of oral tetracycline. Cleocin is an antibiotic gel and is similar to the topical antibiotic the patient has already tried. Isotretinoin (Amnesteem) is generally reserved for severe, diffuse nodular acne, which this patient does not exhibit. Minoxidil does not provide any therapeutic benefit in acne, but instead is used to stimulate hair growth.

11. C) This is a normal finding in some young athletes.
It is common to hear a split S2 heart sound over the pulmonic area of the heart with inspiration. As long as it disappears with expiration, with no other abnormal symptoms, this is a normal finding. The sound is caused by the splitting of the aortic and pulmonic components.

12. A) Colchicine
Colchicine is prescribed to reduce uric acid deposits and ease joint inflammation in the acute phase of a flare-up of gout. Due to the risk of dose-related adverse effects, high doses are no longer recommended, especially in elderly patients or those with impaired liver or kidney function. Celecoxib (Celebrex) is used to reduce joint inflammation and pain in patients with osteoarthritis but has no effect on urate crystal formation in acute gout. Calcium gluconate is used to reverse a negative calcium balance and relieve muscle cramps. A steroid injection is not recommended for the treatment of gout.

13. B) Aortic stenosis
One of the most frequent pathologic systolic murmurs is due to aortic stenosis. The murmur of aortic stenosis is typically a midsystolic ejection murmur, heard best over the "aortic area" or right second intercostal space, with radiation to the right neck. It has a harsh quality and may be associated with a palpably slow rise of the carotid upstroke. Additional heart sounds, such as an S4, may be heard secondary to hypertrophy of the left ventricle, which is caused by the greatly increased work required to pump blood through the stenotic valve.

14. C) Increase chlorthalidone (Hygroton).
The Joint National Committee (JNC) 8 encourages use of chlorthalidone (Hygroton), as it is longer acting and more effective than other options. If a hypertensive patient has blood pressure that is hard to control, consider increasing chlorthalidone (Hygroton) to 25 mg. Decreasing chlorthalidone (Hygroton) will not lower the patient's blood pressure. Propranolol (Inderal; beta-blocker) is contraindicated for a patient with emphysema and should not be prescribed. The patient has a history of breast cancer and may be immunocompromised. Captopril (Capoten) should be avoided as it is associated with agranulocytosis, neutropenia, and leukopenia (rare).

15. B) BMI can be elevated in people with higher muscle mass.
BMI is used to measure patients' weight in comparison to body size. A BMI of 26 for a male adolescent is in the higher-than-normal range (18.5–24.9) but may be attributed to higher muscle mass. BMI alone is not a set parameter used as an indicator of obesity.

16. D) Myxedema coma
Myxedema coma is seen in patients with severe hypothyroidism. It is a medical emergency with a mortality rate of 30% or higher. It is treated with very high doses of thyroid hormone. A thyroid storm occurs when there is extreme elevation of thyroid hormones. Thyroid storm is life-threatening; if left untreated, the mortality rate is about 90%. Call 911 if suspected. Graves disease is associated with thyroid hyperfunction.

17. A) Asthma
Asthma, bronchiectasis, and emphysema are obstructive dysfunctions caused by reduction in airflow rates and would be considered differential diagnoses. Pulmonary fibrosis, pleural disease, and diaphragm obstruction are examples of restrictive dysfunction caused by a reduction in lung volume due to decreased lung compliance.

18. A) Decreased hemoglobin A
Decreased hemoglobin A is associated with beta thalassemia minor. The RBCs in beta thalassemia are hypochromic. A decrease in mean corpuscular volume and mean corpuscular hemoglobin concentration are associated with beta thalassemia.

19. A) Check bilirubin level.
The first intervention is to assess the bilirubin level of the infant before treatment is initiated. If the bilirubin level is >5 mg/dL, phototherapy should be prescribed. The parent should be advised to feed the infant 10 to 12 times per day, and a follow-up visit is indicated once a diagnosis is confirmed.

20. C) Acne rosacea

The patient is presenting with acne rosacea, a chronic inflammatory disease of the cheeks, chin, and nose, with dry, reddened eyes. First-line treatment is to determine triggers such as spicy foods and alcohol. Herpes zoster ophthalmicus affects one side of the head with sudden vesicular lesions on the scalp, nose, and forehead. The patient may also report photophobia, eye pain, and blurred vision. Rocky Mountain spotted fever causes a rash, an abrupt onset of a high fever, chills, severe headache, photophobia, and nausea and vomiting. A petechial rash starts on the wrists, forearms, and feet and then moves up to the trunk. Rocky Mountain spotted fever is caused by the bite of a dog tick that is infected with the parasite *Rickettsia rickettsii*. Actinic keratosis is more common in the elderly. Numerous dry, round, and red-colored lesions do not heal and mostly occur in sun-exposed areas. They may be precancerous lesions to squamous cell carcinoma.

21. B) Delayed puberty

Cushing syndrome is associated with delayed puberty and growth failure in children and adolescents. Patients with Cushing syndrome have an excess of androgens, not estrogen. Gynecomastia, not pseudogynecomastia, occurs with Cushing disease. Pseudogynecomastia is caused by the deposition of fat, whereas gynecomastia is caused by excess cortisol.

22. C) Meniscus tear

A meniscus tear would produce a positive McMurray test. ACL and LCL tears are possible but would result in only a positive Lachman test, not a positive McMurray test. A knee sprain would not elicit a positive McMurray test.

23. B) Smoking

Secondary polycythemia vera is associated with chronic hypoxia. Hypoxia causes an increase in erythropoietin, which stimulates the production of mature red blood cells from the bone marrow. There is a high incidence of secondary polycythemia in chronic cigarette smokers compared with the general population, as they often experience hypoxia. High-fat diet, alcohol misuse, and a sedentary lifestyle are not associated with secondary polycythemia vera.

24. D) *Streptococcus pneumoniae*

The two most common bacteria in community-acquired pneumonia are *S. pneumoniae* and *H. influenzae*. Blood-tinged sputum indicates that *S. pneumoniae* is the more likely of the two in this patient. *Bordetella pertussis* is gram-negative bacteria that causes pertussis (whooping cough). *Treponema pallidum* is a gram-negative spirochete bacterium that causes syphilis.

25. A) Thiazides

Thiazides (hydrochlorothiazide and indapamide) and loop diuretics (furosemide and bumetanide) are contraindicated in patients with sulfa allergies. Potassium-sparing diuretics are a suitable alternative. Beta-blockers and direct renin inhibitors are not diuretics.

26. B) None; normal lung tissue

When a nurse practitioner percusses over the lungs, resonance is heard over normal lung tissue. Hyperresonance is heard with emphysema. Bacterial pneumonia and pleural effusion will percuss a dull tone.

27. B) *Clostridium difficile* colitis

Classic symptoms of *C. difficile* colitis include watery diarrhea after starting an antibiotic treatment. It results from a change in intestinal flora. These symptoms are not associated with hepatitis B. Acute pancreatitis symptoms include upper abdominal pain, nausea and vomiting, and fever. It is not related to antibiotic therapy. Allergic reactions would have signs of rash, compromised respiratory efforts, and/or pruritus.

28. C) >6 mm

In the ABCDE acronym for melanoma screening, the "D" stands for the diameter of a lesion. If the lesion is larger than 6 mm with asymmetry, border irregularity, color variety, and enlargement over time, the patient should be referred to a dermatologist.

29. B) Diabetic ketoacidosis

A patient with serum ketones and serum glucose levels >300 mg/dL is likely experiencing diabetic ketoacidosis. Diabetes insipidus is an overproduction of antidiuretic hormone; it does not create ketones in the blood. Hypoglycemia causes low blood glucose levels. The Somogyi phenomenon is rebound hyperglycemia following an episode of hypoglycemia.

30. C) Lupus erythematosus

Classic symptoms of lupus erythematosus are butterfly rash across both cheeks and the bridge of the nose and fatigue. Risk factors for this patient include being female and 40 years old. Rosacea has a similar rash but is usually not associated with fatigue. Thyroid disease can produce fatigue and dryness of the skin, but it does not cause a facial rash. Atopic dermatitis produces an erythematous and scaling rash that is commonly found on the hands, flexural folds, and neck; however, it does not produce associated fatigue.

31. B) Paroxysmal atrial tachycardia

Signs and symptoms of paroxysmal atrial tachycardia include a rapid, regular heart rate that begins and ends very quickly. The atria are beating at a very fast rate, but this is not life-threatening. Ventricular tachycardia is usually associated with heart disease, occurs when the ventricles are beating rapidly and inefficiently, and can lead to death if not treated. Atrial fibrillation is an irregular heartbeat that can be life-threatening if not treated. Ventricular fibrillation occurs when the heartbeat is rapid and chaotic, and death will occur if the condition is not treated.

32. B) Terazosin (Hytrin)

Terazosin (Hytrin) is a quinazoline used to treat symptoms of BPH and hypertension. Silodosin (Rapaflo) is used to manage the signs and symptoms of BPH. Finasteride (Proscar) is used to treat symptomatic BPH. Phenoxybenzamine (Dibenzyline) is a nonselective alpha-adrenergic blocker used to improve urinary flow; however, because of nonselectivity, it has a high incidence of adverse effects.

33. B, C, D, E) Respiratory; Gastrointestinal; Renal; Cardiovascular

Chronic use of NSAIDs is associated with increased risk of ulcers, perforation, bleeding of the gastrointestinal tract, heart attacks, cardiovascular damage, strokes, acute interstitial nephritis and kidney injury, and liver damage. It can also affect the lungs of those with asthma or underlying aspirin sensitivity, causing bronchospasm. Chronic NSAID use does not adversely affect the endocrine system.

34. C) Sinus tachycardia

The elderly are more prone to accidental overdoses because of changes in metabolism. The EKG reading for someone who took too much amitriptyline (Elavil) would show sinus tachycardia (EKG reading C). EKG reading A is an EKG of atrial fibrillation, EKG reading B is bradycardia, and EKG reading D is normal sinus rhythm.

35. A, B, C) Bedrest with bathroom privileges; Close monitoring of weight and blood pressure; Close follow-up of urinary protein, serum creatinine, and platelet count

Recommended care for patients diagnosed with mild preeclampsia includes bedrest with bathroom privileges; weight and blood pressure monitoring; and closely following urine protein and serum protein, creatinine, and platelet counts. Oral medications are not used as first-line treatment. Magnesium sulfate may be administered for inpatient treatment of eclampsia.

36. C) Hepatitis B vaccination and hepatitis B immunoglobulin

HBsAg is a marker of infectivity. If positive, it indicates either an acute or a chronic hepatitis B infection, so the partner does not have acute or chronic hepatitis B infection. Anti-HBs is a marker of immunity; because this is negative, it indicates that the partner is not immune to hepatitis B. Antibody to hepatitis B core antigen (anti-HBc) is a marker of acute, chronic, or resolved hepatitis B virus (HBV) infection; it may be used in prevaccination testing to determine previous exposure to HBV. The hepatitis B panel results (negative HBsAg, anti-HBc, and anti-HBs) indicate the partner is susceptible (not immune), has not been infected, and is still at risk of future infection, and thus needs vaccine. Hepatitis B immunoglobulin contains antibodies that provide "instant" immunity against hepatitis B, but its action lasts for several days only. It is not a vaccine. It is given to infants and others who are at high risk of becoming infected and are not immune. The hepatitis B vaccine stimulates the body to make its own antibodies, which are permanent. A total of three doses is needed to gain full immunity against hepatitis B. Interpretation of the negative anti-hepatitis C virus (HCV) screening test indicates that the partner is not infected with hepatitis C. The positive anti-hepatitis A virus (HAV) indicates that the individual is immune (either from previous disease or from vaccination) to hepatitis A.

37. D) Hidradenitis suppurativa

Hidradenitis suppurativa is most common in women (3:1). Smoking and obesity are significant risk factors. Lesions are treated with topical antibiotics (or oral antibiotics, warm compresses, and pain medications). Institute diet changes to reduce high glycemic and dairy intake. Refer to a dermatologist for additional treatment options. Impetigo is caused by Group B streptococcus or *Staphylococcus aureus* and is more common in children. Lesions form under the nose and around the mouth. It is very contagious. Dried lesions are honey colored. Carbuncles are a collection of multiple furuncles that are treated with systemic antibiotics. The lesions of shingles present as groups of vesicles and papules with a red base, which rupture and form dermatomal, crusted lesions on one side of the body.

38. B) *Streptococcus pneumoniae*

S. pneumoniae is a gram-positive pathogen that commonly causes meningitis. *Neisseria meningitidis*, *Haemophilus influenzae*, and *Klebsiella pneumoniae* are all gram-negative pathogens that can also cause meningitis.

39. A) Short-acting inhaled beta2-agonist (SABA)

The NP should start the patient on a SABA, such as albuterol, and then reevaluate symptoms. The patient should be instructed to use albuterol 10 to 15 minutes before exercising. The patient is not symptomatic enough at this point to start on step 1 treatment. ICS daily would be used at step 2, and ICS-LABA combination daily would be used at step 3.

40. D) Tissue biopsy

Biopsy and pathology exam of prostate tissue is used to confirm a diagnosis of prostate cancer. CBC is not used to diagnose prostate cancer. A mass can be palpated with DRE; however, this does not confirm a diagnosis of prostate cancer. PSA is a screening test for prostate cancer, but it is not used to confirm final diagnosis.

41. A) Order an MRI scan of the lumbosacral spine as soon as possible.

The patient has new-onset numbness of the perineal area (saddle anesthesia), the sciatica is worsening, and the deep tendon reflexes of the lower extremity are decreased on the affected side. Cauda equina syndrome should be ruled out first as this is an emergent condition. An MRI is the preferred test to evaluate for caudia equina syndrome, nerve root compression, herniated disk, cancer, and spinal stenosis (narrowing of the spinal canal). In addition, the patient would require urgent evaluation with a neurosurgeon, rather than an orthopedist, and should not wait 3 days for follow-up. Physical therapy can be considered only after cauda equina has been ruled out or treated because this will not relieve nerve root compression present in cauda equina syndrome.

42. A) The fundus of the uterus should be at the level of the symphysis pubis.
At 12 weeks' gestation, the fundus of the uterus should be located approximately at the symphysis pubis. The cervix should not be dilated at 12 weeks' gestation. Hegar's sign is positive between 6 and 12 weeks' gestation.

43. B) Warfarin (Coumadin)
Patients with Graves disease hyperthyroidism are at higher risk for osteoporosis and atrial fibrillation. Since atrial fibrillation increases the risk for blood clots and resultant stroke, the most appropriate medication to add to the treatment regimen is warfarin (Coumadin). Furosemide (Lasix) is prescribed for heart failure, which is not a risk factor for a patient with hyperthyroidism. Cholestyramine (Prevalite) is used for hyperlipidemia. A beta-blocker such as metoprolol is normally prescribed when a patient is first diagnosed with Graves disease to lessen hyperstimulation.

44. D) Diabetes mellitus
Persistent urinary and vaginal infections may indicate underlying glucose metabolism disorders and diabetes mellitus. Diabetes insipidus is a rare metabolic disorder affecting fluid balance (excessive fluid intake and urination) in the body and would not be screened for with the symptomatology of this patient. *H. pylori* is a bacterial infection of the digestive tract and would not manifest as vaginal discharge or itching. Anemia is not a possible underlying cause for frequent UTIs or vaginal infections.

45. B) Bullous myringitis
Bullous myringitis is an ear infection in which small, fluid-filled blisters form on the eardrum. This finding distinguishes the diagnosis. Otitis externa, also called swimmer ear, is inflammation of the ear canal. Purulent otitis media is an inflammation of the middle ear in which there is fluid in the middle ear accompanied by signs or symptoms of ear infection: a bulging eardrum usually accompanied by pain or a perforated eardrum, often with drainage of purulent material. In serous otitis media, sterile serous fluid is trapped inside the middle ear.

46. B) Rheumatoid arthritis
When rheumatoid arthritis is active, symptoms can include fatigue, loss of energy, depression, low-grade fever, muscle and joint aches, and stiffness. Muscle and bilateral joint stiffness are common. During flares, joints frequently become red, swollen, painful, and tender. This occurs because the lining of the tissue of the joint (synovium) becomes inflamed, resulting in the production of excessive joint fluid (synovitis). Osteoporosis most commonly produces pain in the spine and loss of height. Osteoarthritis can produce joint pain and stiffness, but the morning stiffness usually lasts only 30 minutes or less. Gout generally presents in a unilateral localized pattern rather than with generalized and diffuse joint pain.

47. B) Initiate daily aspirin therapy.
A patient who is experiencing a TIA can present with focal/one-sided weakness, vertigo, poor balance, and aphasia that is transient or resolves on its own. The patient may be hospitalized for multiple criteria such as duration of >1 hour, first TIA, high risk for atrial fibrillation, carotid stenosis greater than 50%, or crescendo TIAs (two or more in a week). MRI and/or CT should be scheduled within 24 hours of the attack. Prothrombin time (PT), partial thromboplastin time (PTT), international normalized ratio (INR), complete blood count (CBC), glucose, electrolytes, blood urea nitrogen (BUN), and creatinine are indicated diagnostics that can help differentiate a TIA from other medical mimics, such as hypoglycemia, hyponatremia, and infection, as well as determine baseline liver, kidney, and bleeding times. EKG should be placed as soon as possible after symptom onset to evaluate for atrial fibrillation as a possible cause of an embolic TIA. For patients not currently on oral anticoagulation and without a known cardioembolic source for the TIA, aspirin therapy, plus extended-release dipyridamole or clopidogrel, should be initiated. The patient's blood pressure should be maintained at 140/90 mmHg or lower to reduce the risk of future thromboembolic events. High-dose steroids would not be included in the treatment plan for TIA.

48. D) Ophthalmologist
Probable diagnosis is herpes zoster ophthalmicus, a shingles infection of the trigeminal nerve, which is a vision-threatening condition caused by reactivation of the herpes zoster virus on the ophthalmic branch of the trigeminal nerve (cranial nerve V). It is imperative that the patient be seen and treated by an ophthalmologist as soon as possible. The other specialist referrals are not specific for this condition, because there is no indication of cancer or neurologic damage at this point. A dermatologist would be needed if the rash does not respond to treatment.

49. D) "Do you have a history of migraine headaches?"
Abrupt cessation of atenolol (Tenormin), a beta-blocker, can cause rebound hypertension, resulting in potentially severe headache, nausea, and vomiting. Atenolol (Tenormin) should be weaned slowly after chronic use. A patient with a complaint of a "blinding headache" should be asked about a history of migraine and other headaches. The use of fluticasone (Flovent) nasal spray has little effect on blood pressure and is not significant for this patient; nor is a family history of hypercholesterolemia.

50. C) Tetracycline
Tetracyclines (category D) should not be prescribed for patients younger than 9 years. Mupirocin is the preferred first-line therapy for children with impetigo. Dicloxacillin is for penicillinase-producing staph skin infections and is an appropriate antibiotic for impetigo. Amoxicillin (category B), a broad-spectrum penicillin, is also an appropriate antibiotic for impetigo.

51. D) Congenital adrenal hyperplasia

Congenital adrenal hyperplasia is an endocrine disorder that is a RUSP core condition. The RUSP is a list of disorders that the U.S. Department of Health and Human Services (DHHS) recommends for states to screen for as part of their universal newborn screening programs. Disorders on the RUSP are chosen based on evidence that supports the potential net benefit of screening, the ability of states to screen for the disorder, and the availability of effective treatments. It is recommended that every newborn be screened for all disorders on the RUSP. Hypermethioninemia, tyrosinemia type II, and galactokinase deficiency are all secondary conditions. Secondary conditions are believed to be clinically significant, but some may have an unclear natural history or lack appropriate medical therapy that affects long-term outcome. They are detected during screening for core conditions.

52. B) "I should avoid foods that are high in potassium."

Nitrates can precipitate migraines, so patients should avoid consuming them. There is no need to reduce potassium intake. Other potential triggers include cigarette smoke and other strong odors, changes in sleep patterns, emotional or physical stress, alcohol, and caffeine.

53. D) Hordeolum

The patient has a hordeolum, or stye, which is an abscess of a hair follicle and sebaceous gland on the eyelid. A cholesteatoma is an abnormal, noncancerous skin growth that can develop in the middle section of the ear, behind the eardrum. Papilledema is a condition in which increased pressure in or around the brain causes the part of the optic nerve inside the eye to swell. Pinguecula is a yellowish, raised growth on the conjunctiva.

54. A, B, C) Shingles/zoster vaccination; Annual influenza vaccination; Pneumococcal vaccine

Among the vaccinations recommended by the Centers for Disease Control and Prevention (CDC) for individuals age 65 years or older are the shingles/zoster vaccination and annual influenza vaccination. Pneumococcal vaccination is also recommended for those whose previous vaccination histories are unknown. The HPV vaccine is recommended for preteens and persons up to age 26 years. The MMR vaccine is not routinely recommended for those age 65 years or older, although it may be recommended for individuals still employed in healthcare.

55. C) Bacterial pneumonia

The most common cause of bacterial pneumonia is *Streptococcus pneumoniae. Haemophilus influenzae, Chlamydia pneumoniae, Mycoplasma pneumoniae,* and *Legionella pneumophila* are other bacteria that cause pneumonia. Typically, pneumonia comes on very quickly; the patient has high fever/chills, productive cough with yellow or brown sputum, and shortness of breath, and may have chest pain with breathing/coughing. The gold standard for diagnosing bacterial pneumonia is the chest x-ray, which shows infiltrates and/or lobar consolidation. Older people can have confusion or a change in their mental abilities. In patients with bacterial pneumonia, it is important to determine whether bacteria are present in the urine, in order to identify appropriate antibiotics to treat the bacteria.

56. D) Chlamydia

If a pregnant patient is diagnosed with gonorrhea, they should also be evaluated for chlamydia due to the high rate of coinfection; however, the patient should be treated for chlamydia only if the nucleic acid amplification test (NAAT) is positive for chlamydia. Do not cotreat if the test is negative. An individual who is infected with HIV should also be tested for syphilis, a spirochete (bacterium). There is no need to treat genital warts (condyloma acuminata), unless they are present in the vagina, anus, or external glands. HSV-1 is usually an oral infection and would be treated with antiviral medications.

57. C) 29-year-old patient who smokes cigarettes

Cigarette smoking at age 29 years is considered a relative—not absolute—contraindication to oral contraceptive use. However, in a patient aged 35 years or older, smoking is an absolute contraindication. Pregnancy or suspected pregnancy is another absolute contraindication (e.g., in a sexually active patient who presents with amenorrhea). Liver tumors or impaired liver function (hepatitis C infection) is also an absolute contraindication, as is a history of emboli.

58. B) Acute appendicitis

Signs and symptoms of an acute abdomen include involuntary guarding, rebound tenderness, boardlike abdomen, and positive obturator and psoas signs. A positive obturator sign occurs when pain is elicited by internal rotation of the right hip from a 90-degree hip/knee flexion. The psoas sign is positive when pain occurs with passive extension of the thigh while the patient is lying on their side with knees extended, or when pain occurs with active flexion of the thigh at the hip.

59. A) Can see at 20 feet what a person with normal vision sees at 80 feet

The top number is the patient's distance in feet from the chart. The bottom number is the distance at which a person with normal eyesight can read the same line. A patient with 20/80 vision can see at 20 feet what a person with normal vision sees at 80 feet. Presbyopia is caused by loss of elasticity of the lenses, which makes it difficult to focus on close objects.

60. C) Increase of up to 50% of the plasma volume in pregnant patients

Physiologic anemia of pregnancy is caused by the increased volume of plasma during pregnancy when compared with the production of RBCs.

61. B, C, D) Metabolic syndrome; Infertility; Type 2 diabetes mellitus

A diagnosis of PCOS carries with it a risk of developing coronary heart disease, type 2 diabetes mellitus, metabolic syndrome, and infertility because of the high levels of androgens in the body. Endometriosis and congestive heart failure are not complications of PCOS.

62. C) Note on the record to monitor with an annual physical exam.

The findings are indicative of a Still murmur. It is a benign murmur that is common in school-aged children and usually resolves by adolescence. The murmur sound is of musical quality with minimal radiation. Because the condition is benign and usually self-resolves, the most appropriate action is to monitor with an annual physical exam.

63. C) Murphy sign

Murphy sign is performed by pressing deeply on the RUQ during inspiration. Mid-inspiratory arrest is a positive finding that aids in the diagnosis of cholecystitis. Rovsing sign is deep palpation of the lower left quadrant of the abdomen. The Markle test involves having the patient raise their heels and drop them suddenly. The psoas test is positive when the patient experiences abdominal pain while flexing the hip and knee.

64. B) Basal cell carcinoma

This is a classic appearance of a basal cell carcinoma. Lesions are small, translucent papules with a central ulceration, telangiectasia, and rolled borders. They appear as pearly white, light pink, brownish, or flesh colored. Basal cell carcinoma is more common in fair-skinned persons with long-term sun exposure. Acral lentiginous melanoma is a common type of melanoma in African American and Asian patients. These are dark-brown or black lesions located on nail beds. Actinic keratosis is a rough, scaly patch on the skin that develops from years of exposure to the sun. It is most commonly found on the face, lips, and ears; back of the hands; forearms; scalp; or neck. Seborrheic keratoses are soft, wartlike benign lesions that frequently appear on the back and trunk of the elderly.

65. D) Celiac disease

Celiac disease is also known as celiac sprue. Patients should avoid foods containing gluten, which causes malabsorption (diarrhea, gas, bloating, and abdominal pain). Foods to avoid are wheat, rye, and barley. Oats do not damage the mucosa in celiac disease. Antigliadins IgA and IgG are elevated in almost all patients (90%).

66. C) Cholesteatoma

An abnormal skin growth in the middle ear behind the eardrum is called cholesteatoma. Repeated infections and/or a tear or pulling inward of the eardrum can allow skin into the middle ear. Cholesteatomas often develop as cysts or pouches that shed layers of old skin, which build up inside the middle ear. Over time, the cholesteatoma can increase in size and destroy the surrounding delicate bones of the middle ear, leading to hearing loss that surgery can often improve. Permanent hearing loss, dizziness, and facial muscle paralysis are rare, but they can result from continued cholesteatoma growth.

67. D) Amoxicillin-clavulanate (Augmentin)

The patient presents with symptoms associated with *Pasteurella multocida*, which is an anaerobic gram-negative coccobacillus found in the oropharynx of healthy cats, dogs, and other animals. The diagnosis of the bacteria can be made with a gram stain culture; however, a broad-spectrum antibiotic that targets *Pasteurella*, as well as other gram-positive and gram-negative bacteria, is preferred for prescribed prophylaxis. Amoxicillin-clavulanate is a recommended antibiotic for prophylactic treatment. Aminoglycosides such as gentamicin have demonstrated poor activity against *P. multocida*. Tetanus toxoid is necessary only if the patient has received their last tetanus vaccine more than 5 years prior. Rabies prophylaxis is not necessary unless there is a possibility of exposure after a risk assessment.

68. A) Levothyroxine (Synthroid)

The patient is presenting with signs of subclinical hypothyroidism. Free T4 is normal, and TSH is elevated. A normal free T4 ranges between 0.8 and 1.8 ng/dL, and a normal TSH range is 0.4 to 4.0 mU/L. The patient may be started on a low dose of levothyroxine (usually 25 mcg/day). Propylthiouracil (PTU) is used in the treatment of hyperthyroidism. Signs of hyperthyroidism are insomnia, tachycardia, increased blood pressure, and weight loss. Memantine is used to treat severe dementia in Alzheimer's disease. The MMSE results in this case are minimal with a score of 28 (25–30 is questionable significance), so there is no need for memantine. Carbidopa-levodopa (Sinemet) is treatment for Parkinson's disease, which presents with a tremor at rest, muscular rigidity (e.g., shuffling walk), bradykinesia, and depression.

69. B) Osteoarthritis

Heberden nodes are bony nodules on the distal interphalangeal joints, commonly seen in osteoarthritis. In rheumatoid arthritis, patients commonly have swelling of the digits and development of finger shape changes such as swan neck deformity. Psoriatic arthritis does not produce Heberden nodes, but instead can produce finger deformity and characteristic associated psoriatic rash. Septic arthritis also does not produce Heberden nodes, but causes erythema and swelling of the affected joint.

70. C) Age younger than 6 months

The influenza vaccine should not be given before age 6 months because of the immaturity of the immune system. The flu vaccine is recommended for everyone age 6 months or older (with rare exceptions), but especially for children 6 months to 4 years of age; people with congenital heart disease, asthma, cystic fibrosis, sickle cell anemia, heart disease, and chronic obstructive pulmonary disease (COPD); those who will be pregnant during the influenza season; American Indians/Alaska Natives; healthcare personnel; and the elderly.

71. C) HDL
The patient's risk factors for heart disease include low HDL (<40 mg/dL), high triglyceride level (>150 mg/dL), and BMI of 32. Age older than 45 years for men and 55 years for women is considered a risk factor for heart disease. The patient's total cholesterol and blood pressure are within normal limits.

72. A) Paroxetine (Paxil)
Paroxetine (Paxil) is the SSRI most likely to cause erectile dysfunction. Escitalopram (Lexapro) is also an SSRI, but it is more likely to cause serotonin syndrome. Venlafaxine (Effexor) is a serotonin-norepinephrine reuptake inhibitor (SNRI). Amitriptyline is a tricyclic antidepressant (TCA).

73. B) Send the patient for a Doppler study and a d-dimer test.
The patient's symptoms are indicative of a deep vein thrombosis (DVT). A Doppler study and a d-dimer test will be indicative of a DVT. Application of warm compresses, elevation of the affected extremity, and prescription of NSAIDs are appropriate treatment for a superficial thrombophlebitis, not a DVT.

74. B) Tuberculosis (TB)
This is a radiograph of a lung infected by *Mycobacterium tuberculosis*, the causative agent in TB. The upper lobe is the most common location of a TB infection of the lungs. The typical findings are cavitation (round black holes due to local loss of lung tissue), fibrosis, lymphadenopathy, and calcifications.

75. A) Alendronate (Fosamax)
The patient is postmenopausal with osteoporosis, which has led to vertebral compression fractures. Gradual loss of bone density is common in postmenopausal women secondary to estrogen deficiency. Serum alkaline phosphate is elevated in bone fractures. Vertebral compression fractures will cause the spine to lose height. Osteoporosis is treated with bisphosphonates such as alendronate (Fosamax). Supplemental calcium with vitamin D is also recommended. Colchicine is used for an acute gout attack. Allopurinol is used in the treatment of chronic gout. Ferrous sulfate is an essential body mineral that is used to treat iron-deficiency anemia.

76. B) Infective endocarditis
Infective endocarditis (bacterial endocarditis) presents with chills, fever, and malaise, as well as a new murmur. Congestive heart failure symptoms are dyspnea, fatigue, dry cough, and swollen feet and ankles. Dissecting abdominal aortic aneurysm presents as a sudden onset of severe, sharp, excruciating pain in the abdomen, back, or flank area. Acute myocardial infarction generally presents with a gradual onset of intense and heavy chest discomfort that feels like squeezing, tightness, and heavy pressure in the chest.

77. D) Vigorous exercise 3 days prior
PSA levels are elevated in a patient with urinary retention, UTI, or recent stimulation of the prostate (e.g., through sexual activity). Vigorous exercise performed just prior to the exam can also elevate levels, but effects from exercise performed 3 days prior are unlikely to remain.

78. A) Dacryostenosis
Dacryostenosis is an obstruction of the lacrimal duct(s). Any discharge should be cultured and treated with an appropriate antibiotic. Newborn jaundice is a yellowing of an infant's skin and eyes. Newborn jaundice is very common and can occur when infants have a high level of bilirubin, a yellow pigment produced during normal breakdown of red blood cells. Red reflex testing is vital for early detection of vision and potentially life-threatening abnormalities in infants, such as cataracts, glaucoma, retinoblastoma, retinal abnormalities, systemic diseases with ocular manifestations, and high refractive errors. Dark spots in the red reflex, a markedly diminished reflex, the presence of a white reflex, or asymmetry of the reflexes requires referral to an ophthalmologist. Myopia or nearsightedness is when the eyeball is slightly longer than normal from front to back. Light rays focus in front of the retina.

79. A) The spleen is not palpable in the majority of healthy adults.
The spleen is located in the LUQ of the abdomen under the diaphragm and is protected by the lower ribcage. In the majority of adults, it is not palpable. The spleen's longest axis is 11 to 20 cm. Any spleen larger than 20 cm is enlarged. The best test for evaluating splenic (or hepatic) size is the abdominal ultrasound. Disorders that can cause splenomegaly include mononucleosis, sickle cell disease, congestive heart failure, and bone marrow cancers (myeloma, leukemia).

80. A) Acute prostatitis
In the elderly male patient with acute prostatitis, symptoms occur abruptly with a sudden onset of a high fever, chills, and complaints of suprapubic and/or back pain, which sometimes radiates to the rectum. DRE reveals an extremely tender prostate that is warm and boggy. The patient may have an accompanying infection of the bladder, which, given the nature of the sudden onset of symptoms, would be considered an acute UTI, not chronic. Kidney stone pain is described as "renal cholic" with flank pain; there generally is no fever. Urethritis caused by chlamydial infection may be asymptomatic and generally is found in younger adults.

81. C) Renal tubules
The basic functional units of the kidney are nephrons containing glomeruli and renal tubules. Polycystic kidney disease affects the tubules within the nephrons. The loop of Henle is responsible for reabsorption of sodium and is not affected by polycystic kidney disease directly. Likewise,

the glomerulus and Bowman capsules are responsible for filtering blood and reabsorption back into the bloodstream and are affected by disorders such as glomerulonephritis and diabetic nephropathy.

82. D) Ceftriaxone 500 mg IM x one dose plus doxycycline 100 mg twice daily x 14 days plus metronidazole 500 mg twice daily x 14 days

Fitz-Hugh-Curtis syndrome should be treated as a complicated gonorrheal/chlamydial infection: Ceftriaxone 500 mg IM x one dose plus doxycycline 100 mg twice daily x 14 days plus metronidazole 500 mg twice daily x 14 days for anaerobic coverage. Benzathine penicillin G 2.4 mU IM weekly x 3 weeks is used to treat complicated syphilis infections. Doxycycline 100 mg PO twice daily x 14 days is an appropriate regimen to treat complicated chlamydial infections. A pregnant patient with confirmed uncomplicated gonorrheal and chlamydial infections would be prescribed ceftriaxone 500 mg IM x one dose plus azithromycin 1 g PO x one dose.

83. B) Ofloxacin

Ofloxacin ear drops are not considered to be ototoxic. Aminoglycoside otic drops (gentamicin, tobramycin, neomycin) are ototoxic and should not be used to treat otitis media or perforation of the TM. In addition, ear drops with alcohol, benzocaine, or olive oil should be avoided in patients with TM perforation. Swimming and water inside the ear should be avoided until the TM is healed. Topical therapy with quinolone drops may be equivalent to oral therapy, but some experts prefer oral antibiotic therapy, such as amoxicillin or amoxicillin-clavulanate (Augmentin) for 10 days, to treat TM perforations.

84. B) Karyotype

Tanner stage I is prepubertal. At age 14 years, an absence of Tanner stage II characteristics, along with a webbed neck, swollen hands and feet, and short stature, suggests Turner syndrome. Confirmation of Turner syndrome is done with karyotype analysis to confirm the partial or complete absence of the second sex chromosome. Prolactin level would indicate the presence of a tumor in the pituitary as the possible cause of delayed puberty but would need to be confirmed with a CT scan. An x-ray of the hand is used for estimating "bone age." A prolactin level to rule out prolactinoma-induced amenorrhea and a CT scan and x-ray of the hand to determine if true age matches stated age would all be useful for determining the cause of delayed puberty; however, in the presence of a webbed neck, swollen hands and feet, and short stature, Turner syndrome is the primary suspect.

85. C) Edema of the ankles and headache

Common side effects of calcium channel blockers such as nifedipine (Procardia XL) include edema of the ankles, dizziness, headaches, flushing, and weakness. Angiotensin-converting enzyme (ACE) inhibitors tend to have the side effects of angioedema and a dry hacking cough. Diuretics can cause hypokalemia and hyperuricemia.

86. B) Mitral regurgitation

Mitral regurgitation is a pansystolic murmur heard best at the apex or apical area of the heart; it radiates to the axilla and is a loud blowing, high-pitched murmur. Rheumatic fever (a complication of untreated strep throat) can damage the mitral valve, leading to mitral valve regurgitation early or late in life. Aortic stenosis is best heard at the right side of the sternum and is a harsh and noisy murmur. Mitral stenosis is a low-pitched diastolic rumbling murmur. Aortic regurgitation is also a blowing, high-pitched murmur, but it is heard at the right side of the sternum.

87. D) Use an additional method of contraception while on the antibiotic and for one pill cycle after treatment is complete

Patients should be advised to use an additional, alternative form of birth control, such as condoms, when taking tetracycline and for one pill cycle afterward because of reduced efficacy of the oral contraceptive when taken concurrently with the antibiotic. The two medications do not have to be taken separately, as this does not change the effect of the medication. The birth control pill should not be discontinued while taking the antibiotic. It is important that an additional form of birth control be continued for one pill cycle after the course of antibiotic is completed.

88. C) Brown recluse spider bite

This is a classic description of a brown recluse spider bite. These bites begin with burning at the site, followed by blanching with a red halolike center. The central area of the bite becomes necrotic, and black eschar forms. Rocky Mountain spotted fever, a tick-borne disease, starts as a rash on the wrists and hands and rapidly progresses toward the trunk. Early Lyme disease presents as a circular red rash that slowly expands as a "target"or "bull's-eye," which is called erythema migrans. This disease is spread by black-legged ticks that are usually infected with *Borrelia burgdorferi*. It is more common in the northeastern states. A melanoma is a cancerous growth that generally has a dark-brown appearance.

89. B) Chronic obstructive pulmonary disease (COPD)

COPD is a progressive lung disease that includes emphysema and chronic bronchitis. The most common risk factor for COPD is long-term cigarette smoking (80%–90%). Another cause is alpha-1 antitrypsin deficiency and chronic fume exposure. The three cardinal symptoms of COPD are dyspnea, chronic cough, and sputum production. The lungs are hyperinflated, which changes the shape of the chest and diaphragm, making the mechanics of breathing more difficult. Excess mucus and obstructed airflow from progressive thickening and stiffening of the airways diminish breath sounds. COPD creates a high hematocrit percentage because of chronic hypoxemia. Lung cancer is also associated with extended smoking history and can present with pain and fatigue; however, weight loss is also a frequent finding. CHF is less likely given the absence of edema and the described breath sounds; CHF tends to exhibit pulmonary rales.

90. B) Start the patient on levothyroxine (Synthroid) 25 mcg orally daily.

The patient is symptomatic (weight gain, lack of energy, and irregular periods) with low free T4. Even though the TSH level decreased slightly, the free T4 remains low. An elevated TSH and low free T4 are indicative of hypothyroidism. The next step is to start the patient on levothyroxine (Synthroid) 25 mcg daily and recheck the TSH in 6 weeks. The goal is to normalize the TSH (between 1.0 and 3.5) and to ameliorate the patient's symptoms (e.g., increase energy). Armour thyroid (desiccated thyroid) is a natural supplement composed of dried (desiccated) pork thyroid glands. It is used in alternative medicine as a substitute for synthetic levothyroxine (Synthroid). There is no current need for a referral.

91. D) Osteoarthritis

The patient's presentation is a classic case of osteoarthritis. Osteoarthritis of the hip is associated with joint pain that worsens with activity, diminished ROM, joint crepitus, and difficulty arising after long periods of rest. Patients with hip fractures have severe pain in the hip or groin and are unable to bear weight. The leg may also be externally rotated. Rheumatoid arthritis is a systemic autoimmune disorder that presents with inflammation of multiple joints. A medial tibial stress fracture is an injury of the lower extremity and presents with inflammation of muscles, tendons, and bone tissue of the tibia.

92. C) Actinic keratosis

Actinic keratoses are small, raised lesions on skin that has been in the sun for a long period of time. These lesions are usually benign but can develop into skin cancer; therefore, further evaluation is needed to determine whether removal is required. Seborrheic keratosis, lentigo, and rosacea are benign.

93. A) Raised right iliac crest

A raised iliac crest can be a warning sign of curvature secondary to the attachment of the pelvis to the spine. Kyphosis or the kyphotic curve causes the spine to be bent forward. The official medical term for an abnormal curvature of the thoracic spine is *hyperkyphosis*. Lumbar lordosis is the normal inward curvature of the lumbar region of the spine. The curve helps the body to absorb shock and remain stable but flexible. However, if the curve arches too far inward, it is known as an increased lumbar lordosis or "swayback" posture. Osteopenia is a condition where the bones are weaker than normal and is often a precursor to osteoporosis.

94. B) 5

Tuberculin skin tests are tests of delayed hypersensitivity. Purified protein derivative (PPD) tuberculin antigen is injected intradermally to form a 6-mm to 10-mm wheal. The skin test is read within 48 to 72 hours, when the induration is most evident. Erythema without induration is generally considered to be of no significance. An induration that is 5 mm or more in diameter indicates a positive reaction for patients with very high-risk conditions or exposures (e.g., HIV, organ transplant recipient, pharmacologically immunosuppressed, contact with TB patient) and the need for treatment of latent TB infection.

95. C) Impetigo

Impetigo is caused by gram-positive bacteria (streptococcus or *Staphylococcus aureus*) and is very contagious among young children, particularly those age 2 to 5 years. It produces "honey-crusted," pruritic vesiculopustules that rupture and crust. Measles presents with Koplik spots on the mucosa by the rear molars and is also highly contagious. Psoriasis is an inherited disorder in which the squamous epithelial cells rapidly turn over and cause plaques. Psoriasis can be located on the back, knees, antecubital spaces, and gluteal folds. Scabies is caused by an itch mite via skin-to-skin contact and causes a very pruritic rash in the webs of the hands, waist, and genital area.

96. A) Acyclovir

Bell palsy is caused by inflammation in cranial nerve VII. Herpes simplex is a virus, and acyclovir is an antiviral medication that should be prescribed during this visit. Trimethoprim-sulfamethoxazole (Bactrim DS), penicillin, and ciprofloxacin are antibiotics. They will not be effective against a virus.

97. B) Cervical culture

The patient presents with subjective and objective findings associated with endometritis. Endometritis, an infection of the uterus, can be caused by different organisms. It is most commonly associated with pelvic inflammatory disease or invasive gynecologic procedures in the non-obstetric population. To determine the appropriate treatment, the NP will obtain a cervical culture to identify the type of bacteria causing the infection. Vaginal cultures can be easily contaminated and thus may mislead a provider to prescribe inappropriate or inadequate antibiotic coverage. Blood cultures would be obtained if the patient had signs or symptoms of sepsis or bacteremia. Ultrasound imaging would be useful if the patient were postpartum, as it can rule out endometritis caused by retained products of conception, uterine abscesses, or an infected hematoma.

98. C) Shock-like facial pain

Trigeminal neuralgia presents with extreme, shock-like facial pain that lasts from a few seconds to 2 minutes per event. Bilateral stiffness and aching in the posterior neck, shoulders, and upper arms is associated with polymyalgia rheumatica. Shooting pain at the base of the head is a symptom of occipital neuralgia. Severe pain in or around one eye is a symptom of cluster headaches.

99. B) Appendicitis

The patient is exhibiting signs of acute appendicitis. He demonstrates a positive psoas sign, which is indicative of acute appendicitis. Hepatitis is not a viable diagnosis based on the results of the diagnostic testing. Cholecystitis presents with right upper quadrant pain. Nephrolithiasis (kidney stones) does not respond to a psoas test.

100. D) Minimal caffeine consumption

Patients with osteoporosis should limit consumption of caffeine (which can leach calcium from bones), take daily calcium and vitamin D supplements to support normal bone metabolism, limit alcohol consumption, and engage in weight-bearing exercise three times each week. Weight-bearing exercise includes walking, jogging, and other sports; swimming and isometric exercise, while healthy activities, are not weight bearing and so do not provide the necessary stimulus. Adequate protein intake helps slow bone loss, so a low-protein diet would be inappropriate.

101. A) Absent cremasteric reflex

Testicular torsion presents with a sudden onset of pain in the scrotum/ testicles, and initially it may be felt in the abdomen and groin. The scrotum will be swollen, in severe cases acute hydrocele is present, and the affected testicle is higher than the unaffected one. Severe nausea and vomiting are common features. The cremasteric reflex is missing, not present. If not corrected within 24 hours, 100% of testicles become gangrenous and must be surgically removed. Hematuria and pyuria are not symptoms of testicular torsion, and urinalysis is generally normal.

102. A) Iron-deficiency anemia

There is a strong association between lead poisoning and iron deficiency in children as both diagnoses are common in patients of lower socioeconomic status. Iron deficiency has also been shown to increase lead retention in the tissues, leading to increased absorption and toxicity. Thalassemia minor is an inherited blood disorder. Pernicious anemia is a consequence of the inability to absorb vitamin B12. Normocytic anemia results from a long-term chronic disease and generally occurs in the elderly rather than in children.

103. B) The patient is at 50% to 80% of their personal best.

Spirometer readings are used to assess a patient's personal best. The green zone is in the range of 80% to 100% of expected volume, the yellow zone is in the range of 50% to 80% of expected volume, and the red zone is below 50% of expected volume, which would place the patient at risk for hypoxia. The medication would need to be adjusted, but not lowered, to produce the desired effects.

104. C) "I will refer your mother to a psychiatric-mental health NP."

It is a breach of standards of practice if the NP demonstrates a failure to monitor patient outcomes and refer patients to a psychiatric-mental health NP, psychologist, or psychiatrist if symptoms have not improved, if the patient is getting worse (acute decompensation) or is noncompliant, or if family members have raised concerns about a patient. Patients with mental illnesses, such as depression, anxiety, and attention deficit hyperactivity disorder, are often initially treated by primary care providers such as NPs. NPs are well positioned to provide mental healthcare, from mental health screening to initial intervention, which dovetails with the NP philosophy of patient-centered care. However, NP education covers only some aspects of mental healthcare and may not sufficiently prepare providers to treat patients with complex mental illnesses, compared with psychiatric-mental health NPs or other behavioral health specialists. NPs should be aware of potential scenarios where the care they provide could breach their standard operating procedure. Trying a different drug regimen or one-on-one counseling sessions may exceed the scope of practice for an NP. The best response would be to consult with a mental health professional. The nurse practice act does not preclude an NP from continuing to care for the patient; however, the NP should refer the patient to a specialist.

105. B) Quinolones

Patients who are prescribed quinolones are at risk for rupturing their Achilles tendon. They should be educated about this potential complication. Sulfonamides, cephalosporins, and penicillin do not pose this potential risk.

106. D) "Screening has only a small benefit of reducing chance of death from prostate cancer, so you can decide if you want to be screened."

Although the patient has a higher risk of prostate cancer because of his age and ethnicity, the overall recommendation is for patients to choose whether or not they want to be screened. Based on the recommendation, the NP would not instruct the patient to have his prostate-specific antigen checked and/or have a physical exam annually or every 2 years to screen for prostate cancer.

107. C) Abstain from sexual intercourse during treatment.

The patient would be advised to abstain from sexual intercourse until treatment is complete. Douching can alter the normal vaginal pH and be a root cause of overgrowth of bacteria. Bacterial vaginosis is not considered a sexually transmitted infection; therefore, the Centers for Disease Control and Prevention does not recommend treatment of sexual partners.

108. D) Actinic keratosis

Actinic keratosis is considered the most common precancerous lesion of squamous cell carcinoma in the elderly. Actinic keratosis is a rough, scaly patch on the skin that develops from years of exposure to the sun. It is most commonly found on the face, lips, ears, back of the hands, forearms, scalp, or neck. Purpura presents as bright, purple-colored patches located on the forearms and hands and are benign. Lentigines, also known as "liver spots," are brown-colored macules located on the hands and forearms of older adults and are benign. Seborrheic keratoses are soft, wartlike benign lesions that frequently appear on the back and trunk of older adults.

109. C) Oral hairy leukoplakia

Oral hairy leukoplakia presents as elongated papilla of the lateral aspects of the tongue. The EBV is the causative agent of oral hairy leukoplakia. Koplik spots present as clusters of small red papules with white centers located on the buccal mucosa by the lower molars. Koplik spots are a prodromic viral enanthem of measles manifesting 2 to 3 days before the measles rash itself. Geographic tongue is an inflammatory disorder that usually appears on the top and sides of the tongue. Typically, affected tongues have a bald, red area of varying size that is surrounded by an irregular white border that resembles a map. Cheilosis is painful inflammation and cracking of the corners of the mouth.

110. B) *Streptococcus pneumoniae*

Streptococcus pneumoniae is the bacterium *most commonly* associated with CAP. *Chlamydia pneumoniae* and *Mycoplasma pneumonia* are also common causes. *Pseudomonas aeruginosa* is uncommonly associated with CAP, but it is frequently associated with hospital-acquired pneumonia.

111. C) Hypertriglyceridemia

Side effects of thiazide diuretics such as hydrochlorothiazide are hyperglycemia, hyperuricemia, and hypertriglyceridemia and hypercholesterolemia. Patients should also be monitored for hypokalemia, hyponatremia, and hypomagnesemia.

112. A, B, D, E) Treat with nonsteroidal anti-inflammatory drugs (NSAIDs); Prescribe antibiotics to treat infection; Recommend rest and comfort measures; Prescribe a corticosteroid.

Reiter syndrome is an immune-mediated reaction secondary to chlamydia that causes red, swollen joints; ulcers on the skin of the glans penis; and urethritis. It resolves on its own. Treatment usually includes NSAIDs and comfort measures, although corticosteroids may be prescribed for patients with significant pain in the large joints. Treatment with antibiotics will address the underlying cause, which is chlamydia. LNA is used in the treatment of ankylosing spondylitis.

113. C) Insulin lispro (Humalog)

Lispro is a rapid-acting insulin that is used on a sliding scale to work from meal to meal. Insulin isophane and insulin regular is a mixture of intermediate- and short-acting insulins and would not be appropriate for a sliding scale. Insulin glargine is given once a day. NPH is an intermediate-acting insulin that is not appropriate for a sliding scale.

114. A) Azithromycin (Z-Pak) daily x 5 days

The patient presents with signs and symptoms of *Mycoplasma pneumoniae* infection (atypical pneumonia). Because the patient does not have any comorbidities or antibiotic resistance, the most appropriate treatment would be azithromycin (Z-Pak) daily x 5 days. Patients with risk of possible comorbidity (e.g., chronic heart, lung, liver, or renal disease; diabetes mellitus; alcoholism; malignancy; asplenia) and/or those at risk for antibiotic resistance should receive monotherapy with a fluoroquinolone (e.g., levofloxacin, moxifloxacin) or combination therapy of amoxicillin-clavulanate plus a macrolide or doxycycline. Monotherapy with amoxicillin-clavulanate would not be appropriate.

115. D) Report the case to the health department.

The NP is required to report the acute case of hepatitis C to the health department. Isolation is not required, nor is the patient required to wear a mask in public or an identifying bracelet. These actions violate the patient's right to privacy, as hepatitis C is not an airborne-transmitted disease.

116. C) One eye turned inward

During the first 2 months of life, a newborn's eyes may appear crossed or wander at times, which is normal. If one eye is turned in or out consistently, the newborn should be referred to a pediatric ophthalmologist for further evaluation. The lacrimal ducts are immature at birth, but typically a newborn can shed tears by 2 weeks. It is normal for White newborns to be born with bluish-gray eyes, which change as they mature. A newborn will often fixate on their mother's face.

117. A, B, D, E) Conduct Lachman's test; Apply ice to the joint; Support the joint with a compression wrap; Refer to an orthopedic specialist.

Lachman's test should be used to test for anterior cruciate ligament (ACL) damage. An ACL injury is classically associated with a sudden "pop" and swelling. The RICE mnemonic should be followed for musculoskeletal trauma; applying ice and compression are part of the RICE protocol. Referral should be made to an orthopedic specialist for repair and follow-up. Isometric exercises should be avoided during the early phases of recovery from a musculoskeletal injury.

118. A, B) Palmar grasp of objects; Sitting up

At age 6 months, an infant should be able to grasp objects, reach for objects and toys, pass items from one hand to the other, sit up without support, roll over, and bring things to their mouth. Standing independently, moving from one piece of furniture to another, and feeding themselves independently are motor skills expected at a later stage of development.

119. B) 7

Complicated UTIs in male patients, patients with uncontrolled diabetes, pregnant or elderly women, and patients who are immunocompromised require medication treatment for a minimum of 7 days. Three days of treatment is not long enough to remediate any bacteria, and 10 or 14 days would be too long and may cause various other complications, such as antibiotic-related infections (e.g., *Clostridium difficile*).

120. D) Iodine

Iodine is a central component of thyroid hormones, which regulate growth, development, and metabolic rate. Low iodine levels result in hypothyroidism. A patient deficient in iodine will present with weight gain, lethargy, and goiter. If deficient in calcium, a patient will present with impaired growth and osteoporosis. When deficient in fluoride, a patient will present with dental decay and be subject to osteoporosis. A sodium deficiency presents as restlessness, irritability, muscle weakness, cramps, and possibly nausea and vomiting.

121. B) Medial tibial stress syndrome

The patient presents with a classic case of medial tibial stress syndrome. Overuse of the muscles and tendons can cause inflammation of the tibia. It is more common in runners and people with pes planus (flat feet), as well as in female athletes who have eating disorders and amenorrhea. Plantar fasciitis is inflammation of the thick band of tissue at the bottom of the foot that runs from the heel to the toes. Morton neuroma is a painful condition affecting the ball of the foot, most commonly the area between the third and fourth toes. Degenerative joint disease (osteoarthritis) is caused by inflammation and the breakdown and eventual loss of joint cartilage.

122. D) Reticulocyte count

Hemopoietic evaluation of a patient with sickle cell disease who is experiencing a febrile illness includes a complete blood count (CBC) with a differential and reticulocyte count, as well as liver function tests, urinalysis, and blood cultures. The reticulocyte count reflects the efficiency of the bone marrow's response to illness in a patient with sickle cell disease. An elevated B lymphocytic count is associated with an inflammatory condition and is not explicitly evaluated in febrile patients with sickle cell disease. C-reactive protein is produced in the liver and is a marker for inflammation. Prothrombin time is used to assess overall platelet function and evaluate how long it takes for the blood to clot.

123. A) Azithromycin

The patient likely has atypical pneumonia (walking pneumonia), which is an infection of the lungs more common in children and young adults. It is highly contagious and should be treated with a macrolide antibiotic; azithromycin is the drug of choice. The NP will also recommend increased fluids and rest, as well as an antitussive as needed. Amoxicillin–clavulanate is ineffective against the atypical organisms, and albuterol nebulizer is not routinely ordered for atypical pneumonia.

124. D) Raynaud phenomenon

Raynaud phenomenon occurs from vasospasms of the blood vessels, leading to decreased blood supply to the hands and feet, which causes bluish discoloration, with fingertips turning a dark-red color if severe. Stress and cold weather are classic triggers for this syndrome. This degree of circulatory alteration is not a normal phenomenon. Additionally, peripheral vascular disease and chronic arterial insufficiency would produce more consistent symptoms rather than spasms in response to cold and stress.

125. D) IV

Murmurs are graded according to the sound made by vibrations and their intensity. A thrill is a "palpable murmur" that initially presents at the grade IV level. Grades II and III murmurs are audible in progressing sounds upon auscultation. A grade V murmur is very loud with a more obvious thrill than in grade IV.

126. B) V

Cranial nerve (CN) V is the trigeminal nerve. In herpes zoster opthalmicus, it is infected by the shingles virus. CN VII is the facial nerve that provides both sensory and motor functions, such as moving muscles used for facial expressions, providing a sense of taste for most of the tongue, and communicating sensations from the outer parts of the ear. The oculomotor nerve (III) controls muscle function and pupil response. The trochlear nerve (IV) controls the superior oblique muscle.

127. C) Quadrivalent inactivated influenza vaccine (QIV)

A 53-year-old adult with a chronic respiratory disease such as emphysema should receive an annual QIV, which is appropriate to administer in patients age 6 months and older. LAIV is administered via nasal spray in patients age 2 to 49 years; however, it is not recommended for those with a history of wheezing in the last 12 months or for those with underlying lung disease. PPSV23 is administered in one dose at age 65 years. It is also recommended for adults age 19 to 64 years who smoke cigarettes; however, it is administered in one dose, not annually. PCV13 is recommended for children younger than 2 years and in some adults age 65 years or older who do not have an immunocompromised condition, cerebrospinal leak, or cochlear implant.

128. D) Palpable ovary

The ovaries of a postmenopausal patient should not be palpable; this is an abnormal finding that needs to be investigated. A referral to the gynecologist with the order for a pelvic/intravaginal ultrasound is standard to rule out cancer. A positive Pap-smear low-grade squamous intrathecal lesion indicates abnormality of the cervix and would be diagnosed further with colposcopy with conization. A finding of external genital warts would prompt internal examination of the vagina and cervix with colposcopy. Vaginal atrophy is an expected finding in postmenopausal patients.

129. C) Wet mount

A wet mount can be used to diagnose vaginal candidiasis. Vaginal pH is not explicitly used to validate a diagnosis of vaginal candida infection. A whiff test is used to diagnose bacterial vaginitis. Although not commonly used, the Tzanck smear can be used to evaluate a herpetic infection.

130. B) Decreased sperm production

Sperm production decreases as a result of decreased testosterone levels in the aging male. The secretions from the seminal vesicles and prostate gland decrease, resulting in an overall decrease in the volume of the semen produced. Because of the decrease in the production of sperm and secretions from seminal vesicles, the relative concentration of sperm remains consistent in the semen. Low levels of estrogen are associated with low levels of testosterone consistent in the geriatric male.

131. C) Fecal occult blood test

The U.S. Preventive Services Task Force (USPSTF) recommends screening for colorectal cancer in all adults age 45 to 75 years. After age 75 years, screening should be individualized based on the patient's degree of risk. Routine screening should be discontinued at age 85 years. High-sensitivity guaiac fecal occult blood test (gFOBT) or fecal immunochemical test (FIT) should be performed annually, and stool DNA (SDNA) every 1 to 3 years. If positive, colonoscopy is required; otherwise, the patient should have a colonoscopy every 10 years. Flexible sigmoidoscopy or CT colonography would be performed every 5 years.

132. D) Apply nebulizer treatment.

The priority treatment for a patient with an asthma exacerbation is a nebulizer treatment every 20 minutes as needed. Additionally, a short course of oral corticosteroids may be prescribed after an exacerbation or, if the patient is not currently prescribed one, a low-dose inhaled corticosteroid with or without a long-acting beta2-agonist. It is important to ensure that the patient has a rescue inhaler or a short-acting beta2-agonist such as albuterol to decrease morbidity and mortality risks. Assessing triggers and providing teaching on the use of a spacer can be completed after the patient has been stabilized.

133. C) Curettage and electrodessication

The patient has Bowen disease, a squamous cell cancer of the epidermis that has not invaded the dermis yet. Curettage and electrodessication is an efficient, cost-effective method with low complication rates. Surgical treatments such as a standard excision (95% removal) and Moh surgery (100% removal) are more invasive, and there is a greater risk for complications, especially in the elderly. Radiation therapy is not indicated for low-risk lesions.

134. C) Acute viral upper respiratory infection (URI)

Chronic cough can be caused by chronic bronchitis, allergic rhinitis, and GERD. The cough associated with a viral URI is a mild-to-moderate hacking cough. The cough is usually dry (no sputum). With postnasal drip, the cough may bring up some nasal secretions. The cough abates with the viral illness.

135. B) Trimethoprim-sulfamethoxazole (Bactrim DS)

Trimethoprim-sulfamethoxazole (Bactrim DS) is appropriate for treating gram-negative bacteria such as *Escherichia coli*, which is a common cause of urinary tract infections.

It is also appropriate for patients older than 2 months. Ciprofloxacin and levofloxacin are quinolones and should not be administered to children younger than 18 years. Doxycycline should not be prescribed for children younger than 9 years.

136. D) Pterygium

The patient has a pterygium, which is a yellow, triangular thickening of the conjunctiva that extends across the cornea on the nasal side. Pinguecula is a yellowish, raised growth on the conjunctiva next to the cornea. A chalazion is a chronic inflammation of the meibomian gland. A hordeolum, or stye, is an abscess of a hair follicle and sebaceous gland on the eyelid.

137. A) Baseline mammogram should start at age 50 years and repeat every 2 years until age 74 years.

The USPSTF currently recommends mammography every 2 years for women age 50 to 74 years who are at average risk. This recommendation does not apply to those with known genetic mutations, familial breast cancer, or a history of chest radiation at a young age, or to women previously diagnosed with high-risk breast lesion who may benefit from starting screening in their 40s.

138. A) Serum creatinine

When BUN levels are abnormally high, serum creatinine should be performed to determine renal function. If results are normal, renal function is more than likely normal as well. eGFR is an estimated number, based upon multiple factors, and can be falsely elevated in patients who are dehydrated, or have muscle breakdown from exercise. An IVP is a radiographic test that is used to evaluate the urinary system and would be used to determine the cause of renal failure, such as tumor or scarring. An MRI is not required at this time.

139. C) Alzheimer's disease

Alzheimer's disease involves a permanent change to the brain that causes short-term memory loss, agnosia, apraxia, and aphasia. In this case, the patient's physical exam is normal; however, he is having memory loss and difficulty working and carrying out his normal tasks. Delirium is an acute decline in mental status, rather than a gradual permanent process, and is temporary; common causes are fever, shock, drugs, alcohol, and dehydration. Stroke generally produces sudden onset of focal neurologic deficits rather than gradual memory impairment. Tic douloureux produces facial pain and spasms rather than memory impairment.

140. B) Protecting the rights of the human subjects who participate in research done at the institution

Every research institution has an IRB whose job is to review all of the research that is conducted in that institution. The IRB's most important role is to protect the rights of the human subjects who participate in research done at the institution of which the IRB is a part (e.g., research hospitals, universities). Protection of research subjects is done through review of protocols and methodology, but the ultimate goal remains the focus on protecting participants' safety. This, in turn, may protect both the hospital's interest and the researcher; however, the priority is the safety of the research participant rather than the other entities involved.

141. B) It is the value that occurs in the middle when the set is arranged from smallest value to largest.
The median is the middle value in a given set of numbers (arranged from lowest to highest). For example, for a group of numbers that consists of 2, 3, 6, 7, 7, 8, and 10, the number 7 is the median value. The mode is the value that occurs most frequently in the set. The average of the values is referred to as the mean. The difference between the smallest and greatest values is called the range.

142. B) Secondary prevention
The NP is evaluating the patient for major depression. Secondary prevention includes detecting disease at an early stage to halt or slow its progress. All screening tests and lab tests (e.g., mammography, Pap smears) are secondary prevention activities.

143. B) Advise the patient that a peer who is working with the NP can answer the patient's questions more thoroughly.
Discussing personal beliefs is considered unprofessional behavior. Respecting the patient's right to choose is an example of supporting patient autonomy. The best, most appropriate action by the NP is to have a peer answer the patient's questions thoroughly.

144. B) Testify about the standards of nursing care as they apply to the facts in the case
An expert nurse may testify about the laws and standards of practice as they apply to nursing. An expert nurse is not a legal expert. A nurse expert can testify for the prosecution or the defense. As an expert witness, the nurse would provide only facts and would not provide an opinion about the other nurse's actions.

145. B) Collaborative
A collaborative relationship exists when a health caregiver refers a patient to others (e.g., physicians, specialists, physical therapy) to help with patient treatment and management. Consult reports and progress reports are sent to the primary caregiver to report the patient's progress. Consultative relationships are informal, such as talking to a colleague about a patient's treatment.

146. C) Filled-in square
A filled-in square indicates a male who is diseased or affected; a filled-in circle is a female who is diseased or affected. An empty square is a healthy male, and an empty circle is a healthy female.

147. D) Report the child sexual abuse to the department of Child Protective Services (CPS).
There are several "helping" professions (e.g., nurses, teachers, mental healthcare practitioners) who are required to report suspected or actual child/elder abuse to authorities. The NP is legally required to report the case to CPS. If the child is in danger, CPS may ask for a court order to take the child away for protection until the investigation is completed. Talking about the partner's behavior will not be effective and may put the child and/or mother in danger if the partner suspects that he is being watched.

148. C) Triazolam (Halcion)
Triazolam (Halcion) has an average half-life of about 2 hours. Alprazolam (Xanax) has a half-life of 12 hours. Lorazepam (Ativan) has a half-life of 15 hours. Clonazepam (Klonopin) has a half-life of 34 hours.

149. B) Anorexia nervosa
Anorexia nervosa usually has an onset during adolescence and is characterized by an irrational preoccupation with weight gain that presents with a distorted perception of body weight and size. Anorexia nervosa is characterized by marked weight loss, lanugo, thinning hair, and general poor health, as the body is depleted of vital nutrients. Amenorrhea is a common symptom in young female patients. Purging, alopecia, and use of laxatives may be involved in the restriction of food intake, but based on the assessment data, it is not the primary diagnosis.

150. D) Fluoxetine (Prozac)
Fluoxetine (Prozac) is recommended as first-line treatment for children and adolescents with moderate to severe depressive disorders. Second-line therapy includes sertraline (Zoloft); reasonable alternatives include escitalopram, citalopram, or venlafaxine. Third-line pharmacotherapy includes bupropion and duloxetine. However, bupropion (Wellbutrin), an atypical antidepressant, is contraindicated in patients with anorexia nervosa. There appears to be a slightly increased risk of suicidal thoughts and behaviors among children and adolescents who are treated with certain antidepressant medications (including sertraline, fluoxetine, citalopram, duloxetine, venlafaxine, escitalopram, and bupropion, among others). While the evidence is inadequate to conclusively establish an association, the risk of antidepressant-related suicide must be weighed against the benefits of treatment and the risk of suicide in untreated depression. The U.S. Food and Drug Administration requires a boxed warning label regarding the increased risk of suicide, ensuring a discussion with the prescribing NP, patient, and family. Lithium carbonate (Eskalith) is indicated for patients with bipolar disorder.

This practice test is based on the blueprint for the American Academy of Nurse Practitioners Certification Board (AANPCB) Family Nurse Practitioner certification exam.*
It includes 150 questions.

1. The group with the highest percentage of all deaths caused by heart disease is:
   A. American Indian or Alaska Native
   B. African American
   C. Asian
   D. White (non-Hispanic)

2. A patient reports with chest pain and shortness of breath. A 12-lead EKG reveals ST-segment elevation in leads II, III, and aVF. This is suggestive of which type of myocardial infarction (MI)?
   A. Anterior
   B. Lateral
   C. Anteroseptal
   D. Inferior

3. A middle-aged female patient presents with complaints of weight gain, constipation, and alopecia of the eyebrows. Serum cholesterol is 247 mg/dL, thyroid-stimulating hormone (TSH) is 25 mg/dL, and thyroid peroxidase (TPO) is elevated. Which diagnosis is most likely?
   A. Thyroid cancer
   B. Hyperprolactinemia
   C. Pheochromocytoma
   D. Hashimoto's thyroiditis

4. The nurse practitioner is checking a 75-year-old female patient's breast during an annual gynecological exam. The left nipple and areola are scaly and reddened. The patient denies pain or pruritus. She has noticed this scaliness on her left nipple for the past 8 months. Her dermatologist gave her a potent topical steroid, which she used twice a day for 1 month. The patient never went back for follow-up. She still has the rash and wants an evaluation. Which of the following is the best intervention for this patient?
   A. Prescribe another potent topical steroid and tell the patient to use it twice a day for 4 weeks.
   B. Order a mammogram and refer the patient to a breast surgeon.
   C. Advise the patient to stop using soap on her breasts to avoid drying the skin.
   D. Order a sonogram and a fine-needle biopsy of the breast.

5. A 35-year-old female patient who smokes regularly is being evaluated for contraceptive choices. The patient has a history of pelvic inflammatory disease (PID), anorexia nervosa, and a deep vein thrombosis (DVT) after her last pregnancy. The patient reports having multiple sexual partners with inconsistent condom use. Which of the following is the safest option for the nurse practitioner to recommend?
   A. Consistent and correct condom use
   B. Ortho Evra Transdermal patch
   C. Intrauterine device (IUD)
   D. Depo-Provera (depot medroxyprogesterone)

6. A female patient is concerned about her most recent diagnosis. She has been told by her dermatologist that she has an advanced case of actinic keratosis. Which of the following statements is the best explanation for this patient?
   A. It is a benign condition.
   B. It is a precancerous lesion and should be followed up with her dermatologist.
   C. It will diminish with application of hydrocortisone cream 1% twice a day for 2 weeks.
   D. It is important for the patient to follow up with an oncologist.

7. Which of the following laboratory tests is a sensitive test for evaluating renal function?
   A. Electrolyte panel
   B. Estimated glomerular filtration rate (eGFR)
   C. Creatinine
   D. Blood urea nitrogen (BUN)

8. Which of the following is recommended treatment for erythema migrans?
   A. Doxycycline (Vibramycin) 100 mg orally twice a day for 21 days
   B. Ciprofloxacin (Cipro) 250 mg orally twice a day for 14 days
   C. Erythromycin (E-mycin) 333 mg orally three times a day for 10 days
   D. Dicloxacillin (Dynapen) 500 mg orally twice a day for 10 days

---

* AANPCB is the sole owner of its certification programs. It does not endorse this exam preparation resource, nor does it have a proprietary relationship with Springer Publishing.

9. A parent brings their 1-month-old infant to the clinic for evaluation, stating that the infant has poor weight gain despite constant hunger and projectile vomits after eating. The nurse practitioner (NP) notes that the infant has a distended abdomen. Upon palpation, the NP detects an olive-shaped mass in the epigastrium. The NP will:
   A. Refer the patient for ultrasound testing.
   B. Perform blood analysis to determine red blood cell (RBC) status.
   C. Provide the parent with education on infant feeding.
   D. Place the patient on lactose-free feedings.

10. A toddler with congenital heart disease is seen for a 1-week history of facial and lower extremity edema accompanied by shortness of breath. The child's parent reports that the child's appetite has been poor. The chest x-ray reveals that the child has congestive heart failure (CHF). Which of the following heart sounds are found in patients with CHF?
    A. S1 and S2
    B. S1, S2, and S3
    C. S1, S2, and S4
    D. Still murmur and S4

11. The nurse practitioner (NP) is assessing a patient for peripheral arterial disease (PAD). To confirm the diagnosis, the NP will calculate the patient's right ankle-brachial index (ABI) using the following average systolic blood pressures (SBPs): SBP left ankle = 126 mmHg, SBP right ankle = 124 mmHg, SBP left arm = 132 mmHg, SBP right arm = 129 mmHg. What is the patient's right ABI?
    A. 0.96
    B. 0.95
    C. 0.94
    D. 1.04

12. Which class of antibiotics is first-line treatment for an unvaccinated infant diagnosed with pertussis?
    A. Penicillins
    B. Macrolides
    C. Cephalosporins
    D. Quinolones

13. An 84-year-old male patient with a documented history of osteoporosis presents with complaints of worsening back pain. During the physical examination, the nurse practitioner notes a decrease in the last documented height and a C-shaped curvature of the spine. Which diagnosis is most likely?
    A. Sciatica
    B. Avascular necrosis
    C. Hip displacement
    D. Kyphosis

14. The nurse practitioner (NP) is examining a new 3-month-old patient who has not yet received any immunizations. Which immunizations will the NP administer during this visit to bring the child up to date?
    A. Measles, mumps, and rubella (MMR), DTaP, hepatitis B
    B. Inactivated polio vaccine (IPV), DTaP, MMR
    C. Varicella, Haemophilus influenzae type b (Hib), IPV, DTaP
    D. Hib, DTaP, hepatitis B, rotavirus, pneumococcal conjugate vaccine (PCV), IPV

15. In small children with AIDS, which of the following vaccine(s) is(are) contraindicated?
    A. Td
    B. Hepatitis B and mumps
    C. Varicella
    D. Td and oral polio

16. Which statement is true regarding the tetanus and diphtheria vaccine?
    A. Fever occurs in up to 80% of the patients.
    B. A possible side effect is induration on the injection site.
    C. A tetanus and diphtheria toxoid vaccine is given every 12 years.
    D. DPT and DT should not be given beyond the fifth birthday.

17. A 75-year-old female patient presents in the office complaining that her heart "keeps skipping beats and goes very fast." The patient also reports dizziness and shortness of breath, especially with activity. Her pulse is 120 beats/min and irregular. The nurse practitioner (NP) orders a 12-lead EKG and considers an echocardiogram. The NP will likely prescribe:
    A. Chlorthalidone 12.5 mg daily
    B. Warfarin (Coumadin) 5 mg daily
    C. Warfarin (Coumadin) 2.5 mg daily
    D. Chlorthalidone 25 mg daily

18. To prevent treatment-related complications in a patient diagnosed with hepatitis C, the nurse practitioner (NP) will screen for which of the following prior to initiating treatment?
    A. Hepatitis B
    B. Hepatitis A
    C. Osteomyelitis
    D. *Clostridium difficile* colitis

19. A patient with multiple sclerosis (MS) is experiencing intermittent loss of vision in one eye. To which specialist would the nurse practitioner refer the patient?
    A. Neurologist
    B. Ophthalmologist
    C. ED physician
    D. Endocrinologist

20. Which of the following is a true statement regarding the effect of aspirin on a platelet's function?
    A. The effect on platelets is reversible.
    B. The effect on platelets is reversible and lasts 1 week.
    C. The effect on platelet function is minimal.
    D. The effect on platelet function is irreversible and lasts 10 days.

21. The nurse practitioner is seeing a 35-year-old male patient with HIV for follow-up of an initial antiretroviral treatment regimen of 600 mg dolutegravir/50 mg abacavir/300 mg lamivudine. His plasma viral load (PVL) is 25,000 copies/mL, a decrease from 35,000 copies/mL; CD4 is 400 cells/mm3, up from 250 cells/mm3; and assessment reveals that the patient is in no acute distress. Which of the following interventions are indicated for this patient? (Select all that apply.)
    A. Order liver enzyme testing.
    B. Order a follow-up PVL in 2 weeks.
    C. Refer the patient to a nutritionist for low-fat diet counseling.
    D. Order a follow-up CD4 in 3 months.
    E. Monitor cholesterol levels.

22. An 81-year-old patient is brought to the primary care clinic for dysuria, urinary frequency, nocturia, and fever of 100.6°F. The patient is diagnosed with complicated cystitis. Which antibiotic will the nurse practitioner prescribe?
    A. Fosfomycin 3 g x one dose
    B. Levofloxacin 750 mg once daily x 5 to 7 days
    C. Trimethoprim-sulfamethoxazole (Bactrim) twice daily x 3 days
    D. Amoxicillin-clavulanate (Augmentin) 875/125 mg twice daily x 5 to 7 days

23. A 69-year-old male patient who smokes and has chronic gastroesophageal reflux disease (GERD) was diagnosed with Barrett esophagus 5 years ago. He is being seen by the nurse practitioner for a physical exam. The patient reports that he ran out of his proton pump inhibitor (PPI) medication and that he has not taken it for 5 days. He is complaining of severe episodes of daily heartburn. His gastroenterologist is out of town for 1 week. Which of the following is the best plan to follow during this visit?
    A. Write a prescription for the same PPI and give a 1-week supply without refills.
    B. Give the patient free samples of an H2 antagonist.
    C. Prescribe another PPI because worsening symptoms show that the previously prescribed PPI is not effective.
    D. Advise the patient to take over-the-counter antacids as needed.

24. Upon review of the chest x-ray results of a 4-year-old patient, tiny white spots in a distinctive pattern are noted throughout the lungs. Which diagnosis is most likely to manifest in this manner?
    A. Miliary tuberculosis (TB)
    B. Reactivated TB
    C. Latent TB infection
    D. Pleural TB

25. A 67-year-old female patient complains of progressive dyspnea, minimal cough, and a 10-lb weight loss over the past 3 months. The nurse practitioner (NP) notes decreased posterior breath sounds, use of accessory muscles to breathe, temperature of 98.8°F, and respirations of 24 breaths/min. Which condition does the NP suspect?
    A. Emphysema
    B. Chronic bronchitis
    C. Respiratory infection
    D. Pneumonia

26. While auscultating heart sounds, the nurse practitioner (NP) hears an S2 over the pulmonic area during inspiration but not at expiration. How will the NP classify this sound?
    A. Benign S2 variant
    B. Abnormal S2 variant
    C. Atrial kick
    D. Ventricular gallop

27. A 16-year-old female patient who wears contact lenses presents to the clinic with eye pain, redness, and excessive tearing in the right eye. She tells the nurse practitioner (NP) that she frequently sleeps with her contact lenses in because she forgets to take them out. During slit-lamp testing, the NP notes there is an oval-shaped lesion in the right cornea. Which first-line treatment will the NP prescribe?
    A. Oral steroid
    B. Oral antibiotic
    C. Topical steroid
    D. Topical antibiotic

28. Which of the following is first-line therapy for an elderly patient diagnosed with isolated systolic hypertension?
    A. Hydrochlorothiazide (Microzide) 12.5 mg daily
    B. Prazosin (Minipress) 1 mg three times daily
    C. Spironolactone (Aldactone) 40 mg at bedtime
    D. Propranolol (Inderal) 40 mg twice daily

29. Which lab values will the nurse practitioner monitor in a patient taking theophylline (Theo-Dur)?
    A. Liver function test
    B. Complete blood count (CBC)
    C. Serum concentration
    D. Complete metabolic panel

30. A 24-year-old patient presents to the clinic with complaints of weakness, shortness of breath when exercising, and heart palpitations. Significant physical assessment findings include general pallor, heart rate of 98 beats/min, glossitis, splenomegaly, cutaneous paresthesia in the limbs, hyperreflexia, and a positive Romberg sign. Which diagnosis is most likely?
   A. Iron deficiency
   B. Hemolytic anemia
   C. Normocytic anemia
   D. Vitamin B12 deficiency

31. A 29-year-old male patient has a 2-year history of deep depression alternating with periods of high energy levels, which has impacted his ability to keep a job. After changing jobs for the third time in 2 years, he seeks assistance. Which medication will the nurse practitioner prescribe?
   A. Haloperidol (Haldol)
   B. Phenelzine (Nardil)
   C. Diazepam (Valium)
   D. Lithium carbonate (Eskalith)

32. The nurse practitioner finds multiple types of bacteria in a patient's urine sample. Which of the following interventions is most appropriate?
   A. Order an intravenous pyelogram (IVP).
   B. Order an MRI.
   C. Perform a microscopic urine analysis.
   D. Ask the patient to resubmit a clean-catch specimen.

33. In an adolescent with scoliosis, what degree of spinal curvature requires a referral for surgical correction?
   A. 10 to 20 degrees
   B. 20 to 30 degrees
   C. 30 to 40 degrees
   D. >40 degrees

34. The nurse practitioner (NP) suspects possible kidney stones in an elderly male patient. An ultrasound is ordered with no evidence of kidney stones. The patient returns to the clinic with intermittent right-sided flank pain that is severe in intensity. The NP will:
   A. Repeat the renal ultrasound.
   B. Order a noncontrast CT scan.
   C. Order a complete blood count (CBC).
   D. Perform McBurney's test.

35. At what age, in months, should healthy full-term infants be screened for anemia?
   A. 0 to 3
   B. 3 to 6
   C. 6 to 9
   D. 9 to 12

36. The nurse practitioner (NP) is assessing a 14-year-old female patient who is 20% underweight for her height. The NP notes that the patient has thinning hair and brittle nails as well as fine, downy body hair on her back. How will the NP document the body hair finding on the back?
   A. Lanugo
   B. Actinic keratosis
   C. Russell's sign
   D. Telogen effluvium

37. A 15-year-old male patient who became lightheaded and "passed out" in class is being examined by the nurse practitioner (NP). Pulse is tachycardic at 150 beats/min, and EKG exhibits peaked QRS complex with P waves present. The NP will:
   A. Implement vagal maneuvers.
   B. Determine underlying etiology.
   C. Assess blood pressure.
   D. Refer to a cardiologist.

38. A nurse practitioner diagnoses a patient with uncomplicated chlamydia. Which of the following is the treatment recommended by the Centers for Disease Control and Prevention (CDC)?
   A. Acyclovir (Zovirax) 400 mg PO TID x 7 to 10 days
   B. Azithromycin 1 g PO in a single dose (directly observed treatment preferred)
   C. Benzathine penicillin G 2.4 mU intramuscular IM in a single dose
   D. Podofilox (Condylox) 0.5% gel or cream BID x 3 consecutive days

39. A 25-year-old female patient presents to the nurse practitioner (NP) with new symptoms of difficulty urinating, increased frequency of urination, and mild suprapubic discomfort. Urine dipstick identifies a moderate number of leukocytes and nitrates. The NP orders trimethoprim-sulfamethoxazole twice daily for how many days?
   A. 3
   B. 5
   C. 7
   D. 10

40. Which condition will the nurse practitioner monitor for in a geriatric patient taking hydrochlorothiazide and nifedipine (Procardia XL)?
   A. Macrocytosis
   B. Acquired neutropenia
   C. Primary polycythemia
   D. Secondary thrombocythemia

41. Which of the following statements are true regarding herpes zoster? (Select all that apply.)
    A. It occurs secondary to reactivation of the varicella-zoster virus (VZV).
    B. The typical lesions are bullae.
    C. It is usually more severe in immunocompromised individuals.
    D. Infection of the trigeminal nerve ophthalmic branch can cause corneal blindness.
    E. It affects multiple dermatomes simultaneously.

42. A 66-year-old male patient receives lipid panel results from a routine physical. Total cholesterol is 199 mg/dL, high-density lipoprotein (HDL) is 42 mg/dL, low-density lipoprotein (LDL) is 85 mg/dL, and triglycerides are 135 mg/dL. After reviewing the results, the nurse practitioner tells the patient which of the following?
    A. "Everything is normal; I recommend you have the lipid panel repeated in 2 years."
    B. "It is important to reduce the amount of fat in your diet and repeat the test in 90 days."
    C. "I recommend you lose 10 pounds to help reduce your cholesterol."
    D. "It is important for you to increase the amount of soluble fiber in your diet."

43. Which statement is true about Munchausen syndrome?
    A. All illnesses reported by the patient are falsified.
    B. The patient has a medical illness that causes an anxiety reaction and denial.
    C. The patient falsifies illness in a child to gain attention.
    D. The patient may have a past history of frequent hospitalizations.

44. A patient presents for follow-up with the nurse practitioner (NP) after receiving a diagnosis of acute diverticulitis. The NP is educating the patient about how to avoid complications. What instructions should be included? (Select all that apply.)
    A. "Maintain a high-fiber diet."
    B. "Take amoxicillin-clavulanate 875/125 mg twice daily as ordered."
    C. "Take a laxative every other day."
    D. "Use psyllium fiber supplementation daily."
    E. "Report fever to healthcare provider immediately."

45. A 44-year-old female patient who is undergoing treatment for infertility complains of not having had a menstrual period for a few months. The night before, she started spotting and is now having cramplike pains in her pelvic area. Her blood pressure (BP) is 160/80 mmHg, pulse is 110 beats/min, and she is afebrile. Her labs reveal mild anemia with mild leukocytosis. On pelvic exam, the uterine fundus is noted to be above the symphysis pubis. The cervical os is dilated at 3 cm. Which of the following is most likely?
    A. Inevitable abortion
    B. Threatened abortion
    C. Incomplete abortion
    D. Acute pelvic inflammatory disease

46. In the United States, the most common cause of cancer deaths in men is cancer of the:
    A. Lung
    B. Prostate
    C. Colon
    D. Skin

47. A 63-year-old patient with a 10-year history of poorly controlled hypertension presents with a cluster of physical exam findings. Which of the following clusters indicates the target organ damage commonly seen in hypertensive patients?
    A. Pedal edema, hepatomegaly, enlarged kidneys
    B. Arteriovenous (AV) nicking, left ventricular hypertrophy, stroke
    C. Renal infection, S3 heart sound, neuromuscular abnormalities
    D. Glaucoma, jugular vein atrophy, heart failure

48. A patient presents with complaints of acute epigastric pain that is relieved by taking over-the-counter (OTC) antacids. Upon further evaluation, the nurse practitioner (NP) discovers the patient takes ibuprofen three times a day for joint pain. Which of the following diagnostic tests should be ordered to verify the suspected diagnosis? (Select all that apply.)
    A. Fecal occult blood test
    B. Complete blood count
    C. Hemoglobin A1C
    D. Urea breath test
    E. Lower gastrointestinal (GI) series

49. What is the mechanism of action of probenecid (Probalan)?
    A. Increases uric acid excretion
    B. Increases uric acid metabolism
    C. Decreases formation of uric acid
    D. Decreases metabolism of uric acid

50. A left-hand-dominant high-school tennis player presents with a concern of left elbow pain. Which signs and symptoms suggest that the patient is suffering from tennis elbow? (Select all that apply.)
    A. Elbow pain that worsens with pulling activity
    B. Lateral elbow pain with tenderness at the lateral epicondyle
    C. Elbow pain with grasping movement
    D. Medial elbow pain with tenderness at the medial epicondyle
    E. Elbow pain that worsens with extension

51. A 20-year-old male patient is being seen for a physical exam by the nurse practitioner. He complains of pruritic macerated areas in his groin that have been present for the past 2 weeks. Which of the following is the most likely diagnosis?
    A. Tinea cruris
    B. Tinea corporis
    C. Tinea capitis
    D. Tinea pedis

52. The nurse practitioner (NP) is assessing a 56-year-old patient and notes diffuse reddish-brown, pigmented lesions on the back, trunk, abdomen, chest, and arms. A sample of the skin scrapings on a potassium hydroxide (KOH) wet mount reveals short hyphae and budding cells. Which medication will the NP prescribe?
    A. Oral fluconazole (Diflucan)
    B. Oral ketoconazole (Nizoral)
    C. Topical tacrolimus (Protopic)
    D. Topical selenium sulfide

53. The nurse practitioner (NP) is treating a 26-year-old female patient who has been newly diagnosed with systemic lupus erythematosus (SLE). Which instruction will the NP provide to the patient?
    A. "Replace all household lighting with fluorescent bulbs."
    B. "Wear sun-protective clothing."
    C. "Restrict protein in your diet."
    D. "Avoid topical skin products such as lotions."

54. A male teenage patient presents with complaints of fatigue and lethargy. His parent states that he has been falling asleep in school. Upon examination, he is found to be hypertensive with an average blood pressure of 164/92 mmHg. The nurse practitioner suspects secondary hypertension, which likely eliminates disorders of what system as the cause?
    A. Renal
    B. Endocrine
    C. Musculoskeletal
    D. Respiratory

55. Which effect will the nurse practitioner take into consideration when prescribing oral pharmacologic treatment for a 2-week-old infant with omphalitis?
    A. Increased renal excretion
    B. Undeveloped blood-brain barrier
    C. Increased gastric emptying time
    D. Increased ability of protein drugs to bind

56. An adult patient presents after stepping on a nail that punctured their shoe. The patient has a swollen, diffuse pinkish-red, warm foot. Which gram-negative pathogen is most likely the cause of this infection?
    A. *Pseudomonas aeruginosa*
    B. *Vibrio vulnificus*
    C. *Pasteurella multocida*
    D. *Staphylococcus aureus*

57. A 15-year-old female patient in Tanner stage II states, "I had my first period about 6 months ago, but I haven't had one since." Which diagnostic would be ordered first?
    A. CT scan
    B. Prolactin levels
    C. Serum pregnancy test
    D. Examination of chromosomes

58. An adult visits the urgent care clinic with a fever of 104.2°F, vomiting, and petechiae on the hands and feet progressing to the trunk over the past 3 days. The nurse practitioner will prescribe:
    A. Ceftriaxone (Rocephin) 2 g IV every 12 hours
    B. Doxycycline twice daily for 10 days
    C. Rifampin orally every 12 hours for 2 days
    D. Cephalexin (Keflex) four times daily for 10 days

59. An 82-year-old patient sees the nurse practitioner (NP) for an annual physical exam. The patient requests a colonoscopy to screen for colon cancer. Which is the *most* therapeutic response by the NP?
    A. "Tell me what you know about colonoscopy and why you feel it is important."
    B. "Undergoing a colonoscopy at your age could be dangerous and is not typically recommended."
    C. "I will determine which screenings are indicated based upon evidence-based guidelines."
    D. "We should include your spouse in this conversation so you both can make an informed decision."

60. A young adult male patient presents to the clinic after falling and landing on his buttocks. He complains of feeling "electrical impulses" traveling down both legs. He states that he feels as if he needs to void but is unable to do so. Upon physical examination, the nurse practitioner notes decreased lower extremity strength and reflexes. Which diagnosis is most likely?
    A. Cauda equina syndrome
    B. Scoliosis
    C. Fibromyalgia
    D. Paget's disease of bone

61. What is recommended for an infant with noncommunicating hydrocele?
    A. Surgery
    B. Medication
    C. Reassessment in 1 year
    D. Centesis

62. A female patient presents with epigastric pain and intermittent diarrhea that worsens with food. She has a history of multiple ulcers. The nurse practitioner reviews the results of a serum fasting gastrin level and finds there is no inhibition of gastrin levels. Which diagnosis is most likely?
    A. *Helicobacter pylori*
    B. Atrophic gastritis
    C. Zollinger-Ellison syndrome
    D. Meckel diverticulum

63. Which first-line treatment should be administered when treating a patient with chronic obstructive pulmonary disease (COPD), category C?
    A. Long-acting muscarinic agonist (LAMA)
    B. Short-acting beta2-agonist (SABA)
    C. Long-acting beta2-agonist (LABA)
    D. Short-acting muscarinic agonist (SAMA)

64. The nurse practitioner (NP) is considering timolol (Betimol) for a 70-year-old male patient diagnosed with open-angle glaucoma. What would the NP recognize as a contraindication to the medication?
    A. Intraocular pressure (IOP) >25 mmHg
    B. History of asthma
    C. Stinging sensation after first use
    D. Migraine headaches

65. A female patient with Pick disease fell out of bed and hit her head on a bedside table. The patient is not on anticoagulant therapy and is alert and oriented upon arrival to the clinic. The patient's vital signs are blood pressure of 188/90 mmHg, pulse of 43 beats/min, and respirations of 7 breaths/min. Which diagnosis is most likely?
    A. Hypovolemic shock
    B. Increased intracranial pressure (ICP)
    C. Cerebrovascular accident (CVA)
    D. Subdural hematoma

66. Pioglitazone (Actos) is contraindicated in patients with which of the following conditions?
    A. Renal disease
    B. Liver disease
    C. Asthma
    D. Class III or IV heart disease

67. A middle-aged male patient presents with right eyelid pain for 24 hours. He denies vision changes or discharge from the eye. Upon physical examination, the nurse practitioner (NP) notes a painful, swollen red abscess on the upper right eyelid. Which treatment plan will the NP initiate?
    A. Incision and drainage of the abscess
    B. IV antibiotic of ampicillin
    C. Hot compresses three times daily
    D. Application of bacitracin ophthalmic ointment

68. Which initial treatment will the nurse practitioner recommend for a patient experiencing mild allergic conjunctivitis?
    A. Nonsteroidal anti-inflammatory drugs (NSAIDs)
    B. Oral antihistamines
    C. Topical corticosteroids
    D. Topical antihistamines/mast cell stabilizers

69. What type of infection does a potassium hydroxide (KOH) prep help the nurse practitioner diagnose?
    A. Herpes zoster
    B. Fungal
    C. Herpes simplex
    D. Viral

70. The results of a Pap test performed on a 21-year-old patient state, "Atypical squamous epithelial cells present. No endocervical cells present." The nurse practitioner will:
    A. Test for human papillomavirus (HPV).
    B. Perform an endometrial biopsy.
    C. Refer for colposcopy.
    D. Repeat the test as soon as possible.

71. The nurse practitioner is assessing the cerebellar system of an elderly adult with ataxia. During the physical examination, the patient has a positive Romberg test. What does this assessment indicate?
    A. The patient is unable to stand with eyes closed and arms by side without swaying or falling.
    B. The patient is unable to stretch out arms, palms up, with eyes closed without arm movement.
    C. The patient is able to identify a familiar object in the hand with eyes closed.
    D. The patient is able to identify a written letter on the palm with eyes closed.

72. Auscultation of normal breath sounds of the chest will reveal:
    A. Bronchial breath sounds heard at the lower bases
    B. High-pitched vesicular breath sounds heard over the upper lobes
    C. Vesicular breath sounds heard over the trachea
    D. Vesicular breath sounds in the lower lobe

73. A patient diagnosed with eczema was treated with over-the-counter 1% hydrocortisone ointment. During a follow-up visit, the patient reports that the rash does not seem to be improving. The level of steroid the nurse practitioner will prescribe next is Group:
    A. 6
    B. 5
    C. 4
    D. 3

74. An infant has a faun tail nevus at the lumbosacral area. Which diagnostic procedure will the nurse practitioner order first?
    A. CT scan
    B. MRI
    C. Ultrasound
    D. Spinal tap

75. The nurse practitioner (NP) is performing screenings for scoliosis. What will the NP do to accurately perform this screening?
    A. Ask patient to stand firmly on both feet and bend forward at the hips while arms hang free.
    B. Abduct the patient's hips and listen for a clicking sound.
    C. Ask patient to shrug their shoulders as the NP applies pressure to both shoulders.
    D. Ask patient to raise the heel of the right foot and slide the heel down the knee of the left leg while standing.

76. During a breast exam of a 30-year-old nulliparous female patient, the nurse practitioner (NP) palpates several rubbery mobile areas of breast tissue. They are slightly tender to palpation. Both breasts have symmetrical findings. There are no skin changes or nipple discharge. The patient is expecting her menstrual period in 5 days. The NP will:
    A. Refer the patient to a gynecologist for further evaluation.
    B. Advise the patient to return 1 week after her period so her breasts can be rechecked.
    C. Advise the patient to return in 6 months to have her breasts rechecked.
    D. Schedule the patient for a mammogram.

77. A 35-year-old patient is being worked up for microscopic hematuria. This finding likely allows the nurse practitioner to rule out which diagnosis?
    A. Kidney stones
    B. Bladder cancer
    C. Acute pyelonephritis
    D. Renal artery stenosis

78. A 12-year-old child presents with external pain, swelling, and decreased hearing in the left ear. The child is on a swim team and swims every day. Upon physical examination, the child flinches when the affected ear is touched. There are no other abnormal findings. Which diagnosis is most likely?
    A. Otitis media
    B. Rhinosinusitis
    C. Otitis externa
    D. Bullous myringitis

79. The nurse practitioner is treating the male partner of a 22-year-old patient with a positive nucleic acid amplification test (NAAT) for *Chlamydia trachomatis*. Which of the following is the *preferred* treatment for the patient's partner?
    A. Azithromycin 1 g orally in a single dose
    B. Benzathine penicillin 2.4 million units intramuscularly in a single dose
    C. Clindamycin 300 mg twice daily for 7 days
    D. Doxycycline 100 mg orally twice daily for 7 days

80. A female patient receiving thyroid replacement therapy contracts the flu and forgets to take her thyroid replacement medicine. The patient is at risk for which life-threatening complication?
    A. Exophthalmos
    B. Thyroid storm
    C. Myxedema coma
    D. Pretibial myxedema

81. A 4-year-old child presents with a high fever and enlarged lymph nodes in the neck area. The nurse practitioner notes dry, cracked lips and a "strawberry tongue" upon physical assessment. Which diagnosis is most likely?
    A. Pharyngitis
    B. Allergic rhinitis
    C. Kawasaki's disease
    D. Tonsillitis

82. A 22-year-old male athlete presents with knee pain for which the nurse practitioner performs a McMurray test. A positive sign indicates which condition?
    A. Anterior cruciate ligament (ACL) tear
    B. Posterior cruciate ligament (PCL) tear
    C. Patellar tendon rupture
    D. Meniscal tear

83. A 68-year-old female patient has recently been diagnosed with polymyalgia rheumatica (PMR). The nurse practitioner is discussing the treatment options with the patient. Which of the following medications is the first-line treatment for this condition?
    A. Etanercept (Enbrel)
    B. Oral prednisone
    C. Indomethacin
    D. Methotrexate

84. A parent presents with their 4-year-old child and states that the child is unable to attend preschool because of lack of motor skills. Which tactic can be used to determine appropriate growth and development for the patient?
A. Have the child draw a person with six body parts.
B. Toss a ball for the child to catch.
C. Observe the child going up several steps.
D. Ask the child to write their name.

85. The nurse practitioner performs an EKG on a patient before prescribing a calcium channel blocker (CCB). Which EKG reading (which follows) would verify that a CCB is safe to prescribe?

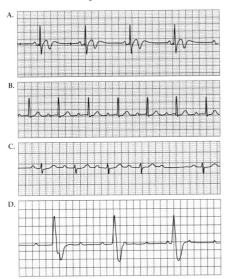

86. During a routine digital rectal exam, a hard, fixed nodule is detected on the prostate gland of a 55-year-old male patient. The patient's prostate-specific antigen (PSA) is 4.1 ng/mL. Which of the following will the nurse practitioner order?
A. CT of the abdomen
B. Radionuclide bone scan
C. Measurement of serum acid phosphatase
D. Transrectal ultrasound-guided needle biopsy

87. The nurse practitioner is reviewing the laboratory results for a female patient who states that she has had one menstrual period over the last year and is experiencing problems sleeping. The patient's lab results include an estradiol level of 200 pg/mL, follicle-stimulating hormone (FSH) of 35 IU/L, and an anti-Müllerian hormone (AMH) level of 0.2 ng/mL. The findings indicate that the patient:
A. Is perimenopausal
B. Is menopausal
C. Is fertile
D. Should be tested for ovarian cancer

88. The nurse practitioner is assessing a 13-year-old male patient who presents with back pain, nausea, and vomiting for the past 24 hours. The patient reports feeling a dull pain and muscle spasms in the back after a direct hit to the side during football practice. His vital signs are blood pressure of 140/84 mmHg, temperature of 99.1°F, pulse of 98 beats/min, and respirations of 26 breaths/min. Which diagnosis is most likely?
A. Appendicitis
B. Bruised kidney
C. Cholecystitis
D. Ruptured vertebral disc

89. A 45-year-old male patient is seen as a walk-in patient in a private clinic. He reports stepping on a nail that morning. He received a Td vaccine 9 years ago. Which of the following vaccines is recommended?
A. Diphtheria, tetanus, acellular pertussis (DTaP)
B. Diphtheria and tetanus (DT)
C. Tetanus diphtheria (Td)
D. Tetanus, diphtheria, acellular pertussis (Tdap)

90. A patient states, "I have had a rash for the past week and cannot stop scratching it." Physical assessment reveals 1-mm papules and pustules, grayish-white burrows on the patient's palms and soles of the feet, and excoriated skin with honey-colored crusting on the face and neck. The nurse practitioner will prescribe:
A. Topical nystatin
B. Oral griseofulvin
C. Oral ketoconazole (Nizoral)
D. Topical permethrin (Elimite)

91. A 22-year-old female patient presents with signs of a broken arm, stating that she fell at home. Upon assessment, the nurse practitioner observes numerous bruises in various stages of healing, and the patient's live-in partner responds aggressively to all questions posed to the patient. Which of the following interventions is most appropriate?
A. Call security and have the partner removed from the examination room.
B. Ask the partner why he will not let the patient answer the questions.
C. Tell the partner that the rest of the exam must be private, show them to the waiting area, and say you will retrieve them when you finish.
D. State your suspicions to the couple and ask them to provide a truthful explanation for the injuries.

92. A female patient diagnosed with irritable bowel syndrome (IBS) tells the nurse practitioner (NP) that over the past few months, she has been experiencing frequent bouts of constipation. Which prescription will the NP add to the treatment plan?
    A. Amitriptyline (Elavil) 50 mg orally once daily
    B. Lubiprostone (Amitiza) 8 mcg orally twice daily
    C. Alosetron (Lotronex) 0.5 mg orally twice daily for 4 weeks
    D. Dicyclomine (Bentyl) 20 mg orally every 6 hours, 30 to 60 minutes before meals

93. What is a common sign of allergic rhinitis?
    A. Transverse nasal crease
    B. Yellow nasal discharge
    C. Cough that worsens with standing
    D. Epistaxis

94. What is a positive Kernig sign?
    A. Flexing of hips and knee to relieve pain
    B. Inability to touch chin to chest
    C. Toes spread like a fan with plantar stroke
    D. Resistance to leg straightening from back pain

95. Which medication can the nurse practitioner include in the treatment plan for a patient with a positive Finkelstein test?
    A. Ibuprofen
    B. Oral prednisone
    C. Lidocaine injection
    D. Corticosteroid injection

96. The nurse practitioner is examining a 56-year-old male patient who presents with a tophus of the right great toe. History reveals a previous attack of gout 2 years ago. The patient was not prescribed preventive medication. What is appropriate *first-line* treatment for the patient?
    A. Tetracycline
    B. Colchicine
    C. Allopurinol
    D. Amoxicillin

97. An infant is born with microcephaly, narrow eyes, a flat nasal bridge, a thin upper lip, and underdeveloped ears. Which diagnosis is most likely?
    A. Down syndrome
    B. Fetal alcohol syndrome
    C. Poor weight gain
    D. Fragile X syndrome

98. Which test will the nurse practitioner order for a patient with symptoms of chronic prostatitis?
    A. Urinalysis
    B. Prostate-specific antigen (PSA)
    C. Meares-Stamey 2-glass test
    D. Gram stain of urethral swab

99. Which assessment finding is associated with Crohn disease (CD)?
    A. Left lower quadrant pain
    B. Weight loss and dehydration
    C. Constipation
    D. Inflammation limited to mucosal layer of colon

100. A 13-year-old male patient visits the clinic. The patient's chief complaint is persistent unilateral knee pain for several weeks. A history reveals no traumatic injury or health issues. He has a painful, bony bump below the affected knee. Upon movement, there is no laxity, but the patient feels pain. The patient's parent reports that a recent x-ray was negative. Which diagnosis is most likely?
    A. Polymyositis
    B. Baker's cyst
    C. Osgood-Schlatter disease
    D. Meniscus tear

101. A female patient presents with complaints of fatigue, cold intolerance, and unexplained weight gain. Which diagnosis is most likely?
    A. Hyperthyroidism
    B. Diabetes mellitus
    C. Hypothyroidism
    D. Heart failure

102. An elderly male patient presents with complaints of severe pain on his left back and a concentrated swath of vesicles. Which diagnosis is most likely?
    A. Herpes zoster
    B. Varicella
    C. Tinea corporis
    D. Plaque psoriasis

103. Which is the most effective way to screen for color blindness?
    A. Snellen chart
    B. Confrontation exam
    C. Extraocular movement test
    D. Ishihara chart

104. Which of the following is a first-line medication for tinea unguium?
    A. Oral terbinafine (Lamisil)
    B. Efinaconazole 10% solution (Jublia)
    C. Azelaic acid (Azelex)
    D. Metronidazole topical gel (Metrogel)

105. A patient presents with fever, fatigue, headache, and joint pain. Upon obtaining a history, the nurse practitioner (NP) notes that the patient has recently returned from a camping trip in the Northeast. On physical examination, the NP notices a large macule on the patient's back with central clearing. Which diagnosis is most likely?
 A. Lyme disease
 B. Brown recluse spider bite
 C. Erythema infectiosum
 D. Rocky Mountain spotted fever

106. The nurse practitioner sees an adult patient who reports frequent headaches over the past few months. The patient has tried acetaminophen and ibuprofen without relief. The patient has a history of a myocardial infarction (MI), bradycardia, and kidney stones. Which medication is most appropriate for this patient?
 A. Topiramate (Topamax)
 B. Sumatriptan (Imitrex)
 C. Imipramine (Elavil)
 D. Atenolol (Tenormin)

107. A patient presents to the clinic complaining of a painful, itchy rash on the elbows and knees that appears as raised erythematous patches of silvery, scaly skin. The patient states that the rash has occurred before but resolved without treatment. For which condition should the nurse practitioner treat?
 A. Impetigo
 B. Psoriasis
 C. Xerosis
 D. Contact dermatitis

108. An adolescent female patient's areola, nipple, and breast tissue develop and become elevated as one mound. Which of the following is the correct Tanner stage for this phase of breast development?
 A. I
 B. II
 C. III
 D. IV

109. An 8-year-old boy with type 1 diabetes is being seen for a 3-day history of urinary frequency and nocturia. He denies flank pain and is afebrile. The urinalysis result is negative for blood and nitrites but is positive for a large amount of leukocytes and ketones. He has a trace amount of protein. Which of the following is the best test to order initially?
 A. Urine culture and sensitivity (C&S)
 B. 24-hour urine for protein and creatinine clearance
 C. 24-hour urine for microalbumin
 D. Intravenous pyelogram

110. Which assessment finding is expected in a 3-year-old male patient with penopubic epispadias?
 A. Fused pelvic bones
 B. Urine leakage with stress
 C. Narrow penis that curves down
 D. Urinary meatus found along shaft of penis

111. A 10-year-old girl who plays on an intramural soccer team has a history of exercise-induced asthma. She wants to know when she should use her albuterol inhaler. The nurse practitioner advises the patient to:
 A. Premedicate 5 to 20 minutes before starting exercise.
 B. Wait until she starts to exercise before using the inhaler.
 C. Premedicate 30 minutes before starting exercise.
 D. Wait until she finishes her exercise before using the inhaler.

112. Which medication will the nurse practitioner prescribe to a 28-year-old female patient newly diagnosed with hypothyroidism?
 A. Levothyroxine T3
 B. Levothyroxine T4
 C. Thyroid-stimulating hormone (TSH)
 D. Combined levothyroxine T3 and T4

113. A patient presents to the office with complaints of asthma 1 or 2 days a week and sleeps routinely 8 to 9 hours a night with rare occurrences of nighttime asthma symptoms. Forced expired volume in 1 second (FEV1) is >80%, and respirations are 20 breaths/min. The asthma classification protocol that the nurse practitioner should follow is Step:
 A. 1
 B. 2
 C. 3
 D. 4

114. A high-school wrestler has been diagnosed with infectious mononucleosis. When can the patient resume participation in the sport?
 A. 2 weeks following onset
 B. 3 weeks following onset
 C. 4 weeks following onset
 D. Never

115. An older adult patient was burned when a large pot of boiling water fell off the stove. According to the Lund-Browder chart, the patient has reddened skin and several bullae on approximately 4% of the abdominal area. The patient is allergic to sulfa products. Which of the following interventions is most appropriate?
 A. Treat with benzocaine spray.
 B. Gently rupture blisters.
 C. Treat with silver sulfadiazine.
 D. Treat with bacitracin zinc.

116. Which of the following is recommended on an annual basis for an elderly patient with type 2 diabetes?
    A. Eye exam with an ophthalmologist
    B. Follow-up visit with a urologist
    C. Periodic visits to an optometrist
    D. Colonoscopy

117. A 65-year-old male patient who works as a carpenter complains of morning stiffness and pain in both his hands and his right knee upon awakening. He feels some relief after warming up. On exam, the nurse practitioner notices the presence of Heberden nodes. Which of the following is most likely?
    A. Osteoporosis
    B. Rheumatoid arthritis
    C. Osteoarthritis
    D. Reiter syndrome

118. Which of the following is considered an objective finding in patients who have a case of suppurative otitis media?
    A. Pale tympanic membrane
    B. Increased mobility of the tympanic membrane as measured by tympanogram
    C. Rinne test showing AC >BC
    D. Bulging of the tympanic membrane

119. A 13-year-old female patient presents with complaints of right lower abdominal pain that began 4 hours ago in volleyball practice. The nurse practitioner assesses rebound tenderness at McBurney's point. What does this assessment finding indicate?
    A. Crohn disease
    B. Ulcerative colitis
    C. Appendicitis
    D. Diverticulitis

120. Which medication will the nurse practitioner include in the treatment plan for a 7-year-old child with acute otitis media?
    A. Cefdinir
    B. Amoxicillin-clavulanate
    C. Erythromycin
    D. Azithromycin

121. A 67-year-old female patient who regularly takes diphenhydramine (Benadryl) as a sleep aid is at risk of which of the following conditions?
    A. Confusion
    B. Bradycardia
    C. Hypertension
    D. Cardiac arrhythmias

122. The nurse practitioner (NP) prescribes an angiotensin-converting enzyme (ACE) inhibitor for a patient with kidney disease. The NP orders which of the following testing to monitor the patient?
    A. Serum potassium
    B. Serum hemoglobin
    C. Ultrasound of kidney
    D. Ultrasound of abdomen

123. A parent presents to the clinic with their newborn. Upon examination, the nurse practitioner (NP) notes black-colored patches on the newborn's lumbosacral area. How will the NP document these findings?
    A. Milia
    B. Erythema toxicum neonatorum
    C. Slate-gray nevi
    D. Port wine stain

124. A 67-year-old female patient comes into the clinic during the first week of November for her annual wellness visit. Her last tetanus diphtheria (Td) booster was 9 years ago. Which immunization(s) would the nurse practitioner recommend for this visit?
    A. Influenza vaccine
    B. Tetanus and influenza vaccine
    C. Pneumococcal (Pneumovax) and influenza vaccines
    D. No vaccines needed

125. A 68-year-old female patient visits the clinic complaining of increasing back pain. Her past medical history reveals a T11 vertebral compression fracture in the last year. Upon physical examination, the nurse practitioner (NP) notes a decrease in height of an inch since the patient's last encounter. The NP will order:
    A. Bone density test (dual-energy x-ray absorptiometry [DEXA])
    B. Colonoscopy
    C. Upper gastrointestinal tract radiography
    D. Nuclear stress test

126. Which child requires assessment and evaluation?
    A. A 7-year-old girl who sucks her thumb when tired
    B. A 2-year-old boy who ignores other children and has never spoken
    C. A 2-year-old boy who refuses attempts at toilet training
    D. A 5-year-old girl who cries most of the day at kindergarten

127. Which of the following burn injuries can be treated by the nurse practitioner without referral to a burn center?
    A. Severe facial burns
    B. Electrical burns
    C. Inhalation injuries
    D. Partial-thickness burns on the lower arm (2% total body surface area [TBSA])

128. A 35-year-old primigravida patient who is at 18 weeks' gestation is expecting twins. What would the nurse practitioner expect the alpha-fetoprotein (AFP) values to be?
A. Normal
B. Higher than normal
C. Lower than normal
D. Variable

129. A 55-year-old male patient has a history of angina and type 2 diabetes. His lipid profile results are total cholesterol of 280 mg/dL, low-density lipoprotein (LDL) of 195 mg/dL, and high-density lipoprotein (HDL) of 25 mg/dL. The nurse practitioner diagnoses the patient with hyperlipidemia and wants to start him on statin therapy. What intensity of treatment is recommended for this patient?
A. Low
B. Moderate
C. High
D. Very high

130. An elderly male patient complains that his central vision appears to be blurred and he cannot see when driving. Which condition is most likely?
A. Macular degeneration
B. Central vision inflammation
C. Blepharitis
D. Conjunctival hemorrhage

131. Which assessment question will the nurse practitioner (NP) ask a 68-year-old patient who has been receiving ongoing treatment with gabapentin after a shingles outbreak?
A. "Have you noticed any new blisters?"
B. "Are you experiencing pain anywhere?"
C. "Have you had a rash over the past month?"
D. "Are you experiencing problems falling asleep?"

132. Which antipsychotic medication is most likely to produce extrapyramidal effects?
A. Sertraline (Zoloft)
B. Citalopram (Celexa)
C. Aripiprazole (Abilify)
D. Haloperidol (Haldol)

133. A 73-year-old male patient presents with bilateral edema in the legs and feet, weight gain of 15 lb, and decreased urine output. The nurse practitioner will order:
A. Hemoglobin testing
B. 24-hour creatinine level
C. Urine culture and sensitivity (C&S)
D. Abdominal ultrasound

134. A possible complication of Bell's palsy is:
A. Corneal ulceration
B. Acute glaucoma
C. Inability to swallow
D. Loss of sensation in the affected side

135. A patient with a history of smoking and estrogen therapy presents with a sudden cough with light pink–tinged sputum, a respiratory rate of 32 breaths/min, a heart rate of 134 beats/min, pallor, and chest pain with deep inspiration. Which diagnosis is most likely?
A. Pulmonary edema
B. Atypical pneumonia
C. Pulmonary emboli
D. Bordetella pertussis

136. A middle-aged male patient presents with swelling of the right leg and pain upon dorsiflexion. Upon examination, the nurse practitioner (NP) finds the right leg to be larger than the left, along with redness and warmth to the calf. Which questions will the NP ask the patient? (Select all that apply.)
A. "Have you traveled recently?"
B. "Do you have any inherited blood disorders?"
C. "Have you broken any bones recently or had surgery?"
D. "Have you recently gained weight?"
E. "Do you walk or exercise regularly?"

137. Which cranial nerve (CN) is measured with a "clicking" stimuli?
A. I
B. II
C. VIII
D. V

138. What is the most common cause of dementia in the elderly?
A. Lewy bodies
B. Delirium
C. Vascular dementia
D. Alzheimer's disease

139. A 65-year-old male patient has been on atorvastatin (Lipitor) 80 mg daily for the past 3 months. The patient now reports significant fatigue for the past 2 weeks with no change in sleeping habits. He has noticed that he has a loss of appetite and his urine has been a darker color for the past 2 weeks. He denies dysuria, frequency, and nocturia. The nurse practitioner (NP) notices that the patient's sclerae have a slight yellow tinge. The NP will:
A. Discontinue atorvastatin (Lipitor) and order a liver function profile.
B. Continue the atorvastatin (Lipitor) but on half the dose.
C. Schedule the patient for a complete physical examination.
D. Schedule the patient for a liver function profile.

140. An elderly patient's bloodwork reveals a diagnosis of hepatitis A. The patient asks the nurse practitioner (NP), "How did I get this disease?" What is the NP's best response?
   A. "Patients often contract hepatitis A by using contaminated needles."
   B. "Some patients who have had a blood transfusion may have received blood that is infected."
   C. "If you have ever engaged in unprotected sex, you may have contracted the virus."
   D. "You may have eaten food that was contaminated with the hepatitis A virus."

141. A patient has a past medical history of childhood chickenpox, which provided which type of immunity?
   A. Herd
   B. Passive
   C. Active
   D. None

142. A 27-year-old male patient reports that he has a strong desire to dress and be treated as a woman and tells the nurse practitioner (NP) that they have never been comfortable with their assigned sex. The NP will: (Select all that apply.)
   A. Refer the patient to a psychiatric-mental health professional.
   B. Explain to the patient that they may be experiencing a hormonal imbalance.
   C. Ask for the patient's preferred gender pronouns and use gender-neutral language in communications and on patient forms.
   D. Maintain respect for the patient's process of disclosure.
   E. Inform the patient that they are experiencing gender dysphoria, which can be treated.

143. A score of 23 on the Folstein Mini-Mental State Exam (MMSE) indicates which of the following?
   A. Severe dementia
   B. Moderate dementia
   C. Mild dementia
   D. Parkinson disease

144. The spouse of an elderly patient with Alzheimer disease tells the nurse practitioner (NP) that they are exhausted and cannot continue to be the sole caregiver. The couple have no children. They both have healthcare coverage with Medicare, but no supplemental insurance. The NP will initially do which of the following to support the caregiver?
   A. Refer to home health services.
   B. Provide a list of qualified in-home caregivers.
   C. Contact an agency that provides skilled respite care.
   D. Provide a brochure for Meals on Wheels.

145. A nurse practitioner's right to practice is regulated under:
   A. Medicare regulations
   B. Board of medicine
   C. Federal government
   D. State board of nursing

146. The nurse practitioner (NP) is examining a child with Down's syndrome brought to the clinic with flu-like symptoms. The caregiver offers conflicting information about the source of bruises on the child's buttocks. The child is quiet and reserved. Which criterion is most important for the NP to consider when evaluating this patient?
   A. Explanation of the injury being inconsistent with the presentation
   B. Behavior of the child during the assessment
   C. Hygiene of the caregiver
   D. Unexplained bruises being common in children with Down syndrome

147. A 37-year-old male patient presents for a follow-up visit after a recent positive HIV diagnosis. Another staff member at the clinic asks the nurse practitioner (NP) if they can see the patient's chart, as the patient is the cousin of a friend. What is the responsibility of the NP? (Select all that apply.)
   A. The NP should inform the staff member of the patient's right to privacy.
   B. The NP should not provide the chart to the staff member.
   C. The NP should remind the staff member not to share the HIV status with anyone.
   D. The NP should ask the staff member to sign a waiver to maintain confidentiality after reviewing the chart.
   E. The NP should report the incident to the supervisor.

148. The nurse practitioner is reviewing evidence regarding the use of a drug used to treat Parkinson's disease. Rank the strength of evidence from strongest (1) to weakest (3).
   A. An editorial that discusses how the drug may impact the advancement of Parkinson's treatment, published in the official journal of the American Academy of Neurology
   B. An experimental study of 300 patients with Parkinson's disease who were randomly assigned to receive either a placebo or the drug daily for 12 months
   C. A meta-analysis that evaluates the effectiveness of the drug, using 25 randomized controlled trials found on Medline and the Cochrane database

149. A nurse practitioner (NP) working in a community health clinic sees a male patient who expresses concern about starting a relationship with a new male partner. Which of the following is the best plan to follow during this visit? (Select all that apply.)
A. Contact the patient's partner to schedule HIV testing.
B. Educate the patient about using barrier devices during sex.
C. Prescribe daily oral preexposure prophylaxis (PrEP).
D. Draw a blood sample for a combination HIV antigen/antibody test.
E. Schedule a follow-up appointment in 1 month to review test results and discuss options for PrEP.

150. An adult male patient is being evaluated for tuberculosis (TB) infection with a Mantoux test. The purified protein derivative (PPD) result is 10.5 mm. The patient denies weight loss, cough, and night sweats, and the results of a chest x-ray are negative. The patient reports that he is an undocumented immigrant to the United States and is fearful about discovery. Which of the following is a true statement?
A. The nurse practitioner (NP) has a legal duty to report the patient to the local federal agency responsible for undocumented immigrants.
B. The NP is legally mandated to report undocumented immigrants to state authorities.
C. The NP should call the state health department to report that the patient has a TB infection.
D. The NP has an ethical duty to provide quality healthcare to all patients.

1. D) White (non-Hispanic)
The percentages of all deaths caused by heart disease in 2020 are White (non-Hispanic; 21.3%), African American (20.7%), Asian (18.9%), and American Indian or Alaska Native (14.2%).

2. D) Inferior
ST-segment elevation in leads II, III, and aVF indicates an inferior wall ST-segment elevation myocardial infarction (STEMI). An EKG characterized by ST-segment elevation or Q waves in precordial leads (V1 to V6) and leads I to aVL suggests anterior wall ischemia or infarction. A lateral MI will present with ST elevation in leads I, aVL, V5, and V6 with reciprocal depression in inferior leads III and aVF. Anteroseptal MI is characterized by the presence of ST elevations in V1 to V3 leads.

3. D) Hashimoto's thyroiditis
Hashimoto's thyroiditis is an autoimmune disorder of the thyroid gland that is more common in women than in men (8:1). Evaluating TPO levels in a patient with hypothyroidism can be useful to confirm an autoimmune cause of the hypothyroidism because elevated levels confirm diagnosis (normal level for TPO antibodies is <35 IU/mL). Patients present with weight gain, cold intolerance, goiter (in most cases), and an elevated cholesterol level. Thyroid cancer presents as hoarseness and problems with swallowing (dysphagia, dyspnea, or cough). Pheochromocytoma causes episodes of headaches, diaphoresis, tachycardia, and hypertension. After an attack, vital signs return to normal. Hyperprolactinemia can be a sign of pituitary adenoma (benign) and has a slow onset. Serum prolactin is elevated, and women can present with amenorrhea. As the tumor grows, it will affect vision and cause headaches.

4. B) Order a mammogram and refer the patient to a breast surgeon.
A scaly, reddened rash on the breast that does not resolve after a few weeks of medical treatment may indicate breast cancer. She should have a mammogram performed and see a breast surgeon for evaluation and treatment. After the mammogram, a sonogram may be ordered to further evalute findings on the mammogram. A needle biopsy may be an appropriate tool for diagnosis, but seeing the breast surgeon should occur first. Paget disease of the breast is a rare type of cancer involving the skin of the nipple and, usually, the areola. It may be misdiagnosed at first because its early symptoms are similar to those caused by some benign skin conditions. Most patients with Paget disease of the breast also have one or more tumors inside the same breast, either ductal carcinoma in situ or invasive breast cancer. Use of another topical steroid is not an appropriate course of action because the patient likely has breast cancer. The patient should not be advised to avoid the use of soap, as skin dryness is not the cause of the symptoms.

5. A) Consistent and correct condom use
Consistent and correct use of condoms reduces the risk of sexually transmitted infections (STIs) and can prevent pregnancy. The patient should be educated on safe sex practices given her report of multiple sexual partners and inconsistent condom use. Consider screening for STIs, as well. Depo-Provera (depot medroxyprogesterone) is an injectable progestin-only form of contraception. It should be avoided in patients with a history of anorexia nervosa because it can further increase their risk of osteopenia/osteoporosis. IUDs are contraindicated in patients with active PID or a history of PID within the past year. The Ortho Evra Transdermal contraceptive patch carries a higher risk of venous thromboembolism compared with oral contraceptive pills and, therefore, should be avoided in those with a history of thromboembolic disorders (e.g., DVT).

6. B) It is a precancerous lesion and should be followed up with her dermatologist.
Actinic keratoses are small, raised skin lesions that result from extended sun exposure. Some actinic keratoses may develop into skin cancer; therefore, further evaluation is needed to determine if removal is required. Patient education is very important, as actinic keratoses can be confusing for the patient. It is not a benign condition and must be monitored regularly. The patient does not need to follow up with an oncologist, unless the lesions become cancerous. Applying hydrocortisone cream does not resolve actinic keratosis; treatment generally includes cryotherapy.

7. B) Estimated glomerular filtration rate (eGFR)
The glomerular filtration rate (GFR) is a sensitive test used to measure and monitor kidney function and evaluate chronic kidney disease (CKD). GFR can be estimated from serum creatinine. The eGFR calculation uses serum creatinine along with age and values assigned for sex and race. The National Kidney Foundation has determined different stages of CKD based on the value of eGFR. An electrolyte panel, creatinine, and BUN are all useful for the evaluation

of a patient with kidney disease, but are not as sensitive as the GFR in evaluating for CKD.

8. A) Doxycycline (Vibramycin) 100 mg orally twice a day for 21 days

Erythema migrans is the rash characteristic of Lyme disease, and it usually appears 7 to 10 days after a tick bite. Lyme disease is caused by *Borrelia burgdorferi*, a spirochete. The rash appears either as a single expanding red patch or as a central spot surrounded by clear skin that is in turn ringed by an expanded red rash (bull's-eye). The choice of antibiotic depends on bacterial sensitivity. Doxycycline 100 mg twice a day for 14 to 21 days is the recommended treatment for adults. Ciprofloxacin, erythromycin, and dicloxacillin are not effective against *Borrelia burgdorferi*. For individuals allergic to doxycycline, alternatives such as ceftriaxone, penicillin G, and cefotaximine are appropriate alternatives.

9. A) Refer the patient for ultrasound testing.

The infant presents with signs and symptoms of pyloric stenosis: abdominal distention, dehydration, projectile vomiting, and failure to thrive. The infant requires an ultrasound to view the pylorus and confirm this diagnosis. Fluid and electrolyte status must be assessed in order to determine hydration and imbalances. The infant will require surgery if pyloric stenosis is confirmed. Educating the parent on feedings is not required until the diagnosis is confirmed. Placing the infant on lactose-free feeding will not treat the condition. Drawing blood is not helpful with this diagnosis, as RBC status does not impact this condition.

10. B) S1, S2, and S3

CHF is the inability of the heart to pump a sufficient amount of blood to the organs to meet the body's requirements. It is common to hear S1, S2, and S3 heart sounds on exam. Common signs and symptoms of CHF include fatigue, shortness of breath with activity, and edema of lower extremities.

11. C) 0.94

The patient's right ABI is 0.94. Right ABI is calculated by dividing the highest SBP of the right ankle by the highest SBP of both arms (right or left). In this case, the arm with the highest average SBP is the left arm, so the right ankle SBP (124 mmHg) is divided by the left arm SBP (132 mmHg), which equals 0.94.

12. B) Macrolides

The first-line antibiotic treatment for an infant with pertussis is macrolides (azithromycin, erythromycin, or clarithromycin). Penicillins are indicated for strep throat and otitis media. Cephalosporins are appropriate for gram-positive cocci bacteria. Quinolones are effective against gram-negative and atypical bacteria.

13. D) Kyphosis

Kyphosis is a degenerative disease caused by an abnormal curvature of the spine. It is common in older patients and contributes to a loss of height in aging adults. Osteoporotic changes in the spine are also present. Sciatica is inflammation of the sciatic nerve that travels down the lower back. It may be painful but does not cause a C-shaped curvature of the spine. Avascular necrosis occurs when a lack of blood flow to the bone(s) causes bone death. Hip displacement creates a physical impairment in mobility but does not cause a C-shaped curvature of the spine.

14. D) Hib, DTaP, hepatitis B, rotavirus, pneumococcal conjugate vaccine (PCV), IPV

The current immunization recommendations for a 2-month-old infant who has not received any are Hib, DTaP, hepatitis B, rotavirus, PCV, and IPV. This child, at 3 months old, is behind schedule but should receive the same immunizations. Since the second dose of all these vaccines can be given in 4 weeks, the infant can be quickly brought up to date on immunizations. The first immunizations for MMR and varicella are recommended when a child is age 12 months.

15. C) Varicella

The data regarding efficacy of the varicella vaccine are insufficient; therefore, varicella vaccine is contraindicated in HIV-infected individuals.

16. B) A possible side effect is induration on the injection site.

Side effects of the Td vaccine include induration at the injection site. Td or Tdap is given in adults every 10 years. DPT and DT should not be given beyond age 7 years. Fever may occur, but studies do not support 80% of patients having fever.

17. C) Warfarin (Coumadin) 2.5 mg daily

The symptoms presented are classic signs of atrial fibrillation. Warfarin (Coumadin) is frequently prescribed to reduce the increased risk for clotting and subsequent stroke associated with the condition. Initial dose in patients older than 70 years is 2.5 mg, which is a lower dose than the 5 mg prescribed for younger patients. Since this patient is 75 years of age, the lower dose (2.5 mg) should be prescribed. Chlorthalidone is prescribed to treat hypertension.

18. A) Hepatitis B

The NP should order blood tests to check for hepatitis B infection. Hepatitis B can reactivate during treatment for hepatitis C and cause serious liver problems. Hepatitis A is a vaccine-preventable, communicable disease of the liver caused by the hepatitis A virus (HAV). It is usually transmitted person-to-person through the fecal–oral route or by consumption of contaminated food or water. Hepatitis A is a self-limiting disease that does not result in chronic infection. Osteomyelitis is an infection in a bone. *C. difficile* is a type of bacteria that lives in many people's intestines. *C. difficile* is part of the normal balance of bacteria in the body. With antibiotic use, changes in the intestinal flora can cause colitis infection.

19. A) Neurologist

A patient with MS with intermittent or new vision loss should see a neurologist because the patient may have optic neuritis. It would not be necessary to refer the patient to the ED for this condition. The patient may be referred to an ophthalmologist after seeing the neurologist. An endocrinologist would not be an appropriate referral, because the condition is not related to the endocrine system.

20. D) The effect on platelet function is irreversible and lasts 10 days.

The use of aspirin affects platelet function by irreversibly inactivating platelet COX-1 enzyme, ultimately affecting platelet aggregation due to lowered levels of thromboxane A2. While the half-life of aspirin is only 15 to 20 minutes, the antiplatelet effect lasts the entire life span of the platelet, which is approximately 10 days. Although it may take 10 days for the total platelet population to be renewed, platelets are renewed at a rate of 10% per day, and partial platelet function can be seen when about one third of the platelets have COX function (~33% or almost 4 days).

21. A, C, D, E) Order liver enzyme testing; Refer the patient to a nutritionist for low-fat diet counseling; Order a follow-up CD4 in 3 months; Monitor cholesterol levels.

An antiretroviral regimen of 600 mg dolutegravir/50 mg abacavir/300 mg lamivudine has a boxed warning for severe hepatomegaly and hepatitis B exacerbation, so monitoring of liver enzymes is crucial. Likewise, steatosis is common with hepatomegaly, so monitoring cholesterol levels and introducing a low-fat diet are important as well. Follow-up PVL should be completed in 4 to 8 weeks and CD4 in 3 months.

22. B) Levofloxacin (Levaquin) 750 mg once daily x 5 to 7 days

An older adult patient with complicated cystitis can be treated for 5 to 7 days with levofloxacin (Levaquin) 750 mg once daily or ciprofloxacin (Cipro) 500 mg twice daily, if there is low risk of multidrug-resistant organisms. Patients with high risk of multidrug-resistant organisms can be treated with oral nitrofurantoin (Macrobid) 100 mg twice daily. Fosfomycin 3 g x 1 dose, trimethoprim-sulfamethoxazole twice a day x 3 days, and amoxicillin-clavulanate (Augmentin) 875/125 mg twice daily x 5 to 7 days are not appropriate treatments for complicated cystitis and should be reserved for patients with uncomplicated cystitis.

23. A) Write a prescription for the same PPI and give a 1-week supply without refills.

This patient is having severe rebound symptoms caused by abrupt cessation of the PPI. In addition, he has Barrett esophagus, which increases the risk of esophageal cancer. Neither an antacid nor an H2 antagonist is likely to be effective in controlling his symptoms.

24. A) Miliary tuberculosis (TB)

Miliary TB (found in children younger than 5 years and in the elderly) is seen on x-ray with milia seed patterns. Reactivated TB is when the infection returns and is noted on x-ray by lesions, nodules, and cavitation. Latent TB is when bacteria is in the lymph nodes and is not infectious. It is noted on x-ray as calcification and fibrosis. Pleural TB is in the pleural space and is very contagious; it is indicated by a mass with obtuse angles on x-ray.

25. A) Emphysema

Emphysema presents with shortness of breath, minimal cough, and decreased heart and lung sounds. Patients use pursed-lip breathing, and use of accessory muscles is prominent. Chronic bronchitis is characterized by a productive cough, wheezing, and coarse crackles. A respiratory infection and/or pneumonia presents with fever and new onset of symptoms.

26. A) Benign S2 variant

A physiologic S2 split is a benign variant that is best heard over the pulmonic area (or second intercostal space [ICS] on the upper left side of the sternum). It is caused by splitting of the aortic and pulmonic components and is considered a normal finding if it appears during inspiration and disappears at expiration. Some healthy elderly patients have an S4 (late diastole) heart sound, also known as the "atrial kick," which is caused by decreased ventricular compliance with age. If there are no signs or symptoms of heart/valvular disease, it is considered a normal variant. The S3 heart sound, which is heard during early diastole, is also called a "ventricular gallop." It is considered abnormal if it occurs after age 40 years.

27. D) Topical antibiotic

Sleeping with contact lenses in is an unhygienic practice that may result in contact lens keratitis. Symptoms include eye pain, redness, excessive tearing, and a lesion on the cornea. Topical antibiotics are the first line of treatment for the condition. Oral steroids, oral antibiotics, and topical steroids are not used as the first line of treatment for contact lens keratitis.

28. A) Hydrochlorothiazide (Microzide) 12.5 mg daily

An elderly patient with isolated systolic hypertension can be started on low-dose hydrochlorothiazide (Microzide). Propranolol (Inderal) should not be used to treat hypertension. Alpha-blockers, such as prazosin (Minipress), are not first-line drugs to manage hypertension unless the patient has preexisting benign prostatic hyperplasia. Spironolactone (Aldactone) is not a first-line therapy for isolated systolic hypertension.

29. C) Serum concentration

It is important to monitor serum concentration when administering theophylline (Theo-Dur). Theophylline can cause adverse effects due to the plasma concentration, especially when it exceeds 20 mg/L. Liver function testing is appropriate for medications that affect the liver such as antibiotics, antipsychotics, and statins. Theophylline does not affect white or red blood cells, so there is no reason for a CBC. Complete metabolic panel lab testing is instrumental in diagnosing disorders such as diabetes, hypertension, and coronary artery disease, but it is not indicated in cases of theophylline use.

30. D) Vitamin B12 deficiency
The patient's history and physical assessment findings correlate with vitamin B12 deficiency. Neurologic manifestations such as paresthesia, hyperreflexia, and balance disorders are common in patients with vitamin B12 deficiency. While many symptoms are similar among anemias, neurologic manifestations are not associated with iron deficiency, hemolytic anemia, or normocytic anemia.

31. D) Lithium carbonate (Eskalith)
The patient is exhibiting signs of bipolar disorder I, including alternating periods of euphoria and high energy levels with periods of extreme depression and exhaustion, so the treatment of choice would be lithium carbonate (Eskalith). Haloperidol (Haldol) is not first-line treatment due to serious side effects such as neuroleptic malignant syndrome and cardiovascular dysfunction. Phenelzine (Nardil) is a monoamine oxidase inhibitor (MAOI) antidepressant that is not used to treat bipolar disorder alone, so it is not first-line treatment. Diazepam (Valium) is a sedative.

32. D) Ask the patient to resubmit a clean-catch specimen.
Multiple bacteria in a urine sample is indicative of a contaminated sample. It should be repeated following appropriate procedure guidelines to obtain a clean-catch specimen. An MRI or IVP would be ordered only if the clean-catch specimen indicates a need, such as with kidney stones or pyelonephritis.

33. D) >40 degrees
A spinal curvature of >40 degrees requires surgical intervention with a Harrington rod. Curvatures between 5 and 20 degrees should be monitored for changes. Bracing is necessary for curvatures between 20 and 40 degrees.

34. B) Order a noncontrast CT scan.
The best imaging test to identify a kidney stone is the noncontrast CT scan. It has the highest sensitivity/specificity for kidney stones. The first initial imaging test is the renal ultrasound; if needed, the noncontrast CT scan is ordered. A CBC and urinalysis will not assist in diagnosis of a kidney stone. There is no reason to repeat the renal ultrasound. McBurney's test would be indicated with signs of appendicitis.

35. D) 9 to 12
Hemoglobin and hematocrit are not routinely screened at birth, because hemoglobin is elevated from maternal red blood cells (RBCs) that are mixed with fetal RBCs. Healthy infants have enough iron stores to last 4 to 6 months after birth. Complementary foods are typically rich in iron, so infants should not be screened until 9 to 12 months.

36. A) Lanugo
The appearance of fine, downy body hair should be documented as lanugo, commonly associated with anorexia nervosa. Actinic keratosis is a rough, scaly patch on the skin that develops from years of exposure to the sun. It is most commonly found on the face, lips, ears, back of the hands, forearms, scalp, or neck. Russell's sign is defined as calluses on the knuckles or back of the hand due to repeated self-induced vomiting over long periods of time. Telogen effluvium is a scalp disorder characterized by the thinning or shedding of hair, resulting from the early entry of hair in the telogen phase (temporary hair loss).

37. B) Determine underlying etiology.
Symptoms describe a paroxysmal supraventricular tachycardia (PSVT), which shows an EKG with tachycardia and a peaked QRS complex with P waves present. The next step for the NP is to determine the underlying etiology so that treatment can be implemented. Treatment may consist of implementing vagal maneuvers: Asking the patient to hold breath and strain hard, massaging carotid sinus, and splashing water on the face. A consult to cardiology is recommended to evaluate and treat after the underlying etiology has been determined. Blood pressure would have been assessed prior to EKG.

38. B) Azithromycin 1 g PO in a single dose (directly observed treatment preferred)
Azithromycin 1 g PO in a single dose is the CDC-recommended treatment for uncomplicated chlamydia. Acyclovir (Zovirax) 400 mg PO TID x 7 to 10 days is the recommended treatment for the first episode of primary genital herpes. Benzathine penicillin G 2.4 mU IM in a single dose is the recommended treatment for primary syphilis (chancre), secondary syphilis, or early latent syphilis (<1 year). Podofilox (Condylox) 0.5% gel or cream BID x 3 consecutive days is the recommended treatment for condylomata acuminata (genital warts), which may appear on the vagina, external genitals, urethra, anus, penis, nasal mucosa, oropharynx, or conjunctivae.

39. A) 3
Healthy women age 18 to 65 years diagnosed with an uncomplicated urinary tract infection may be treated with a 3-day treatment plan. A 5-, 7-, or 10-day course would be excessive and possibly result in antibiotic resistance or other issues involving excess antibiotic use, such as *Clostridium difficile*.

40. B) Acquired neutropenia
Patients taking hydrochlorothiazide and nifedipine (Procardia XL) should be monitored for acquired neutropenia. Hydrochlorothiazide can cause bone marrow suppression, leading to neutropenia. Nifedipine (and other calcium channel blockers) suppress cytokine-induced activation of neutrophils. Macrocytosis is a descriptive term

for macrocytes that are larger than normal. It can occur in the presence of anemia, alcoholism, and sickle cell disease. Primary polycythemia vera is caused by acquired or inherited genetic mutations. It causes abnormally high levels of red blood cell precursors. Excess platelets in the blood cause thrombocythemia. Secondary thrombocythemia can be caused by infection, inflammatory states, hemorrhage, trauma, or splenectomy.

41. A, C, D) It occurs secondary to reactivation of the varicella-zoster virus; It is usually more severe in immunocompromised individuals; Infection of the trigeminal nerve ophthalmic branch can cause corneal blindness.
Herpes zoster (shingles) occurs secondary to reactivation of the VZV. This infection can be more severe in immunocompromised patients because of their inability to fight infection. The typical shingles rash involves groups of papules and vesicles (not bullae) on a red base that rupture and become crusted. The rash is painful and follows one dermatome on one side of the body. When the trigeminal nerve is involved, there is an increased risk of corneal blindness.

42. A) "Everything is normal; I recommend you have the lipid panel repeated in 2 years."
All of the results of the lipid panel are normal. Guidelines recommend lipid screening every 2 to 3 years if the patient is older than 40 years. Reducing the amount of fat in the diet and increasing soluble fiber are lifestyle changes for those patients who need to lower cholesterol. These measures can be effective even if no weight loss occurs.

43. D) The patient may have a past history of frequent hospitalizations.
Munchausen syndrome is a psychiatric disorder in which the patient may falsify or induce illness in themself to gain attention from healthcare providers. Falsifying illness in a child is seen in Munchausen by proxy, which is a related disorder. Given the compulsion to repeatedly seek treatment, individuals with the disorder may have extensive medical histories.

44. B, E) "Take amoxicillin-clavulanate 875/125 mg twice daily as ordered."; "Report fever to healthcare provider immediately."
Uncomplicated acute diverticulitis can be treated on an outpatient basis if the provider educates the patient on the treatment plan. The patient should take amoxicillin-clavulanate 875/125 mg twice daily as ordered and report fever to the healthcare provider immediately so that the patient can be evaluated for abscesses, peritonitis, or sepsis and referred to the ED if necessary. Once the acute episode resolves, the patient should maintain a high-fiber diet with supplemental psyllium fiber. Taking laxatives long term is not recommended for those with diverticulitis, but a stool softener can be added to the regimen, if necessary, to assist with evacuation.

45. A) Inevitable abortion
Inevitable abortion is defined as vaginal bleeding with pain, cervical dilation, and/or cervical effacement. Threatened abortion is defined as vaginal bleeding with absent or minimal pain and a closed, long, and thick cervix. Incomplete abortion involves moderate to diffuse vaginal bleeding, with the passage of tissue and painful uterine cramping or contractions. Acute pelvic inflammatory disease is a sudden onset of inflammation and pain that affects the pelvic area, cervix, uterus, and ovaries, and is caused by infection.

46. A) Lung
Lung cancer is the most common cause of cancer deaths in men. Prostate cancer and colon cancer are the second and third most common causes of cancer death in men.

47. B) Arteriovenous (AV) nicking, left ventricular hypertrophy, stroke
AV nicking and copper wire/silver wire arterioles are signs of hypertensive retinopathy, ventricular hypertrophy affects the heart, and stroke damages the brain. These are all examples of target organ damage seen in hypertensive patients.

48. A, D) Fecal occult blood test; Urea breath test
The NP will order diagnostic testing to verify the likely diagnosis of peptic ulcer disease (PUD). Patients with PUD present with signs and symptoms of epigastric pain often relieved by self-medicating with OTC antacids. The patient reports daily nonsteroidal anti-inflammatory drug (NSAID) use, which is an irritant to the stomach. All patients presenting with PUD symptoms should be tested for *Helicobacter pylori*, so a urea breath test is appropriate. A fecal occult blood test is needed to determine if there is active bleeding. The gold standard for PUD diagnosis is an upper endoscopy (not lower) and biopsy of gastric tissue. A hemoglobin A1C would provide information regarding blood glucose levels and would not be a screening test for PUD.

49. A) Increases uric acid excretion
Probenecid (Probalan) is a uricosuric agent used to increase the excretion of uric acid through the renal system in patients with gout. Probenecid (Probalan) does not affect the formation of uric acid. Uric acid is not metabolized; it is excreted.

50. B, C) Lateral elbow pain with tenderness at the lateral epicondyle; Elbow pain with grasping movement
Tennis elbow, or lateral epicondylitis, is inflammation of the tendon insertion of the extensor carpiradialis brevis muscle. It is associated with lateral tenderness at the insertion site. Pain worsens with grasping or twisting movements. Pulling is associated with medial epicondylitis, or golfer elbow. Elbow pain with extension is indicative of hyperextension.

51. A) Tinea cruris

Tinea cruris (jock itch) is a common skin infection that is caused by a type of fungus called tinea. The fungus thrives in warm, moist areas of the body, and, as a result, infection can affect the genitals, inner thighs, and buttocks. Infections occur more frequently in the summer or warm, wet climates. Tinea cruris appears as a red, itchy rash that is often ring shaped. Tinea corporis involves the body, tinea capitis involves the head, and tinea pedis involves the feet.

52. A) Oral fluconazole (Diflucan)

Pityriasis versicolor, formerly known as tinea versicolor, is a fungal infection caused by a type of yeast that is normally present on the skin but has grown out of control. Pityriasis versicolor is diagnosed by clinical appearance and a sample of the skin scrapings placed on a KOH wet mount, which reveal short hyphae and budding cells. Because of the extent of the patient's fungal infection, oral fluconazole (Diflucan) is the primary prescribed treatment. Oral ketoconazole (Nizoral) is contraindicated in the treatment of pityriasis versicolor because of the risk of adrenal problems, liver damage, and harmful drug interactions. Tacrolimus (Protopic) is an immunosuppressant that demonstrates antimycotic action but is not the most effective in reducing the appearance of hypopigmentation associated with pityriasis versicolor. Topical selenium sulfide for a widespread case of pityriasis versicolor can be expensive, and it is difficult to cover large surface areas of the infected skin.

53. B) "Wear sun-protective clothing."

Patients with SLE have a tendency toward photosensitivity; therefore, the patient should be advised to avoid exposure to sunlight and take precautions, such as wearing sun-protective clothing and sunscreen. The patient should use nonfluorescent bulbs because she is more likely to have a sensitivity reaction to fluorescent bulbs. There is no need to restrict protein in the diet or avoid using lotions with SLE.

54. C) Musculoskeletal

Secondary hypertension can be caused by disorders of the following systems: renal (e.g., renal artery stenosis, polycystic kidneys, chronic kidney disease), endocrine (e.g., hyperthyroidism, hyperaldosteronism, pheochromocytoma), and respiratory (e.g., sleep apnea). Musculoskeletal disorders generally do not cause hypertension.

55. B) Undeveloped blood-brain barrier

The infant's blood-brain barrier is not fully developed for several months; therefore, the infant has an increased risk of central nervous system toxicity and sensitivity to pharmacologic agents that act on the brain. Renal excretion is decreased in infants. Gastric emptying time in infants is prolonged and irregular. Therefore, enhanced absorption of a pharmacologic agent may occur as a result of delayed gastric emptying. Because of the low level of serum albumin, protein-binding drugs are less able to bind in infants, and endogenous compounds that compete with drugs for binding sites result in a higher concentration of free drug levels.

56. A) *Pseudomonas aeruginosa*

Puncture wounds of the foot may become infected with *P. aeruginosa* (gram negative) by the foam material from sneakers, ultimately causing cellulitis. *V. vulnificus* is a gram-negative bacterium that causes infections from consuming raw oysters or clams. *P. multocida* is a gram-negative pathogen that is present in dog and cat bites. *S. aureus* is a gram-positive bacterium that causes a purulent form of cellulitis such as methicillin-resistant *Staphylococcus aureus* (MRSA), especially in the lower leg.

57. C) Serum pregnancy test

Tanner stage II indicates normal physical development congruent with menarche. A serum pregnancy test would be ordered first to determine if the patient is not menstruating because of pregnancy. If there is no pregnancy, further testing would be done. Prolactin levels would be high in pregnancy and during lactation. A CT scan of the abdomen and pelvis would identify tumors in the ovaries or adrenal glands. Examination of chromosomes in a sample of tissue (such as blood) would be performed to check for genetic disorders.

58. B) Doxycycline twice daily for 10 days

The patient likely has Rocky Mountain spotted fever. Doxycycline is the first-line treatment for Rocky Mountain spotted fever, a vector-borne (commonly by ticks) disease caused by the bacterium class *Rickettsia rickettsii*. The treatment is based on empirical diagnosis. To avoid possible complications, treat within 5 days; do not wait for lab results. Rifampin is indicated for treating close contacts of a patient with meningococcemia. If confirmed as having meningococcemia, the patient would be admitted to the hospital and started on ceftriaxone (Rocephin) 2 g IV every 12 hours and vancomycin IV every 8 to 12 hours. Cephalexin (Keflex) is the preferred medication of choice for severe cases of impetigo.

59. A) "Tell me what you know about colonoscopy and why you feel it is important."

The most therapeutic response would be to request more information from the patient. A provider should never scare a patient away from a procedure or take away their autonomy. There is no indication that the patient's partner needs to be involved with the patient's decision, and it devalues the patient's autonomy.

60. A) Cauda equina syndrome

Cauda equina syndrome is an acute-onset saddle anesthesia that affects the nerve roots from L1 to L5 and S1 to S5. Symptoms may include bladder incontinence or retention, fecal incontinence, weakness, and bilateral leg numbness. It results from trauma, disease, or infection that puts pressure on the sacral nerve roots and causes inflammatory changes to the nerves. Scoliosis is a sideways curvature of the spine that is most often noted during the growth spurt just before puberty. Fibromyalgia is a disorder characterized by widespread musculoskeletal pain accompanied by fatigue, sleep, memory, and mood issues. Paget's disease of bone interferes with the body's normal recycling process in which new bone tissue gradually replaces old bone tissue. Over time, the disease can cause affected bones to become fragile and misshapen.

61. C) Reassessment in 1 year
A noncommunicating hydrocele occurs when the sac closes normally around the testicle during development, but the body does not absorb the fluid inside it. This type of hydrocele is common in newborns and usually disappears without treatment by age 1 year. Surgery is recommended for a communicating hydrocele (when the sac does not seal) because the scrotum may swell more over time. There are no drugs available to treat hydrocele. Needle aspiration (centesis) is commonly performed on adult men who are at high risk for complications during surgery.

62. C) Zollinger-Ellison syndrome
Zollinger-Ellison syndrome is a neuroendocrine tumor that leads to gastrin hypersecretion and multiple peptic ulcer formation. These tumors, called gastrinomas, secrete large amounts of the hormone gastrin, which causes the stomach to produce too much acid. The excess acid then leads to peptic ulcers as well as to diarrhea and other symptoms. *H. pylori* is a type of bacteria. These bacteria can enter the body and live in the digestive tract. After many years, they can cause ulcers in the lining of the stomach or the upper part of the small intestine. *H. pylori* is diagnosed with a urea breath test and an upper gastrointestinal examination. Atrophic gastritis develops when the lining of the stomach has been inflamed for several years. The inflammation is most often the result of a bacterial infection caused by the *H. pylori* bacterium. Meckel diverticulum, the remnants of the umbilical cord and the most common congenital defect of the gastrointestinal tract, is an outpouching or bulge in the lower part of the small intestine.

63. A) Long-acting muscarinic agonist (LAMA)
LAMA is the first line of treatment for COPD in category C. For category A, a SABA is recommended. A LABA is used for category B. SAMA blocks only the muscarinic effects.

64. B) History of asthma
Contraindications to timolol (Betimol) include asthma, emphysema, chronic obstructive pulmonary disorder (COPD), heart failure, and second- or third-degree atrioventricular (AV) block. Elevated IOP would be expected with open-angle glaucoma and is an indication for timolol (Betimol), although an IOP of 30 mmHg or above requires urgent referral to an ophthamologist or ED. Stinging sensation is a common side effect of timolol (Betimol) use.

65. B) Increased intracranial pressure (ICP)
The patient's vital signs reveal increased ICP or the Cushing triad. With increased ICP, the systolic blood pressure increases, and the pulse and respirations decrease. In hypovolemic shock, the opposite is true: Blood pressure is decreased, and pulse and respirations increase. A CVA or stroke is caused by an embolus/thrombus or a hemorrhage. The most common risk factors are atrial fibrillation, hypertension, anticoagulant therapy, trauma, and an aneurysm. Embolic stroke signs include sudden dysphasia; unilateral hemiparesis; and weakness of the arms, legs, or both. A hemorrhagic stroke will cause a severe headache, nausea, vomiting, photophobia, nuchal rigidity, and dysphasia. A subdural hematoma is a gradual process, and elderly patients have a history of head trauma by falling or accidents. They are more common in older adults on anticoagulant or aspirin therapies. The bleeding is between the dura and the subarachnoid membranes in the brain.

66. D) Class III or IV heart disease
Pioglitazone (Actos) is contraindicated in patients with class III or IV heart disease and congestive heart failure because it causes water retention. Pioglitazone (Actos) should also be avoided in patients with a history of bladder cancer. Biguanides are contraindicated in patients with renal or kidney disease, alcoholism, and hypoxia. Asthma is not a contraindication for diabetes medications.

67. C) Hot compresses three times daily
The patient has a hordeolum, or stye. The treatment plan should begin with hot compresses to the affected eye until the abscess drains. Many hordeolums will spontaneously drain within the first 48 hours. If infection spreads, the result would be preseptal cellulitis, and antibiotic therapy would be initiated. Incision and drainage would require referral to an ophthalmologist, which is not indicated at this time.

68. D) Topical antihistamines/mast cell stabilizers
Mild allergic conjunctivitis occurs because of a mast cell response to an allergen. An over-the-counter topical antihistamine/mast cell stabilizer can be used to treat the initial symptoms of mild allergic conjunctivitis. NSAIDs are not the first line of treatment for mild allergic conjunctivitis. Patients with allergic conjunctivitis often produce an inadequate amount of tears, which results in dryness of the eyes. Although oral antihistamines can be used for mild allergic conjunctivitis, they may induce dry eye syndrome, which impairs the protective barrier of tears and worsens allergic conjunctivitis. Artificial tears may be needed if oral antihistamines are prescribed. Topical corticosteroids are not the first line of treatment for mild allergic conjunctivitis.

69. B) Fungal
The KOH prep test is performed to evaluate for tinea or candida (yeast) infection of the skin. In vaginal discharge, the yeast organism is outside the skin cells, so KOH is not needed to visualize it. However, for skin cells, yeast is not visible unless the skin cell walls are destroyed by KOH. The test involves placing a sample of skin on a glass slide, with one or two drops of KOH (causes lysis of skin cells) and a cover slip on top. If done correctly, the budding spores and pseudohyphae can be visualized.

70. D) Repeat the test as soon as possible.

A specimen is satisfactory only if both squamous epithelial cells and endocervical cells are present. If lacking either type of cell, the specimen is incomplete, and the test needs to be repeated. Atypical squamous cells are cause for concern in a complete specimen. When atypical squamous cells of undetermined significance are found in women age 25 to 29 years, an HPV test should be performed. An endometrial biopsy is indicated if there are atypical glandular cells in the presence of endometrial cells. A referral for colposcopy is needed only if atypical cells are found in an acceptable specimen in patients age 30 years or older. A colposcopy would be recommended for a 21-year-old patient only if high-grade squamous intraepithelial lesions were found.

71. A) The patient is unable to stand with eyes closed and arms by side without swaying or falling.

A patient who is unable to hold their arms at their sides with feet together and eyes closed, and sways or steps, has a positive Romberg test. The Romberg test assumes that a person needs at least two of the three following senses to maintain balance while standing: proprioception, vestibular function, and vision. A pronator drift exam is positive if the patient is unable to stretch out arms in front of them with palms up and eyes closed and one arm drifts downward. Stereognosis is the ability to recognize a familiar object put in the patient's hand while their eyes are closed. Graphesthesia is the ability for a patient to correctly identify a written letter on the palm while the patient's eyes are closed.

72. D) Vesicular breath sounds in the lower lobe

Normal sounds of the chest wall include vesicular breath sounds in the lower lobes. Bronchial breath sounds are heard best at the second and third intercostal spaces. Tracheal breath sounds are heard over the trachea.

73. A) 6

The patient is currently using a potency Group 7 steroid (OTC topical hydrocortisone, 0.5%–1.0%) for eczema. The NP should prescribe the next level of topical steroids, a Group 6, such as desonide cream or lotion (0.05%) and then reevaluate for effectiveness. The topical steroid strengths range from 7 (least potent) to 1 (very potent). For example, a Group 5 steroid is fluticasone propionate cream (0.05%), a Group 4 steroid is triamcinolone acetonide cream (0.1%), and a Group 3 steroid is amcinonide (0.1%).

74. C) Ultrasound

The infant should be referred for an ultrasound first to assess for any neural tube defects such as spina bifida or spina bifida occulta. A CT scan would be indicated to examine internal organs and structures. MRI is not indicated at this point, but it may be necessary later to view the central nervous system, including the brain and spine. A spinal tap or lumbar puncture would be appropriate if the infant had signs and symptoms of meningitis.

75. A) Ask patient to stand firmly on both feet and bend forward at the hips while arms hang free.

To screen for scoliosis, a lateral curvature of the spine, the patient should stand firmly on both feet with the trunk exposed and arms hanging free. The NP examines the adolescent from behind, checking for asymmetry of the shoulders, scapulae, and hips. The NP should ask the patient to bend forward at the hips and then inspect for a rib hump, which is another sign of scoliosis. The NP would listen for a clicking sound while the patient abducts the hips when screening for congenital hip dysplasia. Having the patient shrug their shoulders against mild resistance helps evaluate the integrity of cranial nerve XI. The heel-to-shin test evaluates cerebellar function.

76. B) Advise the patient to return 1 week after her period so her breasts can be rechecked.

Symptoms of fibrocystic breast disease include cyclic tenderness with prominent breast tissue that is present in both breasts. The symptoms are worse about 1 week before menses. A few days after menses starts, the bloating and breast tenderness resolve. Symptoms are caused by elevated hormone levels (progesterone). Fibrocystic disease is differentiated from breast cancer by the lack of a dominant mass or other symptoms such as peau d'orange, dimpling, retraction, or eczema-like rash on the nipples and areolae.

77. D) Renal artery stenosis

Renal artery stenosis refers to narrowing of the kidney arteries. It is commonly noted in individuals older than 50 years and is associated with atherosclerosis and hypertension. Hematuria is not associated with renal artery stenosis. Evidence of blood in the urine can be seen with kidney stones, bladder cancer, and acute pyelonephritis.

78. C) Otitis externa

The symptoms and history of the patient make otitis externa the most likely diagnosis. Otitis externa, also called swimmer ear, is inflammation of the ear canal. It often presents with ear pain, swelling of the ear canal, and, occasionally, decreased hearing. Typically, there is pain with movement of the outer ear. Otitis media is inflammation or infection located in the middle ear. Otitis media can occur because of a cold, sore throat, or respiratory infection. Rhinosinusitis is defined as inflammation of the sinuses and nasal cavity. Bullous myringitis is a type of ear infection in which small, fluid-filled blisters form on the eardrum. These blisters usually cause severe pain. The infection is caused by the same viruses or bacteria that lead to other ear infections.

79. A) Azithromycin 1 g orally in a single dose

If a patient has a positive NAAT for *Chlamydia trachomatis*, both the patient and their sexual partner should be treated. While azithromycin 1 g orally in a single dose or doxycycline 100 mg orally twice daily for 7 days are recommended regimens, azithromycin is the preferred treatment due to the compliance advantage of a single dose. Clindamycin is not recommended as it is only partially effective in eradicating *C. trachomatis* in men with nongonococcal urethritis. Benzathine penicillin is used to treat syphilis.

80. C) Myxedema coma

Myxedema coma (severe hypothyroidism) is a life-threatening condition that may develop with the abrupt cessation of thyroid replacement therapy. Exophthalmos, protrusion of the eyeballs, is seen with hyperthyroidism. Thyroid storm is life-threatening but is caused by severe hyperthyroidism. Pretibial myxedema, peripheral mucinous edema involving the lower leg, is associated with hypothyroidism but is not life-threatening.

81. C) Kawasaki's disease

Kawasaki's disease classically presents with high fever; enlarged lymph nodes in the neck; conjunctivitis; dry, cracked lips; and a "strawberry" (bright-red) tongue. Most cases occur in children younger than 5 years. Pharyngitis is an acute infection of the pharynx and presents with a stuffy nose, rhinitis with clear mucus, and watery eyes. Allergic rhinitis is inflammatory changes of the nasal mucosa due to an allergy response. Tonsillitis is inflammation of the tonsils, which are two oval-shaped pads of tissue at the back of the throat. Signs and symptoms of tonsillitis include swollen tonsils, sore throat, difficulty swallowing, and tender lymph nodes on the sides of the neck.

82. D) Meniscal tear

A positive McMurray test is suggestive of an injury or tear to the medial or lateral meniscus. An ACL tear is associated with a positive Lachman or anterior drawer test. A PCL tear is associated with a positive posterior drawer test. A patellar tendon rupture is associated with the inability to raise the straightened leg against gravity.

83. B) Oral prednisone

Patients with PMR are treated with oral corticosteroids such as prednisone. One of the hallmarks of the disorder is the dramatic improvement of symptoms after starting treatment with oral prednisone. Usually, the symptoms can be controlled with long-term (2–3 years) low-dose oral prednisone, which can be tapered when symptoms are under control. For most patients, PMR is a self-limiting illness (from a few months to 3 years). Etanercept is a biologic used to treat autoimmune conditions such as ankylosing spondylosis and psoriatic arthritis, but it is not used in PMR. Indomethacin is not used frequently in PMR; however, it is an nonsteroidal anti-inflammatory drug (NSAID) used most commonly for gout flares. Methotrexate is a disease-modifying antirheumatic drug (DMARD) commonly used to treat rheumatoid arthritis rather than PMR.

84. C) Observe the child going up several steps.

A 4-year-old child should be able to trace simple objects, run, climb steps, throw a ball, and perform several activities of daily living with little or no assistance. The child should be able to draw a person with two to four body parts, but not six. The child is likely too young to reliably catch a ball, and the ability to print letters and numbers typically appears around age 5 years.

85. B) It is safe for a patient with first-degree heart block to be prescribed a CCB such as nifedipine (Procardia XL) or verapamil (Calan).

CCBs are contraindicated in patients with bradycardia and second- or third-degree heart blocks. In sinus bradycardia, the heart rate is <60 bpm with a regular rate. The P wave is identical before each QRS complex. A first-degree heart block has a regular rate and rhythm with a PR >0.20 second, and a QRS >0.12 second. In a second-degree heart block, P waves are intermittent, PR is increasingly prolonged, and QRS falls into a repeated pattern. In a third-degree heart block, there is no PR interval, QRS is not applicable, and there is no relationship between P and QRS.

86. D) Transrectal ultrasound-guided needle biopsy

A PSA level greater than or equal to 4 ng/mL is considered an indication for biopsy in men older than 50 years. Although very high levels are significant (suggesting extracapsular extension of the tumor or metastases) and the likelihood of cancer increases with higher PSA levels, there is no cutoff below which there is no risk. CT or MRI of the abdomen and pelvis is commonly done to assess pelvic and retroperitoneal lymph nodes if the Gleason score is 8 to 10 and the PSA is >10 ng/mL. Radionuclide bone scans are rarely helpful for finding bone metastases (they are frequently abnormal because of the trauma of arthritic changes) until the PSA is >20 ng/mL. Elevated serum acid phosphatase correlates well with the presence of metastases, particularly in lymph nodes. However, this enzyme may also be elevated in benign prostatic hyperplasia and is slightly elevated after vigorous prostatic massage.

87. A) Is perimenopausal

The patient's laboratory results indicate that the patient is perimenopausal. The patient's estradiol level reflects a perimenopausal state. The range of estradiol associated with perimenopause is 30 to 400 pg/mL. FSH >30 mIU/mL is indicative of decreased ovarian function, which is associated with perimenopause. An AMH measurement is predictive of ovarian reserve. The level of the AMH declines with age and is a predictor for menopause. An AMH level of <0.5 ng/mL is associated with perimenopause. The patient's laboratory results are not consistent with menopause, which is diagnosed after the menstrual period has been absent for 12 months. The patient does not require testing for ovarian cancer.

88. B) Bruised kidney

The findings (back pain and muscle spasms, nausea with vomiting, and a direct hit to the side of the body) indicate a potential bruised kidney. Appendicitis typically begins with anorexia, nausea, and vomiting for the first 12 to 24 hours. Abdominal pain, a late sign, is usually diffuse at first and gradually localizes to the right lower quadrant. Cholecystitis may cause radiating pain to the back but would not be due to a direct hit and would not manifest as muscle spasms. A ruptured vertebral disc would manifest as pain and muscle spasm but without nausea and vomiting.

89. D) Tetanus, diphtheria, acellular pertussis (Tdap)

The Centers for Disease Control and Prevention (CDC) recommends that one of the tetanus boosters be replaced with the Tdap (once in a lifetime). Thereafter, the Td form of the vaccine is indicated every 10 years. The DTaP and DT forms of the tetanus vaccine are not given after age 7 years. Puncture wounds are at higher risk for tetanus because *Clostridium tetani* bacteria are anaerobes (deep puncture wounds are not exposed to air compared with superficial wounds).

90. D) Topical permethrin (Elimite)

The assessment findings are consistent with scabies and require the application of a scabicide such as topical permethrin (Elimite). Topical nystatin is used to treat candidal infections. Oral griseofulvin is used to treat different fungal infections. Oral ketoconazole (Nizoral) is reserved for severe fungal infections.

91. C) Tell the partner that the rest of the exam must be private, show them to the waiting area, and say you will retrieve them when you finish.

The partner is demonstrating dominant and controlling behavior. This behavior is characteristic in intimate partner violence and abuse. Excuses are being made for injuries, and the victim will not answer questions truthfully in the abuser's presence. Examining the victim privately allows for free therapeutic conversation and truth telling. Challenging the partner with threats or confronting them could escalate violent behavior.

92. B) Lubiprostone (Amitiza) 8 mcg orally twice daily

Lubiprostone (Amitiza) is a chloride channel activator that is approved by the U.S. Food and Drug Administration (FDA) for the treatment of IBS with constipation in adults. Amitriptyline (Elavil) is a tricyclic antidepressant that can be used to treat abdominal pain, mucorrhea, and stool frequency. Dicyclomine (Bentyl) is an anticholinergic and antispasmodic that decreases fecal urgency and pain associated with diarrhea. Alosetron (Lotronex) is administered for IBS associated with diarrhea. It is associated with gastrointestinal toxicity resulting in ischemic colitis and should not be prescribed for patients with constipation.

93. A) Transverse nasal crease

A classic sign of allergic rhinitis is a transverse nasal crease (allergic salute) from frequent rubbing and wiping away of nasal discharge. Allergic rhinitis generally produces clear nasal discharge unless there is also sinusitis. Associated postnasal drip may cause a cough that worsens in the supine position. Epistaxis is not commonly associated with allergic rhinitis.

94. D) Resistance to leg straightening from back pain

A patient with a positive Kernig sign will resist leg straightening when the hip is flexed as a result of painful hamstrings from lumbar nerve root inflammation. A positive Brudzinski sign is seen when the patient's neck is passively flexed and there is flexing of the hips and knees to relieve pressure and pain. Nuchal rigidity is present when touching the chin to the chest causes pain. A positive Babinski reflex is seen when the toes fan when the plantar surface is stroked from the heel to the great toe. Adults should have a negative Babinski reflex.

95. A) Ibuprofen

The Finkelstein test is used to diagnose de Quervain tenosynovitis. De Quervain tenosynovitis occurs from repetitive movement or overuse of the wrist and thumb. The symptoms associated with de Quervain tenosynovitis result from inflammation of the tendons and sheaths located on the thumb side of the wrist, causing pain traveling up the arm and swelling over the thumb and wrist. The patient will be instructed to apply ice packs for a prescribed amount of time daily and take a nonsteroidal anti-inflammatory drug (NSAID) such as ibuprofen for discomfort. Oral prednisone is not used in the treatment of de Quervain tenosynovitis. Doses of 0.5% plain lidocaine and 0.5 mL of a long-acting corticosteroid are injected either simultaneously or subsequentially into the sheath of the first dorsal compartment to reduce tendon inflammation. They are not used singularly for treatment of the condition. Furthermore, the treatments are invasive and increase the risk for complications; therefore, they are not the first line of treatment.

96. B) Colchicine

The patient is experiencing an acute attack of gout and can be treated with anti-inflammatory medications, including colchicine, nonsteroidal anti-inflammatory drugs (NSAIDs), and steroids. Allopurinol is used to treat chronic gout. Tetracycline and amoxicillin are antibiotics that are indicated for the treatment of gout but would not be first line for an acute attack of gout.

97. B) Fetal alcohol syndrome

The classic signs of fetal alcohol syndrome are microcephaly, narrow eyes, thin lips, and a smooth philtrum. Its effects can range from severe intellectual disability to attention deficit hyperactivity disorder in adolescents. Down syndrome causes a flat, round face; low-set ears; macroglossia; and hypotonia. Parents should be educated about high-risk sports and potential spinal cord injuries. Poor weight gain, formerly known as failure to thrive, is most likely diagnosed in the first few months of life when there is a weight decrease over two or more major percentile lines (90th, 75th, 50th, 25th, and 5th). Poor weight gain can be caused by inadequate nutritional intake, neglect, or poor maternal bonding. Fragile X syndrome is an inherited intellectual disability. The face is long and narrow with a prominent forehead and chin and large ears.

98. C) Meares-Stamey 2-glass test

The Meares-Stamey 2-glass test is used to assess for inflammation and the presence of bacteria in the lower urinary tract, findings that are associated with symptoms of chronic prostatitis. Urinalysis may reveal infection, but it may not be related specifically to chronic prostatitis. A PSA level is not a specific test for identifying inflammation or the presence of bacteria associated with chronic prostatitis. A gram stain of a urethral swab can be used to evaluate the patient for a sexually transmitted infection associated with acute bacterial prostatitis.

99. B) Weight loss and dehydration

In CD, fistula formation and anal disease may occur. If the colon is involved, bloody diarrhea with mucus is present; involvement of the ileum is associated with watery diarrhea without blood or mucus. If a mass has developed in the abdomen, anorexia, weight loss, dehydration, and fatigue are commonly found. Periumbilical to right lower quadrant pain occurs more frequently in CD, and left lower quadrant pain is more classically associated with ulcerative colitis (UC). CD is distinguished from UC by its transmural inflammation in skip lesions throughout the intestines versus the mucosal inflammation found throughout the colon in UC.

100. C) Osgood-Schlatter disease

The most likely diagnosis in a 13-year-old male patient with persistent unilateral knee pain is Osgood-Schlatter disease, which causes inflammation of the anterior tibial tubercle. Osgood-Schlatter disease is caused by overuse while the bone is still growing and is most common in prepubescent boys. Polymyositis is caused by immune disorders or disease and presents with bilateral muscle weakness and wasting. Baker's cyst is swelling caused by fluid from the knee joint protruding to the back of the knee. With no history of trauma, a meniscal tear is not likely, particularly in a younger patient.

101. C) Hypothyroidism

Symptoms of hypothyroidism include fatigue, cold intolerance, weight gain, and constipation. A patient with hyperthyroidism would present with weight loss, anxiety, palpitations, warm skin, and insomnia. Diabetes mellitus symptoms include polyphagia, polydipsia, and polyuria. A patient with heart failure would present with respiratory symptoms, weight gain, tachypnea, fatigue, and edema.

102. A) Herpes zoster

Herpes zoster (shingles) is caused by infection with the herpes varicella-zoster virus (VZV), the same virus that causes chickenpox. It commonly causes severe, deep pain along a peripheral nerve on the trunk of the body and red, nodular skin lesions. Fever and malaise typically accompany these findings. Shingles occurs more frequently in the older adult population. Chickenpox, also known as varicella, is a highly contagious infection caused by the VZV. There is a blisterlike rash, which first appears on the face and trunk and then spreads throughout the body. Plaque

psoriasis is a chronic autoimmune condition. It appears on the skin in patches of thick, red, scaly skin. Tinea corporis is a dermatophytosis that causes pink-to-red annular (O-shaped) patches and plaques with raised, scaly borders that expand peripherally and tend to clear centrally.

103. D) Ishihara chart

The Ishihara chart is the most appropriate method for screening a patient for color blindness. The Snellen chart is used to evaluate central distance vision, while the confrontation exam evaluates peripheral vision. The extraocular movement test reveals whether the eyes move together when following an object.

104. A) Oral terbinafine (Lamisil)

Tinea unguium (onychomycosis) is a fungal infection of the nails, usually the great toe. The toenail becomes yellowed and thickened and may even separate from the nail bed. The first-line medication is oral terbinafine (Lamisil) for 12 weeks. For mild-to-moderate infections, efinaconazole 10% solution (Jublia) can be used. Azelaic acid (Azelex) and metronidazole gel (Metrogel) are treatments for rosacea (acne rosacea).

105. A) Lyme disease

The classic lesion in Lyme disease is an expanding red rash with central clearing that resembles a target. This "bullseye" rash (erythema migrans) appears 7 to 14 days after a bite from a deer tick infected with the *Borrelia burgdorferi* bacterium. Lyme disease is accompanied by flu-like symptoms. The bite of a brown recluse spider appears as a reddened skin area that may be followed by a blister that forms at the bite site, and it leads to mild-to-intense pain and itching for 2 to 8 hours following the bite. An open sore (ulcer) with a breakdown of tissue (necrosis) develops a week or more following the bite. Erythema infectiosum is known as fifth disease and generally occurs in children. Rocky Mountain spotted fever is also a tick-borne illness with similar symptoms but has a rash that begins in the extremities and has smaller red spots or macules.

106. C) Imipramine (Elavil)

Based on the patient's medical history, imipramine at half-strength is an appropriate medication to prescribe. Topiramate is not appropriate because of the patient's history of kidney stones. Atenolol and propranolol are not appropriate because of a history of bradycardia. Sumatriptan is not a safe medication because of the patient having a history of MI.

107. B) Psoriasis

Psoriasis causes rapid cell build-up on the skin, causing red, dry, itchy, raised patches covered with silvery lesions. Plaques frequently occur on the elbows and knees but can occur on other body areas. Impetigo is an infection caused by gram-positive bacteria; the lesions are small, red, and pus-filled. Impetigo occurs most frequently in small children. Xerosis is an inherited skin disorder characterized by extremely dry mucosal skin surfaces. Contact dermatitis is an inflammatory skin reaction caused by direct exposure to an irritant. It can occur as a single lesion or generalized rash.

108. C) III
During Tanner stage III, the areola, nipple, and breast grow together in one mound. There is no separation yet. At Tanner stage IV, the areola and the nipple separate to form a distinct mound.

109. A) Urine culture and sensitivity (C&S)
An 8-year-old male patient with the diagnosis of diabetes has a high risk of urinary tract infections (UTIs). A large amount of leukocytes in the urinalysis is abnormal, and he has been having symptoms of frequency and nocturia for the past 3 days. A urine culture would be ordered because he has a high risk of infection. The urine C&S is the best evaluation for diagnosing a UTI.

110. B) Urine leakage with stress
In penopubic epispadias, the urethral meatus is found near the pubic bone. The position of the meatus helps predict how well the bladder stores urine. When the bladder sphincter is shaped more like a horseshoe than a ring, it does not close all the way. Because of this, urine leaks out. Most boys with penopubic epispadias and about two of three with penile epispadias leak urine with stress. In most cases of penopubic epispadias, the bones of the pelvis do not come together in the front. In boys with epispadias, the penis tends to be broad, short, and curved up. In penile epispadias, the urinary meatus is found along the shaft. In penopubic epispadias, it is found on or near the pubic bone.

111. A) Premedicate 5 to 20 minutes before starting exercise.
Exercise-induced asthma is best controlled by using the Proventil inhaler (bronchodilator) approximately 5 to 20 minutes before exercise to prevent vasospasm of the bronchioles and shortness of breath with exercise. The effects of these bronchodilators usually last approximately 4 hours. They also work quickly to open up the bronchioles if an acute attack/shortness of breath occurs.

112. B) Levothyroxine T4
The current treatment for hypothyroidism is levothyroxine T4. Replacement therapy with levothyroxine T3 alone is not recommended. Much of the conversion of T3 comes from T4. T3 has a very short life span in the body, which would require a patient to take the medication several times a day and may result in imbalanced levels causing unpleasant symptoms. Too high of a level can result in injury to the heart and bones. TSH stimulates the release of T3 and T4 from the thyroid gland, which, in hypothyroidism, is not reacting to produce the hormones in response to stimulation of TSH from the anterior pituitary gland. Combined levothyroxine T3 and T4 can be prescribed, but this does not offer any advantage over prescribing T4 alone.

113. A) 1
Step 1 is intermittent asthma with an FEV1 >80% predicted. Albuterol or a short-acting beta2-agonist (SABA) is used as a metered-dose inhaler as needed in patients age 12 years and older. Step 2 would involve a low-dose inhaled corticosteroid (ICS) treatment, and Steps 3 and 4 would involve low-to-medium inhaled corticosteroid treatment plus a long-acting beta2-agonist (LABA).

114. C) 4 weeks following onset
Infectious mononucleosis presents the risk for splenic rupture. Patients who participate in strenuous contact sports are advised to refrain from participation for at least 4 weeks following onset of illness. Athletes who participate in noncontact sports are advised to wait at least 3 weeks. Although most acute symptoms resolve within the first 2 weeks, the risk for splenic rupture may remain elevated for several days beyond that.

115. D) Treat with bacitracin zinc.
The patient has a partial-thickness (second-degree) burn because the patient is older than 50 years and the total body surface area (TBSA) burned is <5%. The treatment is bacitracin zinc and nonadherent dressings. Silver sulfadiazine cream should be avoided because of the patient's allergy to sulfa products. Benzocaine spray or aloe vera gel is the treatment for superficial-thickness (first-degree) burns. Blisters should not be ruptured because it may increase the risk of infection, especially in elderly patients.

116. A) Eye exam with an ophthalmologist
Elderly patients with type 2 diabetes should have a dilated eye exam done annually by an ophthalmologist. They should also see a podiatrist once or twice a year. A diabetes diagnosis does not necessitate routine visits to the urologist or an optometrist, nor does it influence the schedule for colonoscopy.

117. C) Osteoarthritis
Signs of osteoarthritis include stiffness of joints, especially in the morning and after sitting for long periods. Visible signs of osteoarthritis are an element in the diagnosis. Heberden nodes (bony overgrowths) are classic signs of osteoarthritis. They are located at the distal interphalangeal joints. They are felt as hard, nontender nodules that are usually 2 to 3 cm in diameter but sometimes encompass the entire joint. Enlargement of the middle joint of a finger is called a Bouchard node. Rheumatoid arthritis differs in that deformities of the hands and fingers form, and the stiffness of the joints after rest is generally persistent for several hours. Osteoporosis does not commonly cause hand pain or stiffness, but when symptomatic it generally causes loss of height and vertebral pain. It does not cause Heberden nodes. Reiter syndrome is a reactive arthritis that presents in response to arthritis in other areas of the body and generally causes symptoms in the knees and feet more commonly than in the hands. It does not produce Heberden nodes.

118. D) Bulging of the tympanic membrane
Acute suppurative otitis media is an acute infection affecting the mucosal lining of the middle ear and the mastoid air system. In the suppurative stage, the tympanic membrane bulges and ruptures spontaneously through a small perforation in the pars tensa. Ear discharge is usually present. Diagnosis is usually made simply by looking at the eardrum through an otoscope. The eardrum will appear red and swollen, and may appear either abnormally drawn inward or bulging outward. Using the tympanogram with the otoscope allows a puff of air to be blown lightly into the ear. Normally, this should cause movement of the eardrum. In an infection, or when there is fluid behind the eardrum, this movement may be decreased or absent. Conductive hearing loss may be present as evidenced by bone conduction (BC) exceeding air conduction (AC).

119. C) Appendicitis
In up to 50% of presenting cases of appendicitis, local tenderness is elicited at McBurney's point when pressure is applied. Rebound tenderness (i.e., production or intensification of pain when pressure is released) may be present and is considered a positive diagnostic sign. Crohn disease is characterized by bloody diarrhea along with right lower quadrant pain. Ulcerative colitis affects the colon and is characterized by bloody diarrhea with mucus, along with left-sided abdominal pain. Diverticulitis is characterized by pain that may be constant and may persist for several days. The lower left quadrant of the abdomen is the usual site of the pain. Signs and symptoms include nausea and vomiting, fever, and abdominal tenderness.

120. B) Amoxicillin-clavulanate
Amoxicillin-clavulanate is the first line of therapy for the treatment of acute otitis media. A second-generation cephalosporin such as cefdinir may be used in patients with a pencillin allergy. Erythromycin is not prescribed as the first line of treatment for acute otitis media. Azithromycin can be administered as the first line of treatment for acute otitis media if amoxicillin is contraindicated.

121. A) Confusion
Diphenhydramine (Benadryl) is an antihistamine that causes sedation and is used as a hypnotic. Older patients have increased sensitivity to the drug's effects. Diphenhydramine use places the patient at risk for confusion, urinary retention and incontinence, and sedation. Diphenhydramine is not specifically associated with bradycardia, hypertension, or cardiac arrhythmias in older patients.

122. A) Serum potassium
Serum potassium should be monitored upon initiation of an ACE inhibitor or angiotensin-receptor blocker (ARB) in a patient with kidney disease. Potassium may rise initially and begin to taper off 2 to 3 months later, so continued monitoring of serum potassium is recommended. Serum hemoglobin would not be needed, because ACE inhibitors do not affect hemoglobin levels. Likewise, an ultrasound of the kidneys or abdomen would not be needed unless the patient begins to exhibit complications related to kidney function.

123. C) Slate-gray nevi
Slate-gray nevi are the most common type of skin lesions in neonates. The lumbosacral area is a common location for these blue- to black-colored spots that usually fade by age 3 years. Milia are tiny white papules located on the forehead, nose, and cheeks. They contain sebaceous material and keratin and appear during the first week of life. Erythema toxicum neonatorum are small whitish pustules surrounded by a red base. A port wine stain (nevus flammeus) is a pink/red congenital, cutaneous, vascular malformation "birthmark" that usually appears on the face of the newborn.

124. C) Pneumococcal (Pneumovax) and influenza vaccines
The Td immunization is good for about 10 years. October to November is the beginning window of the flu season, and annual influenza vaccination is recommended. The pneumococcal (pneumonia) vaccine is indicated for patients older than 65 years.

125. A) Bone density test (dual-energy x-ray absorptiometry [DEXA])
The patient is postmenopausal and is suffering from osteoporosis. The gradual loss of bone density is common in postmenopausal women secondary to estrogen deficiency. A bone mineral density test is needed to confirm the diagnosis and obtain a baseline for future comparison. A colonoscopy and an upper gastrointestinal tract radiograph examine both the upper and lower gastrointestinal tracts. A nuclear stress test uses radioactive dye and an imaging machine to create pictures that show the blood flow to the heart. The test measures blood flow while at rest and during exertion.

126. B) A 2-year-old boy who ignores other children and has never spoken
A 2-year-old boy who does not speak and shows no interest in other children requires further evaluation because he demonstrates some behaviors associated with autism or other genetic disorders. The other children exhibit behaviors that may be frustrating but do not indicate a behavioral disorder.

127. D) Partial-thickness burns on the lower arm (2% total body surface area [TBSA])
A small, superficial, partial-thickness burn on the forearm can be treated with topical antibiotics and dressing. Criteria for burn center referral include partial-thickness burns greater than 10% of TBSA; burns involving the face, hands, feet, genitalia, perineum, or major joints; full-thickness burns; electrical and chemical burns; inhalation injuries; burn injuries in patients with preexisting comorbidities; burns with concomitant trauma; children in

hospitals without qualified personnel or equipment; and burn injury in patients who require special social or rehabilitative interventions.

128. B) Higher than normal
AFP is produced in the fetal and maternal liver. Higher levels of AFP are commonly seen in multiple gestations because of the growing liver in each fetus, which cumulatively leads to higher AFP levels.

129. C) High
This patient fulfills the criteria for high-intensity statin dosing from guidelines for management of blood cholesterol. He already has heart disease (angina), type 2 diabetes, LDL of 195 mg/dL, and low HDL of 25 mg/dL. This patient is at very high risk for further heart disease and warrants a high-intensity dose of statin. There are only two choices at this level: atorvastatin (Lipitor) 40 to 80 mg or rosuvastatin (Crestor) 20 to 40 mg.

130. A) Macular degeneration
Age-related macular degeneration affects the area of central vision. It creates a blurring or loss of central vision. It is associated with advanced age. "Central vision inflammation" is a generic term. Blepharitis is a chronic condition caused by inflammation of the eyelids. It creates itching, irritation, and eye redness, but does not create blurred vision. Conjunctival hemorrhage is caused by blood trapped underneath the conjunctiva and sclera secondary to broken arterioles and is identified by a red patch in the white of the eye.

131. B) "Are you experiencing pain anywhere?"
The outbreak that occurs with shingles lasts about 3 to 5 weeks. A patient prescribed gabapentin 3 months after an outbreak of shingles is being treated for postherpetic neuralgia. Therefore, the NP will inquire about pain, which is generally confined to the area in which dermatomal involvement occurred. Symptoms associated with postherpetic neuralgia include a sensation of burning, throbbing, sharp pain, and aching at the site of the outbreak. Gabapentin is not prescribed to prevent new lesions, rash, or problems with falling asleep.

132. D) Haloperidol (Haldol)
The conventional, or first-generation, antipsychotic drugs (e.g., haloperidol [Haldol]) are potent antagonists of D2, D3, and D4 receptors. This makes them effective in treating target symptoms, but they also produce many extrapyramidal side effects because of the blocking of the D2 receptors. Newer, atypical, or second-generation antipsychotic drugs and third-generation drugs (e.g., aripiprazole [Abilify]) are relatively weak blockers of D2, which may account for the lower incidence of extrapyramidal side effects. These drugs are thought to stabilize dopamine output that results in control of symptoms without some of the side effects of other antipsychotic medications. Sertraline (Zoloft) and citalopram (Celexa) are antidepressants.

133. B) 24-hour creatinine level
The patient is exhibiting symptoms of acute renal failure. The patient may also complain of lack of appetite, nausea, and lethargy. His serum creatinine level will be elevated. Hemoglobin testing provides information on the level of protein available to carry oxygen in the blood. A urine C&S and abdominal ultrasound are not needed at this time. The patient should first be examined for acute renal failure with 24-hour creatinine level and then MRI or intravenous pyelogram.

134. A) Corneal ulceration
Due to the paralysis caused by cranial nerve (CN) VII damage, the eyelid on the affected side may not close voluntarily. This leads to dryness, which, in turn, can result in ulceration. Glaucoma is caused by damage to the optic nerve, and swallowing is related to CNs IX and X. Although the affected side of the face is paralyzed in Bell's palsy, skin sensation remains intact.

135. C) Pulmonary emboli
Pulmonary emboli would be suspected in a patient with a sudden-onset cough with light pink–tinged sputum, tachycardia, tachypnea, and slight hypoxia. The likely cause is a heart blockage, which can be confirmed with a CT scan revealing right ventricle (RV) enlargement. Pulmonary edema presents with acute-onset dyspnea, crackles, tachycardia, pedal edema, and hypoxia. The diagnosis is confirmed with a chest x-ray revealing pleural effusions and cardiomegaly. When interstitial pressure is higher than pleural pressure, it causes fluid to move across the visceral pleura. Atypical pneumonia presents with gradual onset of a low-grade fever, headache, sore throat, cough, and wheezing. A chest x-ray will show interstitial to patchy infiltrates. Pertussis (B. pertussis) is a gram-negative communicable disease that presents with paroxysmal cough, inspiratory whooping, and posttussive vomiting. Initial symptoms include rhinorrhea and low-grade fever. The cough is present for at least 14 days and can last up to 21 days if not treated with antibiotics.

136. A, B, C, E) "Have you traveled recently?"; "Do you have any inherited blood disorders?"; "Have you broken any bones recently or had surgery?"; "Do you walk or exercise regularly?"
The patient may have a deep vein thrombosis (DVT). Asking the patient if they have traveled recently will identify any prolonged inactivity. Patients with a history of factor C deficiency, Leiden factor, or other inherited coagulation disorders are more prone to DVT. Surgery, trauma, and increased coagulation can also cause DVT. Asking about exercise helps determine the activity level of the patient and thus how much time is spent inactive. A recent weight gain is not significant in the diagnosis of DVT.

137. C) VIII
CN VIII is responsible for auditory function and is tested by using a "clicking" stimuli to test the auditory brainstem response. CN I is the olfactory system (mnemonic: "one nose"). CN II is the optic nerve (mnemonic: "two eyes").

CN V is the trigeminal nerve responsible for chewing and clenching teeth and is the largest CN.

138. D) Alzheimer's disease
Alzheimer's disease is the most common cause of dementia in the elderly, causing a decline in cognition and memory and alterations in personality. Lewy bodies are caused by an alpha-synuclein protein deposited on nerve cells in the brain and lead to cognitive decline, alterations in personality, and a Parkinson-type muscular tremor and rigidity. Delirium is an acute, but temporary and reversible, state of confusion. Vascular dementia is the result of ischemic damage to the brain due to plaques, blood clots, and bleeding.

139. A) Discontinue atorvastatin (Lipitor) and order a liver function profile.
The patient has symptoms of liver damage, including fatigue, anorexia, jaundice, and dark-colored urine. Statin-induced liver injury is a rare complication, occurring generally a few weeks to a few months after initiation of a statin. The statin should be discontinued, and a liver function profile is indicated. Elevated liver enzymes three times the upper limit of normal and an elevated bilirubin are laboratory abnormalities typically seen with statin-induced liver injury. Generally, no other treatment is needed other than statin cessation.

140. D) "You may have eaten food that was contaminated with the hepatitis A virus."
Hepatitis A virus typically is transmitted via the fecal–oral route, commonly by consuming food that was contaminated by infected food handlers. The virus is not transmitted by the IV route, blood transfusions, or unprotected sex. Hepatitis B can be transmitted by IV drug use, unprotected sex, or blood transfusion. Hepatitis C can be transmitted by unprotected sex or contaminated needles.

141. C) Active
Active immunity is acquired by vaccination administration or by infection. Passive immunity is when the antibodies are obtained from another host. Herd immunity occurs when large numbers of the population are resistant to a disease.

142. C, D) Ask for the patient's preferred gender pronouns and use gender-neutral language in communications and on patient forms; Maintain respect for the patient's process of disclosure.
The patient's gender preferences should be acknowledged and respected by the NP. Suggesting that the patient has a medical or psychologic disorder is not an appropriate acknowledgment of the patient's feelings or rights. Explaining a hormone imbalance or informing the patient that they are experiencing treatable gender dysphoria are not appropriate responses.

143. C) Mild dementia
The MMSE measures cognitive decline. A score of 18 to 23 is considered mild dementia, a score of <17 is considered moderate-to-advanced dementia, and a score of <12 is considered severe dementia. Parkinson disease is a progressive neurodegenerative disease caused by decreased dopamine receptors. Depression, resting tremor, and muscular rigidity are common. The disease is not measured by the MMSE.

144. C) Contact an agency that provides skilled respite care.
Contacting an agency that provides skilled respite care is the best intervention because respite care is reimbursed by Medicare and will provide the caregiver with some "break" time. NPs should be knowledgeable regarding resources for patients with these needs. Home health services are not the appropriate level of intervention, as the patient does not need skilled nursing services. Providing a list of qualified in-home caregivers would be helpful if the family has the financial ability to incur the steep costs of private caregivers, but this would not be the best action initially in helping with this problem. Providing a brochure for Meals on Wheels could be useful, but the service would not provide the caregiver with needed rest.

145. D) State board of nursing
APRN practice is typically defined by the state nurse practice act and governed by the state board of nursing, but other laws and regulations may affect practice, and other boards may play a role. For instance, in some states, nurse-midwives are regulated by a board of midwifery or public health. In other states, both the board of medicine and the board of nursing regulate nursing practice.

146. A) Explanation of the injury being inconsistent with the presentation
Incompatibility between the history and the injury is the most important criterion on which to base the decision to report suspected child abuse. Children who are developmentally or physically disabled are at a higher risk for abuse. The behavior of the child may also suggest child abuse but is a less reliable indicator in this case, since the child has a disability. The hygiene of the caregiver and the fact that the child has Down's syndrome (and may have a predisposition for bruising) are less reliable indicators of abuse.

147. A, B, E) The NP should inform the staff member of the patient's right to privacy; The NP should not provide the chart to the staff member; The NP should report the incident to the supervisor.
Under the Health Insurance Portability and Accountability Act (HIPAA), personal health information may not be used for purposes that are not related to healthcare. The staff member is not providing healthcare to the patient and should not have access to the chart. A supervisor should be informed of the incident and will report the infraction to the proper authorities. The obligation of the NP is to protect the patient and all patient information.

148. 1, C; 2, B; 3, A
A meta-analysis study has the highest level of evidence and is considered the gold standard for gathering research evidence for evidence-based practice. Experimental studies are the second level of evidence, and expert opinions and editorials are the lowest level of evidence.

149. B, D, E) Educate the patient about using barrier devices during sex; Draw a blood sample for a combination HIV antigen/antibody test; Schedule a follow-up appointment in 1 month to review test results and discuss options for PrEP.
Education on using barriers during sexual activity (e.g., condom/dental dams) is important. Daily oral PrEP, such as tenofovir emtricitabine, is recommended for sexually active persons who are at risk for HIV. PrEP is used in HIV-negative persons, so the NP must wait for the test results before prescribing. It is appropriate to schedule a 1-month follow-up to review the test results and discuss PrEP options (if the test is negative). It is not appropriate ethically or legally to contact the partner; however, it would be appropriate for the patient to encourage his partner to get tested.

150. D) The NP has an ethical duty to provide quality healthcare to all patients.
Currently, health caregivers are not legally required to report undocumented immigrants to federal, state, or local authorities. This patient does not have the signs and symptoms of active TB disease (cough, weight loss, night sweats) and has a negative chest x-ray. Therefore, he has latent TB infection and is not contagious. Only patients with active TB disease (having signs/symptoms) must be reported to the state public health department.

ABBREVIATIONS AND ACRONYMS

3D-TTE transthoracic 3D echocardiography

AA Alcoholics Anonymous

AAA abdominal aortic aneurysm

AADLs advanced activities of daily living

AAENP American Academy of Emergency Nurse Practitioners

AANP American Association of Nurse Practitioners

AANPCB American Academy of Nurse Practitioners Certification Board

AAP American Academy of Pediatrics

AATD alpha-1 anti-trypsin deficiency

ABCs airway, breathing, and circulation

ABI ankle-brachial index

ABPM ambulatory blood pressure monitoring

ABR auditory brainstem response

ABRS acute bacterial rhinosinusitis

AC air conduction

ACA Affordable Care Act

ACC American College of Cardiology

ACE angiotensin-converting enzyme

ACEI angiotensin-converting enzyme inhibitor

ACE-III Addenbrooke's Cognitive Examination III

ACL anterior cruciate ligament

ACOG American College of Obstetricians and Gynecologists

ACOS asthma–chronic obstructive pulmonary disease overlap syndrome

ACPA anticyclic citrullinated peptide/protein antibodies

ACS acute coronary syndrome

ACTH adrenocorticotropic hormone

AD Alzheimer's disease

ADA American Diabetes Association

ADD attention deficit disorder

ADHD attention deficit hyperactivity disorder

ADLs activities of daily living

AF atrial fibrillation

AFB acid-fast bacilli

AFI amniotic fluid index

AFP alpha-fetoprotein

AGACNP-BC adult-gerontology acute care nurse practitioner

AGC atypical glandular cell

AGNP-C adult-gerontology primary care nurse practitioner

AGS American Geriatrics Society

AHA American Heart Association

AIS adenocarcinoma in situ

AKI acute kidney injury

ALL acute lymphocytic leukemia

ALP alkaline phosphatase

ALS amyotrophic lateral sclerosis

ALT alanine aminotransferase

ALT Ratio alanine aminotransferase ratio

AMA American Medical Association

AMD age-related macular degeneration

AML acute myelogenous leukemia

ANA American Nurses Association

ANA antinuclear antibodies

ANC absolute neutrophil count

ANCC American Nurses Credentialing Center

ANPs adult nurse practitioners

Anti-HCV hepatitis C virus antibody

AOM acute otitis media

aPTT activated partial thromboplastin time

AR aortic regurgitation

ARB angiotensin receptor blocker

ARNI angiotensin receptor-neprilysin inhibitor

ARR absolute risk reduction

ART antiretroviral therapy

AS aortic stenosis

ASA acetylsalicylic acid

ASB asymptomatic bacteriuria

ASC-US atypical squamous cells of undetermined significance

ASCVD atherosclerotic cardiovascular disease

ASD autism spectrum disorder

AST aspartate aminotransferase

ATN acute tubular necrosis

ATS American Thoracic Society

AUA American Urological Association

AUC area under the curve

AUDIT Alcohol Use Disorders Identification Test

AV atrioventricular

AVM arteriovenous malformation

BB beta-blocker

BC bone conduction

BCC basal cell carcinoma

BCG Bacillus Calmette–Guérin

BDTC black dot tinea capitis

BLS basic life support

BMD bone mineral density

BMI body mass index

BNP B-type natriuretic peptide

BON board of nursing

BP blood pressure

BPH benign prostatic hyperplasia

BPPV benign paroxysmal positional vertigo

BSO bilateral salpingo-oophorectomy

BUN blood urea nitrogen

BUN:Cr blood urea nitrogen-to-creatinine

BV bacterial vaginosis

C&S culture and sensitivity

CA carcinoma

CAC coronary artery calcium

CAD coronary artery disease

CAM complementary and alternative medicine

CA-MRSA community-associated methicillin-resistant *Staphylococcus aureus*

CAP community-acquired pneumonia

CBC complete blood count

CBTs computer-based tests

CCB calcium channel blocker

CCNE Commission on Collegiate Nursing Education

CD Crohn's disease

CDAD *Clostridioides difficile*-associated diarrhea

CDC Centers for Disease Control and Prevention

CDSR Cochrane Database of Systematic Reviews

CEA carcinoembryonic antigen

CFU colony-forming units

CGRP calcitonin gene-related peptide

CHD coronary heart disease

CHF congestive heart failure

CHIP Children's Health Insurance Program

CHIPRA Children's Health Insurance Program Reauthorization Act of 2009

CI confidence interval

CIN cervical intraepithelial neoplasia

CINAHL Cumulative Index to Nursing and Allied Health Literature

CKD chronic kidney disease

CKD-EPI Chronic Kidney Disease Epidemiology Collaboration

CMS Centers for Medicare & Medicaid Services

CMV cytomegalovirus

CN cranial nerve

CNS central nervous system

CO cardiac output

COCs combined oral contraceptives

COPD chronic obstructive pulmonary disease

COX-1 cyclooxygenase-1

COX-2 cyclooxygenase-2

CPR cardiopulmonary resuscitation

CPT Current Procedural Terminology

CRAB **C**alcium levels, **R**enal insufficiency, **A**nemia, and **B**one lesions

CRH corticotropin-releasing hormone

CRP C-reactive protein

CSF cerebrospinal fluid

CT/NG *Chlamydia trachomatis/Neisseria gonorrhoeae*

cTnT cardiac troponins

CTS carpal tunnel syndrome

Cu-IUDs copper-bearing intrauterine devices

CV cardiovascular

CVA cerebrovascular accident

CVA costovertebral angle

CVD cardiovascular disease

CXR chest x-ray

DASH Dietary Approaches to Stop Hypertension

DBP diastolic blood pressure

DBT digital breast tomosynthesis

DCIS ductal carcinoma in situ

DEA Drug Enforcement Agency

DES diethylstilbestrol

DEXA dual-energy x-ray absorptiometry

DGI disseminated gonococcal infection

DHEA dehydroepiandrosterone

DHHS U.S. Department of Health and Human Services

DIC disseminated intravascular coagulation

DIP distal interphalangeal

DJD degenerative joint disease

DLB dementia with Lewy bodies

DM diabetes mellitus

DMARD disease-modifying antirheumatic drug

DMDs/DDSs dentists/dental surgeons

DMPA depot medroxyprogesterone acetate

DNP doctor of nursing practice

DOACs direct oral anticoagulants

DOB date of birth

DPP-4 Inhibitors dipeptidyl peptidase-4 inhibitors

DRE digital rectal exam

DT diphtheria–tetanus

DTaP diphtheria, tetanus, acellular pertussis

DTRs deep tendon reflexes

DVP deepest vertical pocket

DVT deep vein thrombosis

E&M Evaluation and Management Service

EBM evidence-based medicine

EBV Epstein–Barr virus

ED erectile dysfunction

EDD estimated date of delivery

EE ethinyl estradiol

EEG electroencephalogram

EES erythromycin estolate

EF ejection fraction

EFT electronic fund transfer

eGFR estimated glomerular filtration rate

EHRs electronic health records

EIB exercise-induced bronchoconstriction

ELISA enzyme-linked immunosorbent assay

ENP-C emergency nurse practitioner

ENT ear, nose, and throat

EOM extraocular movement

EOM extraorbital muscles

EPA Environmental Protection Agency

EPCS electronic prescribing of controlled substances

EPO erythropoietin

EPS extrapyramidal symptoms

EPT expedited partner therapy

ER estrogen receptor

ERT estrogen–progestin replacement therapy

ESR erythrocyte sedimentation rate

ESWL extracorporeal shock wave lithotripsy

EVALI e-cigarette, or vaping, product use–associated lung injury

FBG fasting blood glucose

FBS fasting blood sugar

FDA U.S. Food and Drug Administration

FEV1 forced expiratory volume in 1 second

FH familial hypercholesterolemia

FHTs fetal heart tones

FIT fecal immunochemical test

FNP family nurse practitioner

FNP-BC family nurse practitioner-board certified

FOBT fecal occult blood test

FPG fasting plasma glucose

FSH follicle-stimulating hormone

FTA-ABS fluorescent treponemal antibody absorption

FVC forced vital capacity

FXa factor Xa

G6PD glucose-6-phosphate dehydrogenase

GAD generalized anxiety disorder

GAS Group A *Streptococcus*

GBS Group B *Streptococcus*

GDM gestational diabetes mellitus

GDMT guideline-directed medical therapy

GDS Geriatric Depression Scale

GERD gastroesophageal reflux disease

gFOBT guaiac-based fecal occult blood test

GFR glomerular filtration rate

GGT gamma glutamyl transferase

GH growth hormone

GI gastrointestinal

GINA Global Initiative for Asthma

GNPs gerontological nurse practitioners

GOLD Global Initiative for Chronic Obstructive Lung Disease

H2RAs H2 antagonists

HAV hepatitis A virus

HBIG hepatitis B immunoglobulin

HBPM home blood pressure monitoring

HBsAg hepatitis B surface antigen

HBV hepatitis B virus

HCG human chorionic gonadotropin

HCTZ hydrochlorothiazide

HD-IIV4 high-dose inactivated influenza vaccine

HDL high-density lipoprotein

HDL-C high-density lipoprotein cholesterol

HDV RNA hepatitis D virus RNA

HER2 human epidermal growth factor receptor

HFpEF heart failure with preserved ejection fraction

HFrEF heart failure with reduced ejection fraction

HIPAA Health Insurance Portability and Accountability Act

HITECH Act Health Information Technology for Economic and Clinical Health Act

HMOs health maintenance organizations

HPA hypothalamic–pituitary–adrenal

HPI history of present illness

HPLC high-performance liquid chromatography

HPV human papillomavirus

HRT hormone replacement therapy

HSILs high-grade squamous intraepithelial lesions

HTN hypertension

I&D incision and drainage

IADLs instrumental activities of daily living

IBD inflammatory bowel disease

IBS irritable bowel syndrome

ICD-11 *International Classification of Diseases,* 11th edition

ICP increased intracranial pressure

ICP intracranial pressure

ICS intercostal space

IDA iron-deficiency anemia

IDSA Infectious Diseases Society of America

IEF isoelectric focusing

IFA indirect immunofluorescence assay

IFG impaired fasting blood sugar/ glucose

IGRAs interferon-gamma release assays

IGT impaired glucose tolerance

IHPS infantile hyperpyloric stenosis

IIV influenza

IM intramuscular

INR international normalized ratio

IOP intraocular pressure

IPV inactivated poliovirus vaccine

IRBs institutional review boards

ITP idiopathic thrombocytopenic purpura

IUGR intrauterine growth retardation

IV intravenous

IVF in vitro fertilization

JNC Joint National Committee

JVD jugular vein distention

KDIGO Kidney Disease: Improving Global Outcomes

KOH potassium hydroxide

LABAs long-acting beta-agonists

LAIV live attenuated influenza vaccine

LAMAs long-acting muscarinic antagonists

LCL lateral collateral ligament

LDCT low-dose computed tomography

LDH lactate dehydrogenase

LDL low-density lipoprotein

LEEP loop electrosurgical excision procedure

LFTs liver function tests

LH luteinizing hormone

LLQ left lower quadrant

LNG levonorgestrel

LOC level of consciousness

LP lumbar puncture

LSILs low-grade squamous intraepithelial lesions

LTBI latent tuberculosis infection

LUQ left upper quadrant

LV left ventricular

LVEF left ventricular ejection fraction

LVH left ventricular hypertrophy

MA Medicare Advantage

MAO-B monoamine oxidase-B

MAOI monoamine oxidase inhibitor

MCH mean corpuscular hemoglobin

MCHC mean corpuscular hemoglobin concentration

MCI mild cognitive impairment

MCL medial collateral ligament

MCP metacarpophalangeal

MCV mean corpuscular volume

MDCT multidetector row computed tomography

MDD major depressive disorder

MDRD modification of diet in renal disease

MEE middle ear effusion

MgSO$_4$ magnesium sulfate

MI myocardial infarction

MIC minimum inhibitory concentration

MMR measles, mumps, rubella

MMRV measles, mumps, rubella, varicella

MMSE Mini-Mental State Exam

MODY maturity onset diabetes of the young

MR mitral regurgitation

MRA mineralocorticoid receptor antagonist

MRSA methicillin-resistant *Staphylococcus aureus*

MS mitral stenosis

MS multiple sclerosis

MSM men who have sex with men

MTP metatarsophalangeal

MTSS medial tibial stress syndrome

NAAT nucleic acid amplification test

NAEPP National Asthma Education and Prevention Program

NAFL nonalcoholic fatty liver

NAFLD nonalcoholic fatty liver disease

NASH nonalcoholic steatohepatitis

NAT nonaccidental trauma

NDs naturopaths

NLM National Library of Medicine

NNT number needed to treat

NP nurse practitioner

NPI National Provider Identifier

NPPES National Plan and Provider Enumeration System

NPV negative predictive value

NSAID nonsteroidal anti-inflammatory drug

NSTEMI non–ST-elevation myocardial infarction

NT-proBNP N-terminal pro-BNP

NYHA New York Heart Association

OA osteoarthritis

OCD obsessive-compulsive disorder

OFC occipitofrontal circumference

OGTT oral glucose tolerance test

OHL oral hairy leukoplakia

OME otitis media with effusion

OR operating room

OSHA Occupational Safety and Health Administration

OT occupational therapy

OTC over the counter

PA posterioanterior

PAD peripheral arterial disease

PAs physician assistants

PCC prothrombin complex concentrate

PCI percutaneous coronary intervention

PCL posterior cruciate ligament

PCMH patient-centered medical home

PCOS polycystic ovary syndrome

PCP *Pneumocystis carinii* pneumonia

PCPs primary care providers

PCR polymerase chain reaction

PCSK9 proprotein convertase subtilisin/kexin type 9

PCV13 pneumococcal conjugate vaccine

PD Parkinson's disease

PD pharmacodynamic

PDA patent ductus arteriosus

PDB Paget's disease of the breast

PDE5 phosphodiesterase 5

PDL pulsed-dye laser

PE pulmonary embolism

PEF peak expiratory flow

PEP postexposure prophylaxis

PERCP postendoscopic retrograde cholangiopancreatography

PHI protected health information

PHN postherpetic neuralgia

PHQ-9 Patient Health Questionnaire-9

PID pelvic inflammatory disease

PIP proximal interphalangeal

PK pharmacokinetic

PKU phenylketonuria

PLLR Pregnancy and Lactation Labeling Rule

PMDD premenstrual dysphoric disorder

PMHNP-BC psychiatric–mental health nurse practitioner

PMI point of maximal impulse

PMR polymyalgia rheumatica

POP progestin-only pill

PPD purified protein derivative

PPI proton pump inhibitor

PPOs preferred provider organizations

PPSV23 pneumococcal polysaccharide vaccine

PPV positive predictive value

PR progesterone receptor

PrEP preexposure prophylaxis

PSA prostate-specific antigen

PSVT paroxysmal supraventricular tachycardia

PT physical therapy

PT prothrombin time

PTH parathyroid hormone

PTSD posttraumatic stress disorder

PTT partial thromboplastin time

PUD peptic ulcer disease

PVD peripheral vascular disease

PVR peripheral vascular resistance

RA rheumatoid arthritis

RAAS renin-angiotensin-aldosterone system

RADT rapid antigen detection testing

RAIU radioactive iodine uptake

RAS renin-angiotensin system

RBC red blood cell

RCA root cause analysis

RCT randomized controlled trial

RDW red cell distribution width

REMS Risk Evaluation and Mitigation Strategy

RF rheumatoid factor

RISE Revised Index of Social Engagement

RIV4 recombinant influenza vaccine

RLQ right lower quadrant

RMSF Rocky Mountain spotted fever

ROM range of motion

ROS review of systems

RPR rapid plasma reagent

RRR relative risk reduction

RSV respiratory syncytial virus

RV right ventricular

RV Rotarix

RV5 RotaTeq

RVR rapid ventricular response

SABAs short-acting beta2-agonists

SAH subarachnoid hemorrhage

SAMAs short-acting anticholinergics

SARS-CoV-2 severe acute respiratory syndrome coronavirus 2

SBON state board of nursing

SBP systolic blood pressure

SD standard deviation

SDH subdural hematoma

SDNA stool DNA

SE sentinel event

SERM selective estrogen receptor modulator

SGLT2 sodium-glucose cotransporter 2

SGLT2 inhibitors sodium-glucose cotransporter-2 inhibitors

SGPT serum glutamic pyruvic transaminase

SIDS sudden infant death syndrome

SJS Stevens–Johnson syndrome

SLE systemic lupus erythematosus

SMBP self-measured blood pressure

SNFs skilled nursing facilities

SNRIs serotonin-norepinephrine reuptake inhibitor

SPF sun protection factor

SSRI selective serotonin reuptake inhibitor

STD sexually transmitted disease

STEC shiga toxin–producing *Escherichia coli*

STEMI ST-elevation myocardial infarction

STI sexually transmitted infection

TB tuberculosis

TBG thyroid-binding globulin

TBI traumatic brain injury

TBSA total body surface area

TCA trichloroacetic acid

TCOs test content outlines

TEN toxic epidermal necrolysis

TIA transient ischemic attack

TIBC total iron-binding capacity

TIG tetanus immunoglobulin

TJC The Joint Commission

TM tympanic membrane

TNF tumor necrosis factor

TNM tumor-node-metastasis

TPAs third-party administrators

TP-EIA *Treponema pallidum* enzyme immunoassay

TPO thyroid peroxidase antibody

TPPA *Treponema pallidum* particle agglutination assay

TRAb thyrotropin receptor antibodies

TSH thyroid-stimulating hormone

TSIs thyroid-stimulating immunoglobulins

TSS toxic shock syndrome

TST tuberculin skin test

TTR time in therapeutic range

TZ transformation zone

UA urinalysis

UC ulcerative colitis

ULT urate-lowering therapy

URI upper respiratory infection

USP U.S. Pharmacopeia

USPSTF U.S. Preventive Services Task Force

UTI urinary tract infection

VAR varicella

VDRL Venereal Disease Research Laboratory

VEGF vascular endothelial growth factor

VICP Vaccine Injury Compensation Program

VKA vitamin K antagonist

VTE venous thromboembolism

VZV varicella-zoster virus

WBC white blood cell

WHI Women's Health Initiative

WHO World Health Organization

WIC Women, Infants, and Children

WPW Wolff–Parkinson–White

XOI xanthine oxidase inhibitors

RESOURCES

PRACTICE GUIDELINES AND RECOMMENDATIONS

AIDSinfo
Recommendations for the use of antiretroviral drugs in pregnant women with HIV infection and interventions to reduce perinatal HIV transmission in the United States. (2020). https://aidsinfo.nih.gov/contentfiles/lvguidelines/PerinatalGL.pdf

American Academy of Dermatology
Guidelines of care for the management of acne vulgaris. (2016). https://www.jaad.org/article/S0190-9622(15)02614-6/fulltext

American Academy of Pediatrics
SIDS and other sleep-related infant deaths: Updated 2016 recommendations for a safe infant sleeping environment. (2016). https://pediatrics.aappublications.org/content/138/5/e20162938

American Cancer Society
Recommendations for the early detection of breast cancer. (2020). https://www.cancer.org/cancer/breast-cancer/screening-tests-and-early-detection/american-cancer-society-recommendations-for-the-early-detection-of-breast-cancer.html

American College of Cardiology/American Heart Association
ACC/AHA/AAPA/ABC/ACPM/AGS/APhA/ASH/ASPC/NMA/PCN. (2017). Guideline for the prevention, detection, evaluation, and management of high blood pressure in adults: A report of the American College of Cardiology/American Heart Association Task Force on Clinical Practice Guidelines. https://www.acc.org/latest-in-cardiology/ten-points-to-remember/2017/11/09/11/41/2017-guideline-for-high-blood-pressure-in-adults

ACC/AHA/AAPA/ABC/ACPM/AGS/APhA/ASH/ASPC/NMA/PCNA. (2017). Guideline for the prevention, detection, evaluation, and management of high blood pressure in adults: A report of the American College of Cardiology/American Heart Association Task Force on clinical practice guidelines. *Hypertension, 71*, e13–e115. https://doi.org/10.1161/HYP.0000000000000065

AHA/ACC. (2017). Focused Update of the 2014 AHA/ACC guideline for the management of patients with valvular heart disease: A report of the American College of Cardiology/American Heart Association Task Force on Clinical Practice Guidelines. (2017). https://www.acc.org/latest-in-cardiology/ten-points-to-remember/2017/03/14/18/26/2017-aha-acc-focused-update-of-valvular-heart-disease

AHA/ACC/AACVPR/AAPA/ABC/ACPM/ADA/AGS/APhA/ASPC/NLA/PCNA. (2018). Guideline on the management of blood cholesterol: A report of the American College of Cardiology/American Heart Association Task Force on Clinical Practice Guidelines. (2018). https://www.acc.org/latest-in-cardiology/ten-points-to-remember/2018/11/09/14/28/2018-guideline-on-management-of-blood-cholesterol

American College of Chest Physicians
Antithrombotic therapy for VTE disease: CHEST guideline and expert panel report (9th ed.). (2016). https://www.acc.org/latest-in-cardiology/ten-points-to-remember/2016/03/02/15/45/antithrombotic-therapy-for-vte-disease

American College of Obstetricians and Gynecologists
Cervical cancer screening (Update). (2018). https://www.acog.org/clinical/clinical-guidance/practice-advisory/articles/2018/08/cervical-cancer-screening-update

Menstruation in girls and adolescents: Using the menstrual cycle as a vital sign (Committee Opinion No. 651). (2015; reaffirmed 2017). https://www.acog.org/clinical/clinical-guidance/committee-opinion/articles/2015/12/menstruation-in-girls-and-adolescents-using-the-menstrual-cycle-as-a-vital-sign#:~:text=Clinicians%20should%20convey%20that%20females,is%20considered%20normal%20menstrual%20flow

American College of Rheumatology
American College of Rheumatology/Arthritis Foundation. (2019). Guideline for the management of osteoarthritis of the hand, hip, and knee. (2019). https://www.rheumatology.org/Practice-Quality/Clinical-Support/Clinical-Practice-Guidelines/Osteoarthritis

American College of Rheumatology. (2020). Guideline for the management of gout. (2020). https://www.rheumatology.org/Portals/0/Files/Gout-Guideline-Final-2020.pdf

American Diabetes Association
Standards of medical care in diabetes—2021. https://diabetesjournals.org/care/issue/44/Supplement_1

American Geriatrics Society
Beers Criteria for inappropriate medication use in older patients: An update from the AGS. (2020). https://www.aafp.org/afp/2020/0101/p56.html

Beers Criteria® Update Expert Panel. (2023). American Geriatrics Society 2019 updated AGS Beers Criteria® for potentially inappropriate medication use in older adults. *Journal of the American Geriatrics Society, 67*(4), 674–694. https://doi.org/10.1111/jgs.15767

American Thoracic Society/Infectious Diseases Society of America
Diagnosis and treatment of adults with community-acquired pneumonia. An Official Clinical Practice Guideline of the

American Thoracic Society and Infectious Diseases Society of America. (2019). https://www.idsociety.org /practice-guideline/community-acquired-pneumonia -cap-in-adults/

American Thyroid Association

American Thyroid Association management guidelines for adult patients with thyroid nodules and differentiated thyroid cancer. (2016). https://www.liebertpub.com /doi/full/10.1089/thy.2016.0457

Centers for Disease Control and Prevention

Sexually transmitted diseases treatment guidelines: Summary. (2015). https://www.cdc.gov/std/tg2015/default.htm

Breastfeeding: Vitamin D. (2019). https://www.cdc.gov /breastfeeding/recommendations/vitamin_d.htm

Cervical cancer screening guidelines for average-risk women. (2019). https://www.cdc.gov/cancer/cervical/pdf /guidelines.pdf

Guidelines for the treatment of latent tuberculosis infection: Recommendations from the National Tuberculosis Controllers Association and CDC, 2020. (2020). https:// www.cdc.gov/mmwr/volumes/69/rr/rr6901a1.htm?s_ cid=rr6901a1_w

Immunization schedules. (2020). https://www.cdc.gov /vaccines/schedules/

Influenza (flu): For clinicians—Antiviral medication. (2020). https://www.cdc.gov/flu/professionals/antivirals /summary-clinicians.htm

Pneumococcal vaccine recommendations. (2019). https:// www.cdc.gov/vaccines/vpd/pneumo/hcp /recommendations.html

Recommendations for HIV screening of gay, bisexual, and other men who have sex with men—United States, 2017. (2017). https://www.cdc.gov/mmwr/volumes/66/wr /mm6631a3.htm

Recommendations for providing quality sexually transmitted disease clinical service, 2020. (2020). https://www.cdc .gov/mmwr/volumes/68/rr/rr6805a1.htm

Recommendations of the Advisory Committee on Immunization Practices for use of herpes zoster vaccines. (2018). https:// www.cdc.gov/mmwr/volumes/67/wr/mm6703a5.htm

Rocky Mountain spotted fever (RMSF) research on doxycycline and tooth staining. (2018). https://www.cdc.gov /rmsf/doxycycline/index.html

Shingles vaccination. (2018). https://www.cdc.gov/vaccines /vpd/shingles/public/shingrix/index.html

STD treatment guidelines: Human papillomavirus (HPV) infection. (2015). https://www.cdc.gov/std/tg2015/hpv.htm

Summary chart of U.S. medical eligibility criteria for contraceptive use. (2019). https://www.cdc.gov /reproductivehealth/contraception/pdf/summary -chart-us-medical-eligibility-criteria_508tagged.pdf

Update to CDC's Treatment Guideline for Gonococcal Infection, 2020. (2020). https://www.cdc.gov/std /tg2015/gonorrhea.htm

U.S. selected practice recommendations for contraceptive use. (2016). https://www.cdc.gov/mmwr/volumes/65/rr /rr6504a1.htm?s_cid=rr6504a1_w

Varicella vaccine information. (2019). https://www.cdc.gov /vaccines/vpd/varicella/hcp/recommendations.html

Viral hepatitis: Testing recommendations. (2020). https:// www.cdc.gov/hepatitis/hcv/guidelinesc.htm

Eighth Joint National Committee (JNC 8)

Evidence-based guideline for the management of high blood pressure in adults: Report from the Panel Members Appointed to the Eighth Joint National Committee (JNC 8). (2014). https://doi.org/10.1001/jama.2013.284427

Global Initiative for Asthma

Global strategy for asthma management and prevention. (2020). https://ginasthma.org/wp-content/uploads /2020/04/GINA-2020-full-report_-final-_wms.pdf

Global Initiative for Chronic Obstructive Lung Disease

Global strategy for the prevention, diagnosis, and management of chronic obstructive lung disease. (2020). https:// goldcopd.org/wp-content/uploads/2019/12/GOLD -2020-FINAL-ver1.2-03Dec19_WMV.pdf

GOLD 2023 Global strategy for the prevention, diagnosis, and management of COPD (2023 report). https://goldcopd.org /2023-gold-report-2

Infectious Diseases Society of America

Clinical practice guideline for the management of asymptomatic bacteriuria: 2019 update by the Infectious Diseases Society of America. (2019). https://www.idsociety .org/practice-guideline/asymptomatic-bacteriuria/

Diagnosis and treatment of adults with community-acquired pneumonia. An Official Clinical Practice Guideline of the American Thoracic Society and Infectious Diseases Society of America. (2019). https://www.idsociety.org /practice-guideline/community-acquired-pneumonia -cap-in-adults/

International clinical practice guidelines for the treatment of acute uncomplicated cystitis and pyelonephritis in women: A 2010 update by the Infectious Diseases Society of America and the European Society for Microbiology and Infectious Diseases. (2010). https://www.auanet .org/guidelines/archived-documents/urinary-tract -infection-(uti)-guideline

National Cancer Institute

Cervical cancer screening (PDQ®)–Health professional version. (2020). https://www.cancer.gov/types/cervical /hp/cervical-screening-pdq#_122_toc

National Institutes of Health/National Heart Lung and Blood Institute

Expert panel report 3: Guidelines for the diagnosis and management of asthma. (2007). https://www.nhlbi.nih.gov /health-topics/guidelines-for-diagnosis-management -of-asthma

U.S. Preventive Services Task Force

Final recommendation statement. Abdominal aortic aneurysm: Screening. (2019). https://www .uspreventiveservicestaskforce.org/uspstf /recommendation/abdominal-aortic-aneurysm -screening

Final recommendation statement. Abnormal blood glucose and type 2 diabetes mellitus: Screening. (2015). https:// www.uspreventiveservicestaskforce.org/uspstf /recommendation/screening-for-abnormal-blood -glucose-and-type-2-diabetes

Final recommendation statement. Aspirin use to prevent cardiovascular disease and colorectal cancer: Preventive medication. (2016). https://www .uspreventiveservicestaskforce.org/uspstf

/recommendation/aspirin-to-prevent-cardiovascular
-disease-and-cancer

Final recommendation statement. Breast cancer: Screening.
(2016). http://www.uspreventiveservicestaskforce.org
/Page/Document/UpdateSummaryFinal/breast-cancer
-screening1

Final recommendation statement. Cervical cancer: Screening.
(2018). https://www.uspreventiveservicestaskforce.org
/uspstf/recommendation/cervical-cancer-screening

Final recommendation statement. Colorectal cancer: Screening. (2021). https://www.uspreventiveservicestaskforce.
org/uspstf/recommendation/colorectal-cancer-screening

Final recommendation statement. Depression in adults. (2016).
https://www.uspreventiveservicestaskforce.org/uspstf
/recommendation/depression-in-adults-screening

Final recommendation statement. Depression in children
and adolescents: Screening. (2016). https://www
.uspreventiveservicestaskforce.org/uspstf/document
/RecommendationStatementFinal/depression-in
-children-and-adolescents-screening

Final recommendation statement. Hepatitis C virus infection
in adolescents and adults: Screening. (2020). https://
www.uspreventiveservicestaskforce.org/uspstf
/recommendation/hepatitis-c-screening

Final recommendation statement. Human immunodeficiency virus (HIV) infection: Screening. (2019). https://
www.uspreventiveservicestaskforce.org/uspst
f/document/RecommendationStatementFinal/human
-immunodeficiency-virus-hiv-infection-screening

Final recommendation statement. Hypertension in adults:
Screening. (2021). https://www.uspreventive services-
taskforce.org/uspstf/recommendation/high-blood
-pressure-in-adults-screening

Final recommendation statement. Latent tuberculosis
infection: Screening. (2016). https://www
.uspreventiveservicestaskforce.org/uspstf/document
/RecommendationStatementFinal/latent-tuberculosis
-infection-screening

Final recommendation statement. Lung cancer: Screening.
(2021). https://www.uspreventiveservicestaskforce.org
/uspstf/recommendation/lung-cancer-screening

Final recommendation statement. Obesity in children
and adolescents: Screening. (2017). https://www
.uspreventiveservicestaskforce.org/uspstf/document
/RecommendationStatementFinal/obesity-in-children
-and-adolescents-screening

Final recommendation statement. Osteoporosis to prevent
fractures: Screening. (2018). https://www
.uspreventiveservicestaskforce.org/uspstf/document
/RecommendationStatementFinal/osteoporosis-screening

Final recommendation statement. Ovarian cancer: Screening.
(2018). https://www.uspreventiveservicestaskforce.org
/uspstf/document/RecommendationStatementFinal
/ovarian-cancer-screening

Final recommendation statement. Pancreatic cancer: Screening.
(2019). https://www.uspreventiveservicestasfromkforce.
org/uspstf/document/RecommendationStatementFinal/
pancreatic-cancer-screening

Final recommendation statement. Prostate cancer: Screening.
(2018). https://www.uspreventiveservicestaskforce.org
/uspstf/recommendation/prostate-cancer-screening

Final recommendation statement. Sexually transmitted
infections: Behavioral counseling. (2020). https://www
.uspreventiveservicestaskforce.org/uspstf/document
/RecommendationStatementFinal/sexually-transmitted
-infections-behavioral-counseling

Final recommendation statement. Skin cancer: Screening.
(2016). https://www.uspreventiveservicestaskforce.org
/uspstf/recommendation/skin-cancer-screening

Final recommendation statement. Statin use for the primary
prevention of cardiovascular disease in adults:
Preventive medication. (2016). https://www
.uspreventiveservicestaskforce.org/uspstf/recommendation
/statin-use-in-adults-preventive-medication

Final recommendation statement. Syphilis infection in
pregnant women: Screening. (2018). https://www
.uspreventiveservicestaskforce.org/uspstf/document
/RecommendationStatementFinal/syphilis-infection-in
-pregnancy-screening

ARTICLES AND WEBSITES
Cancer

American Cancer Society. (2020). *Can ovarian cancer be found
early?* https://www.cancer.org/cancer/ovarian-cancer
/detection-diagnosis-staging/detection.html

American Cancer Society. (2020). *Cancer facts & figures 2020.*
https://www.cancer.org/content/dam/cancer-org
/research/cancer-facts-and-statistics/annual-cancer-facts
-and-figures/2020/cancer-facts-and-figures-2020.pdf

American Cancer Society. (2020). *Key statistics for lung cancer.*
https://www.cancer.org/cancer/non-small-cell-lung
-cancer/about/key-statistics.html

American Cancer Society. (2020). *Survival rates for cervical
cancer.* https://www.cancer.org/cancer/cervical-cancer
/detection-diagnosis-staging/survival.html

American Cancer Society. (n.d.). *Skin cancer.* https://www
.cancer.org/cancer/skin-cancer.html

Carlson, K. J. (2020). Patient education: Ovarian cancer screening (beyond the basics). In L. Kunins (Ed.), *UpToDate.*
https://www.uptodate.com/contents/ovarian-cancer
-screening-beyond-the-basics/print

Centers for Disease Control and Prevention. (2020). *Lung cancer
statistics.* https://www.cdc.gov/cancer/lung/statistics
/index.htm

Isaacs, C., & Peshkin, B. N. (2020). Cancer risks and management of BRCA1/2 carriers without cancer. In S. R. Vora
(Ed.), *UpToDate.* https://www.uptodate.com/contents
/cancer-risks-and-management-of-brca1-2-carriers
-without-cancer#H17

Joe, B. N. (2020). Clinical features, diagnosis, and staging of
newly diagnosed breast cancer. In S. R. Vora (Ed.),
UpToDate. https://www.uptodate.com/contents
/clinical-features-diagnosis-and-staging-of-newly
-diagnosed-breast-cancer#H15

Laubach, J. P. (2020). Multiple myeloma: Clinical features,
laboratory manifestations, and diagnosis. In R. F. Connor
(Ed.), *UpToDate.* https://www.uptodate.com/contents
/multiple-myeloma-clinical-features-laboratory
-manifestations-and-diagnosis#H38

National Cancer Institute. (2020). *Cancer stat facts.* https://seer
.cancer.gov/statfacts/

National Cancer Institute. (n.d.). *Cancer treatment*. https://www.cancer.gov/about-cancer/treatment

Peshkin, B. N., & Isaacs, C. (2020). Genetic testing and management of individuals at risk of hereditary breast and ovarian cancer syndromes. In S. R. Vora (Ed.), *UpToDate*. https://www.uptodate.com/contents/genetic-testing-and-management-of-individuals-at-risk-of-hereditary-breast-and-ovarian-cancer-syndromes#H15

Skin Cancer Foundation. (2020). *Skin cancer facts & statistics*. http://www.skincancer.org/skin-cancer-information/skin-cancer-facts

Taghian, A., & Merajver, S. D. (2020). Inflammatory breast cancer: Clinical features and treatment. In S. R. Vora (Ed.), *UpToDate*. https://www.uptodate.com/contents/inflammatory-breast-cancer-clinical-features-and-treatment#H2147235137

Cardiovascular System

Almarshad, F., Alaklabi, A., Bakhsh, E., Pathan, A., & Almegren, M. (2018). *Use of direct oral anticoagulants in daily practice*. https://www.ncbi.nlm.nih.gov/pmc/articles/PMC6334188/

Berul, C. I. (2020). Acquired long QT syndrome. In B. C. Downey (Ed.), *UpToDate*. https://www.uptodate.com/contents/acquired-long-qt-syndrome-definitions-causes-and-pathophysiology

Block, M. J., & Baile, J. (2020). Major side effects and safety of calcium channel blockers. In J. P. Forman (Ed.), *UpToDate*. https://www.uptodate.com/contents/major-side-effects-and-safety-of-calcium-channel-blockers#H15

Carnicelli, A. (2015). *Anticoagulation for valvular heart disease*. https://www.acc.org/latest-in-cardiology/articles/2015/05/18/09/58/anticoagulation-for-valvular-heart-disease

Chobanian, A. V., Bakris, G. L., Black, H. R., Cushman, W. C., Green, L. A., Izzo, J. L., Jr., Jones, D. W., Materson, B. J., Oparil, S., Wright, J. T., Jr., Roccella, E. J., & The National High Blood Pressure Education Program Coordinating Committee. (2003). *Seventh report of the joint national committee on prevention, detection, evaluation, and treatment of high blood pressure*. https://www.ahajournals.org/doi/pdf/10.1161/01.HYP.0000107251.49515.c2

Colucci, W. S. (2020). Overview of the management of heart failure with reduced ejection fraction in adults. In S. B. Yeon (Ed.), *UpToDate*. https://www.uptodate.com/contents/overview-of-the-management-of-heart-failure-with-reduced-ejection-fraction-in-adults

Colucci, W. S. (2020). Treatment of acute decompensated heart failure: Components of therapy. In S. B. Yeon (Ed.), *UpToDate*. https://www.uptodate.com/contents/treatment-of-acute-decompensated-heart-failure-components-of-therapy

Dalman, R. L., & Mell, M. (2020). Overview of abdominal aortic aneurysm. In K. A. Collins (Ed.), *UpToDate*. https://www.uptodate.com/contents/overview-of-abdominal-aortic-aneurysm#H91213842

Desai, N. R., & Cornutt, D. (2019). *Reversal agents for direct oral anticoagulants: Considerations for hospital physicians and intensivists*. https://pubmed.ncbi.nlm.nih.gov/31317796/

Farrer, S. (2018). *Beyond statins: Emerging evidence for HDL-increasing therapies and diet in treating cardiovascular disease*. https://www.ncbi.nlm.nih.gov/pmc/articles/PMC6077683/

Gupta, M., Singh, N., & Verma, S. (2006). *South Asians and cardiovascular risk: What clinicians should know*. https://www.ahajournals.org/doi/full/10.1161/circulationaha.105.583815

Hull, R. D., & Garcia, D. A. (2020). Management of warfarin-associated bleeding or supratherapeutic INR. In J. S. Tirnauer (Ed.), *UpToDate*. https://www.uptodate.com/contents/management-of-warfarin-associated-bleeding-or-supratherapeutic-inr

Hull, R. D., Garcia, D. A., & Vazquez, S. R. (2019). Biology of warfarin and modulators of INR control. In J. S. Tirnauer (Ed.), *UpToDate*. https://www.uptodate.com/contents/biology-of-warfarin-and-modulators-of-inr-control#H13

Hull, R. D., Garcia, D. A., & Vazquez, S. R. (2020). Warfarin and other VKAs: Dosing and adverse effects. In J. S. Tirnauer (Ed.), *UpToDate*. https://www.uptodate.com/contents/warfarin-and-other-vkas-dosing-and-adverse-effects#H46

Lefevre, M. (2018). *ACC/AHA hypertension guideline: What is new? What do we do?* https://www.aafp.org/afp/2018/0315/p372.html#afp20180315p372-t1

Mahajan, R. (2014). *Joint National Committee 8 report: How it differ from JNC 7*. https://www.ncbi.nlm.nih.gov/pmc/articles/PMC4137642/

Mann, J. F. E. (2020). Choice of drug therapy in primary (essential) hypertension. In J. P. Forman (Ed.), *UpToDate*. https://www.uptodate.com/contents/choice-of-drug-therapy-in-primary-essential-hypertension

Mayo Clinic. (2019). *BRCA gene test for breast and ovarian cancer risk*. https://www.mayoclinic.org/tests-procedures/brca-gene-test/about/pac-20384815

OpenAnesthesia. (n.d.). *Herbal medicines: Anticoagulation effects*. https://www.openanesthesia.org/herbal_medicines_anticoagulation_effects

Pignone, M. (2020). Management of elevated low-density lipoprotein-cholesterol (LDL-C) in primary prevention of cardiovascular disease. In G. M. Saperia (Ed.), *UpToDate*. https://www.uptodate.com/contents/management-of-low-density-lipoprotein-cholesterol-ldl-c-in-the-secondary-prevention-of-cardiovascular-disease

Pislaru, S., & Enriquez-Sarano, M. (2020). Definition and diagnosis of mitral valve prolapse. In S. B. Yeon (Ed.), *UpToDate*. https://www.uptodate.com/contents/definition-and-diagnosis-of-mitral-valve-prolapse/print

Prutkin, J. M. (2019). ECG tutorial: Basic principles of ECG analysis. In G. M. Saperia (Ed.), *UpToDate*. https://www.uptodate.com/contents/ecg-tutorial-basic-principles-of-ecg-analysis#H340807881

Reeder, G. S., Awtry, E., & Mahler, S. A. (2020). Initial evaluation and management of suspected acute coronary syndrome (myocardial infarction, unstable angina) in the emergency department. In J. Grayzel (Ed.), *UpToDate*. https://www.uptodate.com/contents/initial-evaluation-and-management-of-suspected-acute-coronary-syndrome-myocardial-infarction-unstable-angina-in-the-emergency-department#H40643584

Rosenson, R. S., & Eckel, R. H. (2020). Hypertriglyceridemia. In G. M. Saperia & J. Givens (Eds.), *UpToDate*. https://www.uptodate.com/contents/hypertriglyceridemia#H302377

Sexton, D. J., & Chu, V. H. (2019). Antimicrobial prophylaxis for bacterial endocarditis. In E. L. Baron & S. B. Yeon (Eds.), *UpToDate*. https://www.uptodate.com/contents

/antimicrobial-prophylaxis-for-the-prevention-of
-bacterial-endocarditis

Sexton, D. J., & Chu, V. H. (2019). Clinical manifestations and evaluation of adults with suspected left-sided native valve endocarditis. In E. L. Baron & S. B. Yeon (Eds.), *UpToDate*. https://www.uptodate.com/contents/clinical -manifestations-and-evaluation-of-adults-with -suspected-left-sided-native-valve-endocarditis#H25

Simons, M., & Alpert, J. S. (2020). Acute coronary syndrome: Terminology and classification. In J. P. Forman (Ed.), *UpToDate*. https://www.uptodate.com/contents/acute -coronary-syndrome-terminology-and-classification#H22

Soos, M. P., & McComb, D. (2020). Sinus arrhythmia. In *Stat-Pearls*. https://www.ncbi.nlm.nih.gov/books/NBK537011/

U.S. Food and Drug Administration. (2016). *FDA Drug Safety Communication: New Warning and Contraindication for blood pressure medicines containing aliskiren (Tekturna)*. https:// www.fda.gov/drugs/drug-safety-and-availability/fda -drug-safety-communication-new-warning-and -contraindication-blood-pressure-medicines-containing

U.S. Food and Drug Administration. (2017). *FDA warns about increased risk of ruptures or tears in the aorta blood vessel with fluoroquinolone antibiotics in certain patients*. https://www .fda.gov/drugs/drug-safety-and-availability/fda-warns -about-increased-risk-ruptures-or-tears-aorta-blood -vessel-fluoroquinolone-antibiotics

U.S. Food and Drug Administration. (2018). *FDA Drug Safety Communication: FDA updates warnings for oral and injectable flouroquinolone antibiotics due to disabling side effects*. https:// www.fda.gov/drugs/drug-safety-and-availability /fda-drug-safety-communication-fda-updates-warnings -oral-and-injectable-fluoroquinolone-antibiotics

Uto-Kondo, H., Ayaori, M., Sotherden, G. M., Nakaya, K., Sasaki, M., Yogo, M., Komatsu, T., Takiguchi, S., Yakushiji, E., Ogura, M., Nishida, T., Endo, Y., & Ikewaki, K. (2014). Ezetimibe enhances macrophage reverse cholesterol transport in hamsters: contribution of hepato-biliary pathway. *Biochimica et Biophysica Acta, 1841*(9), 1247–1255. https://pubmed.ncbi.nlm.nih.gov/24989153/

Vasan, R. S., & Wilson, P. W. F. (2020). Epidemiology and causes of heart failure. In S. B. Yeon (Ed.), *UpToDate*. https://www.uptodate.com/contents/epidemiology -and-causes-of-heart-failure#H7177090

Wang, A., & Holland, T. L. (2020). Overview of management of infective endocarditis in adults. In S. B. Yeon & E. L. Baron (Eds.), *UpToDate*. https://www.uptodate.com/contents /overview-of-management-of-infective-endocarditis-in -adults#H4021937902

Wigley, F. M. (2019). Clinical manifestations and diagnosis of Raynaud phenomenon. In M. R. Curtis (Ed.), *UpToDate*. https://www.uptodate.com/contents /clinical-manifestations-and-diagnosis-of-raynaud -phenomenon#H17

Wigley, F. M. (2019). Treatment of Raynaud phenomenon: Initial management. In M. R. Curtis (Ed.), *UpToDate*. https:// www.uptodate.com/contents/treatment-of-raynaud -phenomenon-initial-management#H10

Endocrine System

Bakris, G. L. (2018). Moderately increased albuminuria (micro-albuminuria) in type 2 diabetes mellitus. In J. P. Forman (Ed.), *UpToDate*. https://www.uptodate.com/contents /moderately-increased-albuminuria-microalbuminuria -in-type-2-diabetes-mellitus

Durnwald, C. (2020). Diabetes mellitus in pregnancy: Screening and diagnosis. In V. A. Barss (Ed.), *UpToDate*. https:// www.uptodate.com/contents/diabetes-mellitus-in -pregnancy-screening-and-diagnosis#H23

ElSayed, N. A., Aleppo, G., Aroda, V. R., Bannuru, R. R., Brown, F. M., Bruemmer, D., Collins, B. S., Hilliard, M. E., Isaacs, D., Johnson, E. L., Kahan, S., Khunti, K., Leon, J., Lyons, S. K., Perry, M. L., Prahalad, P., Pratley, R. E., Seley, J. J., Stanton, R. C., & Gabbay, R. A. (2023). 6. Glycemic targets: Standards of care in diabetes-2023. *Diabetes Care, 46*(Suppl 1), S97–S110. https://doi.org/10.2337/dc23-S006.

ElSayed, N. A., Aleppo, G., Aroda, V. R., Bannuru, R. R., Brown, F. M., Bruemmer, D., Collins, B. S., Das, S. R., Hilliard, M. E., Isaacs, D., Johnson, E. L., Kahan, S., Khunti, K., Kosiborod, M., Leon, J., Lyons, S. K., Perry, M. L., Prahalad, P., Pratley, R. E., . . . Gabbay, R. A. (2023). 10. Cardiovascular disease and risk management: Standards of care in diabetes-2023. *Diabetes Care, 46*(Suppl 1), S158–S190. https://doi.org/10.2337/dc23-S010

Haugen, B. R., Alexander, E. K., Bible, K. C., Doherty, G. M., Mandel, S. J., Nikiforov, Y. E., Pacini, F., Randolph, G. W., Sawka, A. M., Schlumberger, M., Schuff, K. G., Sherman, S. I., Sosa, J. A., Steward, D. L., Tuttle, R. M., & Wartofsky, L. (2016). 2015 American Thyroid Association management guidelines for adult patients with thyroid nodules and differentiated thyroid cancer. *Thyroid, 26*(1), 1–133. https://doi.org/10.1089/thy.2015.0020

Meigs, J. B. (2020). Metabolic syndrome (insulin resistance syndrome or syndrome X). In L. Kunins (Ed.), *UpToDate*. https://www.uptodate.com/contents/metabolic -syndrome-insulin-resistance-syndrome-or-syndrome -x#H2435699

Ross, D. S. (2020). Thionamides in the treatment of Graves' disease. In J. E. Mulder (Ed.), *UpToDate*. https:// www.uptodate.com/contents/thionamides-in-the -treatment-of-graves-disease

Female Reproductive System

Allen, R. H. (2020). Combined estrogen-progestin oral contraceptives: Patient selection, counseling, and use. In K. Eckler & K. A. Martin (Ed.), *UpToDate*. https://www .uptodate.com/contents/combined-estrogen-progestin -oral-contraceptives-patient-selection-counseling-and -use#H3681523291

American Diabetes Association. (2020). Management of diabetes in pregnancy: Standards of medical care in diabetes—2020. *Diabetes Care, 43*(Supplement 1), S183–S192. https://doi.org/10.2337/dc20-S014

Ananth, C. V., & Kinzler, W. L. (2020). Placental abruption: Pathophysiology, clinical features, diagnosis, and consequences. In V. A. Barss (Ed.), *UpToDate*. https://www .uptodate.com/contents/endometriosis-pathogenesis -clinical-features-and-diagnosis#H23

August, P., & Sibai, B. M. (2020). Preeclampsia: Clinical features and diagnosis. In V. A. Barss (Ed.), *UpToDate*. https:// www.uptodate.com/contents/preeclampsia-clinical -features-and-diagnosis#H34

Bachmann, G., & Santen, R. J. (2020). Treatment of genitourinary syndrome of menopause (vulvovaginal atrophy). In A. Chakrabarti (Ed.), *UpToDate*. https://www.uptodate .com/contents/treatment-of-genitourinary-syndrome-of -menopause-vulvovaginal-atrophy#H16

Beloosesky, R., & Ross, M. G. (2020). Polyhydramnios: Etiology, diagnosis, and management. In V. A.

Barss (Ed.), *UpToDate*. https://www.uptodate.com/contents/polyhydramnios-etiology-diagnosis-and-management#H18

Blausen.com staff. (2014). Medical gallery of Blausen Medical 2014. WikiJournal of Medicine, 1(2). https://doi.org/10.15347/wjm/2014.010

Breastcancer.org. (2018). *Fibroadenoma*. https://www.breastcancer.org/symptoms/benign/fibroadenoma

Centers for Disease Control and Prevention. (2016). *U.S. selected practice recommendations for contraceptive use, 2016: Introduction*. https://www.cdc.gov/reproductivehealth/contraception/mmwr/spr/intro.html

Cunningham, F. G. (2023). Normal reference ranges for laboratory values in pregnancy. *UpToDate*. Retrieved [mo/date/year], from https://www.uptodate.com/contents/normal-reference-ranges-for-laboratory-values-in-pregnancy

Dixon, J. M. (2020). Lactational mastitis. In E. L. Baron & K. Eckler (Ed.), *UpToDate*. https://www.uptodate.com/contents/lactational-mastitis#H15

Drugs.com. (2020). *Nitrofurantoin pregnancy and breastfeeding warnings*. https://www.drugs.com/pregnancy/pseudoephedrine.html

Drugs.com. (2020). *Pseudoephedrine pregnancy and breastfeeding warnings*. https://www.drugs.com/pregnancy/nitrofurantoin.html

Drugs.com. (n.d.). *FDA pregnancy categories: FDA pregnancy risk information—An update*. https://www.drugs.com/pregnancy-categories.html

Foley, M. R. (2020). Maternal adaptations to pregnancy: Cardiovascular and hemodynamic changes. In V. A. Barss (Ed.), *UpToDate*. https://www.uptodate.com/contents/maternal-adaptations-to-pregnancy-cardiovascular-and-hemodynamic-changes#H24

Kaunitz, A. M. (2020). Progestin-only pills (POPs) for contraception. In C. A. Schreiber (Ed.), *UpToDate*. http://www.uptodate.com/contents/progestin-only-pills-pops-for-contraception

Laronga, C., Tollin, S., & Mooney, B. (2019). Breast cysts: Clinical manifestations, diagnosis, and management. In W. Chen (Ed.), *UpToDate*. https://www.uptodate.com/contents/breast-cysts-clinical-manifestations-diagnosis-and-management#H14

Lockwood, C. J., & Russo-Stieglitz, K. (2019). Placenta previa: Epidemiology, clinical features, diagnosis, morbidity and mortality. In V. A. Barss (Ed.), *UpToDate*. https://www.uptodate.com/contents/placenta-previa-epidemiology-clinical-features-diagnosis-morbidity-and-mortality#H14

Lukacz, E. S. (2020). Evaluation of females with urinary incontinence. In J. Givens (Ed.), *UpToDate*. https://www.uptodate.com/contents/evaluation-of-females-with-urinary-incontinence#H21991455

Prager, S., Micks, E., & Dalton, V. K. (2020). Pregnancy loss (miscarriage): Risk factors, etiology, clinical manifestations, and diagnostic evaluation. In K. Eckler (Ed.), *UpToDate*. https://www.uptodate.com/contents/pregnancy-loss-miscarriage-risk-factors-etiology-clinical-manifestations-and-diagnostic-evaluation#H1314293314

Rogers, R. G., & Fashokun, T. B. (2020). Pelvic organ prolapse in women: Epidemiology, risk factors, clinical manifestations, and management. In K. Eckler (Ed.), *UpToDate*. https://www.uptodate.com/contents/pelvic-organ-prolapse-in-women-epidemiology-risk-factors-clinical-manifestations-and-management?search=pelvic-organ-prolapse-in-women-an-overview-of-the-epidemiology

%20-risk-factors-clinical-manifestations-and-&source=search_result&selectedTitle=3~150&usage_type=default&display_rank=3#H17

Rosen, H. N., & Drezner, M. K. (2020). Overview of the management of osteoporosis in postmenopausal women. In J. E. Mulder (Ed.), *UpToDate*. https://www.uptodate.com/contents/overview-of-the-management-of-osteoporosis-in-postmenopausal-women#H40

Ross, J., & Chacko, M. R. (2020). Pelvic inflammatory disease: Clinical manifestations and diagnosis. In A. Bloom (Ed.), *UpToDate*. https://www.uptodate.com/contents/pelvic-inflammatory-disease-clinical-manifestations-and-diagnosis

Sable, M. S., & Weaver, D. L. (2020). Paget disease of the breast (PDB). In W. Chen (Ed.), *UpToDate*. https://www.uptodate.com/contents/paget-disease-of-the-breast-pdb#H22

Schenken, R. S. (2020). Endometriosis: Pathogenesis, clinical features, and diagnosis. In K. Eckler (Ed.), *UpToDate*. https://www.uptodate.com/contents/endometriosis-pathogenesis-clinical-features-and-diagnosis#H23

Schmidt, P., Skelly, C. L., & Raines, D. A. (2020). Placental abruption (abruptio placentae). In *StatPearls*. https://www.ncbi.nlm.nih.gov/books/NBK482335/

Sibai, B. M. (2020). HELLP syndrome (hemolysis, elevated liver enzymes, and low platelets). In V. A. Barss (Ed.), *UpToDate*. https://www.uptodate.com/contents/hellp-syndrome-hemolysis-elevated-liver-enzymes-and-low-platelets#H24

Sobel, J. D. (2020). Candida vulvovaginitis: Treatment. In K. Eckler (Ed.), *UpToDate*. https://www.uptodate.com/contents/candida-vulvovaginitis-treatment

Tabrizi, A. D. (2018). Atrophic pap smears, differential diagnosis and pitfalls: A review. *International Journal of Women's Health and Reproduction Sciences, 6*(1), 2–5.

U.S. Department of Health and Human Services. (2019). *Emergency contraception*. https://www.hhs.gov/opa/pregnancy-prevention/birth-control-methods/emergency-contraception/index.html

U.S. Department of Health and Human Services, Office on Women's Health. (2018). *Breastfeeding: Getting a good latch*. https://www.womenshealth.gov/breastfeeding/learning-breastfeed/getting-good-latch

U.S. Preventive Services Task Force. (2018, August 21). *Cervical cancer: Screening*. https://www.uspreventiveservicestaskforce.org/uspstf/recommendation/cervical-cancer-screening

Welt, C. K. (2019). Causes of primary amenorrhea. In K. A. Martin (Ed.), *UpToDate*. https://www.uptodate.com/contents/causes-of-primary-amenorrhea#H272347794

Gastrointestinal System

Allen, J. P., Sillanaukee, P., Strid, N., & Litten, R. Z. (2004). *Biomarkers of heavy drinking*. https://pubs.niaaa.nih.gov/publications/assessingalcohol/biomarkers.htm

Bartelt, L. A. (2020). Giardiasis: Treatment and prevention. In E. L. Baron (Ed.), *UpToDate*. https://www.uptodate.com/contents/giardiasis-treatment-and-prevention

Centers for Disease Control and Prevention. (2020). *Hepatitis C information*. https://www.cdc.gov/hepatitis/hcv/

Fossmark, R., Martinson, T. C., & Waldum, H. L. (2019). *Adverse effects of proton pump inhibitors—Evidence and plausibility*. https://www.ncbi.nlm.nih.gov/pmc/articles/PMC6829383/

Friedman, L. S. (2020). Approach to the patient with abnormal liver biochemical and function tests. In S. Grover (Ed.),

UpToDate. https://www.uptodate.com/contents
/approach-to-the-patient-with-abnormal-liver-biochemical
-and-function-tests#H50

Goldenberg, J. Z., Yap, C., Lytvyn, L., Lo, C. K., Beardsley, J.,
Mertz, D., & Johnston, B. C. (2019). *Probiotics for the prevention of Clostridium difficile-associated diarrhea in adults and
children.* https://pubmed.ncbi.nlm.nih.gov/29257353/

Lai, M., & Chopra, S. (2019). Hepatitis A virus infection in
adults: Epidemiology, clinical manifestations, and diagnosis. In E. L. Baron (Ed.), *UpToDate*. https://www
.uptodate.com/contents/hepatitis-a-virus-infection
-in-adults-epidemiology-clinical-manifestations-and
-diagnosis#H7717987

Oh, R. C., Hustead, T. R., Ali, S. M., & Pantsari, M. W. (2017).
*Mildly elevated liver transaminase levels: Causes and evalua-
tion.* https://www.aafp.org/afp/2017/1201/p709.html

Pemberton, J. H. (2020). Acute colonic diverticulitis: Medical
management. In W. Chen (Ed.), *UpToDate*. https://www
.uptodate.com/contents/acute-colonic-diverticulitis
-medical-management

Sheth, S. G., & Chopra, S. (2019). Epidemiology, clinical features,
and diagnosis of nonalcoholic fatty liver disease in adults.
In S. Grover (Ed.), *UpToDate*. https://www.uptodate.com
/contents/epidemiology-clinical-features-and-diagnosis
-of-nonalcoholic-fatty-liver-disease-in-adults#H11

Vege, S. S. (2019). Clinical manifestations and diagnosis of
acute pancreatitis. In S. Grover (Ed.), *UpToDate*. https://
www.uptodate.com/contents/clinical-manifestations
-and-diagnosis-of-acute-pancreatitis#H24

Vege, S. S. (2019). Etiology of acute pancreatitis. In S. Grover
(Ed.), *UpToDate*. https://www.uptodate.com/contents
/etiology-of-acute-pancreatitis#H24

Wolfe, M. M. (2020). Proton pump inhibitors: Overview of use
and adverse effects in the treatment of acid related disorders. In S. Grover (Ed.), *UpToDate*. https://www
.uptodate.com/contents/proton-pump-inhibitors
-overview-of-use-and-adverse-effects-in-the-treatment
-of-acid-related-disorders#H22

Genitourinary and Renal System

Arihan, O., Wernly, B., Lichtenauer, M., Franz, M., Kabisch,
B., Muessig, J., Masyuk, M., Lauten, A., Schulze, P. C.,
Hoppe, U. C., Kelm, M., & Jung, C. (2018). *Blood Urea
Nitrogen (BUN) is independently associated with mortality in
critically ill patients admitted to ICU.* https://www.ncbi
.nlm.nih.gov/pmc/articles/PMC5784990/

Inker, L. A., & Perrone, R. D. (2020). Assessment of kidney
function. In J. P. Forman (Ed.), *UpToDate*. https://www
.uptodate.com/contents/assessment-of-kidney-function

Liangos, O., & Jaber, B. L. (2020). Kidney and patient outcomes
after acute kidney injury in adults. In S. Motwani (Ed.),
UpToDate. https://www.uptodate.com/contents/kidney
-and-patient-outcomes-after-acute-kidney-injury-in
-adults#H450663

National Institutes of Health. (n.d.). *Estimating glomerular
filtration rate.* https://www.niddk.nih.gov/health-infor-
mation/professionals/clinical-tools-patient-management
/kidney-disease/laboratory-evaluation/glomerular
-filtration-rate/estimating?dkrd=hisce0089

NephCure Kidney International. (n.d.). *Renal diet.* https://
nephcure.org/livingwithkidneydisease/diet-and
-nutrition/renal-diet/

Rovin, B. H. (2020). Assessment of urinary protein excretion
and evaluation of isolated non-nephrotic proteinuria in
adults. In A. Q. Lam (Ed.), *UpToDate*. https://www
.uptodate.com/contents/assessment-of-urinary-protein
-excretion-and-evaluation-of-isolated-non-nephrotic
-proteinuria-in-adults

Thomas-White, K., Brady, M., Wolfe, A. J., & Mueller, E. R.
(2016). *The bladder is not sterile: History and current
discoveries on the urinary microbiome.* https://www.ncbi.nlm
.nih.gov/pmc/articles/PMC4864995/

Gerontology

Administration on Aging, Administration for Community
Living, U.S. Department of Health and Human Services.
(2020). *2019 profile of older Americans.* https://acl.gov
/sites/default/files/Aging%20and%20Disability%20
in%20America/2019ProfileOlderAmericans508.pdf

American Lung Association. (2020). *Lung capacity and aging.*
http://www.lung.org/lung-health-and-diseases/how
-lungs-work/lung-capacity-and-aging.html

Centers for Disease Control and Prevention. (2020). *Older
person's health.* https://www.cdc.gov/nchs/fastats/older
-american-health.htm

Haesler, E. (Ed.). (2019). *Prevention and treatment of pressure
ulcers/injuries: Quick reference guide.* European Pressure
Ulcer Advisory Panel, National Pressure Injury Advisory
Panel & Pan Pacific Pressure Injury Alliance.

Kiehl, D. P. (2020). Falls in older persons: Risk factors and
patient evaluation. In J. Givens (Ed.), *UpToDate*. https://
www.uptodate.com/contents/falls-in-older-persons
-risk-factors-and-patient-evaluation#H30

Larson, E. B. (2019). Evaluation of cognitive impairment and
dementia. In J. Wilterdink (Ed.), *UpToDate*. https://www
.uptodate.com/contents/evaluation-of-cognitive
-impairment-and-dementia#H17

McGrath, K., Hajjar, E. R., Kumar, C., Hwang, C., & Salzman, B.
(2017). Deprescribing: A simple method for reducing polypharmacy. *The Journal of Family Practice*, 66(7), 436–445.

National Institute on Aging. (2019). *Healthy eating: USDA food
patterns.* www.nia.nih.gov/health/usda-food-patterns

Taffet, G. E. (2019). Normal aging. In J. Givens (Ed.), *UpToDate*.
https://www.uptodate.com/contents/normal-aging

Head, Eyes, Ears, Nose, and Throat

Armitage, A. (2015). *Advanced practice nursing guide to the neurological exam.* Springer Publishing Company.

Bhattacharyya, N. (2020). Nasal obstruction: Diagnosis and
management. In L. Kunins (Ed.), *UpToDate*. https://
www.uptodate.com/contents/nasal-obstruction
-diagnosis-and-management#H492107460

Bienfang, D. C. (2019). Overview and differential diagnosis of
papilledema. In J. Wilterdink (Ed.), *UpToDate*. https://
www.uptodate.com/contents/overview-and-differential
-diagnosis-of-papilledema

Bork, J. (2019). Corneal ulcer and ulcerative keratitis in emergency medicine. In B. E. Brenner (Ed.), *Medscape*. https://
emedicine.medscape.com/article/798100-overview

Centers for Disease Control and Prevention. (2016). *Flu vaccine
and people with egg allergies.* https://www.cdc.gov/flu
/prevent/egg-allergies.htm

Centers for Disease Control and Prevention. (2018).
Life expectancy. https://www.cdc.gov/nchs/fastats
/life-expectancy.htm

Centers for Disease Control and Prevention. (2019). *Mumps.*
https://www.cdc.gov/mumps/hcp.html

Chow, A. W., & Doron, S. (2020). Evaluation of acute
pharyngitis in adults. In S. Bond (Ed.), *UpToDate*.
http://www.uptodate.com/contents/evaluation-of
-acute-pharyngitis-in-adults

Ferrer, R. L. (2019). Evaluation of peripheral lymphadenopathy in adults. In L. Kunins (Ed.), *UpToDate*. https://www.uptodate.com/contents/evaluation-of-peripheral-lymphadenopathy-in-adults#H18193923

Ghosh, C., & Ghosh, T. (2020). Eyelid lesions. In J. Givens (Ed.), *UpToDate*. https://www.uptodate.com/contents/eyelid-lesions

Heegaard, W. G. (2019). Skull fractures in adults. In J. Grayzel (Ed.), *UpToDate*. https://www.uptodate.com/contents/skull-fractures-in-adults#H19

Jacobs, D. S. (2020). Corneal abrasions and corneal foreign bodies: Management. In J. Givens (Ed.), *UpToDate*. https://www.uptodate.com/contents/corneal-abrasions-and-corneal-foreign-bodies-management#H7155009

Kaufman, C. A. (2018). Treatment of oropharyngeal and esophageal candidiasis. In J. Mitty (Ed.), *UpToDate*. https://www.uptodate.com/contents/treatment-of-oropharyngeal-and-esophageal-candidiasis

Malloy, K. M. (2020). Assessment and management of auricular hematoma and cauliflower ears. In J. F. Wiley (Ed.), *UpToDate*. https://www.uptodate.com/contents/assessment-and-management-of-auricular-hematoma-and-cauliflower-ear#H3540963

National Eye Institute. (2019). *Facts about retinal detachment*. https://nei.nih.gov/health/retinaldetach/retinaldetach

Park, J. K., Vernick, D. M., & Ramakrishna, N. (2020). Vestibular schwannoma (acoustic neuroma). In A. F. Eichler (Ed.), *UpToDate*. https://www.uptodate.com/contents/vestibular-schwannoma-acoustic-neuroma#H19

Paysse, E. A., & Coats, D. K. (2019). Congenital nasolacrimal duct obstruction (dacryostenosis) and dacryocystocele. In C. Armsby (Ed.), *UpToDate*. https://www.uptodate.com/contents/congenital-nasolacrimal-duct-obstruction-dacryostenosis-and-dacryocystocele#H17

Weber, P. C. (2020). Evaluation of hearing loss in adults. In L. Kunins (Ed.), *UpToDate*. https://www.uptodate.com/contents/evaluation-of-hearing-loss-in-adults

Health Promotion, Screening, and Disease Prevention

Apicella, M. (2020). Treatment and prevention of meningococcal infection. In J. Mitty (Ed.), *UpToDate*. https://www.uptodate.com/contents/treatment-and-prevention-of-meningococcal-infection

Centers for Disease Control and Prevention. (2016). *Flu vaccine and people with egg allergies*. https://www.cdc.gov/flu/prevent/egg-allergies.htm

Centers for Disease Control and Prevention. (2016). *Vaccine information for adults: Healthcare workers*. https://www.cdc.gov/vaccines/adults/rec-vac/hcw.html

Centers for Disease Control and Prevention. (2018). *Life expectancy*. https://www.cdc.gov/nchs/fastats/life-expectancy.htm

Centers for Disease Control and Prevention. (2018). *Rocky Mountain spotted fever (RMSF)*. https://www.cdc.gov/rmsf/index.html

Centers for Disease Control and Prevention. (2019). *Motor vehicle safety*. https://www.cdc.gov/motorvehiclesafety/teen_drivers/teendrivers_factsheet.html

Centers for Disease Control and Prevention. (2019). *Recommendations, scenarios and Q&As for healthcare professionals about PCV13 for adults*. https://www.cdc.gov/vaccines/vpd/pneumo/hcp/PCV13-adults.html

Centers for Disease Control and Prevention. (2019). *Vaccine information statement. Influenza (Flu) Vaccine (Live, Intranasal): What you need to know*. https://www.cdc.gov/vaccines/hcp/vis/vis-statements/flulive.pdf

Centers for Disease Control and Prevention. (2020). *2020 national notifiable conditions (historical)*. https://wwwn.cdc.gov/nndss/conditions/notifiable/2020/

Centers for Disease Control and Prevention. (2020). *Adult obesity facts*. https://www.cdc.gov/obesity/data/adult.html

Centers for Disease Control and Prevention. (2020). *Frequently Asked Influenza (Flu) questions: 2019–2020 season*. https://www.cdc.gov/flu/season/faq-flu-season-2019-2020.htm

Centers for Disease Control and Prevention. (2020). *Health of American Indian or Alaska Native population*. https://www.cdc.gov/nchs/fastats/american-indian-health.htm

Centers for Disease Control and Prevention. (2020). *Influenza (flu): Key facts about flu vaccines*. https://www.cdc.gov/flu/prevent/keyfacts.htm

Centers for Disease Control and Prevention. (2020). *Lyme disease*. http://www.cdc.gov/lyme/healthcare

Centers for Disease Control and Prevention. (2020). *Mortality in the United States, 2018*. https://www.cdc.gov/nchs/products/databriefs/db355.htm

Centers for Disease Control and Prevention. (2020). *What everyone should know about Zostavax*. https://www.cdc.gov/vaccines/vpd/shingles/public/zostavax/index.html

Centers for Disease Control and Prevention. (2023). *Adult immunization schedule by age*. https://www.cdc.gov/vaccines/schedules/hcp/imz/adult.html

Central Intelligence Agency. (2016). *The World Factbook: Obesity—Adult prevalence rate*. https://www.cia.gov/library/publications/the-world-factbook/rankorder/2228rank.html

Donovan, D., & McDowell, I. (2017). *AFMC primer on population health: A virtual textbook on public health concepts for clinicians*. The Association of Faculties of Medicine of Canada. http://phprimer.afmc.ca/Part1-TheoryThinkingAboutHealth/Chapter4BasicConceptsInPreventionSurveillanceAndHealthPromotion/Thestagesofprevention

Harvard T.H. Chan School of Public Health. (n.d.). *Abdominal obesity measurement guidelines for Different Ethnic Groups*. https://www.hsph.harvard.edu/obesity-prevention-source/waist-circumference-guidelines-for-different-ethnic-groups/

Immunization Action Coalition. (2019). *Ask the experts*. https://www.immunize.org/askexperts/experts_inf.asp

Indian Health Service. (2019). *Indian health disparities*. https://www.ihs.gov/sites/newsroom/themes/responsive2017/display_objects/documents/factsheets/Disparities.pdf

Kochanek, K. D., Murphy, S. L., Xu, J., & Arias, A. (2019). Deaths: Final data for 2017. *National Vital Statistics Reports*, 68(9), 1–76. https://www.cdc.gov/nchs/data/nvsr/nvsr68/nvsr68_09-508.pdf?fbclid=IwAR3z03p2bJdu0Q-vqvdMHKDCPtPT_4DePF1xdc39uYlyl3D8sgPtnhAFI3A

Levin, J., Chatters, L. M., & Taylor, J. (2007). Religion, health and medicine in African Americans: Implications for physicians. *Journal of the National Medical Association*, 97(2), 237–247. http://www.baylorisr.org/wp-content/uploads/levin_african.pdf

National Center for Health Statistics. (2020). *Leading causes of death – 2017*. http://www.cdc.gov/nchs/fastats/leading-causes-of-death.htm

National Congress of American Indians. (2020). *Tribal Nations and the United States: An introduction*. http://www.ncai.org/tribalnations/introduction/Indian_Country_101_Updated_February_2019.pdf

National Council of State Boards of Nursing. (2017). *Nurse Practice Acts Guide: Nurse Practice Acts guide and govern nursing practice.* https://www.ncsbn.org/ nurse-practice-act.htm

Population Reference Bureau. (2019). *Fact sheet: Aging in the United States.* https://www.prb.org/aging-unitedstates-fact-sheet/

Sexton, D. J., & McClain, M. T. (2019). Treatment of Rocky Mountain spotted fever. In J. Mitty (Ed.), *UpToDate.* https://www.uptodate.com/contents/treatment-of-rocky-mountain-spotted-fever

U.S. Census Bureau. (n.d.). *QuickFacts.* https://www.census.gov/quickfacts/fact/table/US/PST045217

U.S. Department of Health & Human Services. (n.d.). *Healthy People 2030.* https://health.gov/healthypeople

U.S. Preventive Services Task Force. (n.d.). *A & B recommendations.* Retrieved September 4, 2023, from https://www.uspreventiveservicestaskforce.org/uspstf/recommendation-topics/uspstf-a-and-b-recommendations

World Population Review. (2020). *Obesity rates by Country 2020.* https://worldpopulationreview.com/country-rankings/obesity-rates-by-country

Hematopoietic System

Bacon, B. R. (2019). Clinical manifestations and diagnosis of hereditary hemochromatosis. In J. S. Tirnauer (Ed.), *UpToDate.* https://www.uptodate.com/contents/clinical-manifestations-and-diagnosis-of-hereditary-hemochromatosis#H12535812

Colwell, C. (2020). Initial management of moderate to severe hemorrhage in the adult trauma patient. In J. Grayzel (Ed.), *UpToDate.* https://www.uptodate.com/contents/initial-management-of-moderate-to-severe-hemorrhage-in-the-adult-trauma-patient#H3123328758

Glader, B. (2019). Diagnosis and management of glucose-6-phosphate dehydrogenase (G6PD) deficiency. In J. S. Tirnauer (Ed.), *UpToDate.* https://www.uptodate.com/contents/diagnosis-and-management-of-glucose-6-phosphate-dehydrogenase-g6pd-deficiency#H15

Glader, B. (2019). Genetics and pathophysiology of glucose-6-phosphate dehydrogenase (G6PD) deficiency. In J. S. Tirnauer (Ed.), *UpToDate.* https://www.uptodate.com/contents/genetics-and-pathophysiology-of-glucose-6-phosphate-dehydrogenase-g6pd-deficiency#H22470651

Hoots, W. K., & Shapiro, A. D. (2019). Clinical manifestations and diagnosis of hemophilia. In J. S. Tirnauer (Ed.), *UpToDate.* https://www.uptodate.com/contents/clinical-manifestations-and-diagnosis-of-hemophilia#H23971191

Mount, D. B. (2019). Clinical manifestations and treatment of hypokalemia in adults. In J. P. Forman (Ed.), *UpToDate.* https://www.uptodate.com/contents/clinical-manifestations-and-treatment-of-hypokalemia-in-adults

National Institutes of Health, Office of Dietary Supplements. (2020). *Iron: Fact sheet for health professionals.* https://ods.od.nih.gov/factsheets/Iron-HealthProfessional/

Vinchinsky, E. P., & Mahoney, D. H. (2020). Diagnosis of sickle cell disorders. In J. S. Tirnauer (Ed.), *UpToDate.* https://www.uptodate.com/contents/diagnosis-of-sickle-cell-disorders

Integumentary System

Ackerman, K. E., & Misra, M. (2020). Tinea capitus. In K. A. Martin (Ed.), *UpToDate.* https://www.uptodate.com/contents/functional-hypothalamic-amenorrhea-pathophysiology-and-clinical-manifestations#H573789409

American Cancer Society. (2020). *Cancers facts for men.* https://www.cancer.org/healthy/find-cancer-early/mens-health/cancer-facts-for-men.html

American Cancer Society. (2020). *Cancers in children.* https://www.cancer.org/cancer/cancer-in-children

American Cancer Society. (2022, January 14). *American Cancer Society recommendations for the early detection of breast cancer.* https://www.cancer.org/cancer/breast-cancer/screening-tests-and-early-detection/american-cancer-society-recommendations-for-the-early-detection-of-breast-cancer.html

American Cancer Society. (n.d.). *Skin cancer.* https://www.cancer.org/cancer/skin-cancer.html

Campbell, R. L. (2020). Anaphylaxis: Acute diagnosis. In A. M. Feldweg (Ed.), *UpToDate.* https://www.uptodate.com/contents/anaphylaxis-acute-diagnosis#H3801473448

deLemos, D. M. (2020). Closure of minor skin wounds with sutures. In J. F. Wiley (Ed.), *UpToDate.* https://www.uptodate.com/contents/closure-of-minor-skin-wounds-with-sutures#H44

Ferrell, P. B., & McLeod, H. L. (2008). *Carbamazepine, HLA-B*1502 and risk of Stevens–Johnson syndrome and toxic epidermal necrolysis: U.S. FDA recommendations.* https://www.ncbi.nlm.nih.gov/pmc/articles/PMC2586963/

Furstein, J. S. (2022). *Pediatric anesthesia: A comprehensive approach to safe and effective care.* Springer Publishing Company.

Goldstein, A. O., & Goldstein, B. G. (2020). Dermatophyte (tinea) infections. In A. O. Ofori (Ed.), *UpToDate.* https://www.uptodate.com/contents/dermatophyte-tinea-infections

Graber, E. (2020). Treatment of acne vulgaris. In A. O. Ofori (Ed.), *UpToDate.* http://www.uptodate.com/contents/treatment-of-acne-vulgaris?topicKey?=DERM%2F2&e

Lowy, F. D. (2017). Methicillin-resistant *Staphylococcus aureus* (MRSA) in adults: Treatment of skin and soft tissue infections. In E. L. Baron (Ed.), *UpToDate.* https://www.uptodate.com/contents/methicillin-resistant-staphylococcus-aureus-mrsa-in-adults-treatment-of-skin-and-soft-tissue-infections

Morris, J. G., Jr. (2019). *Vibrio vulnificus* infections. In A. Bloom (Ed.), *UpToDate.* http://www.uptodate.com/contents/vibrio-vulnificus-infections

National Institute of Arthritis and Musculoskeletal and Skin Diseases. (2019). *Questions and answers about vitiligo.* http://www.niams.nih.gov/health_info/vitiligo/#7

Male Reproductive System

Benner, J. S., & Ojo, A. (2020). Causes of scrotal pain in children and adolescents. In J. F. Wiley (Ed.), *UpToDate.* https://www.uptodate.com/contents/causes-of-scrotal-pain-in-children-and-adolescents/print

Brant, W. O., Bella, A. J., & Lue, T. L. (2020). Peyronie's disease: Diagnosis and medical management. In J. Givens (Ed.), *UpToDate.* https://www.uptodate.com/contents/peyronies-disease-diagnosis-and-medical-management#H29

Clemens, J. Q. (2019). Urinary incontinence in men. In J. Givens (Ed.), *UpToDate.* https://www.uptodate.com/contents/urinary-incontinence-in-men

Deveci, S. (2019). Priapism. In J. Givens (Ed.), *UpToDate.* https://www.uptodate.com/contents/priapism#H18

Hooton, T. M., & Gupta, K. (2020). Acute uncomplicated cystitis and pyelonephritis in men. In A. Bloom (Ed.), *UpToDate*. https://www.uptodate.com/contents/acute-complicated-urinary-tract-infection-including-pyelonephritis-in-adults

Khera, M. (2020). Treatment of male sexual dysfunction. In K. A. Martin (Ed.), *UpToDate*. https://www.uptodate.com/contents/treatment-of-male-sexual-dysfunction#H39

Musculoskeletal System

Callahan, L. R. (2020). Overview of running injuries of the lower extremity. In J. Grayzel (Ed.), *UpToDate*. https://www.uptodate.com/contents/overview-of-running-injuries-of-the-lower-extremity#H38751164

Cardone, D. A., & Jacobs, B. C. (2020). Meniscal injury of the knee. In J. Grayzel (Ed.), *UpToDate*. https://www.uptodate.com/contents/meniscal-injury-of-the-knee#H21

Gaffo, A. L. (2019). Clinical manifestations and diagnosis of gout. In P. L. Romain (Ed.), *UpToDate*. https://www.uptodate.com/contents/clinical-manifestations-and-diagnosis-of-gout#H111564623

Gaffo, A. L. (2019). Treatment of gout flares. In P. L. Romain (Ed.), *UpToDate*. https://www.uptodate.com/contents/treatment-of-gout-flares#H20

Helfgott, S. M. (2019). Popliteal (Baker's) cyst. In P. L. Romain (Ed.), *UpToDate*. https://www.uptodate.com/contents/popliteal-bakers-cyst#H104791422

Hicks, B. L., Lam, J. C., & Varacallo, M. (2020). *Piriformis syndrome*. https://www.ncbi.nlm.nih.gov/books/NBK448172/

Johnson, R. (2019). Approach to hip and groin pain in the athlete and active adult. In J. Grayzel (Ed.), *UpToDate*. https://www.uptodate.com/contents/approach-to-hip-and-groin-pain-in-the-athlete-and-active-adult#H283824

Lalani, T., & Schmitt, S. K. (2019). Osteomyelitis in adults: Clinical manifestations and diagnosis. In E. L. Baron (Ed.), *UpToDate*. https://www.uptodate.com/contents/osteomyelitis-in-adults-clinical-manifestations-and-diagnosis#H20

Maughan, K. L. (2019). Ankle sprain. In J. Grayzel (Ed.), *UpToDate*. https://www.uptodate.com/contents/ankle-sprain#H31

The Ottawa Rules. (n.d.). *The Ottawa Ankle rules*. http://www.theottawarules.ca/ankle_rules

Simons, S. M., & Kruse, D. (2018). Rotator cuff tendinopathy. In J. Grayzel (Ed.), *UpToDate*. https://www.uptodate.com/contents/rotator-cuff-tendinopathy#H32

Venables, P. J. W., & Chir, M. B. (2019). Diagnosis and differential diagnosis of rheumatoid arthritis. In P. L. Romain (Ed.), *UpToDate*. https://www.uptodate.com/contents/diagnosis-and-differential-diagnosis-of-rheumatoid-arthritis

Yu, D. T., & van Tubergen, A. (2020). Clinical manifestations of axial spondyloarthritis (ankylosing spondylitis and nonradiographic axial spondyloarthritis) in adults. In P. L. Romain (Ed.), *UpToDate*. https://www.uptodate.com/contents/clinical-manifestations-of-axial-spondyloarthritis-ankylosing-spondylitis-and-nonradiographic-axial-spondyloarthritis-in-adults#H11443893

Yu, D. T., & van Tubergen, A. (2020). Reactive arthritis. In P. L. Romain (Ed.), *UpToDate*. https://www.uptodate.com/contents/reactive-arthritis#H38

Yu, D. T., & van Tubergen, A. (2020). Treatment of axial spondyloarthritis (ankylosing spondylitis and nonradiographic axial spondyloarthritis) in adults. In P. L. Romain (Ed.), *UpToDate*. https://www.uptodate.com/contents/treatment-of-axial-spondyloarthritis-ankylosing-spondylitis-and-nonradiographic-axial-spondyloarthritis-in-adults

Nervous System

Boehme, A. K., Esenwa, C., & Elkind, M. S. V. (2017). *Stroke risk factors, genetics, and prevention*. https://www.ahajournals.org/doi/full/10.1161/CIRCRESAHA.116.308398

Caplan, L. R. (2020). Etiology, classification, and epidemiology of stroke. In J. F. Dashe (Ed.), *UpToDate*. https://www.uptodate.com/contents/etiology-classification-and-epidemiology-of-stroke#H1

Docken, W. P. (2019). Clinical manifestations and diagnosis of polymyalgia rheumatica. In M. R. Curtis (Ed.), *UpToDate*. https://www.uptodate.com/contents/clinical-manifestations-and-diagnosis-of-polymyalgia-rheumatica#H16

Evans, R. W., & Whitlow, C. T. (2019). Acute mild traumatic brain injury (concussion) in adults. In J. L. Wilterdink (Ed.), *UpToDate*. https://www.uptodate.com/contents/acute-mild-traumatic-brain-injury-concussion-in-adults#H25

Furie, K. L. (2020). Initial evaluation and management of transient ischemic attack and minor ischemic stroke. In J. F. Dashe (Ed.), *UpToDate*. https://www.uptodate.com/contents/initial-evaluation-and-management-of-transient-ischemic-attack-and-minor-ischemic-stroke#H19

Garza, I., & Schwedt, T. J. (2020). Medication overuse headache: Etiology, clinical features, and diagnosis. In R. P. Goddeau (Ed.), *UpToDate*. https://www.uptodate.com/contents/medication-overuse-headache-etiology-clinical-features-and-diagnosis#H14

Gelb, D. (2012). The detailed neurologic examination in adults. In J. L. Wilterdink (Ed.), *UpToDate*. https://www.uptodate.com/contents/the-detailed-neurologic-examination-in-adults#H9728271

Hasbun, R. (2019). *Treatment of bacterial meningitis caused by specific pathogens in adults*. https://www.uptodate.com/contents/treatment-of-bacterial-meningitis-caused-by-specific-pathogens-in-adults#H25

Ho, C., Khan, S. A., & Whealy, M. A. (2020). Trigeminal neuralgia. In R. P. Gouddeau (Ed.), *UpToDate*. https://www.uptodate.com/contents/trigeminal-neuralgia#H25

Kothari, M. J. (2020). Carpal tunnel syndrome: Clinical manifestations and diagnosis. In R. P. Gouddeau (Ed.), *UpToDate*. https://www.uptodate.com/contents/carpal-tunnel-syndrome-clinical-manifestations-and-diagnosis#H10

May, A. (2020). Cluster headache: Epidemiology, clinical features, and diagnosis. In R. P. Gouddeau (Ed.), *UpToDate*. https://www.uptodate.com/contents/cluster-headache-epidemiology-clinical-features-and-diagnosis#H16

Olek, M. J., & Howard, J. (2020). Clinical presentation, course, and prognosis of multiple sclerosis in adults. In J. F. Dashe (Ed.), *UpToDate*. https://www.uptodate.com/contents/clinical-presentation-course-and-prognosis-of-multiple-sclerosis-in-adults#H605009573

Olek, M. J., & Mowry, E. (2020). Pathogenesis and epidemiology of multiple sclerosis. In J. F. Dashe (Ed.), *UpToDate*. https://www.uptodate.com/contents/pathogenesis-and-epidemiology-of-multiple-sclerosis#H548441045

Pereira, J. L., de Albuquerque, L. A., Dellaretti, M., de Carvalho, G. T., Vieira, G., Jr., Rocha, M. I., Loures, L. L.,

Christo, P. P., & de Sousa, A. A. (2012). *Importance of recognizing sentinel headache.* https://www.ncbi.nlm.nih.gov/pmc/articles/PMC3551504/

Rothan, M., & Greenstein, P. (2020). Bell's palsy: Pathogenesis, clinical features, and diagnosis in adults. In R. P. Gouddeau (Ed.), *UpToDate.* https://www.uptodate.com/contents/bells-palsy-pathogenesis-clinical-features-and-diagnosis-in-adults

Schwedt, T. J. (2020). Overview of thunderclap headache. In R. P. Goddeau (Ed.), *UpToDate.* https://www.uptodate.com/contents/overview-of-thunderclap-headache#H18

Taylor, F. R. (2018). Tension-type headache in adults: Acute treatment. In R. P. Goddeau (Ed.), *UpToDate.* https://www.uptodate.com/contents/tension-type-headache-in-adults-acute-treatment#H14

Pediatrics

Backeljauw, P. (2020.) Management of Turner syndrome in children and adolescents. In A. G. Hoppin & K. A. Martin (Eds.), *UpToDate.* https://www.uptodate.com/contents/management-of-turner-syndrome-in-children-and-adolescents#H1696801

Brenner, J. S., & Ojo, A. (2020). Causes of painless scrotal swelling in children and adolescents. In J. F. Wiley (Ed.), *UpToDate.* https://www.uptodate.com/contents/causes-of-painless-scrotal-swelling-in-children-and-adolescents#H18

Bull, M. J. (2011). Health supervision for children with Down syndrome. *Pediatrics, 128*(2), 393–406.

Centers for Disease Control and Prevention. (2020). *Milestones.* https://www.cdc.gov/ncbddd/actearly/milestones/index.html

Messerlain, G. M., & Palomaki, G. E. (2019). Laboratory issues related to maternal serum screening for Down syndrome. In V. A. Barss (Ed.), *UpToDate.* https://www.uptodate.com/contents/laboratory-issues-related-to-maternal-serum-screening-for-down-syndrome#H33

Ostermaier, K. K. (2019). Down syndrome: Clinical features and diagnosis. In E. TePas (Ed.), *UpToDate.* https://www.uptodate.com/contents/down-syndrome-clinical-features-and-diagnosis#H12588736

Rice, S. G., & Council on Sports Medicine and Fitness. (2008). Medical conditions affecting sports participation. *Pediatrics, 121*(4), 841–848. http://pediatrics.aappublications.org/content/pediatrics/121/4/841.full.pdf

Vo, N. J., & Sato, T. T. (2020). Intussusception in children. In A. G. Hoppin (Ed.), *UpToDate.* https://www.uptodate.com/contents/intussusception-in-children?

Professional Role

Agency for Healthcare Research and Quality. (n.d.). *Patient centered medical home resource center: Defining the PCMH.* https://pcmh.ahrq.gov/page/defining-pcmh

Centers for Medicare & Medicaid Services (n.d.). (2015). *Palliative care vs. hospice care: Similar but different.* https://www.cms.gov/medicare-medicaid-coordination/fraud-prevention/medicaid-integrity-education/downloads/infograph-palliativecare-%5Bjune-2015%5D.pdf

Centers for Medicare & Medicaid Services. (2020). *List of telehealth services.* https://www.cms.gov/Medicare/Medicare-General-Information/Telehealth/Telehealth-Codes

Centers for Medicare & Medicaid Services. (n.d.). *Welcome to Medicare coverage database.* https://www.cms.gov/medicare-coverage-database

EBSCO Nursing Resources. (n.d.). *CINAHL databases.* https://www.ebscohost.com/nursing/products/cinahl-databases

Epstein, B., & Turner, M. (2015). The nursing code of ethics: Its value, its history. *Online Journal of Issues in Nursing, 20*(2). https://doi.org/10.3912/OJIN.Vol20No02Man04

Frechtling, J., & Sharp, L. (1997). *User-friendly handbook for mixed method evaluations.* Diane Publishing. https://www.nsf.gov/pubs/1997/nsf97153

Guttmacher Institute. (2020). *State laws and policies: Minors' access to contraceptive services.* https://www.guttmacher.org/state-policy/explore/minors-access-contraceptive-services

The Joint Commission. (n.d.). *Patient safety systems chapter, sentinel event policy and RCA2.* https://www.jointcommission.org/sentinel_event.aspx

The Joint Commission. (n.d.). *Sentinel event policy and procedures.* https://www.jointcommission.org/sentinel_event_policy_and_procedures

Medicare Learning Network. (2020). *Evaluation and management services guide.* https://www.cms.gov/Outreach-and-Education/Medicare-Learning-Network-MLN/MLNProducts/Downloads/eval-mgmt-serv-guide-ICN006764.pdf

National Center for Biotechnology Information Resources. (n.d.). *PubMed help. FAQs. PubMed quick start.* https://www.ncbi.nlm.nih.gov/books/NBK3827/#pubmedhelp.FAQs

National Institutes of Health, U.S. National Library of Medicine. (2018). *Fact sheet: MEDLINE.* https://www.nlm.nih.gov/pubs/factsheets/medline.html

O'Brien, J. M. (2003). How nurse practitioners obtained provider status: Lessons for pharmacists. *American Journal of Health-System Pharmacy, 60*(22), 2301–2307. http://www.ajhp.org/content/60/22/2301

Rosenstock, I. M., Strecher, V. J., & Becker, M. H. (1988). Social learning theory and the Health Belief Model. *Health Education Quarterly, 15*(2), 175–183.

Sackett, D. L., Rosenberg, W. M. C., Gray, J. A. M., Haynes, R. B., & Richardson, W. S. (1996). Evidence-based medicine: What it is and what it isn't. *British Medical Journal, 312,* 71. https://doi.org/10.1136/bmj.312.7023.71

Scibella, B. (2015). *Analyzing qualitative data, part 2: Chi-square and multivariate analysis* [Blog post]. http://blog.minitab.com/blog/applying-statistics-in-quality-projects/analyzing-qualitative-data-part-2-chi-square-and-multivariate-analysis

U.S. Food and Drug Administration. (2019). *Institutional review boards frequently asked questions: Information sheet.* http://www.fda.gov/RegulatoryInformation/Guidances/ucm126420.htm

U.S. Food and Drug Administration. (2019). *CFR-code of federal regulations title 21. Part 1308 - Schedule of controlled substances. Schedule II.* https://www.accessdata.fda.gov/scripts/cdrh/cfdocs/cfcfr/cfrsearch.cfm?fr=1308.12

World Health Organization. (2016). *ICD-10: International statistical classification of diseases and related health problems* (10th ed.). http://apps.who.int/classifications/icd10/browse/2016/en

Psychiatric-Mental Health

Center for Substance Abuse Treatment. (1999). Motivational interviewing as a counseling style. In *Enhancing motivation for change in substance abuse treatment* (Treatment Improvement Protocol Series No. 35). Substance Abuse and Mental Health Services Administration (US).https://www.ncbi.nlm.nih.gov/books/NBK64964/

Centers for Disease Control and Prevention. (2019). *Dietary guidelines for alcohol.* https://www.cdc.gov/alcohol/fact-sheets/moderate-drinking.htm

Erlangsen, A., Jeune, B., Bille-Brahe, U., & Vaupel, J. W. (2004). *Loss of partner and suicide risks among oldest old: A population-based register study.* https://pubmed.ncbi.nlm.nih.gov/15151913/

Folstein, M. F., Folstein, S. E., & McHugh, P. R. (1975). "Mini-mental state". A practical method for grading the cognitive state of patients for the clinician. *Journal of Psychiatric Research, 12*(3), 189–198. https://doi.org/10.1016/0022-3956(75)90026-6

Hirsch, M., & Birnbaum, R. J. (2020). Discontinuing antidepressant medications in adults. In S. Solomon (Ed.), *UpToDate.* https://www.uptodate.com/contents/discontinuing-antidepressant-medications-in-adults#H213302

National Institute of Mental Health. (n.d.). *Suicide in America: Frequently asked questions.* https://www.nimh.nih.gov/health/publications/suicide-faq/index.shtml#:~:text=

National Institute for Alcohol Abuse and Alcoholism. (n.d.). What is a standard drink? https://www.niaaa.nih.gov/what-standard-drink

National Institute on Alcohol Abuse and Alcoholism. (2014). *Harmful interactions: Mixing alcohol with medicines.* https://www.niaaa.nih.gov/publications/brochures-and-fact-sheets/harmful-interactions-mixing-alcohol-with-medicines

Press, D., & Alexander, M. (2019). Treatment of dementia. In S. T. DeKosky & K. E. Schmader (Eds.), *UpToDate.* http://www.uptodate.com/contents/treatment-of-dementia

Solomons, H. D. (2012). *Carbohydrate deficient transferrin and alcoholism.* https://www.ncbi.nlm.nih.gov/pmc/articles/PMC3882869/

Respiratory System

Centers for Disease Control and Prevention. (2016). *Tuberculosis (TB). Testing in BCG-vaccinated persons.* https://www.cdc.gov/tb/topic/testing/testingbcgvaccinated.htm

Centers for Disease Control and Prevention. (2018). *Tuberculosis (TB).* https://www.cdc.gov/tb/default.htm

Centers for Disease Control and Prevention. (2019). *Pertussis (Whooping Cough).* https://www.cdc.gov/pertussis/clinical/treatment.html

Fanta, C. H. (2019). Treatment of intermittent and mild persistent asthma in adolescents and adults. In H. Hollingsworth (Ed.), *UpToDate.* https://www.uptodate.com/contents/treatment-of-intermittent-and-mild-persistent-asthma-in-adolescents-and-adults#H36

Fanta, C. H., & Barrett, N. A. (2023). An overview of asthma management (Table 1). Retrieved, from https://www.uptodate.com/contents/an-overview-of-asthma-management

Ferguson, G. T., & Make, B. (2020). Stable COPD: Overview of management. In H. Hollingsworth (Ed.), *UpToDate.* https://www.uptodate.com/contents/stable-copd-overview-of-management

Han, M. K., Dransfield, M. T., & Martinez, F. J. (2020). Chronic obstructive pulmonary disease: Definition, clinical manifestations, diagnosis, and staging. In H. Hollingsworth (Ed.), *UpToDate.* https://www.uptodate.com/contents/chronic-obstructive-pulmonary-disease-definition-clinical-manifestations-diagnosis-and-staging#H17

Hollingsworth, H. (2019). E-cigarette or vaping product use associated lung injury (EVALI). In G. Finley (Ed.), *UpToDate.* https://www.uptodate.com/contents/e-cigarette-or-vaping-product-use-associated-lung-injury-evali#H3095889743

Medscape. (2018). *Latent TB: Updated treatment recommendations.* https://www.medscape.com/viewarticle/905810?src=par_cdc_stm_mscpedt&faf=1

Midthun DE. (2020). Stable COPD: Overview of management. In H. Hollingsworth (Ed.), *UpToDate.* https://www.uptodate.com/contents/overview-of-the-risk-factors-pathology-and-clinical-manifestations-of-lung-cancer#H12

National Institutes of Health, National Heart Lung and Blood Institute. (2012). *Asthma care quick reference: Diagnosing and managing asthma* (NIH Publication No. 12-5075). https://www.nhlbi.nih.gov/files/docs/guidelines/asthma_qrg.pdf

Saag, K. G., Furst, D. E., & Barnes, P. J. (2019). Major side effects of inhaled glucocorticoids. In H. Hollingsworth (Ed.), *UpToDate.* https://www.uptodate.com/contents/major-side-effects-of-inhaled-glucocorticoids#H27

U.S. Food and Drug Administration. (2020). *Lung injuries associated with use of vaping products.* https://www.fda.gov/news-events/public-health-focus/lung-injuries-associated-use-vaping-products

Yealy, D. M., & Fine, M. J. (2019). Community-acquired pneumonia in adults: Assessing severity and determining the appropriate site of care. In S. Bond (Ed.), *UpToDate.* https://www.uptodate.com/contents/community-acquired-pneumonia-in-adults-assessing-severity-and-determining-the-appropriate-site-of-care#H4063445

Sexually Transmitted Diseases and Infections

AIDSinfo. (2019). *Understanding HIV/AIDS.* https://aidsinfo.nih.gov/understanding-hiv-aids#

Carusi, D. A. (2019). Condylomata acuminata (anogenital warts): Treatment of vulvar and vaginal warts. In K. Eckler (Ed.), *UpToDate.* https://www.uptodate.com/contents/ovarian-cancer-screening-beyond-the-basics/print

Centers for Disease Control and Prevention. (2018). *Sexually transmitted disease surveillance 2018.* https://www.cdc.gov/std/stats18/default.htm

Centers for Disease Control and Prevention. (2020). *HIV.* https://www.cdc.gov/hiv/default.html

Centers for Disease Control and Prevention. (2020). *Legal status of expedited partner therapy (EPT).* https://www.cdc.gov/std/ept/legal/default.htm

Gandhi, R. T. (2019). Toxoplasmosis in HIV-infected patients. In J. Mitty (Ed.), *UpToDate.* https://www.uptodate.com/contents/toxoplasmosis-in-hiv-infected-patients#H33

Hsu, K. (2020). Treatment of Chlamydia trachomatis infection. In A. Bloom (Eds.), *UpToDate.* https://www.uptodate.com/contents/treatment-of-chlamydia trachomatis-infection#H49

Johnston, C., & Wald, A. (2019). Epidemiology, clinical manifestations, and diagnosis of herpes simplex virus type 1 infection. In J. Mitty (Ed.), *UpToDate.* https://www.uptodate.com/contents/ovarian-cancer-screening-beyond-the-basics/print

Klausner, J. D. (2020). Disseminated gonococcal infection. In A. Bloom (Ed.), *UpToDate*. https://www.uptodate.com/contents/disseminated-gonococcal-infection#H16637758

Sax, P. E. (2019). Acute and early HIV infection: Clinical manifestations and diagnosis. In A. Bloom (Ed.), *UpToDate*. https://www.uptodate.com/contents/acute-and-early-hiv-infection-clinical-manifestations-and-diagnosis#H956419

Sax, P. E. (2019). Screening and diagnostic testing for HIV infection. In J. Mitty (Ed.), *UpToDate*. https://www.uptodate.com/contents/screening-and-diagnostic-testing-for-hiv-infection#H34

Sax, P. E. (2019). Treatment and prevention of *Pneumocystis* infection in patients with HIV. In J. Mitty (Ed.), *UpToDate*. https://www.uptodate.com/contents/treatment-and-prevention-of-pneumocystis-infection-in-patients-with-hiv#H25052742

Sax, P. E., & Wood, B. R. (2019). The natural history and clinical features of HIV infection in adults and adolescents. In J. Mitty (Ed.), *UpToDate*. https://www.uptodate.com/contents/the-natural-history-and-clinical-features-of-hiv-infection-in-adults-and-adolescents#H25

Seña, A. C., & Cohen, M. S. (2019). Treatment of uncomplicated Neisseria gonorrhoeae infections. In A. Bloom (Ed.), *UpToDate*. https://www.uptodate.com/contents/treatment-of-uncomplicated-neisseria-gonorrhoeae-infections#H7889919

University of Southern California, Clinician Consultation Center. (2020). *PEP quick guide for occupational exposures*. http://nccc.ucsf.edu/clinical-resources/pep-resources/pep-quick-guide

Zachary, K. C. (2019). Management of health care personnel exposed to HIV. In J. Mitty (Ed.), *UpToDate*. https://www.uptodate.com/contents/management-of-health-care-personnel-exposed-to-hiv#H34

BOOKS

AAP Committee on Infectious Diseases. (2018). *Red Book® 2018–2021 Report of the Committee on Infectious Diseases* (31st ed.). American Academy of Pediatrics.

American Psychiatric Association. (2013). *Diagnostic and statistical manual of mental disorders* (5th ed.). American Psychiatric Publishing.

Ball, J. W., Dains, J. E., Flynn, J. A., Solomon, B. S., & Stewart, R. W. (2018). *Seidel's guide to physical examination* (8th ed.). Mosby/Elsevier.

Bickley, L. S. (2017). *Bates' guide to physical examination and history-taking* (12th ed.). Wolters Kluwer.

Centers for Disease Control and Prevention. (2012) *Principles of epidemiology in public health practice: An introduction to applied epidemiology and biostatistics* (3rd ed.). U.S. Department of Health and Human Services.

Colyar, M. R. (2015). *Advanced practice nursing procedures*. F. A. Davis.

Domino, F. J., Baldor, R. A., Golding, J., & Stephens, M. B. (Eds.). (2020). *The 5-minute clinical consult standard 2020* (28th ed.). Lippincott Williams & Wilkins.

Duderstadt, K. G. (2018). *Pediatric physical examination* (3rd ed.). Mosby/Elsevier.

Ferri, F. F. (Ed.). (2020). *Ferri's clinical advisor 2020: 5 books in 1*. Elsevier.

Fishbach, F., & Dunning, M. B. (2017). *A manual of laboratory and diagnostics tests* (10th ed.). Lippincott Williams & Wilkins.

Fowler, M. D. M. (2015). *Guide to the code of ethics for nurses with interpretive statements: Development, interpretation, and application* (2nd ed.). American Nurses Association.

Gabbe, S. G., Niebyl, J. R., Simpson, J. L., Landon, M. B., Galan, H. L., Jauniaux, E. R. M., Driscoll, D. A., Berghella, V., & Grobman, W. A. (Eds.). (2017). *Obstetrics: Normal and problem pregnancies* (7th ed.). Elsevier.

Gawlik, K. S., Melnyk, B. M., Teall, A. M. (Eds.). (2021). *Evidence-based physical examination: Best practices for health and well-being assessment*. Springer Publishing Company.

Gilbert, D. N., Chambers, H. F., Eliopoulos, G. M., Saag, M. S., & Pavia, A. T. (Eds.). (2020). *The Sanford guide to antimicrobial therapy* (46th ed.). Antimicrobial Therapy.

Grove, S. K., Gray, J. R., & Burns, N. (2018). *Understanding nursing research: Building an evidence-based practice* (7th ed.). Saunders/Elsevier.

Innes, J. A. (Ed.). (2020). *Davidson's essentials of medicine* (3rd ed.). Elsevier.

Kersey-Matusiak, G. (2018). *Delivering culturally competent nursing care* (2nd ed.). Springer Publishing Company.

Kleinman, A. (1988). *The illness narratives: Suffering, healing, and the human condition*. Basic Books. https://www.amazon.com/Illness-Narratives-Suffering-Healing-Condition/dp/0465032044

Kleinman, K., McDaniel, L., & Molloy, M. (Eds.). (2020). *The Harriet Lane handbook* (22nd ed.). Saunders/Elsevier.

Kübler-Ross, E. (1969). *On death and dying*. Macmillan.

Myrick, K. M., Karosas, L. M. (Eds.). (2021). *Advanced health assessment: Essentials for clinical practice*. Springer Publishing Company.

Pagana, K. D., Pagana, T. J., & Pagana, T. N. (2018). *Mosby's diagnostic and laboratory test reference* (14th ed.). Elsevier.

Papadakis, M. A., McPhee, S. J., & Rabow, M. W. (Eds.). (2019). *Current medical diagnosis & treatment 2020* (59th ed.). McGraw-Hill.

Reuben, D., Herr, K., Pacala, J. T., Pollock, B. G., Potter, J. F., & Semla, T. P. (2018). *Geriatrics at your fingertips 2018* (20th ed.). American Geriatrics Society.

Suneja, M., Szot, J. F., LeBlond, & Brown, D. D. (Eds.). (2020). *DeGowin's diagnostic examination* (11th ed.). McGraw-Hill.

Taylor, E. J. (Ed.). (2012). *Religion: A clinical guide for nurses*. Springer Publishing Company.

American Nurses Association. (2015). *Code of ethics for nurses with interpretive statements*.

Walter, L. C., & Chang, A. (Eds.). (2020). *Current diagnosis and treatment: Geriatrics* (3rd ed.). McGraw-Hill.

Williamson, M. A., & Snyder, L. M. (Eds.). (2014). *Wallach's interpretation of diagnostic tests* (10th ed.). Lippincott Williams & Wilkins.

Zane, R. D., & Kosowsky, J. M. (2015). *Pocket emergency medicine* (3rd ed.). Wolters Kluwer.

CERTIFICATION INFORMATION

American Academy of Nurse Practitioners. (n.d.). *AANPCP 2018 statistics*. https://www.aanpcert.org/resource/documents/AANPCB%202018%20Pass%20Rate%20Report.pdf

American Academy of Nurse Practitioners National Certification Board. (2020). *Family nurse practitioner. Adult-gerontology nurse practitioner. FNP & AGNP certification. Candidate handbook*. https://www.aanpcert.org/resource/documents/AGNP%20FNP%20Candidate%20Handbook.pdf

American Academy of Nurse Practitioners Certification Board. (n.d.). Adult-gerontology primary care nurse practitioner (AGNP). Retrieved October 18, 2023, from https://www.aanpcert.org/certs/agnp

American Academy of Nurse Practitioners Certification Board. (n.d.). *Family nurse practitioner (FNP)*. Retrieved September 4, 2023, from https://www.aanpcert.org/certs/fnp

American Nurses Association. (2015). *Code of ethics for nurses with interpretive statements.*

American Nurses Credentialing Center. (2017). *Certification: General testing and renewal handbook*. https://www.nursingworld.org/~4ac882/globalassets/certification/renewals/GeneralTestingandRenewalHandbook

American Nurses Credentialing Center. (2019). *2019 ANCC certification data*. https://www.nursingworld.org/~49a2df/globalassets/docs/ancc/ancc-cert-data-website.pdf

American Nurses Credentialing Center. (2019). *Test content outline: Adult-gerontology primary care nurse practitioner board certification examination*. https://www.nursingworld.org/~49eb18/globalassets/certification/certification-specialty-pages/resources/test-content-outlines/exam-61-agpcnp-tco-05-11-2018_for-webposting.pdf

American Nurses Credentialing Center. (2019). *Test content outline: Family nurse practitioner board certification examination*. https://www.nursingworld.org/~49eb18/globalassets/certification/certification-specialty-pages/resources/test-content-outlines/exam-61-agpcnp-tco-05-11-2018_for-webposting.pdf

American Nurses Credentialing Center. (n.d.). *Family nurse practitioner exam sample questions*. https://www.nursingworld.org/certification/our-certifications/study-aids-ce/sample-test-questions/stq-fnp/

American Nurses Credentialing Center. (2022, September 28). *Test content outline: Family nurse practitioner board certification exam*. https://www.nursingworld.org/~496ce3/globalassets/certification/certification-specialty-pages/resources/test-content-outlines/ancc-22-fnp-tco-2021-final-for-webposting_updated-04112022.pdf

American Nurses Credentialing Center. (2023, September 13). Test content outline:Adult-gerontology primary care nurse practitioner board certification exam. https://www.nursingworld.org/~4938be/globalassets/certification/certification-specialty-pages/resources/test-content-outlines/exam-61-agpcnp-tco-03.07.2023-for-webposting.pdf

Page numbers followed by "f" and "t" refer to figures and tables, respectively.

peptic ulcer disease (PUD), 252–257, 597
percussion, 196
percutaneous angioplasty, for peripheral
  arterial disease, 183
perihepatitis, 422, 431. *See also* Fitz-Hugh–
  Curtis syndrome
perimenopausal, 601
perindopril (Aceon), for hypertension, 47
periorbital cellulitis, 459, 460f
peripheral arterial disease, 183
peripheral blood smear, 305
peripheral edema, 351, 410
peripheral neuropathy, 231
peripheral smear, 300, 302, 305
peripheral vascular disease, 27. *See also*
  peripheral arterial disease
peripheral vascular resistance (PVR), and
  blood pressure, 174
peripheral vertigo, 104
peripheral vision, 97
peritonitis, 245
peritonsillar abscess, 92
  and strep throat, 109
peritonsillar cellulitis, 133
perleche, 94
permethrin (Elimite)
  for scabies, 142
pernicious anemia, 302t, 304, 571
pertussis, 203t, 207–208
pessaries, 392f
petit mal seizure, 467
petroleum jelly, for epistaxis, 107
Peyronie's disease, 367
pH, 265
  vaginal, 393
phalanges, 316
Phalen's sign/maneuver, 281, 281f
pharmacodynamics (PD), 41
pharmacogenetics, 41
pharmacogenomics, 41–42
pharmacokinetics (PK), 41, 41f, 42
pharmacology. *See* drugs
pharmacology therapy
  hypertension, 181
pharyngitis, 601
pharynx
  danger signals, 92
  uncomplicated gonorrheal infections
    of, 428
phenazopyridine (Pyridium),
  for uncomplicated UTIs, 269
phenelzine (Nardil), 342
phenobarbital
  drug interactions, 387
  for Stevens–Johnson syndrome, 126
phenoxybenzamine (Dibenzyline), 564
phenylalanine, for otitis media with
  effusion, 103
phenylephrine (Neo-Synephrine), 55
phenylketonuria (PKU), 444
phenytoin (Dilantin), 42, 43t, 44, 197
  drug interactions, 387
  interaction with alcohol, 347t
  for trigeminal neuralgia, 287t
pheochromocytoma, 177, 223, 593
PHI. *See* protected health information
phimosis, 368, 368f
PHN. *See* postherpetic neuralgia
phosphodiesterase-4 inhibitors, for
  chronic obstructive pulmonary
  disease, 202
phosphodiesterase-5 (PDE5) inhibitors
  contraindications to, 45t
  for erectile dysfunction, 366–367

photographs, question dissection and
  analysis of, 166
phototherapy, for jaundice, 452
physical assessment findings, question
  dissection and analysis of, 33
physical examination
  abuse, 344–345
  sprains, 327
physical therapy
  for ankylosing spondylitis, 319
  for Parkinson's disease, 504
  for piriformis syndrome, 324
  for rotator cuff disease, 329
  for urinary incontinence, 505
physicians, collaborative practice
  agreements of NPs with, 525
physiologic anemia of infancy, 453
physiologic anemia of pregnancy, 410
physiologic changes during pregnancy,
  410–411
physiologic changes in older adults,
  485–488
physiologic concerns in infants
  dentition, 445–446
  elimination, 445
  genitourinary anomalies, 446
  head findings, 445
  nutritional intake, 444–445
  reflex testing, 446
  weight gain and length, 445
physiologic jaundice, 452
physiological anemia of pregnancy, 566
Piaget, Jean, 470t
Pick's disease, 500t
PID. *See* pelvic inflammatory disease
pigmentary changes, 411
pimavanserin, 44
pindolol (Visken)
  contraindications to, 45t
  for hypertension, 180
pineal gland, 224
pinguecula, 100, 574
pink puffer, 201
pinna, 93
pioglitazone (Actos), 43t, 599
  for diabetes mellitus, 227–228
pirbuterol (Maxair)
  for asthma, 197, 198, 200
  for chronic obstructive pulmonary
    disease, 202
piriformis muscle, 324
piriformis syndrome, 324
pitavastatin (Livalo), 43t
pituitary gland, 224
pityriasis rosea, 139–140, 139f
pityriasis versicolor, 598. *See* tinea
  versicolor
Pityrosporum orbiculare, 142
Pityrosporum ovale, 142
PK. *See* pharmacokinetics
PKU. *See* phenylketonuria
placenta previa, 403, 403f, 415
placental abruption, 403, 403f, 415
plaintiff, 527
plane xanthomas, 127
plantar fasciitis, 325, 573
plantar reflex (Babinski's sign), 279, 446, 446f
plasma volume, 410
platelets, 299, 301, 346, 595
plecanatide (Trulance),
  for constipation, 496t
pleural effusion, 563
PLLR. *See* Pregnancy and Lactation
  Labeling Rule

PMI. *See* point of maximal impulse
PMR. *See* polymyalgia rheumatic
PND. *See* postnasal drip
pneumococcal conjugate vaccine (PCV13,
  Prevnar), 79, 202, 206, 594
pneumococcal polysaccharide vaccine
  (PPSV23, Pneumovax 23), 79, 202,
  206, 230
pneumococcal vaccines, 78t, 79, 206, 280,
  566, 605
podofilox (Condylox), 596
  for condyloma acuminate (genital
    warts), 428
poikilocytosis (peripheral smear), 301
point of maximal impulse (PMI)
  displacement of, 162
polycarbophil (FiberCon),
  for constipation, 496t
polycystic ovarian syndrome (PCOS), 380,
  392, 566–567
polycythemia, secondary, 301
polyethylene glycol/PEG 3350
  (MiraLAX)
  for constipation, 496t
  for irritable bowel syndrome, 251
polyhydramnios, 411–413
polymyalgia rheumatica (PMR), 284, 601
polymyositis, 603
polymyxin B-neomycin-hydrocortisone,
  for otitis media, 562
polypharmacy, geriatric syndromes
  associated with, 506
polysomnography, 349
poor weight gain, 602
popliteal cyst, 325
POPs. *See* progestin-only pills
port wine stain, 443
position of heart, 162, 410
positive correlation, 535
positive predictive value (PPV), 540
posterior drawer sign, 317, 317f
posterior pharynx, normal findings in, 94
posterior pituitary gland, 224
postexposure prophylaxis (PEP)
  anthrax, 130
  occupationally acquired HIV infection,
    426–427
postherpetic neuralgia (PHN), 143, 606
postnasal drip (PND), 207t
postpartum contraception, 412–413
poststreptococcal glomerulonephritis, 109
posttraumatic stress disorder (PTSD), 351
potassium hydroxide (KOH) prep test,
  383, 599
potassium-sparing diuretics, 42t, 563
  contraindications to, 45t
  for hypertension, 47, 182t
power of attorney, 516
PPD. *See* purified protein derivative
PPIs. *See* proton-pump inhibitors
PPO. *See* preferred provider organization
PPV. *See* positive predictive value
pramipexole (Mirapex), for Parkinson's
  disease, 504
pravastatin (Pravachol), 43t
  for hyperlipidemia, 171t, 173
prazosin (Minipress), for hypertension,
  49, 182t
prediabetes, 226
prednisolone
  for asthma, 198t
  for gout, 320
prednisone, 57, 601
  for asthma, 198t, 200